TINTINALLI'S EMERGENCY MEDICINE
Just the Facts

jason.r.brody@gmail.com

EDITORS

David M. Cline, MD
Professor and Director of Departmental Research
Department of Emergency Medicine
Wake Forest University School of Medicine
Winston-Salem, North Carolina

O. John Ma, MD
Professor and Chair
Department of Emergency Medicine
Oregon Health & Science University
Portland, Oregon

Rita K. Cydulka, MD, MS
Professor and Vice Chair
Department of Emergency Medicine
MetroHealth Medical Center
Case Western Reserve University
Cleveland, Ohio

Stephen H. Thomas, MD, MPH
George Kaiser Family Foundation Professor & Chair
Department of Emergency Medicine
University of Oklahoma School of Community Medicine
Schusterman Center
Tulsa, Oklahoma

Daniel A. Handel, MD
Associate Professor and Vice Chair
Department of Emergency Medicine
Oregon Health & Science University
Portland, Oregon

Garth D. Meckler, MD, MSHS
Associate Professor
Department of Emergency Medicine
Assistant Section Chief and Fellowship Director
Pediatric Emergency Medicine
Oregon Health & Science University
Portland, Oregon

TINTINALLI'S EMERGENCY MEDICINE
Just the Facts

Third Edition

David M. Cline, MD
O. John Ma, MD

Rita K. Cydulka, MD, MS
Stephen H. Thomas, MD, MPH
Daniel A. Handel, MD
Garth D. Meckler, MD, MSHS

American College of Emergency Physicians®
ADVANCING EMERGENCY CARE

McGraw Hill Medical

New York Chicago San Francisco Lisbon London Madrid Mexico City
Milan New Delhi San Juan Seoul Singapore Sydney Toronto

The McGraw-Hill Companies

Tintinalli's Emergency Medicine: *Just the Facts, Third Edition*

7 8 9 10 DSS 20 19 18 17

ISBN 978-0-07-174441-6
MHID 0-07-174441-X

Notice

Medicine is an ever-changing science. As new research and clinical experience broaden our knowledge, changes in treatment and drug therapy are required. The authors and the publisher of this work have checked with sources believed to be reliable in their efforts to provide information that is complete and generally in accord with the standards accepted at the time of publication. However, in view of the possibility of human error or changes in medical sciences, neither the authors nor the publisher nor any other party who has been involved in the preparation or publication of this work warrants that the information contained herein is in every respect accurate or complete, and they disclaim all responsibility for any errors or omissions or for the results obtained from use of the information contained in this work. Readers are encouraged to confirm the information contained herein with other sources. For example and in particular, readers are advised to check the product information sheet included in the package of each drug they plan to administer to be certain that the information contained in this work is accurate and that changes have not been made in the recommended dose or in the contraindications for administration. This recommendation is of particular importance in connection with new or infrequently used drugs.

The book was set in Times New Roman by Cenveo Publisher Services.
The editors were Anne M. Sydor and Christie Naglieri.
The production supervisor was Catherine Saggese.
Project management was provided by Anupriya Tyagi, Cenveo Publisher Services.
RR Donnelley was the printer and binder.

Library of Congress Cataloging-in-Publication Data

Tintinalli's emergency medicine : just the facts / [edited] by David M. Cline ... [et al.].—3rd ed.
p. ; cm.
Emergency medicine
Rev. ed. of: Emergency medicine : just the facts / edited by O. John Ma ... [et al.]. 2nd ed. 2004.
Includes bibliographical references and index.
ISBN 978-0-07-174441-6 (pbk. : alk. paper)—ISBN 0-07-174441-X (pbk. : alk. paper)
I. Cline, David, 1956- II. Emergency medicine. III. Title: Emergency medicine.
[DNLM: 1. Emergency Medicine—Outlines. 2. Emergencies—Outlines. WB 18.2]
616.02'5—dc23

2012012633

CONTENTS

Contributors xv
Preface xxi

Section 1
TEST PREPARATION AND PLANNING 1

1 Facts about Emergency Medicine Board Exams *David M. Cline* 1
2 Test-Taking Techniques *David M. Cline* 4

Section 2
RESUSCITATION TECHNIQUES 6

3 Advanced Airway Support *Robert J. Vissers* 6
4 Arrhythmia Management *James K. Takayesu* 9
5 Resuscitation of Children and Neonates *Marc F. Collin* 20
6 Fluids, Electrolytes, and Acid–Base Disorders *Mary A. Wittler* 23
7 Theraputic Approach to the Hypotensive Patient *John Gough* 32
8 Anaphylaxis, Acute Allergic Reactions, and Angioedema *Alix L. Mitchell* 34

Section 3
ANALGESIA, ANESTHESIA AND PROCEDURAL SEDATION 36

9 Acute Pain Management and Procedural Sedation *Michael S. Mitchell* 36
10 Management of Patients with Chronic Pain *David M. Cline* 44

Section 4
EMERGENCY WOUND MANAGEMENT 48

11 Evaluating and Preparing Wounds *Timothy Reeder* 48
12 Methods for Wound Closure *David M. Cline* 49
13 Lacerations to the Face and Scalp *J. Hayes Calvert* 53
14 Injuries of the Arm, Hand, Fingertip, and Nail *David M. Cline* 56
15 Lacerations of the Leg and Foot *Henderson D. McGinnis* 60
16 Soft Tissue Foreign Bodies *Rodney L. McCaskill* 62
17 Puncture Wounds and Bites *David M. Cline* 64
18 Post Repair Wound Care *David M. Cline* 68

Section 5
CARDIOVASCULAR DISEASE 71

19 Chest Pain: Cardiac or Not *Thomas Rebbecchi* 71
20 Acute Coronary Syndromes: Management of Myocardial Ischemia and Infarction *David M. Cline* 73
21 Cardiogenic Shock *Brian C. Hiestand* 81
22 Low Probability Acute Coronary Syndrome *Chadwick D. Miller* 82
23 Syncope *Bret A. Nicks* 85
24 Congestive Heart Failure and Acute Pulmonary Edema *Lori Whelan* 88
25 Valvular Emergencies *Boyd Burns* 91
26 The Cardiomyopathies, Myocarditis, and Pericardial Disease *N. Stuart Harris* 97
27 Thromboembolism *Christopher Kabrhel* 102
28 Systemic and Pulmonary Hypertension *David M. Cline* 109
29 Aortic Dissection and Aneurysms *David E. Manthey* 112
30 Occlusive Arterial Disease *Carolyn K. Synovitz* 115

Section 6
PULMONARY EMERGENCIES 119

31 Respiratory Distress *Joshua T. Hargraves* 119
32 Pneumonia, Bronchitis, and Upper Respiratory Tract Infection *Jeffrey M. Goodloe* 123
33 Tuberculosis *Amy J. Behrman* 129
34 Spontaneous and Iatrogenic Pneumothorax *Rodney L. McCaskill* 132
35 Hemoptysis *Jeffrey Dixon* 134
36 Asthma and Chronic Obstructive Pulmonary Disease *Joshua Gentges* 136

Section 7
GASTROINTESTINAL EMERGENCIES 140

37 Acute Abdominal Pain *David M. Cline* 140
38 Nausea and Vomiting *Jonathan A. Maisel* 144
39 Disorders Presenting Primarily with Diarrhea *Jonathan A. Maisel* 146
40 Acute and Chronic Constipation *Jonathan A. Maisel* 151
41 Gastrointestinal Bleeding *Mitchell C. Sokolosky* 153
42 Esophageal Emergencies, Gastroesophageal Reflux Disease, and Swallowed Foreign Bodies *Mitchell C. Sokolosky* 154
43 Peptic Ulcer Disease and Gastritis *Matthew C. Gratton* 157
44 Pancreatitis and Cholecystitis *Casey M. Glass* 159
45 Acute Appendicitis *Charles E. Stewart* 163
46 Diverticulitis *James C. O'Neill* 166
47 Bowel Obstruction and Volvulus *Mark Hess* 167
48 Hernia in Adults and Children *Dave W. Lu* 168
49 Anorectal Disorders *Chad E. Branecki* 170
50 Hepatic Disorders, Jaundice, and Hepatic Failure *Joshua A. Gentges* 175
51 Complications of General Surgical Procedures *Daniel J. Egan* 181

Section 8
RENAL AND GENITOURINARY DISORDERS 184

52 Acute Renal Failure *Marc D. Squillante* 184
53 Rhabdomyolysis *Michael Levine* 188
54 Emergencies in Renal Failure and Dialysis Patients *Jonathan A. Maisel* 190
55 Urinary Tract Infections and Hematuria *David M. Cline* 192
56 Acute Urinary Retention *Casey M. Glass* 196
57 Male Genital Problems *Boyd Burns* 197
58 Urologic Stone Disease *Geetika Gupta* 201
59 Complications of Urologic Procedures and Devices *Roy L. Alson* 205

Section 9
OBSTETRICS AND GYNECOLOGY 208

60 Vaginal Bleeding and Pelvic Pain in the Nonpregnant Patient *Thomas W. Lukens* 208
61 Ectopic Pregnancy and Emergencies in the First 20 Weeks of Pregnancy *Robert Jones* 210

62 Comorbid Diseases in Pregnancy
Abigail Hankin-Wei 213
63 Emergencies During the Second Half of Pregnancy
Howard Roemer 216
64 Emergency Delivery *Stacie Zelman* 218
65 Vulvovaginitis *Stacie Zelman* 221
66 Pelvic Inflammatory Disease *Stacie Zelman* 223
67 Complications of Gynecologic Procedures
Anitha Mathew 225

Section 10
PEDIATRICS 228

68 Fever and Serious Bacterial Illness
Milan D. Nadkarni 228
69 Neonate Emergencies and Common
Neonatal Problems *Shad Baab* 232
70 Common Infections of the Ears, Nose, Neck, and
Throat *David M. Spiro* 238
71 Stridor and Drooling *Kathleen M. Adelgais* 242
72 Wheezing in Infants and Children
Donald H. Arnold 249
73 Pneumonia in Infants and Children
Chad D. McCalla 253
74 Pediatric Heart Disease *Garth D. Meckler* 255
75 Vomiting and Diarrhea in Infants and Children
Stephen B. Freedman 260
76 Pediatric Abdominal Emergencies
David I. Magilner 265
77 Urinary Tract Infection in Infants and Children
Justin W. Sales 268
78 Seizures and Status Epilepticus in Children
James C. O'Neill 270
79 Altered Mental Status and Headache in
Children *Kathleen M. Adelgais* 274
80 Syncope and Sudden Death in Children
Derya Caglar 277
81 Hypoglycemia and Metabolic Emergencies in
Infants and Children *Matthew Hansen* 279
82 The Child with Diabetes *Adam Vella* 282
83 Fluid and Electrolyte Therapy in Infants and
Children *Jennifer R. Reid* 284
84 Musculoskeletal Disorders in Children
Mark X. Cicero 287
85 Rashes in Infants and Children *Kim Askew* 293
86 Sickle Cell Disease *Ilene Claudius* 301

87 Oncologic and Hematology Emergencies in Children *Ilene Claudius* 304
88 Renal Emergencies in Infants and Children *Deborah R. Liu* 309

Section 11
INFECTIOUS DISEASES 313

89 Sexually Transmitted Diseases *David M. Cline* 313
90 Toxic Shock Syndrome and Streptococcal Toxic Shock Syndrome *Manoj Pariyadath* 318
91 Septic Shock *John Gough* 321
92 Soft Tissue Infections *David M. Cline* 324
93 Disseminated Viral Infections *Matthew J. Scholer* 328
94 Human Immunodeficiency Virus Infection and Acquired Immunodeficiency Syndrome *David M. Cline* 333
95 Infective Endocarditis *John C. Nalagan* 338
96 Tetanus and Rabies *Vincent Nacouzi* 339
97 Malaria *David M. Cline* 342
98 Foodborne and Waterborne Diseases *David M. Cline* 345
99 Zoonotic Infections *Christopher R. Tainter* 347
100 World Travelers *David M. Cline* 352
101 The Transplant Patient *David M. Cline* 357

Section 12
TOXICOLOGY 363

102 General Management of Poisoned Patients *L. Keith French* 363
103 Anticholinergics *O. John Ma* 368
104 Psychopharmacologic Agents *C. Crawford Mechem* 369
105 Sedative and Hypnotics *L. Keith French* 376
106 Alcohols *Michael P. Kefer* 380
107 Drugs of Abuse *Shana Kusin* 383
108 Analgesics *Joshua Nogar* 388
109 Methylxanthines and Nicotine *L. Keith French* 393
110 Cardiac Medications *D. Adam Algren* 395
111 Anticonvulsants *Alicia B. Minns* 400
112 Iron *O. John Ma* 402
113 Hydrocarbons and Volatile Substances *Allyson A. Kreshak* 404
114 Caustics *Christian A. Tomaszewski* 406
115 Pesticides *Christian A. Tomaszewski* 408

116 Metals and Metalloids *D. Adam Algren* ... 412
117 Industrial Toxins and Cyanide *Christian A. Tomaszewski* ... 415
118 Vitamins and Herbals *Christian A. Tomaszewski* ... 418
119 Dyshemoglobinemias *Kristine L. Bott* ... 420

Section 13
ENVIRONMENTAL EMERGENCIES ... 422

120 Frostbite and Other Localized Cold Injuries *Michael C. Wadman* ... 422
121 Heat Emergencies *T. Paul Tran* ... 424
122 Bites and Stings *Burton Bentley II* ... 426
123 Trauma and Envenomation from Marine Fauna *Christian A. Tomaszewski* ... 430
124 High-Altitude Medical Problems *Shaun D. Carstairs* ... 433
125 Dysbarism and Complications of Diving *Christian A. Tomaszewski* ... 435
126 Drowning *Richard A. Walker* ... 438
127 Thermal and Chemical Burns *Sandra L. Werner* ... 441
128 Electrical and Lightning Injuries *Sachita P. Shah* ... 446
129 Carbon Monoxide *Christian A. Tomaszewski* ... 449
130 Poisonous Plants and Mushrooms *B. Zane Horowitz* ... 451

Section 14
ENDOCRINE EMERGENCIES ... 454

131 Diabetic Emergencies *Michael P. Kefer* ... 454
132 Alcoholic Ketoacidosis *Michael P. Kefer* ... 460
133 Thyroid Disease Emergencies *Katrina A. Leone* ... 461
134 Adrenal Insufficiency and Adrenal Crisis *Michael P. Kefer* ... 463

Section 15
HEMATOLOGIC AND ONCOLOGIC EMERGENCIES ... 466

135 Evaluation of Anemia and the Bleeding Patient *Daniel A. Handel* ... 466
136 Acquired Bleeding Disorders *Aaron Barksdale* ... 471
137 Hemophilias and von Willebrand's Disease *Daniel A. Handel* ... 474
138 Sickle Cell Disease and Other Hereditary Hemolytic Anemias *Jason B. Hack* ... 477
139 Transfusion Therapy *T. Paul Tran* ... 479

140 Anticoagulants, Antiplatelet Agents, and Fibrinolytics *Jessica L. Smith* 484
141 Emergency Complications of Malignancy *Ross J. Fleischman* 486

Section 16
NEUROLOGY 494

142 Headache and Facial Pain *Steven Go* 494
143 Stroke, Transient Ischemic Attack, and Cervical Artery Dissection *Steven Go* 497
144 Altered Mental Status and Coma *C. Crawford Mechem* 505
145 Ataxia and Gait Disturbances *Ross J. Fleischman* 509
146 Vertigo and Dizziness *Steven Go* 510
147 Seizures and Status Epilepticus in Adults *C. Crawford Mechem* 514
148 Acute Peripheral Neurologic Lesions *Jeffrey L. Hackman* 517
149 Chronic Neurologic Disorders *Sarah Andrus Gaines* 519
150 Central Nervous System and Spinal Infections *O. John Ma* 523

Section 17
EYES, EARS, NOSE, THROAT, AND ORAL SURGERY 528

151 Ocular Emergencies *Steven Go* 528
152 Face and Jaw Emergencies *Jeffrey G. Norvell* 538
153 Ear, Nose, and Sinus Emergencies *Medley O. Gatewood* 541
154 Oral and Dental Emergencies *Steven Go* 545
155 Infections and Disorders of the Neck and Upper Airway *Aaron Barksdale* 550

Section 18
SKIN DISORDERS 556

156 Dermatologic Emergencies *Daniel A. Handel* 556
157 Other Dermatologic Disorders *Daniel A. Handel* 560

Section 19
TRAUMA 563

158 Trauma in Adults *Jonathan S. Ilgen* 563
159 Trauma in Children *Matthew Hansen* 564
160 Geriatric Trauma *O. John Ma* 566

161 Trauma in Pregnancy *Nicole M. DeIorio* 568
162 Head Trauma in Adults and Children *O. John Ma* 569
163 Spine and Spinal Cord Trauma *Todd Ellingson* 573
164 Trauma to the Face *Jonathan S. Ilgen* 577
165 Trauma to the Neck *Katrina A. Leone*.............................. 579
166 Cardiothoracic Injuries *Ross J. Fleischman* 580
167 Abdominal Trauma *O. John Ma* 584
168 Penetrating Trauma to the Flank and Buttock *Christine Sullivan* 587
169 Genitourinary Trauma *Matthew C. Gratton* 588
170 Penetrating Trauma to the Extremities *Amy M. Stubbs* 591

Section 20
INJURIES TO BONES AND JOINTS 593

171 Initial Evaluation and Management of Orthopedic Injuries *Michael P. Kefer* 593
172 Hand and Wrist Injuries *Michael P. Kefer*........................ 595
173 Injuries to the Elbow and Forearm *Sandra L. Najarian*.. 598
174 Shoulder and Humerus Injuries *Sandra L. Najarian*......... 601
175 Pelvis, Hip, and Femur Injuries *Jeffrey G. Norvell*........... 604
176 Knee and Leg Injuries *Sandra L. Najarian* 609
177 Ankle and Foot Injuries *Sarah Andrus Gaines*................. 613
178 Compartment Syndrome *Sandra L. Najarian* 615

Section 21
MUSCULOSKELETAL DISORDERS.................................... 617

179 Neck and Thoracolumbar Pain *Amy M. Stubbs* 617
180 Shoulder Pain *Andrew D. Perron*...................................... 620
181 Hip and Knee Pain *Jeffrey L. Hackman*............................ 623
182 Acute Disorders of the Joints and Bursae *Matthew C. DeLaney*... 626
183 Emergencies in Systemic Rheumatic Diseases *Michael P. Kefer*.. 629
184 Infectious and Noninfectious Disorders of the Hand *Michael P. Kefer*... 632
185 Soft Tissue Problems of the Foot *Robert L. Cloutier* 634

Section 22
PSYCHOSOCIAL DISORDERS 639

186 Clinical Features of Behavioral Disorders *Lance H. Hoffman* 639
187 Emergency Assessment and Stabilization of Behavioral Disorders *Lance H. Hoffman* 640

188 Panic and Conversion Disorders *Lance H. Hoffman*......... 643
189 Child and Elderly Abuse *Jonathan Glauser*...................... 645

Section 23
ABUSE AND ASSAULT 648

190 Sexual Assault and Intimate Partner Violence and Abuse *Sara Laskey*... 648

Section 24
PRINCIPLES OF IMAGING 650

191 Principles of Emergency Department Use of Computed Tomography and Magnetic Resonance Imaging *Clare F. Wallner*.. 650
192 Principles of Emergency Department Ultrasonography *Catherine Erickson*............................... 652

Section 25
ADMINISTRATION 655

193 Emergency Medical Services *C. Crawford Mechem*......... 655
194 Emergency Medicine Administration *David M. Cline*...... 657

Index.. 663

CONTRIBUTORS

Kathleen M. Adelgais, MD, MPH, Associate Professor, Section of Pediatric Emergency Medicine, University of Colorado, Denver School of Medicine, Aurora, Colorado

D. Adam Algren, MD, Assistant Professor, Emergency Medicine and Pediatrics, Truman Medical Center, University of Missouri-Kansas City School of Medicine, Kansas City, Missouri

Roy L. Alson, MD, PhD, Associate Professor, Department of Emergency Medicine, Wake Forest School of Medicine, Winston-Salem, North Carolina

Donald H. Arnold, MD, MPH, Associate Professor, Departments of Pediatrics and Emergency Medicine, Vanderbilt University School of Medicine, Nashville, Tennessee

Kim Askew, MD, Assistant Professor, Department of Emergency Medicine, Wake Forest School of Medicine, Winston-Salem, North Carolina

Shad Baab, MD, Assistant Professor, Department of Emergency Medicine, Wake Forest School of Medicine, Winston-Salem, North Carolina

Aaron Barksdale, MD, Assistant Professor, Department of Emergency Medicine, Truman Medical Center, University of Missouri-Kansas City School of Medicine, Kansas City, Missouri

Amy J. Behrman, MD, Associate Professor, Department of Emergency Medicine, Division of Occupational Medicine, Hospital of the University of Pennsylvania, Perelman School of Medicine, Philadelphia, Pennsylvania

Burton Bentley II, MD, Attending Physician, Department Emergency Medicine, Northwest Medical Center, Tucson, Arizona

Kristine L. Bott, MD, Assistant Professor, Department of Emergency Medicine, University of Nebraska Medical Center, Omaha, Nebraska

Chad E. Branecki, MD, Assistant Professor, Department of Emergency Medicine, University of Nebraska Medical Center, Omaha, Nebraska

Boyd D. Burns, DO, Assistant Professor, Residency Director, Department of Emergency Medicine, Oklahoma University School of Community Medicine, Tulsa, Oklahoma

Derya Caglar, MD, Assistant Professor Pediatrics, Division of Emergency Medicine, University of Washington School of Medicine, Seattle, Washington

J. Hayes Calvert, DO, Clinical Instructor, Department of Emergency Medicine, Wake Forest School of Medicine, Winston-Salem, North Carolina

Shaun D. Carstairs, MD, Senior Faculty, Department of Emergency Medicine, Naval Medical Center San Diego, San Diego, California

Mark X. Cicero, MD, Assistant Professor of Pediatrics, Yale University School of Medicine, New Haven, Connecticut

Ilene Claudius, MD, Assistant Professor, Emergency Medicine, Keck School of Medicine, University of Southern California, Los Angeles, California

David M. Cline, MD, Professor, Department of Emergency Medicine, Wake Forest School of Medicine, Winston-Salem, North Carolina

Robert L. Cloutier, MD, Associate Professor, Department of Emergency Medicine and Pediatrics, Oregon Health & Science University, Portland, Oregon

Marc F. Collin, MD, Associate Professor, Pediatrics, Case Western Reserve University School of Medicine, MetroHealth Medical Center, Cleveland, Ohio

Nicole M. DeIorio, MD, Associate Professor, Department of Emergency Medicine, Oregon Health & Science University, Portland, Oregon

Matthew C. DeLaney, MD, Attending Physician, Department of Emergency Medicine, Mercy Hospital, Portland, Maine

Jeffery Dixon, MD, Clinical Associate Professor, Department of Emergency Medicine, University of Oklahoma School of Community Medicine, Hillcrest Medical Center, Tulsa, Oklahoma

Daniel J. Egan, MD, Associate Residency Director, Department of Emergency Medicine, St. Luke's Roosevelt Hospital Center, New York

Todd Ellingson, MD, Assistant Professor, Department of Emergency Medicine, Oregon Health & Science University, Portland, Oregon

Catherine Erickson, MD, Assistant Professor, Department of Emergency Medicine, Oregon Health & Science University, Portland, Oregon

Ross J. Fleischman, MD, MCR, Assistant Professor, Department of Emergency Medicine, Oregon Health & Science University, Portland, Oregon

Stephen B. Freedman, MDCM, MSc, Associate Professor of Pediatrics, Divisions of Pediatric Emergency Medicine and Gastroenterology, Alberta Children's Hospital, University of Calgary, Calgary, Alberta, Canada

L. Keith French, MD, Assistant Professor, Department of Emergency Medicine, Oregon Health & Science University, Portland, Oregon

Sarah Andrus Gaines, MD, Assistant Professor (Clinical), Department of Emergency Medicine, Alpert Medical School of Brown University, Providence, Rhode Island

Medley O. Gatewood, MD, Assistant Professor, Department of Medicine, Division of Emergency Medicine, University of Washington, Seattle, Washington

Joshua A. Gentges, DO, Assistant Professor, Emergency Medicine, University of Oklahoma School Community Medicine, Hillcrest Medical Center, Tulsa, Oklahoma

Casey M. Glass, MD, Assistant Professor, Department of Emergency Medicine, Wake Forest School of Medicine, Winston-Salem, North Carolina

Jonathan Glauser, MD, MBA, Associate Professor, Emergency Medicine, Case Western Reserve University, MetroHealth Medical Center, Cleveland, Ohio

Steven Go, MD, Associate Professor, Department of Emergency Medicine, Truman Medical Center, University of Missouri-Kansas City School of Medicine, Kansas City, Missouri

Jeffrey M. Goodloe, MD, Associate Professor, Department of Emergency Medicine, University of Oklahoma School of Community Medicine, Schusterman Center, Tulsa, Oklahoma

John E. Gough, MD, Professor, Department of Emergency Medicine, East Carolina University, Greenville, North Carolina

Matthew C. Gratton, MD, Associate Professor and Chair, Department of Emergency Medicine, Truman Medical Center, University of Missouri-Kansas City School of Medicine, Kansas City, Missouri

Geetika Gupta, MD, Clinical Faculty, Emergency Medicine, University of Michigan, St. Joseph Mercy Hospital, Ann Arbor, Michigan

Jason B. Hack, MD, Associate Professor, Director, Division of Medical Toxicology, Department of of Emergency Medicine, Alpert Medical School of Brown University, Providence, Rhode Island

Jeffrey L. Hackman, MD, Assistant Professor, Department of Emergency Medicine, Truman Medical Center/University of Missouri-Kansas City, Kansas City, Missouri

Daniel A. Handel, MD, MPH, Associate Professor and Vice Chair, Department of Emergency Medicine, Oregon Health & Science University, Portland, Oregon

Abigail Hankin-Wei, MD, MPH, Assistant Professor, Department of Emergency Medicine, Emory University, Atlanta, Georgia

Matthew Hansen, MD, Fellow, Pediatric Emergency Medicine, Oregon Health & Science University, Portland, Oregon

Joshua T. Hargraves, MD, Assistant Professor, Department of Emergency Medicine, Emory University School of Medicine, Atlanta, Georgia

N. Stuart Harris, MD, MFA, Chief of Division of Wilderness Medicine, Director of Wilderness Medicine Fellowship, Department of Emergency Medicine, Massachusetts General Hospital, Boston, Massachusetts

Mark Hess, MD, Assistant Professor, Department Emergency Medicine, Wake Forest School of Medicine, Winston-Salem, North Carolina

Brian C. Hiestand, MD, MPH, Associate Professor, Department of Emergency Medicine, Wake Forest School of Medicine, Winston-Salem, North Carolina

Lance H. Hoffman, MD, Associate Professor, Department of Emergency Medicine, University of Nebraska Medical Center, Omaha, Nebraska

B. Zane Horowitz, MD, Professor, Department of Emergency Medicine, Medical Director of Oregon Poison Center, Oregon Health & Science University, Portland, Oregon

Jonathan S. Ilgen, MD, MCR, Acting Assistant Professor, Department of Medicine, Division of Emergency Medicine, University of Washington, Seattle, Washington

Robert Jones, DO, Associate Professor, Department of Emergency Medicine, Case Western Reserve University, MetroHealth Medical Center, Cleveland, Ohio

Christopher Kabrhel, MD, MPH, Assistant Professor, Surgery, Harvard Medical School, Boston, Massachusetts, Department of Emergency Medicine, Massachusetts General Hospital, Boston, Massachusetts

Michael P. Kefer, MD, Attending Physician, Oconomowoc, Wisconsin

Allyson A. Kreshak, MD, Clinical Assistant Professor, Department of Emergency Medicine, University of California San Diego, San Diego, California

Shana Kusin, MD, Adunct Clinical Instructor and Toxicology Fellow, Department of Emergency Medicine, Oregon Poison Center, Oregon Health & Science University, Portland, Oregon

Sara Laskey, MD, Associate Professor, Department of Emergency Medicine, Case Western Reserve University School of Medicine, MetroHealth Medical Center, Cleveland, Ohio

Katrina A. Leone, MD, Education Fellow and Instructor, Department of Emergency Medicine, Oregon Health & Science University, Portland, Oregon

Michael Levine, MD, Department of Emergency Medicine, Section of Medical Toxicology, University of Southern California, Keck School of Medicine, Los Angeles, California

Deborah R. Liu, MD, Assistant Professor of Pediatrics, Department of Pediatrics, Keck School of Medicine of USC, Los Angeles, California, Children's Hospital Los Angeles, Division of Emergency Medicine, Los Angeles, California

Dave W. Lu, MD, MBE, Acting Instructor, Department of Medicine, Division of Emergency Medicine, University of Washington School of Medicine, Seattle, Washington

Thomas W. Lukens, MD, PhD, Associate Professor, Emergency Medicine, Case Western Reserve University, MetroHealth Medical Center, Cleveland, Ohio

O. John Ma, MD, Professor and Chair, Department of Emergency Medicine, Oregon Health & Science University, Portland, Oregon

David I. Magilner, MD, MSPH, Assistant Professor, Department of Emergency Medicine, Wake Forest School of Medicine, Winston-Salem, North Carolina

Jonathan A. Maisel, MD, Assistant Clinical Professor, Emergency Medicine, Yale University, New Haven, Connecticut, Department of Emergency Medicine, Bridgeport Hospital, Bridgeport, Connecticut

David E. Manthey, MD, Professor, Department of Emergency Medicine, Associate Dean for Medical Education, Wake Forest School of Medicine, Winston-Salem, North Carolina

Anitha Mathew, MD, Clinical Instructor, Department of Emergency Medicine, Emory University School of Medicine, Atlanta, Georgia

Chad D. McCalla, MD, Assistant Professor, Department of Emergency Medicine, Wake Forst School of Medicine, Winston-Salem, North Carolina

Rodney L. McCaskill, MD, Associate Professor, Department of Emergency Medicine, WakeMed, Raleigh, North Carolina

Henderson D. McGinnis, MD, Assistant Professor, Department of Emergency Medicine, Wake Forest School of Medicine, Winston-Salem, North Carolina

C. Crawford Mechem, MD, MS, Associate Professor, Department of Emergency Medicine, University of Pennsylvania Perelman School of Medicine, Philadelphia, Pennsylvania

Garth D. Meckler, MD, MSHS, Associate Professor, Assistant Section Chief of Pediatric Emergency Medicine, Director of Pediatric Emergency Medicine Fellowship Program, Department of Emergency Medicine, Oregon Health & Science University, Portland, Oregon

Chadwick D. Miller, MD, MS, Associate Professor, Department of Emergency Medicine, Wake Forest School of Medicine, Winston-Salem, North Carolina

Alicia B. Minns, MD, Assistant Professor of Clinical Medicine, Department of Emergency Medicine, University of California, San Diego, California

Alix L. Mitchell, MD, Senior Instructor, Department of Emergency Medicine, Case Western Reserve University School of Medicine, MetroHealth Medical Center, Cleveland, Ohio

Michael S. Mitchell, MD, Assistant Professor, Department of Emergency Medicine, Wake Forest School of Medicine, Winston-Salem, North Carolina

Vincent Nacouzi, MD, Attending Emergency Physician, North Raleigh Medical Center, Raleigh, North Carolina

Milan D. Nadkarni, MD, Associate Professor, Department of Emergency Medicine, Wake Forest Baptist Health, Winston-Salem, North Carolina

Sandra L. Najarian, MD, Assistant Professor, Emergency Medicine, Case Western Reserve University School of Medicine, MetroHealth Medical Center, Cleveland, Ohio

John C. Nalagan, MD, Assistant Professor, Director of Medical Student Education, Department of Emergency Medicine, University of Oklahoma School of Community Medicine, Schusterman Center, Tulsa, Oklahoma

Bret A. Nicks, MD, MHA, Associate Professor, Associate Dean, Department of Emergency Medicine, Wake Forest Baptist Health, Winston-Salem, North Carolina

Joshua Nogar, MD, Clinical Professor, Department of Emergency Medicine & Toxicology, University of California San Diego, San Diego, California

Jeffrey G. Norvell, MD, Assistant Professor, Associate Program Director, Emergency Medicine, University of Kansas School of Medicine, Kansas City, Kansas

James C. O'Neill, MD, Assistant Professor, Department of Pediatrics and Emergency Medicine, Wake Forest Baptist Health, Winston-Salem, North Carolina

Manoj Pariyadath, MD, Assistant Professor, Department of Emergency Medicine, Wake Forest Baptist Health, Winston-Salem, North Carolina

Andrew D. Perron, MD, Professor and Residency Program Director, Department of Emergency Medicine, Maine Medical Center, Portland, Maine

Thomas A. Rebbecchi, MD, Associate Professor, Emergency Medicine, Robert Wood Johnson Medical School/Cooper University Hospital, Camden, New Jersey

Timothy Reeder, MD, MPH, Associate Professor, Emergency Medicine, Brody School of Medicine at East Carolina University, Greenville, North Carolina

Jennifer R. Reid, MD, Assistant Professor of Pediatrics, University of Washington School of Medicine, Seattle, Washington

Howard Roemer, MD, Associate Professor, Department of Emergency Medicine, University of Oklahoma School of Community Medicine, Schusterman Center, Tulsa, Oklahoma

Justin W. Sales, MD, MPH, Attending Physician, Pediatric Emergency Medicine, Randall Children's Hospital, Portland, Oregon

Matthew J. Scholer, MD, PhD, Clinical Associate Professor, Department of Emergency Medicine, University of North Carolina, Chapel Hill, North Carolina

Sachita P. Shah, MD, Assistant Professor, Division of Emergency Medicine, Department of Medicine, University of Washington School of Medicine, Seattle, Washington

Jessica L. Smith, MD, Assistant Professor of Emergency Medicine, Associate Program Director of Emergency Medicine Residency, Emergency Medicine, Alpert Medical School of Brown University, Rhode Island Hospital, Providence, Rhode Island

Mitchell C. Sokolosky, MD, Associate Professor and Residency Program Director, Department of Emergency Medicine, Wake Forest Baptist Health, Winston-Salem, North Carolina

David M. Spiro, MD, MPH, Associate, Department of Emergency Medicine, Oregon Health & Science University, Portland, Oregon

Marc D. Squillante, DO, Associate Professor, Emergency Medicine Residency Program Director, Department of Surgery/Division of Emergency Medicine, University of Illinois College of Medicine at Peoria/OSF St. Francis Medical Center, Peoria, Illinois

Charles E. Stewart, MD, MSc (DM), MPH, Professor of Emergency Medicine, Director of Oklahoma Disaster Institute, Department of Emergency Medicine, University of Oklahoma, School of Community Medicine, Schusterman Center, Tulsa, Oklahoma

Amy M. Stubbs, MD, Assistant Professor of Emergency Medicine, Associate Residency Program Director, Truman Medical Center, University of Missouri-Kansas City School of Medicine, Kansas City, Missouri

Christine Sullivan, MD, Assistant Professor, Department of Emergency Medicine, Truman Medical Center, University of Missouri-Kansas City School of Medicine, Kansas City, Missouri

Carolyn K. Synovitz, MD, MPH, Clinical Associate Professor, Department of Emergency Medicine, University of Oklahoma, School of Community Medicine, Tulsa, Oklahoma

Christopher R. Tainter, MD, Assistant Professor, Department of Emergency Medicine, University of Oklahoma School of Community Medicine, Tulsa, Oklahoma

James K. Takayesu, MD, MSc, Assistant Professor, Emergency Medicine, Harvard Medical School, Boston, Massachusetts, Massachusetts General Hospital, Boston, Massachusetts

Christian A. Tomaszewski, MD, Professor of Clinical Medicine, Department of Emergency Medicine, University of California San Diego Medical Center, San Diego, California

T. Paul Tran, MD, Associate Professor, Department of Emergency Medicine, University of Nebraska College of Medicine, Omaha, Nebraska

Adam Vella, MD, Associate Professor, Emergency Medicine, Mount Sinai Medical Center, New York, New York

Robert J. Vissers, MD, Adjunct Associate Professor, Department of Emergency Medicine, Oregon Health & Sciences University, Portland, Oregon

Michael C. Wadman, Associate Professor, Department of Emergency Medicine, University of Nebraska College of Medicine, Omaha, Nebraska

Richard A. Walker, MD, Associate Professor, Emergency Department, University of Nebraska Medical Center, Omaha, Nebraska

Clare F. Wallner, MD, Adjunct Instructor, Fellow, Department of Emergency Medicine, Oregon Health & Science University, Portland, Oregon

Sandra L. Werner, MD, Assistant Professor, Associate Director of Emergency Medicine Residency Program, Department of Emergency Medicine, Case Western Reserve University, MetroHealth Medical Center, Cleveland, Ohio

Lori Whelan, MD, Assistant Professor, Department of Emergency Medicine, University of Oklahoma School of Community Medicine, Tulsa, Oklahoma

Mary Wittler, MD, Assistant Professor, Department of Emergency Medicine, Wake Forest Baptist Health, Winston-Salem, North Carolina

Stacie Zelman, MD, Assistant Professor, Department of Emergency Medicine, Wake Forest Baptist Health, Winston-Salem, North Carolina

PREFACE

Emergency medicine is a speciality that refuses to sleep and rests only long enough to collect the necessary information to make the next critical move. *Emergency Medicine: Just the Facts*, 3rd edition, is written with the concept that succinct content facilitates the reader's retention of essential information. We hope the reader will immediately see how much this edition has progressed from prior editions. There are now over 100 radiographs/ color images, 93 line drawings/ ECGs, and 300 tables designed to enhance your understanding of the material. This change reflects the development of its award-winning* parent textbook, Tintinalli's *Emergency Medicine: A Comprehensive Study Guide*, 7th edition, as well as advances in diagnostic imaging. Many exams in emergency medicine include a pictorial stimulus section, and the additions to this textbook will greatly facilitate the reader's ability to answer that type of question.

Our goal is to provide the reader with a brief yet comprehensive review of the practice of emergency medicine for the clinician who wishes to update their knowledge of the speciality. While the parent textbook should be regarded as the authority in the field, this book allows the reader to review developments in emergency medicine over several weeks' time, a task that is nearly impossible when facing the 2120 page parent text. We have increased coverage of pediatrics with new chapters on hematologic-oncologic emergencies, and renal emergencies in children. Additionally we have new chapters on low probability coronary syndromes, urinary retention, food- and waterborne diseases, and world travelers as well as increased discussion of toxicology and trauma. Color photographs and diagnostic images are embedded in their respective chapters for instant recognition of challenging and life-threatening disorders.

We would like to express our sincere appreciation to the *Emergency Medicine: Just the Facts* chapter authors for their commitment and work ethic in helping to produce this review book. All authors are experienced clinicians; we thank them for taking time away from their busy practices to summarize these topics. We also are indebted to numerous individuals who assisted us with this project; in particular, we would like to thank Anne M. Sydor and Christie Naglieri at McGraw-Hill Medical. Finally, without the love,

*Tintinalli's *Emergency Medicine*, 7th edition, was awarded first prize in the category for surgical textbooks by the British Medical Association, 2011.

support, and encouragement of our growing families, this book would not have been possible; DMC dedicates this book to Lisa, Jill, Olivia, Paul, and Joseph; OJM dedicates this book to the residents, fellows, and faculty of the OHSU Department of Emergency Medicine; RKC dedicates this book to Marc, Matthew, Lissy, and Noah; GDM dedicates this book to Roo, Padre, and Steve; SHT dedicates this book to Caroline, Sarah Alice, and Cathrine; DAH dedicates this book to Nicole, Zachary, and Logan.

David M. Cline, MD

O. John Ma, MD

Rita K. Cydulka, MD

Stephen H. Thomas MD

Daniel A. Handel, MD

Garth D. Meckler, MD

Section 1

TEST PREPARATION AND PLANNING

1 FACTS ABOUT EMERGENCY MEDICINE BOARD EXAMS

David M. Cline

- The American Board of Emergency Medicine (ABEM) administers three written exams each year: the Qualification Exam (formerly the Certification Exam), the ConCert Exam (formerly the Recertification Exam), and the In-Training Exam. The year 2004 marked the beginning of Emergency Medicine Continuous Certification (ConCert) and the Lifelong Learning and Self-Assessment (LLSA) exams.
- There are requirements for eligibility for initial ABEM certification and maintaining certification in addition to content testing. For up-to-date information concerning these exams, review the ABEM Web site: www.abem.org.
- The American Osteopathic Board of Emergency Medicine (AOBEM) administers one Certification Examination per year in mid to late March. AOBEM implemented a Continuous Certification in Emergency Medicine process, which is termed Continuous Osteopathic Learning Assessment (COLA). There are requirements for eligibility for initial AOBEM certification and maintaining certification in addition to content testing. See www.aobem.org for details.

ABEM WRITTEN QUALIFICATION EXAM

- The ABEM Qualifying Examination is given each year in early November at several locations throughout the country at computer testing centers; check for test site information at www.abem.org.
- The ABEM Qualifying Examination contains approximately 305 single-best-answer, positively worded, multiple-choice questions.
- Between 10% and 15% of the questions will have a pictorial stimulus.
- Each examination appointment is approximately 8 hours in length, with approximately 6 and ½ hours devoted to actual testing time (1.3 minutes per question). There is a break for lunch separating two separately timed testing sessions of 3 hours and 10 minutes.
- The pass/fail criterion for the Qualifying Examination is 75% correct of those test items that are included in the examination for the purpose of scoring.
- Typically, two-thirds to three-fourths of the test are scored, with one-fourth to one-third of the test questions representing new trial content. These investigational questions are compared with standardized questions for reliability and may be included as scored items the following exam cycle. Typically, a question requires 2 years from the time of creation to use as a scored item.
- The pass rate for the Qualifying Exam during the past 20 years has been 90% for first-time takers, and 78% overall.
- Beginning with the 2002 examinations, the subject matter of the written exams is based on The Model of the Clinical Practice of Emergency Medicine and its revisions.
- A percentage breakdown of the exam content compared to the chapters of this book is listed in Table 1-1. Although many of the questions are different, the content percentages are the same for all three ABEM written exams. *Just the Facts in Emergency Medicine* (3rd edition) includes several chapters that include multiple topics; therefore, our chapters do not precisely correlate with the exam question content areas.
- Another consideration for physicians preparing for the written exams is the acuity breakdown. The questions on the exam are rated by patient acuity (or issues surrounding the care of patients in each acuity category) with 27% critical, 37% emergent, 27% lower acuity, and 9% unrelated to acuity. Therefore, when reviewing specific topic areas, the reader should focus on the issues surrounding the assessment and care of critical or emergent patient presentations, as this content represents 64% of the exam.
- Compared to the ConCert Exam (formerly the Recertification Exam), the Qualification Exam has more pathophysiology-based questions. Roughly 60% of the questions are management based, many of which require a diagnosis be made from the clinical description. Diagnostic criteria are covered in 20%, and 10% are pathophysiology based. The remaining

TABLE 1-1 Percentage Distribution of Test Items by Core Content Category Compared to Chapter Listing of *Just the Facts in Emergency Medicine*, 3rd ed.

	WRITTEN EXAM PERCENTAGE DISTRIBUTION	NUMBER OF CHAPTERS (PERCENT)	*JUST THE FACTS IN EMERGENCY MEDICINE* CHAPTERS REPRESENTED
Signs, symptoms, and presentations	9%	14 (7.2+)	7, 9, 10, 19, 31, 37, 51, 59, 67, 68, 69, 102, 119, 172, plus "Clinical Features in all chapters"
Abdominal and gastrointestinal disorders	9%	15 (7.7)	38–50, 75, 76
Cardiovascular disorders	10%	16 (8.2)	4, 5, 20–30, 74, 80, 95
Cutaneous disorders	2%	4 (2.1)	85, 92, 156, 157
Endocrine, metabolic, and nutritional disorders	3%	8 (4.1)	6, 81–83, 131–134
Environmental disorders	3%	11 (5.7)	120–130
Head, ear, eye, nose, and throat disorders	5%	7 (3.6)	70, 71, 151–155
Hematologic disorders	2%	9 (4.6)	86, 87, 135–141
Immune system disorders	2%	4 (2.1)	8, 94, 101, 183
Systemic infectious disorders	5%	9 (4.6)	89–91, 93, 96–100
Musculoskeletal disorders (nontraumatic)	3%	7 (3.6)	179–185
Nervous system disorders	5%	11 (5.7)	78, 79, 142–150
Obstetrics and gynecology	4%	7 (3.6)	60–66
Psychobehavioral disorders	3%	6 (3.1)	13, 186–190
Renal and urogenital disorders	3%	7 (3.7)	52–57, 77, 88
Thoracic-respiratory disorders	8%	7 (3.7)	31–36, 72, 73,
Toxicology	4%	16 (8.2)	103–118
Traumatic disorders	11%	21 (10.8)	84, 158–160, 162–178
Procedures and skills	6%	11 (5.7)	3, 11–18, 191, 192
Other components (including administration and legal aspects)	3%	5 (2.6)	1, 2, 98, 193, 194

10% of questions relate to emergency department administration, emergency medical service (EMS), disaster medicine, and miscellaneous issues.

- Certification expires every 10 years. Recertification requires participation in the Continuous Certification process (see later in this chapter).

■ ABEM CONTINUOUS CERTIFICATION (RECERTIFICATION)

- The recertification process has been renamed Continuous Certification and now requires four components: (1) professional standing, (2) yearly Lifelong Learning Self-Assessment tests that are based on journal articles, (3) assessment of cognitive expertise (the ConCert exam), and (4) assessment of practice performance.
- All diplomates of the boards should check the Web site for information concerning their requirements for recertification, which vary according to the year their current certification expires.
- Information concerning the professional standing requirement (no. 1 above) and assessment of practice performance (no. 4 above) can be found at the ABEM Web site: www.abem.org.
- The yearly required readings for the LLSA tests can be found at the ABEM Web site: www.abem.org. The LLSA tests are based on these readings.
- The new ConCert Exam is a 5.25-hour experience (4.25 hours in the actual exam) and is available at over

200 computer-administered testing centers across the country. See the ABEM Web site for more details: www.abem.org.

- The ConCert Exam consists of approximately 205 multiple-choice questions that are single-best-answer, positively worded questions focused on what the practicing emergency physician needs to know when treating patients.
- Of the test questions, approximately 15% will include a pictorial stimulus, and these are generally during the first portion of the exam.
- The content of the exam comes from The Model of the Clinical Practice of Emergency Medicine and its subsequent revisions.
- For a period of a few years, the ConCert Exam contained questions related to the content of the LLSA articles; however, that is no longer the case, unless the article's recommendations have become standard practice in the specialty.
- The pass/fail criterion for the ConCert Exam has historically been approximately 75% correct of those test items that are included in the examination for the purpose of scoring.
- Typically only two-thirds to three-fourths of the test are scored, with one-fourth to one-third of the test questions representing new trial content. These investigational questions are compared with standardized questions for reliability and may be included as scored items the following exam cycle.
- The pass rate for the ConCert exams since 2004 to date has averaged 95%.
- Compared to the Qualification Exam, the ConCert Exam is more clinically based and has fewer pathophysiology-based questions.
- The content of the LLSA readings is published on the ABEM Web site. In the first decade of their existence, the topics of LLSA readings were chosen from focused areas of the model curriculum. For example, for the year 2013, the topics are thoracic-respiratory disorders, immune system disorders, and musculoskeletal disorders. Beginning in 2014, the readings will be chosen from the broad spectrum of the EM model and will no longer recycle over a 9-year period.
- A percentage breakdown of the exam content compared to the chapters of this book is listed in Table 1-1. Although many of the questions are different, the content percentages are the same for all three ABEM written exams. *Just the Facts in Emergency Medicine* includes several chapters that include multiple topics; therefore, our chapters do not precisely correlate to the exam question content areas.
- Recertification must be accomplished every 10 years to maintain ABEM Board Certification.

ABEM IN-TRAINING EXAM

- The In-Training Exam is given to all emergency medicine residents each year in late February.
- The test consists of approximately 225 questions and lasts 4 hours and 30 minutes (1.1 minutes per question), given in a single session.
- Unlike other ABEM exams, there is no pass/fail criterion; rather, residents are compared to other residents across the country at their same level of training. Scores for individual training programs are compared with other training programs across the country, and this information is provided to residency program directors.
- Subject matter of the exam is based on The Model of the Clinical Practice of Emergency Medicine and its revisions.
- The target at which all questions are aimed is the expected knowledge base and experience of an emergency medicine third-year resident.
- A percentage breakdown of the exam content compared to the chapters of this book is listed in Table 1-1. Although many of the questions are different, the content percentages are the same for all three ABEM written exams. *Just the Facts in Emergency Medicine* includes several chapters that include multiple topics; therefore, our chapters do not precisely correlate to the exam question content areas.

AOBEM WRITTEN CERTIFICATION EXAM

- The AOBEM Certification Exam is given mid-to-late March each year.
- ABEM and AOBEM written test content areas are similar; however, ABEM includes pediatric content throughout its organ-based system categorization as well as administrative and disaster medicine in its other components categorization, and AOBEM includes vital signs and presentations in its similar systems-based categorization. See the AOBEM Web site for details.
- The percentage breakdown of the exam content is similar to the topic areas listed in Table 1-1.
- Like ABEM, AOBEM uses a preset passing score, but it is not currently published. Also, each exam contains non-scored test items that are in the process of evaluation and standardization.

2 TEST-TAKING TECHNIQUES

David M. Cline

- Excellent test performance requires both well-planned study methods and carefully applied test-taking skills.

EXAM PREPARATION AND PHYSICIAN PERFORMANCE

- Exam preparation techniques and successful test completion have not been well studied within the specialty of emergency medicine. Studies from other medical specialties or professional disciplines may or may not pertain to emergency medicine board exams.
- There is only weak evidence to suggest that continuing medical education positively impacts clinical practice.
- Interactive sessions that emphasize practice skills may have a positive impact on physician practice behaviors.
- There is little evidence that routine didactic educational conferences improve test performance.
- It has been shown that an intensive conference series focused on exam content can improve subsequent test performance.
- It has been shown that increased conference attendance by surgery residents improved test performance for residents with higher past performance histories.
- Studies conducted in other specialties have shown several factors that correlate with better test performance: self-directed study, programmed textbook review, and individual resident effort.
- In the specialties of both neurology and surgery, past performances on the in-training exam predicted performance on the certification examination.
- For surgery residents, being on call the night before the exam did not affect in-training exam scores.

STUDY TECHNIQUES

The following techniques are recommended based on commonsense rules of study methods. Supporting studies in emergency medicine have not been conducted.

- Begin by setting a schedule to accomplish your study goals and objectives in the time remaining prior to the test. Allow time for reading this book, using a question-and-answer book to uncover any gaps in your knowledge base and your final review. Your schedule should be written and checked often to document your progress.
- Find a place to study that facilitates concentration, not distraction. It has been shown that a single place of study improves test performance for college students.
- Begin reading each chapter by glancing over the topic headings to get an overview of the material. Formulate questions in your mind such as:
  1. What etiologic information will help me to identify the patient at risk for the disease?
  2. What pathophysiologic concepts will help to treat the disease?
  3. What clinical features will help me to identify the disease?
  4. What criteria confirm the diagnosis of the disease?
  5. What are the recommended treatments for the disease?
- Reading should be an active experience. Don't turn the exercise into a coloring contest with your highlighter. Write in the margins, circle, underline, and identify key points.
- Review your notes and key points at the end. If you find the material confusing or your understanding incomplete, you will need to go to other sources for additional information, such as the parent textbook for this review book: *Emergency Medicine: A Comprehensive Study Guide,* 7th ed. Consider also reviewing a pictorial atlas of disease, an electrocardiogram atlas, and a radiology atlas.
- If you do not have time to read this book in its entirety, review the index to identify gaps in your knowledge. Look for unfamiliar topics or disease-specific treatments you have not previously reviewed.
- Last-minute cramming is an inefficient study method, taxes your energy, and creates anxiety.

PREPARATION IMMEDIATELY BEFORE THE TEST

- Get plenty of sleep the night before the test.
- Arrive at the test site well in advance of the start time to make sure you know where the exam room is located and become familiar with the surroundings and/or the computer-based testing procedure.
- ABEM written exams are conducted at Pearson VUE testing centers; a tutorial can be taken ahead of the exam online: www.pearsonvue.com/sponsors/tutorial.
- A tutorial is available before the actual timed testing session. You should take this tutorial because it may familiarize you with the procedure and does not take time away from the timed testing procedure.
- In addition to those tutorials discussed above, an optional, 20–25 question demonstration test can be taken at the computer center at a date prior to the appointment for the actual test. There is a fee for this

experience, and its purpose is to familiarize candidates with the computer-testing experience. The content and the level of difficulty of this exam experience are not intended to be representative of the actual test.

- Check the temperature of the exam room so that you can anticipate proper attire. Dress comfortably.
- Schedule enough time to wake up, dress, and eat an unhurried breakfast.
- Eat an adequate but not heavy breakfast. Do the same for the lunch break.
- Bring a photo ID to identify yourself and any other specified materials.
- Although anxiety reduction techniques have long been recommended, a certain degree of test anxiety has been shown to improve test performance.

TAKING THE TEST

- Listen carefully to any verbal instructions and read completely any written/on-screen instructions.
- You have between 1.1 and 1.3 minutes per question on the test. Make sure that you maintain this schedule. For example, at the 1-hour mark, you should have answered approximately 60 questions. However, the pictorial stimulus portion of the test is usually first, and these questions take more time than the remaining questions for most test takers.
- There is no penalty for guessing on this multiple-choice exam. Each question is worth 1 point.
- You should answer each question as you work your way through the test the first time, selecting your initial best answer. The program allows you to flag the questions that you wish to return to and reconsider your answer.
- Carefully read the question stem and anticipate the answer before you read the options listed. If you see the choice you anticipate, that answer is most likely correct.
- Read all the answers to check for a more complete or better answer than the one you anticipated.
- Don't waste excessive time on a single question that puzzles you. Simply make your best guess and move on. The computer program facilitates flagging questions so that you can return to the question at the end for further consideration.
- Remember that up to one-third of the test is not scored (see Chap. 1). If you don't know the answer or find the question confusing, it may be a trial question. Don't lose your confidence or your momentum.
- Identify the incorrect options quickly so that if you are forced to guess, you have a better chance of being correct.
- On items that have "all of the above" as an option, if you are certain that two other answers are correct, you should choose "all of the above."
- Options that include broad generalizations are more likely to be incorrect.
- There is no evidence to support the idea that option "C" is more likely to be correct than others on ABEM exams.
- Use every minute of the test time. If you have time left over, review first the questions you have identified as difficult, and then use the remaining time to reread the questions, looking for any misinterpretations that may have occurred the first time through.
- Contrary to popular opinion, your first guess is no more likely to be correct than a carefully considered reevaluation of the answer. If during the review process, you find a better answer to a question stem, do not hesitate to change your choice. You have a 57.8% chance of changing a wrong answer to a correct one, a 22.2% chance of changing a wrong answer to another wrong answer, and only a 20.2% chance of changing a correct answer to an incorrect one. However, students who have a past record of doing well on exams are more likely to make a correct change than those students who have a history of poor test performance.
- Do not spend your lunch break discussing specific test questions with colleagues. This practice could disqualify you from the test, and creates more anxiety, further limiting your performance in the afternoon.
- Relax. The odds are in your favor, and now that you own this book, you have a concise means to review the practice of emergency medicine.

Section 2
RESUSCITATION TECHNIQUES

3 ADVANCED AIRWAY SUPPORT

Robert J. Vissers

INITIAL APPROACH

- Control of the airway is the single most important task for emergency resuscitation.
- The initial approach to airway management is simultaneous assessment and management of the adequacy of airway patency (the A of the ABCs), and oxygenation and ventilation (the B of the ABCs).

PATHOPHYSIOLOLGY

- The upper anatomic airway includes the oral and nasal cavities down to the larynx. The lower airway includes the trachea, bronchi, and lungs.
- Potentially difficult intubations can be predicted by the following:
  1. External features suggestive of difficulty, such as a beard or obesity, short neck, receding chin, or tracheotomy scars.
  2. Inability to open the mouth three fingerbreadths, or a thyromental distance less than three fingerbreadths.
  3. A relatively large tongue for the oral cavity as estimated by the inability to visualize more than the base of the uvula in a cooperative patient opening the mouth in a sniffing position (Fig. 3-1).
  4. Evidence of upper airway obstruction.
  5. Lack of neck mobility. This should be assessed only in patients without potential C-spine injury.

EMERGENCY CARE AND DISPOSITION

- Assess patient's color and respiratory rate; respiratory or cardiac arrest may be an indication for immediate intubation.
- Open the airway with head tilt–chin lift maneuver (use jaw thrust if C-spine injury is suspected). If needed, bag the patient with the bag-valve-mask device that includes an O_2 reservoir. A good seal depends on proper mask size. This technique may require an oral or nasal airway or two rescuers (one to seal the mask with 2 hands and the other to bag the patient).

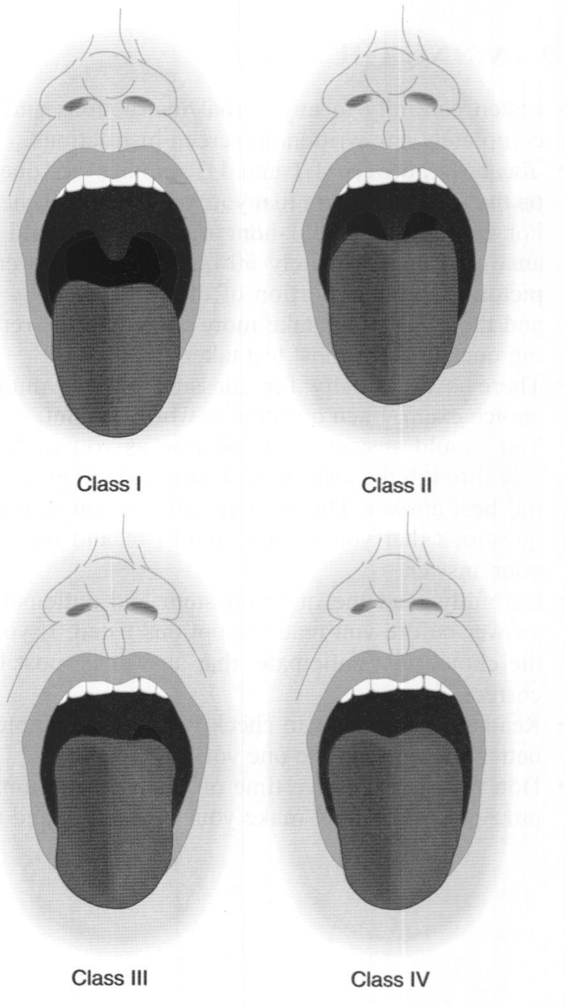

FIG. 3-1. Classification of tongue size relative to the size of the oral cavity as described by Mallampati and colleagues. Class I: Faucial pillars, soft palate, and uvula can be visualized. Class II: Faucial pillars and soft palate can be visualized, but the uvula is masked by the base of the tongue. Class III: Only the base of the uvula can be visualized. Class IV: None of the three structures can be visualized.

- Provide continuous monitoring of vital signs, oxygen saturation, and end-tidal CO_2 (if possible).
- Determine the need for invasive airway management techniques. Do not wait for arterial blood gas analyses if the initial assessment indicates the need for invasive airway management. If the patient does not require immediate airway or ventilation control, administer oxygen by facemask to ensure an O_2 saturation of 95%. Do not remove oxygen to draw an arterial blood gas analysis unless deemed safe from the initial assessment.
- Preoxygenate all patients prior to intubation regardless of saturation. Assess airway difficulty before initiation of advanced airway techniques (see later in the chapter).

OROTRACHEAL INTUBATION

- The most common means used to ensure a patent airway, prevent aspiration, and provide oxygenation and ventilation is orotracheal intubation.
- Rapid sequence intubation (RSI) should be used unless the patient's condition makes it unnecessary (ie, cardiac arrest) or it is contraindicated because of an anticipated difficult airway.

EMERGENCY DEPARTMENT CARE AND DISPOSITION

- Prepare equipment, personnel, and drugs before attempting intubation. Assess airway difficulty and anticipate required airway rescue.
- Ensure adequate ventilation and oxygenation and monitoring while preparing equipment. Preoxygenate with a nonrebreather oxygen mask or with a bag-valve-mask if the patient is not ventilating adequately.
- Select blade type and size (usually a no. 3 or 4 curved blade or a no. 2 or 3 straight blade); test the blade light. Select the tube size (usually 7.5-8.0 mm in women, 8.0-8.5 mm in men) and test the balloon cuff. The use of a flexible stylet is recommended.
- Patient positioning is critical to successful intubation. Position the patient with the head extended and neck flexed, possibly with a rolled towel under the occiput to align the oropharyngolaryngeal axes. If C-spine injury is suspected, maintain the head and neck in a neutral position with an assistant performing inline stabilization.
- Once the vocal cords are visualized, gently pass the tube between the cords. Remove the laryngoscope, check for tube placement by ventilating and listening for bilateral breath sounds and absence of epigastric sounds. Inflate the cuff.
- If the cords are not visualized, manipulate the thyroid cartilage using backward, upward, and rightward pressure (the "burp" maneuver) to help bring the cords into view. If unsuccessful, reoxygenation may need to be performed with bag-valve-mask device. Consider changing the blade, the tube size, or the position of the patient before further attempts. Consider using an intubating stylet (bougie). Three unsuccessful attempts define a failed airway, and other rescue techniques must be considered.
- Confirm placement objectively with an end-tidal CO_2 detector, capnography, or in cardiac arrest, with an esophageal detection device. Check tube length; the usual distance (marked on the tube) from corner of the mouth to 2 cm above the carina is 23 cm in men and 21 cm in women.
- Secure the tube and verify placement with a portable radiograph.
- Immediate complications include unrecognized esophageal intubation or mainstem bronchus intubation. Failure to confirm the position immediately can result in hypoxia and neurologic injury. Endobronchial intubation is usually on the right side and is corrected by withdrawing the tube 2 cm and listening for equal breath sounds.

RAPID-SEQUENCE INTUBATION INDUCTION

- Rapid-sequence intubation is the simultaneous administration of an induction and a neuromuscular blocking agent to facilitate orotracheal intubation. This technique couples sedation with muscular paralysis. Anticipated difficulty in mask ventilation or intubation is a relative contraindication to rapid-sequence intubation.
- If difficulty is anticipated, consider other methods of airway management such as videolaryngoscopy, awake intubation, cricothyrotomy, or an alternative airway device.
- The steps for rapid-sequence intubation are listed in Table 3-1.
- Induction agents are described in Table 3-2.
- Paralytic agents are described in Table 3-3.

ALTERNATIVE AIRWAY DEVICES

- A number of rescue devices are available for management of the difficult airway.
- Intubating stylets (or gum elastic bougies) are semi-rigid stylets with a coude tip, which can be placed by feel, during laryngoscopy, into the trachea, and then guided over the intubating stylet into the trachea.

TABLE 3-1 Rapid-Sequence Intubation

RAPID-SEQUENCE INTUBATION STEPS
1. Set up IV access, cardiac monitor, oximetry, and possibly capnography.
2. Plan procedure incorporating assessment of physiologic status and airway difficulty.
3. Prepare equipment, suction, and potential rescue devices.
4. Preoxygenate.
5. Consider pretreatment agents based on underlying conditions.*
6. Induce with potent sedative agent.
7. Give neuromuscular blocking agent immediately after induction.
8. Bag-mask ventilate only if hypoxic, consider cricoid pressure.
9. Intubate trachea after muscle relaxation has been achieved.
10. Confirm placement and secure tube.
11. Provide postintubation sedation and postintubation management.

*It is unclear if pretreatment improves outcome. **Fentanyl,** 3 micrograms/kg may be used in normotensive patients with possible raised intracranial pressure, cardiac ischemia, or aortic dissection. **Lidocaine,** 1 milligram/kg IV, could be used in patients with possible raised ICP or asthma.

This device is useful for anterior cords that cannot be directly visualized.

- The laryngeal mask airway (LMA) is an airway device that is placed blindly into the supraglottic space. A distal ringed balloon is inflated to seal the glottis above the larynx and allow for ventilation. Aspiration and air leaks may occur. The intubating LMA allows for the placement of a cuffed endotracheal tube through the device.
- Videolaryngoscopy is an excellent option for airway rescue or as a primary intubation technique. These devices can be advantageous in patients with restricted oral opening or cervical spine mobility.
- Crichothyrotomy is performed when intubation, ventilation, and airway rescue have failed. Insert a number-4 cuffed tracheostomy tube (or the largest tube that will fit). Alternatively, use a small cuffed endotracheal

TABLE 3-2 Induction Agents

PREFERRED RAPID-SEQUENCE INTUBATION INDUCTION AGENTS

AGENT	DOSE	INDUCTION	DURATION	BENEFITS	CAVEATS
Etomidate	0.3 milligram/kg IV	<1 min	10–20 min	↓ICP ↓Intraocular pressure Neutral BP	Myoclonic jerking or seizures and vomiting in awake patients No analgesia ↓Cortisol
Propofol	0.5–1.5 milligrams/kg IV	20–40 s	8–15 min	Antiemetic Anticonvulsant ↓ICP	Apnea ↓BP No analgesia
Ketamine	1–2 milligrams/kg IV	1 min	10–20 min	Bronchodilator "Dissociative" amnesia Analgesia	↑Secretions ↑BP Emergence phenomenon

Abbreviations: BP = blood pressure, ICP =intracranial pressure.

TABLE 3-3 Neuromuscular Paralytic Agents

AGENT	ADULT INTUBATING IV DOSE	ONSET	DURATION	COMPLICATIONS
Succinylcholine (short)	1.0–1.5 milligrams/kg	45–60 s	5–9 min	Hyperkalemia in: Burns >5 d old Denervation injury >5 d old Significant crush injures >5 d old Severe infection >5 d old Preexisting myopathies Bradycardia Masseter spasm Increased intragastric, intraocular, and possibly intracranial pressure Malignant hyperthermia Prolonged apnea with pseudocholinesterase deficiency Fasciculations
Rocuronium (intermediate/long)	0.6 milligrams/kg	1–3 min	30–45 min	Tachycardia
Vecuronium (intermediate/long)	0.08–0.15 milligrams/kg 0.15–0.28 milligrams/kg (high-dose protocol)	2–4 min	25–40 min 60–120 min	Prolonged recovery time in the obese or elderly, or if there is hepatorenal dysfunction

TABLE 3-4 Advantages and Adverse Effects of Noninvasive Positive Pressure Ventilation

ADVANTAGES	ADVERSE EFFECTS
Less sedation, noninvasive, patient able to maintain verbalization	Respiratory anxiety and agitation leading to noninvasive positive pressure ventilation failure
Early improvement in hypoxia, acidosis, and hypercapnia	Air trapping, in which exaggerated increased mean intrathoracic pressure can cause marked decreased venous return to the heart, resulting in decreased cardiac output and hypotension
Shorter hospital stay	Abdominal compartment syndrome
Decreased rate of intubation	Pulmonary barotrauma leading to pneumothorax
Decreased mortality	Respiratory alkalosis

tube (No. 6 or the largest tube that will fit). Inflate the cuff. Crichothyrotomy is contraindicated in children younger than 10 to 12 years in whom trans-tracheal jet ventilation is the preferred subglottic technique.
- Formal tracheostomy is not recommended as an emergency surgical airway technique due to increased technical difficulty and time required.

NONINVASIVE POSITIVE PRESSURE VENTILATION

- Noninvasive positive pressure ventilation (NPPV) provides positive pressure airway support using preset volume/pressure of inspiratory air through a face or nasal mask. Noninvasive positive pressure ventilation has been used as an alternative to endotracheal intubation in patients with ventilatory failure due to chronic obstructive pulmonary disease (COPD), and cardiogenic pulmonary edema. Patients need to be cooperative and without cardiac ischemia, hypotension, or dysrhythmia. Table 3-4 lists the advantages and disadvantages of noninvasive positive pressure ventilation.
- Continuous positive airway pressure (CPAP) provides constant positive pressure throughout the respiratory cycle. Continuous positive airway pressures are usually between 5 and 15 cm H_2O and are adjusted to the patients' response to therapy.
- Bilevel positive airway pressure (BiPAP) uses different levels of pressure during inspiration and expiration. Initial settings of 8 to 10 cm H_2O during inspiration and 3 to 4 cm H_2O during expiration are reasonable and can be titrated up based on clinical response.

Alternative drugs for rapid-sequence induction are listed in Chapter 30 of *Emergency Medicine: A Comprehensive Study Guide,* 7th ed. Airway management alternatives to the methods described earlier include blind nasotracheal intubation, digital intubation, transillumination, extraglottic devices, flexible and rigid fiberoptics, retrograde tracheal intubation, and translaryngeal ventilation, These techniques are described in Chapters 28, 30, and 31 of *Emergency Medicine: A Comprehensive Study Guide,* 7th ed.

For further reading in *Emergency Medicine: A Comprehensive Study Guide,* 7th ed., see Chapter 28, "Noninvasive Airway Management," by A. Michael Roman; Chapter 30, "Tracheal Intubation and Mechanical Ventilation," by Robert J. Vissers and Daniel F. Danzl; and Chapter 31, "Surgical Airway Management," by Michael D. Smith.

4 ARRHYTHMIA MANAGEMENT

James K. Takayesu

SINUS ARRHYTHMIA

Some variation in the sinoatrial (SA) node discharge rate is common; however, if the variation exceeds 0.12 second between the longest and shortest intervals, sinus arrhythmia is present. The electrocardiogram (ECG) characteristics of sinus arrhythmia are (a) normal sinus P waves and PR intervals, (b) 1:1 atrioventricular (AV) conduction, and (c) variation of at least 0.12 second between the shortest and longest P-P interval (Fig. 4-1). Sinus arrhythmias are affected primarily by respiration and are most commonly found in children and young adults, disappearing with advancing age. Occasional junctional escape beats may be present during very long P-P intervals. No treatment is required.

PREMATURE ATRIAL CONTRACTIONS

Premature atrial contractions (PACs) have the following ECG characteristics: (a) the ectopic P wave appears sooner (premature) than the next expected sinus beat; (b) the ectopic P wave has a different shape and direction; and (c) the ectopic P wave may or may not be conducted through the AV node (Fig. 4-2). Most PACs are conducted with typical QRS complexes, but some may be conducted aberrantly through the infranodal system, typically with a right bundle branch block (RBBB) pattern. When the PAC occurs during the absolute refractory period, it is not conducted. Since the sinus

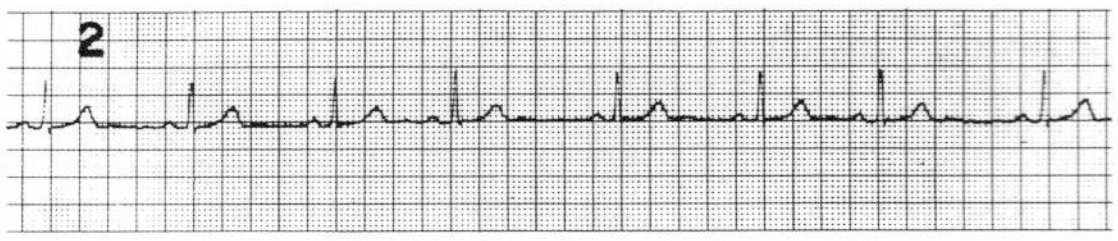

FIG. 4-1. Sinus arrhythmia.

node is often depolarized and reset, the pause is less than fully compensatory. PACs are associated with stress, fatigue, alcohol use, tobacco, coffee, chronic obstructive pulmonary disease (COPD), digoxin toxicity, coronary artery disease, and may also occur after adenosine-converted paroxysmal supraventricular tachycardia (PSVT). PACs are common in all ages, often in the absence of significant heart disease. Patients may complain of palpitations or an intermittent "sinking" or "fluttering" feeling in the chest.

Emergency Department Care and Disposition

1. Discontinue precipitating drugs (alcohol, tobacco, or coffee) or toxins.
2. Treat underlying disorders (stress or fatigue).
3. PACs that produce significant symptoms or initiate sustained tachycardias can be suppressed with agents such as β-adrenergic antagonists (eg, metoprolol 25-50 milligrams PO three times daily), usually in consultation with a follow-up physician.

SUPRAVENTRICULAR BRADYARRYTHMIAS

SINUS BRADYCARDIA

Clinical Features

Sinus bradycardia occurs when the SA node rate becomes slower than 60 beats/min. The ECG characteristics of sinus bradycardia are (a) normal sinus P waves and PR intervals, (b) 1:1 AV conduction, and (c) atrial rate slower than 60 beats/min. Sinus bradycardia represents a suppression of the sinus node discharge rate, usually in response to three categories of stimuli: (a) physiologic (vagal tone), (b) pharmacologic (calcium channel blockers, β-blockers, or digoxin), and (c) pathologic (acute inferior myocardial infarction [MI], increased intracranial pressure, carotid sinus hypersensitivity, hypothyroidism, or sick sinus syndrome).

Emergency Department Care and Disposition

Sinus bradycardia usually does not require specific treatment unless the heart rate is slower than 50 beats/min and there is evidence of hypoperfusion.

1. **Transcutaneous cardiac pacing** is the only Class I treatment for unstable patients.
   a. Attach the patient to the monitor leads of the external pacing device.
   b. When placing transcutaneous pacing pads, place the anterior pad over the left lateral precordium and the posterior pad at the level of the heart in the right infrascapular area. Do not use multifunction pacing defibrillation pads unless the patient is unconscious as they cause a lot of discomfort.
   c. Slowly increase the pacing output from 0 mA to the lowest point where capture is observed, usually at 50 to 100 mA, but may be up to 200 mA. A widened QRS after each pacing spike denotes electrical capture.
   d. If needed, administer a sedative, such as lorazepam, 1 to 2 milligrams IV, or an opiate, such as morphine, 2 to 4 milligrams IV, for pain control.
2. **Atropine** is a Class IIa treatment for symptomatic bradycardia. The dose is 0.5 milligram IV push, repeated every 3–5 minutes as needed up to a total of 3 milligrams IV. If given via endotracheal tube,

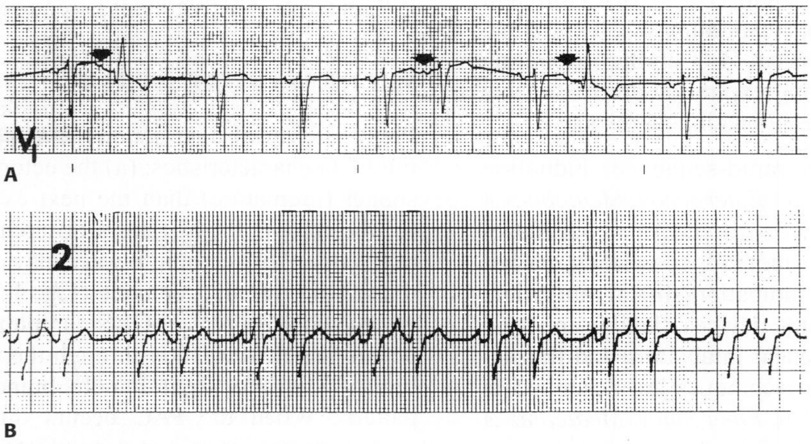

FIG. 4-2. Premature atrial contractions (PACs). **A.** Ectopic P′ waves (arrows). **B.** Atrial bigeminy.

increase the dose by 2–2.5 times over the IV dose. Slow administration or lower doses may cause paradoxical bradycardia. Atropine may not be effective in cardiac transplant patients since the heart is denervated and has no vagal stimulation.

3. **Epinephrine,** 2–10 micrograms/min IV, or **dopamine,** 3–10 micrograms/kg/min IV, may be used if external pacing is not available.
4. Internal pacing will be required in the patient with symptomatic recurrent or persistent sinus bradycardia due to sick sinus syndrome.
5. Isoproterenol, 2–10 micrograms/min IV infusion, may be effective but carries a risk of increased myocardial oxygen demand.

SUPRVENTRICULAR TACHYARRYTHMIAS

SINUS TACHYCARDIA

Clinical Features

The ECG characteristics of sinus tachycardia are (a) normal sinus P waves and PR intervals and (b) an atrial rate usually between 100 and 160 beats/min. Sinus tachycardia is in response to three categories of stimuli: (a) physiologic (pain or exertion), (b) pharmacologic (sympathomimetics, caffeine, or bronchodilators), or (c) pathologic (fever, hypoxia, anemia, hypovolemia, pulmonary embolism, or hyperthyroidism). In many of these conditions, the increased heart rate is an effort to increase cardiac output to match increased circulatory needs.

Emergency Department Care and Disposition

Diagnose and treat the underlying condition.

SUPRAVENTRICULAR TACHYCARDIA

Clinical Features

Supraventricular tachycardia (SVT) is a regular, rapid rhythm that arises from impulse reentry or an ectopic pacemaker above the bifurcation of the His bundle. The reentrant variety is the most common (Fig. 4-3). Patients often present with acute, symptomatic episodes termed paroxysmal supraventricular tachycardia (PSVT). Atrioventricular nodal reentrant tachycardia (AVnRT) can occur in a normal heart or in association with rheumatic heart disease, acute pericarditis, MI, mitral valve prolapse, or preexcitation syndromes. In patients with atrioventricular bypass tracts (AVRT), reentry can occur in either direction, usually (80-90% of patients) in a direction that goes down the AV node and up the bypass tract producing a narrow QRS complex (orthodromic conduction). In the remaining 10% to 20% of patients, reentry occurs in the reverse direction (antidromic conduction). Ectopic SVT usually originates in the atria, with an atrial rate of 100–250 beats/min and may be seen in patients with acute MI, chronic lung disease, pneumonia, alcohol intoxication, or digoxin toxicity.

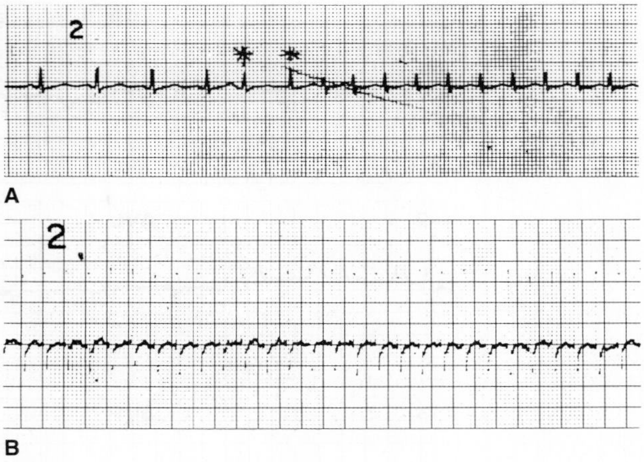

FIG. 4-3. Reentrant supraventricular tachycardia (SVT). **A.** Second (*) initiates run of PAT. **B.** SVT, rate 286.

There is a high incidence of tachyarrhythmias in patients with preexcitation syndromes including PSVT (40-80%), atrial fibrillation (10-20%), and atrial flutter (about 5%). All forms of preexcitation are caused by accessory tracts that bypass part or all of the normal conducting system, the most common form being Wolff–Parkinson–White (WPW) syndrome (Fig. 4-4). The ventricles are activated by an impulse from the atria sooner than would be expected if the impulse were transmitted down the normal conducting pathway. This premature activation causes initial fusion beat morphology with slurring of initial QRS complex, causing the pathognomonic delta wave. Among patients with WPW-PSVT, 80% to 90% will conduct in the orthodromic direction and the remaining 10% to 20% will conduct in the antidromic direction. ECG findings of atrial fibrillation or flutter with antidromic conduction down the bypass tract show a wide QRS complex that is irregular with a rate faster than 180–200 beats/min (see Atrial Fibrillation below).

Emergency Department Care and Disposition

1. Perform synchronized cardioversion in any unstable patient (eg, hypotension, pulmonary edema, or severe chest pain).
2. In stable patients, the first intervention should be vagal maneuvers, including:
   a. Valsalva maneuver: While in the supine position, ask the patient to strain for at least 10 seconds.

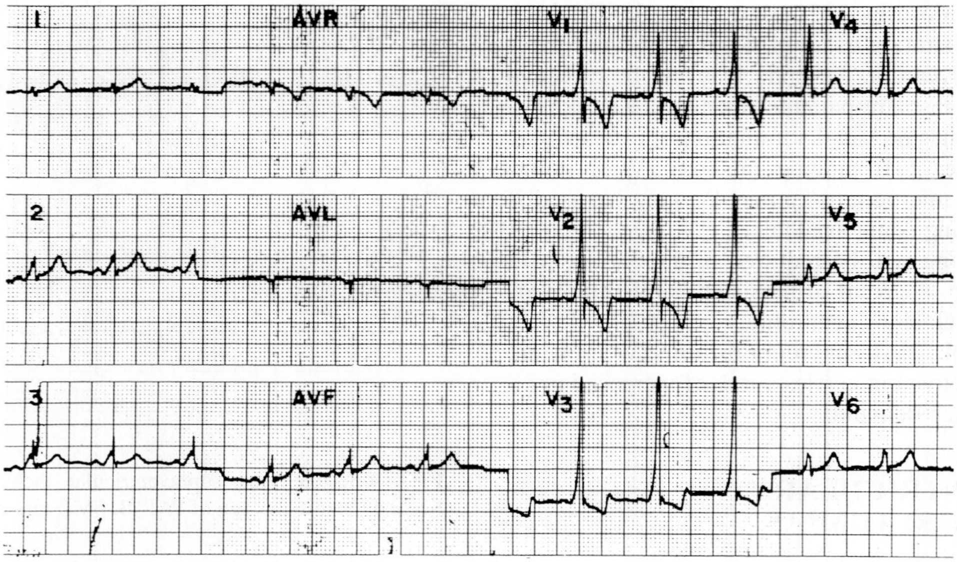

FIG. 4-4. Type A Wolff–Parkinson–White syndrome.

The legs may be lifted to increase venous return and augment the reflex.

b. Diving reflex: Have the patient immerse the face in cold water or apply a bag of ice water to the face for 6–7 seconds. This maneuver is particularly effective in infants.
c. Carotid sinus massage: Auscultate to ensure that there is no carotid bruit and massage the carotid sinus against the transverse process of C6 for 10 seconds at a time, first on the side of the nondominant cerebral hemisphere. This should never be done simultaneously on both sides.

3. Administer **adenosine,** 6 milligrams rapid IV bolus, into a large vein followed by a 20-mL normal saline rapid flush. If there is no effect within 2 minutes, give a second dose of 12 milligrams IV. Most patients experience distressing chest pain, flushing, or anxiety lasting less than 1 minute. Ten percent of patients may experience transient atrial fibrillation or flutter after conversion. This is first-line treatment for WPW-associated SVT with a narrow QRS complex (orthodromic conduction) but is ineffective in cases of anterograde conduction over an accessory pathway. Adenosine may induce bronchospasm in asthmatics requiring treatment with bronchodilators.
4. In patients with narrow-complex SVT (orthodromic conduction) and normal cardiac function, cardioversion may also be achieved with the following second-line agents:
   a. Calcium-channel blockers: **Diltiazem**, 20 milligrams (0.25 milligram/kg) IV over 2 minutes, or **verapamil**, 0.075-0.15 milligram/kg (3-10 milligrams) IV over 15 to 60 seconds with a repeat dose in 30 minutes, if necessary. Verapamil may cause hypotension that can be prevented by pretreatment with calcium chloride or gluconate (500-1000 milligrams).
   b. Beta-blockers: **Esmolol,** 500 micrograms/kg IV bolus, **metoprolol,** 5 milligrams IV, or **propranolol,** 0.1 milligram/kg divided in 3 doses given 2 minutes apart.
   c. **Digoxin,** 0.4 to 0.6 milligram IV.
5. Patients with wide-complex SVT (antidromic conduction across accessory pathway) should be approached as presumed ventricular tachycardia (VT; see Ventricular Tachycardia) unless there is a known history of WPW syndrome. Patients with this type of tachycardia are at risk for rapid ventricular rates and degeneration into ventricular fibrillation (VF); therefore, agents that preferentially block the AV node such as β-blockers, calcium channel blockers, and digoxin should not be used. Treat stable patients with **procainamide**, 17 milligrams/kg IV over 30 minutes up to 50 milligrams/kg, or until 50% QRS widening is noted (contraindicated in patients with myasthenia gravis since it may increase weakness).

ATRIAL FLUTTER

Clinical Features

Atrial flutter is a rhythm that originates from a small area within the atria. ECG characteristics of atrial flutter are (a) a regular atrial rate between 250 and

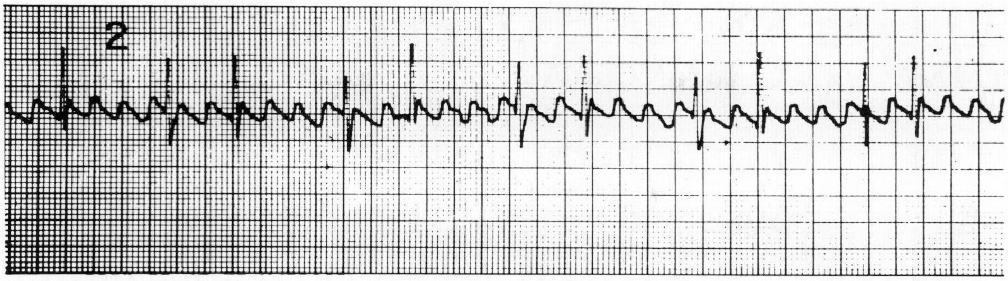

FIG. 4-5. Atrial flutter.

350 beats/min; (b) "sawtooth" flutter waves directed superiorly and most visible in leads II, III, and aVF; and (c) AV block, usually 2:1, but occasionally greater or irregular (Fig. 4-5). One-to-one conduction may occur if a bypass tract is present. Carotid sinus massage or valsalva maneuvers are useful techniques to slow the ventricular response by increasing the degree of AV block, which can unmask flutter waves in uncertain cases. Atrial flutter is seen most commonly in patients with ischemic heart disease as well as congestive heart failure (CHF), acute MI, pulmonary embolus, myocarditis, blunt chest trauma, and digoxin toxicity. Atrial flutter may be a transitional arrhythmia between sinus rhythm and atrial fibrillation. Consider anticoagulation in patients with an unclear time of onset or duration longer than 48 hours before conversion to sinus rhythm due to increased risk of atrial thrombus and embolization.

Emergency Department Care

The treatment is the same as atrial fibrillation and is discussed below.

ATRIAL FIBRILLATION

Clinical Features

Atrial fibrillation (Afib) occurs when there are multiple, small areas of atrial myocardium continuously discharging in a disorganized fashion. This results in loss of effective atrial contraction and decreases left ventricular (LV) end-diastolic volume, which may precipitate CHF in patients with impaired cardiac function. The ECG characteristics of Afib are (a) fibrillatory waves of atrial activity, best seen in leads V_1, V_2, V_3, and aV_F, and (b) an irregular ventricular response, usually between 170 and 180 beats/min in patients with a healthy AV node (Fig. 4-6). Afib may be paroxysmal (lasting for less than 7 days), persistent (lasting for more than 7 days), or chronic (continuous). Afib can be idiopathic (lone Afib) or may be found in association with longstanding hypertension, ischemic heart disease, rheumatic heart disease, alcohol use ("holiday heart"), COPD, and thyrotoxicosis. Patients with LV dysfunction who depend on atrial contraction may suffer acute CHF with Afib onset. Rates of greater than 300 beats/min with a wide QRS complex are concerning for a preexcitation syndrome such as WPW (Fig. 4-7). Patients with Afib who are not anticoagulated have a yearly embolic event rate as high as 5% and a lifetime risk greater than 25%. Conversion from chronic Afib to sinus rhythm carries a 1% to 5% risk of arterial embolism; therefore, anticoagulation for 3 weeks is required before cardioversion in patients with Afib for longer than 48-hour duration and in those patients with an uncertain time of onset who are not on anticoagulation therapy.

Emergency Department Care and Disposition

1. Treat unstable patients with synchronized cardioversion (50–100 J).
2. Stable patients with Afib for longer than 48 hours should be anticoagulated with **heparin** (80 units/kg IV followed by an infusion of 18 units/kg/h IV) before cardioversion. Consider a transesophageal echocardiogram to rule out atrial thrombus before cardioversion.
3. Control rate with diltiazem. Administer 20 milligrams (0.25 milligram/kg) IV over 2 minutes followed by a continuous IV infusion, 5–15 milligrams/h, to maintain rate control. Give a second dose of 25 milligrams (0.35 milligram/kg) in 15 minutes if the first

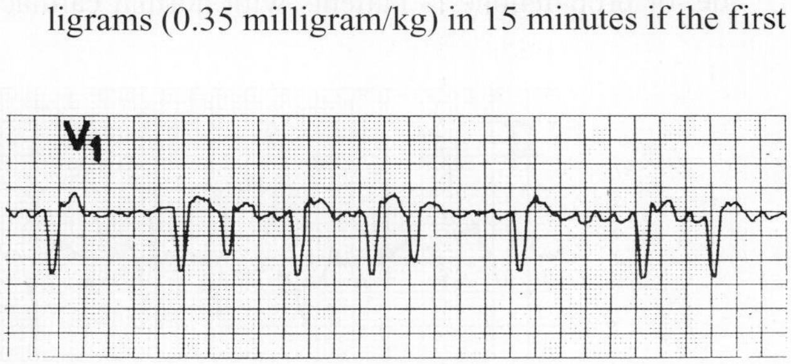

FIG. 4-6. Atrial fibrillation.

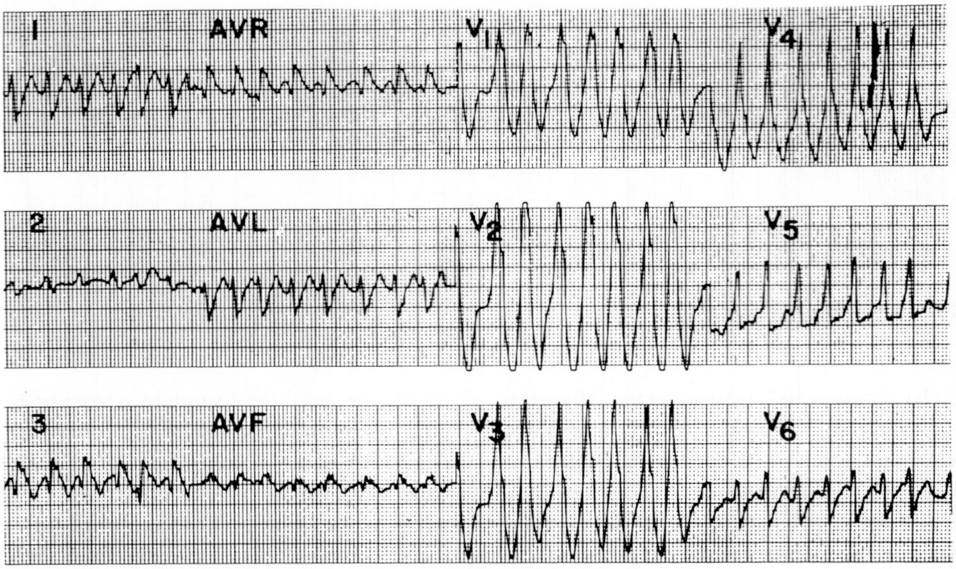

FIG. 4-7. Atrial fibrillation in Wolff–Parkinson–White syndrome.

dose fails to control rate. Alternative rate control agents for patients with normal cardiac function include **verapamil**, 5–10 milligrams IV; **metoprolol**, 5–10 milligrams IV; and **digoxin**, 0.4–0.6 milligram IV. Treat patients with preexcitation syndromes (eg, WPW) with **procainamide,** 17 milligrams/kg IV, over 30 minutes up to 50 milligrams/kg or until 50% QRS widening is noted. Avoid β-adrenergic or calcium channel blockers (ie, verapamil) due to the risk of causing degeneration to VF.

4. In patients with impaired cardiac function (EF <40%), use **amiodarone,** 5 milligrams/kg IV over 30 minutes, followed by 1200 milligrams over 24 hours (contraindicated in patients with iodine or shellfish allergy; increased risk of rhabdomyolysis if coadministered with simvastatin) or **digoxin** 0.4–0.6 milligram IV.
5. Patients with Afib for shorter than 48 hours may be chemically or electrically cardioverted in the emergency department. Use amiodarone, ibutilide (see comments for atrial flutter), procainamide, flecainide, or propafenone in patients with normal cardiac function. **Ibutilide** is dosed at 0.01 milligram/kg IV up to 1 milligram, infused over 10 minutes. A second ibutilide dose may be given if there is no response in 20 minutes. Ibutilide should not be administered to patients with known structural heart disease, hypokalemia, prolonged QTc intervals, hypomagnesemia, or CHF because of the possibility of provoking torsades de pointes. Monitor for 4–6 hours after giving ibutilide. Patients with impaired cardiac function may be cardioverted with amiodarone or electrically.

MULTIFOCAL ATRIAL TACHYCARDIA

Clinical Features

Multifocal atrial tachycardia (MAT) is defined as at least three different sites of atrial ectopy. The ECG characteristics of MAT are (a) three or more differently shaped P waves; (b) changing P-P, PR, and R-R intervals; and (c) atrial rhythm usually between 100 and 180 beats/min (Fig. 4-8). Because the rhythm is irregularly irregular, MAT can be confused with atrial flutter

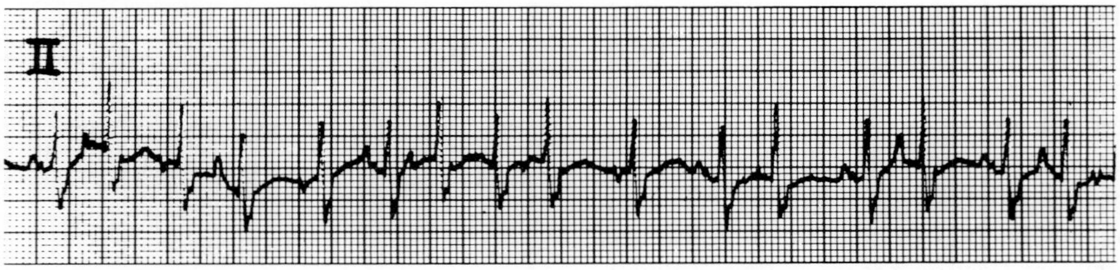

FIG. 4-8. Multifocal atrial tachycardia (MFAT).

or atrial fibrillation (Afib). MAT is found most often in elderly patients with decompensated COPD, but it also may be found in patients with CHF, sepsis, methylxanthine toxicity, or digoxin toxicity.

Emergency Department Care and Disposition

1. Treat the underlying disorder.
2. Specific antiarrhythmic treatment is rarely indicated. Rate control may be achieved with **verapamil,** 5–10 milligrams IV, or **diltiazem,** 10–20 milligrams IV, in patients with acute COPD or CHF exacerbations.
3. **Magnesium sulfate,** 2 grams IV over 60 seconds, followed by a constant infusion of 1–2 grams/h, may decrease ectopy and convert MAT to sinus rhythm in some patients.
4. Replete potassium levels to greater than 4 mEq/L to increase myocardial membrane stability.

JUNCTIONAL RHYTHMS

Clinical Features

In patients with sinus bradycardia, SA node exit block, or AV block, junctional escape beats may occur, usually at a rate between 40 and 60 beats/min, depending on the level of the rescue pacemaker within the conduction system. Junctional escape beats may conduct retrogradely into the atria, but the QRS complex usually will mask any retrograde P wave (Fig. 4-9). When alternating rhythmically with the SA node, junctional escape beats may cause bigeminal or trigeminal rhythms. Sustained junctional escape rhythms may be seen with CHF, myocarditis, acute MI (especially inferior MI), hyperkalemia, or digoxin toxicity ("regularized Afib"). If the ventricular rate is too slow, myocardial or cerebral ischemia may develop. In cases of enhanced junctional automaticity, junctional rhythms may be accelerated (60–100 beats/min) or tachycardic (≥100 beats/min), thus overriding the SA node rate.

Emergency Department Care and Disposition

1. Isolated, infrequent junctional escape beats usually do not require specific treatment.
2. If sustained junctional escape rhythms are producing symptoms, treat the underlying cause.

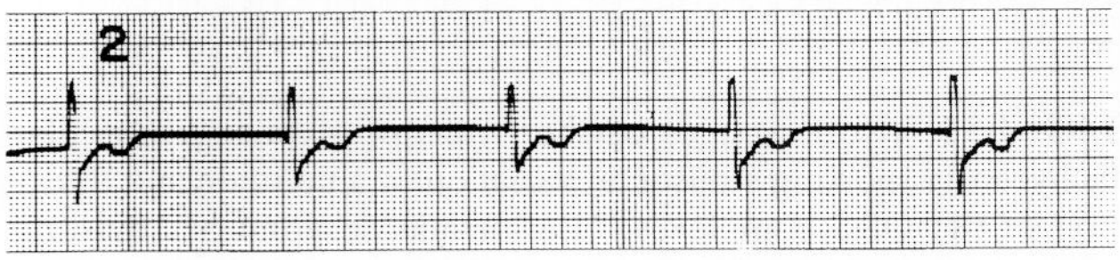

FIG. 4-9. Junctional escape rhythm, rate 42.

3. In unstable patients, give **atropine,** 0.5 milligram IV every 5 minutes to a total of 2 milligrams. This will accelerate the SA node discharge rate and enhance AV nodal conduction.
4. Use transcutaneous or transvenous pacing in unstable patients not responsive to atropine.
5. Manage patients with digoxin toxicity as discussed for SVT.

VENTRICULAR ARRHYTHMIAS

PREMATURE VENTRICULAR CONTRACTIONS

Clinical Features

Premature ventricular contractions (PVCs) are due to impulses originating from single or multiple areas in the ventricles. The ECG characteristics of PVCs are (a) a premature and wide QRS complex; (b) no preceding P wave; (c) the ST segment and T wave of the PVC are directed opposite the preceding major QRS deflection; (d) most PVCs do not affect the sinus node, so there is usually a fully compensatory post-ectopic pause, or the PVC may be interpolated between two sinus beats; (e) many PVCs have a fixed coupling interval (within 0.04 second) from the preceding sinus beat; and (f) many PVCs are conducted into the atria, thus producing a retrograde P wave (Fig. 4-10). If three or more PVCs occur in a row, patients are considered to have nonsustained VT.

PVCs are very common, occurring in most patients with ischemic heart disease and acute MI. Other

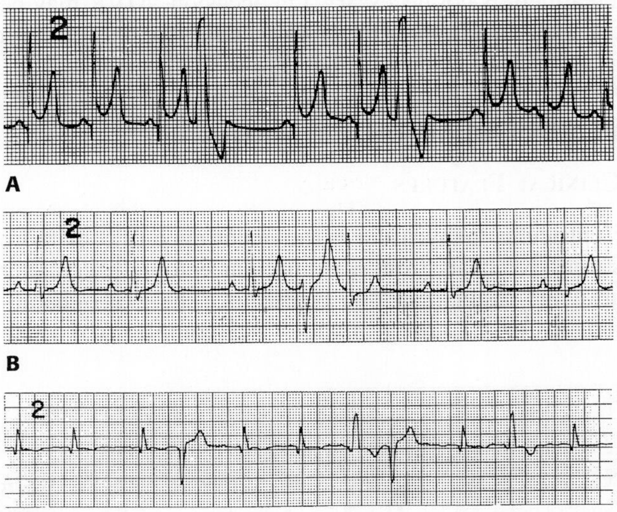

FIG. 4-10. Premature ventricular contractions (PVCs). **A.** Unifocal PVC. **B.** Interpolated PVC. **C.** Multifocal PVC.

common causes of PVCs include digoxin toxicity, CHF, hypokalemia, alkalosis, hypoxia, and sympathomimetic drugs. Pooled data and meta-analyses have found no reduction in mortality from suppressive or prophylactic treatment of PVCs. Ventricular parasystole occurs when the ectopic ventricular focus fires frequently enough to compete with the SA node and is associated with cardiac ischemia, electrolyte imbalance, and hypertensive or ischemic heart disease.

Emergency Department Care and Disposition

1. Stable patients require no treatment.
2. Patients with three or more PVCs occurring in a row should be managed as VT.
3. For hemodynamically unstable patients with PVCs, consider **lidocaine** 1–1.5 milligrams/kg IV (up to 3 milligrams/kg) unless the patient is allergic to amide anesthetics.

ACCELERATED IDIOVENTRICULAR RHYTHM

Clinical Features

The ECG characteristics of accelerated idioventricular rhythm (AIVR) are (a) wide and regular QRS complexes; (b) rate between 40 and 100 beats/min, often close to the preceding sinus rate; (c) most runs of short duration (3–30 beats/min); and (d) an AIVR often beginning with a fusion beat (Fig. 4-11). This condition is found most commonly with an acute MI or in the setting of reperfusion after successful thrombolysis.

Emergency Department Care and Disposition

Treatment is not necessary. On occasion, AIVR may be the only functioning pacemaker, and suppression with lidocaine can lead to cardiac asystole.

VENTRICULAR TACHYCARDIA

Clinical Features

Ventricular tachycardia is the occurrence of 3 or more successive beats from a ventricular ectopic pacemaker at a rate faster than 100 beats/min. The ECG characteristics of VT are (a) a wide QRS complex, (b) a rate faster than 100 beats/min (most commonly 150–200 beats/min), (c) a regular rhythm, although there may be some initial beat-to-beat variation, and (d) a constant QRS axis (Fig. 4-12). The most common causes of VT are ischemic heart disease and acute MI. Because of this fact, patients presenting with VT should be considered candidates for urgent revascularization. Other etiologies include hypertrophic cardiomyopathy, mitral valve prolapse, drug toxicity (digoxin, antiarrhythmics, or sympathomimetics), hypoxia, hypokalemia, and hyperkalemia. In general, all wide-complex tachycardia should be treated as VT regardless of clinical symptoms or initial vital signs. Adenosine appears to cause little harm in patients with VT; therefore, stable patients with wide-complex tachycardia due to suspected SVT with aberrancy (see previous section) may be treated safely with adenosine when the diagnosis is in doubt. Atypical VT (torsade de pointes, or twisting of the points) occurs when the QRS axis swings from a positive to a negative direction in a single lead at a rate of 200–240 beats/min (Fig. 4-13). Drugs that further prolong repolarization—quinidine, disopyramide, procainamide, phenothiazines, and tricyclic antidepressants—exacerbate this arrhythmia.

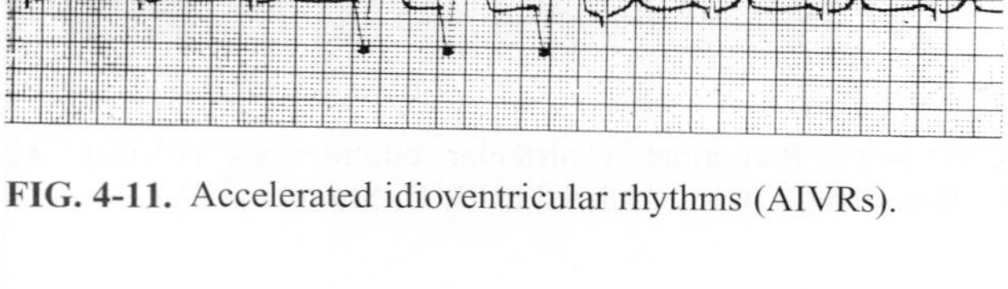

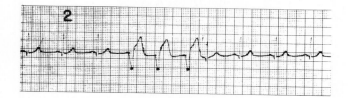

FIG. 4-11. Accelerated idioventricular rhythms (AIVRs).

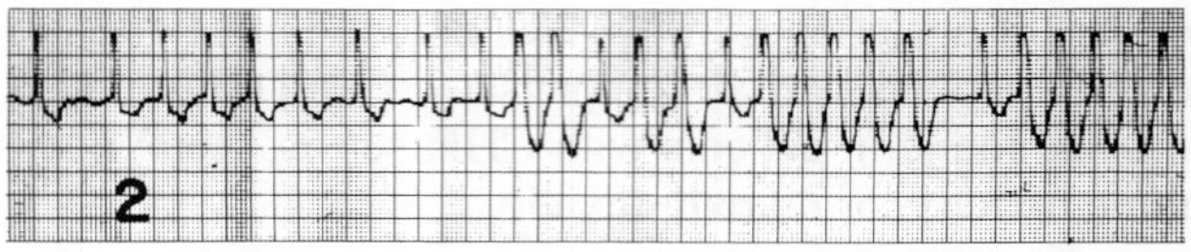

FIG. 4-12. Ventricular tachycardia.

Emergency Department Care and Disposition

1. Defibrillate pulseless VT with unsynchronized cardioversion starting at 100 J. Treat unstable patients who are not pulseless with synchronized cardioversion.

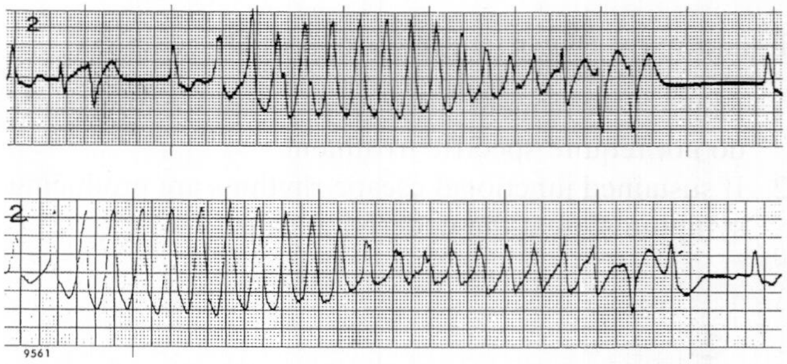

FIG. 4-13. Two examples of short runs of atypical ventricular tachycardia showing sinusoidal variation in amplitude and direction of the QRS complexes: "Le torsade de pointes" (twisting of the points). Note that the top example is initiated by a late-occurring PVC (lead II).

2. Treat hemodynamically stable patients with **amiodarone,** 150 milligrams IV over 10 minutes with repeated boluses every 10 minutes up to a total of 2 grams. Alternatively, an infusion of 0.5 milligram/min over 18 hours may be given after the initial bolus. Second-line agents include procainamide (in patients without suspected MI or LV dysfunction) and lidocaine.
3. For patients with torsades de pointes: Try overdrive pacing set at 90–120 beats/min to terminate torsades de pointes. **Magnesium sulfate,** 1–2 grams IV over 60–90 seconds followed by an infusion of 1–2 grams/h, can be effective.
4. **Isoproterenol,** 2–10 micrograms/min IV infusion, is also in refractory torsades but carries a risk of increased myocardial oxygen demand.

VENTRICULAR TACHYARRHYTHMIAS VERSUS SVT WITH ABERRANCY

Patients with wide-complex tachycardia should be approached as having VT until proven otherwise. Age over 35 years, a history of MI, CHF, or coronary artery bypass grafting strongly favor VT. ECG signs favoring VT include AV dissociation, fusion beats, precordial lead QRS concordance, and a QRS duration longer than 0.14 second.

VENTRICULAR FIBRILLATION

Clinical Features

Ventricular fibrillation (VF) is the totally disorganized depolarization and contraction of small areas of ventricular myocardium during which there is no effective ventricular pumping activity. The ECG shows a fine-to-coarse zigzag pattern without discernible P waves or QRS complexes (Fig. 4-14). VF is seen most commonly in patients with severe ischemic heart disease, with or without an acute MI. It also can be caused by digoxin or quinidine toxicity, hypothermia, chest trauma, hypokalemia, hyperkalemia, or mechanical stimulation (eg, catheter wire). Primary VF occurs suddenly, without preceding hemodynamic deterioration, and usually is due to acute ischemia or peri-infarct scar reentry. Secondary VF occurs after a prolonged period of hemodynamic deterioration due to LV failure or circulatory shock.

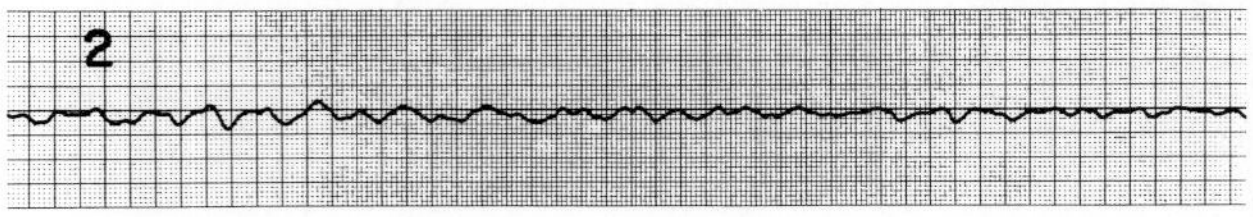

FIG. 4-14. Ventricular fibrillation.

Emergency Department Care and Disposition

1. Perform immediate electrical defibrillation (unsychronized) at 200 J (biphasic) and 360 J (monophasic). If VF persists, do five cycles of CPR, check pulse, and defibrillate again if no pulse is present. Keep defibrillation pads on the patient and in the same location because, with successive countershocks, transthoracic impedance decreases.
2. If the initial 2 cycles of CPR and defibrillation are unsuccessful, administer antiarrhythmic treatment using **amiodarone,** 300 milligrams IV push. **Lidocaine** is second-line and is dosed at 1.5 milligrams/kg IV followed by 0.75 milligram/kg IV for 2 more doses. Repeat the CPR-defibrillation cycle.
3. If no pulse is present after the third CPR-defibrillation cycle, give **epinephrine,** 1 milligram IV push, or **vasopressin,** 40 units IV push (1 time only), followed by a 20-mL normal saline flush and immediate resumption of the CPR-defibrillation cycle.
4. In refractory VF, administer **magnesium sulfate,** 1–2 grams IV over 60–90 seconds followed by an infusion of 1–2 grams/h.

CONDUCTION DISTURBANCES

ATRIOVENTRICULAR (AV) BLOCK

First-degree AV block is characterized by a delay in AV conduction, manifested by a prolonged PR interval (>0.2 second). It can be found in normal hearts and in association with increased vagal tone, digoxin toxicity, inferior MI, amyloid, and myocarditis. First-degree AV block needs no treatment. Second-degree AV block is characterized by intermittent AV nodal conduction: some atrial impulses reach the ventricles, whereas others are blocked, thereby causing "grouped beating." These blocks can be subdivided into nodal blocks, which are typically reversible, and infranodal blocks, which are due to irreversible conduction system disease. Third-degree AV block is characterized by complete interruption in AV conduction with resulting AV dissociation.

SECOND-DEGREE MOBITZ I (WENCKEBACH) AV BLOCK

Clinical Features

Mobitz I AV block is a nodal block causing a progressive prolongation of conduction through the AV node until the atrial impulse is completely blocked. Usually, only one atrial impulse is blocked at a time. After the dropped beat, the AV conduction returns to normal and

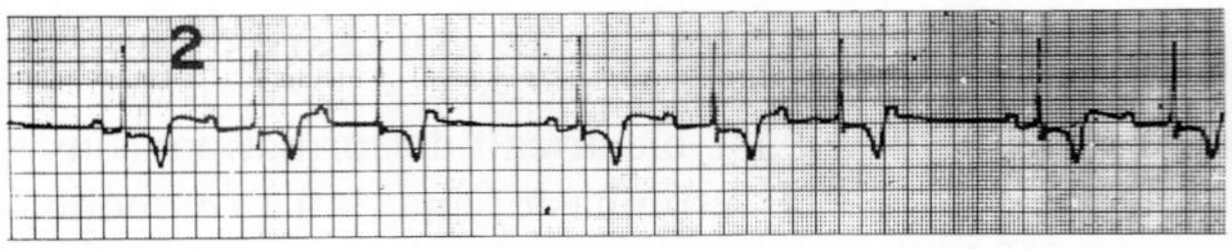

FIG. 4-15. Second-degree Mobitz I (Wenckebach) AV block with 4:3 AV conduction.

the cycle usually repeats itself with the same conduction ratio (fixed ratio) or a different conduction ratio (variable ratio). Although the PR intervals progressively lengthen before the dropped beat, the increments by which they lengthen *decrease* with successive beats, causing a progressive *shortening* of each successive RR interval before the dropped beat (Fig. 4-15). This block is often transient and usually associated with an acute inferior MI, digoxin toxicity, or myocarditis or can be seen after cardiac surgery. Because the blockade occurs at the level of the AV node itself rather than at the infranodal conducting system, this is usually a stable rhythm.

Emergency Department Care and Disposition

1. Specific treatment is not necessary unless slow ventricular rates produce signs of hypoperfusion.
2. In cases associated with acute inferior MI, provide adequate volume resuscitation before initiating further interventions.
3. Administer **atropine,** 0.5 milligram IV repeated every 5 minutes. Titrate to the desired heart rate or until the total dose reaches 2 milligrams.
4. Although rarely needed, transcutaneous pacing may be used.

SECOND-DEGREE MOBITZ II AV BLOCK

Clinical Features

Mobitz II AV block is typically due to infranodal disease, causing a constant PR interval with intermittent non-conducted atrial beats (Fig. 4-16). One or more beats may be non-conducted at a single time. This block indicates significant damage or dysfunction of the infranodal conduction system; therefore, the QRS complexes are usually wide coming from the low His-Purkinje bundle or the ventricles. Type II blocks are more dangerous than type I blocks because they are usually permanent and may progress suddenly to complete heart block, especially in the setting of an acute anterior MI, and almost always require permanent cardiac pacemaker placement. When second-degree AV block occurs with a fixed conduction ratio of 2:1, it is not possible to differentiate between a Mobitz I (Wenckebach) block and a Mobitz II block.

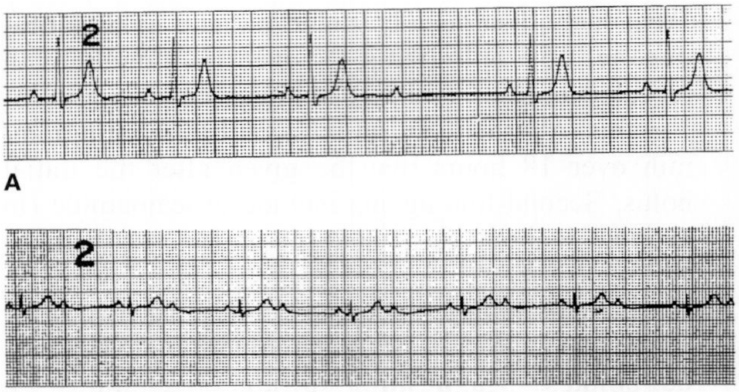

FIG. 4-16. A. Second-degree Mobitz II AV block. **B.** Second-degree AV block with 2:1 AV conduction.

Emergency Department Care and Disposition

1. **Atropine,** 0.5–1 milligram IV bolus, repeated every 5 minutes as needed up to 2 milligrams total dose, is first-line treatment for symptomatic patients. All patients should have transcutaneous pacing pads positioned and ready for use in the case of further deterioration into complete heart block.
2. Initiate transcutaneous cardiac pacing (see Sinus Bradycardia above) in patients unresponsive to atropine.
3. If transcutaneous pacing is unsuccessful, initiate transvenous pacing (0.2–20 mA at 40–140 beats/min via a semi-floating or balloon-tipped pacing catheter).

THIRD-DEGREE (COMPLETE) AV BLOCK

Clinical Features

In third-degree AV block, there is no AV conduction. The ventricles are paced by an escape pacemaker from the AV node or infranodal conduction system at a rate slower than the atrial rate (Fig. 4-17). When third-degree AV block occurs at the AV node, a junctional escape pacemaker takes over with a ventricular rate of 40–60 beats/min; and because the rhythm originates from above the bifurcation of the His bundle, the QRS complexes are narrow. Nodal third-degree AV block may develop in up to 8% of acute inferior MIs, and it is usually transient, although it may last for several days.

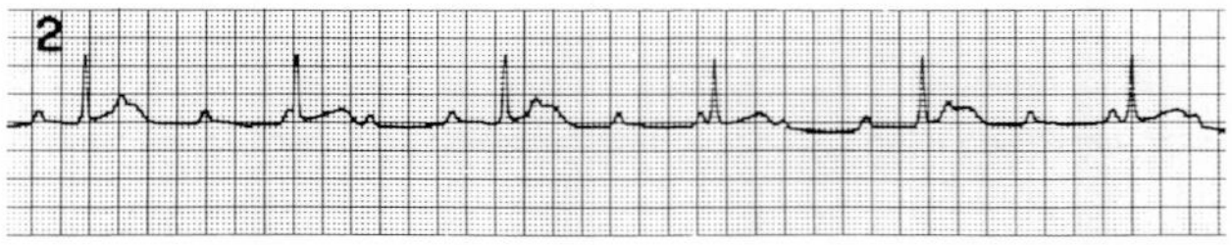

FIG. 4-17. Third-degree AV block.

When third-degree AV block occurs at the infranodal level, the ventricles are driven by a ventricular escape rhythm at a rate slower than 40 beats/min. Third-degree AV block located in the bundle branch or the Purkinje system invariably has an escape rhythm with a wide QRS complex. Like Mobitz II block, this indicates structural damage to the infranodal conduction system and can be seen in acute anterior MIs. The ventricular escape pacemaker is usually inadequate to maintain cardiac output and is unstable with periods of ventricular asystole.

Emergency Department Care and Disposition

1. Perform transcutaneous cardiac pacing in unstable patients until a transvenous pacemaker can be placed.
2. In stable patients, apply transcutaneous pacing pads. Treat the same as second-degree Mobitz II AV block.

FASCICULAR BLOCKS

Conduction blocks may arise in one or more of the three infranodal conduction pathways. Blockage of either of the left fascicles does not prolong the QRS duration, but will change the QRS axis. Left anterior fascicular block (LAFB) causes left axis deviation while left posterior fascicular block (LPFB) causes right axis deviation. Right bundle branch block (RBBB) will prolong the QRS duration (>0.12 second) and cause a RSR′ in the early precordial leads (V1–2). Bifascicular block denotes a combination of any two of these fascicles, the most notable of which is left bundle branch block (LAFB + LPFB). Trifascicular block denotes the presence of first-degree AV block in the presence of a bifascicular block and is indicative of significant conduction system disease that includes the AV node, thus increasing the risk of Mobitz II or third-degree AV block and the potential need for permanent pacemaker placement.

CONDUCTION ABNORMALITIES THAT CAN CAUSE RHYTHM DISTURBANCES

Brugada syndrome and long-QT syndrome increase the risk of spontaneous VT/VF and require evaluation for implantable cardiac defibrillator placement when diagnosed. Brugada syndrome is a genetic disorder of fast sodium channels causing an RBBB pattern in the early precordial leads (V1–2) with a pathognomonic J-point elevation and saddle-shaped or sloped ST segment (Fig. 4-18). Long-QT syndrome is characterized by a QT interval >470 milliseconds in men and >480 milliseconds in women and may be congenital or acquired, leading to an increased risk of torsades de pointes.

PRETERMINAL RHYTHMS

PULSELESS ELECTRICAL ACTIVITY

Pulseless electrical activity is the presence of electrical complexes without accompanying mechanical contraction of the heart. Potential mechanical causes should be diagnosed and treated, including severe hypovolemia, cardiac tamponade, tension pneumothorax, massive pulmonary embolus, MI, and toxic ingestions (eg, tricyclic antidepressants, calcium channel blockers, and

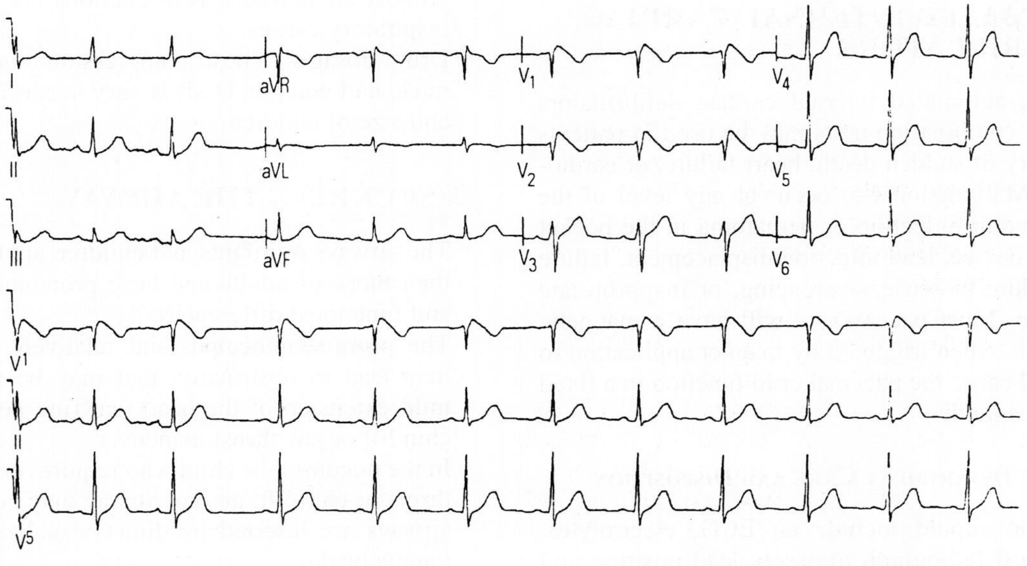

FIG. 4-18. Brugada syndrome.

β-blockers). In addition, profound metabolic abnormalities such as acidosis, hypoxia, hypokalemia, hyperkalemia, and hypothermia also should be considered and treated.

After intubation and initiating CPR, administer **epinephrine,** 1 milligram IV/IO (1:10,000 solution) every 3–5 minutes. If giving via endotracheal tube, increase the dose 2–2.5 times and follow with several rapid ventilations to disperse the drug. Treatment is guided by rapid identification and treatment of the underlying cause. Use agents with α-adrenergic activity, such as norepinephrine and phenylephrine, to improve vascular tone when indicated. Electrical pacing is not effective.

IDIOVENTRICULAR RHYTHM

Idioventricular rhythm is a ventricular escape rhythm at slower than 40 beats/min with a QRS wider than 0.16 second. It is associated with infranodal AV block, massive MI, cardiac tamponade, and exsanguinating hemorrhage.

After intubation and initiating CPR, treatment includes identifying contributing mechanical factors (eg, aggressive volume resuscitation) and α-adrenergic agents.

ASYSTOLE (CARDIAC STANDSTILL)

Asystole is the complete absence of cardiac electrical activity and carries a grim prognosis. Treatment is the same as that for pulseless electrical activity.

CARDIAC PACEMAKERS AND AUTOMATED INTERNAL CARDIAC DEFIBRILLATORS

Pacemakers, automated internal cardiac defibrillators (AICDs), or combination units may be used in patients with a history of sudden death, heart failure, or cardiomyopathy. Malfunction can occur at any level of the device, including infection or hematoma in the pocket housing the device, lead infection/displacement, failure to pace, failure to sense, overpacing, or inappropriate defibrillation. Most pacemakers will have a magnetic switch which, when triggered by magnet application to the unit, will cause the pacemaker to function in a fixed asynchronous mode.

EMERGENCY DEPARTMENT CARE AND DISPOSITION

1. Evaluation should include an ECG, electrolytes, and a chest radiograph to assess lead position and integrity. Arrangements should be made for electrical interrogation of the unit.
2. Patients with pacing failure may require treatment based on their underlying rhythm and associated symptoms.
3. Patients with overpacing may require magnet application to convert the pacemaker to asynchronous mode pacing at a lower rate.

For further reading in *Tintinalli's Emergency Medicine: A Comprehensive Study Guide,* 7th edition, see Chapter 22, "Cardiac Rhythm Disturbances," by Joseph S. Piktel; Chapter 23, "Pharmacology of Antiarrhythmics," by Brad A. Miller and Elizabeth A. Clements; and Chapter 24 "Pharmacology of Vasopressor Agents" by Brad A. Miller and Elizabeth A. Clements.

5 RESUSCITATION OF CHILDREN AND NEONATES

Marc F. Collin

EPIDEMIOLOGY

- Children have very poor survival rates from cardiac arrest.

PATHOPHYSIOLOGY

- Children primarily develop cardiac arrest secondary to hypoxia from respiratory arrest or shock syndromes.
- Almost all newborn resuscitations are secondary to respiratory causes.
- Drug dosages, chest compression and respiratory rates, and equipment sizes vary according to the age and size of children.

SECURING THE AIRWAY

- The airways of infants and children are much smaller than those of adults and have pronounced anatomic and functional differences.
- The prominent occiput and relatively large tongue may lead to obstruction that may be relieved with mild extension of the head (sniffing position) and a chin lift or jaw thrust maneuver.
- In the unconscious child who requires continuous jaw thrust or chin lift, an oral airway may be useful. Oral airways are inserted by direct visualization using a tongue blade.

- Ventilation may be administered using a bag-valve-mask system. The minimum volume for ventilation bags for infants and children is 450 mL. Observe chest rise and auscultate breath sounds to ensure adequate ventilation.
- The large and flaccid epiglottis is best displaced using a straight (Miller) laryngoscope blade. Use Miller 0 blade in preterm newborns and Miller 1 blade in term newborns.
- Endotracheal tube (ET) size can be reasonably estimated using the formula: (16 + age in years)/4. In newborns <1 kg, use 2.5-mm ET; 1–2 kg, use 3.0-mm ET; 2–3 kg, use 3.5-mm ET; and >3 kg, use 3.5- to 4.0-mm ET.
- The position of the tube at the lip is approximately 3 times the size of the tube (eg, 5.0 × 3 = 15 cm at the lip).
- Tidal volume for children is 8–12 mL/kg.
- If the child does not require hyperventilation, then the respiratory rate should be started at 40–60 breaths/min in newborns, 20 breaths/min for infants, 15 breaths/min for young children, and 10 breaths/min for adolescents.
- Confirmation of endotracheal intubation is similar to that in adults: adequate chest rise, symmetric breath sounds, CO_2 readings, vapor steam noted in ET, improved oxygenation, and clinical improvement.
- The laryngeal mask airway (LMA) may be used if endotracheal intubation is not possible.

RAPID SEQUENCE INDUCTION

- Rapid sequence induction is the intravenous administration of an anesthetic and a neuromuscular blocking agent to facilitate endotracheal intubation.
- Preoxygenate the patient with 100% oxygen.
- Atropine (0.02 milligram/kg; minimum dose = 0.1 milligram; maximum dose = 1 milligram) should be given to prevent reflex bradycardia in children less than 5 years old or in the older child or adolescent who requires a second dose of succinylcholine.
- Cricoid pressure should be applied before paralysis and continued until successful intubation is confirmed. As cricoid pressure may occlude the pliable infant trachea, release pressure if intubation is difficult.

VASCULAR ACCESS

- Vascular access is performed in the quickest, least invasive manner possible; peripheral vein (antecubital, hand, foot, or scalp) cannulation should be attempted first.
- Intraosseous cannulation is a rapid, safe, and reliable method and may be used for administration of fluids, resuscitation medications, colloids, and blood.
- Percutaneous central lines or saphenous vein cutdowns may also be used, but are more time consuming.

FLUIDS

- In patients with hypovolemia/shock, intravenous isotonic fluid (ie, normal saline) boluses of 20 mL/kg should be given as rapidly as possible and should be repeated, depending on the clinical response.
- If hypovolemia has been corrected and shock or hypotension persists, a pressor agent should be considered.

DRUGS

- Proper drug dosages in children require knowledge of the patient's weight. The use of a length-based system for estimating the weight of a child in an emergency situation may reduce dosage errors.
- The rule of 6s may be used to quickly calculate continuous infusions of drugs such as dopamine and dobutamine. The amount of drug needed is 6 milligrams times the weight in kilograms added to a total volume of 100 mL D5W. This produces an infusion rate in milliliters per hour that is equal to the micrograms per kilogram per minute rate (ie, an infusion of 1 mL/h = 1 microgram/kg/min or 5 mL/h = 5 micrograms/kg/min).
- Epinephrine is the only drug proven effective in cardiac arrest. It is indicated in pulseless arrest and in hypoxia-induced slow pulse rates that are unresponsive to oxygenation and ventilation.
- The initial dose of epinephrine is 0.01 milligram/kg (0.1 mL/kg of 1:10,000 solution) IV/intraosseous or 0.05–0.1 milligram/kg (0.5–1 mL/kg of 1:10,000 solution) by the endotracheal route. Repeat dosing of epinephrine is recommended every 3–5 minutes for persistent arrest. Intratracheal route of epinephrine is inferior to intravascular route and should be used only if immediate vascular access is unavailable.
- Glucose, 10%, given at 2 mL/kg generally corrects hypoglycemia. Repeat dose if hypoglycemia persists.
- Sodium bicarbonate is no longer considered as a first-line resuscitation drug. It is recommended, if needed, only after effective ventilation is established, epinephrine is administered, and chest compressions to ensure circulation are provided.
- Calcium is also not recommended in routine resuscitation, but may be useful in hyperkalemia, hypocalcemia, and calcium channel blocker overdose.

DYSRHYTHMIAS

- Dysrhythmias in infants and children are most often secondary to respiratory insufficiency and hypoxia, not primary cardiac causes as in adults. Specific attention to oxygenation and ventilation is paramount to dysrhythmia management in pediatrics.
- The most common rhythm seen in a pediatric arrest is bradycardia progressing to asystole. Often, oxygenation and ventilation are sufficient to correct the situation. Epinephrine followed by atropine may be useful in bradycardia unresponsive to ventilation.
- The most common dysrhythmia outside of the arrest situation is supraventricular tachycardia (SVT). It presents as a narrow complex tachycardia with rates typically between 250 and 350 beats/min. The recommended treatment for stable SVT in children is adenosine (0.1 milligram/kg) given simultaneously with a saline flush as rapidly as possible through a well-functioning IV. Treatment for the unstable SVT patient is synchronized cardioversion (0.5–1 J/kg).
- It is often difficult to differentiate between sinus tachycardia (ST) and SVT. Small infants may have ST with rates above 200 beats/min. Patients with ST may have a history of fever, dehydration, or shock. In ST, the heart rate typically varies with activity or stimulation.

DEFIBRILLATION AND CARDIOVERSION

- Ventricular fibrillation is rare in children. It is initially treated with defibrillation at 2 J/kg. If unsuccessful, repeat defibrillation energy is doubled to 4 J/kg.
- If two attempts at defibrillation at 4 J/kg are unsuccessful, epinephrine should be given. Reassessment for treatable causes such as hypoxemia, hypovolemia, and metabolic acidosis should be performed.
- Unstable tachyarrhythmias are treated with cardioversion at a dose of 0.5–1 J/kg.
- The largest paddles that still allow contact of the entire paddle with the chest wall should be used. Electrode cream or paste is used to prevent burns. One paddle is placed on the right of the sternum at the second intercostal space, and the other is placed at the left midclavicular line at the level of the xiphoid.

NEONATAL RESUSCITATION

- The initial decision to resuscitate an infant should be made within the first 30 seconds of delivery.
- The first step is to maintain body temperature. The infant should be immediately dried and placed under a preheated radiant warmer.
- Reserve immediate suctioning for babies who have obvious obstruction to spontaneous breathing or who require positive-pressure ventilation. If needed, the mouth followed by the nose should be gently suctioned with either a bulb syringe or a mechanical suction device.
- The examiner should then rapidly assess heart rate, respiratory effort, color, and activity.
- Infants who are apneic, or who are centrally cyanotic, or whose heart rate is less than 100 beats/min should have positive pressure ventilation initiated with room air ventilation. If the heart rate is below 60 beats/min despite 30 seconds of effective positive-pressure ventilation, increase the oxygen concentration to 100% and begin chest compressions.
- For infants who have not taken an initial breath, pressures over 30 cm H_2O may be required to initially expand the lungs. However, infants, especially if preterm, may be more susceptible to developing pneumothoraces with higher pressures.
- If no improvement is noted or if prolonged bagging is anticipated, endotracheal intubation should be performed.
- If the heart rate is still below 60 beats/min after intubation and assisted ventilation, cardiac massage should be started at 90 compressions/min and coordinated with assisted ventilation in a 3:1 ratio.
- If still unsuccessful in restoring heart rate >60 beats/min after at least another 45–60 seconds, epinephrine therapy should be initiated.
- Drugs may be administered via ET, umbilical vein, or peripheral vein. However, the endotracheal route is not the preferred route and should only be utilized if vascular access cannot be readily achieved.
- Umbilical vein catheterization is a fast, reliable method of obtaining vascular access. The umbilical catheter is placed in the umbilical vein and advanced to 10 to 12 cm or until blood return is noted.
- IV epinephrine (0.01 milligram/kg of 1:10,000 solution) may be used for heart rates less than 60 beats/min despite adequate ventilation and oxygenation.
- Sodium bicarbonate during neonatal resuscitation remains controversial. Adequate ventilation and circulation must be established prior to administration. Sodium bicarbonate (1 mEq/kg of a 4.2% solution = 0.5 mEq/L) should be given intravenously only.

PREVENTION OF MECONIUM ASPIRATION

- Aspiration of meconium-stained amniotic fluid is associated with both morbidity and mortality.

- Ten percent to 20% of all births will have meconium staining of the amniotic fluid.
- If meconium is present, suctioning after delivery of the head and before delivery of the shoulders is no longer recommended.
- If the infant is vigorous after delivery, the mouth and nose may be gently suctioned with no further intervention necessary.
- If the infant is depressed after delivery, direct suctioning of the trachea should be performed by visualizing the trachea with a laryngoscope and suctioning via an endotracheal tube.
- If at any time during this procedure the heart rate drops below 100 beats/min, positive pressure ventilation should be initiated.

For further reading in Tintinalli's *Emergency Medicine: A Comprehensive Study Guide,* 7th ed., see Chapter 14, "Resuscitation of Neonates," by Marc F. Collin; Chapter 15, "Resuscitation of Children," by William E. Hauda II; and Chapter 29, "Pediatric Airway Management," by Robert J. Vissers.

6 FLUIDS, ELECTROLYTES, AND ACID–BASE DISORDERS

Mary A. Wittler

FLUIDS

- An average normal adult requires approximately 2000–3000 mL of water per day to maintain fluid balance.
- When altered, fluids and electrolytes should be corrected in the following order: (1) volume; (2) pH; (3) potassium, calcium, magnesium; and (4) sodium and chloride. Reestablishment of tissue perfusion often re-equilibrates the fluid–electrolyte and acid–base balance.
- Since the osmolarity of normal saline (NS) matches that of the serum, it is an excellent fluid for volume replacement.
- Hypotonic fluids such as 5% dextrose in water (D5W) should never be used to replace volume.
- Lactated Ringer's solution is commonly used for surgical patients or trauma patients; however, only NS can be given in the same line with blood components.
- The more concentrated dextrose solutions, D10W or D20W, are used for patients with compromised ability to mobilize glucose stores, such as patients with hepatic failure, or as part of total parenteral nutrition (TPN) solutions.

CLINICAL ASSESSMENT OF VOLUME STATUS

- Volume loss and dehydration can be inferred from the patient history. Historical features include vomiting, diarrhea, fever, adverse working conditions, decreased fluid intake, chronic disease, altered level of consciousness, and reduced urine output.
- Tachycardia and hypotension are late signs of dehydration.
- Physical exam findings include dry mucosa, shrunken tongue (excellent indicator), and decreased skin turgor. In infants and children, sunken fontanelles, decreased capillary refill, lack of tears, and decreased wet diapers are typical signs and symptoms of dehydration (see Chap. 83).
- Lethargy and coma are more ominous signs and may indicate a significant comorbid condition.
- Laboratory values are not reliable indicators of fluid status. Plasma and urine osmolarity are perhaps the most reliable measures of dehydration. Blood urea nitrogen (BUN), creatinine, hematocrit, and other chemistries are insensitive.
- Volume overload is a purely clinical diagnosis and presents with edema (central or peripheral), respiratory distress (pulmonary edema), and jugular venous distention (in congestive heart failure [CHF]).
- The significant risk factors for volume overload are renal, cardiovascular, and liver disease. Blood pressure (BP) does not necessarily correlate with volume status alone; patients with volume overload can present with hypotension or hypertension.

MAINTENANCE FLUIDS

- Adult: D5½NS at 75 to 125 mL/h + 20 mEq/L of potassium chloride for an average adult (approximately 70 kg).
- Children: D5½NS or D10½NS, 100 mL/kg/d for the first 10 kg (of body weight), 50 mL/kg/d for the second 10 kg, and 20 mL/kg/d for every kilogram thereafter (see Chap. 83 for further discussion of pediatric fluid management).

ELECTROLYTE DISORDERS

- Correcting a single abnormality may not be the only intervention needed, as most electrolytes exist in equilibrium with others.
- Laboratory errors are common. Results should be double-checked when the clinical picture and the laboratory data conflict.

- Abnormalities should be corrected at the same rate they developed; however, slower correction is usually safe unless the condition warrants rapid and/or early intervention (ie, hypoglycemia, hyperkalemia).
- Evaluation of electrolyte disorders frequently requires a comparison of the measured and calculated osmolarity (number of particles per liter of solution). To calculate osmolarity, measured serum values in mEq/L are used:

$$\text{Osmolarity (mOsm/L)} = 2\,[\text{Na}^+] + (\text{glucose}/18) + (\text{BUN}/2.8) + (\text{ETOH}/4.6)$$

HYPONATREMIA ([Na⁺] <135 mEq/L)

CLINICAL FINDINGS

- The clinical manifestations of hyponatremia are more likely to occur when the $[Na^+]$ drops below 120 mEq/L, and include nausea, weakness, headache, agitation, hallucinations, cramps, confusion, lethargy, and seizures.

DIAGNOSIS AND DIFFERENTIAL

- Evaluate volume status, measured serum, and calculated osmolarities.
- True hyponatremia presents with reduced osmolarity in the face of normal volume status and low urine $[Na^+]$. This state results from primary water gain, $[Na^+]$ loss greater than that of water, or alteration in the distribution of water.
- Factitious hyponatremia (false low measurement of the serum sodium) is due to hyperglycemia, hyperproteinemia, hyperlipidemia, and other osmotically active solutes and is associated with a normal-to-high osmolarity.
- The diagnostic criteria for *syndrome of inappropriate secretion of antidiuretic hormone* (SIADH) are (1) hypotonic hyponatremia, (2) inappropriately elevated urinary osmolality (usually >200 mOsm/kg), (3) elevated urinary [Na+] (typically >20 mEq/L), (4) clinical euvolemia, (5) normal adrenal, renal, cardiac, hepatic, and thyroid functions, and (6) correctable with water restriction.
- Isotonic hyponatremia (P_{osm} 275–295) may be due to hyperlipidemia, hyperproteinemia, or hyperglycemia.
- Hypertonic hyponatremia (P_{osm} >295) may be due to hyperglycemia, mannitol excess, or glycerol use.
- Causes of hyponatremia are listed in Table 6-1.

TABLE 6-1 Causes of Hyponatremia

Hypotonic (true) hyponatremia (P_{osm} <275)
Hypovolemic hyponatremia
Extrarenal losses (urinary $[Na^+]$ <20 mEq/L)
Volume replacement with hypotonic fluids
Sweating, vomiting, diarrhea, fistula
Third-space sequestration (burns, peritonitis, pancreatitis)
Renal losses (urinary [Na+] >20 mEq/L)
Diuretic use
Aldosterone deficiency
Salt-wasting nephropathies; renal tubular acidosis
Osmotic diuresis (mannitol, hyperglycemia, hyperuricemia)
Euvolemic hyponatremia (urinary [Na+] usually >20 mEq/L)
Inappropriate ADH secretion (CNS, lung, or carcinoma disease)
Physical and emotional stress or pain
Myxedema, Addison's disease, Sheehan syndrome
Drugs, water intoxication
Hypervolemic hyponatremia
Urinary [Na+] >20 mEq/L
Renal failure (inability to excrete free water)
Urinary [Na+] <20 mEq/L
Cirrhosis
Congestive heart failure
Nephrotic syndrome
Isotonic (pseudo) hyponatremia (P_{osm} 275–295)
Hyperproteinemia, hyperlipidemia
Hypertonic hyponatremia (P_{osm} >295)
Hyperglycemia, mannitol excess, and glycerol use

Abbreviations: ADH = antidiuretic hormone, CNS = central nervous system.

EMERGENCY DEPARTMENT CARE AND DISPOSITION

- Correct existing volume or perfusion deficits with NS.
- In euvolemic or hypervolemic patients, restrict fluids (500–1500 mL of water daily).
- Treat severe hyponatremia ($[Na^+]$ <120 mEq/L) that has developed rapidly with central nervous system (CNS) changes such as coma or seizures with hypertonic saline, **3% NS** (513 mEq/L), at 25–100 mL/h. The $[Na^+]$ should not be corrected faster than 0.5 mEq/L/h in chronic hyponatremia or 1.0 mEq/L/h in acute hyponatremia. The $[Na^+]$ correction should not exceed 12 mEq/L/d.
- The sodium dose can be calculated as follows: weight (kg) × 0.6 × (desired $[Na^+]$ – measured $[Na^+]$) = sodium deficit (mEq).
- Complications of rapid correction include CHF and central pontine myelinolysis, which can cause alterations in consciousness, dysphagia, dysarthria, and paresis.

HYPERNATREMIA ([Na⁺] >150 mEq/L)

CLINICAL FEATURES

- Symptoms of hypernatremia are usually noticeable at a serum osmolarity >350 mOsm/L or $[Na^+]$ >158 mEq/L. Initial symptoms include irritability and ataxia; spasticity, hyperreflexia, lethargy, coma, and seizures occur with osmolarities above 400 mOsm/L.

- An osmolarity increase of 2% stimulates thirst to prevent hypernatremia.
- Morbidity and mortality are highest in infants and the elderly, who may be unable to respond to increased thirst.

DIAGNOSIS AND DIFFERENTIAL

- Hypernatremia is most commonly caused by a decrease in total body water due to decreased intake or excessive loss. It is less often due to an increase in total body [Na^+].
- Common causes are diarrhea, vomiting, hyperpyrexia, and excessive sweating.
- An important etiology of hypernatremia is diabetes insipidus (DI), which results in the loss of hypotonic urine. Central DI (no antidiuretic hormone secreted) results from CNS disease, surgery, or trauma. Nephrogenic DI (unresponsive to antidiuretic hormone) results from congenital disease, drugs, hypercalcemia, hypokalemia, or renal disease.
- The causes of hypernatremia are listed in Table 6-2.

EMERGENCY DEPARTMENT CARE AND DISPOSITION

- Correct existing volume or perfusion deficits with NS or lactated Ringer's solution. Free water deficits are corrected with ½NS. Avoid lowering the [Na^+] more than 10 mEq/L/d.

TABLE 6-2 Causes of Hypernatremia

Loss of water
Reduced water intake
Defective thirst drive
Unconsciousness
Inability to drink water
Lack of access to water
Water loss in excess of sodium
Vomiting, diarrhea
Sweating, fever
Diabetes insipidus
Drugs including lithium, phenytoin
Dialysis
Osmotic diuresis, renal concentrating defects
Thyrotoxicosis
Severe burns
Gain of sodium
Increased intake
Increased salt use, salt pills
Hypertonic saline ingestion or infusion
Sodium bicarbonate administration
Mineralocorticoid or glucocorticoid excess
Primary aldosteronism
Cushing's syndrome

- Each liter of water deficit causes the [Na^+] to increase 3 to 5 mEq/L. Use the formula to calculate the free water deficit: water deficit (L) = (measured [Na^+]/desired [Na^+]) – 1.
- If no urine output is observed after NS or lactated Ringer's solution rehydration, rapidly switch to ½NS: unload the body of the extra sodium by using a diuretic (eg, furosemide 20-40 milligrams IV).
- Central diabetes insipidus DI is treated with desmopressin with careful monitoring of electrolytes, and urine osmolarity and specific gravity. Consult a specialist.

In children with a serum sodium level higher than 180 mEq/L, consider peritoneal dialysis using high-glucose, low-[Na^+] dialysate in consultation with a pediatric nephrologist.

HYPOKALEMIA ([K^+] <3.5 mEq/L)

CLINICAL FEATURES

- The signs and symptoms of hypokalemia usually occur at levels below 2.5 mEq/L and affect the multiple body systems: the central nervous system (weakness, cramps, hyporeflexia, paresthesias), gastrointestinal system (ileus), cardiovascular system (dysrhythmias, worsening of digoxin toxicity, hypotension or hypertension, U waves, ST-segment depression, prolonged QT interval), and renal system (metabolic alkalosis, worsening hepatic encephalopathy). Glucose intolerance can also develop.

DIAGNOSIS AND DIFFERENTIAL

- Causes can be grouped by decreased [K^+] intake, increased [K^+] excretion, or transcellular shift. The most common cause is the use of loop diuretics.
- Table 6-3 lists the causes of hypokalemia.

EMERGENCY DEPARTMENT CARE AND DISPOSITION

- Giving 20 mEq/dose [K^+] will raise the [K^+] by 0.25 mEq/L.
- In stable patients, oral replacement is preferred (safe and rapid); a 20- to 40-mEq [K^+] dose is used.
- In unstable patients, **IV potassium chloride** (KCl) in doses of 10 to 20 mEq/h may be given. Add no more than 40 mEq of KCl to each liter of IV fluid. Infusion rates should not exceed 40 mEq/h.
- Doses greater than 20 mEq/h should be given through a central line. Patients should be monitored continuously for dysrhythmias.

TABLE 6-3 Causes of Hypokalemia

Shift into the cell	
Alkalosis and sodium bicarbonate	
β-Adrenergics	
Administration of insulin and glucose	
Hypokalemic periodic paralysis	
Reduced intake	
Increased loss	
Renal loss	
Primary & secondary hyperaldosteronism, Bartter syndrome	
Diuretics, osmotic disuresis, postobstructive diuresis	
Renal tubular acidosis	
Renal artery stenosis	
Miscellaneous	
Licorice use	
Use of chewing tobacco	
Hypercalcemia	
Liddle syndrome	
Magnesium deficiency	
Acute leukemia	
Drugs and toxins (PCN, lithium, L-dopa, theophylline)	
GI loss (vomiting, diarrhea, fistulas), malabsorption	

Abbreviations: GI = gastrointestinal, PCN = penicillin.

HYPERKALEMIA ($[K^+]$ >5.5 mEq/L)

CLINICAL FEATURES

- The most concerning and serious manifestations of hyperkalemia are the cardiac effects.
- At levels of 6.5 to 7.5 mEq/L the electrocardiogram (ECG) shows peaked T waves (precordial leads—see Fig. 6-1), prolonged PR intervals, and short QT intervals. At levels of 7.5 to 8.0 mEq/L, the QRS widens and the P wave flattens. At levels above 8 mEq/L, a sine-wave pattern, ventricular fibrillation, and heart blocks occur.
- Neuromuscular symptoms include weakness and paralysis. GI symptoms include vomiting, colic, and diarrhea.

DIAGNOSIS AND DIFFERENTIAL

- Beware of pseudohyperkalemia, which is caused by hemolysis associated with blood draws.
- Renal failure with oliguria is the most common cause of true hyperkalemia.
- Appropriate tests for management include an ECG, electrolytes, calcium, magnesium, arterial blood gases (ABGs; check for acidosis), urinalysis, and a digoxin level in appropriate patients.
- Causes of hyperkalemia are listed in Table 6-4.

EMERGENCY DEPARTMENT CARE AND DISPOSITION

- Symptomatic patients are treated in a stepwise approach: stabilize the cardiac membrane with

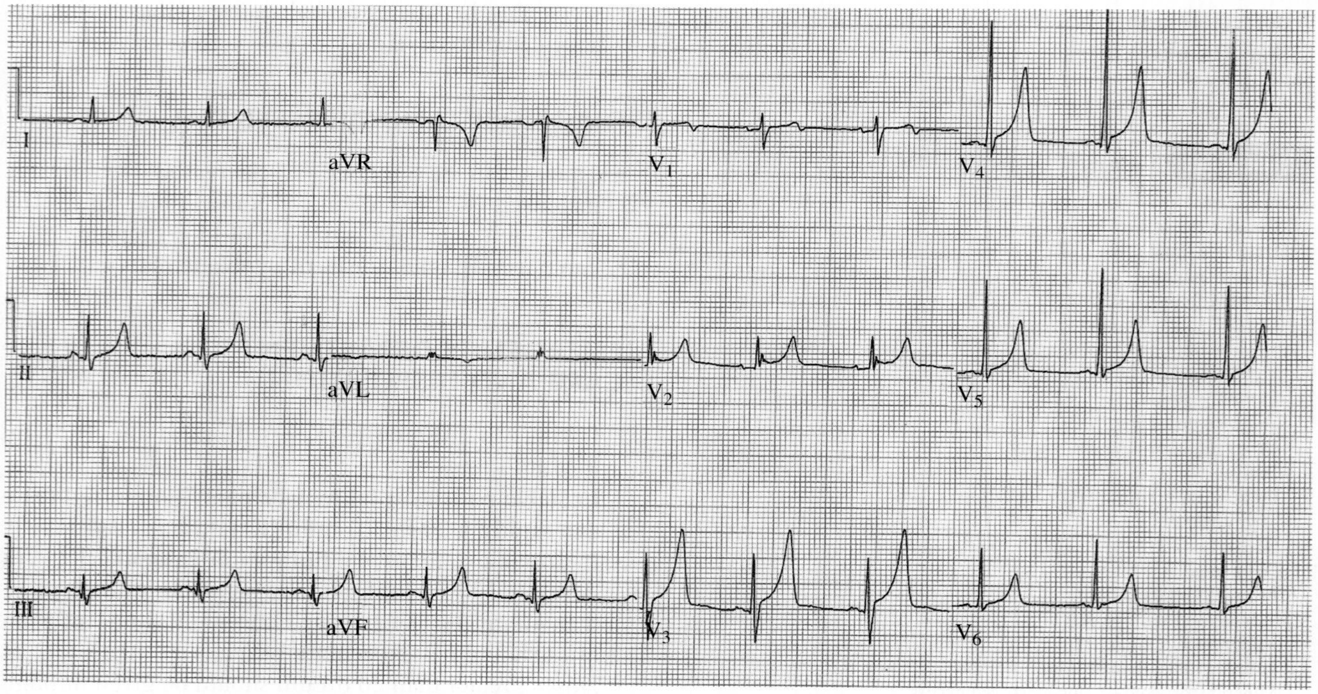

FIG. 6-1. Electrocardiogram of hyperkalemia. Note the narrow, tall, peaked T waves consistent with hyperkalemia. The patient was 3 days overdue for hemodialysis and was found to have a potassium of 7.4 mEq/L. (Figure supplied by David M. Cline, MD, Wake Forest Baptist Health.)

TABLE 6-4 Causes of Hyperkalemia

Factitious
- Laboratory error
- Hemolysis and leukocytosis

Increased plasma [K$^+$] load
- Exogenous: diet, salt substitutes, [K$^+$]-containing medications
- Endogenous: hemolysis, GI bleeding, catabolic states, crush injury

Decreased [K$^+$] excretion
- Renal failure
- Impaired renin–aldosterone axis
  - Addison's disease
  - Primary hypoaldosteronism
- Other (heparin, ACE inhibitors, prostaglandin inhibitors)

Tubular potassium secretory defect
- Sickle cell disease
- Systemic lupus erythematosus
- Postrenal transplantation
- Obstructive uropathy
- Potassium sparing diuretics

Abnormal potassium distribution
- Insulin deficiency
- Hypertonicity (hyperglycemia)
- β-Adrenergic blockers
- Exercise
- Drugs: succinylcholine, β-agonists, digitalis intoxication
- Acidosis

Abbreviations: ACE = angiotensin-converting enzyme, GI = gastrointestinal.

Ca-gluconate or calcium chloride ($CaCl_2$); shift the [K$^+$] into the cell using glucose and insulin and/or bicarbonate and/or albuterol; finally, excrete the [K$^+$] using sodium polystyrene sulfonate, diuretics, or dialysis in severe cases. Table 6-5 summarizes the treatment including medication doses.

- For levels over 7.0 mEq/L or for any ECG changes, give IV $CaCl_2$ or Ca-gluconate (Table 6-5). In children, Ca-gluconate (10%) 0.5 mL/kg is given.
- The presence of digoxin toxicity with hyperkalemia is an indication for digoxin immune Fab (Digibind) therapy (see Chap. 110). Calcium administration should be avoided.
- In acidotic patients, consider giving **sodium bicarbonate** 50–100 mEq slow IV. In children, 1 mEq/kg is given slow IV.
- When treating dialysis/renal failure patients with glucose and insulin, reduce the insulin dose to 5 unit regular insulin. In children, 0.5–1 gram/kg of **glucose as D10W** plus **insulin** 0.1 units/kg is given.
- Diuresis is maintained with **furosemide** 20 to 40 milligrams IV.
- **Sodium polystyrene sulfonate (Kayexalate)** (PO or rectally [PR]) 1 gram binds 1 mEq of [K+]. Administer 15 to 30 grams **Kayexalate** PO with **sorbitol** or 30 to 50 grams PR with sorbitol. Kayexalate can exacerbate CHF. In children, give **Kayexalate** 1 gram/kg PO or PR.
- **Albuterol** 5 to 10 milligrams (by nebulization) may also be used to lower [K$^+$].
- In patients with acute renal failure, consult a nephrologist for emergent dialysis.

HYPOCALCEMIA ([Ca^{2+}] <8.5 mEq/L OR IONIZED LEVEL <2.0 mEq/L)

CLINICAL FEATURES

- The signs and symptoms of hypocalcemia are usually seen with ionized [Ca^{2+}] levels below 1.5 mEq/L. Symptoms include paresthesias, increased deep tendon reflexes (DTRs), cramps, weakness, confusion, and seizures.
- Patients may also demonstrate Chvostek's sign (twitch of the corner of mouth on tapping with a finger over cranial nerve VII at the zygoma) or Trousseau's sign

TABLE 6-5 Emergency Therapy of Hyperkalemia

THERAPY	DOSE AND ROUTE	ONSET OF ACTION	DURATION OF EFFECT	MECHANISM
Albuterol (nebulized)	2.5 milligrams in 4 mL normal saline, nebulized over 20 min	15-30 min	2-4 h	Upregulates cyclic adenosine monophosphate, shifts [K$^+$] into cell
Calcium chloride (10%)*	5-10 mL IV	1-3 min	30-50 min	Membrane stabilization
Calcium gluconate (10%)*	10-20 mL IV	1-3 min	30-50 min	Membrane stabilization
$NaHCO_3$	50-100 mEq IV	5-10 min	1-2 h	Shifts [K$^+$] into cell
Insulin and glucose	5-10 units regular insulin IV 1-2 amps D50W IV	30 min	4-6 h	Shifts [K$^+$] into cell
Furosemide	40 milligrams IV	Varies	Varies	Renal [K$^+$] excretion
Sodium polystyrene sulfonate	25-50 grams PO or PR	1-2 h	4-6 h	GI [K$^+$] excretion
Hemodialysis	–	Minutes	Varies	Removes [K$^+$]

*Calcium chloride is three times as potent as calcium gluconate; 10% calcium chloride=272 milligrams [Ca^{2+}]/ML; 10% calcium gluconate = 9 milligrams [Ca^{2+}]/ML.

(more reliable; carpal spasm when the BP cuff is left inflated at a pressure above the systolic BP for greater than 3 minutes). Low [Ca^{2+}] decreased myocardial contractility, and may precipitate CHF or long QT on the EKG.

DIAGNOSIS AND DIFFERENTIAL

- Causes include shock, sepsis, renal failure, pancreatitis, drugs (usually cimetidine), hypoparathyroidism, hyperphosphatemia, vitamin D deficiency, hypomagnesemia, and fluoride poisoning.
- Alkalosis decreases the ionized [Ca^{2+}] (physiologically active form) without changing the total [Ca^{2+}] level.

EMERGENCY DEPARTMENT CARE AND DISPOSITION

- If asymptomatic, then use **calcium gluconate** tablets, 1–4 grams/d PO divided every 6 hours with or without **vitamin D** (calcitriol 0.2 microgram twice daily). Milk is not a good substitute.
- If symptomatic, then use **calcium gluconate** or calcium chloride, 10 mL of a 10% solution, given over 10 minutes by slow IV injection.
- Replace magnesium in conjunction with [Ca^{2+}].

HYPERCALCEMIA ([Ca^{2+}] >10.5 mEq/L OR IONIZED [Ca^{2+}] >2.7 mEq/L)

- Several factors affect the serum calcium level: parathyroid hormone (PTH) increases calcium; calcitonin and vitamin D metabolites decrease calcium.
- Decreased [H^+] causes a decrease in ionized [Ca^{2+}].
- A decrease in albumin causes a decrease in [Ca^{2+}], but not in the ionized portion.

CLINICAL FEATURES

- Clinical signs and symptoms develop at levels above 12 milligrams/dL.
- A mnemonic to aid recall of common hypercalcemia symptoms is stones (renal calculi), bones (osteolysis), psychic moans (lethargy, weakness, fatigue, confusion), and abdominal groans (abdominal pain, constipation, polyuria, polydipsia).
- ECG changes include depressed ST segments, widened T waves, shortened QT intervals, and heart blocks.

DIAGNOSIS AND DIFFERENTIAL

- Most cases of hypercalcemia are due to hyperparathyroidism or malignancies.
- A mnemonic to aid recall the common causes is PAM P. SCHMIDT: *p*arathyroid hormone, *A*ddison's disease, *m*ultiple myeloma, *P*aget's disease, *s*arcoidosis, *c*ancer, *h*yperthyroidism, *m*ilk-alkali syndrome, *i*mmobilization, excess vitamin *D*, and *t*hiazides.

EMERGENCY DEPARTMENT CARE AND DISPOSITION

- Initiate treatment in patients with severe symptoms, [Ca^{2+}] greater than14 milligrams/dL, or significant dehydration. Treatment therapies include volume repletion, decrease osteoclastic activity, and correct underlying cause.
- Correct fluid deficits with NS; several liters may be required. Consider invasive monitoring.
- Furosemide and other loop diuretics are no longer recommended.
- Drugs that inhibit osteoclastic activity include the bisphosphonates, calcitonin, and glucocorticoids. Recommendations for initiating therapy in the ED are lacking; consultation with a specialist is advised.

HYPOMAGNESEMIA

CLINICAL FEATURES

- [Mg^{2+}], [K^+], and [PO_4^-] move together intra- and extracellularly.
- Hypomagnesemia presents nonspecifically, with CNS symptoms (depression, confusion, vertigo, ataxia, tetany, weakness) or cardiac symptoms (arrhythmias, hypotension, and prolonged PR, QRS, and QT intervals).
- Other clinical manifestations of hypomagnesemia include anemia, hypotension, hypothermia, and dysphagia.

DIAGNOSIS AND DIFFERENTIAL

- The diagnosis should not be based on [Mg^{2+}] levels as severe depletion can occur before any significant laboratory changes; it must therefore be suspected clinically.
- In adults, the most common cause is alcoholism, followed by poor nutrition, cirrhosis, pancreatitis, correction of diabetic ketoacidosis (DKA), excessive GI losses, and renal wasting.

EMERGENCY DEPARTMENT CARE AND DISPOSITION

- Volume deficits and concomitant electrolyte abnormalities should be cautiously corrected.
- Oral [Mg^{2+}] replacement is sufficient for most patients.
- In patients with severe symptoms (delirium tremens, seizure, dysrhythmias) and normal renal function,

magnesium sulfate 2 grams IV is administered over an hour, and may be followed by 6 grams over the first 24 hours. Continuous cardiac monitoring and checking frequent DTRs is recommended.

HYPERMAGNESEMIA

CLINICAL FEATURES

- Signs and symptoms manifest progressively; nausea and somnolence occur initially, muscle weakness develops and DTRs disappear above $[Mg^{2+}]$ 4.0 mEq/L; respiratory depression is noted above $[Mg^{2+}]$ 8 mEq/L; and hypotension and EKG changes occur above $[Mg^{2+}]$ 12 mEq/L.

DIAGNOSIS AND DIFFERENTIAL

- Hypermagnesemia is rare. Common causes are renal failure with concomitant ingestion of $[Mg^{2+}]$-containing preparations (antacids) and lithium ingestion. Serum levels are diagnostic. Suspect coexisting increases in potassium and phosphate.

EMERGENCY DEPARTMENT CARE AND DISPOSITION

- In many patients, stopping $[Mg^{2+}]$ intake is sufficient. More aggressive therapy includes rehydration with NS.
- In severely symptomatic patients, **CaCl (10% solution)** 5 mL IV antagonizes the magnesium effects.

ACID–BASE DISORDERS

CLINICAL FEATURES

- Several conditions should alert the clinician to possible acid–base disorders: a history of renal, pulmonary, or psychiatric disorders (drug ingestion); or signs of acute disease: tachypnea, cyanosis, Kussmaul's respiration, respiratory failure, shock, mental status alteration, vomiting, diarrhea, or other acute fluid losses.
- Acidosis is due to a gain of acid or a loss of base; causes may be metabolic (fall in serum $[HCO_3^-]$) or respiratory (rise in P_{CO2}).
- Alkalosis is due to a loss of acid or an addition of base, and is either metabolic (rise in serum $[HCO_3^-]$) or respiratory (fall in P_{CO2}).
- The lungs and kidneys primarily maintain the acid–base regulation. Compensatory mechanisms of the lungs and kidneys will return the pH toward but not to normal.

DIAGNOSIS AND DIFFERENTIAL

- The diagnosis and differential begins with measurement and analysis (with the stepwise approach below) of serum $[HCO_3^-]$ from the electrolyte panel, and the pH and P_{CO2} from the ABG.
- In a mixed disorder the pH, P_{CO2}, and $[HCO_3^-]$ may be normal, and the only clue to a metabolic acidosis is a wide anion gap (AG; see step 3 in the next section).

STEPWISE METHOD OF ACID–BASE CLINICAL PROBLEM SOLVING

- Use the patient's pre-illness values as a baseline; otherwise, use as normal: pH = 7.4, $[HCO_3^-] = 24$ mm/L, $P_{CO2} = 40$ mm Hg.

1. Examine the pH for acidemia (pH < 7.4) or alkalemia (pH > 7.4).
2. Establish the primary mechanism by evaluating the $[HCO_3^-]$ and P_{CO2}.
   - Metabolic acidosis: pH < 7.4 and $[HCO_3^-]$ < 24 mEq/L
   - Metabolic alkalosis: pH > 7.4 and $[HCO_3^-]$ > 24 mEq/L
   - Respiratory acidosis: pH < 7.4 and P_{CO2} > 40 mm Hg
   - Respiratory alkalosis: pH > 7.4 and P_{CO2} < 40 mm Hg
3. Calculate the AG: $[Na^+] - ([Cl^-] + [HCO_3^-])$ = approximately 10–12 mEq/L is normal.
   - If the AG is greater than 15, then an anion gap metabolic acidosis (AGMA) is present.
   - If the AG is less than 15, and a metabolic acidosis is present (low $[HCO_3^-]$), then a nonwidened anion gap (or hyperchloremic) metabolic acidosis (NAGMA) is present.
4. For AGMA, evaluate for a concomitant hidden metabolic process: each 1 mEq/L decrease in $[HCO_3^-]$ results in a 1 mEq/L increase in the AG. Compare the Δ Gap (= present gap – 12) to the Δ $[HCO_3^-]$ (= 24 – present $[HCO_3^-]$).
   - Δ Gap = Δ $[HCO_3^-]$: pure AGMA
   - Δ Gap > Δ $[HCO_3^-]$: concomitant metabolic alkalosis is likely present
   - Δ Gap < Δ $[HCO_3^-]$: concomitant NAGMA is likely present
5. For a primary metabolic process, estimate the respiratory compensatory response. If the compensatory response is not as expected, then the compensatory mechanism requires more time for complete mobilization or a secondary acid–base disturbance exists.
   - Metabolic acidosis: expected $P_{CO2} = (1.5 \times [HCO_3^-] + 8) \pm 2$. A simpler observation is the

P_{CO2} decreases by 1 mm Hg for every 1-mEq/dL decrease in $[HCO_3^-]$. This process takes 12–24 hours.

- Metabolic alkalosis: expected $P_{CO2} = 0.9\ [HCO_3^-] + 16$.
- Current P_{CO2} = expected P_{CO2}: normal respiratory compensation.
- Current P_{CO2} < expected P_{CO2}: possible concomitant respiratory alkalosis.
- Current P_{CO2} > expected P_{CO2}: possible concomitant respiratory acidosis.

6. For a primary respiratory process, estimate the compensatory metabolic response. If the compensatory response is not as expected, then the compensatory mechanism requires more time for complete mobilization or a secondary acid–base disturbance exists.
   - Respiratory acidosis: clinically judge whether the process is acute (<72 hours) or chronic (>72 hours). The $[HCO_3^-]$ increases 1 mEq/L (acute) or 4 mEq/L (chronic) for every 10-mm Hg increase in P_{CO2}.
   - Respiratory alkalosis: clinically judge whether the process is acute (<72 hours) or chronic (>72 hours). The $[HCO_3^-]$ decreases 2 mEq/L (acute) or 5 mEq/L (chronic) for every 10-mm Hg decrease in P_{CO2}.
   - Current $[HCO_3^-]$ = expected $[HCO_3^-]$: normal metabolic compensation.
   - Current $[HCO_3^-]$ < expected $[HCO_3^-]$: possible concomitant metabolic acidosis.
   - Current $[HCO_3^-]$ > expected $[HCO_3^-]$: possible concomitant metabolic alkalosis.
7. See the later sections in this chapter for determining the etiology and management.

METABOLIC ACIDOSIS

- Metabolic acidosis should be divided into a wide and normal AG acidosis. The term anion gap is misleading because the serum has no gap between total positive and negative ions; however, the unmeasured anions exceed the unmeasured cations.

CLINICAL FEATURES

- No matter the etiology, acidosis can cause nausea and vomiting, abdominal pain, change in sensorium, tachypnea, and sometimes a Kussmaul's respiratory pattern.
- Acidosis causes many negative physiologic effects that result in hypoxia: cardiac contractility decreases; hepatic, renal, and systemic BP decreases; pulmonary vasculature resistance increases; and a catabolic state exists.

TABLE 6-6 Causes of High Anion Gap Metabolic Acidosis

Lactic acidosis
Type A: Decrease in tissue oxygenation
Type B: Normal tissue oxygenation
Renal failure (acute or chronic)
Ketoacidosis
Diabetes
Alcoholism
Prolonged starvation (mild acidosis)
High-fat diet (mild acidosis)
Ingestion of toxic substances
Elevated osmolar gap
Methanol
Ethylene glycol
Normal osmolar gap
Salicylate
Paraldehyde
Cyanide

- Patients may present with nonspecific complaints or shock.

DIAGNOSIS AND DIFFERENTIAL

- Causes of metabolic acidosis can be divided into two main groups: (1) those associated with increased production of organic acids (AGMA; see Table 6-6); and (2) those associated with a loss of $[HCO_3^-]$, failure to excrete $[H^+]$, or addition of $[H^+]$ (NAGMA; see Table 6-7).
- A mnemonic to aid recall the causes of AGMA is *A MUD PILES*: *a*lcohol, *m*ethanol, *u*remia, *D*KA, *p*araldehyde, *i*ron and *i*soniazid, *l*actic acidosis, *e*thylene glycol, *s*alicylates, and *s*tarvation.

TABLE 6-7 Causes of Normal Anion Gap Metabolic Acidosis

With a Tendency to Hyperkalemia	With a Tendency to Hypokalemia
Subsiding DKA Early uremic acidosis	Renal tubular acidosis—type I (classical distal acidosis)
Early obstructive uropathy Renal tubular acidosis—type IV	Renal tubular acidosis—type II (proximal acidosis)
Hypoaldosteronism (Addison's disease)	Acetazolamide Acute diarrhea with losses of HCO_3^- and K^+
Infusion or ingestion of HCl, NH_4Cl, lysine-HCl, or arginine-HCl	Ureterosigmoidostomy with increased resorption of H^+ and Cl^- and losses of HCO_3^- and K^+
Potassium-sparing diuretics	Obstruction of artificial ileal bladder Dilution acidosis

Abbreviation: DKA = diabetic ketoacidosis.

TABLE 6-8 Indications for Bicarbonate Therapy in Metabolic Acidosis

INDICATION	RATIONALE
Severe hypobicarbonatemia (<4 mEq/L)	Insufficient buffer concentrations may lead to extreme increases in acidemia with small increases in acidosis
Severe acidemia (pH <7.20) with signs of shock or myocardial irritability that is not rapidly responsive to support measures	Therapy for the underlying cause of acidosis depends on adequate organ perfusion
Severe hyperchloremic acidemia*	Lost bicarbonate must be regenerated by kidneys and liver, which may require days

*No specific definition by pH exists. The presence of serious hemodynamic insufficiency despite supportive care should guide the use of bicarbonate therapy for this indication.

- A mnemonic that can aid recall the causes of NAMGA is *USED CARP*: *u*reterostomy, *s*mall bowel fistulas, *e*xtra chloride, *d*iarrhea, *c*arbonic anhydrase inhibitors, *a*drenal insufficiency, *r*enal tubular acidosis, and *p*ancreatic fistula.

EMERGENCY DEPARTMENT CARE AND DISPOSITION

- Supportive care is provided by improving perfusion through NS infusion, and improving oxygenation and ventilation.
- Correct the underlying problem. For specific etiologies, consult the appropriate chapters in this handbook.
- Indications for bicarbonate therapy are listed in Table 6-8.
- Giving **bicarbonate** 0.5 mEq/kg for each mEq/L desired rise in [HCO_3^-] is recommended. The goal is to restore adequate buffer capacity ([HCO_3^-] >8 mEq/dL) or achieve clinical improvement in shock or dysrhythmias.
- Bicarbonate should be given as slowly as the clinical situation permits; 75 mEq of **8.4% sodium bicarbonate in 500 mL D5W** produces a nearly isotonic solution for infusion.

METABOLIC ALKALOSIS

- Metabolic alkalosis is classified as [Cl^-] sensitive or [Cl^-] insensitive.
- The two most common causes of metabolic alkalosis are excessive diuresis (with loss of potassium, hydrogen ion, and chloride) and excessive loss of gastric secretions (with loss of hydrogen ion and chloride).

CLINICAL FEATURES

- Symptoms of the underlying disorder (usually fluid loss) dominate the clinical presentation, but general symptoms of metabolic alkalosis include muscular irritability, tachydysrhythmias, and impaired oxygen delivery.
- In most cases, there is also an associated hypokalemia and hypochloremia.

DIAGNOSIS AND DIFFERENTIAL

- [Cl^-]-sensitive causes present with hypovolemia secondary to vomiting, diarrhea, or diuretic therapy.
- [Cl^-]-insensitive causes present with normo- to hypervolemia associated with excess mineralocorticoid activity (renin-secreting tumors, adrenal hyperplasia, hyperaldosteronism, Cushing's syndrome).

EMERGENCY DEPARTMENT CARE AND DISPOSITION

- Treat the underlying disorder.
- Administer NS to treat dehydration.
- Electrolytes should be carefully monitored.
- Potassium is administered as KCl and no faster than 20 mEq/h, unless serum potassium is above 5.0 mEq/L.

RESPIRATORY ACIDOSIS

CLINICAL FEATURES

- Respiratory acidosis secondary to hypoventilation may be life threatening.
- Typically, respiratory acidosis depresses the mental function, which may progressively slow the respiratory rate. Patients may be confused, somnolent, and eventually unconscious.
- In some disorders, the fall in oxygen saturation may lag behind the elevation in P_{CO2}. Pulse oximetry may be misleading, making ABGs essential for the diagnosis.

DIAGNOSIS AND DIFFERENTIAL

- The differential diagnosis includes drug overdose, CNS disease, chest wall disease, pleural or lung disease, and trauma.

EMERGENCY DEPARTMENT CARE AND DISPOSITION

- Increase ventilation. Depressed mental status is an indication for intubation. An exception to this recommendation is in the event of opioid intoxication where rapid treatment with naloxone may improve ventilation.

- Treat the underlying disorder. High-flow oxygen therapy may lead to exacerbation of CO_2 narcosis in patients with COPD and CO_2 retention. Monitor these patients closely when administering oxygen and intubate if necessary.

RESPIRATORY ALKALOSIS

CLINICAL FEATURES

- A number of life-threatening disorders present with tachypnea and anxiety: asthma, pulmonary embolism, DKA, and others.
- Symptoms of respiratory alkalosis often are dominated by the primary disorder promoting the hyperventilation.
- Hyperventilation by virtue of the reduction of P_{CO2}, however, lowers both cerebral and peripheral blood flow, causing distinct symptoms.
- Patients complain of dizziness, carpopedal spasm, and chest tightness or pain.

DIAGNOSIS AND DIFFERENTIAL

- The diagnosis of hyperventilation due to anxiety is a diagnosis of exclusion. ABGs can be used to rule out acidosis and hypoxia.
- Causes of respiratory alkalosis include CNS tumor or stroke, hypoxia, infection or fever, lung disease, hyperthyroidism, toxins (eg, sympathomimetic therapy, aspirin), liver disease, pregnancy, anemia, and anxiety.

EMERGENCY DEPARTMENT CARE AND DISPOSITION

- Treat the underlying cause.
- Only when more serious causes of hyperventilation are ruled out should the treatment of anxiety be considered. Anxiolytics may be helpful, such as **lorazepam**, 1–2 milligrams IV or PO.
- Rebreathing into a paper bag can cause hypoxia and is not recommended.

For further reading in *Tintinalli's Emergency Medicine*: A Comprehensive Study Guide, 7th ed., see Chapter 19, "Acid-Base Disorders," by David D. Nicolaou and Gabor D. Kelen; and Chapter 21, "Fluids and Electrolytes," by Gabor D. Kelen and Edbert Hsu.

7 THERAPUTIC APPROACH TO THE HYPOTENSIVE PATIENT

John E. Gough

PATHOPHYSIOLOGY

- Shock is circulatory insufficiency that creates an imbalance between tissue oxygen supply and demand.
- Tissue hypoperfusion is associated with decreased venous O_2 content and metabolic acidosis.
- Shock is classified into four categories based on etiology: (a) hypovolemic, (b) cardiogenic, (c) distributive (eg, neurogenic and anaphylactic), and (d) obstructive.

CLINICAL FEATURES

- The clinical presentation will depend on the etiology, duration, and severity of the shock state and the underlying medical status of the patient.
- Often the precipitating cause of shock may be apparent; however, nonspecific symptoms are not uncommon.
- A targeted history of the presenting symptoms and existing conditions including drug use (prescribed and nonprescribed) is an essential. Drug toxicity and anaphylactic reactions should be considered.
- Assess vital signs; however, no single vital sign or value is diagnostic.
- The body temperature may be normal, elevated, or subnormal. Hyper- or hypothermia may be a result of endogenous factors or exogenous causes.
- **Cardiovascular:** The heart rate is typically elevated; however, bradycardia may be present, often seen with fit individuals, cardiovascular drug use, hypoglycemia, and preexisting cardiovascular disease. Shock is usually, but not always, associated with arterial hypotension, with a systolic blood pressure (BP) below 90 mm Hg. However, **shock may occur with a normal blood pressure, and hypotension may occur without shock.**
- **Cardiovascular: pulse pressure.** Early in shock, BP may be normal or elevated in response to compensatory mechanisms. As these mechanisms fail, BP typically falls. In hypovolemia, postural changes often precede overt hypotension. The pulse pressure may be an earlier and more sensitive indicator.
- **Cardiovascular: neck veins.** Other cardiovascular manifestations may include neck vein distention or flattening and cardiac dysrhythmias. Decreased coronary perfusion pressures can lead to myocardial ischemia, decreased ventricular compliance, increased left ventricular diastolic pressures, and pulmonary edema.

- **Respiratory.** The respiratory rate is frequently elevated early. As shock progresses, hypoventilation, respiratory failure, and respiratory distress syndrome may occur.
- **Decreased cerebral perfusion** leads to mental status changes such as weakness, restlessness, confusion, disorientation, delirium, syncope, and coma.
- **Cutaneous manifestations** may include pallor, pale or dusky skin, sweating, bruising, petechiae, cyanosis, altered temperature, and delayed capillary refill.
- **GI manifestations** resulting from low flow states may include ileus, GI bleeding, pancreatitis, acalculous cholecystitis, and mesenteric ischemia.
- **Renal manifestations.** Aldosterone and antidiuretic hormone are increased resulting in a reduced glomerular filtration rate and oliguria. In sepsis, a paradoxical polyuria may occur and be mistaken for adequate hydration.
- **Metabolic manifestations.** Respiratory alkalosis is common early. As the shock state continues and compensatory mechanisms begin to fail, anaerobic metabolism occurs, leading to the formation of lactic acid and metabolic acidosis. Other abnormalities that may be seen are hyperglycemia, hypoglycemia, and hyperkalemia.

DIAGNOSIS AND DIFFERENTIAL

- The clinical presentation and presumed etiology of shock will dictate the diagnostic studies, monitoring modalities, and interventions.
- The patient approach must be individualized; however, frequently performed laboratory studies include complete blood count, platelet count, serum lactate levels, electrolytes, blood urea nitrogen, and creatinine determinations; prothrombin and partial thromboplastin times; and urinalysis.
- Other tests commonly used are arterial blood gas, fibrinogen, fibrin split products, D-dimer, and cortisol determinations; hepatic function panel; cerebrospinal fluid studies; and cultures of potential sources of infection.
- A pregnancy test should be performed on all females of childbearing potential.
- Other common diagnostic tests include radiographs (chest and abdominal), electrocardiographs, computed tomography scans (chest, head, abdomen, and pelvis), and echocardiograms. Beside US may also help determine the etiology of shock.
- Continuous monitoring of vital signs should be instituted. Additionally, modalities such as pulse oximetry, end-tidal CO_2, central venous pressure, central venous O_2 saturation, cardiac output, and calculation of systemic vascular resistance and systemic oxygen delivery may be indicated.
- Lack of response to appropriate stabilization should lead to a search for more occult causes. Be certain that basic resuscitation have been carried out including adequate volume replacement. Early use of vasopressors may elevate the central venous pressure and mask the presence of continued hypovolemia. Ensure that all equipment is functioning appropriately.
- Expose and examine for occult wounds.
- Consider less commonly seen diagnoses, such as cardiac tamponade, tension pneumothorax, adrenal insufficiency, toxic or allergic reactions, and occult bleeding (eg, ruptured ectopic pregnancy, or occult intraabdominal or pelvic bleeding).

EMERGENCY DEPARTMENT CARE AND DISPOSITION

- The goal of the interventions is to restore adequate tissue perfusion in concert with the identification and treatment of the underlying etiology.
- Aggressive airway control, best obtained through endotracheal intubation, is indicated. Remember associated interventions such as medications (ie, sedatives can exacerbate hypotension) and positive pressure ventilation may reduce preload and cardiac output and may contribute to hemodynamic collapse.
- All patients should receive supplemental high-flow oxygen. If mechanical ventilation is used, neuromuscular blocking agents should be used to decrease lactic acidosis from muscle fatigue and increased oxygen consumption. Arterial oxygen saturation should be restored to >93% and ventilation controlled to maintain a Pa_{CO2} of 35 to 40 mm Hg.
- Circulatory hemodynamic stabilization begins with IV access through large-bore peripheral venous lines. Central venous access aids in assessing volume status (preload) and monitoring S_{cvO2}. US guidance has proven helpful with these procedures. Central venous access is the preferred route for the long-term administration of vasopressor therapy.
- Early surgical consultation is indicated for internal bleeding.
- Most external hemorrhage can be controlled by direct compression. Rarely, clamping or tying off of vessels may be needed.
- Use isotonic crystalloid intravenous fluids (0.9% NaCl, Ringer's lactate) in the initial resuscitation phase. Standard therapy is 20 to 40 mL/kg given rapidly (over 10-20 minutes). Only about 30% of infused isotonic crystalloids remain in the intravascular space;

therefore, it is recommended to infuse three times the estimated blood loss in acute hemorrhagic shock.

- The benefits of early and aggressive fluid replacement in these trauma patients remain unproven as do the benefits of permissive hypotension.
- Blood remains the ideal resuscitative fluid. When possible, use fully cross-matched PRBCs. If the clinical situation dictates more rapid intervention, type-specific, type O (rhesus negative to be given to females of childbearing years) may be used. The decision to use platelets or fresh frozen plasma (FFP) should be based on clinical evidence of impaired hemostasis and frequent monitoring of coagulation parameters.
- Vasopressors are used after appropriate volume resuscitation, and there is persistent hypotension.
- The goal of resuscitation is to maximize survival and minimize morbidity using objective hemodynamic and physiologic values to guide therapy. A goal-directed approach of urine output >0.5 mL/kg/h, CVP 8 to 12 mm Hg, MAP 65–90 mm Hg, and S_{cvO2} >70% during ED resuscitation of septic shock significantly decreases mortality.
- Acidosis should be treated with adequate ventilation and fluid resuscitation. Sodium bicarbonate (1 mEq/kg) use is controversial. Use only in the setting of severe acidosis refractory to above-mentioned methods. Correct only to arterial pH 7.25.
- Early surgical or medical consultation for admission or transfer is indicated.

For further reading in *Tintinalli's Emergency Medicine: A Comprehensive Study Guide*, 7th ed., see Chapter 25 "Approach to the Patient in Shock," by Ronny M. Otero, H. Bryant Nguyen and Emanuel P. Rivers; Chapter 26 "Fluid and Blood Resuscitation," by José G. Cabañas, James E. Manning and Charles B. Cairns.

8 ANAPHYLAXIS, ACUTE ALLERGIC REACTIONS, AND ANGIOEDEMA

Alix L. Mitchell

EPIDEMIOLOGY

- Allergic reactions range from mild cutaneous symptoms to life-threatening anaphylaxis.
- Common exposures are medications, insect stings, and foods. Many cases are idiopathic.
- Half of the fatalities from anaphylaxis occur within the first hour.

PATHOPHYSIOLOGY

- Mast cell activation caused by histamine, prostaglandin D2, leukotrienes, and other mediators play a role in the progression to anaphylaxis.
- Anaphylactoid reactions, unlike IgE-mediated allergic responses, do not require a previous sensitizing exposure, but both reactions may ultimately progress to anaphylaxis.
- Concurrent use of β-blockers is a risk factor for severe, prolonged anaphylaxis.

CLINICAL FEATURES

- *Anaphylaxis* describes an acute progression of organ system involvement that may lead to cardiovascular collapse.
- Reactions may occur in seconds or may be delayed an hour or more after exposure.
- Up to 20% of reactions are "biphasic," with further mediator release peaking 4 to 8 hours after exposure.
- Symptoms can include dermatologic (flushing, urticaria, angioedema), respiratory (wheezing, cough, dyspnea, stridor), cardiovascular (dysrhythmia, collapse), gastrointestinal (vomiting, diarrhea), and eye (tearing, redness, pruritus) complaints.

DIAGNOSIS AND DIFFERENTIAL

- The diagnosis is clinical. Consider the diagnosis in any rapidly progressing multisystem illness.
- An exposure to an allergen can confirm the diagnosis, but the exposure will not always be identified.
- Work-up should focus on excluding other diagnoses while stabilizing the patient.
- The differential depends on which organ systems are involved. Considerations may include vasovagal reaction, asthma, acute coronary syndrome, epiglottitis or airway foreign body, carcinoid, mastocytosis, and hereditary angioedema.

EMERGENCY DEPARTMENT CARE AND DISPOSITION

- Patients should have intravenous access and be placed on a cardiac monitor with pulse oximetry.
- Angioedema or respiratory distress should prompt early consideration for intubation. Preparations should be made for "rescue" transtracheal jet insufflation or cricothyroidotomy.
- Eliminate the exposure. This may be as simple as stopping a drug or removing a stinger.
- First-line therapy for anaphylaxis is **epinephrine**. In patients without cardiovascular collapse, administer

0.3–0.5 milligrams (0.3–0.5 mL of 1:1000; pediatric dose, 0.01 milligrams/kg to a maximum of 0.5 milligrams) intramuscularly in the thigh; repeat every 5 minutes as needed.

- Patients who are refractory to IM dosing or in significant shock should receive intravenous epinephrine. A bolus of 100 micrograms of 1:100,000 dilution (place 0.1 mL of 1:1000 in 10 mL normal saline) can be given over 5–10 minutes followed by an infusion of 1–4 micrograms/min.
- Hypotensive patients require aggressive fluid resuscitation with **normal saline** 1–2 L (pediatric dose, 10–20 mL/kg).
- Steroids are indicated in all cases of anaphylaxis. Severe cases can be treated with **methylprednisolone** 125 milligrams IV (pediatric dose, 2 milligrams/kg). Mild allergic reactions can be treated with oral **prednisone** 60 milligrams (pediatric dose, 2 milligrams/kg).
- Administer **diphenhydramine** 50 milligrams IV (pediatric dose, 1 milligram/kg). In addition, an H_2 blocker such as **ranitidine** 50 milligrams IV (pediatric dose, 0.5 milligrams/kg) may be helpful.
- Bronchospasm is treated with nebulized β-agonists such as **albuterol** 2.5 milligrams. If refractory, consider an inhaled anticholinergic, **ipratropium bromide** 250 micrograms, and intravenous **magnesium** 2 grams (25-50 milligrams/kg in children) over 20 to 30 minutes.
- For patients on β-blockers with refractory hypotension, use **glucagon** 1 milligram IV every 5 minutes. An infusion of 5 to 15 micrograms/min should be started once blood pressure improves.
- Angiotensin-converting enzyme inhibitors are a common trigger for nonallergic angioedema, which can rapidly lead to airway compromise. Treatment is supportive; epinephrine, steroids, and antihistamines are often given, although benefit has not been proven.
- Patients with hereditary angioedema do not respond to treatment for anaphylaxis and should be treated with C1 esterase inhibitor replacement. Treatment with fresh frozen plasma has been reported as an alternative when C1 esterase inhibitor replacement is not available.
- Unstable or refractory patients merit admission to the intensive care unit.
- Patients with moderate to severe symptoms should be admitted for observation.
- Patients with mild allergic reactions should be observed in the ED and may be sent home if symptoms are stable or improving.
- Patients who received epinephrine are generally felt to be safe for discharge after 4 hours without symptoms.
- Consider observing patients with a history of severe reactions and patients on β-blockers for a longer period.
- Discharge patients on an antihistamine and a short course of prednisone. Counsel all patients about the possibility of a late recurrence of symptoms and about avoiding future exposures to the allergen.
- All patients who have experienced severe allergic reactions should have and know how to use an epinephrine autoinjector. Consider Medic-Alert bracelets and referral to an allergist in these patients.

For further reading in Tintinalli's *Emergency Medicine: A Comprehensive Study Guide*, 7th ed., see Chapter 27, "Anaphylaxis, Acute Allergic Reactions, and Angioedema," by Brian H. Rowe and Theodore J. Gaeta.

Section 3

ANALGESIA, ANESTHESIA, AND PROCEDURAL SEDATION

9 ACUTE PAIN MANAGEMENT AND PROCEDURAL SEDATION

Michael S. Mitchell

EPIDEMIOLOGY

- Acute pain is present in 50% to 60% of patients presenting to the emergency department.
- Factors contributing to inadequate pain control, or oligoanalgesia, include a limited understanding of the related pharmacology, misunderstanding of the patient's perception of pain, and fear of serious side effects.
- Procedural sedation, formerly called conscious sedation, may be indicated for fracture manipulation or joint reduction, abscess drainage, laceration repair, tube thoracostomy, cardioversion, or a diagnostic study.

PATHOPHYSIOLOGY

- Noxious stimuli are first registered peripherally by nociceptors, C fibers, A-σ fibers, and free nerve endings, resulting in the release of glutamate, substance P, neurokinin A, and calcitonin gene-related peptide within the spinal cord.
- Pain is modulated at the level of the dorsal root ganglion, inhibitory interneurons, and ascending pain tracts.
- Cognitive interpretation, localization, and identification of pain occur at the level of the hypothalamus, thalamus, limbus, and reticular activating system.

CLINICAL FEATURES

- The subjective interpretation of pain is variable. Therefore, pain is best assessed using a validated, age-appropriate, objective pain scale.
- Competent patients who are awake and cooperative can often reliably localize pain and determine its quality and severity.
- Patients who have difficulty communicating with their caregivers due to cultural differences, extremes of age, language barriers, or mental illness may not be able to describe and localize pain.
- Physiologic responses to pain and anxiety are nonspecific, but include tachycardia, blood pressure elevation, tachypnea, diaphoresis, flushing or pallor, nausea, and muscle tension.
- Behavioral responses to pain and anxiety include facial expressions, posturing, crying, and vocalization.

EMERGENCY DEPARTMENT CARE AND DISPOSITION

- Nonpharmacologic treatment of pain may be used alone or adjunctively. Examples include application of heat or cold, immobilization or elevation of injured extremities, explanation and reassurance, relaxation, distraction, guided imagery, and biofeedback.
- When pharmacologic intervention is necessary, the desired effect, the route of delivery, and the desired duration of effect should be considered in determining the ideal agent.

ANALGESIA IN ADULTS

NONOPIOIDS

- Nonopioid agents may be used alone for mild pain, or adjunctively with opiates for moderate to severe pain. Nonopioid analgesics cause no respiratory depression or sedation.
- Acetaminophen is an analgesic and anti-inflammatory agent with no antiplatelet effects that is safe in all age groups. Hepatotoxicity may occur in doses above 140 milligrams/kg/d.
- Nonsteroidal anti-inflammatory drugs (NSAIDs) include aspirin, naproxen, indomethacin, ibuprofen, and ketorolac. NSAIDs are analgesics and anti-inflammatory agents with opiate dose-sparing effects,

but may cause platelet dysfunction, impaired coagulation, gastrointestinal irritation, and bleeding.
- Aspirin also may induce bronchospasm and should be avoided in some asthmatic patients.

OPIOIDS

- Opioids have analgesic and sedative effects, but may cause respiratory depression, nausea and vomiting, constipation, urinary retention, pruritus, confusion, and muscle rigidity.
- Morphine is a naturally occurring opiate with a 5- to 20-minute onset of effect, a 10- to 30-minute peak effect, and a 2- to 6-hour duration. The dose of **morphine** is 0.1–0.2 milligram/kg and is commonly administered IV or IM. Morphine may cause hypotension due to histamine release.
- Meperidine is a semisynthetic opiate whose use is discouraged in the ED due to the CNS toxicity of its metabolite normeperidine, significant histamine release, and a higher risk of addiction than other opiates.
- Hydromorphone is a semisynthetic opiate with a 5- to 20-minute onset of effect, a 3- to 4-hour duration of effect, and less sedation and nausea than morphine. The dose of **hydromorphone** is 1–2 milligrams IV (0.015 milligram/kg IV pediatric).

PEDIATRIC PAIN MANAGEMENT

- Pain experienced by pediatric patients is often unrecognized and undertreated.
- The pain these patients feel may be exacerbated by their anxiety, which is oftentimes tied to their developmental stage.
- Infants experience pain.
- Toddlers experience anxiety, greatly exacerbated by their normal developmental phenomenon of "stranger anxiety." It is necessary to involve the parents in all aspects of pain control and procedures.
- School-aged children usually respond well to distraction techniques.
- Adolescents can experience great anxiety with pain and painful procedures, which should be both anticipated and managed.
- Pain is managed similarly as adults, with two important considerations: (1) children require more opioid proportionate to their weight and (2) children may not openly indicate pain; thus their pain should be anticipated and treated.
- NSAIDs are given for mild pain. Ibuprofen is reserved for those children older than 6 months.
- Opioids are given for moderate to severe pain. NSAIDs should be given in conjunction with opioids.
- Meperidine is not recommended for children.

PEDIATRIC ANXIOLYSIS MANAGEMENT

- Anxiety potentiates pain and can be managed with soothing techniques, distraction, and parental assistance during times of pain and during painful procedures.
- Midazolam is a choice agent for use in the ED given its short duration of action and can be used in a variety of routes.
- **Midazolam** can be given PO (0.5 milligram/kg), IV (0.05–0.1 milligram/kg), or intranasally (IN) (0.2 milligram/kg). The oral route takes approximately 20 minutes and can be variable in efficacy. IV and IN routes are generally more predictable. The IN preparation may produce a burning sensation in the nares.
- Be prepared for potential paradoxical reactions to benzodiazepines as well as respiratory depression that can be seen with this medication class.

LOCAL AND REGIONAL ANESTHESIA

- Local anesthesia can be obtained by infiltrating directly into the area, infiltrating into the area of the peripheral nerves supplying the area, or infusing into the venous system supplying the area to be anesthetized.
- Local anesthetics are divided into two classes: amides and esters. Lidocaine is the prototype amide, and procaine the prototype ester. Bupivacaine is an amide anesthetic with duration of action of 2–6 hours, and is preferred for prolonged procedures.
- Local anesthetics work by blocking sodium channels and prohibiting the nerve impulse propagation.
- The injection pain of local anesthetics can be minimized by slow injection of warm, bicarbonate-buffered solution through a 27- or 30-gauge needle. Also, it is recommended to inject through the margins of the wound rather than into the surrounding, intact skin.
- The addition of epinephrine to lidocaine extends the duration of anesthesia and slows systemic absorption. Epinephrine is tolerated for use in end-arterial fields in selected healthy patients, but should be avoided in those with digital vascular injuries, Raynaud disease, or other vascular supply problems.
- Local anesthetic toxicity from excessive total dose or inadvertent IV injection can lead to cardiovascular

depression, arrhythmias, seizures, and death. The maximum dose of **lidocaine** is 4.5 milligrams/kg without epinephrine, and 7 milligrams/kg with epinephrine.

- Aspiration prior to injection of the anesthetic is necessary to prevent inadvertent IV injection.
- In patients who cannot tolerate amides and esters (ie, allergy), both diphenhydramine and benzyl alcohol with epinephrine are alternatives.

TOPICAL ANESTHESIA

- Topical anesthetics reduce the discomfort of painful procedures, decrease the need for local infiltration of anesthetics, and maintain wound edges.
- The most common topical anesthetics for ED use are **lidocaine, epinephrine, tetracaine (LET), liposome-encapsulated lidocaine (LMX), and lidocaine prilocaine (EMLA).**
- EMLA and LMX are reserved for use on intact skin. LET is for nonintact skin.
- Onset of action: EMLA: 30–60 minutes, LMX and LET: 30 minutes.

REGIONAL ANESTHESIA

- The following is a brief discussion of regional blocks. Refer to the Tintinalli's *Emergency Medicine: A Comprehensive Study Guide*, 7th ed. Chapter 40 as well as view videos of each block on the AccessEmergencyMedicine Web site at http://www.accessemergencymedicine.com/multimedia.aspx.
- Regional anesthesia is a technique of infiltrating local anesthetic agents adjacent to peripheral nerves and is ideal for complicated lacerations, fractures, and dislocations. Prior to administering regional anesthesia, neurovascular status must be assessed.
- Topical anesthetic application may reduce the pain of injection of the regional anesthesia. The onset of action is longer than for typical dermal infiltration. Optimal analgesia is obtained in 10–20 minutes with lidocaine and 15–30 minutes with bupivacaine.
- Anatomic variations can distort the usual "landmarks." Ultrasound guidance to locate the nerve may improve the performance.

DIGITAL BLOCKS

- **Digital nerve block**: Provides anesthesia to the entire finger. See Fig. 9-1.
- Application is to the nerves that lie on the lateral aspects of the finger.
- Technique: Inject the finger at the proximal aspect along the lateral edge from the dorsal aspect. Deposit anesthetic and inject additional anesthetic as the needle is withdrawn. Next, insert the needle on the dorsal surface and direct it across the skin to the medial

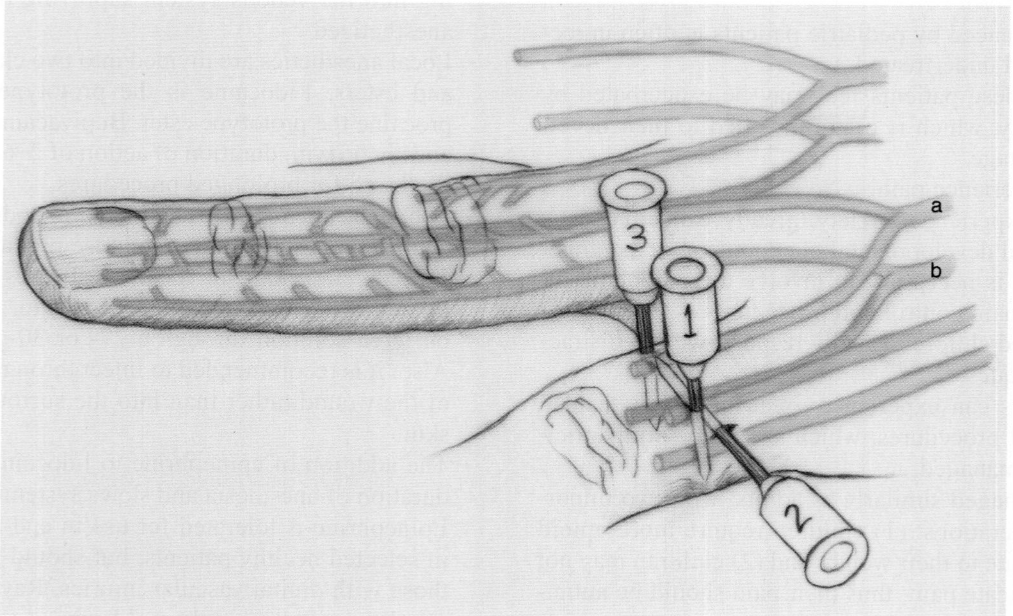

FIG. 9-1. Digital nerve block. Anesthetic placed as shown blocks both the dorsal (a) and palmar (b) digital nerves, ensuring circumferential anesthesia of the finger. By using the sequence shown, the prior injection provides relief from the injection to follow. See Digital Nerve Block for further details. (Courtesy of Timothy Sweeney, MD.)

aspect of the finger. Deposit anesthetic and inject while withdrawing needle. Finally, inject over the medial aspect dorsal surface with the same technique as the other side.

- **Flexor tendon sheath digital nerve block**: Identify the distal palmar crease on the palmar aspect of the hand. Have the patient flex the finger against resistance to improve visualization of the flexor tendon (see Fig. 9-2).
- Technique: Prepare a sterile block site at the distal palmar crease of the digit to be blocked and insert the needle at a 45-degree angle to the palmar plane with the tip pointed distally. Advance the needle until a "pop" is felt, indicating penetration of the flexor tendon sheath. Inject 2–3 mL of anesthetic solution. If bone is struck before the "pop" is felt, withdraw the needle 2–3 mm and inject the solution.

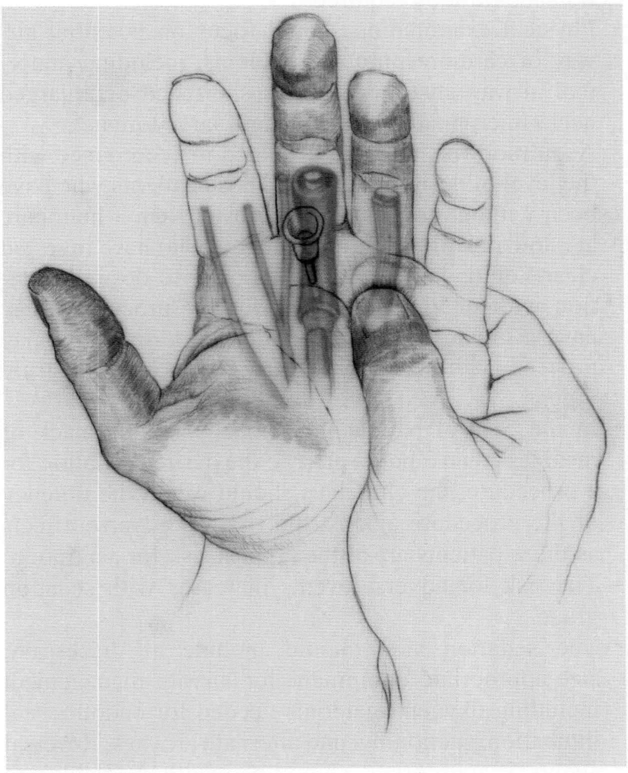

FIG. 9-2. Transthecal (flexor tendon sheath) digital nerve block. The point of injection is in the middle of the flexor tendon sheath at the level of the distal palmar crease. A 25-gauge needle is advanced at 45 degrees, tip directed distally until it enters the flexor tendon sheath (shown in blue) or until bone is encountered. When the needle is properly placed within the flexor tendon sheath, the anesthetic solution is injected. Diffusion out of the tendon sheath blocks adjacent palmar digital nerves. See Transthecal or Flexor Tendon Sheath Digital Nerve Block for further details. (Courtesy of Timothy Sweeney, MD.)

RADIAL NERVE BLOCK

- Provides anesthesia to the dorsal lateral half of the hand and the dorsal aspect of the thumb.
- Technique: Inject a large volume of anesthetic (5 mL) just proximal to the anatomic snuffbox.

ULNAR NERVE BLOCK

- Provides anesthesia to the entire fifth digit, half of the fourth digit, and the medial aspect of the hand and wrist.
- Technique: Deposit anesthetic under the flexor carpi ulnaris tendon just proximal to the distal wrist crease.

DEEP PERONEAL NERVE BLOCK

- Provides anesthesia to the web space of the first and second toes, and a small area proximal to the first and second toes on the plantar aspect.
- Technique: Deposit anesthetic at the medial malleolus between the extensor hallucis longus and the tibialis anterior tendon.

POSTERIOR TIBIAL NERVE BLOCK

- Provides anesthesia to the plantar aspect of the foot.
- Technique: Deposit anesthetic posterior to the posterior tibial artery found at the posterior edge of the medial malleolus.

SUPERFICIAL PERONEAL NERVE BLOCK

- Provides anesthesia to the dorsal lateral aspect of the foot.
- Technique: Deposit anesthetic between the lateral malleolus and the tibialis anterior tendon.

SURAL NERVE BLOCK

- Provides anesthesia to the lateral aspect of the ankle.
- Technique: Deposit anesthetic between the superior portion of the lateral malleolus and the Achilles tendon.

SAPHENOUS NERVE BLOCK

- Provides anesthesia to the medial aspect of the ankle.
- Technique: Deposit anesthetic between the tibialis anterior tendon and the superior border of the medial malleolus.

SUPRAORBITAL AND SUPRATROCHLEAR NERVE BLOCKS

- Provides anesthesia to the forehead from the vertex of the scalp to the bridge of the nose.
- Technique: Deposit anesthetic superior to the eyebrow in line with the pupil. Further, direct needle medially after initial deposit and a wheal is formed to reach the edge of the eyebrow.

INFRAORBITAL NERVE BLOCK

- Provides anesthesia to the lower lid, medial cheek, and both the ipsilateral side of nose and upper lip.
- Technique: Insert needle inside the mouth at the gingival reflection above the maxillary canine and direct needle superiorly.

MENTAL NERVE BLOCK

- Provides anesthesia to the labial mucosa, gingival, and the lower lip adjacent to the incisors and canines.
- Technique: Direct needle and deposit anesthetic from the mouth inferior to the canine at the gingival reflection inferiorly to the mental foramen.

AURICULAR BLOCK

- Provides anesthesia to the entire ear.
- Technique: Deposit anesthetic into several places. From the inferior and superior aspect of the ear, inject anterior and posterior to the ear and deposit anesthetic while withdrawing the needle.

FEMORAL NERVE BLOCK

- Provides anesthesia to the anterior thigh and medial leg.
- Technique: Deposit anesthetic at the level of the femoral nerve. The needle is inserted 1 cm lateral to the femoral artery at the level of the inguinal crease. The needle is directed in the cephalad direction to the femoral nerve, which lies about 2 cm deep. The needle is inserted until the patient experiences paresthesias. The needle is retracted slightly and 20 mL of anesthetic is delivered.

PROCEDURAL SEDATION AND ANALGESIA

- *Sedation* is a pharmacologically induced decrease in environmental awareness. *Analgesia* is relief from the perception of pain.
- Sedation level is on a continuum from minimal sedation (patient can respond to verbal stimuli) to deep sedation (patient has purposeful responses with repeated painful stimuli). Only the lightest level of sedation that is necessary for the planned procedure should be used.
- The risk of adverse respiratory events increase as the patient advances along the continuum from minimal to deep sedation.
- It is imperative to score each patient prior to sedation on the American Society of Anesthesiologists' (ASA) physical classification system in order to predict their risk of adverse events. Class I and II patients have at most a mild systemic illness and have a low risk of adverse events. Class III and higher (Class III is severe systemic disease) patients have a much higher risk of adverse events.
- Assess the Mallampati grading system scale for airways (I–IV) for each patient to assess ease of intubation should it be required.
- Physical examination should focus on potential airway or cardiorespiratory problems, including abnormal airway anatomy such as shortened or enlarged neck, micrognathia, trismus, or a large tongue.
- Aspiration risk must be managed in accordance with the level of desired sedation. Those patients who have been without oral intake for greater than 3 hours are at a low risk of aspiration. Patients who have ingested clear liquids less than 3 hours prior to desired sedation with urgent indications for the procedure may have a greater risk of aspiration, but clinicians may proceed with sedation for procedures that are truly urgent.
- In the case of patient ingestion of a light snack or meal less than 3 hours prior to the desired sedation for a procedure, the clinicians should weigh the urgency of the procedure against the risk for adverse effects as these patients are at the highest risk for aspiration.
- The risk for adverse events increases with sedation grade.
- The sedation area should include all necessary, size-appropriate equipment for airway management including oxygen, materials needed for endotracheal intubation, suctioning, and alternate airways. Reversal agents, if appropriate, should be readily available.
- Minimal sedation requires only direct observation; however, moderate and deep sedation require mechanical monitoring including ongoing cardiorespiratory monitoring, pulse oximetry, and end-tidal CO_2 capnography. Capnography can detect ventilator changes before clinical observation and prior to the ensuing hypoxemia.
- Analgesics are recommended prior to procedural sedation, but may increase the risk of respiratory

adverse events. Ketamine possesses both analgesic and anxiolytic properties.

- Procedural sedation agents often have a narrow therapeutic index. Administer these agents in small incremental doses, allowing adequate time for the development and assessment of peak effect. Continuous reassessment is required.
- Precalculated doses of "rescue" or reversal agents should be at the bedside: **naloxone**, 0.1 milligram/kg every 2–3 minutes to reverse opiate-induced respiratory depression, and **flumazenil**, 0.01–0.02 milligram/kg every 1–2 minutes to reverse benzodiazepine-induced respiratory depression during procedural sedation.
- Flumazenil should not be used on patients with a history of chronic benzodiazepine or tricyclic antidepressant use due to the risk of seizures.

PROCEDURAL SEDATION AGENTS

- For dosing and administration parameters of each agent, see Table 9-1.

NITROUS OXIDE

- Used for minimal sedation in a 50:50 mixture with oxygen.

TABLE 9-1 Sedation Agents for Procedural Sedation and Analgesia

MEDICATION	RECOMMENDED DOSAGE	ROUTE OF ADMINISTRATION	ONSET	DURATION	USE
Nitrous oxide	50:50 mixture with oxygen	Inhalational	2-3 min	15-20 min	Minimal sedation
Midazolam	0.05-0.1 milligram/kg May repeat 0.05 milligram/kg every 2 min until adequately sedated	IV	1-3 min	1 h	Minimal or moderate sedation
	0.1 milligram/kg	IM	15-30 min	1-2 h	Minimal sedation
	Children: 0.1 milligram 0.5 milligram/kg 0.2 milligram/kg	 IM PO/PR Intranasally			
Fentanyl	1-3 micrograms/kg, can be titrated up to 5 micrograms/kg Children: 1-2 micrograms/kg	IV	<1 min	30-60 min	Minimal sedation
Fentanyl and midazolam	1-2 micrograms/kg fentanyl plus midazolam 0.05-0.1 milligram/kg, as needed, up to 2 times	IV	1-2 min	1 h	Moderate and deep sedation
Methohexital	1 milligram/kg	IV	1 min	10 min	Moderate or deep sedation
Pentobarbital	2-2.5 milligrams/kg followed by 1.25 milligrams/kg, as needed, up to 2 times	IV rate should be <50 milligrams/min	30-60 s	15+ min	Minimal and moderate sedation Used frequently for radiological procedures
Ketamine	1-2 milligrams/kg 2-5 milligrams/kg Up to 4 milligrams/kg in children	IV IM	1-3 min 5-20 min	10-20 min 30-60 min	Dissociative sedation Dissociative sedation
Ketamine and midazolam	Ketamine as above plus midazolam 0.05-0.1 milligram/kg	IV	1-3 min	30-60 min	Dissociative sedation
Etomidate	0.15 milligram/kg, followed by 0.1 milligram/kg every 2 min, if needed Children: 0.1-0.3 milligram/kg	IV	30-60 s	5-10 min	Moderate, deep sedation Associated with amnesia
Propofol	1 milligram/kg, followed by 0.5 milligram/kg every 3 min, if needed Children: 1-2 milligrams/kg	IV	1-2 min	5-10 min	Moderate and deep sedation
Propofol and ketamine	Propofol as above plus ketamine 0.3-0.5 milligram/kg Use higher end dose in children	IV	1 min	Propofol—5-10 min ketamine 15-45 min	Moderate and deep sedation

Weight-based medication doses are the same in adults and children unless otherwise noted.

- Relative contraindications to its use include pulmonary hypertension (pulmonary vasoconstricting properties and cardiac depressant), pregnancy (inhibits folate metabolism), and concern for pneumothorax.
- N_2O has opiate agonist properties, and therefore should be used with extreme caution if combined with a sedative or opiate to avoid deep sedation or general anesthesia.

MIDAZOLAM

- Midazolam and other benzodiazepines potentiate the effects of CNS gamma-aminobutyric acid (GABA), resulting in chloride influx, which produces sedation, amnesia, anxiolysis, anticonvulsant effects, and respiratory depression.
- This agent can be used solely or in conjunction with opioids.
- It has a variety of routes, but the IV route is most predictable. Notably, the PO/PR/IM routes can have variable onset and duration secondary to differences in absorption and metabolism.
- Intranasal midazolam is safe, but will irritate the nasal mucosa.
- Midazolam can cause mild cardiovascular depression.

FENTANYL

- This agent is a potent, short-acting opioid.
- Rigid chest syndrome can occur with rapid infusion of fentanyl, but can be prevented by using a slow infusion rate and carefully flushing the IV line. Rigid chest is characterized by spasm of the respiratory muscles and is not overcome with opioid antagonists. Rigid chest is treated by neuromuscular paralysis and intubation.

METHOHEXITAL

- Very short-acting barbiturate that is useful for quick procedures.
- Respiratory depression is noted, especially with subsequent doses after the initial bolus dose.

PENTOBARBITAL

- Short-acting barbiturate that has no analgesic properties.
- Useful for procedures that are not painful (ie, radiologic study).

CHLORAL HYDRATE

- No longer recommended for use in the ED.

KETAMINE

- Ketamine produces analgesia, amnesia, and dissociation with minimal respiratory depression.
- It is a dissociative anesthetic and the dissociative phase is met once a dosing threshold is exceeded (typically above 1 milligram/kg infused).
- Ketamine is a good agent to use for prolonged procedures (ie, hip spica cast placement on a toddler).
- Ketamine has a favorable cardiorespiratory profile, but can cause laryngospasm. This occurs primarily in pediatric patients and usually is overcome with positive pressure ventilation with a bag-valve mask. Those at risk for laryngospasm include infants <3 months of age, those with upper respiratory tract infections, and those undergoing intraoral procedures.
- Vomiting is frequently seen during recovery. Consider giving a pre-sedation dose of ondansetron.
- Another common complication is bronchorrhea, which may be improved with the use of **atropine,** 0.01 milligram/kg IV, or **glycopyrrolate,** 0.004 milligram/kg IV. The use of anticholinergic agents is controversial and may not be necessary.
- Emergence reactions can occur in adolescents and adults. Midazolam can be given as an adjunct or in those patients who develop emergence reactions.
- Ketamine increases intraocular pressure and should be avoided with eye injuries or glaucoma.
- Ketamine may increase intracranial pressure; avoid using in the head-injured patient.

ETOMIDATE

- Etomidate is an ultra-short-acting sedative agent increasingly used for procedural sedation.
- Etomidate has minimal hemodynamic effects and a low risk of apnea.
- Adverse effects may include vomiting, myoclonus, short-term adrenal suppression, and CNS depression.

PROPOFOL

- Propofol is frequently used in the ED for sedation because it is easy to titrate.
- Propofol does not have analgesic properties, thus pre-procedure analgesics are recommended.
- Pain associated with administration of propofol can be attenuated by the coadministration of **lidocaine,** 0.05 milligram/kg.
- Propofol is contraindicated in those with egg allergies, since it contains an egg lecithin emulsion.
- Respiratory depression and apnea can occur, so rescue equipment should be readily available.

- Propofol can induce hypotension. It is essential to attempt to correct hypotension prior to propofol administration.

PROPOFOL AND KETAMINE ("KETOFOL")

- The combination of propofol and ketamine is safe in both adult and pediatric patients.
- The combination may provide benefit in attenuating certain side effects of each other; however, these effects remain controversial. Less propofol is required which may reduce hypotension. Less nausea and vomiting is seen than with ketamine alone. Respiratory depression associated with propofol is not diminished when using this combination.
- Ketofol recovery time falls between propofol (short) and ketamine (long).

POST PROCEDURAL SEDATION CARE

- Patients should be monitored until they return to baseline mental status.
- Patients who vomit are at risk for aspiration until they return to baseline mental status.

SPECIAL CIRCUMSTANCES

CRITICALLY ILL PATIENTS

- Etomidate is the agent of choice for those ASA III and higher.
- Etomidate causes less hypotension than other agents.
- Patients requiring sedation may require general anesthesia in the OR.

ELDERLY

- Procedural sedation in the elderly is associated with more adverse events. The risk of respiratory depression and aspiration events is increased.
- Remove dentures or bridges to prevent aspiration.
- Etomidate may be a good choice for the reasons noted above. An analgesic must be used in addition to etomidate.
- Reduce propofol dose by 50% doses from those recommended for younger adults because of a greater risk of respiratory depression.

EMERGENCY ENDOSCOPY

- Vasovagal reactions can occur with passage of the endoscope causing bradycardia and hypotension.
- There is increased risk of apnea, hypoxia, and aspiration due to the passage of the endoscope.
- Topical anesthesia may be required to suppress the gag reflex, but may not be necessary if adequate IV sedation is achieved.
- Droperidol reduces gagging during upper endoscopy. However, its use is associated with additional side effects including hypotension, dystonic reactions, and rarely, torsades de pointes cardiac dysrhythmia. Avoid using droperidol in patients with prolonged QT interval.
- Promethazine combats nausea. Its strong alpha-adrenergic blocking effect can cause transient hypotension.

PROCEDURAL SEDATION IN CHILDREN

- Involve the parents by allowing them be present for the beginning of the sedation, thereby reducing the child's anxiety.
- Attempt to create a nonstimulating environment for the young child experiencing procedural sedation. Suggestions for this include maintaining a quiet environment in the room prior to the procedural sedation, allowing the family to hold the child during the beginning of procedural sedation, and postponing placing monitoring equipment on the child until under sedation.
- Ketamine and propofol are the most commonly used agents.
- Ketamine can cause unpleasant dreams. This is an important consideration when choosing this agent for young children.
- Reducing pre-sedation anxiety is essential and may reduce unpleasant dreams. Further, suggestions of "good" dreams may allow for the child to avoid the unpleasant dreams.
- Administration of midazolam prior to ketamine is not proven to prevent emergence reactions in children and adolescents.

For further reading in *Tintinalli's Emergency Medicine: A Comprehensive Study Guide,* 7th ed., see Chapter 38, "Acute Pain Management in Adults," by James Ducharme; Chapter 39, "Pain Management in Infants and Children," by William M. Lennarz; Chapter 40, "Local and Regional Anesthesia," by Douglas C. Dillon and Michael A. Gibbs; and Chapter 41, "Procedural Sedation and Analgesia," by James R. Miner.

10 MANAGEMENT OF PATIENTS WITH CHRONIC PAIN

David M. Cline

- Chronic pain is a painful condition that lasts >3 months, pain that persists beyond the reasonable time for an injury to heal, or pain that persists 1 month beyond the usual course of an acute disease.

EPIDEMIOLOGY

- Chronic pain affects at least 116 million American adults—more than the total affected by heart disease, cancer, and diabetes combined. Pain also costs the nation up to $635 billion each year in medical treatment and lost productivity.
- Patients who attribute their chronic pain to a specific traumatic event, experience more emotional distress, more life interference, and more severe pain than those with other causes.
- Chronic pain may be caused by (1) a chronic pathologic process in the musculoskeletal or vascular system, (2) a chronic pathologic process in one of the organ systems, (3) a prolonged dysfunction in the peripheral or central nervous system, or (4) a psychological or environmental disorder.

PATHOPHYSIOLOGY

- The pathophysiology of chronic pain can be divided into three basic types. Nociceptive pain is associated with ongoing tissue damage. Neuropathic pain is associated with nervous system dysfunction in the absence of ongoing tissue damage. Finally, psychogenic pain has no identifiable cause.

CLINICAL FEATURES

- Signs and symptoms of nonneuropathic chronic pain syndromes are summarized in Table 10-1, while signs and symptoms of neuropathic pain syndromes are presented in Table 10-2.
- "Transformed migraine" is a syndrome in which classic migraine headaches change over time and develop into a chronic pain syndrome. One cause of this change is frequent treatment with narcotics.
- Fibromyalgia is classified by the American College of Rheumatology as the presence of 11 of 18 specific tender points, nonrestorative sleep, muscle stiffness, and generalized aching pain, with symptoms present longer than 3 months (see www.rheumatology.org).
- Risk factors for chronic back pain following an acute episode include male gender, advanced age, evidence of nonorganic disease, leg pain, prolonged initial episode, and significant disability at onset. Passive coping strategies (dependence on medication and others for daily tasks) predict significant disability with chronic back pain.
- Patients with complex regional pain type I, also known as reflex sympathetic dystrophy, and complex regional pain type II, also known as causalgia, may be seen in the ED as early as the second week after treatment of an acute injury. These disorders cannot be differentiated from one another on the basis of signs and symptoms. Type I occurs because of prolonged immobilization or disuse, and type II occurs because of a peripheral nerve injury.

TABLE 10-1 Symptoms and Signs of Nonneuropathic Pain Syndromes

DISORDER	PAIN SYMPTOMS	SIGNS
Myofascial headache	Constant dull pain, occasionally shooting pain	Trigger points on scalp, muscle tenderness and tension
Chronic tension headache	Constant dull pain	Diffuse tenderness of the scalp and associated tension
Transformed migraine	Initially migraine like, becomes constant, dull; nausea, vomiting	Muscle tenderness and tension, normal neurologic exam
Myofascial neck pain	Constant dull pain, occasionally shooting pain, pain does not typically follow nerve distribution	Trigger points in area of pain, usually no muscle atrophy, poor ROM in involved muscle
Chronic neck pain	Constant dull pain, occasionally shooting pain, pain does not follow nerve distribution	No trigger points, poor ROM in involved muscle
Fibromyalgia	Diffuse muscular pain, stiffness, fatigue, sleep disturbance	Diffuse muscle tenderness, >11 trigger points
Chronic back pain	Constant dull pain, occasionally shooting pain, pain does not follow nerve distribution	No trigger points, poor ROM in involved muscle
Myofascial back pain syndrome	Constant dull pain, occasionally shooting pain, pain does not typically follow nerve distribution	Trigger points in area of pain, usually no muscle atrophy, poor ROM in involved muscle

Abbreviation: ROM = range of motion.

DIAGNOSIS AND DIFFERENTIAL

- The most important task of the emergency physician is to distinguish an exacerbation of chronic pain from a presentation that heralds a life- or limb-threatening

TABLE 10-2 Symptoms and Signs of Neuropathic Pain Syndromes

DISORDER	PAIN SYMPTOMS	SIGNS
Painful diabetic neuropathy	Symmetric numbness and burning or stabbing pain in lower extremities; allodynia may occur	Sensory loss in lower extremities
Phantom limb pain	Variable: aching, cramping, burning, squeezing, or tearing sensation	May have peri-incisional sensory loss
Trigeminal neuralgia	Paroxysmal, short bursts of sharp, electric-like pain in nerve distribution	Tearing or red eye may be present
Human immunodeficiency virus–related neuropathy	Symmetric pain and paresthesias, most prominent in toes and feet	Sensory loss in areas of greatest pain symptoms
Postherpetic neuralgia	Allodynia; shooting, lancinating pain	Sensory changes in the involved dermatome
Poststroke pain	Same side as weakness; throbbing, shooting pain; allodynia	Loss of hot and cold differentiation
Sciatica (neurogenic back pain)	Constant or intermittent, burning or aching, shooting or electric shock–like pain; may follow dermatome; leg pain > back pain	Possible muscle atrophy in area of pain, possible reflex changes
Complex regional pain type I (reflex sympathetic dystrophy)	Burning persistent pain, allodynia, associated with immobilization or disuse	Early: edema, warmth, local sweating Late: above alternates with cold, pale, cyanosis, eventually atrophic changes
Complex regional pain type II (causalgia)	Burning persistent pain, allodynia, associated with peripheral nerve injury	Early: edema, warmth, local sweating Late: above alternates with cold, pale, cyanosis, eventually atrophic changes

condition. The history and physical examination (see Tables 10-1 and 10-2) should either confirm the chronic condition or point to the need for further evaluation when unexpected signs or symptoms are elicited.

EMERGENCY DEPARTMENT CARE AND DISPOSITION

- The management of chronic pain conditions is listed in Tables 10-3 and 10-4.
- The 1990s saw the rise of pain clinics and the use of opioids for chronic pain by specialists and primary care physicians. The increase in prescribed opioids has been accompanied by increases in opioid misuse, abuse, serious injuries, and overdose-related deaths.
- Use of opioids for chronic pain increases patient disability, the rates of surgery, and the total cost of health care.
- There are two essential points that affect the use of opioids in the ED on which there is agreement:

TABLE 10-3 Management of Nonneuropathic Chronic Pain Syndromes

DISORDER	PRIMARY TREATMENT	SECONDARY TREATMENT	POSSIBLE REFERRAL OUTCOME
Myofascial headache	NSAIDs, phenothiazines IV (acute only)	Cyclic antidepressants	Trigger point injections, optimization of medical therapy
Chronic tension headache	NSAIDs, phenothiazines IV (acute only)	Cyclic antidepressants	Optimization of medical therapy
Transformed migraine	Cyclic antidepressants	Stop prior medications	Optimization of medical therapy, narcotic withdrawal
Myofascial neck pain	NSAIDs	Cyclic antidepressants	Trigger point injections, optimization of medical therapy
Chronic neck pain	Cyclic antidepressants*	NSAIDs, opioids	Optimization of medical therapy
Chronic back pain (no sciatica)	Cyclic antidepressants*	NSAIDs, opioids	Optimization of medical therapy
Myofascial back pain syndrome	NSAIDs	Cyclic antidepressants	Trigger point injections, optimization of medical therapy
Fibromyalgia	Cyclobenzaprine, tramadol	Amitriptyline, pregabalin	Optimization of medical therapy, dedicated exercise program

*Preferred cyclic antidepressants are nortriptyline, starting at 25 milligrams per day PO, or maprotiline, starting at 50 milligrams per day PO.

TABLE 10-4 Typical Features Predicting Difficulties with Opioid Therapy
Unexpected results on toxicologic screening
Frequent requests for dose increases
Concurrent use of nonprescribed psychoactive substances
Failure to adhere to dose schedule
Failure to adhere to concurrently recommended treatments
Frequently reported loss of prescriptions or medications
Frequent visits to the ED for opioid therapy
Missed follow-up visits
Prescriptions obtained from a secondary provider
Tampering with prescriptions

(a) opioids should only be used in chronic pain if they enhance function at home and at work, and (b) a single practitioner should be the sole prescriber of narcotics or be aware of their administration by others.

- A previous narcotic addiction is a relative contraindication to the use of opioids in chronic pain, because when such patients are treated with opioids, addiction relapse rates approach 50%.
- The use of cyclooxygenase 2 (COX-2) inhibitors has been associated with increased cardiovascular complications and several drugs have been removed from the market.
- The need for long-standing treatment of chronic pain conditions may limit the safety of nonsteroidal anti-inflammatory drugs (NSAIDs). Adding a proton pump inhibitor reduces GI complications, and the combination is less expensive than daily use of the COX-2 inhibitors.
- An evidence-based review found antidepressants to be effective in chronic low back pain, fibromyalgia, osteoarthritis, and neuropathic pain. A separate meta-analysis found that tricyclic antidepressants were more effective in states in which symptoms were unexplained, such as fibromyalgia.
- Previous recommendations for bedrest in the treatment of back pain have proven counterproductive. Exercise programs have been found to be helpful in chronic low back pain.
- When antidepressants are prescribed in the ED, a follow-up plan should be in place. The most common drug and initial dose is amitriptyline, 10–25 milligrams, 2 hours prior to bedtime.
- A meta-analysis has found calcitonin to be effective in the treatment of complex regional pain, type I (reflex sympathetic dystrophy). Calcitonin can be given at a dose of 100 IU intranasal spray per day.
- Referral to the appropriate specialist is one of the most productive means to aid in the care of chronic pain patients who present to the ED. Chronic pain clinics have been successful at changing the lives of patients by eliminating opioid use, decreasing pain levels by one-third, and increasing work hours twofold.

MANAGEMENT OF PATIENTS WITH DRUG-SEEKING BEHAVIOR

EPIDEMIOLOGY

- The Drug Abuse Warning Network has tracked drug-related visits in a sampling of U.S. emergency departments and found that the incidence of visits to the ED involving abuse of narcotic-analgesic combinations rose 85% between 1994 and 2000.
- A study conducted in Portland found that drug-seeking patients presented to the ED 12.6 times per year, visited 4.1 different hospitals, and used 2.2 different aliases. Patients who were refused narcotics at one facility were successful in obtaining narcotics at another facility 93% of the time and were later successful at obtaining narcotics from the same facility 71% of the time.

CLINICAL FEATURES

- Because of the spectrum of drug-seeking patients, the history given may be factual or fraudulent.
- Drug seekers may be demanding, intimidating, or flattering.
- In one ED study, the most common complaints of patients who were seeking drugs were (in decreasing order): back pain, headache, extremity pain, and dental pain.
- Many fraudulent techniques are used, including "lost" prescriptions, "impending" surgery, factitious

TABLE 10-5 Characteristics of Drug-Seeking Behavior
Behaviors predictive of drug-seeking behavior*
Sells prescription drugs
Forges/alters prescriptions
Factitious illness, requests opioids
Uses aliases to receive opioids
Current illicit drug addiction
Conceals multiple physicians prescribing opioids
Conceals multiple ED visits for opioids
Less predictive of drug-seeking behavior
Admits to multiple doctors prescribing opioids
Admits to multiple prescriptions for opioids
Abusive when refused
Multiple drug allergies
Uses excessive flattery
From out of town
Asks for drugs by name

*Behaviors in this category are unlawful in many states.

hematuria with a complaint of kidney stones, self-mutilation, factitious injury, and partner waiting near telephone impersonating a doctor to confirm a diagnosis frequently treated with controlled substances.

DIAGNOSIS AND DIFFERENTIAL

- Drug-seeking behaviors can be divided into two groups: predictive and less predictive (Table 10-5). The behaviors listed under "predictive" are illegal in many states and form a solid basis to refuse narcotics to the patient.

EMERGENCY DEPARTMENT CARE AND DISPOSITION

- The treatment of drug-seeking behavior is to refuse the controlled substance, consider the need for alternative medication or treatment, and consider referral for drug counseling.

For further reading in *Tintinalli's Emergency Medicine: A Comprehensive Study Guide*, 7th ed., see Chapter 42, "Adults with Chronic Pain," by David M. Cline.

Section 4
EMERGENCY WOUND MANAGEMENT

11 EVALUATING AND PREPARING WOUNDS

Timothy Reeder

EPIDEMIOLOGY

- Traumatic wounds are common reasons for visits to emergency departments.

PATHOPHYSIOLOGY

- The mechanism of injury will help identify risk of foreign body, contamination, and wound complication.
- A foreign body sensation increases the likelihood of a retained foreign object.
- Predictive factors for infection include: location, depth, configuration, contamination, and patient age.
- Blunt forces compress the skin against underling bone, while sharp objects produce shear forces resulting in skin damage.
- Crush injuries are more likely to cause wound infection due to greater tissue damage.
- Low-energy impact injuries may result in hematoma formation. These require aspiration or incision and drainage if they fail to resorb spontaneously.

CLINICAL FEATURES

- Document important medical conditions such as diabetes, renal disease, immunosuppression, malnutrition, and connective tissue disorders that impact wound healing.
- Most states have regulations requiring reporting of injuries that result from intentional acts.
- Bacterial growth increases from time of injury to wound closure.
- Consider time from injury to presentation, wound etiology, anatomic location, degree of contamination, host risk factors, and the importance of cosmetic appearance in assessing the decision to close wounds.
- Wounds at high risk for infection should be considered for delayed primary closure after 4 days.

DIAGNOSIS AND DIFFERENTIAL

- A complete examination, including neurovascular assessment, should be documented prior to analgesia or anesthesia.
- A thorough visual inspection to the full depth and length of the wound and palpation will minimize missed foreign bodies, tendon and nerve injuries; such missed injuries are a common cause of litigation.
- Consider injecting a wound that extends over a joint to determine the integrity of the joint space.
- Consider radiographs to detect foreign bodies. Ultrasound may be used for non-radiopaque foreign bodies (Fig. 11-1).

EMERGENCY DEPARTMENT CARE AND DISPOSITION

- Wound preparation is the most important step for adequate evaluation of the wound, prevention of infection, and optimal cosmetic outcome.
- Universal precautions and aseptic technique may improve efficiency and cost savings. Full sterile procedures are not required.
- Pain control with consideration of local or regional anesthesia should be provided before any wound manipulation.
- Perform a careful neurovascular examination prior to anesthesia. Two-point discrimination (<6 mm) for digital nerves.

HEMOSTASIS

- Direct pressure is the preferred method to control bleeding to facilitate adequate wound evaluation.
- Epinephrine-containing local anesthetics can be used in distal anatomy such as finger, nose, and ear except in patients with underlying small vessel disease.
- Other measures for control of bleeding include ligation of small vessels, electrocautery, absorbable gelatin foam (Gelfoam), oxidized cellulose (Oxycel), or collagen sponge (Actifoam).

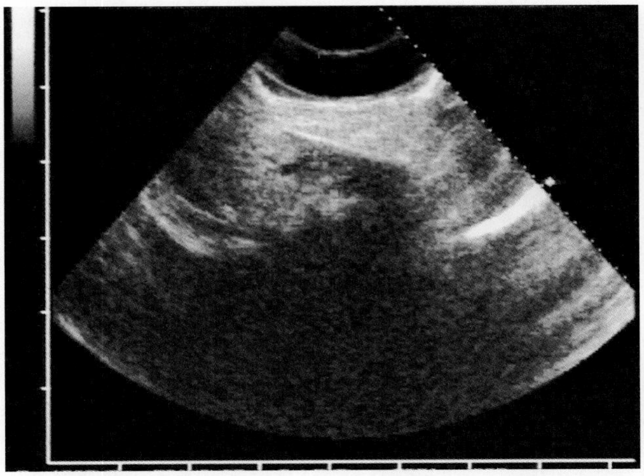

FIG. 11-1. Long-axis sonogram of a wooden foreign body in a patient's foot. The wood fragment is a hyperechoic linear structure that slants to the right; a prominent posterior acoustic shadow is seen beneath the wood fragment. (Reproduced with permission from Dewitz A, Frazee BW. Soft tissue. In: Ma OJ, Mateer JR, Blaivas M. eds. *Emergency Ultrasound*, 2nd ed. Figure 16-50. Copyright © 2008 by the McGraw-Hill Companies, Inc. All rights reserved.)

IRRIGATION AND CLEANING

- Use skin disinfectants only on the wound edges and outward, as these substances may impair host defenses and promote bacterial growth in the wound.
- Wound irrigation reduces infection. Normal saline has lowest toxicity, but tap water is safe and effective.
- Low pressure irrigation (0.5 psi–slow gentle wash) for uncontaminated wounds.
- High pressure irrigation (≥7 psi–18 g catheter) for contaminated wounds.
- Use 60 mL per centimeter of wound length, with a minimum of 200 mL.
- Soaking wounds is not effective in cleaning contaminated wounds and may increase wound bacterial counts.

DEBRIDEMENT AND HAIR REMOVAL

- Debridement of devitalized tissue by elliptical incision removes foreign matter and bacteria, resulting in a decreased infection risk. It also creates a clean wound edge, facilitating repair.
- Clip hair if necessary rather than shaving the skin, as shaving is associated with an increased infection rate. Do not remove hair from eyebrows due to the potential for abnormal or lack of regeneration.

ANTIBIOTICS

- Although there is no clear evidence that antibiotic prophylaxis prevents wound infection in most ED patients, there may be a role in selected high-risk wounds and populations.
- If used, antibiotic prophylaxis should be: (1) initiated before tissue manipulation, (2) effective against predicted pathogens, and (3) administered by routes that quickly achieve adequate blood levels.
- For non-bite infections use a first-generation cephalosporin; cephalexin 25–50 milligrams/kg/day PO qid in children; 500 milligrams PO four times daily in adults. For β-lactam allergic patients use clindamycin 8 to 25 milligrams/kg/day three times daily in children or 150 to 450 four times daily for adults.
- Patients with bites should be treated with amoxicillin-clavulanate, 875 milligrams PO twice daily (25-50 milligrams/kg/day twice daily for children) to cover *Pasteurella, Eikenella,* or *Capnocytophaga*.
- Wounds contaminated by fresh water and plantar puncture wounds of the foot require coverage for Pseudomonas, such as **ciprofloxacin** 500 PO twice daily in adults.
- Prophylactic antibiotics should be given for 3 to 5 days.

For further reading in *Tintinalli's Emergency Medicine: A Comprehensive Study Guide*, 7th ed., see Chapter 43, "Evaluation of Wounds," by Judd Hollander and Adam Singer; and Chapter 44, "Wound Preparation," by Shoma Desai, Susan C. Store and Wallace A. Carter.

12 METHODS FOR WOUND CLOSURE

David M. Cline

- Wounds can be closed primarily in the emergency department (ED) by the placement of sutures, surgical staples, skin-closure tapes, and adhesives.
- All wounds heal with some scarring; however, preferred closure techniques make scars less noticeable.
- In closing a laceration, it is important to match each layer of a wound edge to its counterpart. Care must be taken to avoid having one wound edge rolled inward.
- The rolled-in edge occludes the capillaries, promoting wound infection. The dermal side will not heal to the rolled epidermal side, causing wound dehiscence when the sutures are removed, resulting in an inferior scar appearance.
- The techniques described are an overview of basic wound closure, which should aid the practitioner in achieving acceptable results.

SUTURES

- Sutures are the strongest of all wound closure devices and allow the most accurate approximation of wound edges.
- Sutures are divided into two general classes: nonabsorbable, and absorbable sutures, which lose all their tensile strength within 60 days.
- Monofilament synthetic sutures such as nylon or polypropylene have the lowest rates of infection and are the most commonly used suture materials in the ED.
- Synthetic monofilament absorbable sutures (eg, Monocryl®) are preferred for closure of deep structures such as the dermis or fascia because of their strength and low tissue reactivity.
- Rapidly absorbing sutures (eg, Vicryl Rapide®) can be used to close the superficial skin layers or mucous membranes, especially when the avoidance of removal is desired.
- Sutures are sized according to their diameter. For general ED use, 6-0 suture is the smallest, and it is used for percutaneous closure on the face and other cosmetically important areas.
- Suture sizes 5-0 and 4-0 are progressively larger; 5-0 is commonly used for closure of hand and finger lacerations, and 4-0 is used to close lacerations on the trunk and proximal extremities.
- Very thick skin, such as that of the scalp and sole, may require closure with 3-0 sutures.

SUTURING TECHNIQUES

- Percutaneous sutures that pass through both the epidermal and dermal layers are the most common sutures used in the ED.
- Dermal, or subcuticular, sutures reapproximate the divided edges of the dermis without penetrating the epidermis. These two sutures may be used together in a layered closure as wound complexity demands. Sutures can be applied in a continuous fashion ("running" sutures) or as interrupted sutures.
- Improper tissue handling further traumatizes skin and results in an increased risk of infection and noticeable scarring. Gentle pressure with fine forceps is recommended.

SIMPLE INTERRUPTED PERCUTANEOUS SUTURES

- Percutaneous sutures should be placed to achieve eversion of the wound edges. To accomplish this, the needle should enter the skin at a 90-degree angle. The needle point should also exit the opposite side at 90 degrees. The depth of the suture should be greater than the width. Sutures placed in this manner will encompass a portion of tissue that will evert when the knot is tied (Fig. 12-1).
- An adequate number of interrupted sutures should be placed so that the wound edges are closed without gaping. Generally, the number of ties should correspond to the suture size (ie, 4 ties for 4-0 suture, 5 ties for 5-0 suture).
- Straight, shallow lacerations can be closed with percutaneous sutures only, by sewing from one end toward the other and aligning edges with each individual suture bite. Deep, irregular wounds with uneven, misaligned, or gaping edges are more difficult to suture.
- Certain management principles have been identified for these more difficult wounds.
  - Wounds with edges that cannot be brought together without excessive tension should have dermal sutures placed to partially close the gap.
  - When wound edges of different thickness are to be reunited, the needle should be passed through one side of the wound, and then drawn out before re-entry through the other side, to ensure that the needle is inserted at a comparable level.
  - Uneven edges can be aligned by first approximating the mid-portion of the wound with the initial suture.

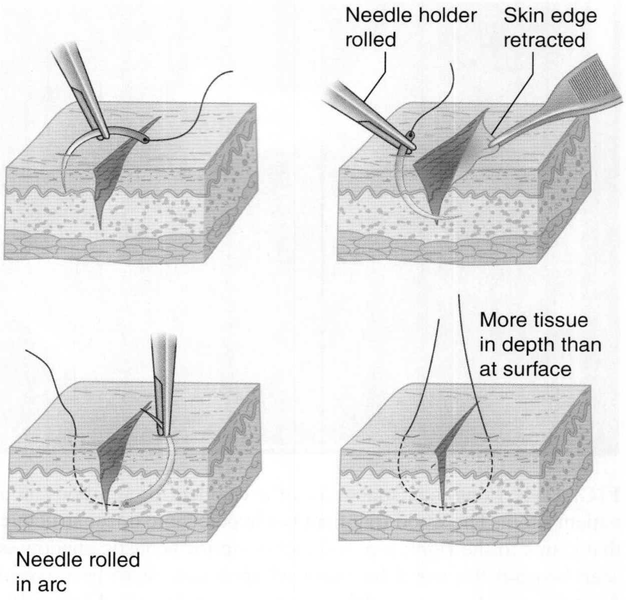

FIG. 12-1. Placement of simple interrupted sutures. The suture path should gather more tissue at its base than at its surface. Therefore, the suture will evert its skin edges when tightened.

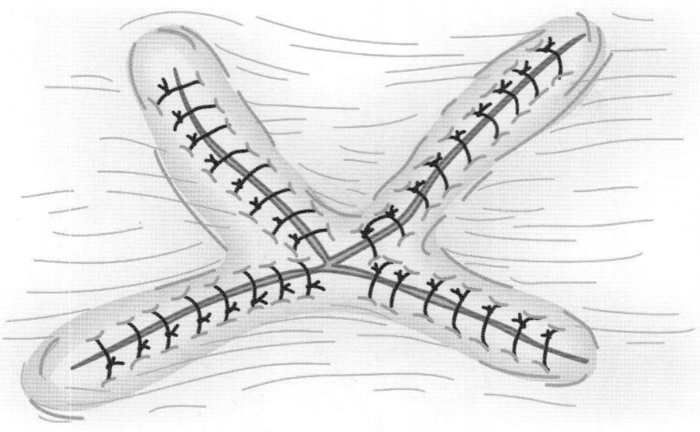

FIG. 12-2. Stellate laceration closed with interrupted sutures.

Subsequent sutures are then placed in the middle of each half until the wound edges are aligned and closed.

- Simple interrupted sutures are the most versatile and effective for realigning irregular wound edges and stellate lacerations (Fig. 12-2). An advantage of interrupted sutures is that only the involved sutures need to be removed in the case of wound infection.

CONTINUOUS (RUNNING) PERCUTANEOUS SUTURES

- Continuous or running percutaneous sutures are best when repairing linear wounds. An advantage of the continuous suture is that it accommodates the developing edema of the wound edges during healing. However, a break in the suture may ruin the entire repair and may cause permanent marks if placed too tightly.
- Continuous suture closure of a laceration can be accomplished by two different patterns. In the first pattern, the needle pathway is at a 90-degree angle to the wound edges and results in a visible suture that crosses the wound edges at a 45-degree angle (Fig. 12-3A).
- In the other pattern, the needle pathway is at a 45-degree angle to the wound edges, so that the visible suture is at a 90-degree angle to the wound edges (Fig. 12-3B). In either case, the physician starts at the corner of the wound farthest away and sutures toward him- or herself.

DEEP DERMAL SUTURES

- The major role of these sutures is to reduce tension. They are also used to close dead spaces.
- However, their presence increases the risk of infection in contaminated wounds.

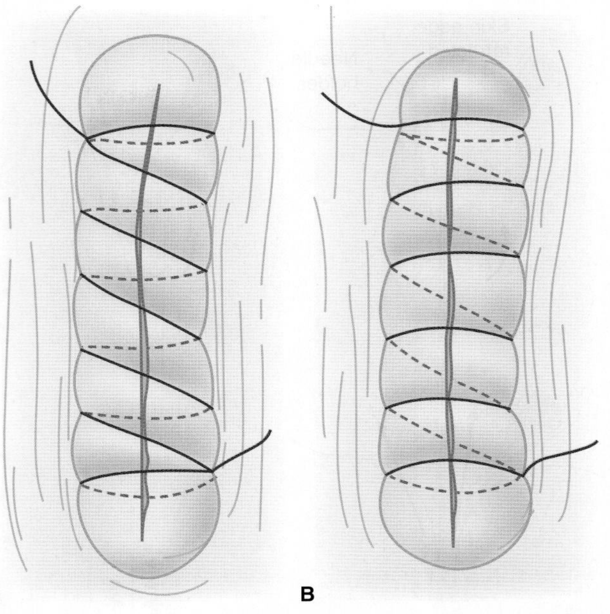

FIG. 12-3. A. Running suture crossing wound at 45 degrees. B. Running suture crossing wound at 90 degrees.

- Sutures though adipose tissues do not hold tension, increase infection rates, and should be avoided.
- With deep dermal sutures, the needle is inserted at the level of the mid-dermis on one side of the wound, and then exits more superficially below the dermal-epidermal junction (Fig. 12-4). The needle is then introduced below the dermal-epidermal junction on the opposite side of the wound and exits at the level of the mid-dermis. Thus, the knot becomes buried in the tissue when tying of the suture is completed.
- The first suture is placed at the center of the laceration, while additional sutures then sequentially bisect the wound. The number of deep sutures should be minimized.

VERTICAL MATTRESS SUTURES

- The vertical mattress suture (Fig. 12-5) is useful in areas of lax skin (eg, the elbow and the dorsum of the hand), where the wound edges tend to fold into the wound. It can act as an "all-in-one" suture, avoiding the need for a layered closure.

HORIZONTAL MATTRESS SUTURES

- Horizontal mattress sutures are faster and better at eversion than vertical mattress sutures.

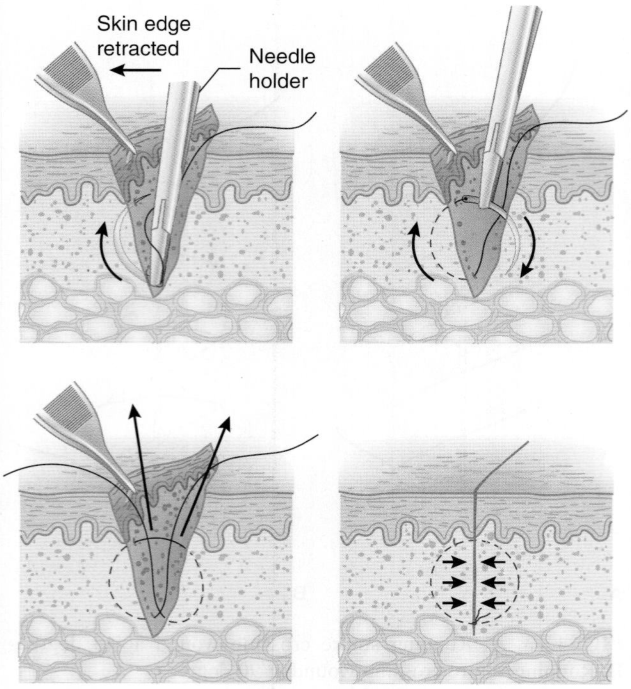

FIG. 12-4. Placement of deep dermal suture. The needle is inserted at the depth of the dermis and directed upward, exiting beneath the dermal-epidermal junction. Then the needle is inserted across the wound and directed downward, exiting at the wound base. The suture knot is then placed deep in the wound.

- They are especially useful in areas of increased tension such as fascia, joints, and callus skin (Fig. 12-6). In order to avoid tissue strangulation, care must be taken not to tie the individual sutures too tightly.

DELAYED CLOSURE

- Delayed primary closure is an option for wounds suspected of contamination, or for wounds presenting beyond 12 hours after injury.
- With this method the wound is left open for a period of 3 to 5 days, after which it may be closed if no infection supervenes.

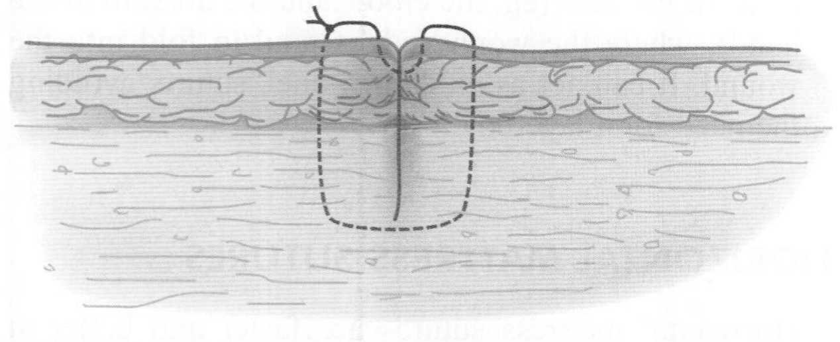

FIG. 12-5. Vertical mattress suture.

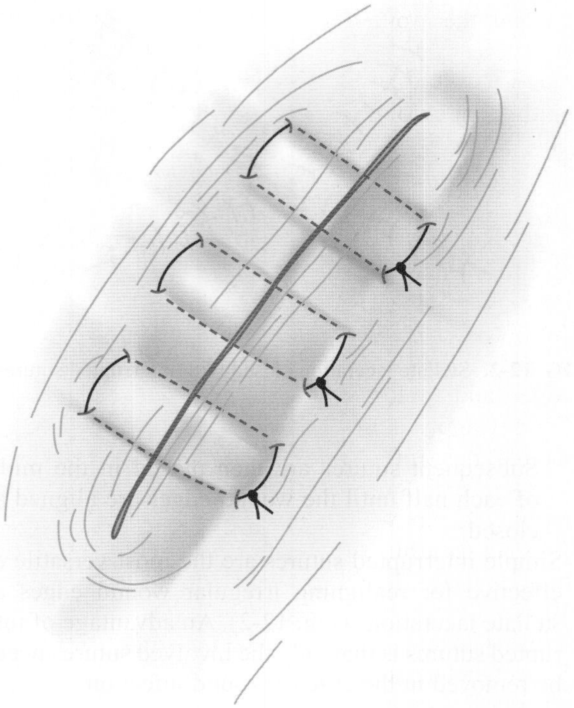

FIG. 12-6. Horizontal mattress suture.

STAPLES

- Skin closure by metal staples is quick and economical, with the added advantage of low tissue reactivity.
- Staples should be reserved for lacerations where the healing scar is not readily apparent (eg, scalp).
- When placing staples, the wound edges should be held together with tissue forceps. Place the device gently against the skin and squeeze the trigger slowly. A properly placed staple should have its topside off the skin surface.

ADHESIVE TAPES

- Adhesive tapes are the least reactive of all wound closure devices.
- Skin-closure tapes are used as an alternative to sutures and staples and for additional support after suture and staple removal.
- Tapes work best on flat, dry, immobile surfaces where the wound edges fit together without tension. Taped wounds are more resistant to infection than sutured wounds.
- Tapes can be used for skin flaps, where sutures may compromise perfusion, and for lacerations with thin, friable skin that will not hold sutures.

- Application of Benzoin to the skin surface 2 to 3 cm beyond the wound edges will enhance adherence. Maintain some space between individual tapes. The tapes will spontaneously detach as the underlying epithelium exfoliates.

CYANOACRYLATE TISSUE ADHESIVES

- Cyanoacrylate tissue adhesives close wounds by forming an adhesive layer on top of intact epithelium.
- Adhesives are most useful when they are used on wounds that close spontaneously, have clean or sharp edges, and are located on clean, immobile areas.
- Do not apply adhesives within wounds, to mucous membranes, infected areas, joints, areas with dense hair (eg, scalp), or on wounds exposed to body fluids.
- Wound closure with adhesives is faster and less painful than suturing and has comparable rates of infection, dehiscence, and cosmetic appearance.
- Wounds with edges separated by more than 5 mm are unlikely to stay closed with tissue adhesives alone.
- Subcutaneous sutures can be inserted to relieve this tension. Lacerations longer than 5 cm are unlikely to remain closed with tissue adhesives alone.
- The adhesive is carefully expressed through the tip of the applicator and gently brushed over the wound surface in a continuous steady motion.
- The adhesive should cover the entire wound in addition to an area covering 5 to 10 mm on either side of the wound edges.
- After allowing the first layer of the adhesive to polymerize for 30 to 45 seconds, 2 to 3 additional layers of the adhesive are similarly brushed onto the surface of the wound, with pauses of 5 to 10 seconds between successive layers.
- Take care to position the patient parallel to the floor, cover the eyes, and use gentle squeezing of the applicator to avoid problematic runoff.
- Once applied, cyanoacrylate should not be covered with ointment, bandage, or dressing.
- Instruct patient not to pick at edges of the adhesive. The area can be gently washed with plain water after 24 hours but should not be scrubbed, soaked, or exposed to moisture for any length of time.
- The adhesive will spontaneously slough off in 5 to 10 days. Should a wound open, the patient should return immediately for closure.

For further reading in *Tintinalli's Emergency Medicine: A Comprehensive Study Guide*, 7th ed., see Chapter 45, "Methods for Wound Closure," by Adam J. Singer and Judd E. Hollander.

13 LACERATIONS TO THE FACE AND SCALP

J. Hayes Calvert

EPIDEMIOLOGY

- Face and forehead wounds are the most cosmetically apparent of all wounds, and therefore warrant careful evaluation and meticulous repair.
- Patients with facial trauma should be questioned about the possibility of domestic violence.

PATHOPHYSIOLOGY

- It takes an average of 10 times fewer bacteria to cause an infection in blunt wounds compared with sharp wounds.
- Lacerations occurring in areas of the lips, nose, and intraorally are more likely to be associated with underlying facial fractures than scalp lacerations.

SCALP AND FOREHEAD

Anatomy

- The scalp and forehead (which includes eyebrows) are parts of the same anatomic structure (Fig. 13-1).

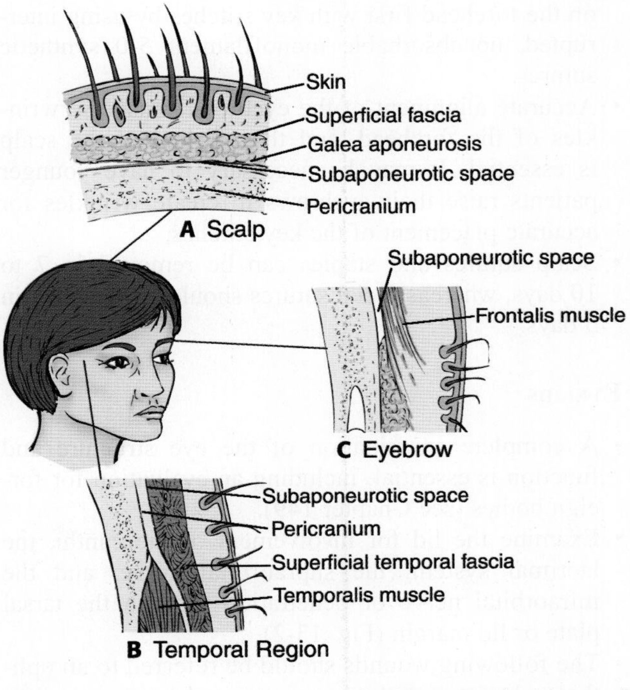

FIG. 13-1. The layers of the **A.** scalp, **B.** temporal region, and **C.** eyebrow.

Evaluation

- Eyebrows are valuable landmarks for the meticulous reapproximation of the wound edges and should never be clipped or shaved.
- The base of the wound always should be palpated for possible skull fracture.

Wound Preperation

- Debride at an angle that is parallel to that of the hair follicles to prevent subsequent alopecia.
- Occasionally direct pressure or vessel clamping may be needed to control hemorrhage at the wound edges.

REPAIR OF SCALP LACERATIONS

- Begin wound closure with approximation of the galea aponeurotica using buried, interrupted absorbable 4-0 sutures.
- Close the divided edges of muscle and fascia with buried, interrupted, absorbable 4-0 synthetic sutures to prevent further development of depressed scars.
- Close the skin with staples or interrupted nylon sutures (consider using sutures of a color different from the patient's hair).

REPAIR OF FOREHEAD LACERATIONS

- Approximate the skin edges of anatomic landmarks on the forehead first with key stitches by using interrupted, nonabsorbable monofilament 5-0 synthetic sutures.
- Accurate alignment of the eyebrow, transverse wrinkles of the forehead, and the hairline of the scalp is essential. It may be necessary to have younger patients raise their eyebrows to create wrinkles for accurate placement of the key stitches.
- Scalp sutures and staples can be removed in 7 to 10 days, whereas facial sutures should be removed in 5 days.

Eyelids

- A complete examination of the eye structure and function is essential, including an evaluation for foreign bodies (see Chapter 149).
- Examine the lid for involvement of the canthi, the lacrimal system, the supraorbital nerve, and the infraorbital nerve or penetration through the tarsal plate or lid margin (Fig. 13-2).
- The following wounds should be referred to an ophthalmologist: (a) those involving the inner surface of the lid, (b) those involving the lid margins, (c) those involving the lacrimal duct, (d) those associated with ptosis, and (e) those extending into the tarsal plate.

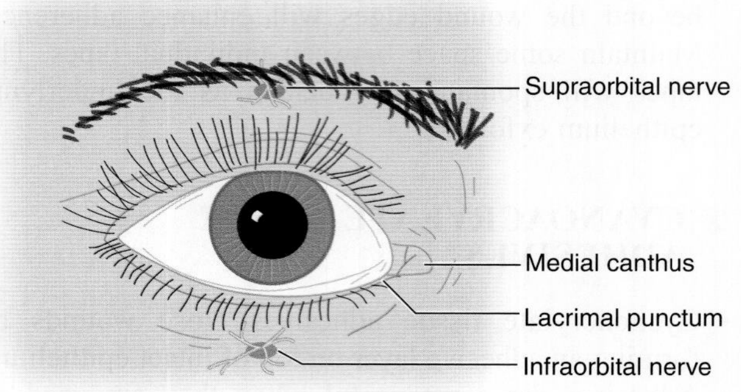

FIG. 13-2. External landmarks.

- Failure to recognize and properly repair the lacrimal system can result in chronic tearing.
- Uncomplicated lid lacerations can be readily closed by using nonabsorbable 6-0 suture, with removal in 3 to 5 days. Do not use tissue adhesive near the eye.

Nose

- Lacerations of the nose may be limited to skin or involve the deeper structures (sparse nasal musculature, cartilaginous framework, and nasal mucous membrane). Each tissue layer must be accurately approximated.
- Local anesthesia of the nose can be difficult because of the tightly adhering skin. Topical anesthesia using lidocaine may be successful.
- When the laceration extends through all tissue layers, begin closure with a nonabsorbable, monofilament 5-0 synthetic suture that aligns the skin surrounding the entrances of the nasal canals to prevent malposition and notching of the alar rim.
- Traction on the long, untied ends of this suture approximates the wounds and aligns the anterior and posterior margins of the divided tissue layers.
- Repair the mucous membrane with interrupted, braided, absorbable 5-0 synthetic sutures, burying the knots in the tissue. Re-irrigate the area gently from the outside.
- Rarely, the cartilage may need to be approximated with a minimal number of 5-0 absorbable sutures.
- In sharply marked linear lacerations, closure of the overlying skin is usually sufficient. Close the cut edges of the skin, with its adherent musculature, using interrupted, nonabsorbable, monofilament 6-0 synthetic sutures. Remove external sutures in 3 to 5 days.

- Inspect the septum for hematoma formation with a nasal speculum. The presence of bluish swelling in the septum confirms the diagnosis of septal hematoma. Treatment of the hematoma is evacuation of the blood clot.
- Drainage of a small hematoma can be accomplished by aspiration of the blood clot through an 18-gauge needle. A larger hematoma should be drained through a horizontal incision at the base.
- Bilateral hematomas should be drained in the operating room (OR) by a specialist. Reaccumulation of blood can be prevented by nasal packing.
- Antibiotic treatment is recommended to prevent infection that may cause necrosis of cartilage. Use an oral penicillin, cephalosporin, or macrolide (in penicillin-allergic patients).

Lips

- Isolated intraoral lesions may not need to be sutured.
- Through-and-through lacerations that do not include the vermilion border can be closed in layers. Begin repair with 5-0 absorbable suture for the mucosal surface, re-irrigate and then close the orbicularis oris muscle with 4-0 or 5-0 absorbable suture. Close skin with 6-0 nonabsorbable suture or tissue adhesive. Remove sutures in 5 days.
- Begin closure of a complicated lip laceration at the junction between the vermilion and the skin with a nonabsorbable, monofilament 6-0 synthetic suture (Fig. 13-3). The orbicularis oris muscle is then repaired with interrupted 4-0 or 5-0 absorbable sutures. Approximate the junction between the vermilion and the mucous membrane with a braided, absorbable 5-0 synthetic suture. Close the divided edges of the mucous membrane and vermilion with interrupted absorbable 5-0 synthetic sutures in a buried knot construction.
- Skin edges of the laceration may be jagged and irregular, but they can be fitted together as the pieces of a jigsaw puzzle by using interrupted, nonabsorbable, monofilament 6-0 synthetic sutures with their knots formed on the surface of the skin.
- Patients with sutured intraoral lacerations should receive prophylactic antibiotics, penicillin or clindamycin.

Ear

- Close superficial lacerations of the ear with 6-0 nylon suture. Cover exposed cartilage.
- Debridement of the skin is not advisable because there is very little excess skin. In most through-and-through lacerations of the ear, the skin can be approximated and the underlying cartilage will be supported adequately (Fig. 13-4).
- After repair of simple lacerations, place a small piece of nonadherent gauze over the laceration only and apply a pressure dressing. Place gauze squares behind the ear to apply pressure, and wrap the head circumferentially with gauze.
- Remove sutures in 5 days.
- Consult an otolaryngologist or plastic surgeon for more complex lacerations, ear avulsions, or auricular hematomas.

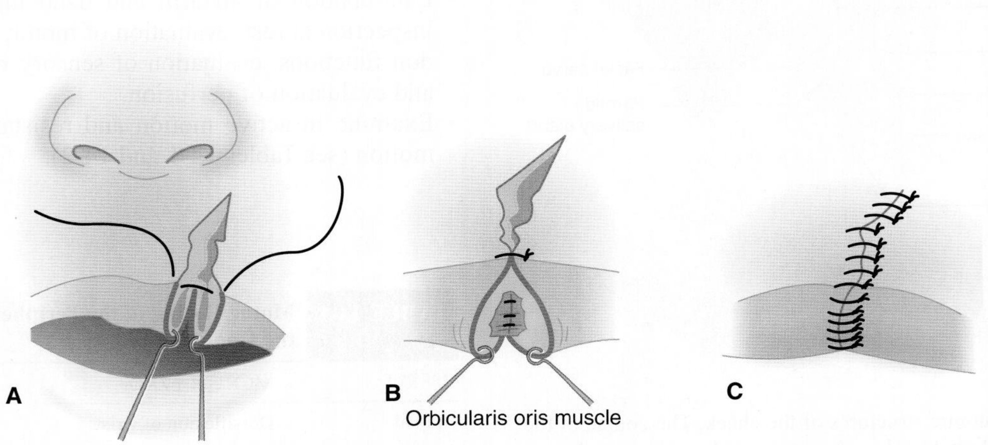

FIG. 13-3. Irregular-edged vertical laceration of the upper lip. **A.** Traction is applied to the lips and closure of the wound is begun first at the vermilion-skin junction. **B.** The orbicularis oris muscle is then repaired with interrupted, absorbable 4-0 synthetic sutures. **C.** The irregular edges of the skin are then approximated.

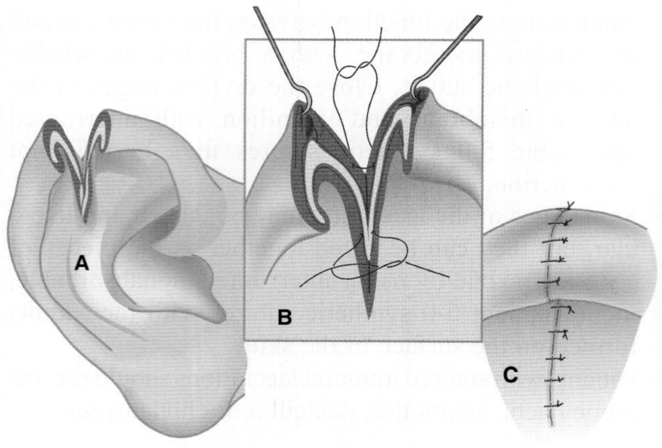

FIG. 13-4. **A.** Laceration through auricle. **B.** One or two interrupted, 6-0 coated nylon sutures will approximate divided edges of cartilage. **C.** Interrupted nonabsorbable 6-0 synthetic sutures approximate the skin edges.

Cheeks and Face

- In general, facial lacerations are closed with 6-0 nonabsorbable, simple interrupted sutures and are removed after 5 days.

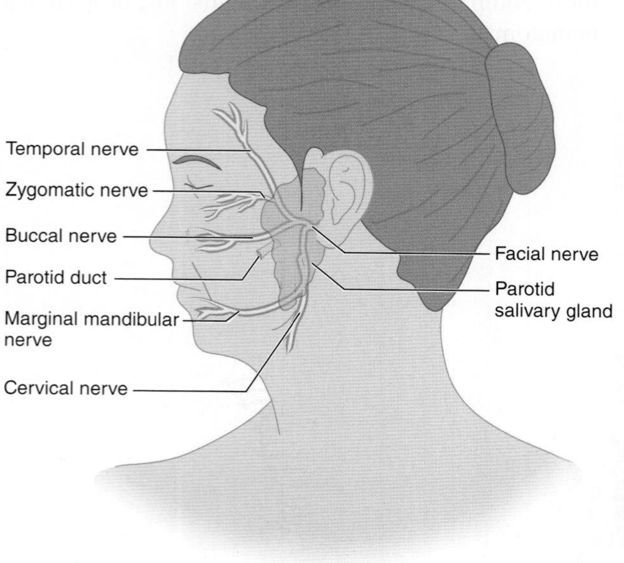

FIG. 13-5. Anatomic structures of the cheek. The course of the parotid duct is deep to a line drawn from the tragus of the ear to the midportion of the upper lip. Branches of the facial nerve: temporal **(T)**, zygomatic **(Z)**, buccal **(B)**, mental **(M)**, and cervical **(C)**.

- Tissue adhesive may also be used.
- Attention to anatomic structures including the facial nerve and parotid gland is necessary (Fig. 13-5). If these structures are involved, operative repair is indicated.

For further reading in *Tintinalli's Emergency Medicine: A Comprehensive Study Guide, 7th ed.*, see Chapter 46, "Lacerations to the Face and Scalp," by Wendy C. Coates.

14 INJURIES OF THE ARM, HAND, FINGERTIP, AND NAIL

David M. Cline

EPIDEMIOLOGY

- Soft tissue upper extremity injuries account for about 35% of the wounds and lacerations evaluated in the ED.

PATHOPHYSIOLOGY

- Injuries may be classified as closed crush, simple lacerations, open crush with partial amputation, and complete amputation.

CLINICAL FEATURES

- History should include occupation and hand dominance.
- Examination of all arm and hand injuries includes inspection at rest, evaluation of motor, nerve and tendon functions, evaluation of sensory nerve function, and evaluation of perfusion.
- Examine in active motion and resistance to passive motion (see Tables 14-1 and 14-2).

TABLE 14-1 Motor Testing of the Peripheral Nerves of the Upper Extremity

NERVE	MOTOR EXAM
Radial	Dorsiflexion of wrist
Median	Thumb abduction away from the palm Thumb interphalangeal joint flexion
Ulnar	Adduction/abduction of digits

TABLE 14-2 Sensory Testing of Peripheral Nerves in the Upper Extremity

SENSORY NERVE	AREA OF TEST
Radial	First dorsal web space
Median	Volar tip of index finger
Ulnar	Volar tip of little finger

- Examine all wounds for evidence of potential artery, nerve, tendon, bone injuries, and the presence of foreign bodies, debris, or bacterial contamination.

DIAGNOSIS AND DIFFERENTIAL

- A bloodless field is needed to achieve adequate visualization.
- If a proximal tourniquet is needed, a Penrose drain can be used for distal finger injures and a manual blood pressure cuff for more proximal injures.
- Once adequate visualization is obtained, examine the wound for foreign bodies and tendon and joint capsule injuries.
- Examine the hand and arm in the position of injury to avoid missing deep structure injuries that may have moved out of the field of view when examined in a neutral position.
- Obtain anteroposterior and lateral radiographs if bony injuries, retained radiopaque foreign bodies, or joint penetration are suspected.

EMERGENCY DEPARTMENT CARE AND DISPOSITION

- All wounds require scrupulous cleaning and irrigation after adequate anesthesia.
- Provide tetanus prophylaxis as indicated (see Chapter 18).
- Consult a plastic or hand surgeon for complex or extensive injuries, injuries requiring skin grafting, injuries requiring technically demanding skills or when the hand is vital to patient's career (eg, a professional musician).
- Additional care instructions of specific injuries are as follows:

FOREARM AND WRIST LACERATIONS

- Injury over the wrist raises the possibility of a suicide attempt. Question the patient about intent and a history of depression.

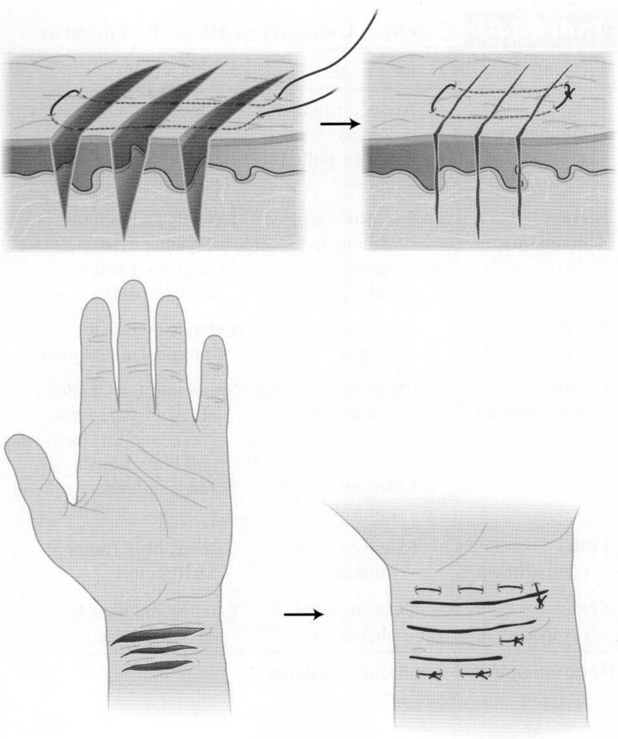

FIG. 14-1. Horizontal mattress sutures for multiple parallel lacerations.

- Injuries that involve more than one parallel laceration, classic for suicide attempts, may require horizontal mattress sutures to cross all lacerations to prevent compromising the vascular supply of the island of skin located between incisions (Fig. 14-1).
- Examine tendons and distal nerves individually (see Tables 14-3 and 14-4).

PALM LACERATIONS

- Injuries to the palm may require a regional anesthetic, for example, a median or ulnar nerve block.
- If no deep injury is suspected, close the wound. Pay particular attention to re-opposing the skin creases accurately.
- Avoid using deep "bites" with the needle because this risks injury to the underlying tendons or tendon sheaths. Interrupted horizontal mattress sutures (see Chapter 12) with 5-0 monofilament suture are recommended.
- Refer patients with deep injuries between the carpometacarpal joints and the distal creases of the wrist ("no-mans' land") to a specialist for exploration and repair.

TABLE 14-3 Extensor Compartments in the Forearm

COMPARTMENT	MUSCLE	FUNCTION
First compartment	Abductor pollicis longus	Abducts and extends thumb
	Extensor pollicis brevis	Extends thumb at MCP joint
Second compartment	Extensor carpi radialis longus	Extends and radially deviates wrist
	Extensor carpi radialis brevis	Extends and radially deviates wrist
Third compartment	Extensor pollicis longus	Extends thumb at interphalangeal joint
Fourth compartment	Extensor digitorum communis	Splits into four tendons at level of the wrist; extends index, long, ring, and little digits
	Extensor indicis proprius	Extends index finger
Fifth compartment	Extensor digiti minimi	Extends little finger at MCP joint
Sixth compartment	Extensor carpi ulnaris	Extends and ulnarly deviates wrist

Abbreviation: MCP = metacarpophalangeal.

Dorsal Hand Lacerations

- Lacerations over the metacarpophalangeal joint suggest a closed fist injury and require special care.
- Polymicrobial infections are the rule; *Staphylococcus aureus*, *Streptococcus* sp., *Corynebacterium* sp., and *Eikenella corrodens* are the most common bacteria.
- Obtain radiographs to rule out fracture or embedded teeth.
- Irrigate thoroughly and débride as needed.
- Infected wounds require IV antibiotics (ampicillin-sulbactam 3 grams every 6 hours), consultation to a hand surgeon, and admission.
- Patients with noninfected, minor closed fist injuries can be treated as outpatients with immobilization in position of function (do not close), amoxicillin-clavulanic acid 875 milligrams PO twice daily (22.5 milligrams/kg per dose two times daily in children), and follow-up in 24–48 hours with strict return instructions in the event of erythema, drainage, or increased pain.
- The pliable skin and extensive movements of the hand may hide tendon injuries.
- Repair skin using 5-0 nonabsorbable sutures.

Extensor Tendon Lacerations

- Experienced emergency physicians may repair (nonbite) extensor tendon injuries over the dorsum of the hand, with the exception of the tendons to the thumb.
- Discuss all tendon injuries with a hand specialist for preferred technique and to arrange follow-up.
- Use a figure-of-eight stitch, tied on the side of the lacerated tendon, using a 4-0 (5-0 for smaller tendons) nonabsorbable suture material such as polypropylene (Fig. 14-2). Close the skin with nonabsorbable suture and splint the limb.
- Lacerations to the extensor tendons over the distal interphalangeal joint may produce a mallet deformity, and if not repaired may result in a swan neck deformity; whereas lacerations over the proximal interphalangeal joint may produce a boutonniere deformity.

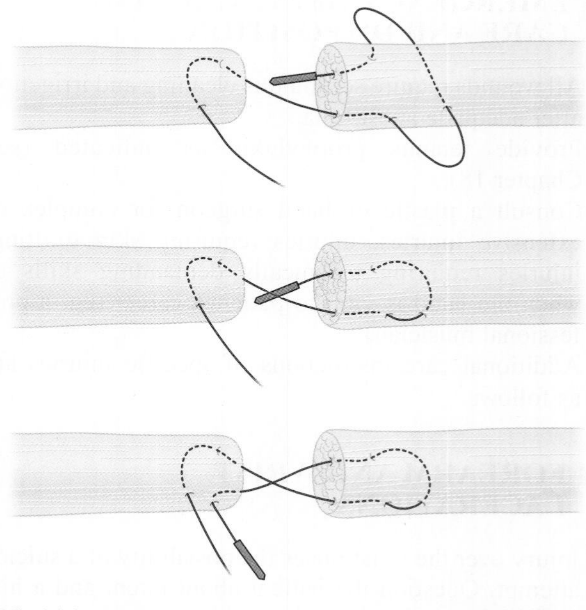

FIG. 14-2. Extensor tendon laceration repair with a figure-of-eight stitch.

TABLE 14-4 Flexor Tendons in the Forearm

FLEXOR TENDON	FUNCTION
Flexor carpi radialis	Flexes and radially deviates wrist
Flexor carpi ulnaris	Flexes and ulnarly deviates wrist
Palmaris longus	Flexes wrist
Flexor pollicis longus	Flexes thumb at MCP and interphalangeal joints
Flexor digitorum superficialis	Flexes index, long, ring, and little digits at MCP and PIP joints
Flexor digitorum profundus	Flexes index, long, ring, and little digits at MCP, PIP, and DIP joints

Abbreviations: DIP = distal interphalangeal; MCP = metacarpophalangeal; PIP = proximal interphalangeal.

- Open tendon lacerations require operative repair; closed tendon injuries are either splinted in extension for up to 6 weeks or until operative repair. Refer to a hand surgeon.

Flexor Tendon Lacerations

- Refer all flexor tendon injuries to a hand specialist.
- Some hand surgeons prefer to repair these injuries within 12 to 24 hours while others delay repair.
- If repair is delayed, clean the wound, repair the skin, splint the limb in a position of function, and arrange follow-up within 2 to 3 days with a hand surgeon.

Finger and Finger Tip Injuries

- Most finger lacerations are straightforward and can be repaired by using 5-0 nonabsorbable suture materials.
- Suspect digital nerve injuries when static two-point discrimination is distinctively greater on one side of the volar pad than on the other, or when it is greater than 10 mm (normal defined as <6 mm).
- Successful repair of fingertip injuries requires knowledge of anatomy (Fig. 14-3) and an understanding of techniques of reconstruction.
- Distal fingertip amputations with skin or pulp loss only are best managed conservatively, with serial dressing change only, especially in children.
- In cases with larger areas of skin loss (>1 cm^2), a skin graft using the severed tip itself or skin harvested from the hypothenar eminence may be required.
- Complications of the skin graft technique include decreased sensation of the fingertip, tenderness at the injury and graft site, poor cosmetic result, and hyperpigmentation in dark-skinned patients.
- Injuries with exposed bone are not amenable to skin grafting. Most of these injuries require specialist advice. If less than 0.5 mm of bone is exposed and the wound defect is small, the bone may be trimmed back and the wound left to heal by secondary intention. Injuries to the thumb or index finger with exposed bone nearly always require specialist attention.
- Subungual hematomas require decompression by simple trephination of the nail plate. Use of heated paper clip delays healing. Use of nail drill, scalpel, or 18-gauge needle is recommended.
- Simple trephination produces an excellent result in patients with subungual hematoma regardless of size, injury mechanism, or presence of simple fracture.
- Injuries to the nail bed require careful repair to reduce scar formation. They are associated with fractures of the distal phalanx in 50% of cases.
- Remove the nail if there is extensive crush injury, associated nail avulsion or surrounding nail fold disruption, or a displaced distal phalanx fracture on radiograph.
- Repair with 6-0 or 7-0 absorbable sutures. If the nail matrix is displaced from its anatomic position at the sulcus, the matrix should be carefully replaced and sewn in place with mattress sutures (Fig. 14-4).
- Alternatively, after nail bed repair, tissue adhesive can be used (dripping it onto the perionychium and into nail fold) to secure the nail, avoiding suturing it in place.
- Apply mild downward pressure on the nail until the adhesive sets.
- If there is extensive injury to the nail bed with avulsed tissue, consult a hand specialist.
- In children with fractures of the distal phalanx, the nail plate may come to lie on the eponychium. After careful cleaning and adequate anesthesia, replace the nail plate under the proximal nail fold.

Ring Tourniquet Syndrome

- Ring removal is required in all injured fingers. Swelling may require that the ring be cut off. If slower

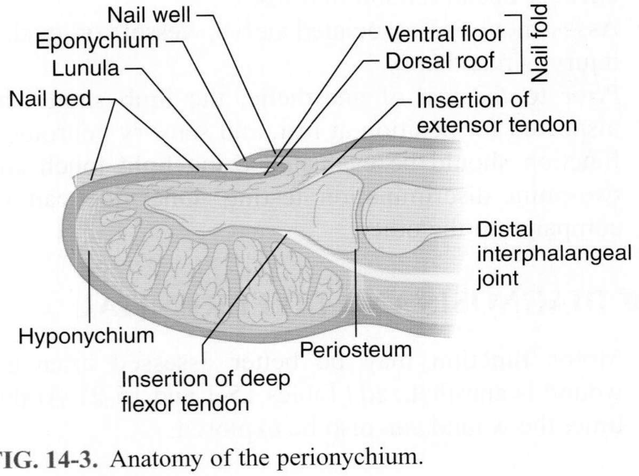

FIG. 14-3. Anatomy of the perionychium.

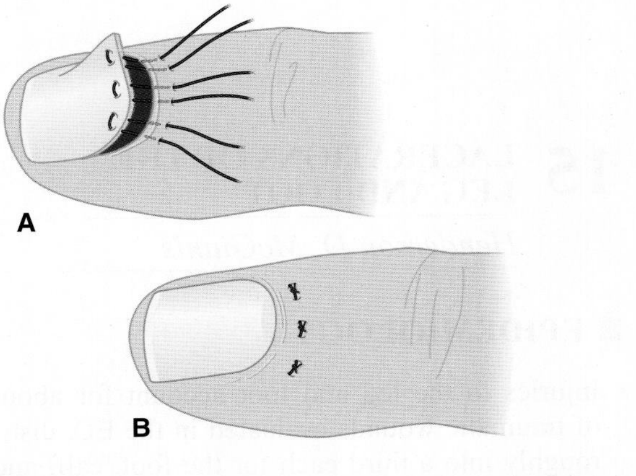

FIG. 14-4 A and B. Technique for repair of an avulsion of the germinal matrix using three horizontal mattress sutures.

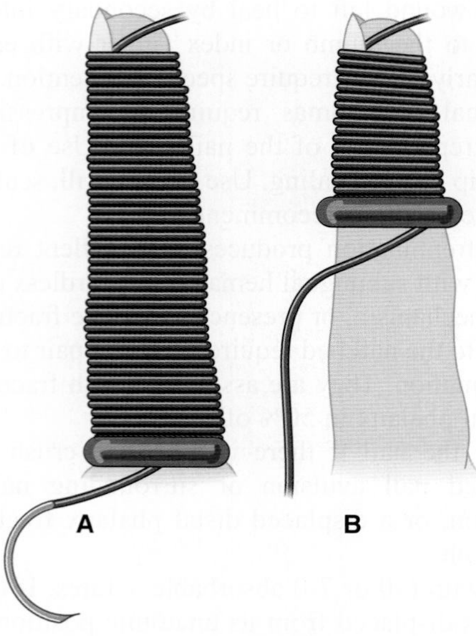

FIG. 14-5. String technique for ring removal. **A.** Completely wrapped. **B.** Unwrapping with ring advancing off with the string.

techniques are appropriate, simple lubrication may suffice.

- The string technique is an alternative method (Fig. 14-5).
  a. String, umbilical tape, or 0-gauge silk may be used.
  b. The string is passed under the ring and then wrapped firmly around the finger from proximal to distal.
  c. The proximal end of the string is then gently pulled, and the ring advances down the finger.

For further reading in *Emergency Medicine: A Comprehensive Study Guide,* 7th ed., see Chapter 44, "Injuries to the arm, hand, fingertip and nail" by Moira Davenport.

15 LACERATIONS OF THE LEG AND FOOT

Henderson D. McGinnis

EPIDEMIOLOGY

- Injuries to the leg and foot account for about 13% of traumatic wounds evaluated in the ED, distributed roughly into a third each for the foot, calf, and knee and thigh regions.
- The foot is commonly injured in sports.
- Many children sustain foot lacerations from broken glass while playing outside.
- Bicycle spoke injuries result in complex lacerations with marked surrounding abrasions and even tissue loss, usually occurring over the lateral malleolus and the base of the fifth metatarsal.
- Lawn mower injuries are usually sustained from the blades of push mowers when being pulled backwards. These wounds are heavily contaminated with multiple organisms.
- Metal lawn and garden edging is associated with plantar and knee injuries.
- Hockey skates are associated with injury to the underlying tibialis anterior tendon, extensor hallucis tendon, and the dorsalis pedis artery and nerve.

PATHOPHYSIOLOGY

- The mechanism of the injury determines the likelihood of disruption to underlying tissue, the risk of a retained foreign body, and the degree of potential contamination.
- The following circumstances are associated with specific pathogens: (1) farming accidents (*Clostridium perfringens*), (2) wading in a freshwater stream (*Aeromonas hydrophila*), and (3) high-pressure water systems used for cleaning surfaces (*Acinetobacter calcoaceticus*).
- Blunt force wounds often have irregular edges and are more likely to be associated with an underlying fracture. These characteristics increase the likelihood of wound infection compared to wounds caused by a sharp object.

CLINICAL FEATURES

- Evaluation of wounds in general is discussed in Chapter 11. It is important to determine the position of the limb at the time of injury, which will help to uncover occult tendon injuries.
- Assessment for associated nerve, vessel, or tendon injury is mandatory.
- Prior to the use of anesthetic, the limb should be inspected for position at rest, and sensory neurologic function should be evaluated using light touch and two-point discrimination testing. One side can be compared to the other.

DIAGNOSIS AND DIFFERENTIAL

- Motor function may be better assessed after the wound is anesthetized (Tables 15-1 and 15-2). At this time, the wound can also be explored.

TABLE 15-1 Motor Function of Lower Extremity Peripheral Nerves

NERVE	MOTOR FUNCTION
Superficial peroneal	Foot eversion
Deep peroneal	Foot inversion Ankle dorsiflexion
Tibial	Ankle plantar flexion

- The limb should be moved through its full range of motion in order to exclude tendon injury.
- Each tendon function should be tested individually, but the tendon should still be visibly inspected to rule out a partial laceration.
- Laboratory studies are usually not indicated.
- Imaging is required if there is a possibility of fracture or radiopaque foreign body. X-ray all injuries caused by glass unless physical examination can reliably exclude a foreign body (see also Chapter 16). Also consider ultrasound or MRI in the evaluation of wounds for foreign bodies.

EMERGENCY DEPARTMENT CARE AND DISPOSITION

General Recommendations

- See Chapter 11 for discussion of wound preparation; thorough irrigation of lower extremity wounds is essential.
- Wounds on the lower extremities are usually under greater tension than those on the upper limb. Consequently, a layered closure with 4-0 absorbable material to the fascia and interrupted 4-0 nonabsorbable sutures to the skin is preferred. The foot is an exception to this guideline.
- Deep sutures should be avoided in diabetics and patients with stasis changes, because of the increased risk of infection.
- Tetanus immunization status should always be considered. The elderly are at particular risk for not being immunized.
- Cyanoacrylate glue is usually not used on the lower extremities because of high wound tension.
- Lacerations involving the joint or tendons should be splinted in a position of function.

TABLE 15-2 Tendon Function of the Lower Extremities

TENDON	MOTOR FUNCTION
Extensor hallucis longus	Great toe extension with ankle inversion
Tibialis anterior	Ankle dorsiflexion and inversion
Achilles tendon	Ankle plantar flexion and inversion

Knee Injuries

- Wounds over the knee, as for all wounds over joints, should be examined throughout the range of movement.
- Injuries over joints should also be evaluated for possible penetration of the joint capsule. Clinical evaluation alone is often insufficient. Radiography may reveal air in the joint.
- An alternative approach to diagnose joint penetration is to inject 60 mL of sterile saline, with or without a few drops of sterile fluorescein, into the joint using a standard joint aspiration technique at a site separate from the laceration. Leakage of the solution from the wound indicates disruption of the joint capsule injury. Consider the use of ultrasound in the evaluation of the injured knee.
- The integrity of the popliteal artery, the popliteal nerve, and the tibial nerve should always be ascertained.
- After closure, the knee should be splinted to prevent excessive tension on the wound edges.

Ankle Injuries

- Lacerations to the ankle can easily damage underlying tendons. The joints should be moved through their full range with direct inspection of the wound to ensure there is no partial injury to the tendon. Particularly at risk are the Achilles tendon, the tibialis anterior, and the extensor hallucis longus.
- Tendon injuries should be formally repaired.
- The Achilles tendon can rupture without a penetrating injury when a tensed gastrocnemius is suddenly contracted. This injury is most common in an athletic middle-aged male. Thompson's test can be utilized to assess the Achilles tendon. While kneeling on a chair, the patient's calf is gently squeezed at the midpoint. Absent plantar flexion of the foot indicates complete Achilles tendon laceration (a partial injury may still yield plantar flexion). Consider ultrasound imaging to evaluate the Achilles tendon.

Foot Injuries

- Lacerations of the sole of the foot must be carefully explored to ensure not only the absence of tendon injury, but also the absence of foreign bodies. The patient lying prone with the foot supported on a pillow or overhanging the bed assists inspection.
- Regional anesthesia is often best for exploration and repair of lacerations in this area.
- Because of the high risk for infection, wounds older than 6 hours at presentation should probably not be repaired primarily.
- Large needles are required in order to adequately penetrate the thick dermis of the sole. Absorbable

material is usually avoided in the foot. Nonabsorbable 3-0 or 4-0 material is used. Injuries to the dorsum of the foot can be repaired with 4-0 or 5-0 nonabsorbable sutures.
- Lacerations between the toes can be difficult to repair. An assistant can hold the toes apart. An interrupted mattress suture is often required to ensure adequate skin apposition.
- Crutches and a walking boot may be required after repair of any laceration on the foot.
- Injuries to the foot caused by lawn mowers and by bicycle spokes may cause extensive soft tissue injury, along with underlying fractures and tendon lacerations. These injuries should be evaluated and treated by an orthopedic specialist.
- Infection occurs in 3% to 8% of lower extremity injuries, and up to 34% of foot lacerations. However, there is no evidence that prophylactic antibiotics reduce the frequency of postrepair wound infections. Therefore, the decision to use antibiotic prophylaxis is made using clinical judgment according to the degree of contamination, the presence of foreign debris, the presence of associated injuries, and host factors that predispose to infection.
- Wounds sustained while wading in fresh water are prone to infection with *Aeromonas* hydrophila. Aeromonas hydrophila should be considered in any rapidly progressive case of cellulitis in the foot after an injury. Treat with fluoroquinolone such as ciprofloxacin 500 milligrams twice daily. In children, trimethoprim-sulfamethoxazole, 5 mL of suspension per 10 kg up to 20 mL twice daily, is used.

HAIR-THREAD TOURNIQUET SYNDROME

- Hair-thread tourniquet syndrome is an unusual type of injury seen in infants. A strand or strands of hair wrap around one of the toes producing vascular compromise.
- The hair must be completely cut to avoid compromising the neurovascular bundle to the toe. This is best accomplished by making an incision on the extensor surface of the toe down to the extensor ligament.

Disposition

- Patients should be instructed to keep wounds clean and dry.
- Sutures should be removed in 10 to 14 days for the lower limb and in 14 days for lacerations over joints.
- Patients should receive routine wound care instructions. Elevation of the affected limb will reduce edema and aid healing.
- Heavily contaminated wounds or those that require complex repair should be rechecked after 48 hours.
- Use crutches 7 to 10 days as needed to prevent additional tension on the wound.

For further reading in *Tintinalli's Emergency Medicine: A Comprehensive Study Guide*, 7th ed., see Chapter 48, "Lacerations of the Leg and Foot," by Timothy F. Platts-Mills.

16 SOFT TISSUE FOREIGN BODIES

Rodney L. McCaskill

EPIDEMIOLOGY

- Only a small percentage of wounds contain a foreign body.
- Most but not all foreign bodies may be discovered with thorough wound examination.

PATHOPHYSIOLOGY

- Retained foreign bodies may lead to a severe local inflammatory response (eg, wood, thorns, spines), chronic local pain (eg, glass, metal, plastic), local toxic reactions (eg, sea urchin spines, catfish spines), systemic toxicity (eg, lead), or infection.
- Infection is the most common complication of a retained foreign body and typically the infection is resistant to antibiotic therapy.

CLINICAL FEATURES

- The mechanism of injury, composition and shape of the wounding object, and the shape and location of the resulting wound may increase the risk of a foreign body.
- Lacerating objects that splinter, shatter, or break increase the risk of a foreign body.
- Discoloration of the skin, palpable mass, sharp well-localized pain with palpation, and limitation of joint movement should heighten suspicion for a foreign body.
- In adults, the perception of a foreign body more than doubles the likelihood of one being present.
- Although all puncture wounds and apparently superficial wounds can hold foreign bodies, wounds deeper than 5 mm and those whose depths cannot be investigated have a higher association with foreign bodies.
- Patients returning to the ED with retained foreign bodies may complain of sharp pain at the wound site with movement, a chronically irritated non-healing wound, or a chronically infected wound.

DIAGNOSIS AND DIFFERENTIAL

- Imaging studies should be ordered if a foreign body is suspected.

- No single imaging modality is ideal for all types of foreign bodies.
- Most foreign bodies (80-90%) can be seen on plain radiographs. Metal, bone, teeth, pencil graphite, glass, gravel, sand, aluminum, and a few types of plastic are visible on plain film while most plastics and organic material specifically wood, thorns, cactus spines, and some fish bones cannot be seen on plain film.
- CT scan is much more sensitive than plain film in detecting foreign bodies.
- Ultrasound is probably less accurate than CT, but it reportedly has a >90% sensitivity for detecting foreign bodies larger than 4 to 5 mm in size.
- MRI can detect radiolucent foreign bodies and is more accurate in identifying wood, plastic, spines, and thorns than the other modalities.
- Fluoroscopy can be useful to detect metal, gravel, glass, and pencil graphite in real time.

EMERGENCY DEPARTMENT CARE AND DISPOSITION

- Careful exploration of the depths of all wounds increases the likelihood of finding a foreign body. Extending the edges of the wound is often necessary to thoroughly investigate for foreign bodies.
- Blind probing with a hemostat is less effective, but may be utilized if the wound is narrow and deep, and extending the wound is not desirable.
- Not all foreign bodies need to be removed. Indications for foreign body removal include potential for infection, toxicity, functional problems, or potential for persistent pain.
- Vegetative material and heavily contaminated objects should always be removed.
- Radiopaque foreign bodies may be localized using skin markers and x-ray or fluoroscopy. Hypodermic needles may be inserted at 90° to each other near the foreign body to help with localization. Alternatively bedside ultrasonograpy may be used.
- Most busy emergency physicians will only be able to dedicate 15 to 30 minutes to removal procedures.
- Needles may be difficult to locate. If the needle is superficial and can be palpated, an incision can be made over one end and the needle removed. If the needle is deeper, then an incision can be made at the midpoint of the needle and the needle grasped with a hemostat and pushed back out through the entrance wound. If the needle is perpendicular to the skin, the entrance wound should be extended. Then pressure applied on the wound edges may reveal the needle so that it can be grasped and removed.
- Wooden splinters and organic spines are difficult to remove because of their tendency to break.
- Only splinters that are superficial should be removed by longitudinal traction. Otherwise the wound should be enlarged and the splinter lifted out of the wound intact. If the splinter is small and localization is difficult, then a block of tissue may be removed in an elliptical fashion and the remaining wound closed primarily. Since infection occurs frequently, subungual splinters should be removed with splinter forceps or by excising a portion of nail over the splinter and then removing the splinter intact.
- Cactus spines may be removed individually or with an adhesive such as facial gel, rubber cement, or household glue.
- Several techniques have been established to remove fishhooks, including the string-pull method, the needle-cover technique, or the advance-and-cut technique. Alternatively, the wound may be enlarged down to the barb and the fishhook removed. When using any of these techniques, anesthesia should be injected around the fishhook entry site.
- After removal of a foreign body, the wound should be adequately cleaned and irrigated.
- If multiple foreign bodies were removed, a post procedure x-ray should be obtained.
- If the potential for infection is low and all foreign bodies were removed, the wound may be closed primarily.
- If there is a significant risk for infection, delayed primary closure is preferred.
- If a foreign body is suspected or identified radiographically but cannot be located even after thorough wound evaluation, or if the foreign body is located in an area that prohibits removal, then the patient should be informed and referred to a surgical specialist for delayed removal. If the foreign body is near a tendon or joint, the limb should be splinted. Prophylactic antibiotics are widely prescribed, but their efficacy has not been determined.

For further reading in Tintinalli's *Emergency Medicine: A Comprehensive Study Guide,* 7th ed., see Chapter 49, "Soft Tissue Foreign Bodies," by Richard L. Lammers.

17 PUNCTURE WOUNDS AND BITES

David M. Cline

PUNCTURE WOUNDS

PATHOPHYSIOLOGY

- The plantar surface of the foot is the most common site for puncture wounds.
- Puncture wounds may injure underlying structures, introduce a foreign body, and plant inoculum for infection.
- Infection occurs in 6% to 11% of puncture wounds, with *Staphylococcus aureus* predominating (including methicillin-resistant *S. aureus*–MRSA). *Pseudomonas aeruginosa* is the most frequent etiologic agent in post-puncture wound osteomyelitis, particularly when penetration occurs through the sole of an athletic shoe.
- Post-puncture wound infections and failure of an infection to respond to antibiotics suggests the presence of a retained foreign body. Organized evaluation and management is necessary to minimize complications.

CLINICAL FEATURES (SEE ALSO CHAPTER 11)

- Wounds older than 6 hours with large and deep penetration and obvious visible contamination, which occurred outdoors with penetration through footwear, carry the highest risk of infectious complications.
- Patients with a history of diabetes mellitus, peripheral vascular disease, immunosuppression, or advanced age are at increased risk of infection.
- On physical examination, the likelihood of injury to structures beneath the skin must be determined. Distal function of tendons, nerves, and vessels should be assessed carefully.
- The site should be inspected for location, condition of the surrounding skin, and the presence of foreign matter, debris, or devitalized tissue.
- Infection is suggested when there is evidence of pain, swelling, erythema, warmth, fluctuance, decreased range of motion, or drainage from the site.

DIAGNOSIS AND DIFFERENTIAL

- Multiple view, "soft tissue," radiographs should be obtained of all infected puncture wounds and of any wound suspicious for a retained foreign body (see Chapter 16 for recommendations on the diagnosis and management of retained foreign bodies).

EMERGENCY DEPARTMENT CARE AND DISPOSITION

Many aspects of the treatment of puncture wounds remain controversial.

- Uncomplicated, clean punctures less than 6 hours after injury require only low-pressure irrigation and tetanus prophylaxis, as indicated.
- Soaking has no proven benefit. Healthy patients do not appear to require prophylactic antibiotics.
- Prophylactic antibiotics "may" benefit patients with peripheral vascular disease, diabetes mellitus, and immunosuppression.
- Plantar puncture wounds, deeper wounds, especially those in high-risk patients, or through athletic shoes should be treated with prophylactic antibiotics.
- Fluoroquinolones (such as **ciprofloxacin** 500 milligrams twice daily) are recommended for plantar wounds and are acceptable alternatives to parenteral administration of a cephalosporin and aminoglycoside.
- For other at risk wounds, **cephalexin** 500 milligrams four times daily, or a macrolide, are recommended. In general, prophylactic antibiotics should be continued for 5 to 7 days.
- Ciprofloxacin is not recommended for routine use in children for prophylaxis. **Cephalexin** 12.5–25 milligrams/kg/dose four times daily up to 500 milligrams/dose can be used with close follow-up.
- Wounds infected at presentation need to be differentiated into cellulitis, abscess, deeper spreading soft tissue infections, and bone or cartilage involvement. Plain radiographs are indicated to detect the possibility of radiopaque foreign body, soft tissue gas, or osteomyelitis. Bedside ultrasound may identify abscess.
- Cellulitis usually is localized without significant drainage, developing within 1 to 4 days. There is no need for routine cultures, and antimicrobial coverage should be directed at gram-positive organisms, especially *S. aureus.* Seven to 10 days of a **cephalexin** (dose above) is usually effective.
- A local abscess may develop at the puncture site, especially if a foreign body remains. Treatment includes incision, drainage, and careful exploration for a retained foreign body. The wound should be rechecked in 48 hours. Serious, deep, soft tissue infections require surgical exploration and debridement in the operating room.

- Any patient who relapses or fails to improve after initial therapy should be suspected of having osteomyelitis, septic arthritis, or retained foreign body. Radiographs, white blood cell count, erythrocyte sedimentation rate, and orthopedic consultation should be obtained. Definitive management frequently necessitates operative intervention for debridement. Pending cultures, antibiotics that cover *Staphylococcus* including MRSA and *Pseudomonas* species are started. A reasonable regimen is parenteral **vancomycin** 1 gram IV every 12 hours (in children, 20 milligrams/kg every 12 hours) and **ceftazidime** 1 to 2 grams IV every 8 hours (in children, 30–50 milligrams/kg/dose every 8 hours, not to exceed adult dose).
- Conditions for admission include wound infection in patients with high risk for complications, immunocompromised states; wounds with progressive cellulitis and lymphangitic spread; osteomyelitis; septic arthritis; and deep foreign bodies necessitating operative removal.
- Tetanus prophylaxis should be provided according to guidelines (see Chapter 18). Outpatients should avoid weight bearing, elevate and soak the wound in warm water, and have follow-up within 48 hours.

NEEDLE-STICK INJURIES

- Needle-stick injuries carry the risk of bacterial infection in addition to the risk of infection with hepatitis B and C, and human immunodeficiency virus (HIV).
- Because recommendations in this area are complex and evolving, each hospital should have a predesigned protocol developed by infectious disease specialists for the expeditious evaluation, testing, and treatment of needle-stick injuries, including hepatitis B and HIV prophylaxis.

HIGH-PRESSURE-INJECTION INJURIES

- High-pressure-injection injuries may present as puncture wounds, usually to the hand or foot. High-pressure-injection equipment is designed to force liquids (usually paint or oil) through a small nozzle under high pressure.
- These injuries are severe owing to intense inflammation incited by the injected liquid spreading along fascial planes.
- Patients have pain and minimal swelling.
- Despite an innocuous appearance, serious damage can develop.
- Pain control should be achieved with parenteral analgesics; digital blocks are contraindicated to avoid increases in tissue pressure with resultant further compromise in perfusion.
- An appropriate hand specialist should be consulted immediately, and early surgical debridement should be implemented for an optimal outcome.

EPINEPHRINE AUTOINJECTOR INJURY

These injuries typically occur when a patient attempts self-injection during a rushed attempt to treat an allergic reaction.

- Patients present with pain due to the needle stick, paresthesias, and epinephrine-induced vasospasm to the injected area; the entire digit may be blanched and cold.
- There is no clear evidence that active treatment is better than observation alone.
- The only treatment that has been shown to be beneficial is phentolamine with lidocaine. A mixture of 0.5 mL of standard **phentolamine solution** (5 milligrams/mL concentration) and 0.5 mL of 1% **lidocaine solution** will produce a 1 mL total volume containing 2.5 milligrams of phentolamine that can be subcutaneously injected directly through the site of autoinjector puncture.
- Once the ischemia is resolved (no blanching, warm digit), the patient can be discharged, as relapse appears very unlikely.

■ HUMAN BITES

Human bites produce a crushing or tearing of tissue, with potential for injury to underlying structures and inoculation of tissues with normal human oral flora.

- Human bites are most often reported on the hands and upper extremities. Infection is the major serious sequelae (see Table 17-1 for common organisms).

CLINICAL FEATURES (SEE ALSO CHAPTER 11)

- Of particular concern is the closed fist injury or clenched fist injury (CFI), or reverse bite injury, which occurs at the metacarpophalangeal (MCP) region as the fist strikes the mouth and teeth of another individual.
- These hand injuries are at increased risk for serious infection, and any questionable injury in the vicinity of the MCP joint should be considered a CFI until proven otherwise (see Chapter 14 for more information).
- The physical examination should include assessment of the direct injury and a careful evaluation of the

TABLE 17-1 Common Bites and First-Line Treatment

ANIMAL	ORGANISM	FIRST-LINE ANTIBIOTIC
Cat	*Pasteurella multocida* *Bartonella henselae* (cat-scratch fever)	Amoxicillin-clavulanate Azithromycin
Dog	*Pasteurella,* streptococci, staphylococci, *Capnocytophaga canimorsus*	Amoxicillin-clavulanate
Human	*Eikenella,* staphylococci, streptococci Herpes simplex (herpetic whitlow)	Amoxicillin-clavulanate Acyclovir or valacyclovir
Rats, mice, squirrels, gerbils	*Streptobacillus moniliformis* (North America) or *Spirillum minus/minor* (Asia)	Amoxicillin-clavulanate
Livestock, large game animals	Multiple organisms *Brucella, Leptospira, Francisella tularensis*	Amoxicillin-clavulanate or specific agent for disease
Bats, monkeys, dogs, skunks, raccoons, foxes (all carnivores and omnivores)	Rabies	Rabies immune globulin, rabies vaccine
Monkeys	Herpes B virus (Cercopithecine herpesvirus)	Acyclovir or valacyclovir
Freshwater fish	*Aeromonas,* staphylococci, streptococci	Fluoroquinolone or trimethoprim-sulfamethoxazole
Saltwater fish	*Vibrio,* staphylococci, streptococci	Fluoroquinolone

underlying structures, including tendons, vessels, nerves, deep spaces, joints, and bone.

- Local anesthesia usually is required to perform a careful wound exploration. In a CFI, the wound must be examined through a full range of motion at the MCP joint to detect extensor tendon involvement, which may have retracted proximally in the unclenched hand.
- The examination also must assess a potential joint-space violation.
- Radiographs are recommended, particularly of the hand, to delineate foreign bodies and fractures.
- Human bites to the hand frequently are complicated by cellulitis, lymphangitis, abscess formation, tenosynovitis, septic arthritis, and osteomyelitis. Infections from human bites are polymicrobial, with staphylococcal and streptococcal species being common isolates in addition to species-specific *Eikenella corrodens.*

DIAGNOSIS AND DIFFERENTIAL

- History and physical examination usually will indicate a straightforward diagnosis.
- There are times, however, when a patient may try to conceal or deny the true etiology of a human bite, and a high degree of suspicion is warranted, particularly when the wound is on the hand.
- It is important to keep in mind that viral diseases also can be transmitted by human bites (eg, herpes simplex, herpetic whitlow, and hepatitis B).
- The potential risk of acquiring HIV through a human bite appears to be negligible due to low levels of HIV in saliva.

EMERGENCY DEPARTMENT CARE AND DISPOSITION

- Copious wound irrigation with a normal saline solution and judicious limited debridement of devitalized tissue are critical to initial management.
- Human bites to the hand initially should be left open. Other sites can undergo primary closure unless there is a high degree of suspicion for infection.
- Prophylactic antibiotics should be considered in all but the most trivial of human bites. **Amoxicillin/clavulanate** 500 to 875 milligrams PO twice daily (12.5–22.5 milligrams/kg/dose twice daily in children) is the antibiotic of choice.
- See Chapter 14 for management of closed/clenched fist injury. Herpetic whitlow is treated with acyclovir or valacyclovir (see Chapter 184 for discussion).
- Wounds that are infected at presentation require systemic antibiotics after cultures are obtained. Local cellulitis in healthy and reliable patients may be managed on an outpatient basis with immobilization, antibiotics, and close follow-up.
- Moderate to severe infections require admission for surgical consultation and parenteral antibiotics. Appropriate coverage includes **ampicillin/sulbactam** 3 grams IV every 6 hours (in children, 25-37.5 milligrams/kg/dose every 6 hours) or **cefoxitin** 2.0 grams IV every 8 hours (in children 27-33 milligrams/kg/dose IV or IM up to 2.0 grams every 8 hours). Penicillin-allergic patients may be treated with **clindamycin** (5-10 milligrams/kg/dose IV four times daily, up to 600 milligrams/dose) *plus* **ciprofloxacin** (10 milligrams/kg/dose every 12 hours IV; maximum: 400 milligrams/dose).
- All patients should receive tetanus immunization according to guidelines.

DOG BITES

CLINICAL FEATURES

- Dog bites account for 80% to 90% of reported animal bites, with school-age children sustaining the majority of reported bites.
- Infection occurs in approximately 5% of cases and is more common in patients older than 50 years, those with hand wounds or deep puncture wounds, and those who delay in seeking initial treatment over a 24-hour period.
- A thorough history and examination as outlined in the section on human bites are required to assess the extent of the wound and the likelihood of infection.
- Infections from dog bite wounds are often polymicrobial and include aerobic and anaerobic bacteria.

DIAGNOSIS AND DIFFERENTIAL

- Radiographs are recommended if there is evidence of infection, suspicion of a foreign body, bony involvement, or large dog intracranial penetration bites to the heads of small children.

EMERGENCY DEPARTMENT CARE AND DISPOSITION

- All dog bite wounds require appropriate local wound care with copious irrigation and debridement of devitalized tissue.
- Primary closure can be used in wounds to the scalp, face, torso, and extremities other than the feet and hands. Lacerations of the feet and hands should be left open initially. Large, extensive lacerations, especially in small children, are best explored and repaired in the operating room.
- Puncture wounds, wounds to the hands and feet, and wounds in high-risk patients should receive 3 to 5 days of prophylactic antibiotics with **amoxicillin/clavulanate** 500 to 875 milligrams PO twice daily (12.5–22.5 milligrams/kg/dose twice daily in children) or **clindamycin** (5 milligrams/kg/dose four times daily, up to 450 milligrams/dose PO) *plus* **ciprofloxacin** (15 milligrams/kg/dose every 12 hours; maximum: 500 milligrams/dose PO).
- **Clindamycin** *plus* **trimethoprim-sulfamethoxazole** can be used for the penicillin-allergic patient.
- Wounds obviously infected at presentation need to be cultured and antibiotics initiated. Reliable, low-risk patients with only local cellulitis and no involvement of underlying structures can be managed as outpatients with close follow-up.
- Significant wound infections require admission and parenteral antibiotics. Examples include infected wounds with evidence of lymphangitis, lymphadenitis, tenosynovitis, septic arthritis, osteomyelitis, systemic signs, and injury to underlying structures, such as tendons, joints, or bones. Cultures should be obtained from deep structures, preferably during exploration in the operating room. Initial antibiotic therapy should begin with **ampicillin/sulbactam** 3 grams IV every 6 hours or clindamycin (5–10 milligrams/kg/dose IV four times daily, up to 600 milligrams/dose) *plus* **ciprofloxacin** (10 milligrams/kg/dose every 12 hours IV; maximum upto 400 milligrams/dose). If the Gram stain reveals gram-negative bacilli, a third- or fourth-generation cephalosporin or aminoglycoside should be added.
- Tetanus prophylaxis should be provided according to standard guidelines.

CAT BITES

- Cat bites account for 5% to 18% of reported animal bites, with the majority resulting in puncture wounds on the arm, forearm, and hand. Up to 80% of cat bites become infected.

CLINICAL FEATURES

- *Pasteurella multocida* is the major pathogen, isolated in 53% to 80% of infected cat bite wounds.
- *Pasteurella* causes a rapidly developing intense inflammatory response with prominent symptoms of pain and swelling.
- It may cause serious bone and joint infections and bacteremia. Many patients with septic arthritis due to *P. multocida* have altered host defenses due to glucocorticoids or alcoholism.

DIAGNOSIS AND DIFFERENTIAL

- Radiographs are recommended if there is evidence of infection, suspicion of a foreign body, or bony involvement.

EMERGENCY DEPARTMENT CARE AND DISPOSITION

- All cat bite wounds require appropriate local wound care with copious irrigation and debridement of devitalized tissue.

- Primary wound closure is usually indicated, except in puncture wounds and lacerations smaller than 1 to 2 cm, because they cannot be adequately cleaned. Delayed primary closure also can be used in cosmetically important areas. Factors favoring delayed closure or avoiding simple primary closure include presentation beyond 6 hours, lack of cosmetic concern, complex repair needed, underlying injury requiring surgical intervention.
- Prophylactic antibiotics should be administered to high-risk patients including those with punctures of the hand; immunocompromised patients; and patients with arthritis or prosthetic joints. The case can be made that all patients with cat bites should receive prophylactic antibiotics because of the high risk of infection. **Amoxicillin/clavulanate** 500 to 875 milligrams PO twice daily (12.5-22.5 milligrams/ kg/dose 2 times daily in children), **cefuroxime** 500 milligrams PO twice daily (10-15 milligrams/kg/dose twice daily in children), or **doxycycline** 100 milligrams PO twice daily in adults (in children, 1–2 milligrams/kg/dose twice daily, up to 100 milligrams/dose) administered 3 to 5 days are appropriate.
- For cat bites that develop infection, evaluation and treatment are similar to those for dog bite infections. **Penicillin** is the drug of choice for *P. multocida* infections.
- Tetanus prophylaxis should be provided according to standard guidelines.

RODENTS, LIVESTOCK, EXOTIC AND WILD ANIMALS

- Rodent bites are typically trivial, rodents are not known to carry rabies, and these bites have a low risk for infection.
- Livestock and large game animals can cause serious injury. There is also a significant risk of infection and systemic illness caused by brucellosis (see Chapter 100), leptospirosis (see Chapter 100), and tularemia (see Chapter 99).
- Aggressive wound care and broad-spectrum antibiotics are recommended. Specific agents are listed in Table 17-1.

For further reading in Tintinalli's *Emergency Medicine: A Comprehensive Study Guide*. 7th ed., see Chapter 50, "Puncture Wounds and Bites," by Robert A. Schwab and Robert D. Powers.

18 POST REPAIR WOUND CARE

David M. Cline

- After repair, proper care is focused on optimized healing and prevention of complications. Considerations include use of dressing, positioning, prophylactic antibiotics, and tetanus prophylaxis.
- Appropriate follow up and patient education regarding cosmetic results are important.

USE OF DRESSINGS

- Wound dressings provide a moist environment that promotes epithelialization and speeds healing.
- Semipermeable films such as OpSite® are available in addition to conventional gauze dressings. The disadvantages of these materials are their inability to absorb large amounts of fluid.
- Alternatively, topical antibiotics may be used to provide a warm, moist environment.
- Topical antibiotics may reduce the rate of wound infection and also may prevent scab formation.
- Wounds closed with tissue adhesives should not be treated with topical antibiotic ointment because it will loosen the adhesive.

PATIENT POSITIONING AFTER WOUND REPAIR

- The injured site should be elevated, if possible, to reduce edema around the wound and speed healing.
- Splints are useful for extremity injuries because they decrease motion and edema and increase attention paid to the body part.
- Pressure dressings minimize the accumulation of fluid and are most useful for ear and scalp lacerations. (see Chapter 13).

PROPHYLACTIC ANTIBIOTICS

- Prophylactic oral antibiotics are only indicated in specific clinical circumstances.
- When deciding whether or not to prescribe antibiotics, consider the mechanism of injury (ie, crush injury), degree of bacterial or soil contamination, and host predisposition to infection.
- Prophylactic antibiotics are recommended for human bites, dog or cat bites on the extremities (see Chapter 17), intraoral lacerations (see Chapter 13),

open fractures, and wounds with exposed joints or tendons (see Chapters 14 and 15).
- Patients with wounds in areas with lymphedema will likely benefit from prophylactic antibiotics as well.
- A 3- to 5-day course is adequate for non-bite injuries and a 5- to 7-day course is adequate for bite wounds.

TETANUS PROPHYLAXIS

- The need for tetanus prophylaxis should be considered for every wounded patient.
- Inquire about the mechanism of injury, age of the wound, and the patient's tetanus immunization status.
- The only contraindication to tetanus toxoid is a history of neurologic or severe systemic reaction after a previous dose.

See Table 18-1 for a summary of recommendations for tetanus prophylaxis.

WOUND CLEANSING

- Sutured or stapled wounds may be cleansed as early as 8 hours after closure without increasing risk of wound infection.
- Wounds should be gently cleansed with soap and water and examined for signs of infection daily.
- Application of topical antibiotics for the first 3 to 5 days decreases scab formation and prevents edge separation.
- Patients with wounds closed with tissue adhesives may shower, but should not immerse the wound, as this will loosen the adhesive bond and cause earlier sloughing of the adhesive.

WOUND DRAINS

- Drains are placed in wounds for removal of interstitial fluid or blood, to keep an open tract for drainage of pus, or to prevent an abscess from forming by allowing drainage from a contaminated area.
- Closed drainage systems have largely replaced open wound drains, especially after surgery, because closed systems prevent bacteria access into the wound.
- Ribbon gauze packing in an abscess cavity after I&D is the most common drain used in the ED. Packing should be changed at each follow-up until the wound stops producing exudate.

PAIN CONTROL

- Inform patients about the expected degree of pain and measures that might reduce pain. Splints help reduce pain and swelling in extremity lacerations.
- Analgesics may be needed although narcotic analgesia is rarely necessary after the first 48 hours.

HEALTH CARE PROVIDER FOLLOW-UP

- Provide specific instructions for wound examination or suture removal.
- Patients with high risk wounds or conditions, or those unable to identify signs of infection should be instructed to return for re-examination, usually in 48 hours.
- Facial sutures should be removed in 3 to 5 days.
- Most other sutures can be removed in 7 to 10 days, except for sutures in the hands or over joints, which should remain for 10 to 14 days.

TABLE 18-1 Recommendations for Tetanus Prophylaxis

	CLEAN MINOR WOUNDS		ALL OTHER WOUNDS*	
HISTORY OF TETANUS IMMUNIZATION	ADMINISTER TETANUS TOXOID†	ADMINISTER TIG‡	ADMINISTER TETANUS TOXOID	ADMINISTER TIG
<3 or uncertain doses	Yes	No	Yes	Yes
≥3 doses				
Last dose within 5 y	No	No	No	No
Last dose within 5–10 y	No	No	Yes	No
Last dose >10 y	Yes	No	Yes	No

*Especially if wound care delayed (>6 h), deep (>1 cm), grossly contaminated, exposed to saliva or feces, stellate, ischemic or infected, avulsions, punctures, or crush injuries.

†Tetanus toxoid: Tdap if adult and no prior record of administration, otherwise tetanus-diphtheria toxoid if >7 years and diphtheria-tetanus toxoid if <7 years, preferably administered into the deltoid.

‡Tetanus immune globulin: adult dose, 250–500 IU administered into deltoid opposite the tetanus-diphtheria toxoid immunization site.

- When removing sutures or adhesive tapes, take care to avoid tension perpendicular to the wound, which could cause dehiscence.
- Tissue adhesives will slough off within 5 to 10 days of application.

PATIENT EDUCATION ABOUT LONG-TERM COSMETIC OUTCOME

- Inform patients that all traumatic lacerations result in some scarring and that the short-term cosmetic appearance is not highly predictive of the ultimate cosmetic outcome.
- Instruct patients to avoid sun exposure while their wounds are healing because it can cause permanent hyperpigmentation.
- Patients should wear sunblock for at least 6 to 12 months after injury.

For further reading in Tintinalli's *Emergency Medicine: A Comprehensive Study* Guide, 7th ed., see Chapter 51. Postrepair Wound Care, by Adam J. Singer and Judd E. Hollander.

Section 5
CARDIOVASCULAR DISEASE

19 CHEST PAIN: CARDIAC OR NOT

Thomas Rebbecchi

EPIDEMIOLOGY

- Chest pain (CP) is a common ED complaint. The management of these patients can be challenging, is of critical importance, and the clinician should systematically determine if CP is cardiac in origin or not.

PATHOPHYSIOLOGY

- CP can be visceral or somatic. Visceral pain originates from vessels or organs, enters the spinal cord at multiple levels, and is thus poorly described, using terms such as heaviness or aching. Somatic pain is dermatomal, from the parietal pleura or structures of the chest wall, and can be more precisely described.
- Ischemia is an imbalance of oxygen supply and demand.
- Cardiac pain is visceral pain due to lack of oxygen to myocytes. Anaerobic metabolism ensues; chemical mediators are released and pain results.

CLINICAL FEATURES

- Typical ischemic CP is felt as tightness, squeezing, crushing, or pressure in the retrosternal/epigastric area. Radiation of pain to the jaw or arm is associated with a higher risk of ischemia; other symptoms also increase the chances of a cardiac etiology (see Table 19-1).
- Factors uncovered in the history and examination (such as pleuritc or positional pain) decrease the likelihood of ischemia or infarction (see Table 19-2), but do not rule out these more concerning conditions.
- Symptoms lasting less than 2 minutes or continuously longer than 24 hours are less likely to be ischemic. Atypical presentations (anginal equivalents) are the rule and are more common in women, diabetics, the elderly, nonwhite minorities, and psychiatric patients.
- Up to a third of patients with acute myocardial infarctions (AMIs) may not have CP. Patients may present with ischemic equivalents of shortness of breath (SOB), nausea, vomiting, shoulder or jaw pain, or palpitations.
- The character of the CP on presentation of the patient may aid in the differentiation of ischemic pain from other diagnostic possibilities.
- Ischemic cardiac pain is typically worsened with exertion and relieved with rest.

DIAGNOSIS AND DIFFERENTIAL

- Diagnosis of cardiac CP is usually based on historical information.

TABLE 19-1 Historical Factors That *Increase* the Likelihood of Acute Myocardial Infarction

PAIN DESCRIPTOR	STUDY	NO. OF PATIENTS STUDIED	POSITIVE LIKELIHOOD RATIO (95% CI)
Radiation to right arm or shoulder	Chun et al.[1]	770	4.7 (1.9-12.0)
Radiation to both arms or shoulders	Goodacre et al.[2]	893	4.1 (2.5-6.5)
Associated with exertion	Goodacre et al.[2]	893	2.4 (1.5-3.8)
Radiation to left arm	Panju et al.[3]	278	2.3 (1.7-3.1)
Associated with diaphoresis	Panju et al.[3]	8426	2.0 (1.9-2.2)
Associated with nausea or vomiting	Panju et al.[3]	970	1.9 (1.7-2.3)
Worse than previous angina or similar to previous myocardial infarction	Chun et al.[1]	7734	1.8 (1.6-2.0)
Described as pressure	Chun et al.[1]	11,504	1.3 (1.2-1.5)

[1]Chun AA, McGee SR: Bedside diagnosis of coronary artery disease: a systematic review. *Am J Med* 117:334, 2004. [PMID: 15336583]
[2]Goodacre S, Locker T, Morris F, Campbell S: How useful are clinical features in the diagnosis of acute, undifferentiated chest pain? *Acad Emerg Med* 9:203, 2002. [PMID: 11874776]
[3]Panju AA, Hemmelgarn BR, Guyatt GH, Simel DL: Is this patient having a myocardial infarction? *JAMA* 280:1256, 1998. [PMID: 9786377]

TABLE 19-2 Historical and Examination Factors That *Decrease* the Likelihood of Acute Myocardial Infarction

PAIN DESCRIPTOR	STUDY	NO. OF PATIENTS STUDIED	POSITIVE LIKELIHOOD RATIO (95% CI)
Described as pleuritic	Chun et al.[1]	8822	0.2 (0.1–0.3)
Described as positional	Chun et al.[1]	8330	0.3 (0.2–0.5)
Described as sharp	Chun et al.[1]	1088	0.3 (0.2–0.5)
Reproducible with palpation	Chun et al.[1]	8822	0.3 (0.2–0.4)
Inframammary location	Everts et al.[2]	903	0.8 (0.7–0.9)
Not associated with exertion	Goodacre et al.[3]	893	0.8 (0.6–0.9)

[1]Chun AA, McGee SR: Bedside diagnosis of coronary artery disease: a systematic review. *Am J Med* 117:334, 2004. [PMID: 15336583]
[2]Everts B, Karlson BW, Wahrborg P, et al: Localization of pain in suspected acute myocardial infarction in relation to final diagnosis, age and sex, and site and type of infarction. *Heart Lung* 25:30, 1996.
[3]Goodacre S, Locker T, Morris F, Campbell S: How useful are clinical features in the diagnosis of acute, undifferentiated chest pain? *Acad Emerg Med* 9:203, 2002. [PMID: 11874776]

- There are many important causes of CP that may not be cardiac in nature (see Table 19-3).
- There are several life-threatening causes of CP which the emergency physician should consider for every CP patient (see Table 19-4).
- The electrocardiogram (ECG) is the most important single test and should be obtained within 10 minutes of arrival to the ED. Only 50% of AMI patients will have a diagnostic ECG. Serial ECGs are imperative in the setting of continued CP.

TABLE 19-3 Important Causes of Acute Chest Pain

CHEST WALL PAIN	PLEURITIC PAIN	VISCERAL PAIN
Costosternal syndrome	Pulmonary embolism	Typical exertional angina
Costochondritis (Tietze syndrome)	Pneumonia Spontaneous	Atypical (nonexertional) angina
Precordial catch syndrome	pneumothorax	Unstable angina
Slipping rib syndrome Xiphodynia	Pericarditis Pleurisy	Acute myocardial infarction
Radicular syndromes		Aortic dissection
Intercostal nerve syndromes		Pericarditis Esophageal reflux or spasm
Fibromyalgia		Esophageal rupture Mitral valve prolapse

- Serum cardiac markers are useful for ischemia and infarction. Creatine Kinase (CK), specifically the MB fraction, measured over 24 hours historically has been considered the gold standard for AMI. However, CK-MB may be elevated by as many as 37 other varied conditions including extreme exercise, head trauma, and febrile disorders.
- Troponin I and T are specific to cardiac muscle and have a high specificity and sensitivity for AMI. Troponins have thus replaced CK as the preferred cardiac marker. Troponins can also be elevated in noncardiac ischemic disorders (see Table 19-5).
- Myoglobin rises predictably in AMI, but there is a high false-positive rate due to its presence in all muscle tissue.

TABLE 19-4 Life-Threatening Causes of Chest Pain: Classic Symptoms Compared*

DISORDER	PAIN (LOCATION)	PAIN (CHARACTER)	PAIN (RADIATION)	ASSOCIATED SYMPTOMS
Angina pectoris	Retrosternal or epigastric	Crushing, tightness, squeezing, pressure	R or L shoulder, R or L arm/hand, jaw	Dyspnea, diaphoresis, nausea
Massive pulmonary embolism	Whole chest	Heaviness, tightness	None	Dyspnea, unstable vital signs, feeling of impending doom
Segmental pulmonary embolism	Focal chest	Pleuritic	None	Tachycardia, tachypnea
Aortic dissection	Midline, substernal	Ripping, tearing	Intrascapular area of back	Secondary arterial branch occlusion
Pneumothorax	One side of chest	Sudden, sharp, lancinating, pleuritic	Shoulder, back	Dyspnea
Esophageal rupture	Substernal	Sudden, sharp, after forceful vomiting	Back	Dyspnea, diaphoresis, may see signs of sepsis
Pericarditis	Substernal	Sharp, constant or pleuritic	Back, neck, shoulder	Fever, pericardial friction rub
Pneumonia	Focal chest	Sharp, pleuritic	None	Fever, may see signs of sepsis
Perforated peptic ulcer	Epigastric	Severe, sharp	Back, up into chest	Acute distress, diaphoresis

Abbreviations: L = left, R = right.
*Atypical presentations are common with all listed life-threatening disorders.

TABLE 19-5	Conditions Associated with Elevated Troponin Levels in the Absence of Ischemic Heart Disease
Cardiac contusion	
Cardioinvasive procedures (surgery, ablation, pacing, stenting)	
Acute or chronic congestive heart failure	
Aortic dissection	
Aortic valve disease	
Hypertrophic cardiomyopathy	
Arrhythmias (tachy- or brady-)	
Apical ballooning syndrome	
Rhabdomyolysis with cardiac injury	
Severe pulmonary hypertension, including pulmonary embolism	
Acute neurologic disease (eg, stroke, subarachnoid hemorrhage)	
Myocardial infiltrative diseases (amyloid, sarcoid, hemochromatosis, scleroderma)	
Inflammatory cardiac diseases (myocarditis, endocarditis, pericarditis)	
Drug toxicity	
Respiratory failure	
Sepsis	
Burns	
Extreme exertion (eg, endurance athletes)	

- The relationship between elevations of CK-MB, myoglobin, and troponin can be seen in Fig. 19-1.
- Various additional diagnostic tools can aid in the detection of cardiac CP. These are mentioned in detail in other chapters in this section but include echocardiography and stress testing (exercise, echo, and nuclear). These tests may aid in the diagnosis of cardiac CP; additionally, echocardiography can facilitate diagnosis of other conditions (eg, pericarditis, aortic dissection, hypertrophic cardiomyopathy) that can mimic ischemic disease.

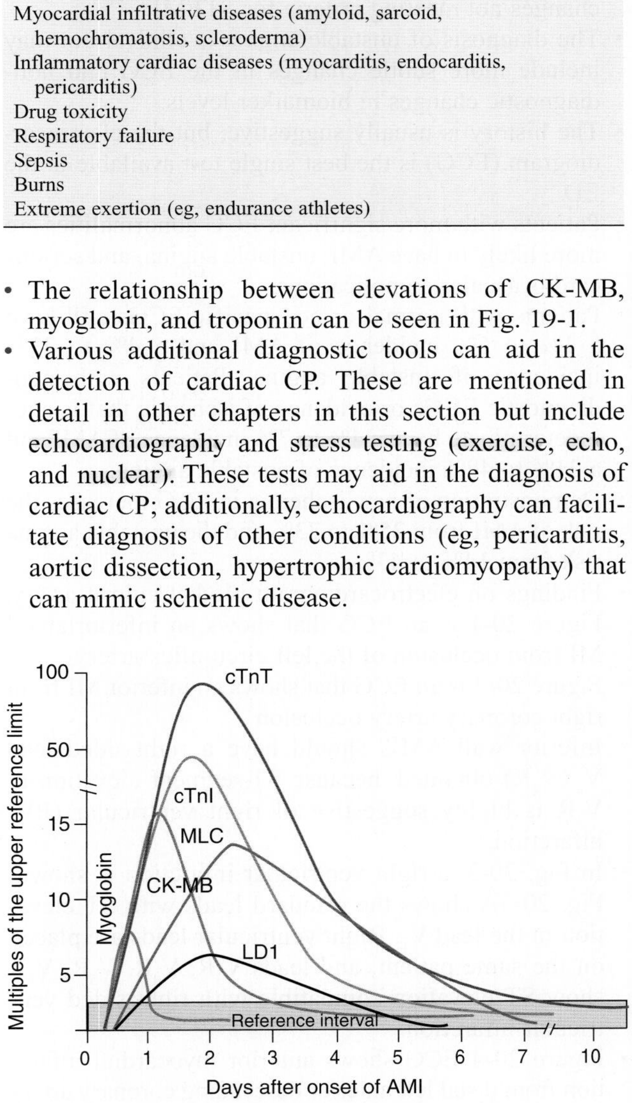

FIG. 19-1. Typical pattern of serum marker elevation after acute myocardial infarction (AMI). CK-MB = MB fraction of creatine kinase; cTnI = cardiac troponin I; cTnT = cardiac troponin T; LD1 = lactate dehydrogenase isoenzyme 1; MLC = myosin light chain.

- The use of chest x-ray usually provides limited information with cardiac CP, but chest x-ray can aid in the diagnosis of other serious conditions.

EMERGENCY DEPARTMENT CARE AND DISPOSITION

- Place the patient on a cardiac monitor, administer oxygen, and obtain IV access. Obtain an ECG. The initial focus should be on immediate life threats.
- The patient should be treated aggressively if the clinical suspicion is high, even if the initial ECG is nondiagnostic of cardiac ischemia. Admit the patient to a high-acuity setting in the presence of an acute coronary syndrome.
- The combination of ECG, clinical history, and cardiac markers should be used for both diagnostic purposes (ie, "is this pain cardiac?") and for risk stratification that guides management and disposition decisions.

For further reading in *Tintinalli's Emergency Medicine: A Comprehensive Study Guide*, 7th edition., see Chap. 52, "Chest Pain: Cardiac or Not," by Gary B. Green and Peter M. Hill.

20 ACUTE CORONARY SYNDROMES: MANAGEMENT OF MYOCARDIAL ISCHEMIA AND INFARCTION

David M. Cline

EPIDEMIOLOGY

- Ischemic heart disease is the number one killer of adults in the United States, with 204.3 deaths per 100,000 population.
- Acute coronary syndrome (ACS) is a spectrum of disease ranging from acute episodes of intermittent angina to acute myocardial infarction (AMI).

PATHOPHYSIOLOGY

- Coronary plaque forms on coronary vessel walls after repetitive injury. With plaque rupture, thrombogenic substances are exposed to platelets.
- Platelet response involves adhesion, activation, and aggregation. Platelet adhesion molecules are strongly thrombogenic and bind to von Willebrand's factor (VWF). Thrombin, collagen, shearing forces, adenosine diphosphate (ADP), thromboxane A2, and

serotonin are potent platelet activators. Platelet glycoprotein IIb/IIIa receptors cross-link fibrinogen or VWF as the common pathway of aggregation.

- The severity of ACS depends upon the extent of O_2 deprivation by thrombus, with complete occlusion resulting in cell death.
- AMI results in injury to both the conduction system, leading to ectopy and dysrhythmia, and left ventricle (LV) pump function, leading to increased filling pressures.
- Cocaine is directly toxic to the myocardium and chronic use accelerates atherosclerosis; acute use may prompt AMI.

CLINICAL FEATURES

- Cardiac risk factors are modestly predictive of CAD in asymptomatic patients, but poor emergency department (ED) predictors for AMI or other ACS.
- The physical examination of a patient with an ACS can range from normal to profound illness.
- Silent (painless)/atypical presentations of ischemia are common. Women and the elderly are more likely to present in this way and may complain of easy fatigability and/or shortness of breath.
- Ischemic/anginal pain is similar to AMI pain. AMI pain usually resolves only with aggressive intervention, whereas anginal pain can resolve with rest or nitroglycerin (NTG).
- Extent and location of myocardial loss determines prognosis and predicts complications. A 25% loss of the LV leads to congestive heart failure (CHF). A 40% LV loss leads to shock. Right ventricle (RV) infarct leads to hypotension.
- Anterior injury leads to tachydysrhythmia. Inferior injury leads to increased vagal tone and first-degree and Mobitz I blocks.
- Mobitz II block is usually associated with anterior AMI and may lead to complete heart block. Anterior and/or inferior injury may lead to complete heart block.
- Fifteen to twenty percent of AMI patients have some degree of CHF.
- Free wall myocardial rupture accounts for 10% of AMI fatalities and occurs 1 to 5 days post-AMI.
- Interventricular wall rupture is signified by pain, shortness of breath (SOB), and a holosystolic murmur.
- Papillary muscle rupture occurs in 1% of all MIs, typically a day into the event and up to 14 days later.
- Pericarditis is seen in up to 20% of all MIs 2 to 4 days after the event. Dressler's syndrome occurs 2 to 10 weeks post-AMI.
- Thirty percent of inferior AMIs involve the right ventricle, and are associated with increased mortality and complications.

DIAGNOSIS AND DIFFERENTIAL

- The diagnosis of ST-segment elevation myocardial infarction (STEMI) is made when criteria on the ECG are met in the setting of symptoms suggestive of MI: ≥ than 1 mm ST elevation in two or more contiguous leads.
- The diagnosis of non-ST-segment elevation myocardial infarction (NSTEMI) depends on abnormal elevation of biologic markers but may include ECG changes not meeting criteria for STEMI.
- The diagnosis of unstable angina is clinical but may include more subtle changes in the ECG and nondiagnostic changes in biomarker levels.
- The history is usually suggestive, but the electrocardiogram (ECG) is the best single test available in the ED.
- Patients with more significant ECG abnormalities are more likely to have AMI, unstable angina, and serious cardiovascular complications.
- Patients with normal or nonspecific ECGs still have a 1% to 5% incidence of AMI and a 4% to 23% incidence of unstable angina. Patients with nondiagnostic ECGs or evidence of ischemia that is age-indeterminate have a 4% to 7% incidence of AMI and a 21% to 48% incidence of unstable angina.
- Demonstration of new ischemia in ECG increases the risk of AMI from 25% to 73% and the unstable angina risk from 14% to 43%.
- Findings on electrocardiogram predict culprit artery. Figure 20-1 is an ECG that shows an inferiorlateral MI from occlusion of the left circumflex artery.
- Figure 20-2 is an ECG that shows an inferior MI from right coronary artery occlusion.
- Inferior wall AMIs should have a right-sided lead V_4 (V_4R) obtained, because ST-segment elevation in V_4R is highly suggestive of right ventricular (RV) infarction.
- In Fig. 20-3, a right ventricular infarction is shown; Fig. 20-3A shows the standard leads with ST elevation in the lead V_1. Right ventricular leads are placed on the same patient, and leads V_3R, V_4R, V_5R, V_6R show ST elevation compatible with right-sided ventricular infarction.
- Figure 20-4 ECG shows anterior myocardial infarction from distal left anterior descending coronary artery occlusion.
- Figure 20-5 shows an ECG demonstrating anterior myocardial infarction due to occlusion of the left anterior descending coronary artery.

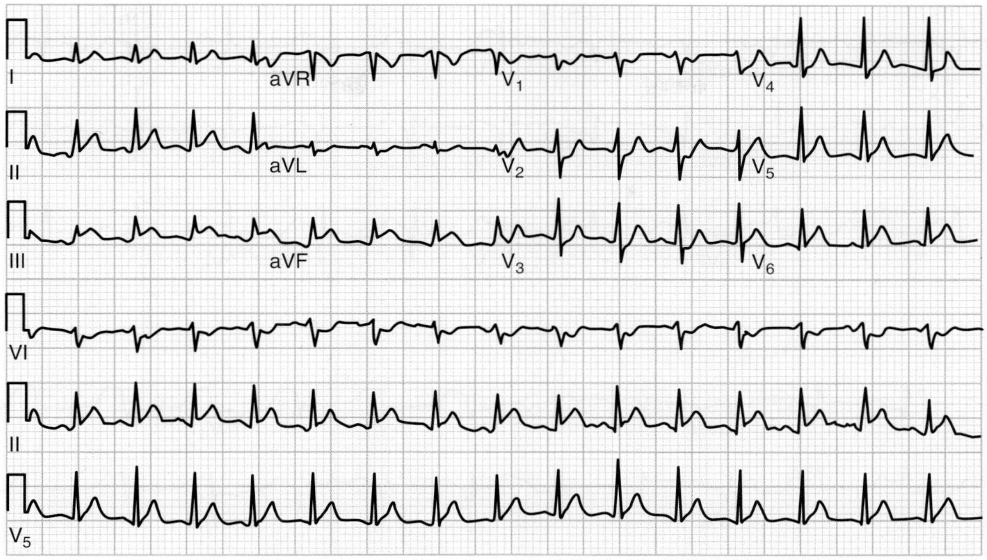

FIG. 20-1. ECG showing inferiorlateral myocardial infarction from left circumflex coronary artery occlusion. (ECG from a 42-year-old man presenting with chest pain. ECG shows ST-segment elevation in limb leads II, III [inferior], and aVF, as well as lead V_6 [lateral]. ST-segment depression is evident in leads V_1, V_2, and V_3, reflecting reciprocal changes in the anterior leads. The patient was found to have 100% occlusion of the left circumflex coronary artery at cardiac catheterization. (*Courtesy of David M. Cline, MD, Wake Forest Baptist Health.*)

- In the setting of AMI, the ECG can range from normal (up to 5%) to distinct ST-segment elevation (Table 20-1).
- Although the cardiac troponins are useful for both diagnosis and risk stratification of patients with chest pain, ACS, and AMI, cardiac marker testing in the ED will not identify most ED patients who subsequently develop adverse events.
- Chest radiography may be useful in determining other causes of ischemic-like pain.

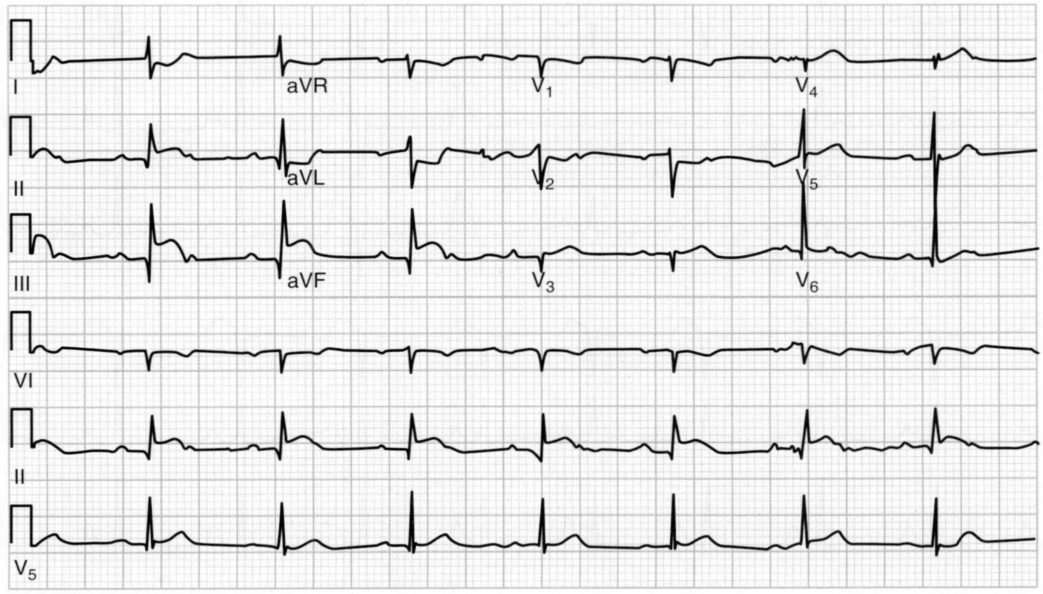

FIG. 20-2. ECG showing inferior myocardial infarction from right coronary artery occlusion. (ECG from an 80-year-old man presenting with acute chest pain. The ECG shows ST-segment elevation in lead III greater than in lead II plus ST-segment depression of >1 mm in lead I and lead aVL. The patient was found to have 100% occlusion of the right coronary artery at cardiac catheterization.) (*Courtesy of David M. Cline, MD, Wake Forest Baptist Health.*)

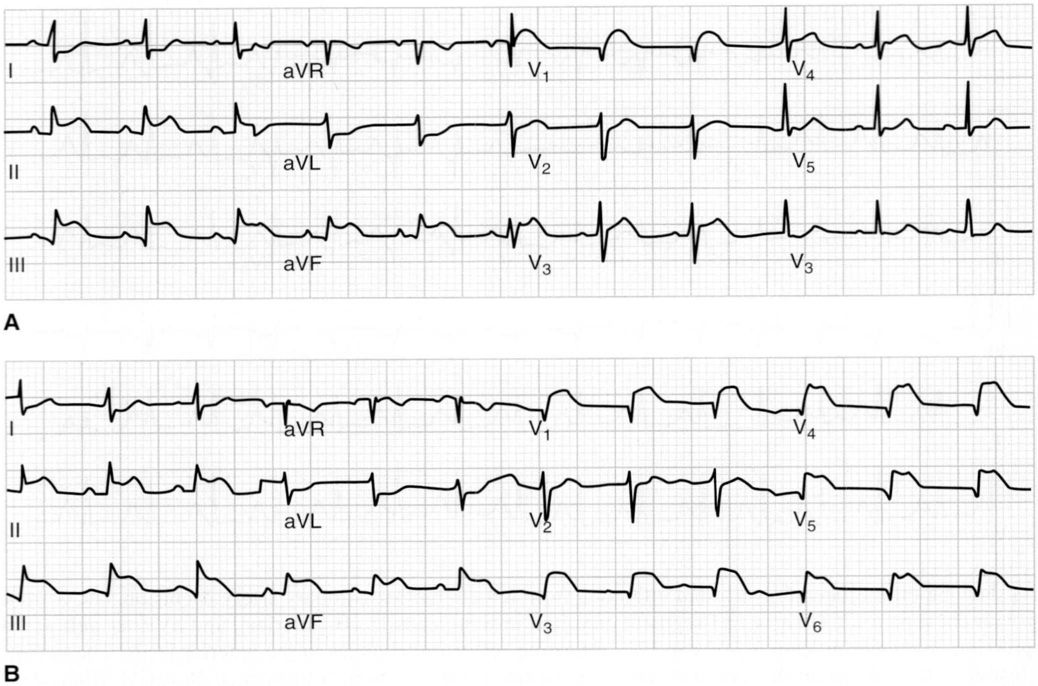

FIG. 20-3. Right ventricular infarction. **A.** Inferior wall myocardial infarction with ST elevation in lead V_1. ECG showing inferior ST-segment elevation myocardial infarction, also with ST-segment elevation in lead V_1 suggestive of right ventricular infarction. **B.** Inferior wall myocardial infarction with right ventricular leads. Same patient with placement of right ventricular leads, showing ST-segment elevation in V_3R, V_4R, V_5R, and V_6R compatible with right ventricular infarction. (*Courtesy of J. Stephan Stapczynski, Maricopa Medical Center.*)

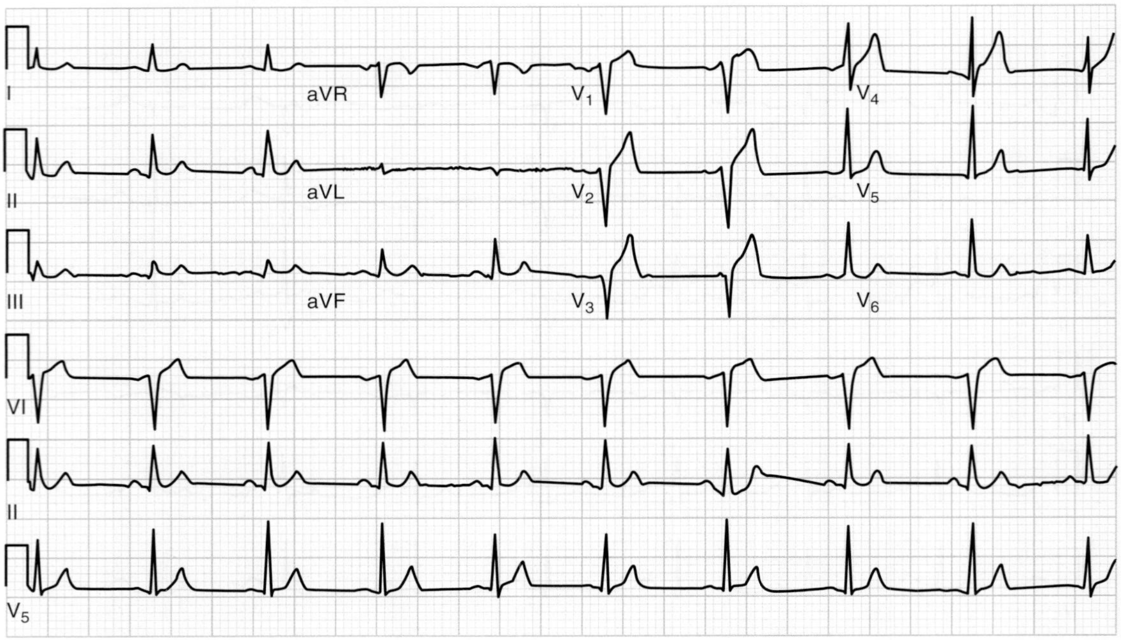

FIG. 20-4. ECG showing anterior myocardial infarction from distal left anterior descending coronary artery occlusion. (ECG from a 52-year-old man presenting with chest pain. ECG shows ST-segment elevation in V_1, V_2, and V_3, with the absence of ST-segment epression in leads II, III, and aVF. The patient was found to have 100% occlusion of the distal left anterior descending coronary artery at cardiac catheterization. (*Courtesy of David M. Cline, MD, Wake Forest Baptist Health.*)

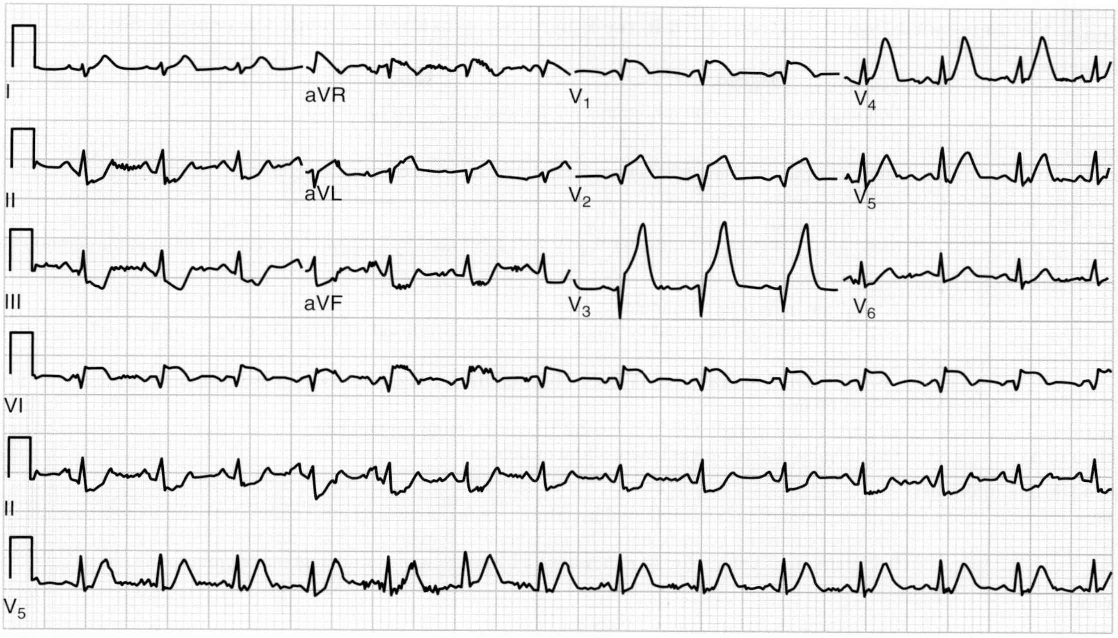

FIG. 20-5. ECG showing anterior myocardial infarction from proximal left anterior descending coronary artery occlusion. (ECG from a 65-year-old man presenting with chest pain. ECG shows ST-segment elevation in V_1, V_2, and V_3, and >1 mm of ST-segment depression in leads II, III, and aVF. The patient was found to have 100% occlusion of the proximal left anterior descending coronary artery at cardiac catheterization. (*Courtesy of David M. Cline, MD, Wake Forest Baptist Health.*)

- The differential diagnosis of cardiac ischemia is particularly broad (see Chapter 19). Entities that should be considered include pericarditis, cardiomyopathies, cardiac valvular disease, pulmonary embolism, pneumonia, pneumothorax, asthma or chronic obstructive pulmonary disease, gastrointestinal disorders (especially esophageal disease), chest trauma, chest wall disorders, hyperventilation, aortic aneurysm, and dissection.

TABLE 20-1	Electrocardiographic Q-Wave-Based Criteria for AMI
Anterior	rS deflection in V_1 with Q waves in $V_{2\text{-}4}$ or decrease in amplitude of initial R waves in $V_{1\text{-}4}$
Inferior	Q waves in II, III, aVF
Anteroseptal	QS deflections in V_1-V_3, and possibly V_4
Lateral	Q waves in I and aVL
Anterolateral	Q waves in V_4-V_6, I, and aVL
Inferolateral	Q waves in II, III, aVF, and V_5 and V_6
Right ventricular	Q waves in II, III, and aVF, and ST elevation in right-side V_4
True posterior*	Initial R waves in V_1 and V_2 >0.04 s and R/S ratio ≥1

*Posterior wall infarction does not produce Q wave abnormalities in conventional leads and is diagnosed in the presence of tall R waves in V_1 and V_2.

EMERGENCY DEPARTMENT CARE AND DISPOSITION

- The primary goal of initial treatment is early reperfusion, achieved by the preferred modality, percutaneous coronary intervention (PCI), or fibrinolytics.
- Institutional goals for reperfusion are PCI within 90 minutes of ED arrival, or fibrinolysis within 30 minutes of ED arrival. Patients ineligible for fibrinolytic therapy should be considered for transfer to a PCI facility, even if arrival at the cardiac center will be delayed beyond the target time frame.
- Measures given to maintain coronary artery patency through anticoagulation and antiplatelet activity are discussed below. Table 20-2 lists agents and doses.
- Dysrhythmias should be treated if their effect on heart rate exacerbates oxygen supply-demand imbalance, or if the dysrhythmia seems capable of electrical deterioration (eg, to a nonperfusing rhythm; see Chapter 4). The process of risk stratification using tools such as the Thrombolysis in Myocardial Infarction (TIMI) Risk Score should be rapidly undertaken.
- Immediate management includes IV access, O_2, cardiac monitoring, and obtaining an ECG.
- Patients meeting criteria for STEMI should receive the following treatments: aspirin, clopidogrel, nitroglycerin, oral beta blocker, an antithrombin, and PCI if available or fibrinolysis if PCI is not

TABLE 20-2 Recommended Doses* of Drugs Used in the Emergency Treatment of Acute Coronary Syndromes

Antiplatelet agents	
Aspirin	160–325 milligrams PO
Clopidogrel	Loading dose of 300-600 milligrams PO followed by 75 milligrams/d
Anticoagulants	
Heparin	60 units/kg bolus (max, 4000 units) followed by infusion of 12 units/kg/h (max, 1000 units/h) titrated to aPTT 1.5–2.5 times control
Enoxaparin (LMWH)	1 milligrams/kg SC q12h
Bivalirudin	(dose prior to PCI) 0.75 milligram/kg IV bolus followed by 1.75 milligrams/kg/h infusion for duration of procedure
Fibrinolytic agents	
Streptokinase	1.5 million units over 60 minutes
Alteplase (tPA)	>67 kg: 15 milligrams initial IV bolus; 50 milligrams infused over next 30 min; 35 milligrams infused over next 60 min <67 kg: 15 milligrams initial IV bolus; 0.75 milligrams/kg infused over next 30 min; 0.5 milligrams/kg infused over next 60 min
Reteplase (rPA)	10 units IV bolus followed by a second 10 unit IV bolus 30 min later
Tenecteplase (tPA)	Single bolus that is weight based, 30-50 milligrams
Glycoprotein IIb/IIIa inhibitors	
Abciximab	0.25 milligrams/kg bolus followed by infusion of 0.125 micrograms/kg/min (max, 10 micrograms/min) for 12–24 h
Eptifibatide	180 micrograms/kg bolus followed by infusion of 2.0 micrograms/kg/min for 72–96 h
Tirofiban	0.4 micrograms/kg/min for 30 min followed by infusion of 0.1 micrograms/kg/min for 48–96 h
Other therapies	
Nitroglycerin	SL: 0.4 milligrams q5 min × 3 PRN for pain IV: start at 10 micrograms/min, titrate to 10% reduction in MAP if normotensive, 30% reduction in MAP if hypertensive
Morphine	2–5 milligrams IV q5–15 min PRN for pain
Metoprolol	50 milligrams PO
Atenolol	25-50 milligrams PO

**Dosage may vary by indication such as presence or absence of ST-segment elevation.*

Abbreviations: LMWH = low-molecular-weight heparin; MAP = mean arterial pressure; max = maximum; PCI = percutaneous coronary intervention; PTT = partial thromboplastin time; q = every; rPA = recombinant plasminogen activator; SL = sublingual; tPA = tissue-type plasminogen activator.

available within a reasonable time frame (within 90 minutes is the goal, times in practice are longer on average, especially for transferred patients). Glycoprotein IIb/IIIa inhibitors can be delayed until arrival in the catheterization laboratory.

- Patients who do not meet criteria for STEMI who have positive markers, or meet otherwise high-risk criteria should be given aspirin, clopidogrel, nitroglycerin, oral beta-blockers, an antithrombin, and should be considered for early intervention with PCI.
- Aspirin should be administered in a dose of 160 to 325 milligrams (chewed) in patients with suspected ACS, unless contraindicated or already taken by the patient.
- Oral and transdermal nitroglycerin (NTG) are useful in treating angina. A sublingual dose should be repeated twice, for a total of three tablets, administered at 2- to 5-min intervals. If there is no improvement with sublingual NTG, intravenous NTG should be started at 5 to 10 micrograms/min.
- IV NTG is recommended for MI or recurrent ischemia. The dose should be adjusted by 5 to 10 micrograms/min increments every 3 to 5 minutes, titrated to pain level and blood pressure reduction up to 200 micrograms/min maximum. NTG should be used cautiously in the setting of borderline-low blood pressure, as hypotension may worsen ischemia.
- NTG is contraindicated in the setting of RV infarction, due to risk of hypotension related to loss of preload. A common side effect of NTG is headache.
- Morphine sulfate can be used if there is uncontrolled ischemic chest discomfort despite NTG. Morphine may decrease cardiac output, and should be used with caution in the presence of hypotension, and in patients with inferior MI.
- The thienopyridine clopidogrel, when added to ASA, reduces the composite risk of cardiovascular death, MI, or stoke. Thienopyridines bind to the ADP receptor and inhibit platelet aggregation.
- Clopidogrel should be considered in addition to standard care (ASA, anticoagulants) for patients with moderate-to high-risk NSTEMI and STEMI, and in patients in whom PCI is planned.
- Clopidogrel is used without aspirin in patients allergic to aspirin. Clopidogrel increases risk of bleeding,

and should be withheld at least 5 days before coronary artery bypass grafting (CABG).

- Prasugrel is an oral thienopyridine prodrug and should not be used in patients with prior stroke or age > 74 years.
- Unfractionated heparin (UFH) is used for its anticoagulant properties. UFH has several disadvantages, including: (1) the need for IV administration, (2) the requirement for frequent monitoring of the activated partial thromboplastin time (aPTT) (3) an unpredictable anticoagulant response in individual patients, (4) heparin-induced thrombocytopenia (HIT), and (5) increased risk of bleeding.
- Anticoagulation due to UFH can be reversed with protamine. The dosage is 1 milligram of protamine per 100 U of UFH infused in the previous 4 hours.
- As compared to UFH, low molecular weight heparins (LMWH) offer greater bioavailability, lower protein binding, longer half-life, improved safety, and more reliable anticoagulant effect.
- LMWH are administered in fixed subcutaneous doses and do not require laboratory monitoring. As compared to UFH, LMWH administration for ACS is associated with decreased ischemia and MI although there is an increase in minor bleeding complications.
- For patients with UA/NSTEMI, enoxaparin (a LMWH) or UFH are both reasonable choices for patients undergoing PCI revascularization. Improved outcomes are demonstrated with consistent therapy (use of a single antithrombin from the ED through the catheterization laboratory) and increased bleeding is seen when patients are switched from one antithrombin to another.
- In patients in whom CABG is planned, LMWH should be avoided (due to its half-life) in favor of UFH. In patients > 75 years of age, enoxaparin must be used with caution due to an increased risk of ICH. Enoxaparin dosing adjustments are recommended in patients with impaired renal function (creatinine clearance < 30 mL/min).
- Factor Xa Inhibitors such as fondaparinux**,** a synthetic pentasaccharide, have similar efficacy to UFH in patients with UA/NSTEMI; bleeding risk is lower than that with enoxaparin.
- Current ACC/AHA guidelines consider fondaparinux an option as an antithrombin. In STEMI patients lacking renal impairment, fondaparinux may be considered for those patients treated with thrombolytics that are not fibrin-specific (ie, streptokinase).
- Direct thrombin inhibitors bind directly to thrombin in clot and are resistant to agents that degrade heparin. Comparison of bivalirudin with UFH found no outcomes benefit in NSTEMI patients, but less bleeding occurred and no dosage adjustment is required in renal impairment. For patients with STEMI, bivalirudin may be considered as an alternative to UFH and GP IIb/IIIa inhibitors.
- Percutaneous Coronary Intervention (PCI), coronary angioplasty with or without stent placement, is the treatment of choice for the management of STEMI when PCI can be performed within 90 minutes of initial ED presentation.
- PCI may be offered to patients presenting to a non-PCI facility when prompt transfer can result in acceptable door-to-balloon times. Early invasive therapy (PCI) within 48 hours is recommended in high-risk patients with UA/STEMI, in patients with recurrent angina/ischemia, and in those who have elevated troponin, new or presumably new ST-segment depression, or high-risk findings on stress testing.
- PCI is also more likely to be beneficial in the setting of depressed LV function, hemodynamic instability, sustained ventricular tachycardia, PCI within the previous 6 months, or prior CABG.
- In treatment settings without timely access to PCI, fibrinolytics are indicated for patients with STEMI if time to treatment is <6 to 12 hours from symptom onset, and the ECG has at least 1-mm ST-segment elevation in two or more contiguous leads.
- The dosages of individual fibrinolytic agents are listed in Table 20-2. STEMI patients who have received fibrinolytics should receive full-dose anticoagulants, started in the ED and maintained for a minimum of 48 hours.
- Similar efficacy and safety profiles have been demonstrated for tissue plasminogen activator (tPA), reteplase (rPA), and tenecteplase (TNK). Contraindications for fibrinolytics are listed in Table 20-3. Before administering thrombolytics, informed consent should be obtained (with particular attention paid to an understanding of the risks). Arterial puncture should be avoided, as should venipuncture or central line placement in areas which are not readily compressible.
  - (a) Tissue plasminogen activator (tPA) is a naturally occurring human protein and is not antigenic. This is fibrin-specific and has a half-life of 5 minutes. When compared with traditional dosing, front-loaded tPA has been shown to have superior 90-minutes patency rates and reocclusion rates, with no increase in bleeding risk.
  - (b) Reteplase (rPA) is a non-fibrin–specific deletion mutant of tPA with a prolonged half-life of 18 minutes (as compared to tPA's half-life of 3 minutes). Reteplase may have a faster time to perfusion. The main advantage of reteplase is that it is given as a (double) bolus rather than infusion.

TABLE 20-3 Contraindications to Fibrinolytic Therapy in ST-segment Elevation Myocardial Infarction

Absolute
Any prior intracranial hemorrhage
Known structural cerebral vascular lesion (e.g., AVM)
Known malignant intracranial neoplasm (primary or metastatic)
Ischemic stroke within 3 months EXCEPT acute stroke within 3 hours
Suspected aortic dissection
Active bleeding or bleeding diathesis (excluding menses)
Significant closed head trauma or facial trauma within 3 months
Relative
History of chronic, severe, poorly controlled hypertension
Severe uncontrolled hypertension on presentation (SBP >180 mm Hg or DBP >110 mm Hg
History of prior ischemic stroke > 3 months, dementia, or known intracranial pathology not covered in contraindications
Traumatic or prolonged (>10 minutes) CPR or major surgery (< 3 weeks)
Recent (within 2 to 4 weeks) internal bleeding
Non-compressible vascular punctures
Current use of anticoagulants: the higher the INR, the higher the risk of bleeding
Pregnancy
Active peptic ulcer
Streptokinase/anistreplase should not be given a second time

(c) Tenecteplase (TNK) is a fibrin-specific substitution mutant of tPA that is given as a single weight-based bolus.

(d) Streptokinase (SK) activates circulating plasminogen, is not fibrin-specific, and is capable of generating an allergic reaction (minor: 5-5.7%, anaphylaxis: < 0.2-0.7%). Hypotension occurs in up to 15% of patients and is usually responsive to fluids and slowing of SK infusion. Contraindications to SK include hypotension, prior SK administration (within 6 months), and streptococcal infection within a year. SK's half-life is 23 minutes, but systemic fibrinolysis persists for 24 hours. Heparin must be given within 4 hours of starting SK.

(e) The most significant complication of thrombolytics is hemorrhage, particularly ICH. Significant bleeding, especially internal, requires cessation of thrombolytics, heparin, and aspirin. Crystalloid and red blood cell infusion may be necessary. Cryoprecipitate (cryo) and fresh frozen plasma (FFP) may be used in an attempt to reverse fibrinolysis due to thrombolytics. Initially, 10 U of cryo are given, and fibrinogen levels are obtained. If the fibrinogen level is < 1 gram/L, the dose of cryo should be repeated. If bleeding continues despite a fibrinogen > 1 gram/L, or if the fibrinogen level is < 1 gram/L after 20 U of cryo, then 2 U of FFP should be administered. If this does not control hemorrhage, then platelets or antifibrinolytic agents (aminocaproic acid or tranexamic acid) are indicated.

- Recent evidence shows no particular benefit to the early IV administration of β-blockers on cardiac rhythm, infarct size, reinfarction, or mortality. Oral β-blocker therapy does not need to be initiated in the ED unless there is a specific indication (eg, tachycardia), but β-blockers may be initiated within the first 24 hours of hospitalization for patients lacking contraindications, alternatives include metoprolol and atenolol among others.
- Glycoprotein IIb/IIIa (GP IIb/IIIa) antagonists bind to platelets and inhibit their aggregation. Abciximab, eptifibatide, and tirofiban are currently available.
- There is no current evidence supporting the routine use of GP IIb/IIIa inhibitor therapy *prior* to angiography in patients with STEMI, and the use of these agents upstream is uncertain. Use of GP IIb/IIIa inhibitors should be guided by local interdisciplinary review of ongoing clinical trials, guidelines, and recommendations.
- AMI patients with continued hemodynamic instability and pain or those who have not reperfused after administration of thrombolytics are candidates for rescue angioplasty.
- Emergent CABG may also be indicated for these patients. Patients in refractory cardiogenic shock should undergo emergent angioplasty. Intraaortic balloon pump or other LV-assisting devices may also be indicated for these patients.
- Patients with AMI or UA who have ongoing chest pain, ECG changes, dysrhythmias, or hemodynamic compromise require cardiac intensive care. Patients with UA and resolved chest pain, normal or nonspecific ECG changes, and no complications should be admitted to a monitored bed. Certain patients, usually those with low risk, may undergo rule-out protocols in chest pain observation units (see Chapter 22).

For further reading in *Tintinalli's Emergency Medicine: A Comprehensive Study Guide*, 7th ed., see Chapter 53, "Acute Coronary Syndromes: Unstable Angina, Myocardial Ischemia, and Infarction," by Judd E. Hollander and Deborah B. Dierck.

21 CARDIOGENIC SHOCK

Brian C. Hiestand

EPIDEMIOLOGY

- Cardiogenic shock is the most common cause of in-hospital mortality from acute myocardial infarction (AMI).
- Approximately 6% to 8% of patients with AMI will develop cardiogenic shock.
- Cardiogenic shock usually occurs early in the course of AMI, with a median onset time of 8 hours.
- Risk factors for developing cardiogenic shock after AMI are related to the likelihood of having widespread myocardial dysfunction, and include advanced age, large or anterior MI, preexisting heart failure, and diabetes mellitus.
- With medical treatment alone, mortality from cardiogenic shock is high (70-90%). Mechanical revascularization improves mortality to ~50%.

PATHOPHYSIOLOGY

- Cardiogenic shock occurs when there is insufficient pumping ability of the heart to support the metabolic needs of the tissues.
- Cardiogenic shock most commonly occurs secondary to extensive myocardial infarction.
- Reduction in cardiac output leads to diffuse tissue hypoperfusion and organ failure. Further myocardial dysfunction results from the subsequent release of systemic inflammatory mediators.
- Cardiogenic shock can occur in a wide variety of presentations of ejection fraction, degree of ventricular involvement, and systemic vascular resistance. Unfortunately, the full mechanism of cardiogenic shock is incompletely understood (see Table 21-1)

TABLE 21-1 Causes of Cardiogenic Shock

Acute myocardial infarction
Pump failure
Mechanical complications
Acute mitral regurgitation secondary to papillary muscle rupture
Ventricular septal defect
Free-wall rupture
Right ventricular infarction
Severe depression of cardiac contractility
Sepsis
Myocarditis
Myocardial contusion
Cardiomyopathy
Mechanical obstruction to forward blood flow
Aortic stenosis
Hypertrophic cardiomyopathy
Mitral stenosis
Left atrial myxoma
Pericardial tamponade
Regurgitation of left ventricular output
Chordal rupture
Acute aortic insufficiency

CLINICAL FEATURES

- Patients may complain of chest pain or anginal equivalent.
- Cardiogenic shock usually presents with hypotension (systolic blood pressure <90 mm Hg), although systolic blood pressure may be higher if there is pre-existing hypertension.
- Heart rate may be fast (compensatory), slow (right or inferior MI with nodal dysfunction), or normal (tachycardia blunted by beta blocker or calcium channel blocker use).
- Skin may be cool, clammy, or mottled.
- Diminished perfusion may lead to altered mentation and oliguria.
- LV failure may result in tachypnea, rales, and frothy sputum.
- It is crucial to listen for a murmur that may represent acute valvular dysfunction (eg, chordae rupture) or ventricular septal defects, conditions warranting immediate surgical intervention.
- Jugular venous distension and abdominal jugular reflex are usually present.

DIAGNOSIS AND DIFFERENTIAL

- The diagnosis of cardiogenic shock should be suspected from the initial history and physical exam. The key task is to differentiate cardiogenic shock from shock due to hypovolemia or distributive causes (sepsis, neurogenic).
- Ancillary tests, used to assist with determining the shock etiology and complications, may include:
  - Electrocardiogram (ECG) to detect ischemia and the need for reperfusion. Right ventricular infarction can be detected using right precordial ECG leads (see Figure 20-3 in Chapter 20 Acute Coronary Syndromes).
  - Chest radiograph for evidence of pulmonary edema, abnormal mediastinum, and evaluation of the cardiac silhouette.
  - Lab studies including cardiac biomarkers, coagulation parameters, serum lactate, and serum chemistries (including liver function tests) may also help establish the diagnosis and detect secondary organ damage.

  - A normal B-type natriuretic peptide (BNP) or N-terminal pro-BNP should suggest a different diagnosis other than cardiogenic shock due to a high negative predictive value.
  - Transthoracic echocardiography done at the bedside can be helpful when evaluating a patient in shock with an unclear etiology.
- Disease processes to be considered in the differential diagnosis include aortic dissection, pulmonary embolism, pericardial tamponade, acute valvular insufficiency, cardiotoxic drugs, hemorrhage, and sepsis.

EMERGENCY DEPARTMENT CARE

- ED care is a temporizing measure while arranging for revascularization in the cardiac catheterization laboratory or surgical intervention for mechanical catastrophe.
- Airway management, circulatory stabilization, and arrangements for definitive cardiac care must occur simultaneously. Cardiology and cardiac surgery should be consulted early. Transfer should be arranged if indicated.
- Percutaneous coronary intervention (PCI) or surgical bypass is preferred over fibrinolysis in the setting of AMI complicated by shock. However, fibrinolysis is preferred over supportive treatment alone and should be delivered should PCI not be available in a timely fashion.
- Stabilize the patient; perform endotracheal intubation if necessary, attain intravenous access, provide high-flow oxygen, place the patient on a monitor and pulse oximeter, and obtain an ECG and rhythm strip.
- Identify rhythm disturbances, hypovolemia, hypoxemia, and electrolyte abnormalities early and treat accordingly.
- Especially with concomitant right ventricular ischemia, anti-anginal therapies may precipitate cardiovascular collapse. For chest pain, titrated intravenous nitroglycerin 5 to 100 micrograms/min or morphine sulfate given in 2-milligrams increments may be administered with caution. Do not give β-blockers in cardiogenic shock.
- For mild hypotension without pulmonary congestion, a small fluid challenge (250-500 mL) may be considered. For hypotension in the setting of right ventricular ischemia, a more robust fluid resuscitation is warranted.
- Norepinephrine may be considered for severe hypotension as a vasopressor and positive inotrope.
- For mild to moderate hypotension without hypovolemia, dobutamine may be administered. Dobutamine may cause peripheral vasodilatation, requiring the concomitant use of dopamine titrated to the desired effect with the lowest dose possible.
- Milrinone may be considered as a positive inotrope. It is less arrhythmogenic than dobutamine, although a comparative survival advantage has not been demonstrated.
- As a temporizing measure, intraaortic balloon pump counter pulsation (if available) should be considered to decrease afterload and to augment coronary perfusion.
- In the setting of acute mitral regurgitation, afterload reduction through intravenous sodium nitroprusside 0.5 to 10.0 micrograms/kg/min should be combined with inotropic support via dobutamine 2.5 to 20.0 micrograms/kg/min. An intraaortic balloon pump may also be indicated to augment forward blood flow (contraindicated in severe aortic regurgitation).
- All patients with cardiogenic shock require admission to an intensive care unit.

For further reading in *Emergency Medicine: A Comprehensive Study Guide,* 7th edition., see Chapter 54, "Cardiogenic Shock," by James Edward Weber and W. Frank Peacock.

22 LOW PROBABILITY ACUTE CORONARY SYNDROME

Chadwick D. Miller

- This chapter discusses the features of low-probability, or possible, acute coronary syndrome (ACS). Patients classified into this group have no objective evidence of acute coronary ischemia or infarction: there is no characteristic electrocardiogram (ECG) ST-segment elevation or depression, and cardiac markers are not elevated.

EPIDEMIOLOGY

- Chest pain accounts for approximately 6 million ED visits annually. Only 15% to 25% of patients tested for ACS will have this condition.

PATHOPHYSIOLOGY

- ACS is a constellation of signs and symptoms resulting from an imbalance of myocardial oxygen supply and demand.
- ACS can be further classified as unstable angina, ST-segment elevation myocardial infarction (STEMI),

and non-ST-segment elevation myocardial infarction (NSTEMI).

- Unstable angina (UA) is characterized by myocardial ischemia but not infarction; as a result, no elevation of biomarkers and no pathologic ST-segment elevation occur.
- Acute myocardial infarction (AMI) occurs when myocardial tissue is devoid of oxygen and substrate for a sufficient period of time to cause myocyte death.
- NSTEMI is characterized by biomarker elevation and no pathologic ST-segment elevation.
- STEMI is characterized by ST-segment elevation and biomarker elevation, although biomarker elevation is not required at onset to make this diagnosis.
- The vast majority of ACS is caused by intraluminal coronary arterial obstruction, usually associated with atherosclerosis.
- Atherosclerotic plaques can slowly enlarge, leading to progressive exertional angina. Or, more commonly, plaques become unstable and rupture, leading to coronary artery thrombosis. If the thrombus is completely occlusive, STEMI occurs, but partial occlusion may result in intermittent angina, rest angina, or NSTEMI.
- Plaque rupture is unpredictable and commonly occurs in plaques previously demonstrated to be "nonocclusive."

CLINICAL FEATURES

- A key determination by the emergency physician is whether to pursue further evaluation for possible ACS. From 3% to 6% of patients thought to have noncardiac chest pain or a clear-cut alternative diagnosis, will have a short-term adverse cardiac event.
- High-risk historical features include chest pain with any of the following descriptors: radiation to shoulders or arms, occurrence with exertion, pressure sensation, similarity to previous cardiac pain, or accompanying nausea or diaphoresis.
- Low-risk historical features include pain that is pleuritic, positional, reproducible, and sharp or stabbing.
- Patients with low-risk features, or without high-risk features, may still have a clinically significant risk of ACS. Therefore absence of high-risk, or presence of low-risk historical features should not solely be used to exclude ACS. The clinical features of patients with possible ACS are the same as discussed in Chapter 20.
- A previous negative cardiac stress test should not prevent an appropriate evaluation for ACS in a patient with concerning history or ECG findings. Previous stress testing results cannot determine whether the patient's current symptoms represent new ischemia from a recent plaque rupture.
- Previous cardiac catheterization results can be of benefit in determining whether a patient should undergo stress testing after exclusion of myocardial infarction. It is unlikely that a patient with previously normal or near-normal coronary arteries has developed significant epicardial stenosis within 2 years of the procedure.

DIAGNOSIS AND DIFFERENTIAL

- The evaluation of patients with possible ACS can be conceptualized into a primary and secondary assessment. The primary evaluation must detect patients with ST-segment elevation that require emergent revascularization and distinguish between patients with definite ACS, possible ACS, and those with symptoms that are definitely not ACS. Alternative causes of chest pain should be considered (see Chapter 19).
- The primary evaluation should include a history, physical examination, ECG, chest radiography, and cardiac biomarkers if ACS remains in the differential diagnosis. Serial ECGs should be obtained in patients with ongoing symptoms. All available data are used to create a composite picture for decision making.
- The pretest ACS probability below which further testing is not indicated is a subject of debate; current recommendations are in the 1% to 2% range.
- At the conclusion of the primary evaluation, patients should be classified as having AMI, possible acute ischemia, or definitely not ischemia.
- Patients with possible acute ischemia are further stratified into high, intermediate, and low risk for adverse events based on the pattern of symptoms, clinical features, and ECG findings (Table 22-1).

TABLE 22-1 Risk Stratification Scheme for Patients with Possible Acute Coronary Syndrome

I. Acute myocardial infarction: immediate revascularization candidate
II. Probable acute ischemia: high risk for adverse events Clinical instability, ongoing pain thought to be ischemic, pain at rest associated with ischemic ECG changes
III. Possible acute ischemia: intermediate risk for adverse events History suggestive of ischemia with absence of high-risk features, and any of the following: Pain at rest, new onset of pain, crescendo pattern of pain, ischemic pattern on ECG not associated with pain (may include ST depression < 1 mm or T-wave inversion > 1 mm)
IV. Possible acute ischemia: low risk for adverse events History not strongly suggestive of ischemia, ECG normal, unchanged from previous, or nonspecific changes
V. Definitely not ischemia: very low risk for adverse events Clear objective evidence of non-ischemic symptom etiology, ECG normal, unchanged from previous, or nonspecific changes, clinician estimate of ACS probability ≤ 2%

- The TIMI risk score may inform risk assessment decision making, but this score should not be used as the sole determinant as to whether a patient is above or below the testing threshold.
- The secondary assessment can be conducted in an observation unit or in the inpatient arena. This assessment should exclude both components of ACS, AMI, and UA.
- AMI is excluded through the use of serial troponin measurements to detect myocardial necrosis. Serum troponin levels can take as long as 8 hours from the time of infarction to become elevated. Therefore, a cardiac biomarker approach should take into account the time from symptom onset, and generally should include multiple measurements. A traditional approach is to obtain troponin measurements at the time of arrival and 6 to 8 hours after arrival. An interim 3 to 4 hour measurement may be added depending on clinical circumstances.
- Normal serial myocardial marker measurements reduce the likelihood of AMI but do not exclude UA, which if diagnosed still puts the patient at high risk for a subsequent adverse cardiac event. Therefore, patients with possible ACS should undergo some form of objective cardiac testing.
- Objective cardiac testing defines either the patient's coronary anatomy, cardiac function, or both.
- Common cardiac testing modalities include stress electrocardiography, stress echocardiography, resting and/or stress nuclear imaging, stress cardiac magnetic resonance imaging (MRI), and computed tomography coronary angiography (CTCA).
- Most patients undergo cardiac testing during the hospitalization associated with the ED presentation. Outpatient testing is an option for low-risk patients in whom AMI has been excluded. This option is most useful in reliable patients presenting to a facility where a mechanism exists to arrange this testing.
- Selection of an objective cardiac testing strategy needs to take into account the modalities available at each institution. The first determination is whether stress testing or coronary imaging with CTCA is desired.
- The most promising application of CTCA is the exclusion of coronary disease in low-risk patients, and its use in this population is supported in the 2007 ACC/AHA Guidelines. At this time, it appears that in patients likely to have, or known to have coronary atherosclerosis, a functional assessment with stress testing is preferable.
- If a stress testing approach is desired, the method of stress (exercise or pharmacologic) should be determined based on ability to exercise; those who cannot walk receive pharmacologic stress.
- Options for the method of cardiac assessment during stress testing include ECG, nuclear imaging, echocardiography, or MRI-based strategies. Selection from these strategies is often based on institutional expertise and equipment availability. Decision making is informed by matching pretest disease probability with imaging modality sensitivity; radiation exposure risks are also included in decision making.
- ECG-based exercise treadmill testing is the least costly and most widely available modality, but has the lowest sensitivity (68%) of the imaging options; it should not be used in patients with high pretest probability for disease. Further, ECG-based exercise treadmill testing should not be used in patients with abnormal baseline ECGs due to difficulties in interpretation.
- Stress echocardiography has the advantages of no radiation exposure, improved sensitivity (80%), and wide availability.
- Nuclear imaging, also widely available, allows assessment of myocardial perfusion and has high accuracy. However, it is associated with radiation exposure and delays in readying radio-isotopes.

EMERGENCY DEPARTMENT CARE AND DISPOSITION

- While testing is ongoing for possible ACS, patients should receive aspirin 160 to 325 milligrams PO, and nitroglycerin 0.4 milligrams spray or sublingual.
- If symptoms continue, administer anti-ischemic therapy using β-blockers (metoprolol 25-50 milligrams PO in the first 24 hours) and/or morphine sulfate 1 to 5 milligrams IV. There are several contraindications to β-blockade; they include heart failure, low cardiac output, heart blocks, active reactive airway disease, tachycardia, and hypotension (see Chapter 20, Acute Coronary Syndrome, for further details).
- There are other adjunctive treatment options for patients at intermediate risk. The decision to administer these medications should be institution-specific, balanced with the patient's bleeding risk and potential benefit, and determined through multidisciplinary discussions. These options include: (1) dual antiplatelet therapy: a common regimen is clopidogrel 300 to 600 milligrams PO in addition to aspirin, (2) anti-thrombin therapy: common regimens are heparin 60 units/kg IV bolus (maximum bolus 4000 units) 12 units/kg/h IV infusion (maximum infusion

1000 units/h) or enoxaparin 1 milligrams/kg SC every 12 hours.

- Patients with negative serial cardiac markers, without diagnostic ECG changes, and who have normal objective cardiac testing are unlikely to have ACS as a cause of their symptoms.
- Consideration should be given to alternative life-threatening causes with further evaluation conducted as appropriate.
- Those with positive cardiac markers, diagnostic ECG changes, or diagnostic testing supporting ACS are admitted to the hospital for cardiology care.
- Those with nondiagnostic testing should be handled on a case-by-case basis and most should be discussed with a cardiologist.

For further reading in *Tintinalli's Emergency Medicine: A Comprehensive Study Guide,* 7th edition., see Chapter 55, "Low Probability Acute Coronary Syndromes," by Chadwick D. Miller.

TABLE 23-1 Causes of Syncope

CARDIAC*	NEURAL/REFLEX-MEDIATED
Structural cardiopulmonary disease	Vasovagal
Valvular heart disease	Situational
Aortic stenosis	Cough
Tricuspid stenosis	Micturition
Mitral stenosis	Defecation
Cardiomyopathy	Swallow
Pulmonary hypertension	Neuralgia
Congenital heart disease	Carotid sinus syndrome
Myxoma	Orthostatic hypotension
Pericardial disease	Psychiatric
Aortic dissection	Neurologic
Pulmonary embolism	Transient ischemic attacks
Myocardial ischemia	Subclavian steal
Myocardial infarction	Migraine
Dysrhythmias	Medications
Bradydysrhythmias	Antihypertensives
Stokes-Adams attack	Antiparkinsonism drugs
Sinus node disease	Beta-blockers
Second- or third-degree heart block	Diuretics
Pacemaker malfunction	Cardiac glycosides
Tachydysrhythmias	Antidysrhythmics
Ventricular tachycardia	Antipsychotics
Torsades de pointes	Antidepressants
Supraventricular tachycardia	Phenothiazines
Atrial fibrillation or flutter	Nitrates
	Cocaine
	Alcohol

*See also Chapter 80, Syncope and Sudden Death in Children, Chapter 78, Seizures and Status Epilepticus in Children, and Chapter 147, Seizures and Status Epilepticus in Adults.

23 SYNCOPE

Bret A. Nicks

EPIDEMIOLOGY

- Syncope accounts for 1% to 2% of ED visits each year.
- The elderly have the highest incidence and risk for morbidity.
- Cause remains idiopathic in 40% of patients.

PATHOPHYSIOLOGY

- The final common pathway of syncope is lack of blood flow or vital nutrient delivery to the brain stem reticular activating system, leading to loss of consciousness and postural tone.
- The most common causes of syncope are vasovagal reflex, cardiac-related (structural and dysrhythmias), and orthostatic hypotension (Table 23-1).
- An inciting event causes a drop in cardiac output, which decreases oxygen and substrate delivery to the brain. The reclined posture and the response of autonomic autoregulation centers re-establish cerebral perfusion, leading to a spontaneous return of consciousness.
- In patients with reflex-mediated (vasovagal) syncope, a stimulus produces an abnormal autonomic response: vagal tone increases. Vasodilatory hypotension with or without bradycardia ensues. Less commonly, the stimulus leads directly to vagal hyperactivity.

CLINICAL FEATURES

- The most common cause of syncope is reflex-mediated, which leads to inappropriate vagal tone with hypotension and/or bradycardia.
- Less common causes of syncope include cerebrovascular disorders, subarachnoid hemorrhage, and subclavian steal syndrome. Patients with a loss of consciousness with persistent neurologic deficits or altered mental status do not have true syncope.

- The hallmark of vasovagal syncope is the slow progressive prodrome of dizziness, nausea, diminished vision, pallor, and diaphoresis.
- Carotid sinus hypersensitivity, a form of reflex-mediated syncope, may result in bradycardia, asystole (for over 3 seconds), or hypotension. This diagnosis should be considered in older patients with recurrent syncope and negative cardiac evaluations (only 25% of these patients have spontaneous symptoms due to true carotid sinus syndrome).
- Orthostatic syncope results from a sudden change to an upright posture, combined with inability to mount an adequate increase in heart rate and/or peripheral vascular resistance. Orthostasis can be associated with medications, aging, volume depletion, and autonomic dysfunction.
- Cardiac-related syncope is due to dysrhythmia or structural heart disease and is a harbinger of sudden death. Syncope from dysrhythmia is typically sudden, usually without prodromal symptoms. Structural heart disease is usually unmasked as syncope during exertion or vasodilation. In the elderly this is most commonly due to aortic stenosis. In the young it is most commonly hypertrophic cardiomyopathy (Table 23-1).
- Ten percent of patients with pulmonary embolism will present with syncope.
- Hyperventilation, classically used as a provocative maneuver in diagnosing panic disorders, can lead to hypocarbia, cerebral vasoconstriction, and subsequent syncope.
- Patients with syncope associated with a concurrent psychiatric disorder are likely to be young, with repeated episodes of syncope, multiple prodromal symptoms, and a generally positive review of systems.
- Multiple medications, such as antidepressants and antihypertensives (eg, β-blockers, calcium channel antagonists, diuretics), are frequent causes of syncope, especially in the elderly.

DIAGNOSIS AND DIFFERENTIAL

- The most important tools in the work-up of syncope are the history, physical examination, and ECG.
- The history is aimed at identifying any high-risk features, including age, history of structural heart disease, and prodromal events.
- Syncope without warning suggests a dysrhythmia; exertional syncope suggests outflow obstruction.
- The cardiac examination may uncover a murmur such as due to aortic stenosis or hypertrophic cardiomyopathy.
- An ECG may identify evidence of previous unknown myocardial infarction, acute ischemia, dysrhythmia, heart block, prolonged QT, or evidence of Wolff–Parkinson–White (WPW) syndrome.
- Selective laboratory testing directed by the history may consist of a hematocrit, pregnancy test, or electrolytes and glucose.
- Seizure, the most common disorder mistaken for syncope, can often be distinguished by the identification of a postictal phase. A tongue laceration is strong evidence for seizure, but occurs in a minority of seizures.

EMERGENCY DEPARTMENT CARE AND DISPOSITION

- The goal of ED evaluation is to identify those at risk for immediate decompensation and future risk of serious morbidity or sudden death.
- If the cause of syncope can be determined by the initial history, physical examination, and ECG, the disposition can be made accordingly.
- The algorithm in Fig. 23-1 provides a framework for the assessment, management, and disposition of syncope patients.
- Additional or post-ED testing, inpatient or outpatient, is defined by syncope's cause or related symptoms (Table 23-2).
- Patients who are not at high risk, are unlikely to have a cardiac etiology and therefore are appropriate for outpatient follow-up.
- Common outpatient evaluations may include 24-hour ambulatory or event monitoring and tilt testing.
- Discharge recommendations may include advising patients not to drive, work at heights, or place themselves in situations that would be dangerous in the event of another syncopal episode.

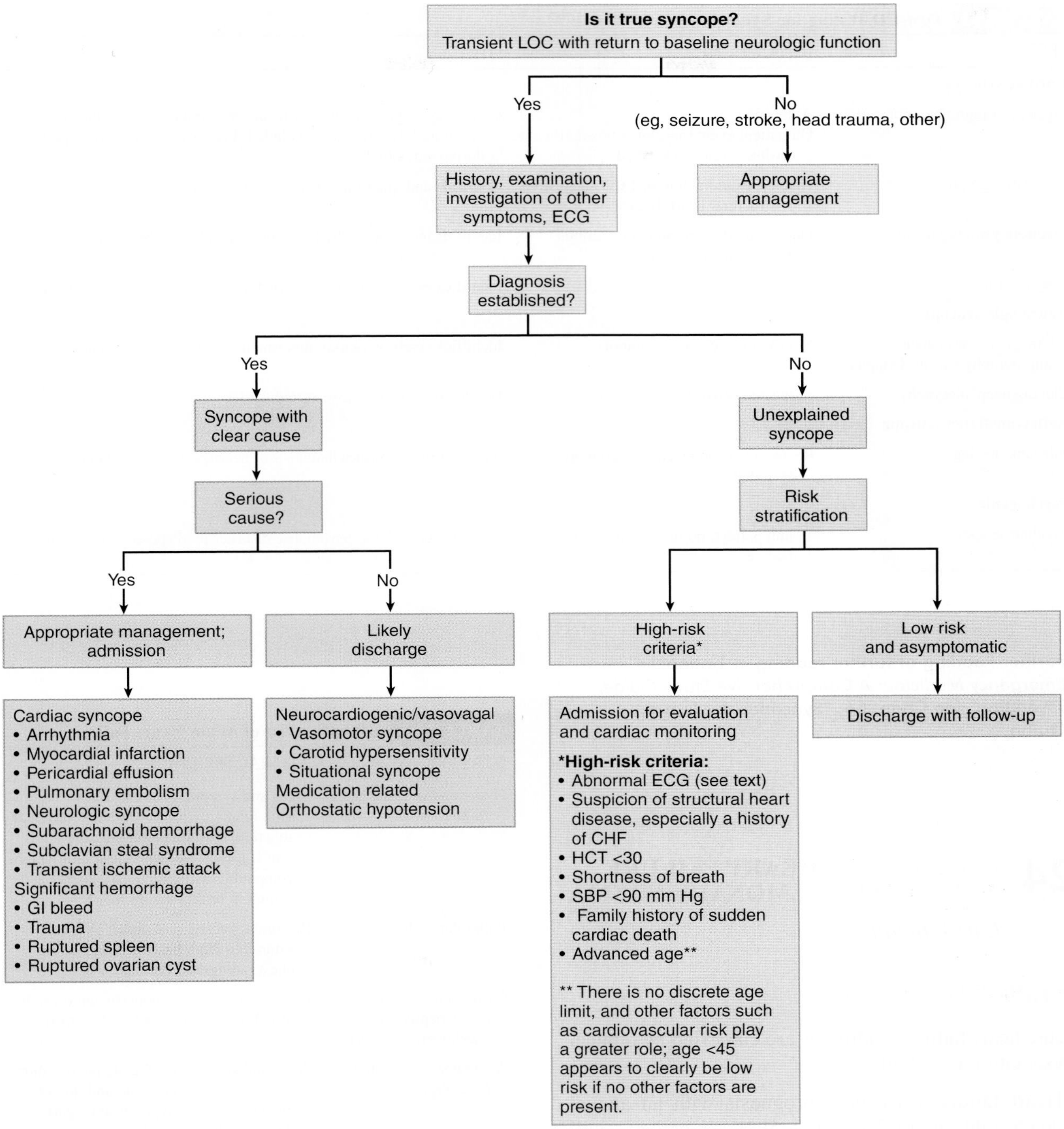

FIG. 23-1. ED evaluation of syncope provides a general management strategy. CHF = congestive heart failure; HCT = hematocrit; LOC = loss of consciousness; SBP = systolic blood pressure.

TABLE 23-2 Post-ED Testing for Syncope

TEST	INDICATION	UTILITY
Cardiac syncope		
Electrocardiographic monitoring	Admission Outpatient event monitor if no significant cardiac disease suspected	Cardiac syncope confirmed if recurrent symptoms occur during monitored dysrhythmia; excluded if recurrent symptoms reported during sinus rhythm
Echocardiography	History, examination, or ECG suggestive of structural heart disease	Confirms and quantifies suspected structural heart disease
Electrophysiology testing	Documented dysrhythmia or serious underlying heart disease	Identifies inducible tachydysrhythmias and some bradydysrhythmias
Stress testing	Exercise-related syncope	Identifies exercise-induced dysrhythmias and postexercise syncope
Neurologic syncope		
CT/magnetic resonance angiography/carotid Doppler	Neurologic signs or symptoms	Identifies cerebrovascular abnormality or subclavian stenosis
Electroencephalography	Suspected seizure	Documents underlying seizure disorder
Reflex-mediated syncope		
Tilt-table testing	Recurrent syncope, cardiac etiology excluded	Positive test establishes diagnosis of neurocardiogenic syncope
Psychogenic		
Psychiatric testing	Young patient, no underlying heart disease	Identifies underlying psychiatric disorder predisposing to syncope

Further Reading or further reading in Tintinalli's *Emergency Medicine: A Comprehensive Study Guide*, 7th edition, see Chap. 56, "Syncope," by James Quinn.

24 CONGESTIVE HEART FAILURE AND ACUTE PULMONARY EDEMA

Lori Whelan

EPIDEMIOLOGY

Acute heart failure syndromes are classified by clinical presentation (see Table 24-1).

- Heart failure has a poor prognosis with an annual death rate of 18.7%. Only 50% of patients will survive 1 year after the development of pulmonary edema.
- The majority of acute heart failure patients have arterial hypertension (53-73%) and ischemic heart disease (46-68%): many have diabetes (27-42%) and atrial fibrillation (21-42%).
- One-quarter to one-third of patients with acute heart failure present with new onset of symptoms, most commonly with acute coronary artery syndrome.

TABLE 24-1 Classification of Acute Heart Failure

CLASSIFICATION	CHARACTERISTICS
Hypertensive acute heart failure	Signs and symptoms of acute heart failure with relatively preserved left ventricular function, systolic blood pressure >140 mm Hg, typically with chest radiograph compatible with pulmonary edema and symptom onset over 48 h or less
Pulmonary edema	Respiratory distress, reduced oxygen saturation from baseline, verified by chest radiograph findings
Cardiogenic shock (see Chapter 54, Cardiogenic Shock)	Evidence of tissue hypoperfusion (systolic blood pressure typically <90 mm Hg)
Acute decompensated heart failure	Signs and symptoms of acute heart failure that are mild to moderate and do not meet criteria for hypertensive heart failure, pulmonary edema, or cardiogenic shock, systolic blood pressure <140 mm Hg and >90 mm Hg, typically associated with increased peripheral edema and symptom onset over days
High output failure	High cardiac output, typically with tachycardia, warm extremities, and pulmonary congestion
Right heart failure	Low-output syndrome with jugular venous distention, hepatomegaly, and may have hypotension

PATHOPHYSIOLOGY

- Three factors, preload, afterload, and contractility, determine ventricular stroke volume. Coupled with heart rate, stroke volume determines cardiac output.
- Low-output heart failure is due to an inherent problem in myocardial contraction.
- High-output heart failure occurs when functionally intact myocardium cannot meet excess systemic demands. The causes of high-output failure are relatively few and include anemia, thyrotoxicosis, large arteriovenous shunts, beriberi, and Paget's disease of the bone.
- Systolic dysfunction, defined as an ejection fraction of less than 40%, is most commonly due to ischemic heart disease, leads to afterload sensitivity, and manifests as increased cardiac pressures with circulatory stress (eg, during exercise). Mechanically, the ventricle has difficulty ejecting blood. Impaired contractility leads to increased intra-cardiac volumes and pressure and afterload sensitivity.
- Diastolic dysfunction represents impaired ventricular relaxation with preserved ejection fraction which results in a left ventricle (LV) that has difficulty in receiving blood. Decreased LV compliance necessitates high atrial pressures to ensure adequate diastolic LV filling and results in preload sensitivity. Chronic hypertension and LV hypertrophy often lead to this condition.
- The most common cause of right-sided failure is left-sided failure.
- Once heart failure has developed, several neurohormonal compensatory mechanisms occur.
- The reduction in cardiac output results in increased stimulation of the renin-angiotensin-aldosterone axis and secretion of antidiuretic hormone. The end result is enhanced sodium and water retention by the kidneys, which leads to fluid overload and the clinical manifestations of congestive heart failure (CHF). The increased adrenergic tone leads to arteriolar vasoconstriction, a significant rise in afterload, and finally, to increased cardiac work.

CLINICAL FEATURES

- Acute pulmonary edema or congestion is the cardinal manifestation of left-sided heart failure, and patients usually present with severe respiratory distress, frothy pink or white sputum, moist pulmonary rales, and an S3 or S4.
- Patients frequently have tachycardia, cardiac dysrhythmias such as atrial fibrillation or premature ventricular contractions (PVCs), and are hypertensive.
- Symptoms of left-sided heart failure include dyspnea (especially with exertion), paroxysmal nocturnal dyspnea, orthopnea, nocturia, fatigue, and weakness.
- Patients with right-sided heart failure commonly have dependent edema of the extremities, and may have jugular venous distention, hepatic enlargement, and a hepatojugular reflex.

DIAGNOSIS AND DIFFERENTIAL

- The correct diagnosis of CHF and/or acute pulmonary edema is very challenging because neither history nor physical examination is accurate. The diagnosis is clinically based using multiple data points including x-rays, laboratories, and echocardiography with "clinical gestalt" frequently outperforming diagnostic tests available in the ED.
- Chest x-ray may reveal vascular redistribution to the upper lung fields, cardiomegaly (cardiothoracic ratio >0.6 on a posteroanterior [PA] film), interstitial edema, enlarged pulmonary artery, pleural effusions, alveolar edema, prominent superior vena cava, and Kerley B lines (short linear markings at the periphery of the lower lung fields) (see Fig. 24-1). Keep in mind, up to 18% of patients with acute heart failure syndromes have no findings on chest x-ray. Although a chest x-ray cannot exclude abnormal left ventricular function, it can confirm other diagnoses, such as pneumonia.
- B-type natriuretic peptide (BNP) is synthesized in the ventricular myocardium in response to elevated ventricular pressures or volume stimulus. BNP measurement is recommended to aid in the diagnosis or exclusion of acute heart failure and in patients with

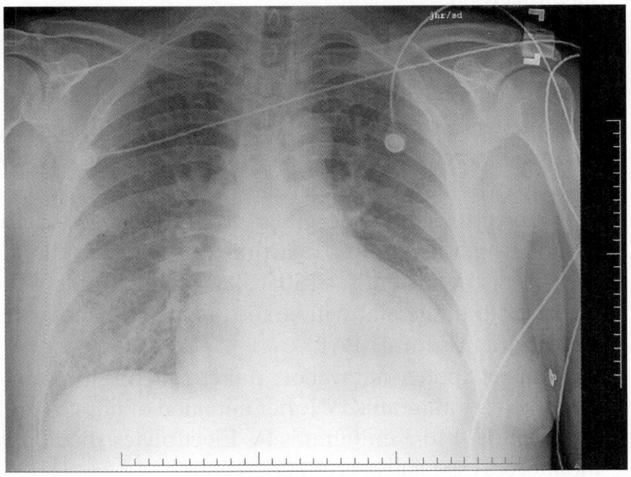

FIG. 24-1. Chest radiograph with findings of congestive heart failure. Chest radiograph demonstrating cardiomegaly, interstitial edema, and left-sided pleural effusion.

acute dyspnea, but it has limitations and it should not be used as a stand-alone test.

- If the BNP level is low (BNP <100 picograms/mL or N-terminal pro-BNP of 300 picograms/mL) then an alternative diagnosis should be considered.

If the BNP level is markedly elevated (BNP >500 picograms/mL or N-terminal pro-BNP >1000 picograms/mL) then there is strong evidence for the diagnosis of congestive heart failure. Normal ranges increase with age.

- Intermediate values should prompt consideration of other confounding diagnoses such as pulmonary embolism, myocardial infarction or primary pulmonary hypertension and additional testing directed by the clinical presentation should be obtained.
- Other limitations include: (1) higher levels than clinically predicted in renal failure/insufficiency, (2) lower levels in obesity and in the patient who presents acutely as the release of BNP may lag behind by an hour.
- Differential diagnosis for acute pulmonary edema includes the common causes of acute respiratory distress: asthma, chronic obstructive pulmonary disease (COPD), pneumonia, pulmonary embolus, allergenic reactions, and other causes of respiratory failure.

EMERGENCY DEPARTMENT CARE AND DISPOSITION

- Administer 100% oxygen by non-rebreather to achieve an oxygen saturation of 95% by pulse oximetry in cases of acute pulmonary edema.
- If the patient is in any respiratory distress, consider applying continuous positive airway pressure (CPAP) or biphasic positive airway pressure (BiPAP) through face mask.
- Immediate intubation is indicated for patients who are visibly tiring, uncooperative with non-invasive ventilation, unconscious, or hemodynamically unstable.
- Administer nitroglycerin sublingually 0.4 milligram (may be repeated up to every 1-5 minutes) to all patients who are hypertensive.
- Nitroglycerin should be given as an IV drip, 0.2 to 0.4 micrograms/kg/min (starting dose) if the blood pressure is persistently >150/100 as the IV route will be easier to titrate and will be the only route accessible if the patient is on BiPAP.
- Administer a potent intravenous diuretic such as furosemide 40 to 80 milligrams IV (after initiation of nitrates), or bumetanide, 1 to 3 milligrams IV. Electrolytes should be monitored, especially serum potassium.
- For patients with resistant hypertension, or those who are not responding well to nitroglycerin, nitroprusside may be used, starting at 0.3 microgram/kg/min (starting dose) and titrated for blood pressure and symptom improvement.
- For hypotensive patients or patients in need of additional inotropic support, begin dopamine at 5 to 10 micrograms/kg/min and titrate to a systolic BP of 90 to 100.
- Assess ECG for ST elevation myocardial infarction (see Chapter 20). Dobutamine can be given in combination with dopamine or as a single agent, provided the patient is not in severe circulatory shock. Start dobutamine at 2.5 micrograms/kg/min and titrate to the desired response (see Chapter 21, Cardiogenic Shock).
- Consider thrombolytic agents for heart failure caused by myocardial infarction.
- Treat coexisting dysrhythmias (see Chapter 4) or electrolyte disturbances (see Chapter 6), avoiding those therapies that impair the inotropic state of the heart.
- Morphine can be given (2-5 milligrams IV) and repeated as needed for pain control. It may cause respiratory depression and adds no benefit to that of oxygen, diuretics, and nitrates for the treatment of the underlying heart failure.
- A randomized controlled trial of 7141 patients showed no benefit in the use of nesiritide for its use in acute decompensated heart failure compared to standard therapy.
- Digoxin acts too slowly to be of benefit in acute situations.
- For anuric (dialysis) patients, emergent dialysis is the treatment of choice in these patients who prove resistant to nitrates.
- Long-term treatment of congestive heart failure includes dietary salt reduction, preload reduction through chronic use of diuretics (eg, furosemide) and afterload reduction via β-blockers (eg, metoprolol), angiotensin-converting enzyme (ACE) inhibitors (eg, captopril), and digoxin.
- Most patients with heart failure require inpatient management or at least observation to monitor kidney function during diuresis and to rule out AMI as a cause of acute decompensation. Patients requiring IV NTG and/or BiPAP will need ICU admission.
- Candidates for outpatient management include those with mild symptoms due to a clearly correctable precipitant that have resolved. These patients must have a normal diagnostic evaluation and a strong social network.

For further reading in *Tintinalli's Emergency Medicine: A Comprehensive Study Guide*, 7th edition, see Chap. 57, "Congestive Heart Failure and Acute Pulmonary Edema," by W. Frank Peacock.

25 VALVULAR EMERGENCIES

Bo Burns

- Ninety percent of valvular disease is chronic, with decades between the onset of the structural abnormality and onset of symptoms.
- Through chronic adaptation by dilation and hypertrophy, cardiac function can be preserved for years, which may delay the diagnosis for one to two decades until a murmur is detected on auscultation.
- The four heart valves prevent retrograde flow of blood during the cardiac cycle, allowing efficient ejection of blood with each contraction of the ventricles. The mitral valve has two cusps, while the other three heart valves normally have three cusps. The right and left papillary muscles promote effective closure of the tricuspid and mitral valves, respectively.
- Compared to the general population, patients with hemodynamically significant valvular heart disease have a 2.5-fold increased rate of death and a 3.2-fold increased rate of stroke.

MITRAL STENOSIS

EPIDEMIOLOGY

- Despite its declining frequency, rheumatic heart disease is still the most common cause of mitral valve stenosis.
- Women are twice as likely as men to have mitral stenosis.

PATHOPHYSIOLOGY

- The majority of patients eventually develop atrial fibrillation because of progressive dilation of the atria.
- Although the valvular obstruction is slowly progressive, symptoms tend to appear acutely, when obstruction becomes sufficient to prevent compensatory increase in cardiac output (eg, during exercise).

CLINICAL FEATURES

- As with all valvular diseases, the most common presenting symptom is exertional dyspnea (seen in 80% of patients with mitral stenosis).
- Hemoptysis, historically the second most common presenting symptom, has become less common due to earlier recognition and treatment of valvular disease.
- Systemic emboli may result in myocardial, renal, central nervous system, or peripheral infarction.
- The classic murmur and signs of mitral stenosis are listed in Table 25-1.

DIAGNOSIS AND DIFFERENTIAL

- The electrocardiogram (ECG) may demonstrate notched or biphasic P waves and right axis deviation (see Figure 25-1).
- On the chest radiograph, straightening of the left heart border, indicating left atrial enlargement, is a typical early radiographic finding. Eventually, there are findings of pulmonary congestion: redistribution of flow to the upper lung fields, Kerley B lines, and an increase in vascular markings.

TABLE 25-1 Comparison of Heart Murmurs, Sounds, and Signs

VALVE DISORDER	MURMUR	HEART SOUNDS AND SIGNS
Mitral stenosis	Mid-diastolic rumble, crescendos into S_1	Loud snapping S_1, apical impulse is small, tapping due to underfilled ventricle
Mitral regurgitation	Acute: harsh apical systolic murmur that starts with S_1 and may end before S_2 Chronic: high-pitched apical holosystolic murmur that radiates into S_2	S_3 and S_4 may be heard
Mitral valve prolapse	Click may be followed by a late systolic murmur that crescendos into S_2	Mid-systolic click; S_2 may be diminished by the late systolic murmur
Aortic stenosis	Harsh systolic ejection murmur	Paradoxic splitting of S_2, S_3, and S_4 may be present; pulse of small amplitude; pulse has a slow rise and sustained peak
Aortic regurgitation	High-pitched blowing diastolic murmur immediately after S_2	S_3 may be present; wide pulse pressure

Abbreviations: S_1 = first heart sound, S_2 = second heart sound, S_3 = third heart sound, S_4 = fourth heart sound.

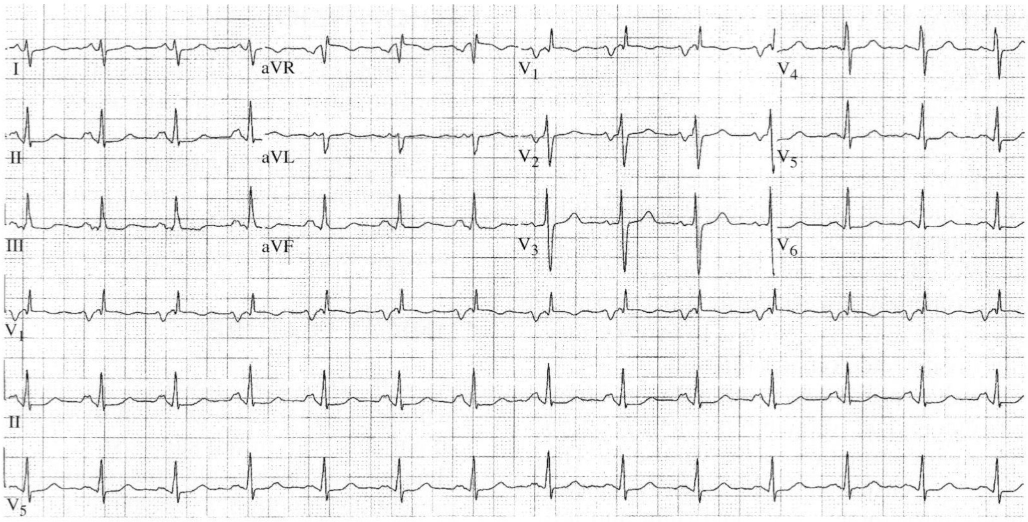

FIG. 25-1. An ECG demonstrating left atrial enlargement and right axis deviation in a patient with mitral stenosis. Note abnormal P waves in lead V_2. (Courtesy of David Cline, Wake Forest University).

- The diagnosis of mitral stenosis should be confirmed with echocardiography and/or cardiology consultation. Symptom severity determines the urgency of ascertaining an accurate diagnosis and arranging for appropriate referral.

EMERGENCY DEPARTMENT CARE AND DISPOSITION

- The medical management of mitral stenosis includes intermittent diuretics, such as furosemide 40 milligrams IV, to alleviate pulmonary congestion; treatment of atrial fibrillation (see Chapter 4); and anticoagulation for patients at risk for arterial embolic events.
- Patients with mitral stenosis and paroxysmal or chronic atrial fibrillation or a history of an embolic event should be on long-term anticoagulation. The goal of warfarin therapy is an international normalized ratio (INR) goal of 2 to 3.2.
- Frank hemoptysis may occur in the setting of mitral stenosis and pulmonary hypertension.
- Bleeding may be sufficiently severe to require blood transfusion, consultation with a thoracic surgeon, and emergency surgery.

MITRAL INCOMPETENCE

EPIDEMIOLOGY

- Infective endocarditis or myocardial infarction can cause acute rupture of the chordae tendineae or papillary muscles or cause perforation of the valve leaflets.
- Inferior myocardial infarction due to right coronary occlusion is the most common cause of ischemic mitral valve incompetence.
- Although an association between aortic regurgitation and appetite suppressant drugs (fenfluramine and phentermine, or dexfenfluramine alone) has generally been accepted, the suspected association of mitral incompetence with appetite suppressants remains unclear.

PATHOPHYSIOLOGY

- Acute regurgitation into a noncompliant left atrium quickly elevates pressures and causes pulmonary edema. In contrast, in the chronic state the left atrium dilates so that left atrial pressure increases little, even with a large regurgitant flow.

CLINICAL FEATURES

- Acute mitral incompetence presents with dyspnea, tachycardia, and pulmonary edema. Patients may quickly deteriorate to cardiogenic shock or cardiac arrest.
- Intermittent mitral incompetence usually presents with acute episodes of respiratory distress due to pulmonary edema, and can be asymptomatic between attacks.

- Chronic mitral incompetence may be tolerated for years or even decades. The first symptom is usually exertional dyspnea, sometimes prompted by atrial fibrillation. Systemic emboli (often asymptomatic) occur in 20% of patients who are not anticoagulated.
- The classic murmur and signs of mitral incompetence are listed in Table 25-1.

DIAGNOSIS AND DIFFERENTIAL

- In acute rupture, the ECG may show evidence of acute inferior wall infarction (more common than anterior wall infarction in this setting).
- On the chest radiograph, acute mitral incompetence from papillary muscle rupture may be manifest by a minimally enlarged left atrium and pulmonary edema, with less cardiac enlargement than expected.
- In chronic disease, the ECG may demonstrate findings of left atrial and left ventricular hypertrophy (LVH). On chest radiography, chronic mitral incompetence produces left ventricular and atrial enlargement proportional to the degree of regurgitant volume.
- Echocardiography is essential to make the diagnosis with certainty and determine severity (see Fig. 25-2). Bedside technique may be mandatory in the acutely ill patient. However, transthoracic echocardiography may underestimate lesion severity, and transesophageal imaging should be undertaken as soon as the patient is adequately stable. In stable patients, echocardiography can be scheduled electively.

EMERGENCY DEPARTMENT CARE AND DISPOSITION

- Pulmonary edema should be treated initially with oxygen, non-invasive positive pressure ventilation, diuretics, as-tolerated nitrates, and intubation for failing respiratory effort.
- Nitroprusside increases forward output by increasing aortic flow and partially restoring mitral valve competence as left ventricular size diminishes. Consider nitroprusside at 5 micrograms/kg/min IV unless the patient is hypotensive.
- There may be a subset of patients in whom mitral regurgitation is worsened by nitroprusside (those patients who respond with dilation of the regurgitant orifice), so careful monitoring is essential.
- Hypotensive patients should receive inotropic agents such as dobutamine 2.5 to 20 micrograms/kg/min in addition to nitroprusside.
- Aortic balloon counterpulsation increases forward flow and mean arterial pressure while diminishing regurgitant volume and left ventricular filling pressure; this intervention can be used to stabilize a patient while awaiting surgery.
- Emergency surgery should be considered in cases of acute mitral valve rupture.

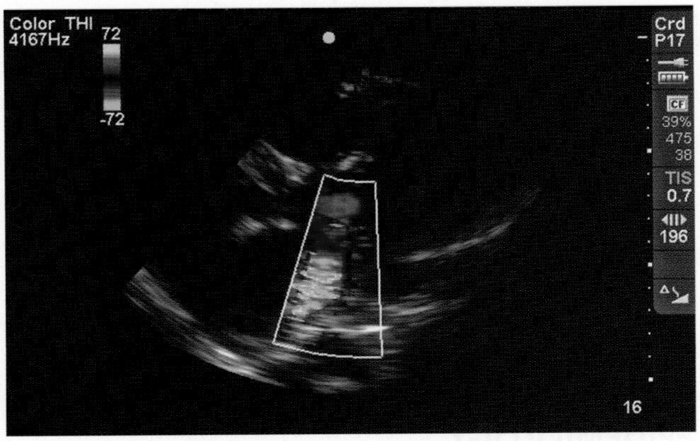

FIG. 25-2. An echocardiogram demonstrating severe mitral regurgitation. Color flow Doppler shows regurgitant flow back into left atrium. (Courtesy of S. Mahler)

MITRAL VALVE PROLAPSE

EPIDEMIOLOGY

- Mitral valve prolapse is the most common valvular heart disease in industrialized countries, affecting about 2.4% of the population.
- Population studies comparing patients with mitral valve prolapse to those without the disorder have found no increased risk of atrial fibrillation, syncope, stroke, or sudden death.

PATHOPHYSIOLOGY

- The etiology of mitral valve prolapse, or the click-murmur syndrome, is unknown but the condition may be congenital.
- Male sex, age over 45, and the presence of regurgitation (recognized clinically by a short systolic murmur), are associated with higher risk for complications.

CLINICAL FEATURES

- Most patients are asymptomatic. Symptoms include atypical chest pain, palpitations, and fatigue and dyspnea unrelated to exertion.
- The abnormal heart sounds are listed in Table 25-1.
- In patients with mitral valve prolapse without mitral regurgitation at rest, exercise-induced mitral regurgitation (which occurs in 32% of cases) predicts a higher risk for morbid events.

DIAGNOSIS AND DIFFERENTIAL

- Echocardiography is recommended to confirm the clinical diagnosis of mitral valve prolapse and to identify any associated mitral regurgitation. Echocardiography and/or consultation with a cardiologist can be performed on an outpatient basis.

EMERGENCY DEPARTMENT CARE AND DISPOSITION

- Initiating treatment for mitral valve prolapse is rarely required for patients seen in the ED. Patients with palpitations, chest pain, or anxiety frequently respond to β-blockers, such as atenolol 25 milligrams qd. Avoiding alcohol, tobacco, and caffeine may also relieve symptoms.

AORTIC STENOSIS

EPIDEMIOLOGY

- Degenerative heart disease (or calcific aortic stenosis) is the most common cause of aortic stenosis in adults residing in the United States.
- Congenital heart disease is the most common cause of aortic stenosis in young adults, with the presence of a bicuspid valve accounting for 50% of cases. Rheumatic heart disease, the third most common cause in the United States, remains the most common cause worldwide.

PATHOPHYSIOLOGY

- Blood flow into the aorta is obstructed, producing progressive LVH and low cardiac output.

CLINICAL FEATURES

- The classic triad is dyspnea, chest pain, and syncope.
- Dyspnea is usually the first symptom, followed by paroxysmal nocturnal dyspnea, syncope on exertion, angina, and myocardial infarction.
- The classic murmur and associated signs of aortic stenosis are listed in Table 25-1.
- Blood pressure is normal or low, with a narrow pulse pressure.
- Brachioradial delay is an important finding in aortic stenosis. The examiner simultaneously palpates the right brachial artery of the patient with the thumb and the right radial artery of the patient with the middle or index finger. Any palpable pulse delay between the brachial artery and radial artery is considered abnormal.

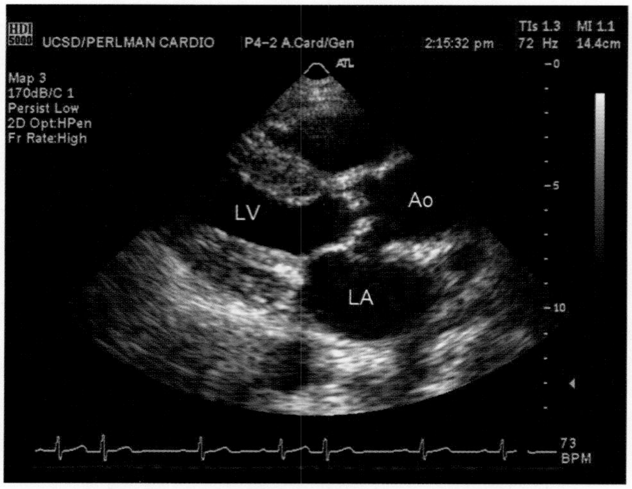

FIG. 25-3. Parasternal long-axis plane demonstrating a thickened, stenotic aortic valve. Ao = aorta; LA = left atrium; LV = left ventricle. (Reproduced with permission from Fuster V, O'Rourke RA, Walsh RA, Poole-Wilson P. eds. *Hurst's The Heart*, 12th edition. New York: McGraw-Hill. 2008.)

DIAGNOSIS AND DIFFERENTIAL

- The ECG usually demonstrates criteria for LVH and, in 10% of patients, left or right bundle-branch block.
- The chest radiograph is normal early, but patients who do not receive valve replacement eventually manifest LVH and findings of congestive heart failure.
- Echocardiography should be undertaken to confirm the suspected diagnosis of aortic stenosis in the hospital if the murmur is associated with syncope (see Fig. 25-3).

EMERGENCY DEPARTMENT CARE AND DISPOSITION

- Patients presenting with pulmonary edema can be treated with oxygen and diuretics, but nitrates should be used with caution since preload reduction may cause significant hypotension. Nitroprusside is not well tolerated in patients with aortic stenosis.
- New-onset atrial fibrillation may severely compromise cardiac output, and therefore require anticoagulation with heparin and cardioversion.
- Patients with profound aortic stenosis-related symptoms (eg, syncope) should be admitted to the hospital.

AORTIC INCOMPETENCE

EPIDEMIOLOGY

- In 20% of patients, the cause of aortic incompetence is acute in nature. Infective endocarditis accounts for the majority of acute cases; the remainder are cased by dissection at the aortic root. Calcific degeneration, congenital disease (most notably bicuspid valves), systemic hypertension, myxomatous proliferation, and rheumatic heart disease cause the majority of chronic cases.

- Marfan syndrome, syphilis, ankylosing spondylitis, Ehlers-Danlos syndrome, and Reiter syndrome are less frequent causes.
- An association between the appetite suppressant drugs (fenfluramine and phentermine or dexfenfluramine alone) has been found for aortic incompetence.

PATHOPHYSIOLOGY

- In acute cases, a sudden increase in backflow of blood into the ventricle raises left ventricular end-diastolic pressure, which may cause acute heart failure.
- In chronic disease, the ventricle progressively dilates to accommodate the regurgitant blood volume. Wide pulse pressures result from the fall in diastolic pressure, and marked peripheral vasodilatation is seen.

CLINICAL FEATURES

- In acute disease, the most common presenting symptom is dyspnea, seen in 50% of patients. Many patients have acute pulmonary edema with pink frothy sputum. Patients may complain of fever and chills if endocarditis is the cause.
- Dissection of the ascending aorta typically produces a "tearing" chest pain that may radiate between the shoulder blades.
- The classic murmur and signs of aortic incompetence are listed in Table 25-1.
- In the chronic state, about one-third of patients will have palpitations associated with a large stroke volume and/or premature ventricular contractions. Frequently these sensations are noticed in bed.
- In the chronic state, signs include a wide pulse pressure with a prominent ventricular impulse, which may be manifested as head bobbing.
- "Water hammer pulse" may be noted; this is a peripheral pulse that has a quick rise in upstroke followed by a peripheral collapse.
- Other classic findings may include accentuated precordial apical thrust, pulsus bisferiens, Duroziez sign (a to-and-fro femoral murmur), and Quincke pulse (capillary pulsations visible at the proximal nail bed, while pressure is applied at the tip).

DIAGNOSIS AND DIFFERENTIAL

- ECG changes may be seen with aortic dissection, including ischemia or findings of acute inferior myocardial infarction, suggesting involvement of the right coronary artery.
- In patients with acute regurgitation, the chest radiograph demonstrates acute pulmonary edema with less cardiac enlargement than expected.
- In chronic aortic incompetence, the ECG demonstrates LVH, and the chest radiograph shows LVH, aortic dilation, and possibly evidence of congestive heart failure.
- Echocardiography is essential for confirming the presence and evaluating the severity of valvular regurgitation. Bedside transthoracic echocardiography should be undertaken in the unstable patient potentially in need of emergency surgery. Transesophageal echocardiography is recommended when aortic dissection is suspected, but this approach may not be feasible in acutely unstable patients.

EMERGENCY DEPARTMENT CARE AND DISPOSITION

- Pulmonary edema should be treated initially with oxygen and intubation for failing respiratory effort. Diuretics and nitrates can be used, but are often ineffective.
- Nitroprusside (start at 5 micrograms/kg/min) along with inotropic agents such as dobutamine (start at 2.5 micrograms/kg/min) or dopamine can be used to augment forward flow and reduce left ventricular end-diastolic pressure in an attempt to stabilize a patient prior to emergency surgery.
- Intra-aortic balloon counterpulsation is contraindicated.
- Although β-blockers are often used in treating aortic dissection, these drugs should be used with great caution, if at all, in the setting of acute aortic valve rupture because they will block the compensatory tachycardia.
- Emergency surgery may be life-saving.
- Chronic aortic regurgitation is typically treated with vasodilators such as angiotensin-converting enzyme (ACE) inhibitors or nifedipine (initiated by a patient's longitudinal care physician).

PROSTHETIC VALVE DISEASE

EPIDEMIOLOGY

- Prosthetic valves are implanted in 40,000 patients per year in the United States. There are approximately 80 types of artificial valves, each with advantages and disadvantages. Patients who receive prosthetic valves are instructed to carry a descriptive card in their wallet.
- Patients with artificial valves develop endocarditis at a rate of 0.5% per year. Infections occur more

frequently during the first 2 months after operation. The most common organisms during this period are *Staphylococcus epidermidis* and *S. aureus*. Gram-negative organisms and fungi are also frequent causes of endocarditis during this early period.
- The most important complications of mechanical heart valves, bleeding, and systemic embolism originating from a thrombus on the prosthetic valve, occur at rates of 1.4% and 1% per year, respectively, for patients on warfarin.

PATHOPHYSIOLOGY

- Prosthetic valves tend to be slightly stenotic, and a very small amount of regurgitation is common because of incomplete closure.
- Patients with mechanical valves require continuous anticoagulation. Some bioprostheses do not require long-term anticoagulation, unless atrial fibrillation is coexistent.
- Thrombi can form on a prosthetic valve and may become large enough to obstruct flow or prevent closure. The dysfunction due to thrombi can be acute or slowly progressive.
- Bioprostheses may gradually degenerate, undergoing gradual thinning, stiffening, and possible tearing, which result in valvular incompetence.
- The sutures that secure the prosthetic valve may become disrupted, leading to perivalvular regurgitation as a fistula forms at the periphery of the valve.
- Mechanical models may suddenly fracture or fail. These failures usually bring sudden symptoms and often cause death before corrective surgery can be accomplished.

CLINICAL FEATURES

- Many patients have persistent dyspnea and reduced effort tolerance after successful valve replacement. This is more common in the presence of pre-existing heart dysfunction or atrial fibrillation.
- Large paravalvular leaks usually present with congestive heart failure. Patients with new neurologic symptoms may have thromboembolism associated with the valve thrombi or endocarditis.
- Patients with prosthetic valves usually have abnormal cardiac sounds. Mechanical valves have loud, metallic closing sounds.
- Systolic murmurs are commonly present with mechanical models. Loud diastolic murmurs are generally not present with mechanical valves.
- Patients with bioprostheses usually have normal S_1 and S_2, with no abnormal opening sounds.
- The aortic bioprostheses are usually associated with a short midsystolic murmur.

DIAGNOSIS AND DIFFERENTIAL

- New or progressive dyspnea of any form, new onset or worsening of congestive heart failure, decreased exercise tolerance, or a change in chest pain compatible with ischemia all suggest valvular dysfunction.
- Persistent fever in patients with prosthetic valves should be evaluated for possible endocarditis with blood cultures.
- Blood studies that may be helpful include a blood count with red blood cell indices and coagulation studies if the patient is on warfarin.
- Emergency echocardiographic studies should be requested if there is any question about valve dysfunction. Ultimately, echocardiography and/or cardiac catheterization may be required for diagnosis.

EMERGENCY DEPARTMENT CARE AND DISPOSITION

- It is critical that patients suspected of having acute prosthetic valvular dysfunction have immediate referral to a cardiac surgeon for possible emergency surgery.
- The intensity of anticoagulation therapy varies with each type of mechanical valve, but ranges from an INR goal of 2 to 3.5.
- Acute prosthetic valvular dysfunction due to thrombotic obstruction has been successfully treated with thrombolytic therapy, but the diagnosis generally requires consultation with a cardiologist. Lesser degrees of obstruction should be treated with optimization of anticoagulation.
- Disposition of patients with worsening symptoms can be problematic, and consultation with the patient's longitudinal care physician may be needed prior to consideration for discharge.

PROPHYLAXIS FOR INFECTIVE ENDOCARDITIS

- See Chapter 95 for recommendations on prophylaxis prior to procedures performed in the emergency department.

For further reading in *Emergency Medicine: A Comprehensive Study Guide,* 7th edition., see Chapter 58, "Valvular Emergencies" by Simon A. Mahler.

26 THE CARDIOMYOPATHIES, MYOCARDITIS, AND PERICARDIAL DISEASE

N. Stuart Harris

- The term *cardiomyopathy* is used to describe a heterogeneous group of diseases that directly alter cardiac structure, impair myocardial function, or alter myocardial electrical properties.
- Cardiomyopathies are the third most common form of heart disease in the United States and are the second most common cause of sudden death in the adolescent population.
- In a patient with CHF and associated cardiomegaly or cardiomegaly in an asymptomatic patient, one of the following five disease entities will usually be diagnosed: ischemic heart disease (see Chapters 20 and 21), hypertensive heart disease (see Chapter 24), valvular heart disease (see Chapter 25), myocarditis, or idiopathic cardiomyopathy.
- Patients with cardiomyopathy may manifest primarily diastolic dysfunction (hypertrophic cardiomyopathy and restrictive cardiomyopathy) or both systolic dysfunction and diastolic dysfunction (dilated cardiomyopathy, inflammatory cardiomyopathy, or myocarditis).

DILATED CARDIOMYOPATHY

PATHOPHYSIOLOGY

- Dilation and compensatory hypertrophy of the myocardium result in depressed systolic function and pump failure leading to low cardiac output.
- Eighty percent of cases of dilated cardiomyopathy (DCM) are not associated with specific cardiac or systemic disorders and are considered idiopathic. Idiopathic DCM is the primary indication for cardiac transplant in the United States.
- Blacks and males have a 2.5-fold increased risk compared to whites and females. The age range at time of diagnosis is typically 20 to 50 years.

CLINICAL FEATURES

- Systolic pump failure leads to signs and symptoms of congestive heart failure (CHF) including dyspnea on exertion, orthopnea, and paroxysmal nocturnal dyspnea.
- Chest pain due to limited coronary vascular reserve may also be present.
- Mural thrombi can form from diminished ventricular contractile force, and there may be signs of peripheral embolization (eg, acute neurologic deficit, flank pain, hematuria, or a pulseless, cyanotic extremity).
- A holosystolic regurgitant murmur of the tricuspid and mitral valve may be heard along the lower left sternal border or at the apex. Other findings include a summation gallop, an enlarged and pulsatile liver, bibasilar rales, and dependent edema.

DIAGNOSIS AND DIFFERENTIAL

- Chest x-ray usually shows an enlarged cardiac silhouette, biventricular enlargement, and pulmonary vascular congestion ("cephalization of flow" and enlarged hila).
- The electrocardiogram (ECG) shows left ventricular hypertrophy, left atrial enlargement, Q or QS waves, and poor R wave progression across the precordium. Atrial fibrillation and ventricular ectopy are frequently present.
- Echocardiography confirms the diagnosis and demonstrates ventricular enlargement, increased systolic and diastolic volumes, and a decreased ejection fraction.
- Differential diagnosis includes acute myocardial infarction, restrictive pericarditis, acute valvular disruption, sepsis, or any other condition that results in a low cardiac output state.

EMERGENCY DEPARTMENT CARE AND DISPOSITION

- Patients with newly diagnosed, symptomatic DCM require admission to a monitored bed or intensive care unit.
- Intravenous diuretics (eg, furosemide 40 milligrams intravenously) and digoxin (maximum dose 0.5 milligram intravenously) can be administered. These drugs have symptomatic benefit, but have not been shown to increase survival.
- Angiotensin-converting enzyme (ACE) inhibitors (eg, enalaprilat 1.25 milligrams intravenously every 6 hours) and β-blockers (eg, carvedilol 3.125 milligrams orally) can be administered. These drugs have been shown to improve survival in DCM with CHF.
- Amiodarone (loaded 150 milligrams intravenously over 10 minutes, then 1 milligram/min for 6 hours) for complex ventricular ectopy can be administered.
- Anticoagulation should be considered to reduce mural thrombus formation.

MYOCARDITIS (INFLAMMATORY CARDIOMYOPATHY)

PATHOPHYSIOLOGY

- Inflammation of the myocardium may be the result of a systemic disorder or an infectious agent.
- Viral etiologies include coxsackie B, echovirus, influenza, parainfluenza, Epstein-Barr, and HIV.
- Bacterial causes include *Corynebacterium diphtheriae, Neisseria meningitidis, Mycoplasma pneumoniae,* and beta-hemolytic streptococci.
- Pericarditis frequently accompanies myocarditis.

CLINICAL FEATURES

- Patients are usually young, have no significant past cardiac history, have few risk factors for atherosclerotic coronary arterial disease, and present with a recent, abrupt onset of symptoms during or immediately after a systemic or viral illness.
- Systemic signs and symptoms predominate, and include myalgias, headache, rigors, fever, and tachycardia out of proportion to the fever.
- Chest pain due to coexisting pericarditis is frequently present.
- A pericardial friction rub may be heard in patients with concomitant pericarditis.
- In severe cases, there may be symptoms of progressive heart failure (eg, CHF, pulmonary rales, pedal edema).

DIAGNOSIS AND DIFFERENTIAL

The diagnosis is primarily clinical with testing that may support but may not confirm the diagnosis; confirmation of a suspected infectious cause (such as appropriate viral serology) is rarely completed in the ED if done at all.

- The chest radiograph is usually normal or nondiagnostic. Cardiomegaly and pulmonary venous hypertension or pulmonary edema are present with severe disease.
- ECG changes include nonspecific ST-T-wave changes, ST-segment elevation from associated pericarditis, atrioventricular block, and QRS interval prolongation.
- Cardiac enzymes may be elevated.
- Differential diagnosis includes cardiac ischemia or infarction, valvular disease, and sepsis.
- Echocardiographic studies are also nonspecific, with myocardial depression and wall motion abnormalities in severe cases.
- Newer imaging modalities include nuclear imaging with gallium^{67}- or indium^{111}-labeled anti-myosin antibodies. Both of these radionuclides are taken up by injured or necrotic myocytes.

EMERGENCY DEPARTMENT CARE AND DISPOSITION

- Treatment for idiopathic or viral myocarditis is supportive.
- Antibiotics are needed for myocarditis complicating rheumatic fever, diphtheria, or meningococcemia; treatment in these cases is guiding by the total clinical picture not simply symptoms suggesting myocarditis.
- Immunosuppressive therapy may be of value in selected patients, but large trials have not consistently demonstrated benefit.
- Admission is usually indicated if the patient presents with CHF symptoms.

HYPERTROPHIC CARDIOMYOPATHY

PATHOPHYSIOLOGY

- This illness is characterized by left ventricular and/or right ventricular hypertrophy that is usually asymmetrical and involves primarily the intraventricular septum without ventricular dilation.
- The result is abnormal compliance of the left ventricle leading to impaired diastolic relaxation and diastolic filling. Cardiac output is usually normal.
- Fifty percent of cases are hereditary. Molecular genetics demonstrate that HCM is a heterogeneous disease of the sarcomere with many mutations, most commonly involving the beta-myosin heavy chain.
- The prevalence is 1 in 500; the mortality rate is 1% overall, but 4% to 6% in childhood and adolescence.

CLINICAL FEATURES

- Symptom severity progresses with age.
- Dyspnea on exertion is the most common symptom, followed by angina-like chest pain, palpitations, and syncope.
- Patients may be aware of forceful ventricular contractions and call these palpitations.
- Physical examination may reveal a fourth heart sound (S4), hyperdynamic apical impulse, a precordial lift, and a systolic ejection murmur best heard at the lower left sternal border or apex.
- The murmur may be increased with Valsalva maneuver or standing after squatting. The murmur can be decreased by squatting, forceful hand gripping,

or passive leg elevation with the patient supine (see Chapter 25 for contrasting murmurs).

DIAGNOSIS AND DIFFERENTIAL

- The ECG demonstrates left ventricular hypertrophy in 30% of patients and left atrial enlargement in 25% to 50%. Large septal Q waves (> 0.3 mV) are present in 25%. Another ECG finding is upright T waves in those leads with QS or QR complexes (T-wave inversion in those leads would suggest ischemia).
- Chest x-ray is usually normal. Echocardiography is the diagnostic study of choice, and will demonstrate disproportionate septal hypertrophy.

EMERGENCY DEPARTMENT CARE AND DISPOSITION

- Symptoms of HCM may mimic ischemic heart disease and treatment of those symptoms is covered in Chapter 20. Otherwise, general supportive care is indicated. Patients who present complaining of exercise intolerance or chest pain in whom the typical murmur of HCM is heard should be referred for echocardiographic evaluation. β-blockers are the mainstay of treatment for patients with HCM and chest pain.
- Patients should be discouraged from engaging in vigorous exercise. Those with suspected HCM who have syncope should be hospitalized.

■ RESTRICTIVE CARDIOMYOPATHY

EPIDEMIOLOGY AND PATHOPHYSIOLOGY

- *Restrictive cardiomyopathy* is heart muscle disease that results in restricted ventricular filling, with normal or decreased diastolic volume of one or both ventricles.
- Most causes are idiopathic, but systemic disorders have been implicated, including amyloidosis, sarcoidosis, hemochromatosis, scleroderma, carcinoid, hypereosinophilic syndrome, and endomyocardial fibrosis. The idiopathic form is sometimes familial.
- Systolic function is usually normal, and ventricular wall thickness may be normal or increased, depending on the underlying cause.
- The hemodynamic hallmarks include: (1) elevated LV and RV end-diastolic pressure, (2) normal LV systolic function (ejection fraction >50%), and (3) a marked decrease followed by a rapid rise and plateau in early-diastolic ventricular pressure.
- The rapid rise and abrupt plateau in the early diastolic ventricular pressure trace produce a characteristic "square-root sign" or "dip-and-plateau" filling pattern.
- This filling pattern may also be seen in constrictive pericarditis, with which restrictive cardiomyopathy is commonly confused. Differentiation between the two is critical because constrictive pericarditis can be cured surgically.
- The diagnosis of restrictive cardiomyopathy should be considered in a patient presenting with CHF but no evidence of cardiomegaly or systolic dysfunction.

CLINICAL FEATURES

- Symptoms of CHF predominate, including dyspnea, orthopnea, and pedal edema. Chest pain is uncommon.
- Physical examination may reveal an S_3 or S_4 cardiac gallop, pulmonary rales, jugular venous distension, Kussmaul's sign (inspiratory jugular venous distension), hepatomegaly, pedal edema, and ascites.

DIAGNOSIS AND DIFFERENTIAL

- Chest x-ray may show signs of CHF without cardiomegaly.
- Nonspecific ECG changes are most likely. However, in cases of amyloidosis or sarcoidosis, conduction disturbances and low-voltage QRS complexes are common.
- Differential diagnosis includes constrictive pericarditis and diastolic left ventricular dysfunction (most commonly due to ischemic or hypertensive heart disease). Differentiating between restrictive cardiomyopathy and constrictive pericarditis is critical, because constrictive pericarditis can be cured surgically.
- Doppler echocardiographic studies and cardiac catheterization with hemodynamic assessment are often required for specific diagnosis. CT and MRI of the heart can differentiate constrictive pericarditis from restrictive cardiomyopathy.

EMERGENCY DEPARTMENT CARE AND DISPOSITION

- Treatment is symptom-directed with the use of diuretics and ACE inhibitors.
- Corticosteroid therapy is indicated for sarcoidosis. Chelation is used for the treatment of hemochromatosis.
- Admission is determined by the severity of the symptoms and the availability of prompt subspecialty follow-up.

ACUTE PERICARDITIS

PATHOPHYSIOLOGY

- The pericardium consists of a loose fibrous membrane (visceral pericardium) overlying the epicardium, and a dense collagenous sac (parietal pericardium) surrounding the heart. The space between these layers may contain up to 50 mL of fluid under normal conditions. Intrapericardial pressure is usually subatmospheric.
- Inflammation of the pericardium may be the result of viral infection (eg, coxsackie virus, echovirus, HIV), bacterial infection (eg, *Staphylococcus, Streptococcus pneumoniae,* beta-hemolytic *Streptococcus, Mycobacterium tuberculosis*), fungal infection (eg, *Histoplasma capsulatum*), malignancy (leukemia, lymphoma, melanoma, metastatic breast cancer), drugs (procainamide and hydralazine), radiation, connective tissue disease, uremia, myxedema, postmyocardial infarction (Dressler's syndrome), or may be idiopathic.

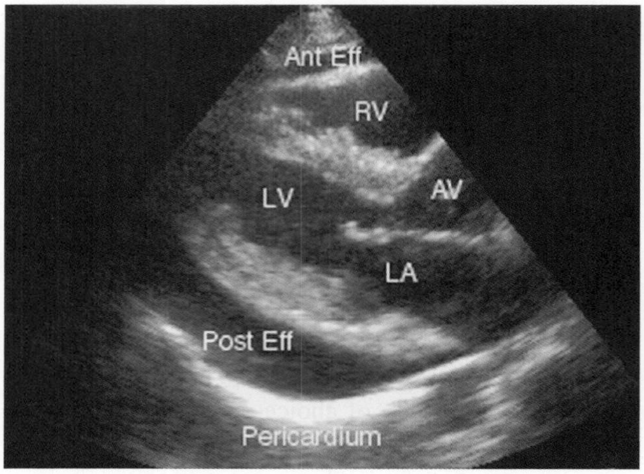

FIG. 26-1. Pericardial effusion on parasternal long-axis view. Ant Eff = anterior effusion; AV = aortic valve; LA = left atrium; LV = left ventricle; Post Eff = posterior effusion; RV = right ventricle. (Reprinted with permission from Reardon RF, Joing SA: Cardiac. In: Ma OJ, Mateer JR, Blaivas M. eds. *Emergency Ultrasound,* 2nd edition. The McGraw-Hill Companies, Inc., all rights reserved. Figure 6-24A. 2008.)

CLINICAL FEATURES

- The most common symptom is sudden or gradual onset of sharp or stabbing chest pain that radiates to the back, neck, left shoulder, or arm. Radiation to the left trapezial ridge (due to inflammation of the adjoining diaphragmatic pleura) is particularly distinguishing.
- The pain may be aggravated by movement or inspiration. Typically, chest pain is made most severe by lying supine and is often relieved by sitting up and leaning forward.
- Associated symptoms include low-grade intermittent fever, dyspnea, and dysphagia.
- A transient, intermittent friction rub heard best at the lower left sternal border or apex is the most common physical finding. This rub is characteristically transient (eg, heard one hour and not the next).

DIAGNOSIS AND DIFFERENTIAL

- ECG changes of acute pericarditis and its convalescence have been divided into four stages. During stage 1, or the acute phase, there is ST-segment elevation in leads I, V_5, and V_6, with PR-segment depression in leads II, aVF, and V_4 through V_6. As the disease resolves (stage 2), the ST segment normalizes and T-wave amplitude decreases. In stage 3, inverted T waves appear in leads previously showing ST elevations. The final phase, stage 4, is characterized by the resolution of repolarization abnormalities and a return to a normal ECG.
- When sequential ECGs are not available, it can be difficult to distinguish pericarditis from the normal variant with "early repolarization." In these cases, a simple criterion offers considerable diagnostic utility: an ST segment: T-wave amplitude ratio greater than 0.25 in leads I, V_5, or V_6 is indicative of acute pericarditis.
- Pericarditis without other underlying cardiac disease does not typically produce dysrhythmias.
- Chest x-ray is of limited value. It is usually normal, but should be done to rule out other disease.
- Echocardiography is the best diagnostic test (Fig. 26-1) to assess for pericardial effusion.
- Other tests that may be of value in establishing etiologic diagnosis include complete blood cell count with differential, blood urea nitrogen and creatinine levels (to rule out uremia), streptococcal serology, appropriate viral serology, other serology (eg, antinuclear and anti-DNA antibodies), thyroid function studies, erythrocyte sedimentation rate, and creatinine kinase levels with isoenzymes (to assess for myocarditis).

EMERGENCY DEPARTMENT CARE AND DISPOSITION

- Patients with idiopathic or presumed viral etiologies are treated as outpatients with nonsteroidal anti-inflammatory agents (eg, ibuprofen 400-600 milligrams orally four times daily) for 1 to 3 weeks.

- Patients should be treated for a specific cause if one is identified.
- Indicators of a poor prognosis include: temperature >38°C (100.4°F), subacute onset over weeks, immunosuppression, history of oral anticoagulant use, associated myocarditis (elevated cardiac biomarkers, symptoms of CHF), and a large pericardial effusion (an echo-free space >20 mm).
- In general, patients with these risk factors or with an enlarged cardiac silhouette on chest radiograph should be admitted for early echocardiography and monitoring.

NONTRAUMATIC CARDIAC TAMPONADE

PATHOPHYSIOLOGY

- Tamponade occurs when the pressure in the pericardial sac exceeds the normal filling pressure of the right ventricle, resulting in restricted filling and decreased cardiac output.
- Causes include metastatic malignancy, uremia, hemorrhage (over-anticoagulation), idiopathic disorders, bacterial or tubercular disorders, chronic pericarditis, and others (eg, systemic lupus erythematosus, postradiation, myxedema).

CLINICAL FEATURES

- The most common complaints are dyspnea and decreased exercise tolerance. Other nonspecific symptoms include weight loss, pedal edema, and ascites.
- Physical findings include tachycardia, low systolic blood pressure, and a narrow pulse pressure. Pulsus paradoxus (apparent dropped beats in the peripheral pulse during inspiration), neck vein distension, distant heart sounds, and right upper quadrant pain (due to hepatic congestion) may also be present. Pulmonary rales are usually absent.

DIAGNOSIS AND DIFFERENTIAL

- Low-voltage QRS complexes and ST-segment elevation with PR-segment depression may be present on the ECG. Electrical alternans (beat-to-beat variability in the amplitude of the P and R waves unrelated to inspiratory cycle) is a classic but uncommon finding (about 20% of cases). Chest x-ray may or may not reveal an enlarged cardiac silhouette. Echocardiography is the diagnostic test of choice.

EMERGENCY DEPARTMENT CARE AND DISPOSITION

- An intravenous fluid bolus of 500 to 1000 mL of normal saline will increase intravascular volume, facilitate right heart filling, and increase cardiac output and arterial pressure. However, it is a temporary measure.
- Pericardiocentesis is both therapeutic and diagnostic. This procedure is optimally performed in the cardiac catheterization laboratory using echocardiographic guidance to avoid cardiac perforation and coronary artery laceration. In addition, a pigtail catheter can be inserted to allow continuous fluid drainage and prevention of re-accumulation.
- If there is hemodynamic instability, emergency pericardiocentesis is indicated in the ED.
- These patients require admission to an intensive care unit or monitored setting.

CONSTRICTIVE PERICARDITIS

PATHOPHYSIOLOGY

- Constriction occurs when fibrous thickening and loss of elasticity of the pericardium results in interference with diastolic filling. Cardiac trauma, pericardiotomy (open-heart surgery), intrapericardial hemorrhage, fungal or bacterial pericarditis, and uremic pericarditis are the most common causes.

CLINICAL FEATURES

- Symptoms develop gradually and mimic those of restrictive cardiomyopathy, including CHF, exertional dyspnea, and decreased exercise tolerance. Chest pain, orthopnea, and paroxysmal nocturnal dyspnea are uncommon.
- On physical examination, patients may have pedal edema, hepatomegaly, ascites, jugular venous distension, and Kussmaul's sign. A pericardial "knock" (an early diastolic sound) may be heard at the apex. There is usually no friction rub.

DIAGNOSIS AND DIFFERENTIAL

- The ECG is not usually helpful, but may show low-voltage QRS complexes and inverted T waves.
- Pericardial calcification is seen in up to 50% of patients on the lateral chest x-ray, but is not diagnostic of constrictive pericarditis.
- Doppler echocardiography, cardiac CT, and MRI are diagnostic.

- Other diseases that should be considered include acute pericarditis or myocarditis, exacerbation of chronic ventricular dysfunction, or a systemic process resulting in decreased cardiac performance (eg, sepsis).

EMERGENCY DEPARTMENT CARE AND DISPOSITION

- General supportive care is the initial treatment. Symptomatic patients will require hospitalization and pericardiectomy.

For further reading in *Emergency Medicine: A Comprehensive Study Guide*, 7th edition., see Chapter 55, "The Cardiomyopathies, Myocarditis, and Pericardial Disease," by James T. Niemann.

27 THROMBOEMBOLISM

Christopher Kabrhel

EPIDEMIOLOGY

- Venous thromboembolism (VTE) includes two main disease entities: deep vein thrombosis (DVT) and pulmonary embolism (PE).
- There are approximately 2 million cases of VTE diagnosed in the United States every year.
- Between 1 to 2/1000 emergency department (ED) patients are diagnosed with PE annually.
- PE is the third most common cause of cardiovascular death in the United States, with an annual incidence similar to stroke. However, approximately 18 ED patients are evaluated for possible PE for every PE diagnosed, making negative workups for PE extremely common.
- Major risk factors for VTE include advanced age (>50 years), venous stasis, hypercoagulable states, and endothelial injury (Table 27-1).
- Venous stasis may result from general immobility (eg, obesity, sedentary lifestyle, neurologic disorders, debilitating illness, general anesthesia) or limb immobility (eg, trauma, surgery, neurologic paralysis).
- Hypercoagulable states may be inherited (eg, factor V Leiden, prothrombin 20210A mutation, protein C or S deficiency) or acquired (eg, malignancy, pregnancy, estrogen use, antiphospholipid antibody syndrome).
- Endothelial injury may be a result of trauma, surgery, vascular access, indwelling catheters, or prior deep venous thrombosis (DVT).

TABLE 27-1 Risk Factors for Venous Thromboembolism (VTE) that are Generally Relevant to Emergency Medicine

FACTOR	COMMENT
Age	Risk becomes significant at 50 y and increases with each year of life until age 80 y.
Obesity	Risk starts at BMI >35 kg/m^2 and increases with increasing BMI.
Pregnancy	Risk increases with trimester (but overall risk remains low throughout pregnancy).
Solid cancers	Risk greatest with adenocarcinomas and metastatic disease. A history of remote, inactive cancer probably does not increase risk.
Hematologic cancers	Acute leukemias confer the greatest risk.
Inherited thrombophilia	Factor V Leiden and familial protein C deficiency have the strongest risk.
Recent surgery or major trauma	Risk continues at least 4 wk postoperatively or after trauma intensive care.
Immobility	Acute limb immobility confers the highest risk.
Bed rest	Becomes a risk factor at approximately 72 h.
Indwelling catheters	Cause approximately one half of arm deep venous thromboses.
Long-distance travel	Published data are controversial.
Smoking	Not a risk factor itself, but may increase risk of other factors such as oral contraceptives.
Congestive heart failure	Related primarily to severity of systolic dysfunction.
Stroke	Risk greatest in first month after deficit.
Estrogen	All contraceptives containing estrogen increase risk of VTE.
Noninfectious inflammatory conditions	Examples are inflammatory bowel disease, lupus, nephrotic syndrome. Risk of VTE increases roughly in proportion to severity of underlying disease.

Abbreviation: BMI = body mass index.

PATHOPHYSIOLOGY

DEEP VEIN THROMBOSIS

- DVT forms most commonly at the venous cusps of deep veins and at sites of endothelial injury, though

DVT may also propagate from thrombosed superficial veins. Thromboses are composed mostly of erythrocytes, fibrin, and platelets.
- The majority (90%) of DVT occur in the lower extremities, though thrombosis of the upper extremities can also occur, especially in the presence of indwelling venous catheters.
- DVT may propagate, dissolve, or embolize, depending on the balance between thrombogenesis and thrombolysis.
- Most (80%) symptomatic DVT will be located in or proximal to the popliteal vein, though 20% of isolated calf DVT will extend proximally within a week of diagnosis.
- Proximal DVTs are more likely to cause PE than distal DVT.

PULMONARY EMBOLISM

- PE occurs when a portion of a venous clot breaks off, traverses the right ventricle, and lodges in a pulmonary artery.
- The pathophysiologic effects of PE are the result of mechanical obstruction of right ventricular outflow and the release of inflammatory mediators from thrombus in the pulmonary vasculature.
- Depending on the degree of mechanical obstruction, PE may cause minimal symptoms, tachycardia, right heart failure, or complete cardiovascular collapse.
- The mechanism of the dyspnea and hypoxia in PE is unclear and unpredictable. It is likely related to V/Q mismatch caused by vasoactive mediators combined with the relative shunting of blood away from oxygenated alveoli.

CLINICAL FEATURES

DEEP VEIN THROMBOSIS

- The classic symptoms of DVT include calf or leg pain, redness, swelling, tenderness, and warmth. Unfortunately, fewer than 50% of patients with confirmed lower extremity DVT present with these symptoms, making the clinical examination for DVT challenging.
- The signs and symptoms of DVT may also be seen with cellulitis, congestive heart failure, venous stasis without thrombosis, ruptured Baker's cysts, and musculoskeletal injuries. DVT may also coexist with these entities. Thus, ruling out DVT without diagnostic testing can be challenging.
- Homans' sign, pain in the calf with forced dorsiflexion of the ankle with the leg straight, is unreliable for DVT.
- Uncommon but severe presentations of DVT include *phlegmasia cerulea dolens* and *phlegmasia alba dolens.*
- *Phlegmasia cerulea dolens* is a high-grade obstruction that elevates compartment pressures and can compromise limb perfusion. It presents as a massively swollen, cyanotic limb.
- *Phlegmasia alba dolens* is usually associated with pregnancy and has a similar pathophysiology but presents as a pale limb secondary to arterial spasm.

PULMONARY EMBOLISM

- The clinical presentation of PE varies considerably. Patients with similar co-morbidities and clot burden can present very differently.
- PE should be suspected in patients with dyspnea unexplained by findings on auscultation, ECG, or chest x-ray.
- Common symptoms include dyspnea (the most common symptom, seen in 75% of PE patients) and chest pain (the second most common symptom, seen in 50% of PE patients). Chest pain may be pleuritic (worse with breathing or coughing). Other symptoms include cough, syncope, palpitations, and anxiety.
- Approximately 30% of patients with demonstrated DVT, but no symptoms of PE, will have subclinical PE found upon further study.
- Common signs include tachypnea, tachycardia, hypoxemia (S_aO_2 <95% on room air), hemoptysis, diaphoresis, and fever (>38°C).
- Signs of DVT (calf pain, tenderness, swelling, erythema) occur in about 50% of patients. DVT is diagnosed in only 40% of ambulatory patients with demonstrated PE.
- Massive PE results in hypotension and severe hypoxia. Cardiac arrest occurs in about 2% of diagnosed PE, though it is estimated that 20% to 25% of sudden cardiac death may be secondary to PE.

DIAGNOSIS AND DIFFERENTIAL

PRETEST PROBABILITY ASSESSMENT

- Estimating the patient's pretest probability for VTE is the first step in selecting a diagnostic pathway. The importance of determining the pretest probability should not be underestimated.
- Pretest probability can be subjectively determined by the clinician, though accuracy requires experience. Alternatively, clinical scores that incorporate symptoms, signs, and risk factors can group patients into low, intermediate, and high probability categories.

TABLE 27-2 Wells Score for Deep Vein Thrombosis

PREDICTOR OF DEEP VEIN THROMBOSIS:	POINTS*
Active cancer	1
Paralysis or immobilization of lower extremity	1
Bed ridden (>3 days) after recent surgery	1
Tenderness along distribution of deep veins	1
Swelling of entire leg	1
Unilateral calf swelling of (>3 cm)	1
Unilateral pitting edema of leg	1
Collateral superficial veins	1
Alternative diagnosis as or more likely than DVT	−2

*Risk score interpretation (probability of deep venous thrombosis): ≥3 points: high risk (75%); 1 or 2 points: moderate risk (17%); <1 point: low risk (3%).

TABLE 27-4 Wells Score for Pulmonary Embolism (PE)

OBJECTIVE CRITERIA	POINTS	SUBJECTIVE CRITERIA	POINTS
Heart rate >100 beats/min	1.5	Clinician considers alternative diagnosis to be less likely than PE	3
Hemoptysis	1		
History of thromboembolism	1.5		
Malignancy (active)	1		
Leg swelling, pain with palpation of deep veins (clinical signs of DVT)	3		
Immobilization within prior 4 weeks	1.5		

Risk score interpretation (probability of PE): >6 points: high risk (78.4%); 2-6 points: moderate risk (27.8%); <2 points: low risk (3.4%).

Deep Vein Thrombosis

- Decision instruments, such as the scoring system developed by Wells and colleagues, have been developed to categorize patients as having low, moderate, or high probability of DVT before diagnostic testing (Table 27-2). The system is scored as follows: a score of 3 or more represents high probability; a score of 1 to 2 corresponds to moderate probability; and a 0 score indicates low probability.

Pulmonary Embolism

- The pulmonary embolism rule-out criteria (PERC Rule) can be used to define a group of patients whose probability of PE is below the test threshold (ie, the risk of testing outweighs the risk of a missed PE) (see Table 27-3). When combined with a low clinical probability, a negative PERC rule reduces the likelihood of PE to about 1%. These patients need not undergo objective testing (eg, d-dimer) for PE.

TABLE 27-3 Pulmonary Embolism Rule-Out Criteria (PERC Rule)

Age <50
Pulse oximetry >94% (breathing room air)
Heart rate <100 beats/min
No prior venous thromboembolism
No recent surgery or trauma (requiring hospitalization, intubation, or epidural anesthesia within 4 wk prior)
No hemoptysis
No estrogen use
No unilateral leg swelling

- For patients with non-low clinical probability or a positive PERC Rule, the pretest probability of PE guides the clinician's choice of diagnostic modality and helps determine when it is safe to terminate ancillary testing.
- For an experienced clinician, clinical gestalt and published clinical decision rules have similar accuracy for defining the pretest probability of PE. The PE scoring system developed by Wells is well validated and can categorize patients as having low, moderate, or high probability of PE (Table 27-4). The system is scored as follows: a score of 6 or more represents high probability; a score of 2 to 6 corresponds to moderate probability; and less than 2 score indicates low probability. A modified Wells score can also be used, with a score of greater than 4 defining high probability, and a score of less than or equal to 4 defining low probability.

ANCILLARY TESTING

Deep Vein Thrombosis

- Quantitative d-dimer assays are highly sensitive for DVT. Patients with a low pretest probability (eg, Wells DVT score ≤1) can be safely considered to be without DVT if the d-dimer result is negative. Patients with a positive d-dimer result should undergo venous ultrasound in the ED to rule out DVT.
- Diagnostic algorithms can help guide appropriate diagnostic testing for DVT, though it is important to acknowledge that no diagnostic algorithm is perfect (see Fig. 27-1).

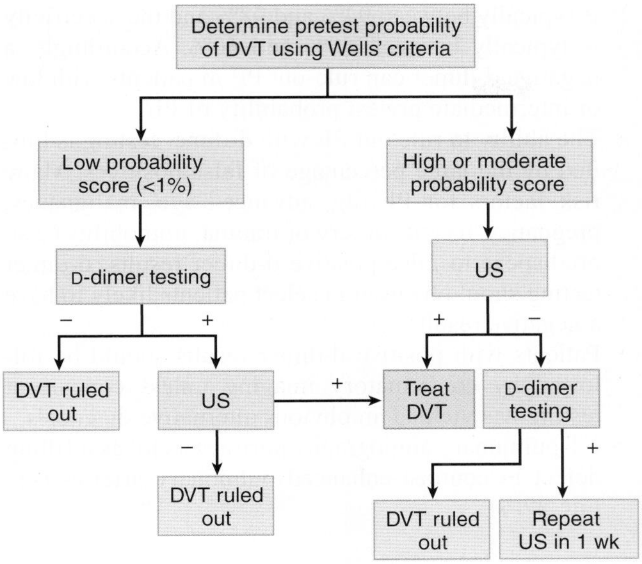

FIG. 27-1. Diagnostic algorithm for deep venous thrombosis (DVT). This algorithm is to be applied in patients with leg symptoms compatible with DVT + = positive test result; – = negative test result.

- Venous ultrasonography is the imaging test of choice for evaluating DVT in the ED. Duplex ultrasonography (real time B-mode imaging combined with Doppler flow imaging) has high sensitivity (97%) and specificity (94%) for lower extremity DVT. Sensitivity is lower for pelvic and isolated calf DVT (73%), and for upper extremity DVT (56%–100%).
- For patients with moderate or high pretest probability for DVT, both venous ultrasound and d-dimer testing should be performed.

If both tests are negative, DVT can be considered ruled-out in the ED, with no further testing necessary.

- If the ultrasound is negative but d-dimer is positive, a repeat ultrasound should be scheduled for a week later. Two negative duplex scans 1 week apart translate into a risk of <1%, for DVT or PE within 3 months. Several studies have demonstrated the safety of withholding anticoagulation pending repeat evaluation.
- A positive ultrasound confirms the diagnosis of DVT (Fig. 27-2).
- The traditional gold standard for DVT is contrast venography. However, the technique is invasive and impractical, and thus rarely performed. Other tests, such as CT and MRI venography, may be useful in diagnosing DVT when ultrasound cannot be performed, or when pelvic vein thrombosis is suspected. However, the diagnostic accuracy of these tests is not well defined, and availability in the ED may be limited.

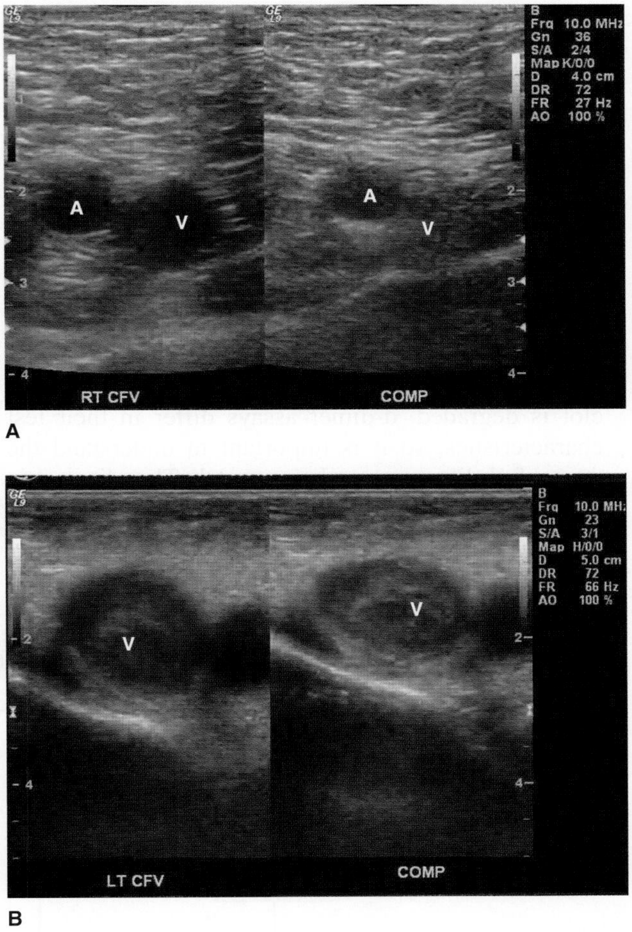

FIG. 27-2. Compression venous US images showing normal findings and findings indicating deep venous thrombosis. **A.** Compression venous US of the common femoral vein and femoral artery. The left view shows a sonographic image of the right femoral artery (**A**) and common femoral vein (V) obtained immediately inferior to the inguinal ligament. The image on the right shows the same view after manual compression by the operator. The image demonstrates obliteration of the vein while the artery remains open. This is a normal US finding for the vein. **B**. Venous US image showing evidence of common left femoral vein thrombosis after compression (right panel). The common femoral vein (V) does not compress. Echogenic thrombolytic material can be observed within the vein.

Pulmonary Embolism

- Most patients presenting with symptoms/signs suggestive of PE will undergo basic cardiopulmonary testing including electrocardiography (ECG), pulse oximetry, and chest radiography. However, these tests are insensitive and nonspecific for PE.
- The classic EKG findings of an S wave in lead I, a Q wave in lead III, and T-wave inversions in lead III ($S_1Q_3T_3$) are seen in a minority of PE patients.

- Chest radiographs are typically normal or nonspecific in PE. Classically described findings such as Westermark's sign and Hampton's hump are infrequently seen.
- Arterial blood gas testing (ABG) cannot be used alone to diagnose or exclude PE. The sensitivity of an abnormal P_aO_2 or A-a gradient for PE is about 90%; specificity of either of these findings is only 15%.
- Diagnostic algorithms can help guide appropriate diagnostic imaging for PE, though it is important to acknowledge that no diagnostic algorithm is perfect (Fig. 27-3).
- d-dimer testing is an important adjunct in exclusion of PE. d-dimers are released into the blood as fibrin clot is degraded. d-dimer assays differ in their test characteristics, so it is important to understand the type of d-dimer assay being used. The diagnostic sensitivity of automated quantitative d-dimer assays is typically between 94% and 98% and the specificity is typically between 50% and 60%. Accordingly, a negative d-dimer can rule-out PE in patients with low or intermediate pretest probability of PE.
- The ability to rule out PE with d-dimer testing is limited by the large percentage of false positives. Many risk factors for PE (eg, advanced age, malignancy, pregnancy, recent surgery or trauma, immobility) also predispose to false positive d-dimer results. d-dimer testing should be used in select patients likely to have a negative result.
- Patients with positive d-dimer results should be followed by confirmatory imaging unless concurrent testing has yielded an obvious alternative diagnosis.
- CT pulmonary angiography portrays a clot as a filling defect in contrast-enhanced pulmonary arteries (see Fig. 27-4).

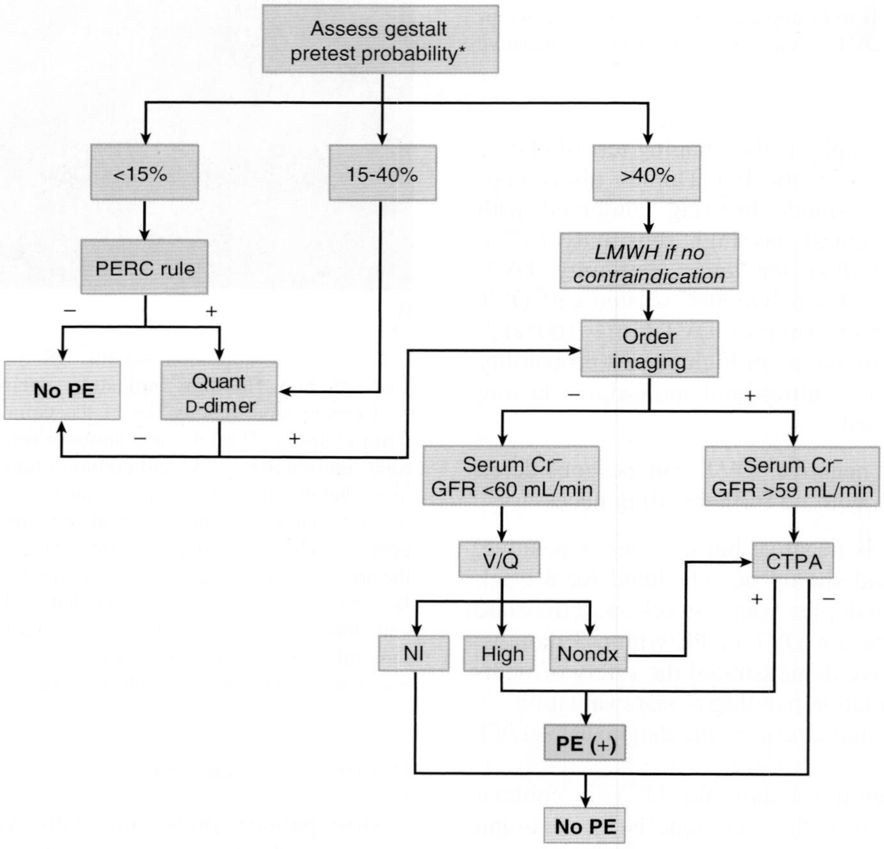

FIG. 27-3. Charlotte diagnostic algorithm for pulmonary embolism (PE). *Some physicians prefer to start with a clinical decision rule such as the Wells score (where <2, 2-6, and >6 are used instead of <15%, 15%-40%, and >40%, respectively). Note: Renal function should be determined by clinical picture (healthy, no risk factors for reduced glomerular filtration rate [GFR]) or calculated using known formulas. Nondiagnostic ventilation–perfusion (V/Q) scan findings require confirmation from results of another test, such as CT pulmonary angiography (CTPA), if benefits outweigh risks. + = positive for PE; – = negative for PE; Cr = creatinine; high = high probability scan findings; LMWH = low-molecular-weight heparin; Nl = normal; Nondx = nondiagnostic (any reading other than normal or high probability); PERC = pulmonary embolism rule-out criteria; quant = quantitative.

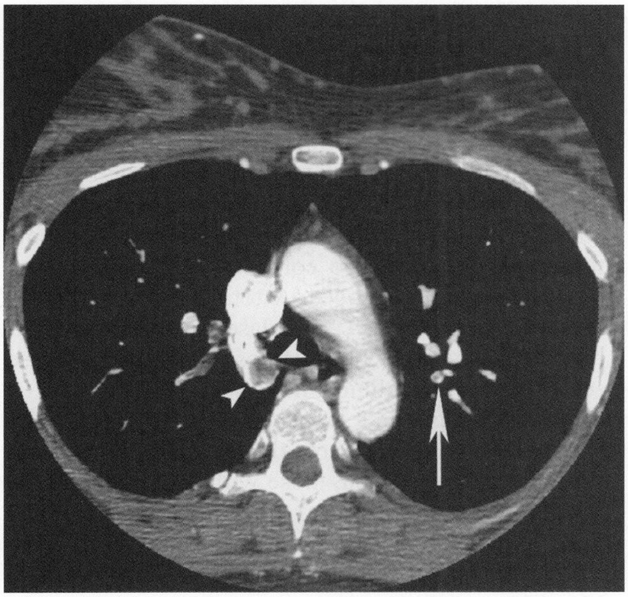

FIG. 27-4. Axial image from a chest CT angiogram demonstrating a filling defect consistent with acute pulmonary embolism. Two white arrowheads outline a circular filling defect in the right middle lobar pulmonary artery. The long white arrow projecting in the left lung points to a filling defect in a segmental artery in the posterior medial segmental artery.

- Images are obtained in 1.25 to 3.0-mm slices from the diaphragm to the apex of the lung.
- This may be followed by indirect venography to evaluate the lower extremity vasculature.
- The diagnostic sensitivity and specificity of a technically adequate CT scan, performed on a multidetector CT scanner in an ED population independently of pretest probability, is about 85% to 90%.
- CT pulmonary angiography has the advantage of demonstrating alternative diagnoses in about 20% of studies in which no PE is found.
- CT pulmonary angiography carries risks of radiation exposure, anaphylactoid reactions to contrast dye, and contrast-induced nephropathy; it is contraindicated in patients with impaired renal function.
- Ventilation-perfusion (V/Q) scanning compares the density of scintillations emitted from radionucleotides injected during a perfusion phase to those inspired during a ventilation phase.
- A V/Q scan that demonstrates homogeneous scintillation throughout the lung in the perfusion portion has nearly 100% accuracy for ruling out PE, regardless of the appearance of the ventilation portion.
- A V/Q scan that demonstrates two or more apex central wedge-shaped defects in the perfusion phase with normal ventilation in these regions indicates >80% probability of PE.
- All other V/Q scan findings are nondiagnostic.
- Catheter-based pulmonary angiography is the traditional gold-standard diagnostic test for PE, but this test requires expertise and carries risks associated with contrast and radiation exposure, dysrhythmias, and pulmonary artery perforation. It has been largely supplanted by CT pulmonary angiography.
- Lower extremity venous ultrasound can be accomplished at the bedside and without ionizing radiation. However, venous US has a sensitivity of only 40% as a surrogate method to diagnose PE. Venous ultrasound can be a useful adjunct in patients with symptoms/signs of PE who have contraindications to CT pulmonary angiography (eg, pregnancy, renal insufficiency).
- PE remains a common cause of pregnancy-related mortality and special consideration should be given to the evaluation of PE in these patients.
- For pregnant patients undergoing V/Q scanning, Foley catheter placement and IV hydration can reduce fetal exposure to ionizing radiation.
- In the case of a normal perfusion scan, the ventilation phase of the study can be avoided, thus limiting radiation exposure.
- For pregnant patients undergoing CT scanning, lead shielding may decrease fetal radiation exposure.
- With appropriate precautions in place, V/Q and CT probably expose the fetus to similarly low levels of ionizing radiation and should be considered safe techniques.

EMERGENCY DEPARTMENT CARE AND DISPOSITION

BASIC ED CARE

- As always, attention to airway stabilization, respiratory and circulatory support is paramount. Administer crystalloid IV fluids to augment preload and correct hypotension. Administer oxygen as necessary to correct hypoxia secondary to PE.

ANTICOAGULATION

- The specific objectives in treating VTE are to eliminate the clot burden and prevent recurrent thrombosis and embolization.
- Anticoagulation with a form of heparin is standard ED treatment for most cases of VTE. Heparin therapy inhibits thrombin and prevents thrombus extension. Heparin has no intrinsic thrombolytic activity, but by allowing unopposed action of plasmin, it accelerates clot removal over 48 to 72 hours.

- Low molecular weight heparins (LMWH) are safe and effective for the treatment of DVT. The three most commonly used LMWHs are dalteparin (200 units/kg subcutaneously every 24 hours, maximum 18,000 units), enoxaparin (1.5 milligrams/kg subcutaneously every 24 hours, maximum 180 milligrams), and tinzaparin (175 units/kg subcutaneously every 24 hours, maximum 18,000 units).
- There are no treatment guidelines for thromboses isolated to the calf veins (soleal or gastrocnemius) or the saphenous vein. Isolated calf vein thrombosis has been reported to have varying risk levels of PE; estimates for PE development in these cases range from 0.3% to 8.0%. Options include no acute treatment with repeat US in a week to identify progression of clot, and outpatient treatment with LMWH.
- Systematic reviews also favor the use of LMWH over unfractionated heparin (UFH) for treatment of PE, although the magnitude of benefit is not large. However, LMWH should be avoided in severe renal insufficiency and when absorption may be unreliable (eg, obesity).
- When UFH is used, dosing should be weight based, with 80 units/kg given as an initial bolus followed by 18 units/kg/h. The activated partial thromboplastin time (aPTT) should be maintained between 55 and 80 seconds (1.5-2.5 times normal). Traditional dosing using a 5000-units bolus and 1000 units/h infusion will underdose two-thirds of patients.
- There are few absolute contraindications to anticoagulation with heparin for acute VTE, though patients with recent intracranial hemorrhage or active gastrointestinal hemorrhage may have anticoagulation withheld.
- For patients with documented heparin-induced thrombocytopenia (HIT), a direct thrombin inhibitor or factor Xa inhibitor may be considered.
- Oral anticoagulation with warfarin can be initiated simultaneously with heparin therapy. However, because of a transient hypercoagulable state caused by a relative deficiency in protein C in the first days of warfarin therapy, treatment should always be accompanied by heparin anticoagulation. Initial dosing of warfarin is usually 5 milligrams/day with a target INR of 2 to 3. Anticoagulation is typically continued for 3 to 6 months, but may be life-long in patients with persistent risk factors. Warfarin is absolutely contraindicated in pregnancy.

THROMBOLYSIS

- Thrombolytic therapy should be considered for patients who require more aggressive treatment for VTE.
- For DVT, there is no evidence showing a survival benefit of thrombolytic therapy over heparin and warfarin.
- DVT that causes phlegmasia can lead to loss of limb. In these cases, catheter-directed thrombolysis should be discussed with an interventional radiologist or vascular surgeon. If no such service is available, and emergency transfer cannot be arranged, systemic thrombolysis should be considered if there are no absolute contraindications. A total IV dose of 50 to 100 milligrams of tPA (alteplase) infused over four hours is suggested, with this dosing based upon case series and limited clinical trials.
- Patients who might realize substantial benefit from active thrombolysis are those with significant iliofemoral clot burden, those with acute phlegmasia (symptom onset <10 days) requiring aggressive and urgent intervention to decrease compartment pressures, and patients with occluded veins as a result of May-Thurner (iliac vein compression) syndrome.
- Currently, the only patients with a demonstrated mortality benefit from thrombolytic therapy are those with massive PE, defined as a large PE associated with hemodynamic instability.
- Thrombolysis also does not appear to reduce mortality in submassive PE, defined as near-normal blood pressure with other evidence of cardiovascular strain (eg, echocardiographic evidence of right ventricular dysfunction, positive troponin, elevated brain natriuretic peptide). However, these patients may benefit from thrombolytic therapy in terms of functional capacity and quality of life.
- Best-evidence practice is consideration of systemic fibrinolysis only in the following carefully selected patients as long as there is no increased risk of bleeding: patients with cardiac arrest at any point; patients with arterial hypotension and massive PE; patients with respiratory failure, evidenced by severe hypoxemia despite oxygen administration together with evidence of increased work of breathing; and patients with evidence of right-sided heart strain on echocardiography or elevated levels of troponin.
- The FDA has approved three regimens for treatment of PE: streptokinase, urokinase, and tissue plasminogen activator (tPA). The recommended dosage of tPA, or alteplase, for PE is 100 milligrams infused over 2 hours. However, in emergent cases where a 2-hour infusion is impractical, 100 milligrams of tPA may be given as an off-label bolus over 10 to 15 minutes.

ADJECTIVE THERAPY

- An inferior vena cava filter can be placed to prevent PE when anticoagulation is contraindicated, a major complication occurs, or when DVT continues to propagate despite adequate anticoagulation.

- Surgical or catheter-based thrombectomy may be considered for patients with severe VTE (massive PE or DVT with persistently ischemic limb secondary to *phlegmasia cerulea dolens*). This procedure is typically only available in specialized centers.

DISPOSITION

- Outpatient treatment of DVT is favored over inpatient treatment if the patient does not have complicating factors favoring admission. Admission should be considered in patients with: extensive iliofemoral thrombosis, increased risk of bleeding, limited cardiorespiratory reserve, risk of poor compliance with home therapy, a contraindication to use of LMWH, a high suspicion of HIT, or renal insufficiency.
- Stable patients with PE can be admitted to a telemetry bed. Patients who exhibit signs of circulatory compromise and all patients who receive thrombolytic therapy should be admitted to an intensive care unit.

For further reading in Tintinalli's *Emergency Medicine: A Comprehensive Study Guide*, 7th ed., see Chapter 60, "Thromboembolism," by Jeffrey A. Kline.

28 SYSTEMIC AND PULMONARY HYPERTENSION

David M. Cline

- Classification of acute systemic hypertension into categories facilitates management.
- Hypertensive emergency: elevated blood pressure (BP) associated with target organ dysfunction such as aortic dissection, acute pulmonary edema, acute coronary syndrome, acute renal failure, severe preeclampsia, hypertensive encephalopathy, subarachnoid hemorrhage, intracranial hemorrhage, acute ischemic stroke, and sympathetic crisis.
- Immediate recognition and treatment are required for the conditions above but therapeutic goals (percentage reduction or target pressures) for hypertensive emergencies vary considerably.
- Hypertensive urgency: a clinical presentation associated with severe elevations in blood pressure without progressive target organ dysfunction. The arbitrary numerical criterion of ≥180/110 mm Hg is often cited as an indication for treatment, when in fact the clinical benefit of such treatment not well defined (see Emergency Department Care section).
- The clinician must ensure that the BP cuff size is appropriate for the patient's size; a small cuff relative to the arm size produces a falsely elevated reading.

PATHOPHYSIOLOGY

- Although poorly understood, one mechanism of severe hypertension is a sudden increase in systemic vascular resistance secondary to circulating humoral vasoconstrictors.
- There appears to be a critical arterial pressure that overwhelms the target organ's ability to compensate for the increased arterial pressure, which limits blood flow.
- These initial events trigger mechanical wall stress and endothelial injury, leading to increased permeability, activation of the coagulation cascade and platelets, and deposition of fibrin. Ultimately fibrinoid necrosis of the arterioles ensues, which potentially can be recognized clinically by hematuria (when the kidney is involved) or arterial hemorrhages or exudates on fundus examination (when the eye is involved).
- The renin-angiotensin system is activated, which leads to further vasoconstriction. Volume depletion may occur through pressure natriuresis, prompting further release of vasoconstrictors from the kidney.
- These combined effects produce hypoperfusion of the end-organs with ischemia and dysfunction.

CLINICAL FEATURES

- Essential historic features include a prior history of HTN; noncompliance with BP medications; cardiovascular, renal, or cerebrovascular disease; diabetes; hyperlipidemia; chronic obstructive pulmonary disease or asthma; and a family history of HTN.
- Precipitating causes such as pregnancy, illicit drug use (cocaine and methamphetamines), or decongestants should be considered.
- Patients should be asked about central nervous system symptoms (headaches, visual changes, weakness, seizures, and confusion), cardiovascular symptoms (chest pain, palpitations, dyspnea, syncope, pedal edema, or tearing pain radiating to the back or abdomen), and renal symptoms (anuria, edema, or hematuria).
- The patient should be examined for evidence of papilledema, retinal exudates, neurologic deficits, seizures, or encephalopathy; the presence of these findings may constitute a hypertensive emergency in the setting of elevated blood pressure.
- The patient also should be assessed for carotid bruits, heart murmurs, gallops, asymmetrical pulses

or unequal blood pressures (coarctation vs aortic dissection), pulsatile abdominal masses, and pulmonary rales.

- Hypertensive encephalopathy is characterized by altered mental status in the setting of acute hypertension, and may be accompanied by headache, vomiting, seizures, visual disturbances, papilledema, or hematuria.
- In the pregnant (or postpartum) patient, the clinician should look for hyperreflexia and peripheral edema, suggesting preeclampsia.

DIAGNOSIS AND DIFFERENTIAL

- Testing should be guiding by presenting symptoms, the most cost effective test is urinalysis.
- Renal impairment may present as hematuria, proteinuria, red cell casts, or elevations in blood urea nitrogen, creatinine, and potassium levels.
- An electrocardiogram may show ST- and T-wave changes consistent with coronary ischemia (see Chapter 20), electrolyte abnormalities, or left ventricular hypertrophy.
- A chest x-ray may help identify congestive heart failure (see Chapter 24), or aortic dissection (see Chapter 29).
- In patients with neurologic compromise, computed tomography of the head may show ischemic changes, edema, or blood (see Chapter 143).
- A urine or serum drug screen may identify illicit drug use. A pregnancy test should be done on all hypertensive women of childbearing potential.

EMERGENCY DEPARTMENT CARE AND DISPOSITION

- Patients with hypertensive emergencies require O_2 supplementation, cardiac monitoring, and intravenous access. After attention to the ABCs of resuscitation, the treatment goal is to reduce arterial pressure gradually in the following clinical situations, with attention to the therapeutic goal.

Aortic Dissection

- For aortic dissection reduce force of contraction and sheer forces first with β-blockers, reduce heart rate to approximately 60 beats per minute, reduce BP below 140 mm Hg systolic, and ideally, below 120 systolic (100-120 mm Hg) if tolerated by the patient.
- Recommended first agents include esmolol (300 micrograms/kg IV bolus followed by a 50 micrograms/kg per min infusion) or labetalol (20 milligrams IV over 2 min followed by subsequent doses of 20-40 milligrams IV g over 10 min as needed up to 300 milligrams maximum).
- If β-blockers are contraindicated, use verapamil 5 to 10 milligrams IV, or diltiazem 0.25 milligrams/kg IV over 2 minutes, to reduce heart rate. Follow β-blockers with vasodilators as needed to achieve desired blood pressure reduction.
- Nicardipine can be started by IV infusion: start at a rate of 5 milligrams/h. If target BP is not achieved in 5 to 15 minutes, increase dose by 2.5 milligrams/h every 5 to 15 minutes until target pressure or the maximum dose of 15 milligrams/h is reached.
- Alternatively, use nitroprusside IV infusion: 0.3 to 0.5 micrograms/kg/min initial infusion, increase by increments of 0.5 micrograms/kg/min; titrate to desired effect.

Acute Hypertensive Pulmonary Edema

- For acute hypertensive pulmonary edema, reduce BP by no more than 20% to 30%.
- First agent of choice is nitroglycerin, sublingual 0.4 milligrams, up to three doses, paste 1 to 2 inches, or IV infusion, start 5 micrograms/min, increase by 5 micrograms/min every 3 to 5 minutes to 20 micrograms/min; if no response at 20 micrograms/min, increase by 10 micrograms/min every 3 to 5 minutes, up to 200 micrograms/min.
- Alternatives include enalaprilat IV, 0.625 to 1.25 milligrams over 5 minutes every 4 to 6 hours, titrate at 30 minutes intervals to a maximum of 5 milligrams every 6 hours, nicardipine (see dose above) or nitroprusside (see dose above).

Acute Coronary Syndrome

- For acute coronary syndrome, if BP is above 160 mm Hg systolic, reduce BP no more than 20% acutely.
- Start with nitroglycerin (see dose above) or metoprolol 50 to 100 milligrams PO every 12 hours, or 5 milligrams IV every 5 to 15 minutes up to 15 milligrams. Avoid IV β-blockers if patient is at risk for cardiogenic shock.

Acute Sympathetic Crisis

- In acute sympathetic crisis, treat to relieve symptoms, start with benzodiazepines first.
- Follow with nitroglycerin (see dose above), or phentolamine, bolus load: 5 to 15 milligrams IV.

Acute Renal Failure

- For BP above 180/110 mm Hg, reduce BP by no more than 20% acutely.
- Recommend agents include labetalol (see dose above), nicardipine (see dose above) or fenoldopam, start

0.1 microgram/kg/min, titrate to desired effect every 15 minutes, range 0.1 to 1.6 micrograms/kg/min.

Preeclampsia

For preeclampsia with BP above 160/110 mm Hg, use labetalol (see dose above). Hydralazine, 5 to 10 milligrams IV, is less predictable, but commonly used.

Hypertensive Encephalopathy

- For BP above 180/110 (in the setting of immunosuppressive drugs, symptomatic BP may be lower), reduce BP by no more than 20% acutely.
- Recommended agents include nicardipine (see dose above), labetalol (see dose above), fenoldopam (see dose above), or nitroprusside (see dose above).

Subarachnoid Hemorrhage

- Reduce systolic pressure below 160 mm Hg or MAP below 130 mm Hg to prevent rebleeding.
- Recommended agents include nicardipine (see dose above), labetalol (see dose above), or esmolol (see dose above).

Intracranial Hemorrhage

- To reduce hemorrhage growth, for patients with evidence of increased intracranial pressure (decreased level of consciousness, evidence of midline shift, or hematoma volume >30 mL on CT imaging), reduce MAP to 130 mm Hg.
- In patients for whom there is no suspicion of increased intracranial pressure, treatment may be intensified to a MAP of 110 mm Hg, or a systolic pressure of 150 to 160 mm Hg.
- Recommended agents include nicardipine (see dose above), labetalol (see dose above), or esmolol (see dose above).

Acute Ischemic Stroke

- If fibrinolytic therapy is planned, reduce BP below 185/110 mm Hg; if no fibrinolytic therapy is planned and BP remains elevated on repeat measures, reduce BP below 220/120 mm Hg. More intensive lowering can be accomplished safely (however, pharmacologic reduction below 160/100 is not advised).
- Recommended agents include labetalol (see dose above), nicardipine (see dose above), or nitroglycerin paste, 1 to 2 inches.

Hypertensive Urgency

- For hypertensive urgency, useful agents include oral labetalol 200 to 400 milligrams, repeated every 2 to 3 hours; oral captopril 25 milligrams every 4 to 6 hours; sublingual nitroglycerin spray or tablets (0.3–0.6 milligrams); or clonidine, 0.2 milligrams oral loading dose, followed by 0.1 milligrams/h until the DBP is below 115 mm Hg, or a maximum of 0.7 milligrams.
- For asymptomatic patients with severe hypertension, with BP above the 180/200 systolic range, or above 110/120 diastolic range, starting an oral agent at discharge should be considered.
- The choice of the oral agent should be based on coexisting conditions, if any. Diuretics, such as hydrochlorothiazide 25 milligrams/d, should be used in most patients with uncomplicated HTN.
- For patients with angina, postmyocardial infarction, migraines, or supraventricular arrhythmias, a β-blocker should be considered, such as metoprolol 50 milligrams orally 2 times daily.
- Angiotensin-converting enzyme inhibitors such as lisinopril, start at 10 milligrams daily, can be used in those with heart failure, renal disease, recurrent strokes, or diabetes mellitus.
- Restarting a noncompliant patient on a previously established regimen is a recommended strategy.

CHILDHOOD HYPERTENSIVE EMERGENCIES

- Children often will have nonspecific complaints such as throbbing frontal headache or blurred vision.
- Physical findings associated with HTN are similar to those found in adults.
- The most common etiologies in pre-teenage children are renovascular lesions and pheochromocytoma.
- The decision to treat a hypertensive emergency in a child is based on the BP and associated symptoms.
- Urgent treatment is required if the BP exceeds prior measurements by 30%.
- Alternatively, if prior measurements are not known, childhood hypertension is defined as diastolic or systolic blood pressure ≥ the 95th percentile on a standardized table.
- The goal is to reduce the BP by 25% within an hour in acutely symptomatic patients.
- Preferred medications for the control of hypertensive emergencies in children include labetalol, 0.2 to 1.0 milligram/kg per dose, up to 40 milligrams/dose, or an infusion of 0.25 to 3.0 milligrams/kg/h; nicardipine, 1 to 3 micrograms/kg/min; or, if prior drugs fail, nitroprusside, 0.5 to 10.0 micrograms/kg/min.
- The treatment of pheochromocytoma is surgical excision and managing the BP with α-adrenergic blockers such as phentolamine. Pediatric HTN that requires intervention in the emergency department will likely require admission.

PULMONARY HYPERTENSION

- Although the diagnosis of pulmonary hypertension cannot be made in the ED, suspicion of primary or secondary pulmonary hypertension as a cause of dyspnea, chest pain, or syncope can affect ED evaluation, consultation, or disposition.
- Pulmonary hypertension is a pathologic condition characterized by elevation of the pulmonary vascular pressure, which compromises right ventricular function.
- There can be an isolated increase in pulmonary arterial pressure or an elevation of both arterial and venous pressure.
- The hemodynamic parameter that defines pulmonary hypertension is a median pulmonary artery pressure of >25 mm Hg at rest or >30 mm Hg during effort.
- The most common symptoms are dyspnea, fatigue, syncope, and chest pain.
- Typically, this disorder will be seen in association with other cardiovascular or pulmonary disorders such as chronic obstructive pulmonary disease, left ventricular dysfunction, or disorders associated with hypoxemia.
- Treatment of the underlying disorder is the only management indicated in the emergency setting, for example, oxygen for conditions producing hypoxia.
- Patients may be on calcium channel blockers chronically, or for primary pulmonary hypertension, patients may have arrangements for home infusions of epoprostenol (prostacyclin).

For further reading in *Emergency Medicine: A Comprehensive Study Guide,* 7th edition., see Chapter 61, "Systemic and Pulmonary Hypertension," by David M. Cline, and Alberto J. Machado.

29 AORTIC DISSECTION AND ANEURYSMS

David E. Manthey

ABDOMINAL AORTIC ANEURYSMS

EPIDEMIOLOGY

- The incidence of abdominal aortic aneurysm (AAA) increases with age.
- Most patients are older than 60.
- Males are at increased risk.
- Eighteen percent of patients have a family history of aneurysm in a first-degree relative.
- Other risk factors include connective tissue disease, Marfan's syndrome, and atherosclerotic risk factors (smoking, hypertension, hyperlipidemia, and diabetes).

PATHOPHYSIOLOGY

- Thinning of the media of the aorta with a reduction in elastin, collagen, and fibrolamellar units results in a decrease in tensile wall strength.
- Laplace's law (wall tension = [pressure × radius]) dictates that as the aorta dilates, the force on the aortic wall increases, causing further aortic dilation.
- The rate of aneurysmal dilation is variable, with larger aneurysms expanding more quickly. An average rate may be 0.25 to 0.5 cm per year.

CLINICAL FEATURES

- Asymptomatic AAAs may be found on physical examination or during an unrelated radiologic evaluation. Those larger than 5 cm are at higher risk of rupture.
- Three clinical scenarios exist for symptomatic aneurysms: acute rupture, aortoenteric fistula, and chronic contained rupture.
- Sudden death most commonly occurs with intraperitoneal rupture of the aneurysm.
- The classic presentation is an older male with severe back or abdominal pain who presents with syncope or hypotension.
- Pain, described as abrupt and severe at onset, is the most common presenting symptom; 50% describe this pain as "tearing" or "ripping."
- Many patients present with a complaint of unilateral flank or groin pain, hip pain, or abdominal pain localized to a specific quadrant. An AAA is most commonly misdiagnosed as renal colic.
- The presence of an AAA does not alter the femoral arterial pulsations.
- Lack of tenderness does not imply an intact aorta.
- There may be signs of retroperitoneal hemorrhage such as periumbilical (Cullen's sign) or flank ecchymosis (Grey-Turner's sign) or scrotal hematoma.
- Aortoenteric fistulas may present with a deceptively minor "sentinel" bleed or massive GI hemorrhage. This is classically seen after prior aortic grafting.
- Chronic contained rupture is uncommon, but is seen when an AAA ruptures retroperitoneal with significant fibrosis that limits blood loss.

DIAGNOSIS AND DIFFERENTIAL

- The differential for AAA depends on its presentation. The key is to keep AAA in your differential when evaluating patients for symptoms such as back pain, syncope, and renal colic.
- Diagnostic studies should never unnecessarily delay the surgical repair of an AAA. They are only needed when the diagnosis of AAA is unclear.
- In the unstable patient, bedside abdominal ultrasound has >90% sensitivity for demonstrating the presence of an aneurysm and measuring its diameter. Ultrasound cannot reliably determine the presence of retroperitoneal hemorrhage and rupture (see Fig. 29-1).
- Computed tomographic (CT) scanning, approximately 100% accurate in determining the presence or absence of an AAA, is preferred in the stable patient as it better delineates the anatomic details of the aneurysm and any associated rupture (see Fig. 29-2).

EMERGENCY DEPARTMENT CARE AND DISPOSITION

- Stabilize the patient with volume resuscitation with isotonic fluids and/or blood transfusion through multiple large-bore IV lines.
- Immediate surgical consultation or transfer to an appropriate institution is warranted for suspected rupturing AAA or aortoenteric fistula.
- Symptomatic aneurysms of any size should be considered emergent.
- Control pain appropriately with narcotics. Utilize a short acting β-blocker if elevated BP remains after pain control.

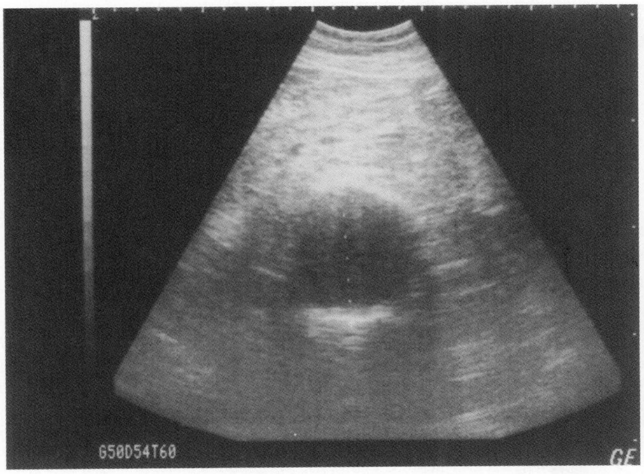

FIG. 29-1. Bedside US image of an abdominal aortic aneurysm. This aneurysm measures 6.5 cm.

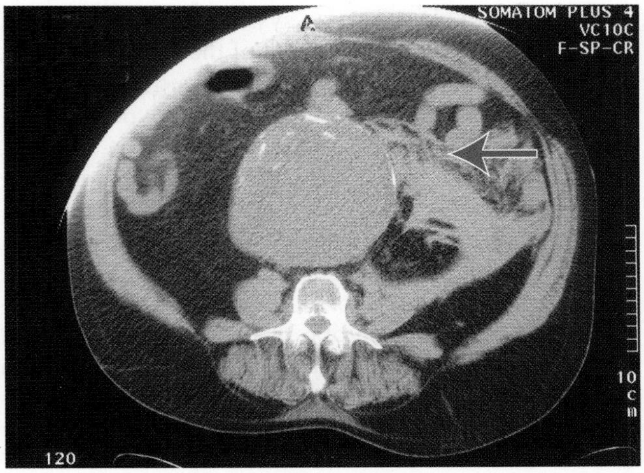

FIG. 29-2. CT scan of a patient with a 12-cm abdominal aortic aneurysm. Calcification of the aortic wall is seen anterior to the spinal column. Evidence of hemorrhage and surrounding inflammation (*arrow*) is seen in the left side of the abdomen.

- Type and cross patient with rupturing AAA or aortoenteric fistula for several units of blood.
- Consult a vascular surgeon for urgent repair of chronically contained ruptured AAAs.
- For an incidentally discovered AAA, consultation with a vascular surgeon for admission or close outpatient follow-up based on the size of the aneurysm is appropriate.

AORTIC DISSECTION

EPIDEMIOLOGY

- Aortic dissection has a bimodal distribution. First peak is of younger patients with predisposing conditions, and a larger number in the second peak with age > 50 years.
- A major risk factor for the older group is chronic hypertension.
- Younger patients have identifiable risk factors such as bicuspid aortic valve, connective tissue disease, and familial history of aortic dissection.

PATHOPHYSIOLOGY

- Aortic dissection occurs when the intima is violated, allowing blood to enter the media and dissect between the intimal and adventitial layers, developing a false lumen.
- The false lumen may dissect proximally and/or distally and may rupture back through the intima or out through the adventitia.

- The Stanford classification system categorizes type A dissections as any involvement of the ascending aorta, and type B dissections as restricted to the descending aorta. The DeBakey system classifies type I dissections as those that involve the ascending aorta, the arch, and the descending aorta. Type II involves only the ascending aorta, and type III only the descending aorta.
- Intramural hematomas result from injury to the vasa vasorum with subsequent infarction of the media. They are often precursors to aortic dissection.
- Penetrating atherosclerotic ulcers involve the intima and can lead to hematomas, dissection, or perforation of the aorta.

CLINICAL FEATURES

- More than 85% of patients have abrupt onset of severe or the worst pain ever. It is more commonly described as "sharp" followed by tearing or ripping.
- Type A dissection presents with chest pain (80%), more commonly anterior (71% of those with chest pain). Patients also report back (47%) and abdominal pain (21%). Type B dissections present with back pain (64%), chest pain (63%), and abdominal pain (43%).
- Syncope occurs in up to 10% of patients.
- Interruption of blood supply may alter the presentation by the area affected such as coronary artery occlusion with MI, stroke symptoms with carotid involvement, or paraplegia with occlusion of the vertebral blood supply. The dissection may progress distally, causing abdominal or flank pain or limb ischemia.
- Proximal retrograde dissection into the aortic root may lead to cardiac tamponade.
- An aortic insufficiency murmur may be heard in 32%. Fifteen percent of patients have decreased radial or femoral pulse deficits.
- Hypertension (49%) and tachycardia are common, but hypotension (18%) may also be present.
- Very few patients with aortic dissection have involvement of a coronary artery (6%). The ratio of acute coronary syndrome to aortic dissection is about 3000:5.

DIAGNOSIS AND DIFFERENTIAL

- Ischemic end-organ manifestations associated with dissections may confuse the differential diagnosis, including myocardial infarction, pericardial disease, and spinal cord injuries.
- Rupture of the dissection back through the intima into the true lumen may cause a cessation of symptoms, leading to false reassurance.
- Most patients with a thoracic dissection will have an abnormal chest x-ray, but up to 37% will be normal. More common findings include a widening of the mediastinum, abnormal aortic contour, pleural effusion, apical capping, and depression of the left main stem bronchus (see Fig. 29-3).
- CT scanning, with and without contrast, is the imaging modality of choice. It can reliably diagnose dissection as well as location of flap and extension into great vessels (see Fig. 29-4).
- CT scanning will also diagnose intramural hematomas and penetrating atherosclerotic ulcers.
- Transesophageal echocardiography may be as sensitive and specific as CT in experienced hands.

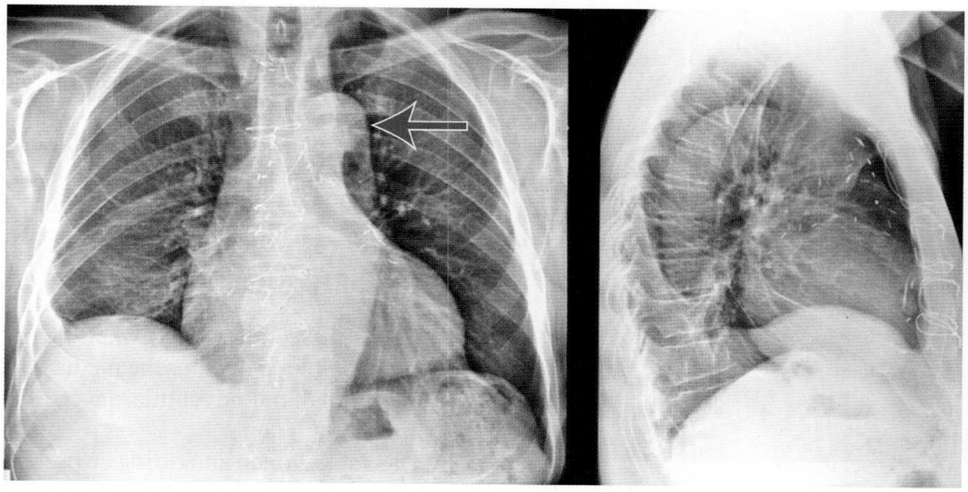

FIG. 29-3. Abnormal aortic contour on chest radiography. Frontal and lateral radiographs of the chest in a patient with type B aortic dissection reveal an abnormal aortic contour (*arrow*). A right pleural effusion is present, and multiple postoperative clips and wires are also seen.

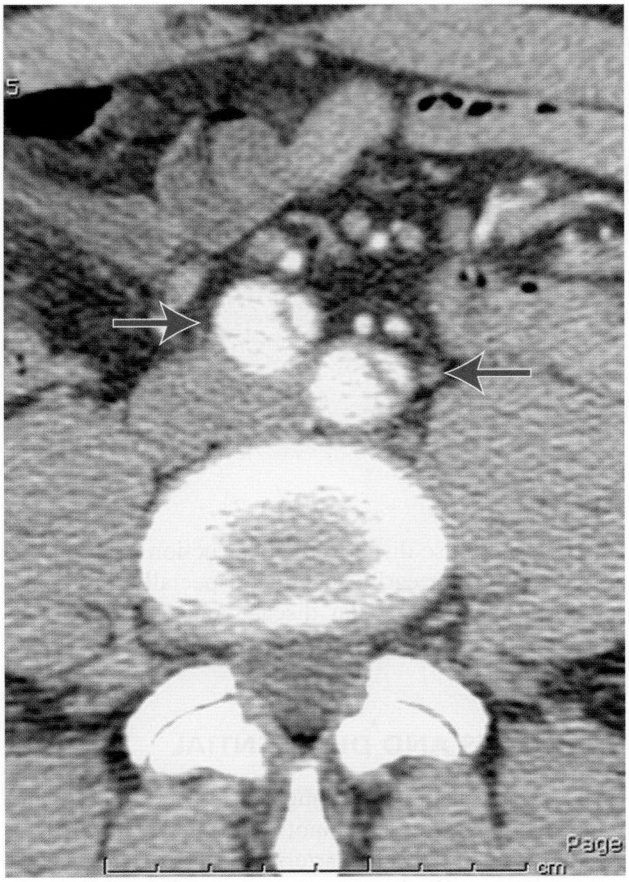

FIG. 29-4. Type B dissection into the iliac arteries. Contrast CT image of dissection extending into the iliac arteries (anterior to vertebral body). True and false lumens are visible in both arteries (*arrows*).

EMERGENCY DEPARTMENT CARE AND DISPOSITION

- Patients with suspected aortic dissection require prompt radiographic confirmation of the diagnosis and early consultation with the CT surgeon.
- Hypertension must be controlled with drugs that will not increase the shear force on the intimal flap. β-Blockers are the first-line choice, with nitroprusside added if the blood pressure remains elevated. Calcium channel blockers can be used if there is a contraindication to β-blockers.
- Dissection of the ascending aorta requires prompt surgical repair. Repair may include surgical repair, endovascular treatment or fenestration of the intimal flap.
- As acute coronary syndrome and dissection may present with anterior chest pain, a chest radiograph should be assessed for signs of dissection before administering heparin or fibrinolytics.

For further reading in *Emergency Medicine: A Comprehensive Study Guide*, 7th ed., see Chapter 62, "Aortic Dissection and Related Aortic Syndromes," by Gary A. Johnson and Louise A. Prince. Please also see Chapter 63, "Aneurysms of the Aorta and Major Arteries", by Louise A. Prince and Gary A. Johnson.

30 OCCLUSIVE ARTERIAL DISEASE

Carolyn K. Synovitz

EPIDEMIOLOGY

- The disease prevalence is 4.3% in Americans under age 40 years; prevalence climbs to 15.5% in those >70 years of age. High-risk individuals include those over 70 years of age, or those over age 50 with risk factors such as diabetes or tobacco use. At least half of these patients also have coronary or cerebrovascular disease.
- Acute arterial occlusion secondary to thrombosis or embolism is potentially life-threatening (mortality 25%). In survivors of this condition, limb amputation is necessary in 25%.
- The most frequently involved arteries, in descending order, are the femoropopliteal, tibial, aortoiliac, and brachiocephalic.

PATHOPHYSIOLOGY

- In the lower extremities, thrombotic arterial occlusion is more common than embolic arterial occlusion (20% of cases).
- In the upper extremities, thrombosis also accounts for the largest proportion of arterial occlusion, but here, one-third of cases are embolic and a quarter are secondary to arteritis.
- Arteritis can be secondary to Takayasu's arteritis, Raynaud's disease, thromboangiitis obliterans (Buerger's disease), or collagen vascular disease such as rheumatoid arthritis, lupus, or polyarteritis nodosa.
- The embolus usually originates in the heart and atrial fibrillation is responsible for two-thirds of these emboli. A mural thrombus after myocardial infarction is the second most common source of emboli. Noncardiac sources of emboli include tumor, vegetations, prosthetic devices, and thrombi from aneurysms or atheromatous plaques.

TABLE 30-1 Brief Differential Diagnoses of Intermittent Claudication

CONDITION	LOCATION	PREVALENCE	CHARACTERISTIC	EFFECT OF EXERCISE	EFFECT OF REST	EFFECT OF POSITION
Calf/thigh foot IC	Calf/thigh/foot	3-5% to Rare	Cramping	Reproducible	Quick relief	None
Venous claudication	Entire Leg	Rare	Tight, bursting pain	After walking	Subsides slowly	Relief with elevation
Nerve root compression	Radiates down leg	Common	Sharp pain	Induced by sitting, standing, or walking	Often present at rest	Improved by change in position
Hip arthritis	Lateral hip, thigh	Common	Aching discomfort	After exercise	Subsides slowly	Improved with non weight bearing
Spinal stenosis	Bilateral buttocks	Common	Pain and weakness	Mimics IC	Variable relief	Improved by lumbar flexion

- The most common location for an embolus in the leg is the bifurcation of the common femoral artery, followed by the popliteal artery. The brachial artery is the most common site in the upper extremity. Thrombosis can occur at any site of vessel injury.
- Decreased pulse distal to the obstruction is an unreliable finding for early ischemia, especially in patients with peripheral vascular disease and well-developed collateral circulation.

CLINICAL FEATURES

- Patients with acute arterial limb ischemia typically present with one of the "six P's": Pain, Pallor, Polar (coldness), Pulselessness, Paresthesias, and Paralysis.
- Patients with embolism will have unilateral disease; however, those with thrombosis will have occlusive arterial disease bilaterally.
- Pain and muscle weakness can be the earliest symptoms and pain may increase with elevation of the limb. Commonly seen skin changes include discoloration, mottling, and temperature differences.

DIAGNOSIS AND DIFFERENTIAL

- History of claudication suggests a thrombosis, and many times a source cannot be located (Table 30-1). Other causes of acute arterial occlusion are vasculitis, Raynaud's disease, thromboangiitis obliterans, blunt or penetrating trauma, catheter complications, or low-flow shock states such as sepsis. A history of an abruptly ischemic limb in a patient with atrial fibrillation or recent myocardial infarction is strongly suggestive of an embolus; in these cases a source can often be identified (Table 30-2).

TABLE 30-2 Comparison of Disorders Associated with Acute Arterial Occlusion

DISORDER	CAUSE	SYMPTOMS/SIGNS	MANAGEMENT
Thrombus	Atherosclerosis or thrombosis of bypass grafts	Intermittent claudication	Medical vs surgical
Embolism	Cardiac source: atrial fibrillation, rheumatic heart disease, mechanical valves, post-MI thrombus	Sudden onset of territorial arterial symptoms	Preventive anticoagulation, embolectomy
Catheterization complication (brachial or femoral)	Can occur during standard angioplasty, angiography, or arterial puncture (eg, for blood gas)	Expanding hematoma, pain, temperature, and pulse changes	Conservative therapy vs operative repair
Trash foot or blue toe syndrome	Cholesterol/platelet aggregate emboli	Painful cyanotic discoloration of isolated portion of foot, remainder of foot warm, dorsalis pedis pulse intact	Conservative therapy

- A hand-held Doppler transducer can document flow (or demonstrate its absence) over the dorsalis pedis, posterior tibial, popliteal, or femoral arteries in the lower extremity, and over the radial, ulnar, and brachial arteries in the upper extremity.
- The ankle-brachial index (ABI) is the ratio of systolic blood pressure measured in the lower extremity, to the brachial systolic pressure. With arterial occlusion the ABI is usually markedly diminished (<0.5). A pressure difference of >30 mm Hg between any two adjacent levels can localize the site of obstruction (see Fig. 30-1).
- Duplex ultrasonography can detect an obstruction to flow with a sensitivity greater than 85%.
- The diagnostic gold standard is the arteriogram, which can define the anatomy of the obstruction and direct treatment.

EMERGENCY DEPARTMENT CARE AND DISPOSITION

- Patients with acute arterial occlusion should be treated with unfractionated heparin, though there is no equivocal evidence demonstrating benefit of this practice (see DVT treatment section for dosing guidelines). Aspirin should also be administered. Use of thrombolytics is controversial, with no clear benefit.

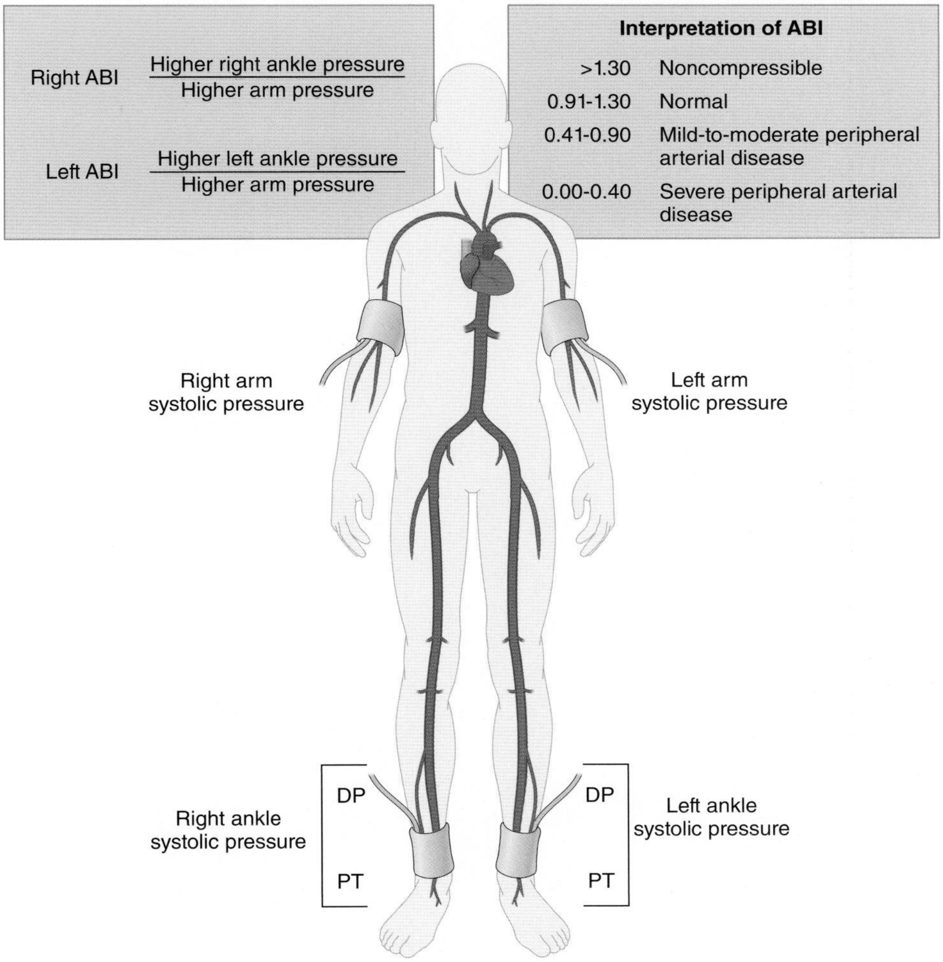

FIG. 30-1. Measurement of the ankle-brachial index (ABI). Measure the systolic blood pressure using Doppler US in each arm and in the dorsalis pedis (DP) and posterior tibial (PT) arteries in each ankle. Select the higher of the two arm pressures (right vs left) and the higher of the two pressures in the ankle (DP vs PT). Determine the right and left ABI values by dividing the higher ankle pressure in each leg by the higher arm pressure. The ranges of the ABI and the interpretation are shown in the figure. In the case of a noncompressible calcified vessel, the true pressure at that location cannot be obtained, and alternative tests are required to diagnose peripheral arterial disease. Patients with claudication typically have ABI values ranging from 0.41 to 0.90, and those with critical leg ischemia have values <0.41.

- Fluid resuscitation and treatment of heart failure may augment perfusion to the ischemic limb.
- Definitive treatment should be performed in consultation with a vascular surgeon and an interventional radiologist. Catheter embolectomy using a Fogarty balloon is the preferred approach. Other options include thrombolysis and surgery.
- All patients with an acute arterial occlusion should be admitted to a telemetry bed or to the ICU, depending on the stability of the patient and the planned course of therapy.
- Reperfusion injury after revascularization of the injury can result in myoglobinemia, renal failure, hyperkalemia, and metabolic acidosis—these complications account for a third of deaths from occlusive arterial disease.

For further reading in *Tintinalli's Emergency Medicine: A Comprehensive Study Guide*, 7th edition, See Chapter 64, "Occlusive Arterial Disease," by Anil Chopra and David Carr.

Section 6
PULMONARY EMERGENCIES

31 RESPIRATORY DISTRESS

Joshua T. Hargraves

DYSPNEA

PATHOPHYSIOLOGY

- Dyspnea is a subjective feeling of difficult, labored, or uncomfortable breathing. It is a complex sensation, without a defined neural pathway.
- Mechanical factors include a sense of skeletal muscle effort dependent on work of breathing and intraparenchymal stretch receptors.
- Chemoreceptors in the central medulla and carotid body respond to changes in CO_2 and O_2, respectively. Receptors in the atria and pulmonary arteries contribute, but in a poorly defined manner.
- Central and peripheral receptors send afferent neurons to the central nervous system (CNS), where the information is integrated in a complex manner.

CLINICAL FEATURES

- Patients may present with complaints of shortness of breath, air hunger, or dyspnea on exertion.
- Signs include tachypnea, tachycardia, difficulty speaking, use of accessory respiratory muscles, and/or stridor.
- The complaint of dyspnea must be rapidly evaluated with immediate identification of abnormal vital signs and abnormalities in the primary survey (airway, breathing, and circulation). Airway obstruction, poor respiratory effort, and altered mental status mandate immediate intervention.

DIAGNOSIS AND DIFFERENTIAL

- A detailed history and physical examination will often lead to an accurate diagnosis of dyspnea.
- Pulse oximetry provides an immediate assessment of oxygenation, but has poor sensitivity.
- Arterial blood gas analysis (ABG) is invasive, but has improved sensitivity over pulse oximetry. ABG results must be interpreted with consideration of the patient's work of breathing.
- Chest radiograph (CXR), electrocardiogram (EKG), peak expiratory flows, and hematocrit may prove helpful.
- Elevated D-dimer and B-natriuretic peptide (BNP) may lead to specific diagnoses.
- Other ancillary tests, not usually available in the ED, include spirometry, cardiac and exercise stress testing, echocardiography, ventilation–perfusion scans, and lung biopsies.
- Table 31-1 lists a focused differential diagnosis of dyspnea.

EMERGENCY DEPARTMENT CARE AND DISPOSITION

- Immediate priorities include maintaining the airway and supporting respiratory function. Supplemental oxygen is given to anyone in respiratory distress. Patients with chronic obstructive pulmonary disease (COPD) may tolerate lower Pa_{O_2} levels and must be treated symptomatically.
- Noninvasive positive pressure ventilation including continuous positive airway pressure (CPAP) and biphasic positive airway pressure (BiPAP) ventilation may be initiated.
- Bag-valve-mask ventilation followed by endotracheal intubation with mechanical ventilation can be used for critically ill patients, and allows for long-term support.
- Definitive treatment depends on the etiology.
- All patients with an unclear cause of their dyspnea and hypoxia require admission to a monitored bed. Admission otherwise depends on the exact cause of dyspnea.

HYPOXIA

PATHOPHYSIOLOGY

- Hypoxia, the inadequate delivery of oxygen to the tissues, is arbitrarily defined as a Pa_{O_2} <60 mm Hg. Hypoxia is caused by one of five mechanisms:

TABLE 31-1 Differential Diagnosis of Consequence: Dyspnea

MOST COMMON CAUSES	MOST IMMEDIATELY LIFE-THREATENING
Obstructive airway disease: asthma, chronic obstructive pulmonary disease	Upper airway obstruction: foreign body, angioedema, hemorrhage
Heart failure/cardiogenic pulmonary edema	Tension pneumothorax
Ischemic heart disease: unstable angina and myocardial infarction	Pulmonary embolism
Pneumonia	Neuromuscular weakness: myasthenia gravis, Guillain-Barré syndrome, botulism
Psychogenic	Fat embolism

- Hypoventilation: Rising $Paco_2$ displaces O_2 from the alveoli, decreasing the diffusion gradient across the pulmonary membrane.
- Right-to-left shunt: Unoxygenated blood enters the systemic circulation; this occurs with congenital heart abnormalities or perfusion of unoxygenated lung segments.
- Ventilation-perfusion mismatch: From abnormalities of ventilation or perfusion.
- Diffusion impairment: Caused by abnormalities of the alveolar-blood barrier.
- Low inspired O_2: Only a factor at high altitudes.

CLINICAL FEATURES

- Signs and symptoms are nonspecific, ranging from tachycardia and tachypnea to CNS manifestations such as lethargy, seizures, and coma.
- At a Pao_2 <20 mm Hg, there is a paradoxical depression of the respiratory drive.
- Dyspnea does not always occur with hypoxia, and cyanosis is a poor indicator of oxygenation.

DIAGNOSIS AND DIFFERENTIAL

- Pulse oximetry is quick and frequently useful, but direct ABG analysis of arterial oxygen levels defines the diagnosis.
- Tests used to determine the cause of dyspnea are also useful to elucidate the cause of hypoxia.

EMERGENCY DEPARTMENT CARE AND DISPOSITION

- Support, identify, and aggressively treat hypoxia, and try to maintain a Pao_2 >60 mm Hg. Lower Pao_2 levels may be tolerated in COPD.
- All patients require hospitalization in a monitored bed, until the underlying process is stabilized and/or a definitive diagnosis made.
- Frequent ABGs may require an arterial line for patient comfort and reduction of complications of multiple arterial punctures.

HYPERCAPNIA

PATHOPHYSIOLOGY

- Hypercapnia, defined as a $Paco_2$ >45 mm Hg, is caused by a decrease in minute ventilation. Minute ventilation is dependent on respiratory rate and tidal volume; changes in either may lead to hypoventilation and hypercapnia.
- Hypercapnia is almost never due to increased CO_2 production.
- Alveolar ventilation per minute is calculated as [respiratory rate] × [tidal volume minus the dead space volume]. Alveolar minute ventilation is an accurate ventilatory measure, but its calculation is impractical in the ED.
- Minute ventilation is controlled via a neural chemoreceptor in the medulla. Efferent outputs control the respiratory rate and tidal volume.

CLINICAL FEATURES

- Signs and symptoms of hypercapnia depend on $Paco_2$'s absolute value and its rate of increase.
- Acute elevations of $Paco_2$ cause an increase in intracranial pressure, leading to confusion, lethargy, seizures, and coma. Asterixis may be found on physical examination.
- Acute elevations in $Paco_2$ >100 mm Hg may lead to cardiovascular collapse.
- In acute hypercapnia, for every 10-mm Hg increase in CO_2, the pH will decrease 0.1 unit.
- In chronic hypercapnia, patients may tolerate high levels of CO_2. For every 10-mm Hg increase in CO_2, the [HCO_3^-] increases 0.35 mEq/L (see Chap. 6).

DIAGNOSIS AND DIFFERENTIAL

- The diagnosis is made by clinical suspicion and confirmed on ABG analysis. Pulse oximetry plays no role in the identification of hypercapnia. Table 31-2 lists a focused differential diagnosis of hypercapnia.

EMERGENCY DEPARTMENT CARE AND DISPOSITION

- Aggressively support, treat, and identify causes of hypercapnia.
- Early identification of the etiology may make treatment options easier. For example, a patient with

TABLE 31-2 Differential Diagnosis of Consequence: Hypercapnia

Depressed central respiratory drive
Structural central nervous system disease: brain stem lesions
Drug depression of respiratory center: opioids, sedatives, anesthetics
Endogenous toxins: tetanus
Thoracic cage disorders
Kyphoscoliosis
Morbid obesity
Neuromuscular impairment
Neuromuscular disease: myasthenia gravis, Guillain–Barré syndrome
Neuromuscular toxin: organophosphate poisoning, botulism
Intrinsic lung disease associated with increased dead space
Chronic obstructive pulmonary disease
Upper airway obstruction

respiratory depression, pinpoint pupils, and altered mental status may have a heroin overdose that will respond to naloxone, while a patient with amyotrophic lateral sclerosis may require early assisted ventilation.

- Oxygen should be given to every patient with respiratory distress and not withheld over concern for decreasing the respiratory drive. Hypoxia will kill a patient, while only extreme hypercapnia will do the same.
- BiPAP or CPAP may be used to increase tidal volume and thus increase minute ventilation. However, if there is profound hypoxia or inability to control the airway, endotracheal intubation and mechanical ventilation may be required.
- Disposition depends on the underlying cause and frequently requires admission to a monitored bed or intensive care setting.

CYANOSIS

PATHOPHYSIOLOGY

- Cyanosis is a bluish color of the skin and mucous membranes resulting from an increased level of deoxyhemoglobin.
- The level of deoxyhemoglobin necessary for development of cyanosis is variable, but is in the range of 5 grams/mL.
- Lighting and temperature affect the ability to detect cyanosis.
- Other factors that affect the ability to identify cyanosis include skin thickness, pigmentation, and microcirculation.

CLINICAL FEATURES

- The presence of cyanosis usually indicates hypoxia, but this is not always the case.
- The tongue is very sensitive for identifying cyanosis. The earlobes, nail beds, and conjunctiva are less reliable.
- Cyanosis may be central or peripheral. Central cyanosis is usually the result of deoxyhemoglobin. Peripheral cyanosis is the result of poor peripheral circulation, leading to increased oxygen extraction by the peripheral tissues.

DIAGNOSIS AND DIFFERENTIAL

- The presence of cyanosis must be taken in the context of the clinical situation (see Table 31-3).
- ABG analysis will confirm the presence of hypoxia as a cause of cyanosis.
- Other useful tests include a hematocrit to detect anemia or polycythemia vera, a CXR, and an EKG.
- Pseudocyanosis should be considered in any asymptomatic patient, but it should be a diagnosis of exclusion. Pseudocyanosis is caused by abnormal skin pigmentation, giving the skin a bluish or silver hue. Causative agents include heavy metals (iron, gold, lead, and silver) and certain drugs (phenothiazines, minocycline, amiodarone, and chloroquine).
- Methemoglobinemia, carboxyhemoglobin, and other acquired hemoglobinopathies, although rare, must be considered in certain clinical situations. Methemoglobinemia will turn blood a chocolate brown that will not normalize to red upon exposure to air.

TABLE 31-3 Differential Diagnosis of Consequence: Cyanosis

CENTRAL CYANOSIS	PERIPHERAL CYANOSIS
Hypoxemia	Reduced cardiac output
Decreased fraction of inspired oxygen: high altitude	Cold extremities
Hypoventilation	Maldistribution of blood flow: distributive forms of shock
Ventilation–perfusion mismatch	Arterial or venous obstruction
Right-to-left shunt: congenital heart disease, pulmonary arteriovenous fistulas, multiple intrapulmonary shunts	
Abnormal skin pigmentation	
Heavy metals: iron, gold, silver, lead, arsenic	
Drugs: phenothiazine, minocycline, amiodarone, chloroquine	
Hemoglobin abnormalities	
Methemoglobinemia: hereditary, acquired	
Sulfhemoglobinemia: acquired	
Carboxyhemoglobinemia (not true cyanosis)	

Carboxyhemoglobin will cause an atypical cherry-pink cyanosis. It is important to identify these acquired hemoglobinopathies because they can be quickly and easily treated.

EMERGENCY DEPARTMENT CARE AND DISPOSITION

- Aggressive support, treatment, and identification of cyanosis are always indicated. Supplemental oxygen is an appropriate first-line treatment. If the patient is unresponsive to supplemental oxygen, poor perfusion, acquired hemoglobinopathies, or large right-to-left shunts may be present.
- Specific antidotes for acquired hemoglobinopathies include methylene blue (1-2 milligrams/kg IV) for methemoglobinemia, and supplemental oxygen (possibly including hyperbaric therapy) for carboxyhemoglobin poisoning.
- All patients with an unknown cause of cyanosis require admission until the condition is stabilized and/or definitively identified.

PLEURAL EFFUSION

PATHOPHYSIOLOGY

- Pleural effusions result from the collection of fluid between the visceral and parietal pleura.
- Effusions are categorized as exudates or transudates.
- Exudative effusions have increased protein content and typically result from increased fluid production due to inflammatory process or neoplasm.
- Transudative effusions are due to imbalance in hydrostatic pressure and have low protein content.

CLINICAL FEATURES

- Effusions may be clinically silent or may cause dyspnea as fluid accumulates.
- Physical findings include percussion dullness and decreased breath sounds.

DIAGNOSIS AND DIFFERENTIAL

- Approximately 150 to 200 mL of pleural fluid are required to identify an effusion on upright CXR (see Fig. 31-1).
- A listing of the differential diagnosis of pleural effusion is listed in Table 31-4.
- Significant pleural effusions will be large enough to produce a >10-mm strip on a lateral decubitus CXR, or on thoracic ultrasound.

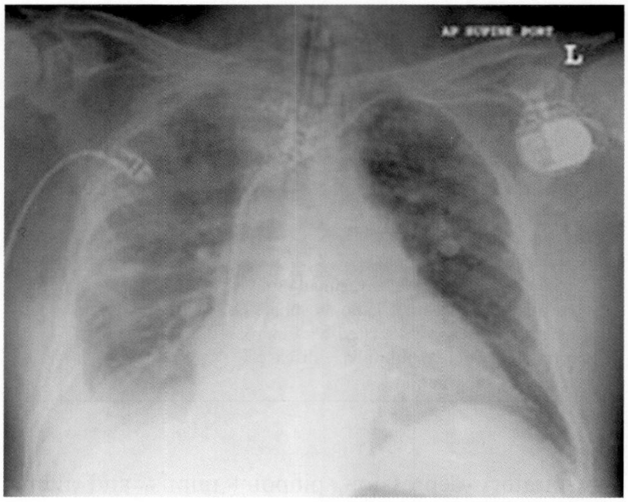

A

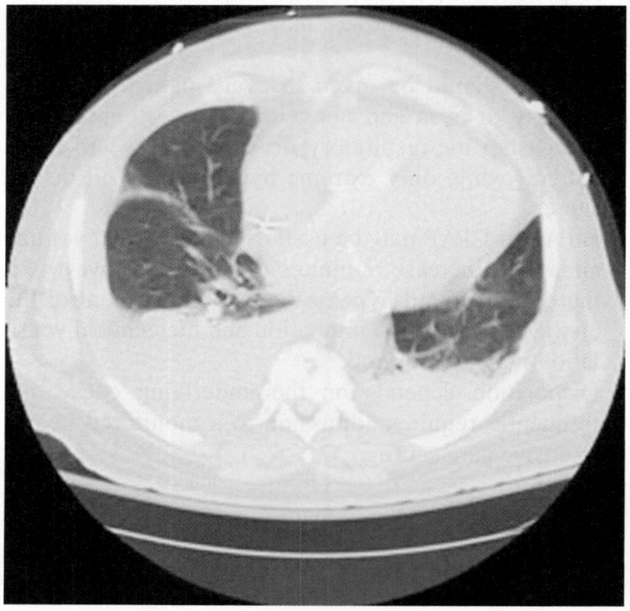

B

FIG. 31-1. **A**. This is a supine radiograph showing a right-sided pleural effusion. The right lung field is hazy compared to the left, and a small layer of fluid is noted inferiorly. **B**. CT scan of the patient in (A). A moderate pleural effusion is noted in the right lung field, and a small effusion not seen in the left lung field of the plain film is noted on the CT scan.

- Diagnostic thoracentesis can be performed on patients without an obvious cause of effusion.
- An effusion is considered an exudate if it has one or more of the following criteria:
  - Pleural fluid/serum protein ratio >0.5 and/or
  - Pleural fluid/serum LDH ratio >0.6 and/or
  - Pleural fluid LDH > two-thirds of the upper limit of serum LDH

TABLE 31-4 Differential Diagnosis of Consequence: Pleural Effusion

COMMON	LESS COMMON
Transudates	
Heart failure	Cirrhosis with ascites Peritoneal dialysis Nephrotic syndrome
Exudates	
Cancer: primary or metastatic	Viral, fungal, mycobacterial, or parasitic infection
Bacterial pneumonia with parapneumonic effusion	Systemic rheumatologic disorders: systemic lupus erythematosus, rheumatoid arthritis
Pulmonary embolism	Uremia, pancreatitis Postcardiac surgery or radiotherapy Drug-related: amiodarone
Either transudates or exudates	
Transudates after diuretic therapy	Pulmonary embolism

EMERGENCY DEPARTMENT CARE AND DISPOSITION

- A therapeutic thoracentesis with drainage of 1.0 to 1.5 L is indicated if a patient has dyspnea at rest.
- Drainage of larger volumes has been associated with reexpansion pulmonary edema and should be avoided.
- Treatment of effusions varies widely. Empyema requires a large-bore thoracostomy tube, while treatment of parapneumonic effusions is controversial.

For further reading in Tintinalli's *Emergency Medicine: A Comprehensive Study Guide,* 7th ed., see Chapter 65, "Respiratory Distress," by John Sarko and J. Stephan Stapczynski.

32 PNEUMONIA, BRONCHITIS, AND UPPER RESPIRATORY TRACT INFECTION

Jeffrey M. Goodloe

BRONCHITIS

EPIDEMIOLOGY

- Acute bronchitis is a commonly encountered, typically viral infection of the lower respiratory tract airways that often follows an upper respiratory infection.
- Incidence of acute bronchitis predominates in fall and winter, affecting up to 5% of the adult population in the United States.

PATHOPHYSIOLOGY

- Respiratory viruses cause the vast majority of cases of acute bronchitis. Influenza A or B, parainfluenza, respiratory syncytial virus (RSV), and coronavirus are amongst the more common viral etiologies (Table 32-1).
- Atypical bacteria, specifically *Mycoplasma pneumoniae*, *Chlamydia pneumoniae*, and *Bordetella pertussis* may cause acute bronchitis in otherwise healthy individuals (Table 32-2).

CLINICAL FEATURES

- Early acute bronchitis B manifestations may closely mimic the common cold with symptoms of nasal congestion, rhinorrhea, and sore throat.
- Acute bronchitis symptoms, including the primary manifestation of cough with or without sputum, typically resolve within 3 weeks.
- Sputum purulence may accompany the hallmark persistent cough of acute bronchitis and is indicative of sloughed inflammatory airway cells; taken alone, sputum does not indicate a bacterial etiology.
- Acute bronchitis typically presents *without* fever >38°C (100.4°F), heart rate >100 beats/min, or respiratory rate >24 breaths/min. These vital signs, particularly in patients older than 64 years of age, should lead to investigation for other respiratory ailments, including pneumonia.

DIAGNOSIS AND DIFFERENTIAL

- Clinical diagnosis of acute bronchitis is supported with (1) acute cough (less than 2–3 weeks duration), (2) no history of chronic lung disease, and (3) absence of focal consolidation, egophony, or fremitus by chest auscultation.
- Pulse oximetry is indicated if the patient describes dyspnea or appears short of breath.
- Sputum Gram's stain and culture are not recommended in the routine diagnosis of acute bronchitis.
- A chest radiograph is not required in nonelderly patients who appear nontoxic, unless symptoms exceed 3 weeks in duration.
- Consider pertussis in adolescents and young adults, particularly if eliciting a known contact with a confirmed pertussis case or coughing paroxysms with prominent post-tussive emesis.

TABLE 32-1 Viral Causes of Acute Bronchitis and Upper Respiratory Infections: Presentation and Management

PATHOGEN	CLINICAL PRESENTATION*	MANAGEMENT
Influenza and avian influenza	Abrupt onset of fever, chills, myalgias, headache, and cough. May have myositis with elevated serum creatine phosphokinase and myoglobinuria. May cause pneumonia.	If symptoms <48 h: oseltamivir, 75 milligrams twice daily for 5 d; zanamivir, two puffs (5 milligrams/puff) twice daily for 5 d (see CDC Web site for most recent recommendations, including H1N1: http://www.cdc.gov/flu).
Parainfluenza virus	Epidemics occur autumn to winter, most commonly causes croup in children but may lead to bronchitis or pneumonia; mild symptoms in adults.	See Chapter 71, Stridor and Drooling, for management of croup; symptomatic treatment† in adults.
Respiratory syncytial virus	Outbreaks in winter or spring, 45% of adults exposed to infants with bronchiolitis experience cold-like symptoms, ear pain in 20% of adults.	Symptomatic treatment.†
Coronavirus	May present as common cold but also may cause severe respiratory distress in the elderly, epidemics with high attack rates have been reported in military recruits.	Supportive care for severe symptoms; symptomatic treatment† for mild symptoms.
Adenovirus	May be similar to influenza with abrupt onset of fever.	Symptomatic treatment.†
Rhinovirus	Mild cold symptoms, fever uncommon.	Symptomatic treatment.†
Enterovirus	Acute undifferentiated febrile illness most common, may cause rhinitis and pharyngitis and rarely pneumonia.	Symptomatic treatment.†
Severe acute respiratory syndrome—coronavirus	Acute onset.	Supportive care for severe symptoms.

*Incubation for respiratory syncytial virus is 2-7 d; potential for respiratory viruses to cause pneumonia in children, elderly, and immunocompromised patients.
†See text for discussion of symptomatic treatment of bronchitis.

EMERGENCY DEPARTMENT CARE AND DISPOSITION

- Although predominantly viral in etiology, acute bronchitis is strongly associated with the prescribing of antibiotics in acute care environments. Although antibiotics are commonly requested by acute bronchitis patients, in non-atypical bacterial cases, antibiotics do *not* confer clinically relevant benefits and contribute to medication side effects and future pathogen resistance.
- For strongly suspected pertussis, treat with azithromycin to decrease coughing paroxysms and limit disease transmission.
- Airflow obstruction findings (eg, wheezing) should be treated with bronchodilators. Albuterol by a metered dose inhaler, 2 puffs q4h to q6h, is usually effective.

TABLE 32-2 Known Bacterial Causes of Bronchitis

PATHOGEN	CLINICAL PRESENTATION	MANAGEMENT*
Bordetella pertussis	Incubation is 1-3 wk, most common in adolescents and young adults, 10%-20% have cough for over 2 wk, "whooping" occurs in a minority of patients, fever is uncommon, may have leukocytosis with lymphocytic predominance.	Treatment does not shorten course of illness, but may prevent transmission to contacts; azithromycin, 500 milligrams day 1, 250 milligrams days 2–5 or similar macrolide; second-line therapy is trimethoprim/sulfamethoxazole, 1 double strength tablet twice daily.
Mycoplasma pneumoniae	Incubation is 2-3 wk, onset over 2-3 d, outbreaks common in adolescents or young adults in sequestered environments (military recruits, boarding school residents).	No specific therapy, or consider azithromycin, 500 milligrams day 1, 250 milligrams days 2-5 or similar macrolide.
Chlamydophila pneumoniae	Incubation is 3 wk, gradual onset of symptoms with hoarseness before cough, outbreaks common in those living in sequestered environments (college students, nursing home residents).	No specific therapy, or consider azithromycin, 500 milligrams day 1, 250 milligrams days 2-5, or similar macrolide.

*Symptomatic treatment should also be considered; see text.

- Additional agents for cough suppression, mucolysis, or other symptom relief should be considered on an individual basis, factoring comorbidities, drug interactions, and potential side effects.

PNEUMONIA

EPIDEMIOLOGY

- Community-acquired pneumonia (CAP) is a common medical problem, accounting for about 4 million cases and 1 million hospitalizations per year in the United States.
- Pneumonia is the sixth leading cause of death in the United States. Bacterial causes are the most common.

PATHOPHYSIOLOGY

- Pneumonia is an infection of the alveolar or gas exchange portions of the lung. Some forms of pneumonia produce an intense inflammatory response within the alveoli that leads to filling the air space with organisms, exudate, and white blood cells.
- Patients most at risk for pneumonia are those with a predisposition to aspiration, impaired mucociliary clearance, or risk of bacteremia.
- Pneumococcus (*Streptococcus pneumonia*) remains the classic bacterial etiology.
- Besides pneumococcus, other prevalent bacterial pneumonias are caused by *Staphylococcus aureus*, *Klebsiella pneumoniae*, *Pseudomonas aeruginosa*, and *Haemophilus influenza*.
- Incidence from atypical and opportunistic agents, particularly if pneumonia is acquired in the health care setting, is increasing.
- *Legionella pneumophila*, *M. pneumoniae*, *C. pneumoniae*, and a spectrum of respiratory viruses account for the bulk of atypical pneumonia.
- Multiple risk factors exist for pneumonia and include chronic diseases, such as cancer, bronchiectasis, chronic obstructive pulmonary disease (COPD), diabetes, sickle-cell anemia, AIDS, and other immunodeficiencies, as well as smoking.
- Aspiration pneumonia occurs more frequently in alcoholics and patients with seizures, stroke, or other neuromuscular diseases. Anaerobic agents must be suspected in aspiration.
- Lung abscesses are frequently related to aspiration pneumonia. Other causes of abscess in the lower respiratory tract include bacteremia from a remote source, pulmonary infarction, neoplasm, or pulmonary trauma.

CLINICAL FEATURES

- Patients with undifferentiated bacterial pneumonia generally present with some combination of cough, fatigue, fever, dyspnea, sputum production, and pleuritic chest pain.
- Physical findings of pneumonia vary with the offending organism and the type of pneumonia each causes, although most are associated with some degree of tachypnea and tachycardia (Table 32-3).
- Pneumococcal pneumonia classically presents with abrupt fever, rigor, and rusty brown sputum. Pleural effusion occurs in 25% of patients.
- Lobar pneumonias (see Fig. 32-1), such as those caused by pneumococcus and *K. pneumoniae*, exhibit signs of consolidation, including bronchial breath sounds, egophony, increased tactile and vocal fremitus, and dullness to percussion.
- Bronchial pneumonias, such as those caused by *H. influenzae*, reveal rales and rhonchi on examination, without signs of consolidation. A parapneumonic pleural effusion may occur in either setting; empyemas are most common with *S. aureus*, *K. pneumoniae*, and anaerobic infections.
- Interstitial pneumonias, such as those caused by *M. pneumoniae*, *C. pneumoniae*, and a host of respiratory viruses may exhibit fine rales, rhonchi, or normal breath sounds.
- Pneumonia due to *Legionella* is spread via airborne aerosolized water droplets rather than by person-to-person contact. This particular agent creates patchy bronchopneumonia (see Fig. 32-2), which may progress to frank consolidation and be associated with relative bradycardia and confusion.
- Clinical features of aspiration pneumonitis depend on the volume and pH of the aspirate, the presence of particulate matter in the aspirate, and bacterial contamination. Although acid aspiration results in the rapid onset of symptoms of tachypnea, tachycardia, and cyanosis, and often progresses to frank pulmonary failure, most other cases of aspiration pneumonia progress more insidiously.
- Physical signs of aspiration pneumonia develop over hours and include rales, rhonchi, wheezing, and copious frothy or bloody sputum. The right lower lobe is most commonly involved due to the anatomy of the tracheobronchial tree and gravity.
- Hypoxemia quantified by pulse oximetry may result from any agent of pneumonia, depending upon extent of disease and comorbidities.

DIAGNOSIS AND DIFFERENTIAL

- Uncomplicated presentations in otherwise healthy patients may not require use of radiology, laboratory,

TABLE 32-3 Clinical Characteristics of Common Bacterial Pneumonias

ORGANISM	SYMPTOMS	SPUTUM	CHEST RADIOGRAPH
Streptococcus pneumoniae	Sudden onset, fever, rigors, pleuritic chest pain, productive cough, dyspnea	Rust-colored; gram-positive encapsulated diplococci	Lobar infiltrate, occasionally patchy, occasional pleural effusion
Staphylococcus aureus	Gradual onset of productive cough, fever, dyspnea, especially just after viral illness	Purulent; gram-positive cocci in clusters	Patchy, multilobar infiltrate; empyema, lung abscess
Klebsiella pneumoniae	Sudden onset, rigors, dyspnea, chest pain, bloody sputum; especially in alcoholics or nursing home patients	Brown "currant jelly"; thick, short, plump, gram-negative, encapsulated, paired coccobacilli	Upper lobe infiltrate, bulging fissure sign, abscess formation
Pseudomonas aeruginosa	Recently hospitalized, debilitated, or immunocompromised patient with fever, dyspnea, cough	Gram-negative coccobacilli	Patchy infiltrate with frequent abscess formation
Haemophilus influenzae	Gradual onset, fever, dyspnea, pleuritic chest pain; especially in elderly and COPD	Short, tiny, gram-negative encapsulated coccobacilli	Patchy, frequently basilar infiltrate, occasional pleural effusion
Legionella pneumophila	Fever, chills, headache, malaise, dry cough, dyspnea, anorexia, diarrhea, nausea, vomiting	Few neutrophils and no predominant bacterial species	Multiple patchy nonsegmented infiltrates, progresses to consolidation, occasional cavitation, and pleural effusion
Moraxella catarrhalis	Indolent course of cough, fever, sputum, and chest pain; more common in COPD patients	Gram-negative diplococci found in sputum	Diffuse infiltrates
Chlamydophila pneumoniae	Gradual onset, fever, dry cough, wheezing, occasionally sinus symptoms	Few neutrophils, organisms not visible	Patchy subsegmental infiltrates
Mycoplasma pneumoniae	Upper and lower respiratory tract symptoms, nonproductive cough, bullous myringitis, headache, malaise, fever	Few neutrophils, organisms not visible	Interstitial infiltrates, (reticulonodular pattern), patchy densities, occasional consolidation
Anaerobic organisms	Gradual onset, putrid sputum, especially in alcoholics	Purulent; multiple neutrophils and mixed organisms	Consolidation of dependent portion of lung; abscess formation

Abbreviation: COPD = chronic obstructive pulmonary disease.

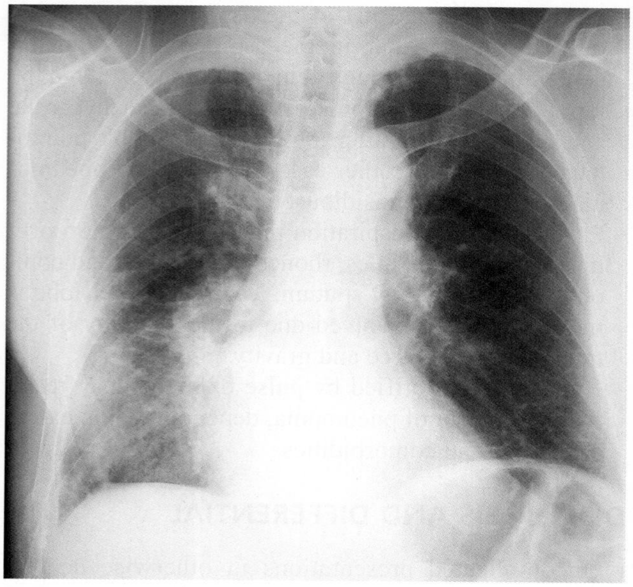

FIG. 32-1. Lobar pneumonia.

or pathology resources, although chest radiography is most commonly used in diagnosis (see Figs. 32-1 and 32-2).

- Additional diagnostic tests can include white blood count with differential and pulse oximetry. In patients with serious consideration for intensive care unit admission, obtaining blood gas analysis and cultures of blood and sputum may provide benefit to the continued treatment course.
- Sputum Gram's stain rarely changes therapy in the emergency department.
- If *Legionella* is being considered, serum chemistry studies and liver function tests should be performed, as hyponatremia, hypophosphatemia, and elevated liver enzymes are commonly found. Urine can also be tested for *Legionella* antigen.
- Most patients do not require identification of a specific organism for clinical resolution of disease.
- Given a multitude of significant pneumonia-causing organisms and special patient populations, the parent

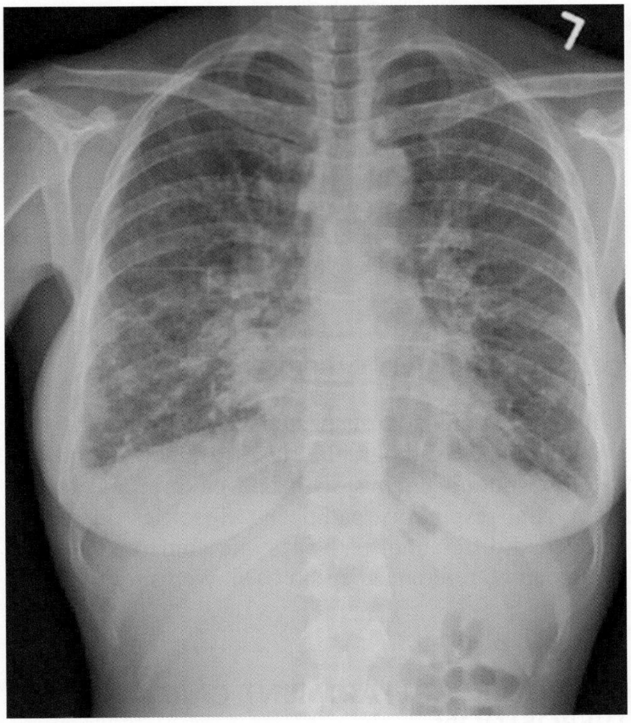

FIG. 32-2. Pneumonia suggesting *Legionella*.

text should often be consulted for additional guidance in complicated cases.

- The differential diagnosis includes noninfectious atelectasis; acute tracheobronchitis; pulmonary embolus or infarction; exacerbation of COPD; pulmonary vasculitides, including Goodpasture's disease or Wegener's granulomatosis; bronchiolitis obliterans; and endocarditis.

EMERGENCY DEPARTMENT CARE AND DISPOSITION

- The emergency department treatment and disposition of pneumonia depends primarily on the severity of the clinical presentation and radiographic findings.
- Vital respiratory function (oxygenation and ventilation) should be supported as indicated, up to and including intubation and mechanical ventilation.
- While historical features and clinical examination can prove helpful in predicting a causative organism, the treatment of pneumonia has shifted to empiric therapy based upon the patient's environment.
- The emergency clinician should differentiate between CAP and healthcare-associated pneumonia with its risk for organisms that require specific and/or broadened antibiotic coverage, such as *P. aeruginosa* or methicillin-resistant *S. aureus*.
- The complexity of pneumonia severity scoring as a means to determine discharge or admission prevents inclusion in this review. In general, progressive degrees of abnormal vital signs, comorbidities, and advancing age are associated with need for inpatient management.
- Specialty society guidelines and infectious disease consultation advice change with advent of antimicrobials and resistance patterns. The antimicrobials listed here represent a summary of current and generally accepted antibiotic regimens for adults with the indicated clinical situations. Dosages may require adjustment for renal insufficiency. Refer to parent text for more details.
- Outpatient CAP management for otherwise healthy patients who present in nontoxic states: azithromycin 500 milligrams on day 1 followed by 250 milligrams daily for 4 additional days *or* doxycycline 100 milligrams twice daily for 10 days (a low-cost alternative). The Centers for Disease Control and Prevention (CDC) recommends reserving oral fluoroquinolones for those failing macrolide or tetracycline class therapy to minimize resistance.
- Outpatient CAP management for patients with significant comorbidities (and without healthcare-associated pneumonia suspected): levofloxacin 750 milligrams orally daily for 5 days *or* amoxicillin-clavulanate 875/125 milligrams orally twice daily for 10 days *plus* azithromycin 500 milligrams orally on day 1, followed by 250 milligrams orally on days 2 to 5.
- Inpatient CAP management for patients not requiring ICU admission: initiate levofloxacin 750 milligrams IV *or* ceftriaxone 1 gram IV *plus* azithromycin 500 milligrams IV. Implement antibiotics early in the course of any patient with pneumonia requiring admission.
- Inpatient CAP management for patients requiring ICU admission: initiate ceftriaxone 1 gram IV *plus* levofloxacin 750 milligrams IV. If methicillin-resistant *S. aureus* (MRSA) is suspected, add vancomycin 10 to 15 milligrams/kg IV to the regimen.
- Inpatient management of suspected healthcare-associated pneumonia: initiate double coverage against *Pseudomonas* with levofloxacin 750 milligrams IV *plus* cefepime 1 to 2 grams IV every 8 to 12 hours *or* piperacillin/tazobactam 4.5 grams IV every 6 hours. Also, initiate coverage against MRSA with vancomycin 10 to 15 milligrams/kg IV *or* linezolid 600 milligrams IV every 12 hours.
- Aspiration: In aspiration-induced pneumonitis, prophylactic antibiotics are not recommended and their indiscriminate use may contribute to organism resistance. For witnessed aspirations, immediate tracheal

suction followed by bronchoscopy (if needed to remove large particles) is indicated. In pneumonitis that has already progressed to pneumonia prior to or shortly after emergency department presentation, initiate levofloxacin 750 milligrams IV *plus* clindamycin 600 milligrams IV every 6 hours.

- Empyema: Initiate piperacillin/tazobactam 4.5 grams IV every 6 hours. If MRSA suspected, add vancomycin 10 to 15 milligrams/kg IV to the regimen. The patient should be admitted with early consultation with a pulmonologist or thoracic surgeon for further consideration of definitive diagnostic measures and treatment options to promote drainage.
- Lung abscess: Initiate clindamycin 600 milligrams IV every 6 hours for anaerobic coverage *plus* ceftriaxone 1 gram IV every 12 hours. Inpatient medical management successfully treats a significant majority of lung abscesses; surgical consultation is required in only a minority of cases.
- Discharge instructions should, at a minimum, include close follow-up with a primary care physician, smoking cessation (when applicable), and delineation of symptoms that should prompt a return visit to the emergency department.

SEVERE ACUTE RESPIRATORY SYNDROME

Up-to-date information regarding severe acute respiratory syndrome (SARS) can be found at the CDC Web site.

EPIDEMIOLOGY

- SARS came to worldwide attention in the winter of 2002 to 2003. Numerous deaths were reported in Asia, North America, and Europe.

PATHOPHYSIOLOGY

- The etiologic agent is a coronavirus, SARS-CoV, spread by "droplet infection."

CLINICAL FEATURES

- SARS should be considered in symptomatic individuals who have traveled to an area with current suspected community transmission of SARS or who have had close contact within 10 days of symptom onset with a person known or suspected to have SARS.
- In the appearance of SARS, clinical findings included temperature >100.4°F (>38°C) and one or more findings of cough, shortness of breath, difficult breathing, or hypoxia, with advanced cases indicating radiographic evidence of pneumonia or respiratory distress syndrome. Future outbreak symptoms can be referenced at the CDC Web site.

DIAGNOSIS AND DIFFERENTIAL

- Initial testing for suspected SARS patients may include chest radiograph, pulse oximetry, blood cultures, sputum Gram's stain and culture, and testing for viral respiratory pathogens. Specifics on recommended differential pathways and confirmatory testing can be referenced at the CDC Web site.

EMERGENCY DEPARTMENT CARE AND DISPOSITION

- No specific SARS treatment recommendations can be made at the time of this text's creation.
- Clinicians evaluating suspected SARS cases should use standard precautions (eg, hand hygiene) together with airborne (eg, N-95 respirator or greater), and contact (eg, gowns and gloves) isolation precautions. Consider eye protection.
- Empiric therapy should include coverage for organisms associated with any CAP of unclear etiology, including agents with activity against both typical and atypical respiratory pathogens. Treatment choices may be influenced by severity of the illness. See section above.
- Infectious disease consultation is recommended.

For further reading in Tintinalli's *Emergency Medicine: A Comprehensive Study Guide,* 7th ed., see Chapter 67, "Acute Bronchitis and Upper Respiratory Tract Infections," by Thomas A. Tallman; Chapter 68, "Community-Acquired Pneumonia, Aspiration Pneumonia, and Noninfectious Pulmonary Infiltrates," by Charles L. Emerman, Eric Anderson, and David M. Cline; and Chapter 69, "Empyema and Lung Abscess," by Eric Anderson and Sharon E. Mace.

33 TUBERCULOSIS

Amy J. Behrman

EPIDEMIOLOGY

- Tuberculosis (TB) remains a major global problem. More than 30% of the world's population is infected with latent or active TB, which causes 2 million deaths yearly.
- The incidence of TB in the United States rose sharply between 1984 and 1992. The rise was driven by increases in rates of risk factors such as incarceration, human immunodeficiency virus (HIV) infection, drug-resistant TB, and immigration from areas with endemic TB. TB control programs targeting high-risk groups have reversed this trend progressively since 1993.
- TB case rates remain highest among U.S. residents born in high-prevalence foreign countries, who also account for the majority of multidrug-resistant TB (MDR-TB) cases. Other populations with increased prevalence include immune-compromised patients (particularly those with HIV infection), the elderly, and nursing home residents, alcoholics and illicit drug users, and residents and staff of prisons and homeless shelters.
- Patients with unrecognized TB frequently present to EDs for evaluation and care, presenting challenges for diagnosis, treatment, and infection control.

PATHOPHYSIOLOGY

- *Mycobacterium tuberculosis* is a slow-growing obligate anaerobic rod with a complex multi-lipid cell wall (responsible for its characteristic acid-fast staining property).
- Transmission occurs through inhalation of droplet nuclei, although only 30% of patients become infected after exposure. Patients with stainable mycobacteria in saliva or sputum are the most infectious.
- The organism survives best in areas with high oxygen content and blood flow, including (in the lung) the apical and posterior segments of the upper lobe and the superior segment of the lower lobe. TB organisms also survive well in the renal cortex, the meninges, the epiphyses of long bones, and the vertebrae.
- After inhalation of infectious particles, organisms that survive initial host defenses may cause granuloma formation in regional lymph nodes. The granulomas may progress to central caseating necrosis and calcification, identifiable on chest radiograph (CXR) as characteristic Ghon complexes.
- If the granuloma does not contain the primary infection, TB can spread by hematogenous, lymphatic, or direct routes.
- Progression of early active infection is most likely in immune-compromised patients.

In immune-competent hosts, initial TB infection often becomes latent and asymptomatic.

- Latent TB infection (LTBI) is manifested by positive tuberculin skin tests (TSTs, also known as purified protein derivative [PPD] testing), or interferon gamma release assays (IGRAs), in the absence of active radiologic or clinical disease.
- Untreated LTBI will progress to active disease in 5% of cases within 2 years of primary infection; an additional 5% will reactivate over their host-patient lifetimes. Reactivation rates are higher in the young, the elderly, persons with recent primary infection, those with immune deficiency (particularly HIV), and those with chronic diseases such as diabetes, silicosis, and renal failure.

CLINICAL FEATURES

- Primary TB infection is usually asymptomatic, presenting most frequently with only a new positive TST. Presenting symptoms of active primary TB infection often include fever, malaise, weight loss, and chest pain.
- Most active TB cases manifest as reactivation of LTBI. Patients usually present subacutely with systemic or pulmonary symptoms of fever, night sweats, malaise, weight loss, and fatigue. As lung infection progresses, patients may develop productive cough, hemoptysis, dyspnea, and/or chest pain.
- Rales and rhonchi may be found, but the pulmonary examination is usually nondiagnostic.
- Extrapulmonary TB develops in up to 20% of cases, most often presenting as painless lymphadenitis, with possible draining sinuses.
- Pleural effusion may occur when a peripheral parenchymal focus or local lymph node ruptures.
- TB peritonitis and pericarditis often require biopsy to diagnose as the exudates are often stain-negative.
- CNS infection may lead to TB meningitis, generally presenting with fever, headache, meningeal signs, mental status changes, and/or cranial nerve deficits. Presentation is usually acute in children and subacute in adults.
- Miliary TB is a multisystem disease caused by massive hematogenous dissemination during primary infection or secondary seeding in immune-compromised and pediatric patients. Miliary TB from primary infection often presents as acute severe

illness, which may include shock, adult respiratory distress syndrome (ARDS), and multiorgan failure. Reactivation miliary TB may present with chronic and nonspecific constitutional symptoms and signs of multisystem illness such as fever, cough, sweats, weight loss, adenopathy, hepatosplenomegaly, and cytopenias.

- Extrapulmonary TB may also involve bone, joints, skin, kidneys, adrenals, and eyes.
- Immunocompromised patients (HIV patients in particular) are extremely susceptible to TB and far more likely to develop active infections with atypical presentations. Disseminated extrapulmonary TB is also more common in HIV patients and should be considered in the evaluation of nonpulmonary complaints. **Patients with suspected TB should be offered HIV testing.**
- Prior partially treated TB is a risk factor for drug-resistant TB. It should be considered when TB is diagnosed, especially among those with suboptimal prior care (eg, immigrants from endemic areas, prisoners, homeless persons, drug users).
- As compared to the general population, HIV patients more commonly have MDR-TB, and the disease is more likely fatal in this group.

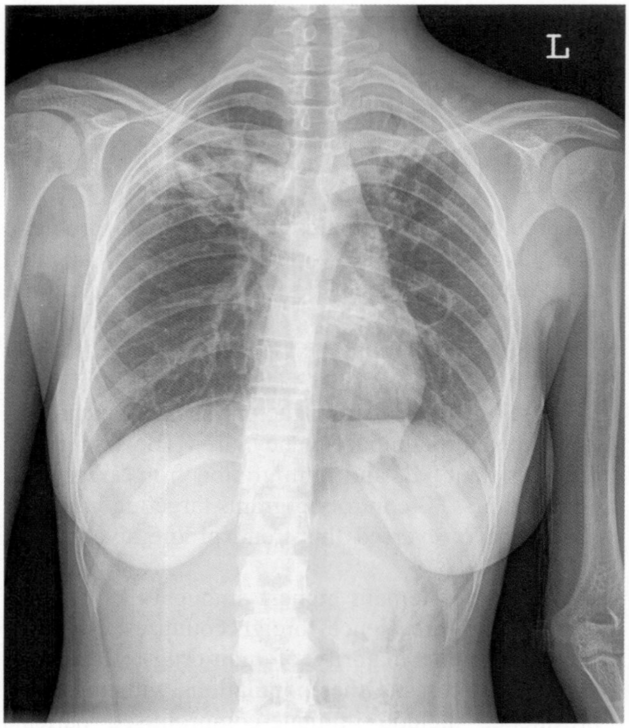

FIG. 33-1. Cavitary tuberculosis of the right upper lobe.

DIAGNOSIS AND DIFFERENTIAL

- TB infection is difficult to diagnose because of its variable presentations. Early consideration of TB in any patient with respiratory or systemic complaints facilitates early diagnosis, appropriate disposition, and protection of staff.
- CXRs remain the most useful diagnostic tool for active TB in the ED. Although atypical (or even normal) CXRs are common in immune-compromised hosts, the clinician should be familiar with common findings. Active primary TB usually presents with parenchymal infiltrates in any lung area. Hilar and/or mediastinal adenopathy may occur with or without infiltrates. Lesions may calcify.
- Reactivation TB typically presents with lesions in the upper lobes or superior segments of the lower lobes. Cavitation, calcification, scarring, atelectasis, and effusions may be seen (Fig. 33-1). Cavitation is associated with increased infectivity.
- Miliary TB may cause diffuse small (1- to 3-mm) nodular infiltrates.
- Acid-fast staining of sputum can detect mycobacteria in 60% of patients with pulmonary TB, although the yield is lower in HIV patients. Atypical mycobacteria can cause false-positive stains. Many patients will have false-negatives on a single sputum sample. Microscopy of non-sputum samples (eg, pleural fluid, cerebrospinal fluid [CSF]) is even less sensitive.
- Definitive cultures generally take weeks, but new genetic tests employing DNA probes or polymerase chain reaction technology can confirm the diagnosis sooner.
- TST using the Mantoux method (intradermal tuberculin skin testing with PPD) identifies most patients with latent, prior, or active TB infection. Results are read 48 to 72 hours after placement, limiting the usefulness of this test for ED patients. Persons with positive PPDs and no active TB disease should be evaluated for prophylactic treatment with isoniazid (INH) to prevent reactivation TB (see Fig. 33-2).
- Patients with HIV or other immunosuppressive conditions and patients with disseminated TB may have false-negative skin tests even if these individuals are not fully anergic.
- IGRAs may be helpful in diagnosing latent, and potentially active, TB infection, but results are also unlikely to be available in time for ED management needs.

EMERGENCY DEPARTMENT CARE AND DISPOSITION

- To prevent drug resistance, TB infection is treated with combination antimicrobials. Initial therapy

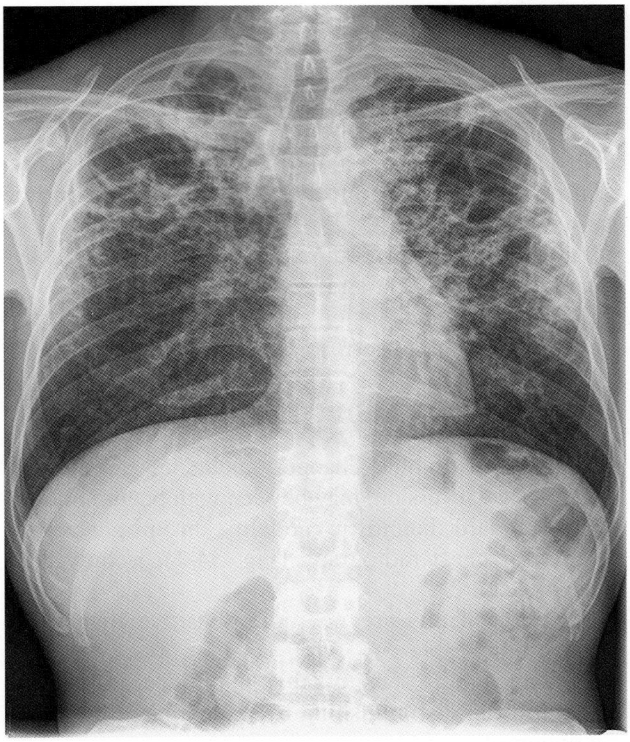

FIG. 33-2. Reactivation tuberculosis. Multiple fine nodular densities are seen throughout the central and peripheral lungs bilaterally, overlying residual scaring from prior active infection.

should include at least four drugs until susceptibility profiles are available for the patient.

- Initial therapy usually includes INH, rifampin, pyrazinamide, and ethambutol for 2 to 8 weeks; this should be followed by administration of at least two drugs (usually INH and rifampin) for at least 18 weeks (see Table 33-1).
- Patients with immune compromise, extrapulmonary TB, or MDR-TB may require more drugs or longer treatment periods.
- Table 33-1 summarizes usual initial daily drug doses and side effects.
- Most TB infection is treated in an outpatient setting. Ambulatory treatment for TB should not be initiated in the ED unless coordinated with or directed by the providers who will manage ongoing care.
- Patients with active TB who are discharged from the ED must have documented immediate referral to a public health department or qualified physician for long-term treatment and monitoring of drug toxicity. Patients should be educated about home isolation, follow-up, and screening of household contacts.
- Directly observed treatment (DOT) improves treatment outcomes for patients at high risk for noncompliance and the development of MDR-TB.
- Admission is indicated for clinical instability, diagnostic uncertainty, unreliable outpatient follow-up or compliance, and active known MDR-TB. Physicians should know local laws regarding involuntary hospitalization and treatment.

TABLE 33-1 Dosages and Common Side Effects of Some Drugs Used in Tuberculosis (Adults)*

DRUG	DAILY (MAXIMUM)	THREE TIMES WEEKLY DOT (MAXIMUM)	TWO TIMES WEEKLY DOT (MAXIMUM)	POTENTIAL SIDE EFFECTS AND COMMENTS
Isoniazid	5 milligrams/kg PO* (300 milligrams)	15 milligrams/kg PO (900 milligrams)	15 milligrams/kg PO (900 milligrams)	Hepatitis, peripheral neuropathy, drug interactions.
Rifampin (RIF)	10 milligrams/kg PO* (600 milligrams)	10 milligrams/kg PO (600 milligrams)	10 milligrams/kg PO (600 milligrams)	Hepatitis, thrombocytopenia, GI disturbances, drug interactions.
Rifapentine	Not given daily	Not given three times weekly	600 milligrams PO twice weekly in adults; not approved in children <12 y old	Hepatitis, thrombocytopenia, exacerbation of porphyria. Centers for Disease Control and Prevention recommended for continuation therapy only for human immunodeficiency virus–negative patients.
Rifabutin	5 milligrams/kg PO (300 milligrams)	5 milligrams/kg PO (300 milligrams)	5 milligrams/kg PO (300 milligrams)	Similar to RIF, used for patients who cannot tolerate RIF.
Ethambutol	15-20 milligrams/kg PO (1.6 grams)	25-30 milligrams/kg PO (2.5 grams)	50 milligrams/kg PO (2.5 grams)	Retrobulbar neuritis, peripheral neuropathy.
Pyrazinamide	15-30 milligrams/kg PO (2 grams)	50 milligrams/kg PO (3 grams)	50 milligrams/kg PO (2 grams)	Hepatitis, arthralgia, hyperuricemia.

Abbreviation: DOT = directly observed therapy.
*See http://www.cdc.gov/tb for more accurate weight-based protocols and dosages for children.

- Admission to airborne isolation is mandatory for all cases of suspected TB to protect staff and other patients.
- Prehospital and ED staff should be trained to identify patients at risk for active TB as early as possible in their presentation. Patients with suspected TB should be masked or placed in respiratory isolation. TB should be considered in all immune-compromised or high-risk patients with respiratory symptoms.
- Staff caring directly for patients with suspected TB should wear National Institute of Occupational Safety and Health (NIOSH)-approved respiratory protection such as N95 or powered air-purifying respirators.
- ED staff should receive regular TST or IGRA testing to detect new primary infections, rule out active disease, and guide decisions for INH prophylaxis.

For further reading in Tintinalli's *Emergency Medicine: A Comprehensive Study Guide*, 7th ed., see Chapter 70, "Tuberculosis" by Vu D. Phan and Janet M. Poponick.

34 SPONTANEOUS AND IATROGENIC PNEUMOTHORAX

Rodney L. McCaskill

EPIDEMIOLOGY

- The most common risk factor for spontaneous pneumothorax is smoking, although chronic lung disease and infections are predisposing factors.
- History of prior pneumothorax is common since 20% to 30% of patients experience recurrence.
- Iatrogenic pneumothorax occurs secondary to invasive procedures such as transthoracic needle biopsy (50%), subclavian line placement (25%), nasogastric tube placement, or positive pressure ventilation; post-procedure chest radiograph should always be performed to assess for this complication.

PATHOPHYSIOLOGY

- Pneumothorax likely occurs after rupture of a subpleural bulla allows air to enter the potential space between the parietal and visceral pleura, leading to partial lung collapse.
- Tension pneumothorax is caused by positive pressure in the pleural space leading to decreased venous return, hypotension, and hypoxia.

CLINICAL FEATURES

- Symptoms resulting from a pneumothorax are directly related to the size, rate of development, and underlying lung disease.
- Most patients complain of acute onset pleuritic pain and have diminished breath sounds on the affected side.
- Large volume pneumothoraces cause dyspnea, tachycardia, hypotension, and hypoxia.
- Clinical signs of tension pneumothorax include tracheal deviation, hyperresonance, and hypotension.

DIAGNOSIS AND DIFFERENTIAL

- Electrocardiographic changes, including ST changes and T-wave inversion, may be seen with pneumothorax.
- The standard diagnostic modality, an upright posteroanterior chest radiograph (Fig. 34-1), is only 83% sensitive.
- Expiratory films are no more sensitive than a PA chest radiograph.
- CT scan is more sensitive than plain radiography, and is helpful in distinguishing between a large bulla and a pneumothorax.
- The sensitivity of ultrasound is near 100%. Sonographic signs include absence of lung sliding,

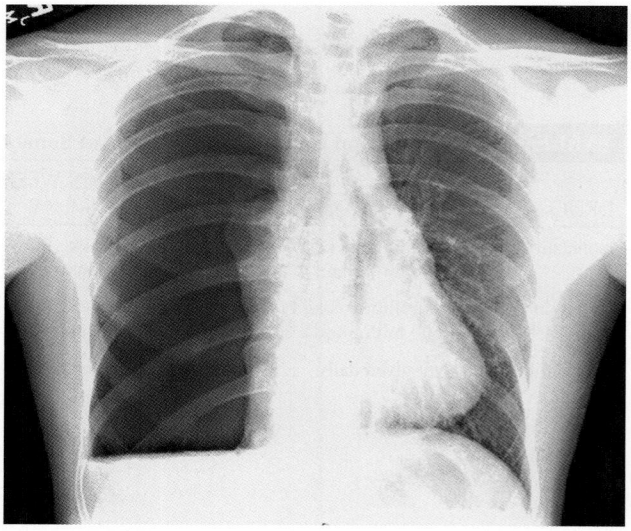

FIG. 34-1. Spontaneous hemopneumothorax. Upright chest radiograph of a 19-year-old male college student with spontaneous hemopneumothorax. Note the large air-fluid level in the inferior portion of the right hemithorax in addition to the complete collapse of the entire right lung. In spite of reexpansion of the collapsed lung after thoracostomy tube placement, the patient experienced persistent bleeding. After 1 L of blood loss from the chest, emergent thoracotomy was required for control of hemorrhage from a vessel along the apical parietal pleura.

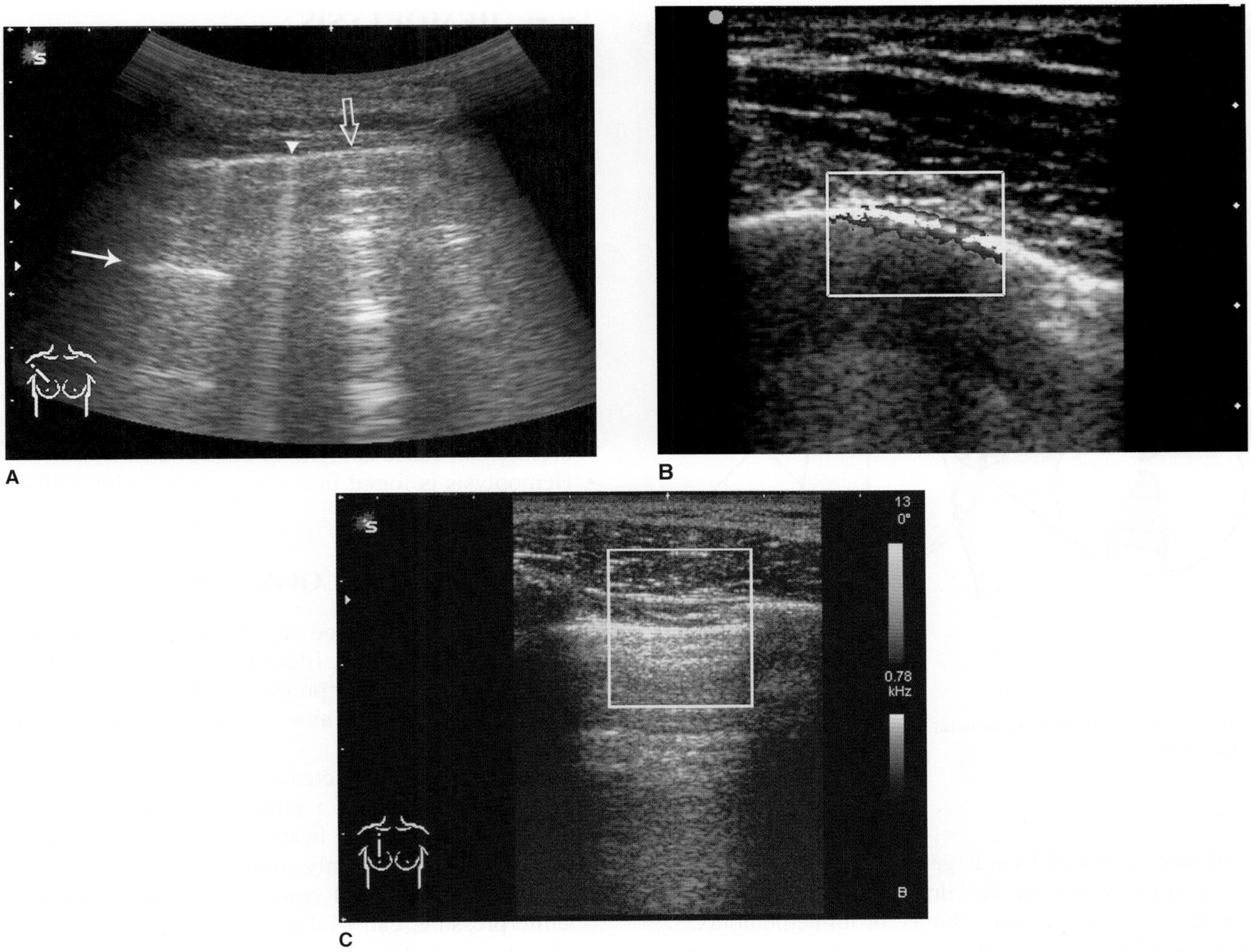

FIG. 34-2. Ultrasonography (US) of normal lung and pneumothorax. **A.** Normal lung artifacts. The A-line (*arrow*) represents the horizontal reverberation artifact generated by the parietal pleura (line shown by *arrowhead* and *open arrow*). Comet-tail artifacts arise from the pleura and project to the depth of the image. They move back and forth along the pleura in real time and may vary between a narrow (*arrowhead*) and a wider (*open arrow*) appearance. **B.** Power Doppler with color gain set low, normal lung appearance. Color highlights the movement of the parietal and visceral pleura interface. **C.** US of pneumothorax. Absence of lung movement on power Doppler. No sliding movement seen in real time; comet-tail artifacts replaced by horizontal airy artifacts.

demonstration of a "lung point," and absence of normal vertical comet-tail artifacts (Fig. 34-2).

- Differential diagnosis includes costochondritis, angina, myocardial infarction, pulmonary embolism, pericarditis, pleurisy, pneumonia, and aortic dissection.

EMERGENCY DEPARTMENT CARE AND DISPOSITION

- Oxygen 3 to 10 L by nasal cannula helps increase resorption of pleural air.
- For patients with small pneumothoraces and *no* known lung disease treatment, options include the following:

1. Observation for 6 hours and outpatient surgical follow-up within 24 hours if there is no enlargement on radiograph.
2. Aspiration using a needle or catheter (<14 gauge) followed by immediate removal of the device, 6 hours of observation, and surgical follow-up if there is no recurrence. This method has a success rate reported as 37% to 75%.
3. Placement of a small catheter (<14 F) or chest tube (10-14 F) and admission. Consider use of Heimlich valve with this approach (see Fig. 34-3).

- In patients with small pneumothoraces and known lung disease, a small catheter (<14 F) or chest tube (10-22 F) should be placed. Consider use of Heimlich valve (see Fig. 34-3).

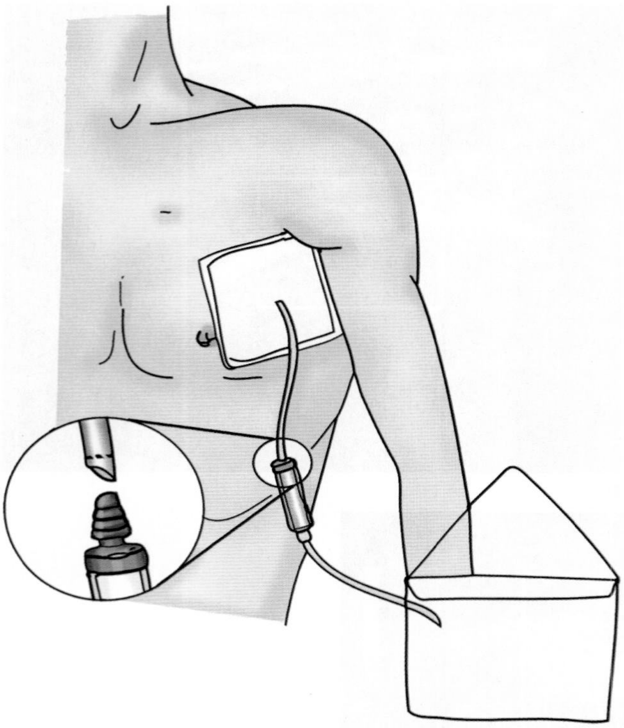

FIG. 34-3. Illustration of catheter or tube with Heimlich valve placement.

- Moderate- (16-22 F) or large- (24-36 F) sized tube thoracostomy with water seal drainage is indicated for any large or bilateral pneumothorax, or for hemothorax.
- In unstable patients (those with tension pneumothorax or pneumothorax with severe underlying lung disease), needle thoracostomy followed by tube thoracostomy should be performed before radiography.
- Helicopter transport, general anesthesia, or mechanical ventilation may also be indications for tube thoracostomy.
- Treatment for iatrogenic pneumothorax follows the above general principles.
- The treatment complication of reexpansion pulmonary edema is rare; it tends to occur more commonly in those aged 20 to 39 years, those with large pneumothoraces, and those with a pneumothorax that has been present for more than 72 hours prior to lung reexpansion.

For further reading in Tintinalli's *Emergency Medicine: A Comprehensive Study Guide*, 7th ed., see Chapter 71, "Spontaneous and Iatrogenic Pneumothorax," by Roger L. Humphries and William Franklin Young, Jr.

35 HEMOPTYSIS

Jeffrey Dixon

EPIDEMIOLOGY

- Hemoptysis is defined somewhat arbitrarily as mild (less than 20 mL of blood loss in 24 hours), moderate, or massive (greater than 600 mL of blood loss in 24 hours).
- Most cases are not life threatening—but all require careful evaluation.
- The most common causes include infection (eg, tuberculosis or TB), neoplasm, and cardiovascular disease. No cause is found in 28% of cases.
- Hemoptysis is found in all age groups, with a 60:40 male predominance.

PATHOPHYSIOLOGY

- The lung has dual blood supply from the pulmonary and bronchial arteries. Bleeding may result (1) from increased intravascular pressure, (2) from erosion into a blood vessel, or (3) as a complication of a coagulopathy.
- Hemoptysis due to increased intravascular pressure generally arises from a primary cardiac abnormality such as congestive heart failure (75% of cardiac cases) or, less commonly, mitral stenosis.
- Erosion into bronchial vessels, which are under systemic pressure, can lead to severe hemoptysis. This often is due to TB, bronchiectasis, or malignancy.

CLINICAL FEATURES

- The acute onset of fever, cough, and bloody sputum suggests pneumonia or bronchitis. A more indolent productive cough may represent bronchitis or bronchiectasis.
- Dyspnea and pleuritic chest pain are hallmarks of pulmonary embolism.
- Fever, night sweats, and weight loss often reflect TB or malignancy. Chronic dyspnea and minor hemoptysis may represent mitral stenosis or alveolar hemorrhage syndromes (often associated with renal disease).
- Smoking, male gender, and age greater than 40 years are the main risk factors for neoplasm.
- The physical examination is aimed at assessing the severity of hemoptysis and the underlying disease process, but is unreliable in localizing the site of bleeding.
- Commonly associated findings include fever and tachypnea. Hypotension is rare except in massive hemoptysis. Cardiac examination may reveal signs of

mitral stenosis. Lung auscultation, often normal, may reveal rales, wheezes, or signs of focal consolidation. Adenopathy or muscle wasting should increase concern for malignancy.

- Careful inspection of the oral and nasal cavities is warranted to help exclude an extrapulmonary source of bleeding.

DIAGNOSIS AND DIFFERENTIAL

- The differential diagnosis of hemoptysis includes infection (bronchitis, pneumonia, TB, fungal pneumonia, and lung abscess), malignant lesions (primary lung neoplasms or metastatic tumors), cardiogenic causes (left ventricular failure or mitral stenosis), inflammatory causes (bronchiectasis or cystic fibrosis), trauma, foreign body aspiration, pulmonary embolism, primary pulmonary hypertension, vasculitis, and bleeding diathesis.
- Testing should include pulse oximetry and chest radiography (see Fig. 35-1). While 15% to 30% of all patients presenting with hemoptysis will have a normal chest radiograph, an abnormal chest radiograph is seen in the vast majority (80%-90%) of those with underlying malignancy; chest computed tomography (CT) should be considered in hemoptysis patients with abnormal chest radiographs.
- A hematocrit and type and crossmatch should be obtained in major hemoptysis. Other testing should be ordered as indicated by the clinical situation.

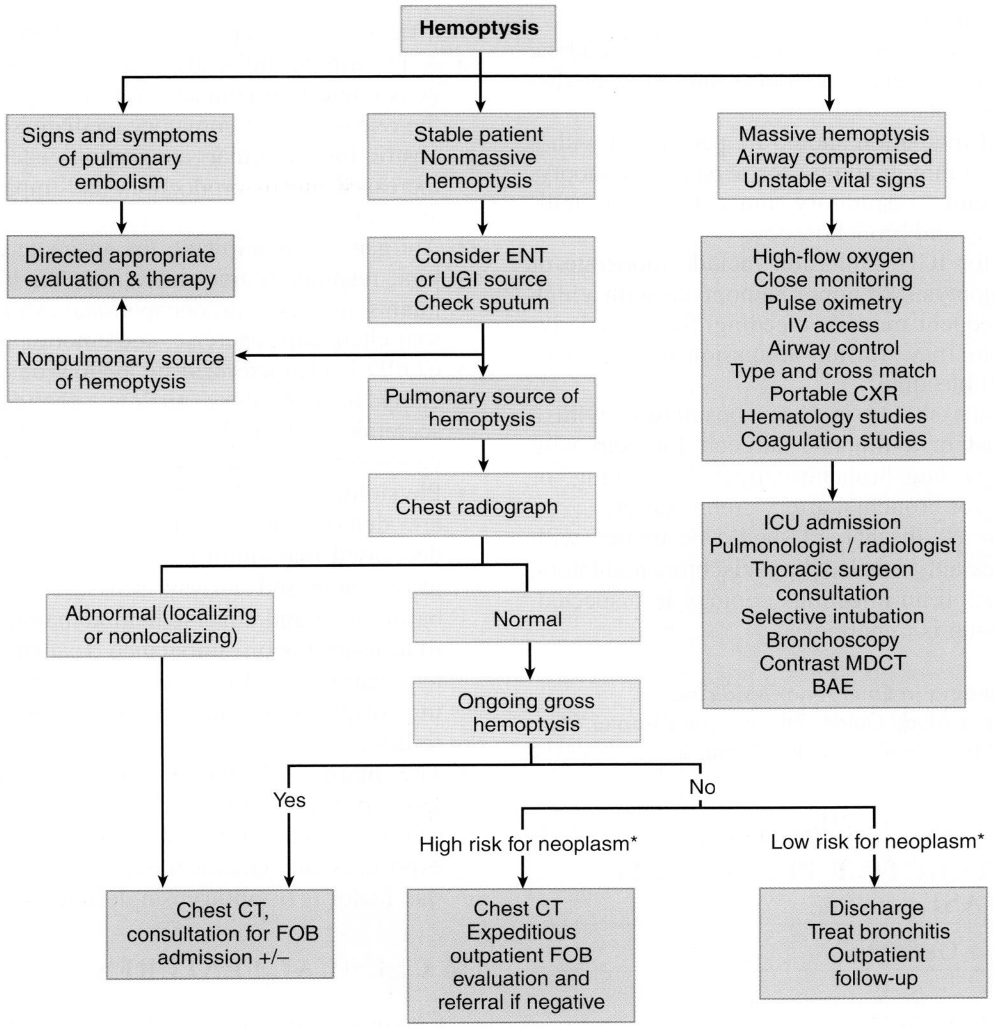

FIG. 35-1. Evaluation of hemoptysis. *High risk for neoplasm: age >40 years old, >40 pack-year smoking history, recurrent bleed, or no history consistent with lower respiratory tract infection. BAE = bronchial artery embolization; CXR = chest radiograph; ENT = ear, nose, and throat; FOB = fiber-optic bronchoscopy; ICU = intensive care unit; MDCT = multidetector CT; UGI = upper GI.

EMERGENCY DEPARTMENT CARE AND DISPOSITION

- ED treatment is based on hemoptysis severity and associated signs and symptoms. Initial management focuses on airway, breathing, and circulation. Cardiac and noninvasive blood pressure monitoring, along with pulse oximetry, should be utilized. Large-bore IV lines should be placed in patients with more severe presentations.
- Administer supplemental oxygen as needed.
- Administer normal saline or lactated Ringer's solution initially for hypotension. Packed red blood cells should be transfused as needed.
- Fresh frozen plasma (two units) should be given to those patients with coagulopathies; platelets should be administered to those with thrombocytopenia.
- Patients with ongoing massive hemoptysis may benefit from being placed in the decubitus position with the bleeding side down.
- Cough suppression with opioids (eg, hydrocodone 5-15 milligrams every 4-6 hours) may prevent dislodgement of clots.
- Endotracheal intubation should be performed with a large tube (8.0 mm in adults) for persistent hemoptysis and worsening respiratory status. This will facilitate suctioning and bronchoscopy.
- Indications for ICU admission include moderate or massive hemoptysis, or minor hemoptysis with a high risk of subsequent massive bleeding. Some underlying conditions may warrant admission regardless of the degree of bleeding.
- All admissions should include consultation with a pulmonologist or a thoracic surgeon for help with decisions regarding bronchoscopy, CT scanning, or angiography for bronchial artery embolization.
- Patients who are discharged should be treated with cough suppressants, inhaled β-agonist bronchodilators, and antibiotics if an infectious etiology is suspected. Close follow-up is important.

For further reading in *Emergency Medicine: A Comprehensive Study Guide*, 7th ed., see Chapter 66, "Hemoptysis," by William Franklin Young, Jr.

36 ASTHMA AND CHRONIC OBSTRUCTIVE PULMONARY DISEASE

Joshua Gentges

EPIDEMIOLOGY

- Asthma is a common, chronic respiratory complaint. Increased incidence is associated with a Western lifestyle, increased environmental pollutants, and exposure to allergens.
- Chronic obstructive pulmonary disease (COPD) is a worldwide respiratory health problem. It is the only major cause of death that is increasing.
- COPD is more common and more severe in the elderly. The incidence of and mortality from COPD is rising in women. Worldwide, COPD prevalence is rising and is closely associated with cigarette use.

PATHOPHYSIOLOGY

- The pathophysiologic hallmark of asthma is the reduction in airway diameter caused by smooth muscle contraction, vascular congestion, bronchial wall edema, and thick secretions. The inflammatory reaction that triggers the decrease in airway diameter results in increasing work of breathing and has a significant effect on pulmonary function.
- Acute airway inflammation is triggered when antigens come into contact with mast cells, resulting in the release of inflammatory mediators and bronchoconstriction, vascular congestion, edema formation, increased mucus production, and impaired mucociliary transport.
- Antigens or precipitants of an acute attack include viral respiratory tract infections, environmental pollutants, medications, occupational exposures to industrial chemicals, exercise, and emotional stress.
- COPD is characterized by airflow obstruction, especially in expiratory airflow secondary to airway secretions, mucosal edema, bronchospasm, and bronchoconstriction due to impaired lung elasticity.
- Physiologic consequences of airflow obstruction are demonstrated in increased airway resistance, decreased maximum expiratory flow rates, air trapping, increased airway pressures (with resultant barotrauma and adverse hemodynamic effects), ventilation-perfusion imbalance (causing hypoxemia/hypercarbia), and increased work of breathing causing respiratory muscle fatigue with ventilatory failure.
- The major risk factor for developing COPD is tobacco smoke. Other risk factors associated with COPD include respiratory infections, occupational exposures, and chemical exposures. The only genetic risk factor is α_1-antitrypsin deficiency.

CLINICAL FEATURES

- Classically, asthma and COPD exacerbations present with dyspnea, chest tightness, wheezing, and cough.
- Physical examination findings of a mild asthma attack include wheezing and a prolonged expiratory phase.

Wheezing does not correlate with the degree of airflow obstruction, as a quiet chest may indicate severe airflow obstruction.
- A patient with a severe asthma exacerbation may present in a tripod position gasping for air with audible wheezing, diaphoresis, and accessory muscle use. Other signs of severe exacerbation include tachycardia, tachypnea, hypertension, and hypoxia. Paradoxical respirations, altered mental status, lethargy, and a quiet chest are all indicative of severe airflow obstruction and impending respiratory failure.
- The two dominant clinical forms of COPD are pulmonary emphysema and chronic bronchitis. Emphysema is characterized by abnormal permanent enlargement and destruction of the air spaces distal to terminal bronchioles. By contrast, excess mucus secretion in the bronchial tree with a chronic productive cough occurring on most days for at least 3 months, in the year for two consecutive years, is characteristic of chronic bronchitis. Elements of both clinical forms are often present, although one may predominate.
- Signs of hypercapnia include confusion, tremor, plethora, stupor, hypopnea, and apnea.
- Risk factors for death from asthma include past history of intubation, multiple hospitalizations or recent emergency room visits, heavy use of inhaled β_2-agonists, illicit drug use, and chronic psychiatric disease.
- Respiratory failure from COPD is associated with severe dyspnea refractory to initial treatment, worsening hypoxemia or hypercapnia, or respiratory acidosis.

DIAGNOSIS AND DIFFERENTIAL

- Diagnosis of asthma or COPD is based on the history and physical examination. Investigate possible causes of decompensation.
- Spirometry is commonly used to determine the severity of airflow obstruction and the effectiveness of therapy by measuring the peak expiratory flow rate (PEFR). Sequential measurements of PEFR assess the response of treatment and can be used to predict need for hospitalization. PEFR less than 40% of predicted is associated with severe airway obstruction.
- Pulse oximetry is a noninvasive means for assessing and monitoring oxygen saturation during treatment. It does not provide information about acid-base disturbances and hypercapnia.
- Arterial blood gases (ABGs) may be used in asthma and COPD to assess for hypercapnia and respiratory acidosis. These are ominous findings and indicate extreme airway obstruction and fatigue with possible onset of acute respiratory failure.

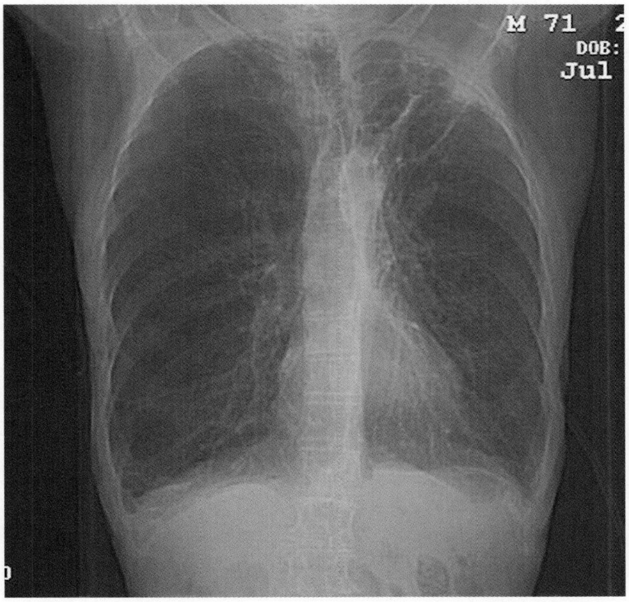

FIG. 36-1. Posterior-anterior chest radiograph in a patient with chronic obstructive pulmonary disease.

- A chest radiograph should be obtained if there is clinical suspicion of pneumothorax, pneumomediastinum, pneumonia, or other medical concerns such as congestive heart failure (CHF), pleural effusions, or pulmonary neoplasia (see Fig. 36-1).
- Electrocardiograms (ECGs) are helpful in asthma and COPD to assess for cardiac ischemia, myocardial infarction, and arrhythmias such as multifocal atrial tachycardia. ECG findings in moderate to severe pulmonary disease may reveal right ventricular strain, abnormal P waves, or nonspecific ST-T wave abnormalities, which may resolve with treatment (see Fig. 36-2).
- The differential diagnosis of decompensated asthma and COPD includes CHF, upper airway obstruction, aspiration, pulmonary neoplasia, pleural effusions, interstitial lung diseases, pneumonia, pulmonary embolism, and exposure to asphyxiants. COPD is a major risk factor for pneumothorax. CHF, pneumonia, and acute coronary syndrome commonly coexist with decompensated COPD.

EMERGENCY DEPARTMENT CARE AND DISPOSITION

- All patients should be placed on a cardiac monitor, pulse oximeter, and noninvasive blood pressure monitor, and patients with moderate to severe attacks should have IV access.

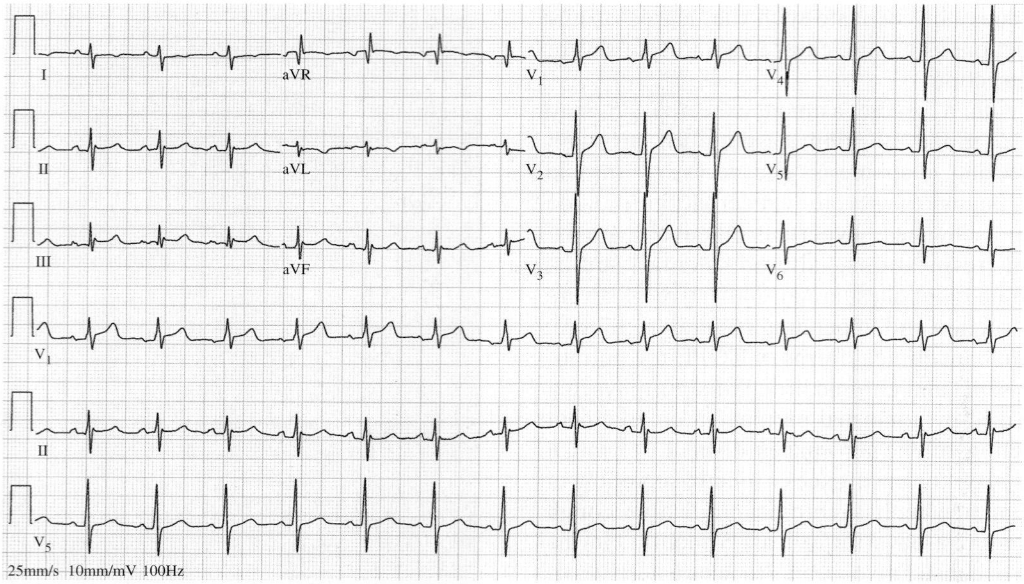

FIG. 36-2. ECG findings of right ventricular hypertrophy in a patient with chronic obstructive pulmonary disease: rightward axis, R wave taller than the S wave in lead V_1, and a persistent S wave into the lateral precordial leads. Findings of right ventricular hypertrophy, not demonstrated here, are an incomplete right bundle branch block pattern, and a strain pattern (asymmetric ST-segment depression and T-wave inversion) in right ventricular leads.

- Empiric supplemental oxygen should be administered to correct Sao_2 above 90%. Oxygen may exacerbate hypercapnia in the setting of COPD. Perform an ABG measurement if there is concern for symptomatic hypercapnia.
- β-Adrenergic agonists are first-line agents used to treat acute bronchospasm in COPD and asthma. Aerosolized forms minimize systemic toxicity and are preferred. Albuterol sulfate 2.5 to 5 milligrams is the most common agent. Deliver doses every 20 minutes or as continuous nebulization (10-15 milligrams/h), continuing treatment based on clinical response and signs of toxicity (tachycardia, hypertension, and palpitations). Levalbuterol can be given at one-half of the dose of albuterol, but has not been studied by continuous nebulization. Terbutaline sulfate (0.25-0.5 mL) or epinephrine 1:1000 (0.1-0.3 mL) SC may be administered to patients not tolerating aerosolized therapy. Epinephrine should be avoided in the first trimester of pregnancy and in patients with underlying cardiovascular disease.
- Anticholinergics are useful adjuvants when given with other therapies. Nebulized ipratropium (500 milligrams = 2.5 mL) may be administered alone or mixed with albuterol. The effects of ipratropium peak in 1 to 2 hours and last 3 to 4 hours. Dosages may be repeated every 1 to 4 hours.
- Steroids should be given immediately to patients with exacerbations of asthma and COPD. The initial dose is the equivalent of 40 to 60 milligrams of oral prednisone. If the patient is unable to take oral medication, intravenous methylprednisolone 60 to 125 milligrams may be used. Additional doses may be given every 4 to 6 hours. Inhaled steroids are not indicated for the treatment of acute symptoms. A 5- to 10-day course of oral steroids (prednisone 40-60 milligrams/d) is beneficial for discharged patients with a significant exacerbation of asthma or COPD.
- COPD exacerbations with change in sputum color or volume should be administered antibiotic therapy directed at respiratory pathogens. No specific agents are shown to be superior. Reserve antibiotic use in asthma for concurrent bacterial infections.
- Magnesium sulfate (1-2 grams IV) may be used in severe asthma attack due to its bronchodilatory properties.
- Heliox (80% helium and 20% oxygen) can be used in severe asthma exacerbations to lower airway resistance in patients with no supplemental oxygen requirement.
- Patients with respiratory muscle fatigue, respiratory acidosis, altered mental status, or hypoxia refractory to standard therapies need mechanical ventilation. Noninvasive partial pressure ventilation (NPPV) is a

useful alternative to intubation and invasive ventilation. It lowers intubation rates, short-term mortality, and length of hospitalization in COPD. NPPV can be given by continuous positive airway pressure (CPAP) or bi-level positive airway pressure (BiPAP). BiPAP has the advantage of reducing the work of breathing. CPAP is titrated up to 15 cm H_2O, while BiPAP settings are between 8 and 20 cm H_2O for inspiration and 4 and 15 cm H_2O for expiration. Evidence for NPPV in severe asthma is promising but less compelling than that for COPD. NPPV should not be used for patients with a suspected pneumothorax.

- Patients that are uncooperative or obtunded, cannot clear airway secretions, are hemodynamically unstable, in respiratory arrest, have had recent facial or gastroesophageal surgery, facial burns, extreme obesity, or poor NPPV mask fit are not candidates for NPPV and require invasive ventilation. Oral intubation is the preferred method. Using rapid inspiratory flow rates at a reduced respiratory frequency (12-14 breaths/min) and allowing for an adequate expiratory phase may help reduce air trapping and subsequent barotrauma. Therapy should be guided by pulse oximetry and ABG results. Sedation and continued therapy for bronchospasm should continue after the patient has been placed on artificial ventilation.
- In patients being discharged, continued treatment with β_2-agonists and oral steroids is important. In addition, patient education and close medical follow-up is essential.

For further reading in Tintinalli's *Emergency Medicine: A Comprehensive Study Guide*, 7th ed., see Chapter 72, "Acute Asthma in Adults," by Rita K. Cydulka, and Chapter 73, "Chronic Obstructive Pulmonary Disease," by Craig G. Bates and Rita K. Cydulka.

Section 7
GASTROINTESTINAL EMERGENCIES

37 ACUTE ABDOMINAL PAIN

David M. Cline

EPIDEMIOLOGY

- Data from the United States National Center for Health Statistics indicate that abdominal pain was the single most frequently mentioned reason offered by patients for visiting the ED in 2006 (6.7% of ED visits—8.04 million patient encounters).
- Admission rates for abdominal pain vary markedly, ranging from 18% to 42%, with rates as high as 63% reported in patients over 65 years of age.

PATHOPHYSIOLOGY

- Visceral abdominal pain is usually caused by stretching of fibers innervating the walls or capsules of hollow or solid organs, respectively. Less commonly it is caused by early ischemia or inflammation.
- Foregut organs (stomach, duodenum, and biliary tract) produce pain in the epigastric region; midgut organs (most of the small bowel, and the appendix and cecum) cause periumbilical pain; and hindgut organs (most of the colon, including the sigmoid) as well as the intraperitoneal portions of the genitourinary system tend to cause pain initially in the suprapubic or hypogastric area.
- Visceral pain is usually felt at the midline.
- Parietal or somatic abdominal pain is caused by irritation of fibers that innervate the parietal peritoneum, usually the portion covering the anterior abdominal wall.
- In contrast to visceral pain, parietal pain can be localized to the dermatome directly above the site of the painful stimulus. As the underlying disease process evolves, the symptoms of visceral pain give way to the signs of parietal pain, with tenderness and guarding. As localized peritonitis develops further, rigidity and rebound appear.
- Referred pain is felt at a location distant from the diseased organ.

CLINICAL FEATURES

- Consider immediate life threats that might require emergency intervention.
- Elicit time of pain onset; character, severity, location of pain (Fig. 37-1), and its referral; aggravating and alleviating factors; and similar prior episodes.
- Cardiorespiratory symptoms, such as chest pain, dyspnea, and cough; genitourinary symptoms, such as urgency, dysuria, and vaginal discharge; and any history of trauma should be elicited.
- In older patients it is also important to obtain a history of myocardial infarction, dysrhythmias, coagulopathies, and vasculopathies.
- Past medical and surgical histories should be elicited, and a list of medications, particularly steroids, antibiotics, or nonsteroidal anti-inflammatory drugs (NSAIDs), should be noted.
- A thorough gynecologic history is indicated in female patients.
- The physical examination should include the patient's general appearance. Patients with peritonitis tend to lie still.
- The skin should be evaluated for pallor or jaundice.
- The vital signs should be inspected for signs of hypovolemia due to blood loss or volume depletion. Due to medications or the physiology of aging, tachycardia may not always occur in the face of hypovolemia.
- A core temperature should be obtained; however, absence of fever does not rule out infection, particularly in the elderly.
- The abdomen should be inspected for contour, scars, peristalsis, masses, distention, and pulsation. The presence of hyperactive or high-pitched or tinkling bowel sounds increases the likelihood of small bowel obstruction.
- Palpation is the most important aspect of the physical examination.
- The abdomen and genitals should be assessed for tenderness, guarding, masses, organomegaly, and hernias.
- "Rebound" tenderness, often regarded as the clinical criterion standard of peritonitis, has several important limitations. In patients with peritonitis, the

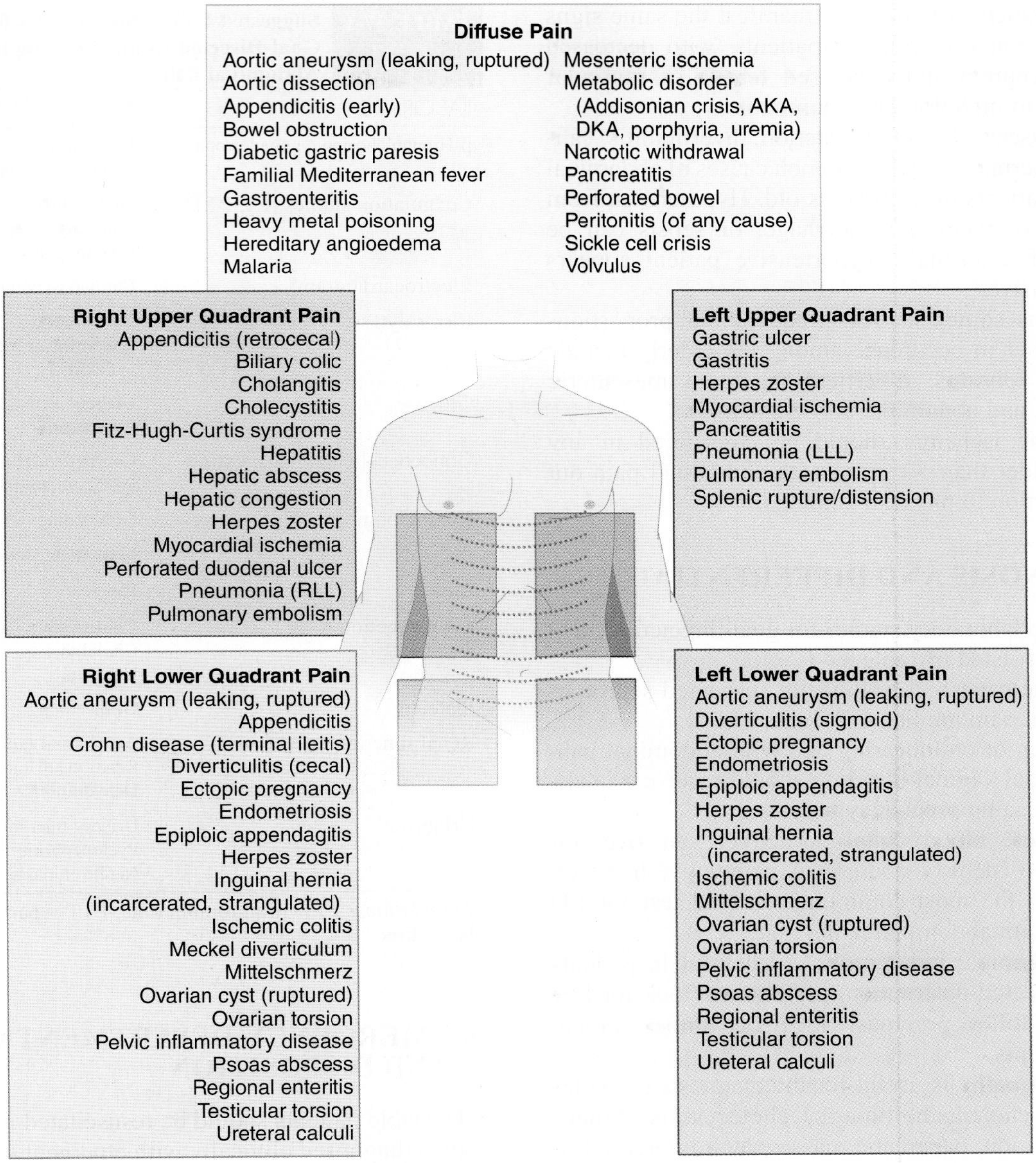

FIG. 37-1. Differential diagnosis of acute abdominal pain by location. AKA = alcoholic ketoacidosis; DKA = diabetic ketoacidosis; LLL = lower left lobe; RLL = right lower lobe.

combination of rigidity, referred tenderness, and, especially, "cough pain" usually provides sufficient diagnostic confirmation; false-positive rebound tenderness occurs in about one patient in four without peritonitis.

- The false-positive rate of rebound tenderness (up to 25%) has led some investigators to conclude that rebound tenderness, in contrast to cough pain, is of "no predictive value."
- A useful and underused test to diagnose abdominal wall pain is the sit-up test, also known as the *Carnett sign.* After identification of the site of maximum abdominal tenderness, the patient is asked to fold his or her arms across the chest and sit up halfway. The examiner maintains a finger on the tender area, and if palpation in the semisitting position produces the same or increased tenderness, the test is said to be positive for an abdominal wall syndrome.
- Perform a pelvic examination in all postpubertal females.
- During the rectal examination, the lower pelvis should be assessed for tenderness, bleeding, and masses.

- Elderly patients often fail to manifest the same signs and symptoms as younger patients, with decreased pain perception and decreased febrile or muscular response to infection or inflammation.
- Biliary disease, bowel obstruction, diverticulitis, cancer, and hernia are more common causes of abdominal pain in patients over 50 years old. Hypotension from volume contraction, hemorrhage, or sepsis can be missed if a normally hypertensive patient appears normotensive.
- Conditions somewhat less frequent but proportionately higher in occurence among the elderly include sigmoid volvulus, diverticulitis, acute mesenteric ischemia, and abdominal aortic aneurysm.
- Mesenteric ischemia should be considered in any patient older than 50 years with abdominal pain out of proportion to physical findings.

DIAGNOSIS AND DIFFERENTIAL

- Suggested laboratory studies for goal-directed clinical testing are listed in Table 37-1.
- Diagnostic caveats for clinically suspected source of abdominal pain are listed in Table 37-2.
- All women of childbearing age with abdominal pain or abnormal vaginal bleeding should receive a qualitative screening pregnancy test.
- A complete blood count is neither sensitive nor specific to identify abdominal pathology; however, it remains the most commonly ordered test for ED patients with abdominal pain.
- Plain abdominal radiographs are helpful in patients with suspected obstruction, perforation (look for free air), or to follow previously identified stones in renal colic patients.
- Ultrasonography is useful for the diagnosis of cholelithiasis, choledocholithiasis, cholecystitis, biliary duct dilatation, pancreatic masses, hydroureter, intrauterine or ectopic pregnancies, ovarian and tubal pathologies, free intraperitoneal fluid, suspected appendicitis (institution specific), and abdominal aortic aneurysm.
- Computed tomography (CT) is the preferred imaging method for mesenteric ischemia, pancreatitis, biliary obstruction, aortic aneurysm, appendicitis, and urolithiasis and is superior for identifying virtually any abnormality that can be seen on plain films.
- Intravenous contrast is essential to identify vascular lesions, is helpful to identify inflammatory conditions (ie, appendicitis), but is not needed for urolithiasis.
- Oral contrast aids in the diagnosis of bowel obstruction, but otherwise is less useful.

TABLE 37-1 Suggested Laboratory Studies for Goal-Directed Clinical Testing in Acute Abdominal Pain

LABORATORY TEST	CLINICAL SUSPICION
β-Human chorionic gonadotropin	Pregnancy Ectopic or molar pregnancy
Coagulation studies (PT, PTT)	GI bleeding End-stage liver disease Coagulopathy
Electrocardiogram	Cardiac ischemia
Electrolytes	Dehydration Endocrine or metabolic disorder
Glucose	Diabetic ketoacidosis Pancreatitis
Gonococcal/chlamydia testing	Cervicitis/urethritis Pelvic inflammatory disease
Hemoglobin	GI bleeding
Lactate	Mesenteric ischemia
Lipase	Pancreatitis
Liver function tests	Cholecystitis Cholelithiasis Hepatitis
Platelets	GI bleeding
Renal function tests	Acute renal failure Renal insufficiency Dehydration
Urinalysis	Urinary tract infection Pyelonephritis Nephrolithiasis

Abbreviations: PT = prothrombin time, PTT = partial thromboplastin time.

EMERGENCY DEPARTMENT CARE AND DISPOSITION

- Unstable patients should be resuscitated immediately, then diagnosed clinically with emergent surgical consultation.
- The most common resuscitation need for abdominal pain patients is intravenous hydration with normal saline or lactated Ringer solution. During the initial evaluation, the patient should have nothing by mouth.
- The judicious use of analgesics is appropriate and may facilitate the ability to obtain a better history and more accurate physical examination. Consider **morphine** 0.1 milligram/kg IV, which can be reversed by **naloxone** (0.4-2 milligrams SC/IV) if necessary. NSAIDs are useful in patients with renal colic, but their use in other conditions is controversial and they can mask peritoneal inflammation.
- Antiemetics, such as **ondansetron** 4 milligrams IM/IV, or **metoclopramide** 10 milligrams IM or

TABLE 37-2 Diagnostic Caveats for Clinically Suspected Source of Abdominal Pain

DIAGNOSIS	DIAGNOSTIC CAVEATS
Appendicitis	No single test will exclude all cases; RLQ pain LR + 8; pain migrated from periumbilical area to RLQ: LR + 3; pain before vomiting 99% sens, 66% spec; CT preferred in adults and nonpregnant women; CT 93%-95% sens if appendix seen.
Bowel obstruction	Pain colicky; vomiting and distension increase likelihood; prior surgery most common risk factor; plain radiographs 77% sens; CT 93% sens.
Cholecystitis	Pain initially colicky, becomes continuous; (+) Murphy's sign increases likelihood of cholecystitis (OR 2.5); jaundice suggests obstruction; no single test can exclude diagnosis; elevated bilirubin/aspartate aminotransferase/alkaline phosphatase each only 70% sens and 42% spec; US: 91% sens; hepatobiliary iminodiacetic acid scan: 97% sens, 90% spec.
Diverticulitis	Incidence increases with age; 50% report previous episode of similar pain; sigmoid (85%): LLQ; cecal/Meckel: RLQ; CT: sens 93%-100%, spec 100%.
Ectopic pregnancy	Risks are previous ectopic, PID, infertility treatment, intrauterine device; pain is sudden onset and severe; pelvic examination may be normal; pregnancy test +, transvaginal US preferred.
Mesenteric ischemia	Pain out of proportion to physical findings; nausea: 56%-93%; vomiting: 38%-80%; diarrhea: 31%-48%; lactate: 75%-90% sens; not specific; elevated WBC: 90% sens; selective CT angiography: 96% sens.
Myocardial ischemia	ECG may be normal; troponin: 80% sens at 4 h from symptom onset; abdominal-related sepsis may give noncardiac troponin elevations.
Pancreatitis	Risks: alcohol; biliary disease; drugs; endoscopic retrograde cholangiopancreatography; lipase: 90% sens first 24 h; US may show edema; CT: 78% sens, 86% spec.
Pelvic inflammatory disease/TOA	Sexually transmitted diseases; prior PID; multiple partners; vaginal discharge, dyspareunia, cervical motion tenderness suggestive; fever or elevated WBC not necessary for diagnosis; transvaginal US preferred imaging modality; MRI more sensitive.
Perforated viscus	Pain is typically severe; upright chest radiograph 80% sens while CT is 87%-98% sens for free air.
Ovarian torsion	Pain is sudden, severe, sharp; may have nausea/vomiting; pelvic US with Doppler flow preferred.
Renal/ureteral colic	Pain is severe, colicky; nausea and vomiting common; 85%-90% have hematuria; only 30% have gross hematuria; noncontrast spiral CT preferred.
Ruptured abdominal aortic aneurysm	Pain location is mid-abdomen or flank, back, groin, or thigh, pain of severe; sudden onset, constant; pulsatile mass detected: 22%-96% sens; only 50% are hypotensive at presentation, normal pulses do not exclude diagnosis; bedside US 100% sens for enlarged aorta.

Abbreviations: + = positive; LLQ = left lower quadrant; LR = likelihood ratio; OR = odds ratio; PID = pelvic inflammatory disease; RLQ = right lower quadrant; sens = sensitivity; spec = specificity; TOA = tubo-ovarian abscess; WBC = white blood cell count.

slow IV, also increase the patient's comfort and facilitate assessment of the patient's signs and symptoms.

- When appropriate, antibiotic treatment (ie, **gentamicin** 1.5 milligrams/kg IV plus **metronidazole** 1 gram IV; or **piperacillin-tazobactam**, 3.375 grams IV) should be initiated, depending on the suspected source of infection. See specific chapters that follow in this section for additional guidelines.
- Surgical or obstetric and gynecologic consultation should be obtained for patients with suspected acute abdominal or pelvic pathology requiring immediate intervention, including, but not limited to, abdominal aortic aneurysm, intraabdominal hemorrhage, perforated viscus, intestinal obstruction or infarction, and ectopic pregnancy. Historically, the "acute abdomen" or "surgical abdomen" has been identified by the presence of pain, guarding, and rebound as indicating a likely need for emergent surgery.
- Indications for admission include toxic appearance, unclear diagnosis in elderly or immunocompromised patients, inability to reasonably exclude serious etiologies, intractable pain or vomiting, altered mental status, and inability to follow discharge or follow-up instructions. Continued observation with serial examinations is an alternative.
- Many patients with nonspecific abdominal pain can be discharged safely with 24 hours of follow-up and instructions to return immediately for increased pain, vomiting, fever, or failure of symptoms to resolve.

For further reading in Tintinalli's *Emergency Medicine: A Comprehensive Study Guide*, 7th ed., see Chapter 74, "Acute Abdominal Pain," by Mary Claire O'Brien.

38 NAUSEA AND VOMITING

Jonathan A. Maisel

EPIDEMIOLOGY

- Although nausea and vomiting is typically caused by gastrointestinal disorders, the clinician must consider systemic causes as well.
- Neurologic, infectious, cardiac, endocrine, renal, obstetric, pharmacologic, toxicologic, and psychiatric disorders may all be the cause of nausea and vomiting.
- A comprehensive history and physical examination, as well as the use of various diagnostic modalities, are needed to determine the cause and its complications.

PATHOPHYSIOLOGY

- Vomiting is a complex, highly coordinated activity involving the gastrointestinal tract, the central and autonomic nervous system, and the vestibular system.
- Three stages of vomiting have been described: nausea, retching, and emesis. With nausea comes hypersalivation and tachycardia. Retching occurs with gastric relaxation and repetitive simultaneous contraction of the diaphragm and abdominal muscles, which allows for the development of a pressure gradient. Finally, in response to changes in intra-abdominal and intrathoracic pressure, emesis occurs, expelling gastric contents from the stomach.

CLINICAL FEATURES

- History is essential in determining the cause of vomiting. Important features to elicit include the following:
  - The onset and duration of symptoms
  - The frequency and timing of episodes
  - The content of the vomitus (eg, undigested food, bile-tinged, feculent)
  - Associated symptoms (eg, fever, abdominal pain, diarrhea)
  - Exposure to foodborne pathogens
  - The presence of sick contacts
- A thorough past medical and abdominal surgical history can also be valuable.
- The physical examination should initially focus on determining the presence or absence of a critical, life-threatening condition.
- Hypotension, tachycardia, lethargy, poor skin turgor, dry mucous membranes, and delayed capillary refill suggest significant dehydration.
- A careful abdominal examination will help clarify the presence or absence of a primary GI etiology.
- The extent to which the balance of the physical examination will be of value will be dictated by the history. In the event that a reliable history is not available (eg, drug overdose, cognitive impairment), a comprehensive physical examination is warranted.

DIAGNOSIS AND DIFFERENTIAL

- Vomiting with blood could represent gastritis, peptic ulcer disease, or carcinoma. However, aggressive nonbloody vomiting followed by hematemesis is more consistent with a Mallory–Weiss tear.
- The presence of bile rules out gastric outlet obstruction, as from pyloric stenosis or strictures.
- The presence of abdominal distension, surgical scars, or an incarcerated hernia suggests a small bowel obstruction.
- The presence of fever suggests an infectious (eg, gastroenteritis, appendicitis, cholecystitis) or inflammatory cause.
- Vomiting with chest pain suggests myocardial infarction.
- Post-tussive vomiting suggests pneumonia.
- Vomiting with back or flank pain can be seen with aortic aneurysm or dissection, pancreatitis, pyelonephritis, or renal colic.
- Headache with vomiting suggests increased intracranial pressure, such as with subarachnoid hemorrhage, tumor, or head injury.
- The presence of vertigo and nystagmus suggests either vestibular or CNS pathology.
- Vomiting in a pregnant patient is consistent with hyperemesis gravidarum in the first trimester; but in the third trimester, could represent preeclampsia if accompanied by hypertension.
- Associated medical conditions are also useful in discerning the cause of vomiting: diabetes mellitus suggests ketoacidosis, peripheral vascular disease suggests mesenteric ischemia, and medication use or overdose (eg, lithium or digoxin) suggests toxicity.
- The physical examination in a vomiting patient includes a careful assessment of hydration status; the gastrointestinal, pelvic, and genitourinary systems; and selected additional systems as dictated by the history. The potential causes of vomiting, based on physical examination findings, are summarized in Table 38-1.
- All women of childbearing age warrant a pregnancy test.
- In vomiting associated with abdominal pain, liver function tests, urinalysis, and lipase or amylase determinations may be useful.
- Electrolyte determinations and renal function tests are usually of benefit only in patients with severe dehydration or prolonged vomiting. In addition, they may confirm the presence of Addisonian crisis, with hyperkalemia and hyponatremia.

TABLE 38-1 Differential Diagnosis Based on Physical Examination Findings

PHYSICAL EXAMINATION	ABNORMAL SIGNS OR SYMPTOMS	SOME DIAGNOSTIC CONSIDERATIONS
General	Toxic appearing Generalized weakness Weight loss	Dehydration Chronic malnutrition Malignancy
Vital signs	Fever Tachycardia Hypotension Hypertension	Infection (gastroenteritis, appendicitis, cholecystitis) Bowel perforation, secondary peritonitis Severe volume depletion Intracranial hemorrhage or stroke
Head, eyes, ears, nose, throat	Nystagmus Exophthalmos Pin-point pupils Fixed-dilated pupil, eye pain Dry mucous membranes Poor dental enamel Parotid gland enlargement Lymphadenopathy	Peripheral vs. central causes (benign positional vertigo, cerebellar infarct) Thyroid disorders (Graves disease) Opiate abuse Acute glaucoma Dehydration Bulimia
Abdomen	Distention ↓ bowel sounds Surgical scars Hernias or palpable masses Abdominal rigidity	Small bowel obstruction, gastroparesis, gastric outlet obstruction Ileus Incarcerated hernia, tumors Peritonitis
Neurologic	Mental status Cranial nerve findings or neurologic deficits Papilledema	Dehydration, intracranial lesion or pathology, brain stem tumor, elevated intracranial pressure
Extremities	Scarring on dorsal surface of the hands	Bulimia
Skin	Jaundice Poor skin turgor Hyperpigmentation Decreased elasticity Track marks	Hepatobiliary disease (hepatitis, choledocholithiasis) Dehydration Addison disease Scleroderma Drug abuse/withdrawal

- Obtain specific drug levels for acetaminophen, salicylates, and digoxin when toxicity is suspected, and urine and/or serum toxicology screens when ethanol or illicit drug use is suspected.
- The electrocardiogram and chest radiograph can be reserved for patients with suspected cardiac ischemia or pulmonary infection.
- Abdominal radiograph can be used to confirm the presence of intestinal obstruction.
- If plain radiographs are unrevealing, CT scan of the abdomen and pelvis with IV and PO contrast is helpful for revealing the location of a mechanical obstruction and may also clarify alternative explanations for the patient's symptoms.
- CT scan of the brain will be helpful if a CNS lesion is suspected.
- Measuring intraocular pressure is useful if glaucoma is suspected.

EMERGENCY DEPARTMENT CARE AND DISPOSITION

- The treatment of nausea and vomiting consists of correcting fluid and electrolyte problems. In addition, one must initiate specific therapy for any life-threatening cause identified in the initial workup.
- Resuscitation of seriously ill patients requires intravenous boluses of **normal saline** 20 mL/kg. Boluses may be repeated as necessary, targeting euvolemia. Caution should be used in the elderly, and those with compromised left ventricular function.
- Mildly dehydrated patients may tolerate an oral rehydration solution containing sodium, as well as glucose to enhance fluid absorption. Many commercial products (eg, **Pedialyte**) are available. The World Health Organization advocates a mixture of **4 oz orange juice, 8 tsp sugar,** and **1 tsp salt in 1 L boiled water**.
- Nutritional supplementation should be started as soon as nausea and vomiting subside. Patients can quickly advance from clear liquids to solids, such as rice and bread. Patients may benefit from avoiding raw fruit, caffeine and lactose, and sorbitol-containing products.
- Antiemetic agents are useful in actively vomiting patients with dehydration.
  - **Ondansetron** 4 to 8 milligrams IV or ODT (children 0.15 milligram/kg) is very effective and well tolerated, and can be administered to pregnant women (category B).
  - **Promethazine** 25 milligrams (0.25-1 milligram/kg in children over 2 years) IM or PR every 4 to 6 hours can be effective.
  - **Prochlorperazine** 5 to 10 milligrams IM every 6 hours, or 25 milligrams PR every 12 hours is effective.
  - **Metoclopramide** 10 milligrams (children 0.1 milligram/kg) IV/IM every 6 to 8 hours is useful and can be administered to pregnant women (category B).
  - **Meclizine** 25 milligrams PO every 6 hours is effective for vomiting associated with vertigo.
- Patients with a life-threatening cause of vomiting require admission. In addition, toxic or severely dehydrated patients, particularly infants and the elderly, or those still intolerant of oral fluids following hydration, warrant admission.

- Patients with an unclear diagnosis, but favorable examination findings following hydration, can be discharged home safely with antiemetic medication.
- Work excuses are indicated for patients in the food, day care, and health care industries.

For further reading in Tintinalli's *Emergency Medicine: A Comprehensive Study Guide*, 7th ed., see Chapter 75, "Nausea and Vomiting," by Susan Bork, Jeffrey Ditkoff, and Bophal Sarha Hang.

39 DISORDERS PRESENTING PRIMARILY WITH DIARRHEA

Jonathan A. Maisel

DIARRHEA

EPIDEMIOLOGY

- Diarrhea is defined as three or more watery stools per day.

PATHOPHYSIOLOGY

- There are four basic mechanisms:
  - Increased intestinal secretion (eg, cholera)
  - Decreased intestinal absorption (eg, enterotoxins, inflammation, or ischemia)
  - Increased osmotic load (eg, laxatives, lactose intolerance)
  - Abnormal intestinal motility (eg, irritable bowel syndrome, neuropathy)
- Approximately 85% of cases are infectious in etiology.

CLINICAL FEATURES

- Determine if the diarrhea is acute (<3-week duration) or chronic (>3 weeks). Acute diarrhea is more likely to represent a serious problem, such as infection, ischemia, intoxication, or inflammation.
- Inquire about associated symptoms. Features such as fever, pain, presence of blood, or type of food ingested may help in the diagnosis of infectious gastroenteritis, food poisoning, diverticulitis, or inflammatory bowel disease.
- Neurological symptoms can be seen in certain diarrheal illnesses, such as seizure with shigellosis or hyponatremia, or paresthesias and reverse temperature sensation with ciguatoxin.
- Details about the host can also better define the diagnosis. Malabsorption from pancreatic insufficiency or HIV-related bowel disorders need not be considered in a healthy host.
- Dietary practices, including frequent restaurant meals, exposure to day care centers, consumption of street-vendor food or raw seafood, overseas travel, and camping with the ingestion of lake or stream water, may isolate the vector and narrow the differential diagnosis for infectious diarrhea (eg, lakes or streams—*Giardia*, oysters—*Vibrio;* rice—*Bacillus cereus*; eggs—*Salmonella;* and meat—*Campylobacter, Staphylococcus*, *Yersinia*, *Escherichia coli*, or *Clostridium).*
- Certain medications, particularly antibiotics, colchicine, lithium, and laxatives, can all contribute to diarrhea.
- Travel may predispose the patient to enterotoxigenic *E. coli* or *Giardia*.
- Social history, such as sexual preference, drug use, and occupation, may suggest diagnoses such as HIV-related illness or organophosphate poisoning.
- The physical examination begins with assessment of hydration status.
- Abdominal examination can narrow the differential diagnosis as well as reveal the need for surgical intervention. Even appendicitis can present with diarrhea in up to 20% of cases.
- Rectal examination can rule out impaction or presence of blood, the latter suggesting inflammation, infection, or mesenteric ischemia.

DIAGNOSIS AND DIFFERENTIAL

- The most specific tests in diarrheal illness all involve examination of the stool in the laboratory.
- Stool culture testing should be limited to severely dehydrated or toxic patients, those with blood or pus in their stool, immunocompromised patients, and those with diarrhea lasting longer than 3 days. Consider testing for *Salmonella*, *Shigella*, *Campylobacter*, Shiga toxin-producing *E. coli*, or amoebic infection. Make the laboratory aware of which pathogens you suspect.
- In patients with diarrhea >7 days, those who have traveled abroad, or consumed untreated water, an examination for ova and parasites may be useful to rule out *Giardia* or *Cryptosporidium*. Multiple samples may be required.

- Assay for *Clostridium difficile* toxin may be useful in ill patients with antibiotic-associated diarrhea or recent hospitalization.
- Because most diarrheal illnesses are viral or self-limited, laboratory testing in routine cases is not indicated. However, in extremely dehydrated or toxic patients, electrolyte determinations and renal function tests may be useful. (Hemolytic-uremic syndrome, characterized by acute renal failure, thrombocytopenia, and hemolytic anemia, may complicate *E. coli 0157:H7* infections in children and the elderly.)
- If toxicity is suspected, tests for levels for theophylline, lithium, or heavy metals will aid in the diagnosis.
- Radiographs are reserved for ruling out intestinal obstruction or pneumonia, particularly *Legionella*.
- CT scanning or angiography may be indicated to diagnose acute mesenteric ischemia.

EMERGENCY DEPARTMENT CARE AND DISPOSITION

- The treatment of diarrhea consists of correcting fluid and electrolyte problems.
- Initiate specific therapy for any life-threatening cause identified in the initial workup.
- Replacement of fluids can be intravenous (boluses of 500 mL IV in adults, 20 mL/kg in children) with **normal saline solution** in seriously ill patients.
- Mildly dehydrated patients who are not vomiting may tolerate an **oral rehydrating solution-containing sodium** (eg, Pedialyte) as well as glucose to enhance fluid absorption (glucose transport unaffected by enterotoxins). The World Health Organization advocates a mixture of **4 oz orange juice, 8 tsp sugar, and 1 tsp salt in 1 L boiled water**. The goal is 50 to 100 mL/kg over the first 4 hours.
- As patients tolerate, introduce a "BRAT" diet (bananas, rice, apples, toast).
- Patients should avoid raw fruit, caffeine, and lactose and sorbitol-containing products.
- Antibiotics are recommended for adult patients with severe or prolonged diarrhea. (See section on acute infectious and traveler's diarrhea.) Antibiotics should be avoided in infectious diarrhea due to *E. coli* O157:H7.
- Antidiarrheal agents, especially in combination with antibiotics, have been shown to shorten the course of diarrhea. (See section on acute infectious and traveler's diarrhea.)
- Antibiotic-associated diarrhea often responds to withdrawal of the offending drug. Metronidazole or vancomycin may be indicated in selected situations (see section on *Clostridium difficile* infection).
- Almost all true diarrheal emergencies (eg, GI bleed, adrenal insufficiency, thyroid storm, toxicologic exposures, acute radiation syndrome, and mesenteric ischemia) are of noninfectious origin. Patients with these conditions require intensive treatment and hospitalization.
- Toxic or severely dehydrated patients, particularly infants and the elderly, warrant admission.
- Patients with an unclear diagnosis, but favorable examination findings after hydration, can be discharged home safely.

ACUTE INFECTIOUS AND TRAVELER'S DIARRHEA

EPIDEMIOLOGY

- *Norovirus* causes 50% to 80% of all infectious diarrheas in the United States, followed much less frequently by non-Shiga toxin-producing *E. coli*, *C. difficile*, invasive bacteria (*Campylobacter*, *Shigella*, *Salmonella*), Shiga toxin-producing *E. coli*, and protozoa.
- A history of foreign travel, with consumption of contaminated food or drink, is associated with an 80% probability of bacterial diarrhea, primarily toxin and non-toxin-producing strains of *E. coli*.

PATHOPHYSIOLOGY

- Intestinal absorption occurs through the villi, and secretion occurs through the crypts. Fluids are absorbed passively with the transport of sodium, and actively with the absorption of glucose.
- Selected enterotoxins disrupt the structure of intestinal villi preferentially, with less involvement of the crypts. As a result, diarrhea occurs because of diminished intestinal villi absorption and unopposed crypt secretion. The glucose dependent mechanism of water reabsorption is unaffected by these toxins, allowing for therapeutic oral rehydration.

DIAGNOSIS AND DIFFERENTIAL

- Patients with severe abdominal pain, fever, and bloody stool should undergo stool studies for specific pathogens, including culture for *Salmonella*, *Shigella*, *Campylobacter*, and *E. coli* O157:H7; assay for Shiga toxin; and microscopy or antigen assay for *Entamoeba histolytica*.
- Exposure of a traveler or hiker to untreated water, and illness that persists for more than 7 days, should prompt an evaluation for a protozoal pathogen.

Stool should be tested by enzyme immunoassay for *E. histolytica* antigen, *Giardia intestinalis* antigen, and *Cryptosporidium parvum* antigen.

EMERGENCY DEPARTMENT CARE AND DISPOSITION

- Treatment of moderately severe infectious diarrhea (including viral causes) includes antibiotics, antimotility agents, fluid resuscitation (oral or parenteral), and dietary modification (BRAT diet—bananas, rice, apples, toast).
- **Ciprofloxacin** 500 milligrams as a single dose, or 500 milligrams twice daily for 3 days will shorten the duration of illness by approximately 24 hours. (Similar dosing for culture proven *Shigella* or enterotoxigenic, enteropathogenic, or enteroinvasive *E. coli*. However, both antibiotics and antimotility agents should be avoided in cases of Shiga toxin-producing *E. coli* O157:H7).
- **Trimethoprim/sulfamethoxazole**, TMP 10 milligrams/kg/day:SMX 50 milligrams/kg/day (maximum dose TMP 160 milligrams:SMX 800 milligrams) for 3 days is indicated for children or nursing mothers.
- **Metronidazole** 750 milligrams PO three times per day for 5 to 10 days is indicated for *Giardia* or *Entamoeba* infection. Add **iodoquinol** 650 milligrams three times per day for 20 days, or **paromomycin** 500 milligrams three times per day for 5 to 10 days, for the latter.
- Antimotility agents, such as **loperamide** 4 milligrams initially, then 2 milligrams following each unformed stool (16 milligrams/d maximum), will shorten the duration of symptoms when combined with an antibiotic. Alternative agents include **bismuth subsalicylate** 30 mL or 2 tablets every 30 minutes for 8 doses, or **diphenoxylate and atropine** 4 milligrams four times per day.
- Avoid antimotility agents in the subset of patients with bloody or suspected inflammatory diarrhea because of the potential for prolonged fever, toxic megacolon in *C. difficile* patients, and hemolytic uremic syndrome in children infected with Shiga-toxin producing *E. coli*.
- Most patients can be discharged home. Educate patients regarding the need for frequent hand washing to minimize transmission.
- Provide work excuses to patients employed in the food, day care, and health care industries.
- Any toxic-appearing patient should be admitted. Consider admission for those at extremes of age as well.
- Individuals should be counseled about the proper selection of food and beverages consumed when traveling abroad, as well as the use of water for drinking, brushing teeth, and the preparation of food and infant formula.

CLOSTRIDIUM DIFFICILE-ASSOCIATED INFECTION, DIARRHEA, AND COLITIS

EPIDEMIOLOGY

- Broad-spectrum antibiotics—most notably clindamycin, cephalosporins, ampicillin, amoxicillin, and fluoroquinolones—alter gut flora in such a way that *C. difficile* can flourish within the colon, causing enteropathy.
- Transmission of the organism can occur from contact with humans and fomites.
- *Clostridium difficile* is the most common cause of infectious diarrhea in hospitalized patients, and is now reported to affect healthy adults who were not exposed to a hospital setting.

PATHOPHYSIOLOGY

- *Clostridium difficile* is an anaerobic bacillus which secretes two toxins that interact in a complex manner to cause illness ranging from secretory diarrhea to pseudomembranous colitis.
- Recent antibiotic use, GI surgery or manipulation, severe underlying illness, chemotherapy, and advanced age are risk factors for developing pseudomembranous colitis.
- Pseudomembranous colitis is an inflammatory bowel disorder in which membrane-like yellowish plaques of exudate overlay and replace necrotic intestinal mucosa.

CLINICAL FEATURES

- Onset is typically 7 to 10 days after initiating antibiotic treatment, but may occur up to several weeks following treatment.
- Clinical manifestations can vary from frequent, watery, mucoid stools to a toxic picture, including profuse diarrhea, crampy abdominal pain, fever, leukocytosis, and dehydration.

DIAGNOSIS AND DIFFERENTIAL

- The diagnosis is confirmed by the demonstration of *C. difficile* toxin in stool. Colonoscopy is not routinely needed to confirm the diagnosis.

EMERGENCY DEPARTMENT CARE AND DISPOSITION

- Mild *C. difficile* infection in an otherwise healthy patient can be treated with discontinuing the offending antibiotic, confirmation of infection, and clinical monitoring.

- **Metronidazole** 500 milligrams PO every 6 hours for 10 to 14 days is the treatment of choice in patients with mild to moderate disease who do not respond to conservative measures.
- Patients with severe diarrhea, those with a systemic response (eg, fever, leukocytosis, or severe abdominal pain), and those whose symptoms persist despite appropriate outpatient management, must be hospitalized and should receive **vancomycin** 125 to 250 milligrams PO four times daily for 10 to 14 days. The symptoms usually resolve within a few days.
- Patients with pseudomembranous colitis complicated by toxic megacolon or intestinal perforation require immediate surgical consultation. Rarely, emergency colectomy may be required for fulminant colitis.
- Use of antidiarrheal agents is controversial. Relapses occur in 10% to 25% of patients.

CROHN'S DISEASE

EPIDEMIOLOGY

- Crohn's disease is a chronic, idiopathic, granulomatous inflammatory disease, characterized by segmental ulceration of the gastrointestinal (GI) tract anywhere from the mouth to the anus.

PATHOPHYSIOLOGY

- Pathologically, one sees intermittent, longitudinal, deep ulcerations penetrating all layers of the bowel wall, resulting in fissures, fistulas, and abscesses.

CLINICAL FEATURES

- The clinical course is variable and unpredictable, with multiple remissions and exacerbations.
- Patients commonly report a history of recurring fever, abdominal pain, and diarrhea over several years before a definitive diagnosis is made. Abdominal pain, anorexia, diarrhea, and weight loss occur in most cases.
- Patients may also present with complications of the disease, such as intestinal obstruction, intra-abdominal abscess, or a variety of extra-intestinal manifestations.
- One-third of patients develop perianal fissures, fistulas, abscesses, or rectal prolapse. Fistulas occur between the ileum and sigmoid colon, the cecum, another ileal segment, or the skin, or between the colon and the vagina. Abscesses can be intraperitoneal, retroperitoneal, interloop, or intramesenteric.
- Obstruction, hemorrhage, and toxic megacolon also occur. Toxic megacolon can be associated with massive GI bleeding.
- Up to 50% of patients develop extraintestinal manifestations, including arthritis, uveitis, nephrolithiasis, and skin disease (eg, erythema nodosum, pyoderma gangrenosum). Hepatobiliary disease, including gallstones, pericholangitis, and chronic active hepatitis is commonly seen, as is pancreatitis.
- Some patients develop thromboembolic disease as a result of a hypercoaguable state.
- Malabsorption, malnutrition, and chronic anemia develop in long-standing disease, and the incidence of GI tract carcinoma is triple that of the general population.
- The recurrence rate for those with Crohn's disease is 25% to 50% when treated medically; higher for patients treated surgically.

DIAGNOSIS AND DIFFERENTIAL

- The definitive diagnosis of Crohn's disease is usually established months or years after the onset of symptoms. A careful and detailed history for previous bowel symptoms that preceded the acute presentation may provide clues to the correct diagnosis.
- Abdominal CT scanning is the most useful diagnostic test, potentially revealing bowel wall thickening, mesenteric edema, abscess formation, and fistulas, as well as extra-intestinal complications (eg, gallstones, renal stones, sacroiliitis).
- Colonoscopy can detect early mucosal lesions, define the extent of colonic involvement, and identify colon cancer.
- The differential diagnosis of Crohn's disease includes lymphoma, ileocecal amebiasis, sarcoidosis, chronic mycotic infections, tuberculosis, Kaposi's sarcoma, *Campylobacter* enteritis, and *Yersinia* ileocolitis. Most of these conditions are uncommon, and the latter two can be differentiated by stool cultures.
- When confined to the colon, ischemic colitis, infectious colitis, pseudomembranous enterocolitis, irritable bowel syndrome, and ulcerative colitis should be considered.

EMERGENCY DEPARTMENT CARE AND DISPOSITION

- Initial evaluation should determine the severity of the attack and identify significant complications.
- Laboratory evaluation should include complete blood count, chemistries, and type and cross match when indicated.
- Plain abdominal x-rays may identify obstruction, perforation, and toxic megacolon, which may appear as

a long, continuous segment of air-filled colon greater than 6 cm in diameter.

- CT of the abdomen is the most useful test to confirm the diagnosis, and identify both intra and extra-intestinal manifestations.
- Initial ED management includes intravenous fluid replacement, parenteral analgesia, bowel rest, correction of electrolyte abnormalities, and nasogastric suction if obstruction, ileus, or toxic megacolon is present.
- Additional treatment may include:
  - **Sulfasalazine** 3 to 5 grams/d is effective for mild to moderate Crohn's disease, but has multiple toxic side effects, including GI and hypersensitivity reactions. **Mesalamine**, up to 4 grams/d, is equally effective, with fewer side effects.
  - Glucocorticoids (**prednisone**) 40 to 60 milligrams/d provides symptom relief, but does not alter the course of the disease.
  - Immunosuppressive drugs, **6-mercaptopurine** 1 to 1.5 milligrams/kg/d or **azathioprine** 2 to 2.5 milligrams/kg/d, are used as steroid-sparing agents, in healing fistulas, and in patients with serious surgical contraindications.
  - Antibiotics can help induce remission. **Ciprofloxacin** 500 milligrams every 8 to 12 hours, **metronidazole** 500 milligrams every 6 hours, and **rifaximin** 800 milligrams twice daily, are effective.
  - Patients with medically resistant, moderate to severe Crohn's disease may benefit from the anti-tumor necrosis factor antibody **infliximab** 5 milligrams/kg IV.
  - Diarrhea can be controlled by **loperamide** 4 to 16 milligrams/d, **diphenoxylate** 5 to 20 milligrams/d, or **cholestyramine** 4 grams 1 to 6 times daily.
- Hospital admission is recommended for those who demonstrate signs of fulminant colitis, peritonitis, obstruction, significant hemorrhage, severe dehydration, or electrolyte imbalance, or those with less severe disease who fail outpatient management.
- Surgical intervention is indicated in patients with intestinal obstruction or hemorrhage, perforation, abscess or fistula formation, toxic megacolon, or perianal disease, and in some patients who fail medical therapy.
- Alterations in therapy should be discussed with a gastroenterologist, and close follow-up must be ensured for patients discharged from the ED.

ULCERATIVE COLITIS

EPIDEMIOLOGY

- Ulcerative colitis is an idiopathic chronic inflammatory and ulcerative disease of the colon and rectum, characterized clinically by intermittent episodes of crampy abdominal pain and bloody diarrhea, with complete remission between bouts.

PATHOPHYSIOLOGY

- The illness is characterized by mucosal inflammation, with the formation of crypt abscesses, epithelial necrosis, and mucosal ulceration. The deeper layers of bowel are typically spared. The disease increases in severity more distally, with rectal involvement in nearly every case.

CLINICAL FEATURES

- Patients with mild disease (>50%), typically limited to the rectum, have fewer than four bowel movements per day, no systemic symptoms, and few extraintestinal manifestations.
- Patients with moderate disease (25%) have colitis extending to the splenic flexure.
- Severe disease (pancolitis) is associated with frequent daily bowel movements, weight loss, fever, tachycardia, anemia, and more frequent extraintestinal manifestations, including peripheral arthritis, ankylosing spondylitis, episcleritis, uveitis, pyoderma gangrenosum, erythema nodosum, hepatobiliary disease, thromboembolic disease, renal stones, and malnutrition.
- Complications include GI hemorrhage (most common), abscess and fistula formation, obstruction secondary to stricture formation, and acute perforation.
- There is a 10- to 30-fold increase in the risk of developing colon carcinoma.
- The most feared complication is toxic megacolon, which presents with fever, tachycardia, dehydration, and a tender, distended abdomen. Radiograph reveals a long, continuous segment of air-filled colon > 6 cm in diameter. Perforation and peritonitis are life-threatening complications.

DIAGNOSIS AND DIFFERENTIAL

- The diagnosis of ulcerative colitis may be considered with a history of abdominal cramps, diarrhea, and mucoid stools.
- Laboratory findings are nonspecific, and may include leukocytosis, anemia, thrombocytosis, decreased serum albumin levels, abnormal liver function test results, and negative stool studies for ova, parasites, and enteric pathogens.
- Abdominal CT scanning is important for the diagnosis of nonspecific abdominal pain or for suspected colitis.
- Colonoscopy can confirm the diagnosis and define the extent of colonic involvement.

- The differential diagnosis includes infectious, ischemic, radiation, anti-neoplastic agent induced, pseudomembranous, and Crohn's colitis.
- When the disease is limited to the rectum, consider sexually acquired diseases, such as rectal syphilis, gonococcal proctitis, lymphogranuloma venereum, and inflammation caused by herpes simplex virus, *Entamoeba histolytica, Shigella*, and *Campylobacter*.

EMERGENCY DEPARTMENT CARE AND DISPOSITION

- Patients with severe disease should be admitted for intravenous fluid replacement, parenteral analgesia, bowel rest, correction of electrolyte abnormalities, and nasogastric suction if obstruction, ileus, or toxic megacolon are present.
- Consultation with both gastroenterology and surgery should be arranged for patients with significant GI hemorrhage, toxic megacolon, and bowel perforation.
- The following interventions should be considered:
  - Intravenous antibiotics, such as **ciprofloxacin** 400 milligrams every 8 to 12 h, and **metronidazole** 500 milligrams every 6 h.
  - Parenteral steroid treatment with either **hydrocortisone** 100 milligrams every 8 h, **methylprednisolone** 16 milligrams every 8 h, or **prednisolone** 30 milligrams every 12 h.
- The majority of patients with mild and moderate disease can be treated as outpatients.
- Therapy listed below should be discussed with a gastroenterologist, and close follow up must be ensured.
  - For mild active proctitis and left sided colitis, **mesalamine** suppositories or enemas are effective. However, topical steroid preparations (**beclomethasone**, **hydrocortisone**) may be better tolerated.
  - For patients who do not respond to or tolerate topical therapy, oral **mesalamine** is an effective alternative.
  - If topical therapy or oral mesalamine is unsuccessful, **prednisone** 40 to 60 milligrams/d can induce a remission. Once clinical remission is achieved, steroids should be slowly tapered and discontinued.
  - In refractory cases, a combination of glucocorticoids and immunomodulators, such as **6-mercaptopurine** 1 to 1.5 milligrams/kg per day or **azathioprine** 2 milligrams/kg per day should be considered.
- Supportive measures include a nutritious diet, physical and psychological rest, replenishment of iron stores, dietary elimination of lactose, and addition of bulking agents, such as psyllium.
- Antidiarrheal agents can precipitate toxic megacolon and should be avoided.

For further reading in Tintinalli's *Emergency Medicine: A Comprehensive Study Guide*, 7th ed., see Chapter 76, "Disorders Presenting Primarily with Diarrhea," by Nicholas E. Kman and Howard A. Werman.

40 ACUTE AND CHRONIC CONSTIPATION

Jonathan A. Maisel

EPIDEMIOLOGY

- Constipation is the most common digestive complaint in the United States.
- Criteria for the diagnosis of constipation include the following:
  - Less than three bowel movements per week
  - Hard stools, straining at defecation, and/or incomplete evacuation at least 25% of the time

PATHOPHYSIOLOGY

- Fluid intake, fiber intake, exercise, medications, toxins, anatomic lesions, gut flora, hormone levels, and a host of medical and psychiatric conditions can affect gut motility.

CLINICAL FEATURES

- Several historical features may be helpful in eliciting the cause, including new medications or dietary supplements, a decrease in fluid or fiber intake, or a change in activity level.
- Acute onset implies obstruction until proven otherwise. Associated symptoms, such as vomiting, abdominal distention, and inability to pass flatus, further suggest obstruction.
- A history of unexplained weight loss, rectal bleeding, change in stool caliber, or unexplained iron deficiency anemia suggests colon cancer. A family history of colon cancer would escalate one's suspicion.
- Associated illnesses can help disclose the underlying diagnosis: cold intolerance (hypothyroidism), diverticulitis (inflammatory stricture), or nephrolithiasis (hyperparathyroidism).

- Diarrhea alone does not rule out constipation/obstruction, as liquid stool can pass around an obstructive source.
- Physical examination should focus on detection of hernias or abdominal masses.
- Bowel sounds will be decreased in the setting of slow gut transit, but increased in the setting of obstruction.
- Rectal examination will detect masses, foreign bodies, hemorrhoids, abscesses, fecal impaction, anal fissures, or fecal blood. The latter, accompanied by weight loss or decreasing stool caliber, may confirm the presence of colon cancer.
- Fecal impaction itself can cause rectal bleeding from stercoral ulcers.
- The presence of ascites in postmenopausal women raises suspicion of ovarian or uterine carcinoma.

DIAGNOSIS AND DIFFERENTIAL DIAGNOSIS

- The differential diagnosis of constipation is extensive, as noted in Table 40-1.
- Directed testing in acute constipation, based on level of suspicion, can include a complete blood count (to rule out anemia), thyroid panel (to rule out hypothyroidism), and electrolyte determinations (to rule out hypokalemia or hypercalcemia).
- Flat and erect abdominal radiographs may be useful in confirming obstruction or assessing stool burden.
- CT scan of the abdomen and pelvis with IV and PO contrast may be necessary to identify bowel obstruction or other organic causes of constipation.

TABLE 40-1 Differential Diagnosis of Constipation

Acute causes:
GI: quickly growing tumors, strictures, hernias, adhesions, inflammatory conditions, and volvulus
Medicinal: narcotic analgesic, antipsychotic, anticholinergic, antacid, antihistamine
Exercise and nutrition: decrease in level of exercise, fiber intake, fluid intake
Painful anal pathology: anal fissure, hemorrhoids, anorectal abscesses, proctitis
Chronic causes:
GI: slowly growing tumor, colonic dysmotility, chronic anal pathology
Medicinal: chronic laxative abuse, narcotic analgesic, antipsychotic, anticholinergic, antacid, antihistamine
Neurologic: neuropathies, Parkinson disease, cerebral palsy, paraplegia
Endocrine: hypothyroidism, hyperparathyroidism, diabetes
Electrolyte abnormalities: hypomagnesia, hypercalcemia, hypokalemia
Rheumatologic: amyloidosis, scleroderma
Toxicologic: lead, iron

- Chronic constipation is usually a functional disorder that can be worked up on an outpatient basis. However, complications of chronic constipation, such as fecal impaction and intestinal pseudo-obstruction, will require either manual, colonoscopic, or surgical intervention.

EMERGENCY DEPARTMENT CARE AND DISPOSITION

- Treatment of functional constipation is directed at symptomatic relief, as well as addressing lifestyle issues.
- Occasionally, specific treatment is required for complications of constipation, or for underlying disorders that can lead to organic constipation.
- The most important prescription for functional constipation is a dietary and exercise regimen that includes fluids (1.5 L daily), fiber (10 grams daily), and exercise. Fiber in the form of bran (one cup daily) or **psyllium** (**Metamucil** at one teaspoon three times a day) increases stool volume and gut motility.
- Medications can provide temporary relief.
  - Stimulants can be either given PO, as with **anthraquinones** (eg, **Peri-Colace** 1-2 tablets PO daily or twice daily), or PR, as with **bisacodyl** (eg, **Dulcolax** 10 mg PR three times daily in adults or children).
  - In the absence of renal failure, saline laxatives such as **milk of magnesia** 15 to 30 mL PO once or twice a day, or **magnesium citrate** 240 mL PO once a day, are useful.
  - Hyperosmolar agents, such as **lactulose** or **sorbitol** 15 to 30 mL PO once or twice a day may be helpful, as is **polyethylene glycol** (eg, **MiraLAX** 17 grams PO).
  - In children, **glycerine rectal suppositories**, or **mineral oil** (age 5-11 years : 5-15 mL PO daily; age >12 years : 15-45 mL PO daily) have been advocated.
- **Enemas of soapsuds** (1500 mL PR) or **phosphate** (eg, **Fleets** 1 unit PR, 1 oz/10 kg in children) are generally reserved for severe cases or after fecal disimpaction. Use care to avoid rectal perforation.
- Fecal impaction should be removed manually using local anesthetic lubricant and parenteral analgesia or sedation as required. In female patients, transvaginal pressure with the other hand may be helpful. An enema or suppositories to complete evacuation can follow. Following disimpaction, a regimen of medication should be prescribed to reestablish fecal flow.
- All patients with apparent functional constipation can be managed as outpatients. Early follow-up is indicated in patients with recent severe constipation; chronic

constipation associated with systemic symptoms, such as weight loss, anemia, or change in stool caliber; refractory constipation; and constipation requiring chronic laxative use.
- Patients with organic constipation from obstruction require hospitalization and surgical evaluation. Intestinal pseudo-obstruction and sigmoid volvulus can sometimes be corrected colonoscopically.

For further reading in Tintinalli's *Emergency Medicine: A Comprehensive Study Guide*, 7th ed., see Chapter 77, "Acute and Chronic Constipation," by Vito Rocco and Paul Krivickas.

41 GASTROINTESTINAL BLEEDING

Mitchell C. Sokolosky

EPIDEMIOLOGY

- Acute upper gastrointestinal (UGI) bleeding.
- Lower GI bleeding has an annual incidence of 20 per 100,000.
- Both upper GI bleeding and lower GI bleeding are more common in males and the elderly.

PATHOPHYSIOLOGY

- UGI bleeding originates proximal to the ligament of Treitz.
- Peptic ulcer disease is the commonest cause of UGI bleeding followed by erosive gastritis and esophagitis, esophageal and gastric varices, and Mallory–Weiss tear.
- Predisposing factors for UGI bleeding include alcohol, salicylates, and NSAIDs.
- The most common cause of lower GI bleeding is diverticular disease, followed by colitis, adenomatous polyps, and malignancies.
- Lower GI bleeding may be due to an UGI source 10% to 14% of the time.
- It is estimated that 80% of lower GI bleeding will resolve spontaneously.

CLINICAL FEATURES

- Most patients will volunteer complaints of hematemesis (UGI source), hematochezia (bright red or maroon-colored bleeding usually from lower GI source), or melena (dark or black stools usually from UGI source).
- Hypotension and tachycardia suggests severe bleeding.
- Some patients will have more subtle presentations of hypotension, tachycardia, angina, syncope, weakness, and confusion.
- Vomiting and retching followed by hematemesis is suggestive of a Mallory–Weiss tear.
- A history of aortic graft should suggest the possibility of an aortoenteric fistula.
- Spider angiomata, palmar erythema, jaundice, and gynecomastia suggest underlying liver disease.
- Weight loss and changes in bowel habits are classic symptoms of malignancy.

DIAGNOSIS AND DIFFERENTIAL

- The diagnosis may be obvious with the finding of hematemesis, hematochezia, or melena.
- A careful ear, nose, and throat (ENT) examination can exclude swallowed blood as a source.
- A rectal examination is mandatory to detect the presence of blood, its appearance (bright red, maroon, or melanotic), and the presence of masses.
- Ingestion of iron or bismuth can simulate melena, and certain foods such as beets can simulate hematochezia; however, stool guaiac testing will be negative.
- Nasogastric (NG) tube placement may have both diagnostic (identify occult UGI source and assess for ongoing active bleeding) and therapeutic (prepare patient for endoscopy) benefits. A negative NG aspirate does not conclusively exclude a UGI source of bleeding. Concerns that NG tube passage may provoke bleeding in patients with varices are unwarranted.
- Guaiac testing of NG aspirate can yield both false-negative and false-positive results. Most reliable is gross inspection of the aspirate for bloody, maroon, or coffee-ground appearance, reserving guaiac testing to confirm that what appears to be blood actually is blood.
- In patients with significant GI bleeding, the most important laboratory test is the type and crossmatch of blood.
- Other important tests include a complete blood count, blood urea nitrogen (BUN), creatinine, electrolytes, glucose, coagulation studies, and liver function tests. The initial hematocrit level often will not reflect the actual amount of blood loss. UGI bleeding may elevate the BUN.
- UGI endoscopy is the diagnostic study of choice in the evaluation of UGI bleeding.

- Where available, angiography should be considered for the evaluation (detect site of bleeding) and management (embolization or infusion of vasoactive substances) of cases of severe lower GI bleeding.
- Scintigraphy has been used to localize the site of bleeding in obscure hemorrhage.
- Endoscopy is more accurate than angiography or scintigraphy, but the timing of colonoscopy is controversial for lower GI bleeding.
- Multidetector CT's role in the emergent evaluation of lower GI bleeding remains in evolution.

EMERGENCY DEPARTMENT CARE AND DISPOSITION

- Emergency stabilization of the airway, breathing, and circulation takes priority.
- Oxygen, large-bore IVs, and monitors should be applied. Immediately replace volume loss with IV crystalloids.
- The decision to start blood should be based on clinical factors (continued active bleeding and no improvement in perfusion after infusion of 2 L of crystalloids) rather than initial hematocrit.
- An NG tube should be placed in all patients with significant bleeding, regardless of presumed source. Room temperature water is the preferred irrigant for gastric lavage if performed.
- Where available, early therapeutic endoscopy should be considered the treatment of choice for significant UGI bleeding. Endoscopic therapeutic interventions include injection therapy, coaptive therapy, endoscopic clips, and band ligation.
- Proton pump inhibitors should be considered for the treatment of bleeding peptic ulcers. **Pantoprazole** and **esomeprazole**, 80 milligram IV bolus followed by 8 milligram/h infusion, or **lansoprazol**, 60 milligram IV bolus followed by 6 milligram/h infusion, may be used.
- **Octreotid,** 25 to 50 microgram IV bolus followed by 25 to 50 microgram/h infusion, may be considered for patients with uncontrolled UGI bleeding awaiting endoscopy or when endoscopy is unsuccessful, contraindicated, or unavailable.
- Histamine-2 antagonists are not beneficial in acute GI bleeding.
- Balloon tamponade with the Sengstaken–Blakemore tube or its variants can control documented variceal hemorrhage, but because of adverse reactions, it should be considered only a temporizing measure until therapeutic endoscopy.
- Emergency surgical intervention may be necessary with patients who do not respond to medical or endoscopic therapy.
- Patients with significant GI hemorrhage will require hospital admission and early referral to an endoscopist.
- Clinical features predicting adverse outcomes include initial hematocrit <30%, initial systolic BP <100 mm Hg, red blood in the NG lavage, history of cirrhosis or ascites on examination, and a history of vomiting red blood.

For further reading in Tintinalli's *Emergency Medicine: A Comprehensive Study Guide,* 7th ed., see Chapter 78, "Upper Gastrointestinal Bleeding," by David T. Overton, and Chapter 79, "Lower Gastrointestinal Bleeding," by Bruce M. Lo.

42 ESOPHAGEAL EMERGENCIES, GASTROESOPHAGEAL REFLUX DISEASE, AND SWALLOWED FOREIGN BODIES

Mitchell C. Sokolosky

DYSPHAGIA

PATHOPHYSIOLOGY

- Dysphagia is defined as difficulty in swallowing.
- Most patients will have an identifiable, organic process causing their symptoms.
- Dysphagia can be grouped into two broad classification schemes: (1) transfer dysphagia (difficulty in initiating swallowing) and (2) transport dysphagia (feeling of food getting "stuck").

CLINICAL FEATURES

- Historical information is the key to the diagnosis of dysphagia.
- Transport dysphagia that is present for solids only generally suggests a mechanical or obstructive process.
- Motility disorders typically cause transport dysphagia for solids and liquids.
- A poorly chewed meat bolus may obstruct the esophagus and be the presenting sign for a variety of underlying esophageal pathologies.
- Physical examination of patients with dysphagia should focus on the head and neck and the neurologic examination. Unfortunately, the examination is often normal.
- The patient should be watched taking a sip of water.

DIAGNOSIS AND DIFFERENTIAL

- The diagnosis of the underlying pathology of dysphagia is most often made outside the emergency department (ED).
- Initial evaluation may include anteroposterior (AP) and lateral neck and chest radiographs.
- Barium swallow is usually the first test for patients with transport dysphagia.
- Direct laryngoscopy can be used to identify structural lesions.
- Oropharyngeal dysphagia is best worked up using videoesophagography.
- Structural or obstructive causes of dysphagia include neoplasms (squamous cell carcinoma is most common), esophageal strictures and webs, Schatzki ring, and diverticula.
- Motor lesions causing dysphagia include neuromuscular disorders (cerebrovascular accident [CVA] is most common), achalasia, and diffuse esophageal spasm.

EMERGENCY DEPARTMENT CARE AND DISPOSITION

- Protection of the airway and breathing is vital since aspiration is a major concern with most causes of dysphagia.
- Most causes of dysphagia can be further evaluated and managed in the outpatient setting.
- Many of the structural lesions will ultimately require dilatation as definitive therapy.

CHEST PAIN OF ESOPHAGEAL ORIGIN

EPIDEMIOLOGY

- The incidence of esophageal disease in patients with chest pain and normal coronary arteries ranges from 20% to 60%.
- Gastroesophageal reflux disease (GERD) affects up to 20% of the US population, with higher rates in elderly populations.

PATHOPHYSIOLOGY

- Reflux of gastric contents into the esophagus causes a wide array of symptoms and long-term effects.
- Transient relaxation of the lower esophageal sphincter (LES) complex (with normal tone in between periods of relaxation) is the primary mechanism causing reflux.
- Hiatal hernia, prolonged gastric emptying, agents that decrease LES pressure, and impaired esophageal motility predispose to reflux.
- Inflammatory esophagitis can be caused by GERD and medications. Patients with immunosuppression can develop infectious esophagitis.
- Esophageal dysmotility is the excessive, uncoordinated contraction of esophageal smooth muscle.

CLINICAL FEATURES

- Heartburn is the classic symptom of GERD, and chest discomfort may be the sole manifestation of the disease.
- The association of pain with meals, postural changes in pain, and relief of symptoms with antacids are more consistent with GERD.
- Less obvious presentations of GERD also occur such as pulmonary symptoms, especially asthma exacerbations, and multiple ear/nose/throat symptoms.
- GERD has also been implicated in the etiology of dental erosion, vocal cord ulcers and granulomas, laryngitis with hoarseness, chronic sinusitis, and chronic cough.
- Over time, GERD can cause complications such as strictures, inflammatory esophagitis, and Barrett's esophagus (a premalignant condition).
- Esophagitis can cause prolonged periods of chest pain and almost always causes odynophagia as well.
- Esophageal dysmotility often presents with chest pain, onset usually in fifth decade.

DIAGNOSIS AND DIFFERENTIAL

- Diagnosis is often made by history and favorable response to antacid treatment.
- Unfortunately, like cardiac pain, esophageal pain may be squeezing, be pressure-like, and include a history of onset with exertion and rest. Both types of pain may be accompanied by diaphoresis, pallor, radiation, and nausea and vomiting.

EMERGENCY DEPARTMENT CARE AND DISPOSITION

- Comprehensive treatment of reflux disease involves decreasing acid production in the stomach, enhancing upper tract motility, and eliminating risk factors for the disease.
- Mild disease is often treated empirically with an H_2 blocker or proton pump inhibitor. A prokinetic drug may also greatly decrease symptoms.
- Patients should avoid agents that exacerbate GERD (ethanol, caffeine, nicotine, chocolate, fatty foods), sleep with the head of the bed elevated 30 degrees, and avoid eating within 3 hours of going to bed at night.

- Pain from spasm may respond to nitroglycerin. Calcium channel blockers and anticholinergic agents can also be employed.

ESOPHAGEAL PERFORATION

EPIDEMIOLOGY

- Perforation of the esophagus is associated with a high mortality rate regardless of the underlying cause.

PATHOPHYSIOLOGY

- Iatrogenic injury is the most common cause of esophageal perforation.
- Other causes include Boerhaave's syndrome (up to 15%), trauma (10%), and foreign body ingestion.
- Boerhaave's syndrome is a full-thickness perforation of the esophagus after a sudden rise in intraesophageal pressure, often due to forceful emesis. Alcohol consumption is frequently an antecedent to this syndrome.

CLINICAL FEATURES

- Pain is classically described as acute, severe, unrelenting, and diffuse, and is reported in the chest, neck, and abdomen.
- Pain can radiate to the back and shoulders, or back pain may be the predominant symptom.
- Swallowing often exacerbates pain.
- Physical exam varies with the severity of the rupture and the elapsed time between the rupture and presentation.
- Tachycardia and tachypnea are common.
- Abdominal rigidity with hypotension and fever often occur early.
- Mediastinal emphysema takes time to develop. It is less commonly detected by examination or radiography in lower esophageal perforation, and its absence does not rule out perforation.
- Hammon's crunch, caused by air in the mediastinum being moved by the beating heart, can sometimes be auscultated.
- Pleural effusions develop in half of patients with intrathoracic perforations and are uncommon in cervical perforations.

DIAGNOSIS AND DIFFERENTIAL

- Chest radiographs can suggest the diagnosis.
- CT of the chest or endoscopy is most often used to confirm the diagnosis; the choice depends upon clinical setting and the local resources available.
- Esophageal perforation is often ascribed to acute myocardial infarction (MI), pulmonary embolus, peptic ulcer disease, aortic catastrophe, or acute abdomen, resulting in critical delays in diagnosis, the most important factor in determining morbidity and mortality.

EMERGENCY DEPARTMENT CARE AND DISPOSITION

- Rapid, aggressive management is key to minimizing the morbidity and mortality associated with esophageal perforation.
- In the ED, resuscitation of shock (see Chapter 7) and broad-spectrum parenteral antibiotics should be given to cover both aerobic and anaerobic organisms. Examples include single-drug coverage such as **piperacillin-tazobactam** 3.375 grams IV, or double-drug coverage with **cefotaxime** 2 grams IV, or **ceftriaxone** 2 grams IV plus **clindamycin** 600 milligrams IV or **metronidazole** 1 gram IV.
- Emergent surgical consultation should be obtained as soon as the diagnosis is seriously entertained.
- All patients require admission to the hospital.

SWALLOWED FOREIGN BODIES

EPIDEMIOLOGY

- Children from 18 to 48 months of age account for 80% of all cases of ingested foreign bodies.
- Adult candidates for swallowed foreign bodies are those with esophageal disease, prisoners, and psychiatric patients.

PATHOPHYSIOLOGY

- Small objects, such as coins, toys, and crayons, typically lodge in the anatomically narrow proximal esophagus. In adults, most impactions are distal.
- In children and adults, once an object has traversed the pylorus, it usually continues through the GI tract and is passed without issue.
- Irregular, sharp, wide (>2.5 cm), or long objects (>6 cm) may become lodged distal to the pylorus.
- Esophageal impaction can result in airway obstruction, stricture, or perforation.
- Esophageal mucosal irritation can be perceived as a foreign body by the patient.

CLINICAL FEATURES

- Adults with an esophageal foreign body generally provide unequivocal history. Patients often complain of retrosternal pain, dysphagia, vomiting, choking, and inability to tolerate pooled secretions.

- In children, the history can be unclear. Signs and symptoms include refusal or inability to eat, vomiting, gagging and choking, stridor, neck or throat pain, and drooling.
- A high degree of suspicion is necessary for unwitnessed ingestions in children, especially in those <2 years of age.
- Examination starts with assessment of the airway. Occasionally, a foreign body can be directly visualized in the oropharynx.

DIAGNOSIS AND DIFFERENTIAL

- Plain films are used to screen for radiopaque objects. Coins in the esophagus present their circular face on anteroposterior films, as opposed to coins in the trachea, which show that face on lateral films.
- Plain films are <50% sensitive for detecting impacted bones, so lack of visualization does not exclude bone impaction. Plain films are often not necessary for patients with food impaction.
- Contrast radiographs (barium or meglumine diatrizoate...*Gastrograffin*) have low yields; the contrast material can impair endoscopy and present an aspiration risk.
- CT scanning is a very high-yield test for esophageal foreign bodies and has replaced the contrast radiographs to evaluate possible nonradiopaque objects.
- If endoscopy is clearly indicated, performing advanced imaging studies delays definitive intervention and adds little value to care.

EMERGENCY DEPARTMENT CARE AND DISPOSITION

- Patients in extremis or those with pending airway compromise are resuscitated in standard fashion.
- Emergent endoscopy is indicated for complete esophageal obstruction due to distal food impaction.
- Circumstances warranting urgent endoscopy for esophageal foreign bodies are shown in Table 42-1.

TABLE 42-1 Circumstances Warranting Urgent Endoscopy for Esophageal Foreign Bodies

Ingestion of sharp or elongated objects (including toothpicks, aluminum soda can tabs)
Ingestion of multiple foreign bodies
Ingestion of button batteries
Evidence of perforation
Coin at the level of the cricopharyngeus muscle in a child
Airway compromise
Presence of a foreign body for >24 h

- Success rates of glucagon therapy to relax the LES are poor. The use of proteolytic enzymes (meat tenderizer containing papain) to dissolve a meat bolus is contraindicated.
- Very proximally lodged objects may be removed by indirect laryngoscopy or fiber-optic scope.
- Coin removal with a Foley catheter is institution dependent. Complications include aspiration, airway compromise, and mucosal laceration.
- A button battery lodged in the esophagus is a true emergency requiring prompt removal because of the possibility of perforation.
- Sharp objects should be removed by endoscopy while they are in the stomach or duodenum in order to prevent intestinal perforation (up to 35%).
- Endoscopy is contraindicated for the removal of ingested narcotic packets ingested by narcotic couriers (body packers) because of the risk of iatrogenic packet rupture. Observation until the packet reaches the rectum is the favored treatment. Whole-bowel irrigation may aid the process.
- Consult surgery for worrisome foreign bodies that are in the more distal GI tract or if signs or symptoms of intestinal injury (eg, pain, emesis, fever, GI bleeding) are present.

For further reading in Tintinalli's *Emergency Medicine: A Comprehensive Study Guide,* 7th ed., see Chapter 80, "Esophageal Emergencies, Gastroesophageal Reflux Disease, and Swallowed Foreign Bodies," by Moss H. Mendelson.

43 PEPTIC ULCER DISEASE AND GASTRITIS

Matthew C. Gratton

EPIDEMIOLOGY

- Peptic ulcer disease (PUD) is a chronic illness manifested by recurrent ulcerations in the stomach and proximal duodenum. The great majority of peptic ulcers are directly related to infection with *Helicobacter pylori* or NSAID use.
- Gastritis is acute or chronic inflammation of the gastric mucosa.
- Dyspepsia is continuous or recurrent upper abdominal pain or discomfort with or without associated symptoms.

PATHOPHYSIOLOGY

- Hydrochloric acid and pepsin destroy gastric and duodenal mucosa while mucus and bicarbonate ion secretions protect mucosa. Prostaglandins protect mucosa by enhancing mucus and bicarbonate production. The balance between these protective and destructive forces determines whether ulceration occurs.
- *Helicobacter pylori* is a spiral, gram-negative, flagellated bacterium that produces urease, cytotoxins, proteases, and other compounds that disturb the mucous gel and cause tissue injury and ulceration.
- *Helicobacter pylori* infection is present in about 95% of patients who develop duodenal ulcer and about 70% of those who develop gastric ulcer.
- Traditional ulcer treatment heals most ulcers, but eradication of *H. pylori* reduces recurrence rates from 35% to 2% for duodenal ulcers and from 39% to 3% for gastric ulcers.
- NSAIDs inhibit prostaglandin synthesis, thereby decreasing mucus and bicarbonate production and mucosal blood flow, which allows ulcer formation.
- Acute gastritis is generally caused by ischemia due to severe illness (burns, trauma, shock, etc.), direct toxic effects (NSAIDs, alcohol, etc.), or *H. pylori* infection.
- Dyspepsia has multiple causes including esophagitis, endoscopically negative reflux disease, and PUD, but about 50% of dyspepsia patients have no cause found and are said to have "functional dyspepsia."

CLINICAL FEATURES

- Burning epigastric pain that is relieved with food, milk, or antacids and recurs at night as the stomach empties is the most classic presentation of PUD. Pain tends to occur daily for weeks and then resolve and then recur in weeks to months.
- Atypical presentations are common, especially in the elderly.
- A change in the character of the pain may indicate a complication: abrupt onset of severe pain in perforation with peritonitis; rapid onset of back pain associated with posterior perforation and pancreatitis; nausea and vomiting from gastric outlet obstruction; and vomiting blood or passing blood per rectum from a GI bleed.
- The only physical sign of PUD may be epigastric tenderness, and this is neither sensitive nor specific. Physical examination findings of complications include rigid abdomen (perforation), abdominal distention and vomiting (gastric outlet obstruction), or GI bleeding.
- Acute gastritis may present with epigastric pain and nausea and vomiting, although the most common presentation is GI bleeding (microscopic to gross blood).

DIAGNOSIS AND DIFFERENTIAL

- The classic history with epigastric tenderness may suggest PUD, but definitive diagnosis cannot be made clinically.
- The differential diagnosis of PUD includes gastritis, functional dyspepsia, gastroesophageal reflux disease (GERD), pancreatitis, hepatitis, cholelithiasis, cardiac ischemia, abdominal aortic aneurysm (AAA), gastroparesis, and gastric cancer.
- The "gold standard" for diagnosis is the visualization of an ulcer via upper GI endoscopy. The sensitivity and specificity are both >95%, and this test also allows visualization of other potential abnormalities and biopsy of appropriate lesions.
- Although not all patients with epigastric pain require endoscopy, those with "alarm" features suggestive of esophageal or gastric cancer or other serious diseases do (see Table 43-1).
- Ancillary tests to consider include complete blood cell count (CBC) to look for anemia in chronic GI blood loss, abdominal ultrasound for cholelithiasis and AAA, electrocardiogram and cardiac enzymes for cardiac ischemia, liver function tests to look for hepatitis and cholelithiasis, lipase to look for pancreatitis, and acute abdominal series to look for perforation.
- *Helicobacter pylori* infection could be investigated in the ED via serologic tests or stool antigen tests, but there is no evidence from the literature describing this in an ED setting and it is probably best deferred to the primary care provider follow-up visit.

EMERGENCY DEPARTMENT CARE AND DISPOSITION

- After PUD is diagnosed, the goal of treatment is to heal the ulcer while relieving pain and preventing complications and recurrence. H_2 receptor antagonists (H_2RAs) and proton pump inhibitors (PPIs) are the mainstay of treatment, while a variety of antibiotic regimens can be used to eradicate *H. pylori*.

TABLE 43-1 "Alarm Features" Suggesting Need for Endoscopy Referral

Age >55 y
Unexplained weight loss
Early satiety
Persistent vomiting
Dysphagia
Anemia or GI bleeding
Abdominal mass
Persistent anorexia
Jaundice

- PPIs (such as **omeprazole**, 20-40 milligrams PO daily, or **lansoprazole**, 15-30 milligrams PO daily) will generally heal ulcers faster than H_2RAs and have an inhibitory effect against *H. pylori*.
- H_2RAs (such as **cimetidine**, 300 milligrams IV or 800 milligrams PO at bedtime, or **ranitidine**, 50 milligrams IV or 300 milligrams PO at bedtime) can be instituted for ongoing therapy to promote ulcer healing.
- If acute infection with *H. pylori* is found, antimicrobial and antisecretory therapy is instituted with cure rates of 70% to 90%. Such a regimen might include a PPI, clarithromycin, and amoxicillin or metronidazole for 14 days.
- Patients with PUD complications always require consultation, and most require admission to an appropriate inpatient unit based on the diagnosis and hemodynamic stability.
- Most patients with epigastric pain do not receive a definitive diagnosis in the ED, but if a critical diagnosis (ie, abdominal aortic aneurysm or myocardial infarction) is still in the differential, then consultation for admission and further evaluation is indicated.
- When uncomplicated PUD, gastritis, or dyspepsia is strongly suspected, the great majority of patients can be discharged with acid-suppressive therapy with a PPI or H_2RA and instructions to follow-up with their primary care physician.
- All patients should receive discharge instructions that include avoidance of NSAIDs, alcohol, tobacco, caffeine, and non-enteric-coated aspirin. Early follow-up should be sought for patients with "alarm" features.

For further reading in Tintinalli's *Emergency Medicine: A Comprehensive Study Guide*, 7th ed., see Chapter 81, "Peptic Ulcer Disease and Gastritis," by Matthew C. Gratton.

44 PANCREATITIS AND CHOLECYSTITIS

Casey M. Glass

EPIDEMIOLOGY

- Cholelithiasis or alcohol abuse account for 90% of all cases of acute pancreatitis in the United States.
- Many other causes account for the remaining cases of acute pancreatitis (Table 44-1).

TABLE 44-1 Causes of Acute Pancreatitis

Gallstones (including microlithiasis)
Alcohol (acute and chronic alcohol consumption)
Hypertriglyceridemia
Endoscopic retrograde cholangiopancreatography
Drugs
Autoimmune disease (eg, systemic lupus erythematosus, Sjögren syndrome)
Genetic factors (PRSS1, SPINK1, CFTR)
Abdominal trauma
Postoperative complications (abdominal or cardiac surgery)
Bacterial infections (*Legionella, Leptospira, Mycoplasma, Salmonella*)
Viral infections (mumps virus, coxsackievirus, cytomegalovirus, echovirus, hepatitis B virus)
Parasitic infections (*Ascaris, Cryptosporidium, Toxoplasma*)
Hypercalcemia
Hyperparathyroidism
Ischemia
Posterior penetrating ulcer
Scorpion venom
Organophosphate insecticide
Pancreatic or ampullary tumor
Pancreas divisum with ductular narrowing on pancreatogram
Oddi sphincter dysfunction
Idiopathic

Abbreviations: CFTR = cystic fibrosis transmembrane conductance regulator; PRSS1 = protease, serine, 1 (trypsin 1); SPINK1 = serine peptidase inhibitor, Kazal type, 1.

- The cause of up to 20% of acute pancreatitis cases remains unclear after evaluation.
- Biliary colic is pain related to intermittent gallbladder obstruction from stones, typically lasting less than 5 hours. Gallstones are usually clinically silent with only 1% to 4% of affected persons developing symptoms in any year or 10% and 20% in 5 and 20 years, respectively.
- Cholecystitis is inflammation of the gallbladder, most often due to obstruction from gallstones. Up to 10% of cases of acute cholecystitis are complicated by perforation.
- Acalculous cholecystitis occurs in the absence of gallstones. Advanced age, critical illness, long-term total parenteral nutrition (TPN), diabetes, immunosuppression, and childbirth are risk factors.
- Cholangitis is bacterial infection of the biliary tree as a result of biliary obstruction. It is a serious illness with a high mortality rate if untreated.
- Choledocholithiasis is the presence of stones in the common bile duct.

PATHOPHYSIOLOGY

- The central cause of acute pancreatitis is believed to be unregulated intracellular activation of trypsin. Trypsin activates digestive enzymes leading to pancreatic inflamation and necrosis.

- In severe cases of acute pancreatitis, local activation of inflammatory mediators can cause systemic symptoms, systemic inflamatory response syndrome, organ failure, and death (Table 44-2).
- The causes of the gallstone formation are unclear. Large fasting and residual gallbladder volumes are associated with increased risk for stone formation. Cholesterol stones (70%) form from increased concentration of cholesterol in the bile. Mixed pigment stones (20%) form from bilirubin-calcium salts and are assoicated with biliary sludge, enteric infection, cholangitis, and parasites. Pure pigment stones (10%) form from bilirubin polymers and are associated with hemolysis, advnaced age, alcoholism, pancreatitis, cirrhosis, and TPN.
- Gallstone passage from the gallbladder to the cystic duct and common bile duct causes pain and nausea seocndary to increased luminal pressure in the obstructed gallbladder or duct.

TABLE 44-2 Complications of Acute Pancreatitis

LOCAL	SYSTEMIC
Pancreatic necrosis	Cardiovascular
Sterile	Hypotension
Infected	Hypovolemia
Pancreatic fluid collection	Myocardial depression
Pancreatic abscess	Pericardial effusion
Pancreatic pseudocyst	Pulmonary
Pleural effusion and fistula	Hypoxemia
Pancreatic ascites	Atelectasis
Involvement of peripancreatic tissues with necrosis	Pleural effusion
Hemorrhage	Pulmonary infiltrates
Pancreatic pseudocyst	Acute respiratory distress syndrome
Pseudoaneurysm	Respiratory failure
Thrombosis—splenic vein, portal vein	Hematologic
Bowel infarction	Disseminated intravascular coagulation
Biliary obstruction with jaundice	GI
	Peptic ulcer disease/erosive gastritis
	GI perforation
	GI bleeding
	Obstruction of duodenum or stomach
	Inflammation of the transverse colon
	Splenic infarct
	Renal
	Oliguria
	Azotemia
	Acute renal failure
	Renal artery and/or vein thrombosis
	Metabolic
	Hyperglycemia
	Hypocalcemia
	Hypertriglyceridemia

- Persistent biliary obstruction leads to visceral ischemia, transmural inflammation, and peritoneal irritation.
- Polymicrobial infection as a component of acute cholecystitis is common. Pathogens include gram-negative bacteria (*Escherichia coli*, 36%; and *Klebsiella*, 15%) and gram-positive bacteria (*Enterococcus*, 6%; *Staphylococcus*, 3%; and *Streptococcus*, 2%).

CLINICAL FEATURES

- Patients suffering from acute pancreatitis typically present with nausea, vomiting, and epigastric pain. Pain may localize to the right or left upper quadrant or radiate to the back.
- Pain from acute pancreatitis usually begins abruptly and lasts for days.
- In the setting of acute pancreatitis, vital sign abnormalities are variably present and correlate with severity of disease.
- In patients with acute pancreatitis, physical examination typically demonstrates epigastric tenderness. Bowel sounds may be diminished. Cullen or Turner signs are present only in the most severe cases.
- Jaundice is not typically present in acute pancreatitis and, when noted, is associated with gallstone pancreatitis.
- Patients suffering from biliary colic complain of RUQ pain associated with nausea and vomiting. The pain may radiate to the right back or shoulder or occasionally the left back. The pain does not persist for more than 5 to 6 hours.
- Patients with acute cholecystitis complain of similar pain as those with biliary colic but with more persistent symptoms. They may exhibit Murphy's sign (respiratory arrest with palpation of the RUQ).
- Patients with chronic cholecystitis have milder symptoms that may occur frequently.
- Patients with choledocholithiasis often note pain radiating to the middle of the back and have epigastric tenderness to palpation.
- Ascending cholangitis is associated with RUQ pain, fever, and jaundice (Charcot triad), although all three are present in less than half of cases.

DIAGNOSIS AND DIFFERENTIAL

- Differential diagnosis of acute pancreatitis, acute cholecystitis, cholangitis, and choledocholithasis includes lower lobe pneumonia, rupture of a pseudocyst, peritonitis, peptic ulcer disease, referred cardiac pain, small bowel obstruction, renal colic, dissecting aortic aneurysm, diabetic ketoacidosis, and gastroenteritis.

- The diagnosis of acute pancreatitis is based on history and examination findings consistent with the diagnosis.
- Objective criteria for acute pancreatitis require two of the following three components: (1) characteristic abdominal pain, (2) serum amylase/lipase levels greater than three times the upper limit of normal, or (3) computed tomography (CT) or ultrasonography (US) findings consistent with pancreatitis.
- Lipase is the laboratory test of choice for diagnosis of acute pancreatitis. At cutoff levels of 600 IU/L, the specificity is above 95% and sensitivity is 55% to 100%. A normal lipase does not exclude the diagnosis of pancreatitis, especially in patients with chronic pancreatitis.
- Amylase is less accurate than lipase in the diagnosis of acute pancreatitis. Amylase is found in many tissues throughout the body including the pancreas and salivary glands. Amylase greater than 3 times the upper limit of normal has a specificity of 95% and a sensitivity of 61% for acute pancreatitis.
- Abnormal liver function tests suggest a biliary cause of acute pancreatitis.
- CBC, serum chemistries, and serum lactate dehydrogenase (LDH) can be helpful in determining the severity of acute pancreatitis. Prospective scoring systems to predict severe pancreatitis include the acute pancreatitis APACHE II score or Ranson's criteria (Table 44-3).
- No single laboratory or radiographic test is effective at ruling in or ruling out cholecystitis.
- The most sensitive finding for acute cholecystitis is a positive Murphy's sign.

TABLE 44-3 Ranson's Criteria*

AT ADMISSION	WITHIN NEXT 48 H
Age >55 y (>70 y) White blood cell count >16,000/mm³ (>18,000/mm³) Blood glucose level >200 milligrams/dL (>220 milligrams/dL) Serum lactate dehydrogenase level >350 IU/L (>400 IU/L) Serum aspartate aminotransferase level >250 IU/L (same)	Decrease in hematocrit by >10% (same) Estimated fluid sequestration >6 L (>4 L) Serum calcium level <8.0 milligrams/dL (same) Partial pressure of arterial oxygen <60 mm Hg (omitted) Increase in blood urea nitrogen level >5 milligrams/dL after IV fluid hydration (>2 milligrams/dL) Base deficit of >4 mmol/L (>6 mmol)

*The criteria for nongallstone (alcoholic) acute pancreatitis are listed first; the changes (if any) in the criteria for gallstone pancreatitis are in parentheses.

- Leukocytosis is neither sensitive nor specific for cholecystitis.
- Abnormal liver function tests are suggestive of common bile duct stone, cholangitis, or Mirizzi's syndrome (compression of the common hepatic duct by a common bile duct stone).
- Plain radiographs of the abdomen are usually not helpful in the evaluation of pancreatitis or biliary pathology.
- US is helpful in the identification of gallstones or dilatation of the biliary tree. It is the test of choice for diagnosis of biliary pathology. It has a sensitivity up to 94% and specificity of 78% for the diagnosis of acute cholecystitis. Common US findings in acute cholecystitis are a sonographic Murphy's sign (pain over the gallbladder), gallstones, wall thickening (>3-5 mm), and pericholecystic fluid (Fig. 44-1). US is also helpful for identifying common duct pathology. The normal diameter of the common bile duct is approximately 7 mm.
- CT is the study of choice for visualizing the pancreas, the confirmation of pancreatic inflammation, and the identification of phlegmons, abscesses, or pseudocysts. It cannot be used to rule out acute pancreatitis as it may be normal in mild pancreatitis (Fig. 44-2). CT scanning scores can be used to estimate the severity of acute pancreatitis. CT has a sensitivity of up to 95% and specificity of 96% for detection of acute cholecystitis (Fig. 44-3).
- Hepatobiliary iminodiacetic acid (HIDA) scan is an adjunctive test when initial studies for gallbladder disease are indeterminate.
- Endoscopic retrograde cholangiopancreatography (ERCP) is rarely used in the ED, but can be useful when the etiology of acute pancreatitis remains unclear after initial evaluation. ERCP can be therapeutic for common duct stones or gallstone pancreatitis.
- The utility of magnetic resonance imaging (MRI) in acute pancreatitis is unclear. MRI can be an alternative diagnostic imaging method for acute cholecystitis with high sensitivities for identifying wall thickening, pericholecystic fluid, and adjacent fat stranding.

EMERGENCY DEPARTMENT CARE AND DISPOSITION

- The mainstays of acute pancreatitis treatment are pain and nausea control, hydration, and bowel rest.
- All patients with acute pancreatitis should have regular reassessment of vital signs and oxygen saturation.
- Adminster IV hydration to maintain urine output greater than 0.5 cc/kg/h.
- Patients with acute pancreatitis and mild symptoms who are tolerating clear fluids may be discharged

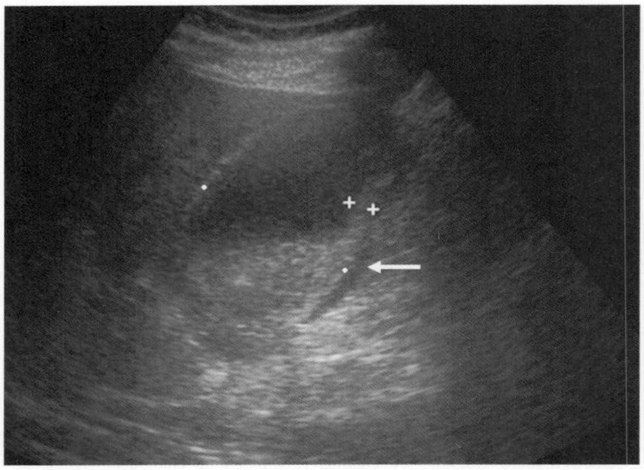

FIG. 44-1. Abdominal US image showing acute cholecystitis with pericholecystic fluid (white *arrow*), gallbladder wall thickening (white *pluses*), and enlarged short-axis dimension (white *dots*). (Courtesy of Mustafa Secil, MD.)

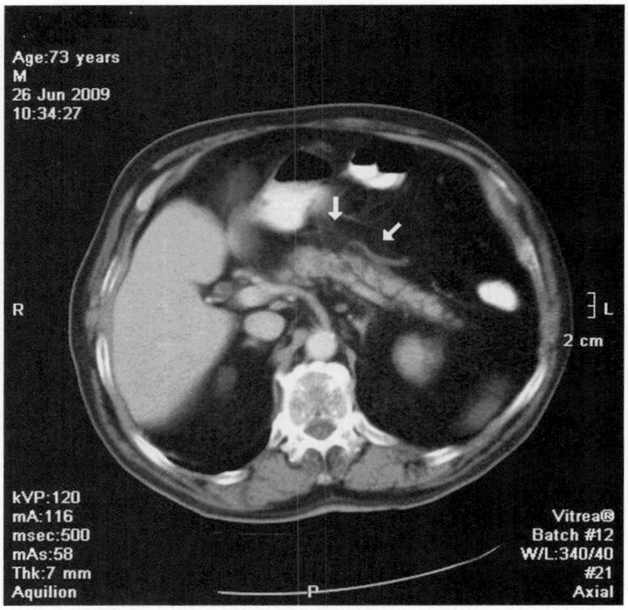

FIG. 44-2. Abominal CT scan showing mild pancreatitis with the borders of the gland becoming indistinct, with hazy soft tissue stranding consistent with inflammation surrounding the pancreas (*arrows*).

home, provided they have minimal laboratory abnormalities and normal vital signs.

- Acute pancreatitis associated with organ dysfunction, respiratory distress, and hypotension should be treated aggressively.
- Gallstone pancreatitis is an indication for urgent ERCP.
- Antibiotics are not indicated for acute pancreatitis unless a specific source of infection is suspected. If associated infection is noted (infected phlegmon, pseudocyst, sepsis), treatment with **imipenem-cilastin** 500 milligrams IV or **meropenem** 1 gram IV is appropriate. Alternative treatment may include **ciprofloxacin** 400 milligrams IV with **metronidazole** 500 milligrams IV.

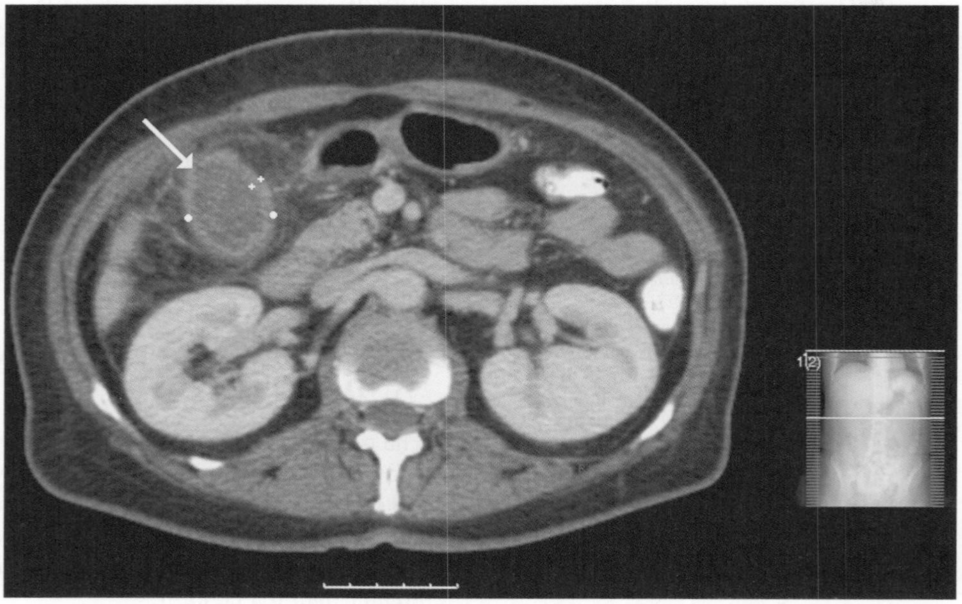

FIG. 44-3. Enhanced abdominal CT image showing acute cholecystitis with enlarged gallbladder with fluid (white *arrow*), gallbladder wall thickening (white *pluses*), and enlarged short-axis dimension (white *dots*). (Courtesy of Mustafa Secil, MD.)

- Patients with acute pancreatitis and significant systemic complications, shock, or extensive pancreatic necrosis will necessitate an intensive care setting.
- Incidental identification of gallstones requires no treatment. Patients should be warned about symptoms of biliary colic and cholecystitis.
- Patients with biliary colic require outpatient referral to a general surgeon.
- Patients with acute cholecystitis require surgical consultation and admission for choelcstectomy or percutaneous drainage.
- Antibiotics should be given as soon as acute cholecystitis is confirmed. Initial treatment regimens include **ceftriaxone** or **cefotaxime** 1 gram IV in conjunction with **metronidazole** 500 milligrams IV, or a **quinolone** plus **metronidazole** IV for patients who are beta-lactam allergic. Patients with severe disease require extended coverage with medications such as **piperacillin/tazobactam** 3.75 grams IV.
- Patients with ascending cholangitis require fluid resuscitation, broad-spectrum antibiotics, and emergent consultation for surigcal or endoscopic decompression of the biliary tract.
- Patients with choledocholithiasis or gallstone panreactitis require urgent ERCP for stone removal.

For further reading in Tintinalli's *Emergency Medicine: A Comprehensive Study Guide,* 7th ed., see Chapter 82, "Pancreatitis and Cholecystitis," by Ridvan Atilla and Cem Oktay.

45 ACUTE APPENDICITIS

Charles E. Stewart

EPIDEMIOLOGY

- Appendicitis is common. Always consider appendicitis in the patient with abdominal pain who has not had an appendectomy. The lifetime incidence of appendicitis is about 7% to 9%, making appendicitis the most common abdominal surgical emergency. The lifetime risk for appendicitis is slightly higher for men than for women (8.6% and 6.7%, respectively).
- Preoperative diagnosis of acute appendicitis has improved due to imaging techniques, but misdiagnosis remains an important cause of successful malpractice claims against emergency physicians.

PATHOPHYSIOLOGY

- Acute appendicitis develops from obstruction of the appendiceal lumen. Increased luminal pressure leads to vascular compromise, bacterial invasion, inflammatory response, and resultant tissue necrosis with possible perforation and peritoneal contamination.
- Classically, appendicitis is associated with the migration of pain from the periumbilical area to the right lower quadrant (RLQ). However, there are many atypical presentations, often affected by variability of the anatomic location (eg, retrocecal, retroileal) of the appendix.

CLINICAL FEATURES

- The most reliable symptom in acute appendicitis is abdominal pain.
- RLQ pain is 81% sensitive and 53% specific for the diagnosis of acute appendicitis. Migration of periumbilical pain to the RLQ is 64% sensitive and 82% specific for the diagnosis of acute appendicitis.
- After the onset of vague abdominal pain, the classic triad of symptoms in appendicitis includes anorexia, nausea, and vomiting. Sixty percent of patients with appendicitis will have some combination of these symptoms, but they are by themselves neither specific nor sensitive for appendicitis.
- McBurney's point tenderness, Rovsing's sign, psoas sign, obturator sign, rectal examination tenderness, and rebound tenderness are all clinical examination findings that may be present. In children, the most reliable sign on physical examination is rebound tenderness.
- Fever in appendicitis is a relatively late finding and rarely exceeds 39°C (102.2°F) unless rupture or other complications occur. As might be expected, fever is unreliable as an indicator for appendicitis. A temperature >99.0°F had a sensitivity of 47% (95% CI = 36%-57%) and a specificity of 64% (95% CI = 57%-71%).

DIAGNOSIS AND DIFFERENTIAL

- The diagnosis of appendicitis is primarily clinical. Factors that increase the likelihood of appendicitis, listed in decreasing order of importance, are RLQ pain, rebound tenderness and/or rigidity, migration of pain to the RLQ, pain before vomiting, positive psoas sign, fever, and guarding. None of these factors are specific for appendicitis.
- The differential diagnosis of appendicitis can include other RLQ GI complaints including volvulus, colitis, ileitis, bowel obstruction, diverticulitis, Crohn's disease, intrabdominal abscess, intussusception, incarcerated hernias, gut malrotation, and mesenteric

lymphadenitis. Genitourinary (GU) complaints that can mimic appendicitis include ovarian torsion, ectopic or hetertopic pregnancy, ovarian vein thrombosis and tubo-ovarian abscess or salpingitis in the female. In the male, testicular pain can be referred to the RLQ. Pyelonephritis or renal colic may cause RLQ pain in both women and men. Abdominal wall or rectus sheath hematomas and abscess within the psoas can also mimic appendicitis. Again, if the patient has right-sided abdominal pain, appendicitis should be considered unless a prior appendectomy has been done.

- If the diagnosis is unclear, additional studies such as complete blood count, urinalysis, pregnancy test, and radiologic imaging should be considered.
- Elevation of the white blood cell count is sensitive, but has a very low specificity for appendicitis.
- Obtaining a urinalysis is important to rule out other diagnoses, such as urolithiasis or urinary tract infection; however, pyuria and hematuria can occur when an inflamed appendix overlies a ureter. Obtain a pregnancy test in every female of childbearing age who has a uterus.

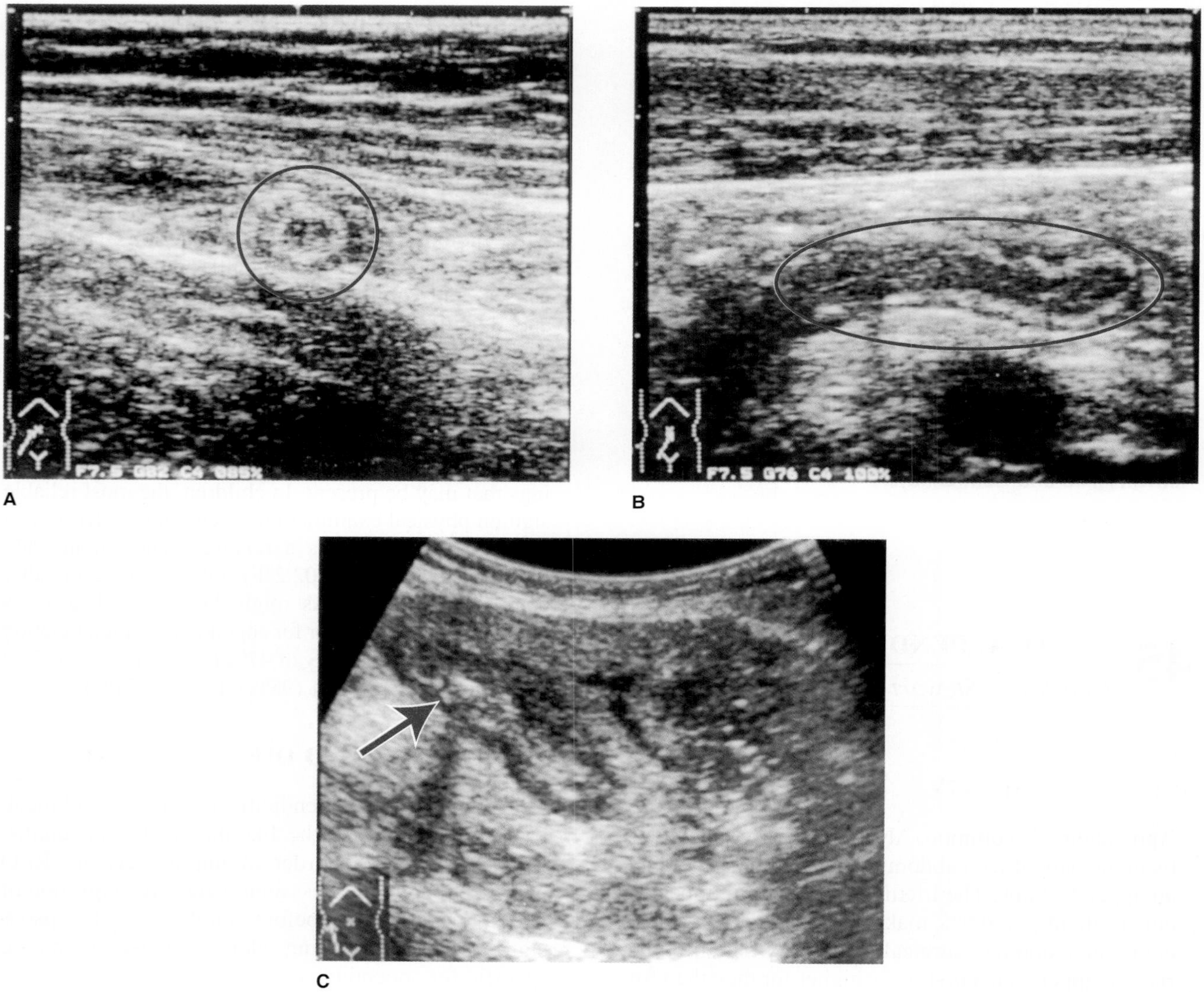

FIG. 45-1. Ultrasonographic demonstration of acute appendicitis. A noncomprehensible inflamed appendix (*red circles*) is shown in a cross-sectional view (**A**; 7.5 MHz) and a longitudinal section (**B**; 7.5 MHz). Mural lamintion of the swollen appendix is maintained in the early stages of acute appendicitis. **C**. An appendicolith (*arrow*) with acoustic shadowing is demonstated (5 MHz). (Reprinted with permission from Ma OJ, Mateer JR, Blaivas M: *Emergency Ultrasound, 2nd ed*. Copyright © The McGraw-Hill Companies, 2008. All rights reserved. Chaper 9: General Surgery Applications, Figure 9-23, Parts A-C.)

- Plain radiographs of the abdomen often have nonspecific abnormalities. Radiographic findings of possible acute appendicitis include appendiceal fecalith, appendiceal gas, localized paralytic ileus, blurred right psoas muscle, and free air.
- Ultrasound is operator dependent and is significantly better in institutions where it is routinely used. Ultrasonography is limited in evaluating a ruptured appendix or an abnormally located (eg, retrocecal) appendix and in the obese patient. Ultrasound should be considered as an initial study for females and children as a means to limit radiation exposure (see Fig. 45-1).
- Computed tomography (CT) is sensitive (98%) and quite specific (95%). Debate exists whether focused appendiceal CT or traditional nonfocused abdominal CT is the better choice and whether contrast need be used. CT findings suggesting acute appendicitis include pericecal inflammation, abscess, and periappendiceal phlegmon or fluid collections. Recent increases in use of CT scan have led to concerns about radiation risks to the patient (see Fig. 45-2).
- Magnetic resonance imaging (MRI) may be useful for pregnant patients as there is no radiation involved in the diagnosis of appendicitis. Although MRI avoids any ionizing radiation and is deemed to be safe in pregnancy, it is more costly, time consuming, and of limited availability in most emergency departments. This significantly limits its usefulness in other patients.
- In order to avoid premature surgical intervention or discharge of the patient with an uncertain diagnosis, patients with atypical presentations may be observed with serial abdominal examination.

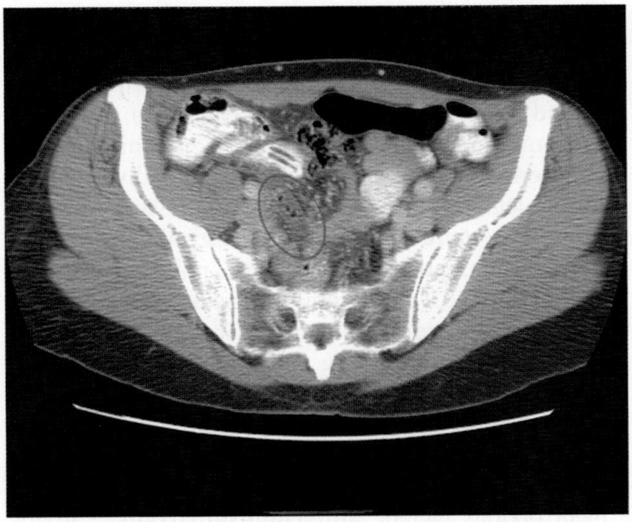

FIG. 45-2. Acute appendicitis on contrast CT scan as evidenced by dilated and inflamed appendix (*red circle*).

- The overall mortality rate for appendicitis is less than 1%, but it increases to 3% if the appendix is ruptured and approaches 15% in the elderly. The diagnosis of appendicitis is more difficult in the extremely young and the elderly, resulting in a higher incidence of delayed diagnosis and rupture with subsequent increases in mortality in these populations.
- Appendicitis is the most common extrauterine surgical emergency in pregnancy, and occurs with an incidence equal to that of nonpregnant patients; if perforation and peritonitis occur, then fetal mortality rates are high.

EMERGENCY DEPARTMENT CARE AND DISPOSITION

- In the United States, prompt surgical removal of the appendix is considered the most appropriate therapy.
- Prior to surgery, patients should have nothing by mouth, and should have IV access, analgesia, and antibiotic therapy started.
- Short-acting narcotic analgesics such as fentanyl (0.01-0.02 milligram/kg) are preferred, since they can be reversed by time or naloxone if necessary.
- Antibiotics should cover anaerobes, enterococci, and gram-negative intestinal flora. Antibiotics given before surgery decrease the incidence of postoperative wound infection or, in cases of perforation, postoperative abscess formation. Several antibiotic regimens to cover anaerobes, enterococci, and gram-negative intestinal flora have been recommended, including **piperacillin/tazobactam** 3.375 grams IV or **ampicillin/sulbactam** 3 grams IV.
- If no precise diagnosis is determined after evaluation and observation, the patient should be diagnosed as having nonspecific abdominal pain rather than be given a more specific diagnosis.
- Patients who have no contraindication to discharge should be given specific instructions to obtain close follow-up with their primary care physician, and to return if their condition worsens or if they develop increased pain, fever, or nausea. The physician should ensure that a responsible party: parent or patient, understands that reevaluation can prevent serious complications and that diagnostic tests are not infallible.

For further reading in Tintinalli's *Emergency Medicine: A Comprehensive Study Guide*, 7th ed., see Chapter 84, "Appendicitis," by E. Paul DeKoning.

46 DIVERTICULITIS

James C. O'Neill

Diverticulitis is a common GI disorder that occurs when small herniations through the wall of the colon, or diverticula, become inflamed or infected.

EPIDEMIOLOGY

- Clinical diverticulitis occurs in 10% to 25% of patients with diverticulosis. One-third of the population will have acquired the disease by age 50 years, and two-thirds by age 85 years.

PATHOPHYSIOLOGY

- Clinical diverticulitis results from high colonic pressures, resulting in erosion and microperforation of the diverticular wall, leading to inflammation of pericolonic tissue.

CLINICAL FEATURES

- The most common symptom is a steady, deep discomfort in the left lower quadrant of the abdomen. Other symptoms include tenesmus and changes in bowel habits, such as diarrhea or increasing constipation.
- The involved diverticulum can irritate the urinary tract and cause frequency, dysuria, or pyuria.
- Paralytic ileus with abdominal distension, nausea, and vomiting may develop secondary to intra-abdominal irritation and peritonitis. Small bowel obstruction and perforation can also occur.
- Right lower quadrant pain, which may be indistinguishable from acute appendicitis, can occur with ascending colonic diverticular involvement and in patients with a redundant right-sided sigmoid colon.
- Physical examination frequently demonstrates a low-grade fever, but the temperature may be higher in patients with generalized peritonitis and in those with an abscess.
- Physical findings range from mild abdominal tenderness to severe pain, obstruction, and peritonitis. A fullness or mass may be appreciated over the affected area of colon.
- Occult blood may be present in the stool.

DIAGNOSIS AND DIFFERENTIAL

- Diverticulitis can be diagnosed by clinical history and examination alone. In stable patients with past similar acute presentations, no further diagnostic evaluation is necessary unless the patient fails to improve with conservative medical treatment.
- If a patient does not have a prior diagnosis or the current episode is different from past episodes, diagnostic imaging should be performed to rule out other intra-abdominal pathology and evaluate for complications. CT scan is the preferred imaging modality for its ability to evaluate the severity of disease and the presence of complications. CT with IV and oral contrast has documented sensitivities of 97% and specificities approaching 100%.
- Laboratory tests, such as a CBC, liver function tests, and urinalysis, are rarely diagnostic but may help exclude other diagnoses.
- Abdominal radiographs may be normal or may demonstrate an associated ileus, partial small bowel obstruction, colonic obstruction, free air indicating bowel perforation, or extraluminal collections of air, suggesting a walled-off abscess.
- The differential diagnosis includes acute appendicitis, colitis (ischemic or infectious), inflammatory bowel disease (Crohn disease or ulcerative colitis), colon cancer, irritable bowel syndrome, pseudomembranous colitis, epiploic appendagitis, gallbladder disease, incarcerated hernia, mesenteric infarction, complicated ulcer disease, peritonitis, obstruction, ovarian torsion, ectopic pregnancy, ovarian cyst or mass, pelvic inflammatory disease, sarcoidosis, collagen vascular disease, cystitis, kidney stone, renal pathology, and pancreatic disease.

EMERGENCY DEPARTMENT CARE AND DISPOSITION

- Emergency department (ED) care begins with fluid and electrolyte replacement, and pain and nausea control. Ill-appearing patients; those with uncontrolled pain, vomiting, peritoneal signs, signs of systemic infection, comorbidities, or immunosuppression; and those with complicated diverticulitis (eg, phlegmon, abscess, obstruction, fistula, or perforation) require admission and surgical consultation.
- Place the patient on complete bowel rest. Opiates, such as **morphine** 0.1 milligram/kg IV, may be required for pain. Nasogastric suction may be indicated in patients with bowel obstruction or adynamic ileus.
- Administer IV antibiotics to patients requiring admission. Options include **metronidazole** 500 milligrams IV with either **ciprofloxacin** 400 milligrams IV or **levofloxacin** 750 milligrams IV. Alternate single-agent treatment options include **ampicillin-sulbactam**, 3 grams IV; **piperacillin-tazobactam**, 3.35 grams IV; **ertapenem**, 1 gram IV; **ticarcillin-clavulanate**, 3.1 grams IV;

or **moxifloxacin**, 400 milligrams IV. Patients with very severe disease may require extended broad-spectrum antibiotics such as **imipenem** 500 milligrams IV, **meropenem** 1 gram IV, or **doripenem** 500 milligrams IV.

- Immunocompetent patients with uncomplicated diverticulitis who look well have mild findings on physical examination and in whom pain is controlled with oral analgesia may be managed as outpatients with oral antibiotics for 7 to 14 days, on a clear liquid diet that is advanced as tolerated, and close follow-up (2-3 days). Patients should contact their physicians or return to the ED if they develop increasing abdominal pain or fever or are unable to tolerate oral intake.
- Oral antibiotic regimens include **metronidazole** 500 milligrams every 8 hours plus either **ciprofloxacin** 500 milligrams every 12 hours or **clindamycin** 300 milligrams every 6 hours or **trimethoprim-sulfamethoxazole DS**, one tablet every 12 hours. Monotherapy includes **amoxicillin-clavulanate**, 875 milligrams every 12 hours, and **moxifloxacin**, 400 milligrams PO once a day.

For further reading in Tintinalli's Emergency Medicine: A Comprehensive Study Guide, 7th ed., see Chapter 85, "Diverticulitis," by Autumn Graham.

47 BOWEL OBSTRUCTION AND VOLVULUS

Mark Hess

EPIDEMIOLOGY

- Small bowel obstruction (SBO) is more common than large bowel obstruction (LBO).
- Intestinal obstruction is due to mechanical obstruction or functional (adynamic or paralytic ileus) obstruction, with ileus being more common. Mechanical obstruction may be due to either intrinsic or extrinsic mechanisms.
- Adhesions following surgery are the most common cause of SBO. Incarcerated inguinal hernias are the second most common cause of SBO. Other causes of bowel obstruction are listed in Table 47-1.
- LBO is most commonly due to neoplasm. Fecal impaction is common in elderly and debilitated patients. Sigmoid volvulus is common in the elderly, especially those taking anticholinergic medications. Cecal volvulus is more common in gravid patients.

TABLE 47-1 Common Causes of Intestinal Obstruction

DUODENUM	SMALL BOWEL	COLON
Stenosis	Adhesions	Carcinoma
Foreign body (bezoars)	Hernia	Fecal impaction
Stricture	Intussusception	Ulcerative colitis
Superior mesenteric artery syndrome	Lymphoma	Volvulus
	Stricture	Diverticulitis (stricture, abscess)
		Intussusception
		Pseudo-obstruction

- Complications and mortality rise in those over 60 years of age. Mortality also increases dramatically if corrective surgery is delayed beyond 24 hours.
- Ileus may be due to injury, infection, medications, or electrolyte abnormalities.

PATHOPHYSIOLOGY

- Blockage prevents passage of luminal contents and results in dilatation due to accumulation of gastric, biliary, and pancreatic secretions.
- With distention, intraluminal pressure rises, decreasing bowel wall blood flow. When pressure exceeds capillary pressure, absorption ceases and leakage of fluids (third-spacing) may occur. Microvascular changes may allow entry of gut flora into the circulation, resulting in bacteremia and sepsis. Necrosis and bowel perforation may follow.
- With obstruction, oral fluid intake stops and vomiting occurs. This fluid loss, coupled with the third space losses mentioned above, leads to hypovolemia and shock.
- Closed loop obstruction (LBO in presence of closed ileocecal valve) has a more rapid progression.

CLINICAL FEATURES

- Classic history includes vomiting, abdominal distention, and pain, with a past history of abdominal surgery or hernia.
- Abdominal pain is usually crampy and intermittent. SBO results in primarily periumbilical pain versus hypogastric pain for LBO. Pain with ileus may be constant.
- Emesis is often bilious early and may be feculent with late SBO or with LBO.
- Early in the disease course, bowel sounds have high-pitched rushes, but this finding diminishes with time.
- The patient may have surgical scars, hernias, or intra-abdominal masses.

- Peritoneal signs suggest perforation.
- Clinical signs of dehydration and/or shock may be present (tachycardia, hypotension).
- Rectal examination may reveal impaction, occult blood, or carcinoma. Passage of stool does not rule out obstruction.
- Women may have palpable gynecologic neoplasms on pelvic examination.

DIAGNOSIS AND DIFFERENTIAL

- Radiographs help localize SBO versus LBO. Plicae circulares are linear densities that traverse the small bowel lumen. Haustra in the large bowel do not extend fully across the lumen.
- Dilated loops of bowel on supine film with stepladder air-fluid levels on upright film are diagnostic. Look on the upright or decubitus film for free air suggesting perforation, and for pneumonia or pleural effusions on the chest film.
- Contrast-enhanced abdominal CT has been advocated to identify partial versus complete bowel obstruction. It also can differentiate between bowel obstruction and ileus as well as identify the site and cause of the obstruction.
- Laboratory tests include complete blood count (CBC), blood urea nitrogen (BUN), serum electrolytes, and urinalysis. Liver function tests as well as crossmatch and coagulation studies may also be needed.
- Leukocytosis with a left shift may suggest peritonitis, gangrene of the bowel, or an abscess. Serum lactate may be useful in assessing the presence of mesenteric vascular occlusion or severe dehydration.
- As dehydration and shock develop, elevated urine specific gravity and metabolic acidosis may be seen along with hemoconcentration.
- Sigmoidoscopy or barium enema may be useful in localizing the site of LBO.
- Pseudo-obstruction (Ogilvie's syndrome) is most commonly seen in the low colonic region. Intestinal motility is depressed (often due to tricyclic antidepressants or anticholinergic agents), resulting in large volumes of retained gas. Air-fluid levels are rarely seen on radiographs. Pseudo-obstruction is treated by colonoscopy.

EMERGENCY DEPARTMENT CARE AND DISPOSITION

- With mechanical bowel obstruction, prompt surgical consultation is required.
- A nasogastric tube is used to decompress the bowel, especially if vomiting or distension is present.
- Fluid resuscitation should be started using crystalloid. Monitor vital signs and urine output to measure response to fluids.
- Appropriate antibiotic therapy (such as **piperacillin-tazobactam** 3.375 grams, or **ampicillin-sulbactam** 3.0 grams IV) should be started if perforation is suspected or surgery is anticipated.
- For adynamic ileus, conservative treatments including nasogastric decompression, fluid replacement, and observation are usually effective.

For further reading in *Emergency Medicine: A Comprehensive Study Guide*, 7th ed., see Chapter 86, "Bowel Obstruction and Volvulus," by Salvator J. Vicario and Timothy G. Price.

48 HERNIA IN ADULTS AND CHILDREN

Dave W. Lu

A hernia is a protrusion of any viscus from its normal cavity.

EPIDEMIOLOGY

- Nearly 10% of the population develops a hernia during their lifetime.
- Hernias are classified by anatomic location, hernia contents, and the status of those contents (eg, reducible, incarcerated, or strangulated).
- The most common abdominal hernias are inguinal, ventral, and femoral hernias (Fig. 48-1).
- Seventy-five percent of all hernias are inguinal hernias, with two-thirds of these being indirect hernias. Although inguinal hernias occur more frequently in men, they are also the most common hernias in women. There is no gender predilection in ventral hernias, but femoral hernias occur much more commonly in women.
- Predisposing factors include family history, lack of developmental maturity, undescended testes, genitourinary abnormalities, conditions that increase intra-abdominal pressure (eg, ascites or pregnancy), and surgical incision sites.

PATHOPHYSIOLOGY

- Hernias occur in structural areas with inherent weakness, including penetration sites for extraperitoneal structures, areas lacking strong multilayer support, and wound sites (either surgical or traumatic).

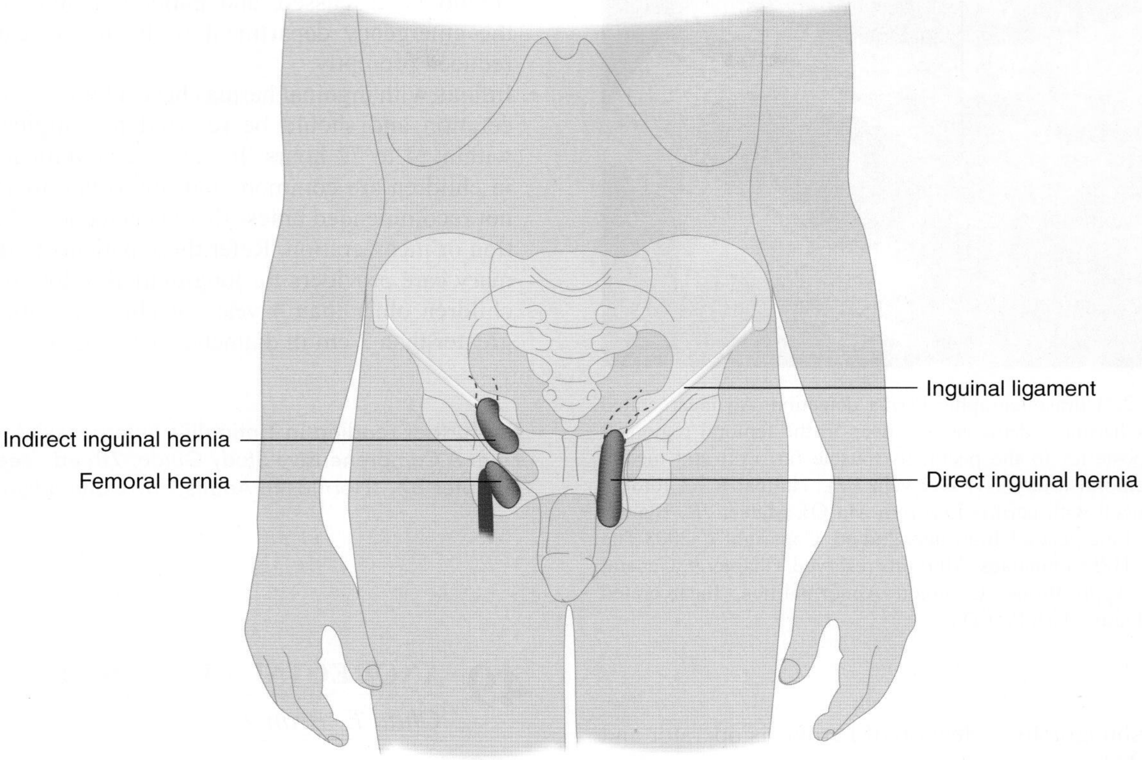

FIG. 48-1. Groin hernias.

- Specific hernia types include (1) direct inguinal hernias, which project directly through a weakness in the transversalis fascia in Hesselbach triangle; (2) indirect inguinal hernias, which pass through the internal inguinal ring and present as a groin mass upon exiting the external inguinal ring; (3) incisional hernias, which occur as a result of excess wall tension or inadequate wound healing and are associated with wound infections; (4) umbilical hernias, which commonly are seen in infants but can be found in adults as a result of conditions that increase intra-abdominal pressure; and (5) femoral hernias, which travel through the femoral canal and protrude below the inguinal ligament.

CLINICAL FEATURES

- Most hernias are detected on routine physical examination.
- When the contents of a hernia can be easily returned to their original cavity by manipulation, the hernia is *reducible*.
- A hernia becomes *incarcerated* when its contents are not reducible. Incarcerated hernias may lead to bowel obstruction and strangulation. *Strangulation* refers to vascular compromise of the incarcerated contents and is an acute surgical emergency. When not relieved, strangulation may lead to gangrene, perforation, peritonitis, and septic shock.
- Symptoms other than a protruding mass include localized pain, nausea, and vomiting. Children may exhibit irritability and poor feeding.

DIAGNOSIS AND DIFFERENTIAL

- Physical examination is the predominant means of diagnosis.
- Laboratory testing has no reliable indicators; however, leukocytosis and acidosis may indicate ischemic bowel.
- An acute abdominal series can reveal signs of intestinal obstruction and free air if perforation is suspected.

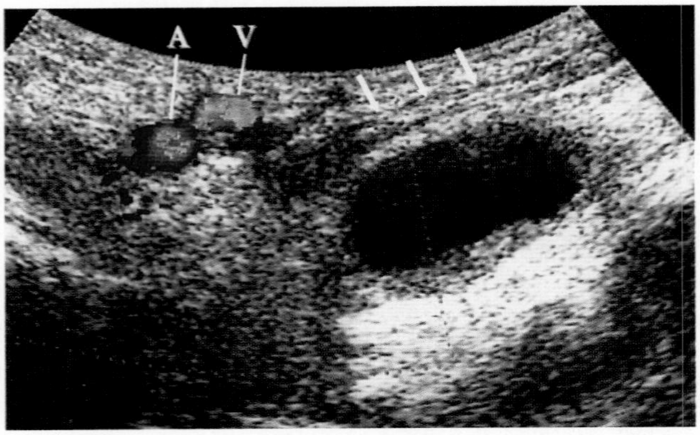

FIG. 48-2. Ultrasonographic hernia detection. An incarcerated obturator hernia is demonstrated deep in the femoral region. It locates posterior to the pectineus muscle (arrows) and medial to the femoral artery (A) and vein (V). Tintinall's 7th edition. [Reproduced with permission from Ma OJ, Mateer JR, Blaivas M (eds): Emergency Ultrasound, 2nd ed. Copyright © 2008 The McGraw-Hill Companies, All rights reserved. Chapter 9, General Surgery Applications, Common Abnormalities, Incarcerated Hernia. Figure 9-16 Part D.]

- Ultrasonographic detection of hernias is operator and body habitus dependent, but can be helpful in pediatric and pregnant patients when radiation exposure is a concern (Fig. 48-2).
- Computed tomography remains the best radiographic test for the evaluation of hernias.
- The differential diagnosis of a groin mass includes direct or indirect hernia, testicular torsion, tumor, groin abscess, hydrocele, varicocele, and hidradenitis. In children, retracted or undescended testes may be mistaken for inguinal hernias.

EMERGENCY DEPARTMENT CARE AND DISPOSITION

- An attempt to reduce a recently incarcerated hernia should be made. If there is question of the duration of the incarceration, reduction should not be attempted so as to not introduce dead bowel into the abdomen. General surgery should be consulted immediately.
- Emergent surgical intervention is the treatment of choice for incarcerated hernias that cannot be reduced or are strangulated. Patients should be made NPO, have intravenous fluid resuscitation, and receive adequate analgesia. Broad-spectrum antibiotics, such as **cefoxitin** 2 grams IV or **piperacillin/tazobactam** 3.375 grams IV, are indicated if there is evidence of perforation or strangulation.
- In adults with reducible hernias, refer for outpatient surgical evaluation and repair. Signs of obstruction should be discussed, and patients should return to the emergency department if the hernia cannot be reduced promptly.
- Infants with inguinal hernias have a high risk of incarceration and should be referred for surgical repair within 24 to 72 hours. In contrast, umbilical hernias in children are common, and immediate treatment is not recommended unless there is evidence of obstruction or incarceration. Refer these patients to their primary care providers for longitudinal follow-up. Refer children older than 4 years or children with hernias greater than 2 cm in diameter to a surgeon.

For further reading in Tintinalli's *Emergency Medicine: A Comprehensive Study Guide,* 7th ed., see Chapter 87, "Hernias in Adults," by Donald Byars.

49 ANORECTAL DISORDERS

Chad E. Branecki

HEMORRHOIDS

EPIDEMIOLOGY

- Hemorrhoids are associated with constipation, straining at stool, frequent diarrhea, advanced age, and pregnancy. Chronic liver disease, portal hypertension, obesity, and tumors or the rectum and colon may contribute to the formation of hemorrhoids.

PATHOPHYSIOLOGY

- Internal hemorrhoid veins are proximal to the dentate line, and drain into the portal venous system.
- External hemorrhoid veins are distal to the dentate line, therefore have sensory innervation, and can be viewed on external inspection (Fig. 49-1).

CLINICAL FEATURES

- Internal hemorrhoids are best visualized through an anoscope and frequently located at the 2-, 5-, and 9-o'clock positions in a prone patient.
- External hemorrhoids cause severe pain, discomfort, and bleeding at the time of defecation.
- Thrombosis of external hemorrhoids may appear as a bluish-purple mass protruding from the rectum and is exquisitely tender to palpation.

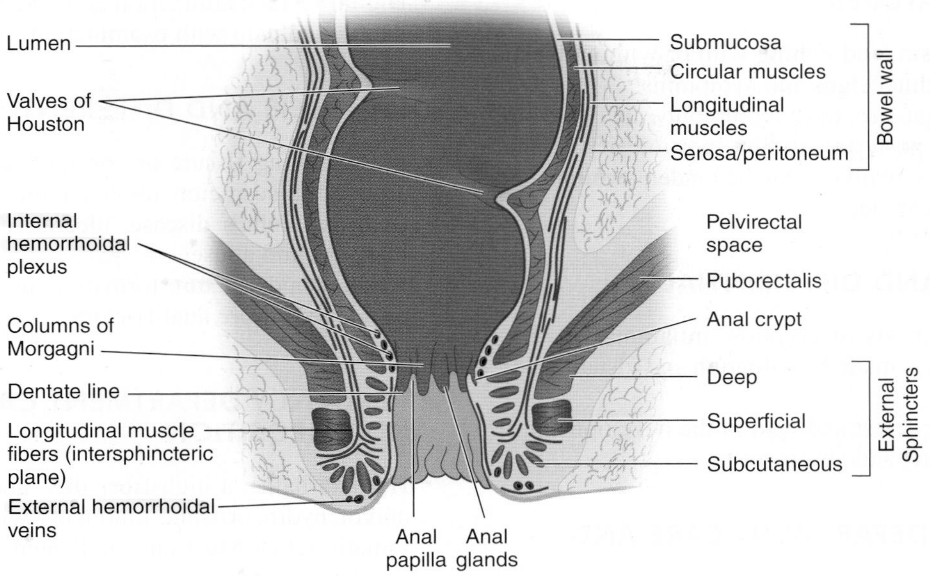

FIG. 49-1. Coronal section of the anorectum.

- Prolapse can occur with large hemorrhoids, requiring manual reduction by the patient or clinician. The hemorrhoid may become incarcerated causing mucous drainage, pruritus ani, heavy bleeding, urinary retention, gangrene, or even sepsis. Surgical intervention may be required.

DIAGNOSIS AND DIFFERENTIAL

- Other causes of rectal pain and bleeding may include malignancy, abscess, cryptitis, anal fissure, trauma, foreign bodies, rectal prolapse, or venereal proctitis.

EMERGENCY DEPARTMENT CARE AND DISPOSITION

- Treatment is usually nonsurgical. Most hemorrhoids can be relieved by hot sitz baths, topical steroids, analgesics, and bulk laxatives (psyllium seed compounds, stool softeners) after the acute phase has subsided.
- Acute (<48 hours), non-tolerable painful thrombosed external hemorrhoids can be managed by clot excision. The thrombosed vein should be unroofed by an elliptical incision that allows evacuation of the clot (Fig. 49-2).
- Surgical referral and intervention is indicated for continued bleeding, intractable pain, or incarceration and strangulation.

CRYPTITIS

EPIDEMIOLOGY

- Cryptitis is associated with repetitive sphincter trauma from spasm, recurrent diarrhea, or passage of large, hard stools.

PATHOPHYSIOLOGY

- Anal crypts are superficial mucosal pockets that lie between the columns of Morgagni. This tissue becomes hypertrophied from the repeated puckering action of the sphincter muscles, resulting in local inflammation or infection (cryptitis).

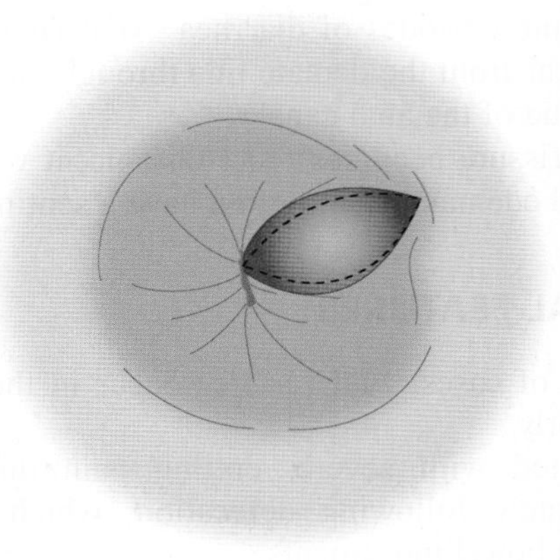

FIG. 49-2. Elliptical incision of thrombosed external hemorrhoid.

CLINICAL FEATURES

- Anal pain, spasm, and itching with or without bleeding are the cardinal signs and symptoms.
- The Crypts that are most commonly involved are located in the posterior midline portion of the anal ring. The crypts involved may be tender, swollen, and nodular in appearance.

DIAGNOSIS AND DIFFERENTIAL

- Definitive diagnosis of cryptitis, inflammation, erythema, and pus is made by palpation and visualization by anoscopy.
- Cryptitis may coexist and lead to the development of fissures, fistulae, and abscesses.

EMERGENCY DEPARTMENT CARE AND DISPOSITON

- Bulk laxatives, a high-fiber diet, and sitz baths will enhance passage of stool and healing by keeping the anus clean and crypts empty.
- Refractory cases or deep large crypts may require surgical intervention.

ANAL FISSURES

EPIDEMIOLOGY

- Anal fissures are the most common cause of painful rectal bleeding.
- Anal fissures are common among infants, children, young adults, and postpartum women.

PATHOPHYSIOLOGY

- Traditional midline anal fissures are caused by the passage of hard, large fecal masses, but can be seen after acute episodes of diarrhea. Anal fissures are a linear tear from the dentate line through the anodermal tissue of the anal canal.
- As the fissure becomes more chronic, it will appear pale and edematous, and often have a sentinel pile.

CLINICAL FEATURES

- In 90% of cases, anal fissures occur in the midline posteriorly.
- Associated with severe, cutting pain during and immediately following defecation, which subsides between bowel movements.
- Digital rectal examination and anoscopy may be limited due to pain with examination.

DIAGNOSIS AND DIFFERENTIAL

- A nonhealing fissure or non-midline location should arouse the suspicion for other more serious causes, such as Crohn's disease, ulcerative colitis, carcinomas, or child abuse.
- Abscess and stricture formation are complications of prolonged severe anal fissures.

EMERGENCY DEPARTMENT CARE AND DISPOSITION

- Hot sitz baths, a high-fiber diet, and local analgesic and/or hydrocortisone ointments will provide symptomatic relief. Most uncomplicated fissures will heal in a few weeks.

FISTULA IN ANO

EPIDEMIOLOGY

- A fistula in ano most commonly results as a complication of perianal or ischiorectal abscesses.
- Fistulas can also be associated with ulcerative colitis, Crohn's disease, malignancies, STDs, trauma, or TB.

PATHOPHYSIOLOGY

- An anal fistula is an abnormal inflammatory tract, connecting the anal canal with external skin.
- Anterior opening fistulas tend to follow a simple direct course to the anal canal (Goodsall rule), whereas posterior opening fistulas tend to follow a more curving path to the posterior midline.

CLINICAL FEATURES

- Malodorous, blood-stained discharge will be present as long as the tract remains open.
- Throbbing constant pain worsened by sitting, moving, and stooling will be present when the tract is blocked and abscess formation occurs.

DIAGNOSIS AND DIFFERENTIAL

- Abscess may be the initial presenting symptom.
- Ultrasound using 7-MHz endoprobe with hydrogen peroxide may aid in the diagnosis.

EMERGENCY DEPARTMENT CARE AND DISPOSITION

- Non-ill-appearing patients can be treated with analgesia, antipyretics, and oral antibiotics (**ciprofloxin** 750 milligrams BID and **metronidazole** 500 milligrams QID for 7 days).
- Surgical excision is the definitive treatment.

ANORECTAL ABCESSES

EPIDEMIOLOGY

- Abscesses originate from infected anal crypts and spread to the perianal and deep rectal spaces.
- Perianal abscess is the most common type and is located close to the anal verge.
- Anorectal abscesses are most common among middle-aged men.

PATHOPHYSIOLOGY

- The mechanism involves the obstruction of an anal gland, resulting in a polymicrobial abscess formation.
- Infection can progress to any potential spaces that are normally filled with fatty areolar tissue.
- Other diseases that are associated with rectal abscess should be investigated, including Crohn's disease, ulcerative colitis, carcinomas, TB, venereal disease, and trauma.

CLINICAL FEATURES

- Persistent dull, aching, throbbing pain that increases prior to defecation is typical.
- As the abscess progresses, pain may interfere with walking or sitting.
- Fever, leukocytosis, and a painful tender mass on digital rectal examination may be observed.

DIAGNOSIS AND DIFFERENTIAL

- Deep space abscesses can be difficult to detect on physical examination alone.
- Endorectal ultrasonography, CT, MRI, or needle localization may be needed to confirm the diagnosis of deep space abscess.

EMERGENCY DEPARTMENT CARE AND DISPOSITION

- Simple perianal abscess without systemic illness is the only abscess that should be drained in the ED. Other deep space abscess should be drained in the operating room.
- After adequate local anesthesia, a cruciate incision is made over the abscess and the "dog ears" are excised. Packing is usually not necessary.
- Antibiotics usually are not necessary unless systemic infection or toxicity is present.
- The patient should have follow-up care in 24 hours, and surgical referral.

PROCTITIS

EPIDEMIOLOGY/PATHOPHYSIOLOGY

- Proctitis is inflammation of the rectal mucosa.
- Common causes include prior radiation treatments, autoimmune disorders, vasculitis, ischemia, and infections.
- STDs of the anorectum can be seen in individuals who engage in anal sex.

CLINICAL FEATURES

- Symptoms include anorectal pain, itching, discharge, diarrhea, bleeding, and lower abdominal cramping.
- Mucosal inflammation, erythema, ulcers, or discharge may be noted using anoscopy.

DIAGNOSIS AND DIFFERENTIAL

- Condylomata acuminata, gonorrhea, syphilis, herpes, and AIDS-related infections should be investigated in patients presenting with proctitis.

EMERGENCY DEPARTMENT CARE AND DISPOSITION

- Obtain cultures if infectious etiology is suspected.
- Sitz bath, stool softeners, good anal hygiene, and analgesics will provide some relief.
- Empiric therapy aimed at eradicating infection should be started while cultures are pending.
- Referral for appropriate follow-up and further evaluation should be recommended.

RECTAL PROLAPSE

EPIDEMIOLOGY

- Prolapse of the rectal mucosa only is most commonly seen in children under the age of 2 years. Mucosal prolapse can also occur in adults with third- and fourth-degree hemorrhoids.

- Complete rectal prolapse occurs with extremes of age, most commonly in elderly women.

PATHOPHYSIOLOGY

- There are three classes of rectal prolapse based on anatomic differences: (1) prolapse of rectal mucosa only; (2) prolapse of all three layers of mucosa; (3) intussusception of the upper rectum through the lower rectum.
- Occurs due to both laxity in the pelvic floor and weakening of the sphincter muscles.

CLINICAL FEATURES

- Most patients detect as mass, accompanied by bloody mucous discharge, and/or fecal incontinence.
- Mucosal prolapse will only extrude few centimeters from the dentate line.
- Complete rectal prolapse can extend up to 15 cm outside the anus, and appears as a red, ball-like mass.

EMERGENCY DEPARTMENT CARE AND DISPOSITION

- Manual reduction with gentle steady pressure should be attempted to prevent edema, strangulation, or ischemia.
- Analgesia, sedation, and application of generous amounts of granulated sugar to the prolapsed segment may aid in reduction if tissue is edematous.
- Surgical correction is often required; however, the patient can be discharged from the ED with stool softeners to prevent constipation.

ANORECTAL TUMORS

EPIDEMIOLOGY

- Factors such as smoking, anal intercourse, HIV, and genital warts have been associated with anorectal cancers.
- Anal canal neoplasms are more common, and have a poorer prognosis.

PATHOPHYSIOLOGY

- Classification depends on location in respect to dentate line. Anal canal neoplasms are proximal to the dentate line; whereas anal margin neoplasms are distal to the dentate line.
- Anal canal neoplasms include adenocarcinoma, melanoma, and Kaposi's sarcoma.

CLINICAL FEATURES

- Patients present with nonspecific symptoms including sensation of a mass, pruritus, and bloody stools. As the neoplasm progresses, anorexia, bloating, weight loss, diarrhea, constipation, and narrowing of the stool caliber develop.

DIAGNOSIS AND DIFFERENTIAL

- All anorectal tumors can be detected by careful visual examination, anoscopy, or sigmoidoscopy.
- Tumors may be misdiagnosed as hemorrhoids.
- Complications of anorectal tumors include rectal prolapse, prolonged blood loss, abscess, or fistula formation.

EMERGENCY DEPARTMENT CARE AND DISPOSITION

- Referral for proctoscopic or sigmoidoscopic examination with biopsy is mandatory.

RECTAL FOREIGN BODIES

EPIDEMIOLOGY

- Not all patients may be forthcoming with accurate history of rectal foreign-body insertion.

PATHOPHYSIOLOGY

- Most foreign bodies are in the rectal ampulla.
- Peritoneal reflection determines where presence of free air on radiography will be found. Below the peritoneal reflection causes air along the psoas muscles, whereas above the peritoneal reflection causes air under the diaphragm.

CLINICAL FEATURES

- Patient may complain of pain, cramping, bleeding, or discharge.
- Perforation of the rectum may cause fever, leukocytosis, peritoneal signs, and bleeding.

DIAGNOSIS AND DIFFERENTIAL

- Radiographs must be obtained to determine the position, shape, and number of foreign bodies and perforation.

EMERGENCY DEPARTMENT CARE AND DISPOSITION

- Most of the foreign bodies in the distal rectum can be removed in the ED with adequate sedation.
- Objects that are made of glass, have sharp edges, or cannot be easily removed may require surgery or gastroenterology consultation.
- Broad-spectrum antibiotics (**piperacillin/tazobactam** 3.375 grams every 6 hours) should be administered if perforation is suspected.

PRURITUS ANI

EPIDEMIOLOGY

- Common causes include diet, infectious agents, and irritants.
- This disorder is most common in males during the fifth and sixth decades of life.
- Pinworms (*Enterobius vermicularis*) are the most common cause in children.

CLINICAL FEATURES

- Rectal itching, with a reddened, excoriated, and moist perianal area.

DIAGNOSIS AND DIFFERNTIAL

- Atopic dermatitis, lichen planus, psoriasis, and anal margin neoplasms need to be considered in the differential diagnosis of puritus ani.

EMERGENCY DEPARTMENT CARE AND DISPOSITION

- Increased fiber, sitz bath, anti-histamines, zinc oxide, and 1% hydrocortisone creams can be used for acute symptoms and enhance healing.
- Consider referral to proctologist or dermatologist for refractory cases.

PILONIDAL SINUS

EPIDEMIOLOGY

- Most commonly affects males before the fourth decade of life.

PATHOPHYSIOLOGY

- Pilonidal sinus is an acquired problem, formed by a recurring foreign-body granulomatous reaction to an ingrown hair.

CLINICAL FEATURES

- A pilonidal cyst can present as a painless, cyst, an acute infected abscess, or chronic drainage in the midline part of the natal cleft, which overlies the lower sacrum and coccyx.
- Ultrasound may be helpful in determining the extent of the abscess.

DIAGNOSIS AND DIFFERENTIAL

- Pilonidal disease is often mistakenly diagnosed as perirectal abscesses.

EMERGENCY DEPARTMENT CARE AND DISPOSITION

- Acute abscesses should be incised, drained, and packed in the ED.
- Antibiotics are not usually necessary unless the patient is immune compromised or surrounding cellulitis is present.
- Surgical referral is necessary to prevent recurrence.

For further reading in Tintinalli's *Emergency Medicine: A Comprehensive Study Guide,* 7th ed., see Chapter 88, "Anorectal Disorders," by Brian E. Burgess.

50 HEPATIC DISORDERS, JAUNDICE, AND HEPATIC FAILURE

Joshua A. Gentges

JAUNDICE

PATHOPHYSIOLOGY

- Jaundice, a yellowish discoloration of the skin, sclerae, and mucous membranes, is a symptom that results from hyperbilirubinemia (breakdown of hemoglobin) and thus the deposition of bile pigments.
- Hyperbilirubinemia can be divided into two types. The unconjugated form results from increased bilirubin production (eg, hemolysis) or a liver defect in its uptake or conjugation. The conjugated form occurs in the setting of intra- or extrahepatic cholestasis, resulting in decreased excretion of conjugated bilirubin via the intestinal tract.

- The total serum bilirubin should be elevated in a jaundiced patient. The clinical assessment of jaundice can be unreliable, with only 70% sensitivity and specificity.

CLINICAL FEATURES

- Sudden onset of jaundice in a previously healthy young person, together with a prodrome of fever, malaise, myalgias, and a tender enlarged liver, points to hepatitis (probably viral) as a likely cause.
- Heavy ethanol use suggests alcoholic hepatitis. In the setting of alcoholic liver disease and cirrhosis, jaundice usually develops gradually (discussed later).
- A family history of jaundice or a history of recurrent mild jaundice that spontaneously resolves usually accompanies inherited causes of jaundice such as Gilbert's syndrome.
- Cholecystitis in itself may not cause jaundice unless there is acute biliary obstruction present such as with a retained common bile duct gallstone.
- Painless jaundice in an older patient classically suggests pancreatic or hepatobiliary malignancy.
- Patients with a known prior malignancy and a hard, nodular liver accompanied by jaundice may be found to have liver metastases.
- Biliary tract scarring or strictures must always be suspected as a cause of jaundice in patients with a prior history of biliary tract surgery, pancreatitis, cholangitis, or inflammatory bowel disease.
- Hepatomegaly with jaundice, accompanied by pedal edema, jugular venous distention, and a gallop rhythm, suggests chronic heart failure.

DIAGNOSIS AND DIFFERENTIAL

- Initial laboratory tests that should be obtained in the work-up of a jaundiced patient include total and direct serum bilirubin level, serum aminotransferases and alkaline phosphatase (AP) levels, urinalysis to check for bilirubin and urobilinogen, and a complete blood count (CBC).
- Additional laboratory tests may be indicated based on the clinical setting (serum amylase and lipase levels, prothrombin time [PT], electrolytes and glucose levels, blood urea nitrogen [BUN] and creatinine levels, viral hepatitis panels, drug levels, and pregnancy test).
- PT is the most sensitive measure of hepatic synthetic function and, if elevated, suggests significant hepatocellular dysfunction or necrosis.
- With normal liver enzyme levels, the jaundice is more likely to be caused by sepsis or systemic infection, inborn errors of metabolism, or pregnancy, rather than by primary hepatic disease.
- With abnormally elevated liver enzymes, the pattern of abnormalities may suggest the etiology. Aminotransferase elevation, if predominant, suggests hepatocellular diseases such as viral or toxic hepatitis or cirrhosis, whereas markedly elevated AP levels (two to three times normal) and GGT (γ-glutamyl transferase) point to intra- or extrahepatic obstruction (gallstones, stricture, or malignancy).
- A Coombs' test and hemoglobin electrophoresis may be useful if anemia is present, along with normal liver aminotransferase levels (to look for hemolysis and hemoglobinopathy).
- If clinical features and initial laboratory results reveal conjugated hyperbilirubinemia, ultrasound studies of the biliary tract, liver, and pancreas should be performed to rule out gallstones, dilated extrahepatic biliary ducts, or mass/tumor in the liver, pancreas, and portal region.
- A computed tomography (CT) scan may also be considered, but is more costly and is not as sensitive as ultrasound for detection of gallstones in the gallbladder.

EMERGENCY DEPARTMENT CARE AND DISPOSITION

- Hemodynamically stable patients with new-onset jaundice may be appropriate for discharge and outpatient follow-up if there is no evidence of liver failure or acute biliary obstruction, if appropriate laboratory studies have been ordered, if the patient has timely follow-up readily available, and is reliable and has adequate social support.
- If extrahepatic biliary obstruction is suspected, surgical consultation should be obtained in the emergency department (ED).

HEPATITIS

EPIDEMIOLOGY

- In the USA, 33% of the population has acquired immunity to hepatitis A (HAV). New hepatitis B (HBV) and hepatitis C (HCV) infections total approximately 50,000 and 20,000, respectively.
- The incidence of HAV and HBV has fallen dramatically due to effective vaccination programs.
- Acetaminophen is the most common cause of acute liver failure in the USA.

PATHOPHYSIOLOGY

- Hepatitis is liver inflammation from toxic, metabolic, or infectious insult. It follows a spectrum from asymptomatic infection to fulminant liver disease and chronic cirrhosis.

- Hepatocellular death leads to disruption of liver metabolic and synthetic function, leading to toxin accumulation, coagulopathy, and nutritional deficiencies. Ongoing disease can cause scarring and disruption of liver anatomy. This leads to ascites, esophageal varices, and portal hypertension.

CLINICAL FEATURES

- There is a continuum of disease from acute hepatitis to chronic hepatitis, cirrhosis, and liver failure (Table 50-1).
- Consider acute hepatitis in patients with right upper quadrant or epigastric abdominal pain, nausea, vomiting, diarrhea, jaundice, or pruritis. Patients may report anorexia, fatigue, or malaise.
- A few days of generalized pruritus, clay-colored stools, and dark urine may precede the onset of gastrointestinal (GI) symptoms and jaundice. Malaise usually persists while the other prodromal symptoms resolve.
- Rarely, fulminant hepatic failure develops with a clinical picture of encephalopathy, coagulopathy, and rapidly worsening jaundice.
- HAV is transmitted predominantly by the fecal-oral route and is commonly seen in Americans. Children and

TABLE 50-1 Clinical Features of Hepatitis

DIAGNOSIS	ACUTE HEPATITIS (HEPATITIS A VIRUS, HBV, HCV, TOXIC)	CHRONIC HEPATITIS/ CIRRHOSIS (HBV, HCV, ALCOHOL LIVER DISEASE)	LIVER FAILURE (END-STAGE HBV/HCV, TOXIC)
Symptoms			
Nausea/vomiting	+	+	+
Fever	+	−	−
Pain	+	+	±
Altered mental status	−	+	+
Bruising/bleeding	−	+	+
Physical examination			
Jaundice	+	+	+
Hepatomegaly	+	−	±
Ascites	−	+	+
Edema	−	+	+
Spider nevus	−	+	±
Lab abnormalities			
Elevated ALT/AST	+	+	±
AST/ALT >2	+	±	±
Elevated prothrombin time/ international normalized ratio	−	±	+
Elevated ammonia	−	±	+
Low albumin	−	+	+
Direct bilirubinemia	−	+	±
Indirect bilirubinemia	+	+	±
Urobilinogen	+	+	+
Elevated blood urea nitrogen/ creatinine	−	−	±
Radiologic findings			
Ascites	−	±	+
Fatty liver	+	−	−
Cirrhosis	−	+	+

Abbreviations: ALT = alanine aminotransferase; AST = aspartate aminotransferase; HBV = hepatitis B virus; HCV = hepatitis C virus; + = typically present; − = typically absent; ± = variable.

adolescents are more commonly affected, but often subclinically, whereas most adults are symptomatic with a longer, more severe course. Symptom onset is often more abrupt than with other viruses. Epidemic outbreaks have been seen in children at day care centers, institutionalized patients, and in patients exposed to a common source case via contaminated food or water.

- HBV is acquired primarily via a percutaneous exposure to infected blood or body fluids. Most cases are subclinical without jaundice. Often symptom onset is insidious and, in 5% to 10% of cases, is preceded by a serum sickness–like syndrome with polyarthritis, proteinuria, and angioneurotic edema. Symptomatic patients usually have a more severe and protracted course than those with HAV.
- HCV is the most common of all blood-borne infections in the United States, and may be contracted via parenteral, sexual, and perinatal contact. Most patients remain asymptomatic or have milder symptoms than those with HBV or HAV.
- Between 6% and 10% of HBV and over 50% of HCV patients progress to chronic liver disease and cirrhosis, and these patients are at increased risk of hepatocellular carcinoma.
- Patients with alcoholic liver disease can present with acute hepatitis. Common findings are tender hepatomegaly, jaundice, nausea, fever, anorexia, and generalized weakness. Alcoholic liver disease follows a continuum from asymptomatic fatty liver, to hepatitis, to cirrhosis, and to end-stage liver disease.
- Many medications cause liver disease, including hepatocellular necrosis (acetaminophen, phenytoin), cholestasis (oral contraceptives, anabolic steroids), steatohepatitis (valproic acid, amiodarone), and chronic disease (nitrofurantoin, minocycline).
- Acetaminophen accounts for over 40% of the liver failure cases in the United States and is the most common fatal toxic ingestion. Toxic mushrooms are an uncommon but important cause of hepatitis and acute liver failure. See Chapters 108 and 130.

DIAGNOSIS AND DIFFERENTIAL

- Initial laboratory tests for suspected liver disease include a serum bilirubin level (total and direct fractions; indirect fraction can be deduced by simple subtraction), aspartate aminotransferase, alanine aminotransferase, and γ-glutamyl transpeptidase (AST/ALT/GGT), AP levels, and a CBC.
- AST/ALT values in the hundreds of units per liter are consistent with mild viral inflammation, but elevations into the thousands suggest extensive acute hepatocellular necrosis and more fulminant disease.
- In acute and chronic viral hepatitis, the ratio of AST to ALT is usually <1. A ratio >2 is more suggestive of alcoholic hepatitis.
- Mild to moderate elevations of AP are seen in virtually all hepatobiliary disease. Suspect cholestasis if levels are elevated greater than four times normal. A concurrently elevated GGT supports this.
- Isolated significant elevation of AP without marked hyperbilirubinemia (AP:bilirubin ratio of 1000:1) suggests an infiltrative or granulomatous disease such as lymphoma, tuberculosis, sarcoidosis, or fungal infection.
- Total serum bilirubin along with its direct fraction may also be useful since a conjugated (direct) fraction of 30% or higher is consistent with viral hepatitis.
- A persistent total bilirubin level >20 mg/dL or a PT prolonged by more than a few seconds indicates significant disruption of liver function.
- Serum electrolytes, BUN, and creatinine should be checked if there is clinical suspicion of volume depletion or electrolyte abnormalities.
- Abnormal mental status should prompt an immediate determination of serum glucose level, which may be low due to poor oral intake or hepatic failure. Other causes of abnormal mental status such as hypoxia, sepsis, intoxication, structural intracranial process, or encephalopathy must also be considered.
- A CBC may be useful, as an early transient neutropenia followed by a relative lymphocytosis with atypical forms is often seen with viral hepatitis. Anemia, if present, may be more suggestive of alcoholic hepatitis, decompensated cirrhosis, GI bleeding, or a hemolytic process.
- Viral hepatitis panels are useful for definitive diagnosis but generally not immediately available in the ED.
- Important differential diagnoses include alcohol- or toxin-induced hepatitis, infectious mononucleosis, cholecystitis, ascending cholangitis, sarcoidosis, lymphoma, liver metastases, and pancreatic or biliary tumors.

EMERGENCY DEPARTMENT CARE AND DISPOSITION

- Most patients can be successfully managed as outpatients with emphasis on rest, adequate oral intake, strict personal hygiene, and avoidance of hepatotoxins (ethanol and drugs). Close follow-up arrangements should be made.
- Admission is warranted in high-risk populations, including the elderly or pregnant patient, or patients with serum bilirubin greater than 20 milligrams/dL, elevated PT, hypoglycemia, hypoalbuminemia,

encephalopathy, GI bleeding, or suspected toxic ingestion, especially acetaminophen.

- Patients with mild alcohol-induced hepatitis may be managed as outpatients with emphasis on nutritional supplementation, including thiamine, folate, magnesium, and potassium supplements; adequate oral intake; and strict avoidance of alcohol and other hepatotoxins. Patients should be instructed to return for worsening symptoms, in particular vomiting, fever, jaundice, or abdominal pain. Follow-up arrangements should be made.
- Patients who require admission for alcoholic hepatitis should receive thiamine 100 milligrams PO or IV and also be given prophylactic treatment for alcohol withdrawal.
- Volume depletion and electrolyte imbalances should be corrected with intravenous crystalloid. Hypoglycemia should be initially treated with 1 amp of 50% dextrose in water intravenously followed by the addition of dextrose to intravenous fluids and careful monitoring.
- Fulminant hepatic failure should warrant admission to the intensive care unit, with aggressive support of circulation and respiration, monitoring and treatment of increased intracranial pressure if present, correction of hypoglycemia and coagulopathy, and administration of **lactulose** (20 grams PO or 300 mL of **lactulose solution** diluted with 700 mL of water or saline rectally as a 30-minute retention enema) for hepatic encephalopathy. Patients requiring ventilatory support with hepatic failure generally require intubation, as they are obtunded and not candidates for bilevel positive pressure ventilation. Consultations with a hepatologist and liver transplant service are indicated.

CIRRHOSIS AND CHRONIC HEPATITIS

PATHOPHYSIOLOGY

- Longstanding hepatocellular injury leads eventually to the widespread fibrosis and isolation of functional hepatocytes into parenchymal nodules of chronic liver failure.
- The metabolic and mechanical functions of the liver are compromised, leading to metabolic derangement and the manifestations of portal hypertension, including ascites, esophageal varices, and portal-systemic shunting.

CLINICAL FEATURES

- Patients with cirrhosis may present with abdominal pain and distention, nausea and vomiting, peripheral edema, upper or lower GI bleeding, or jaundice. They may complain of altered mental status, weakness, and malaise.
- Hepatomegaly is usually absent. Jaundice, pedal edema, ascites, palmar erythema, caput medusa, gynecomastia, splenomegaly, and spider angiomata are also common.
- Hepatic encephalopathy, characterized by a progression from altered mental status to hyperreflexia, spasticity, seizures, and coma, may also be present. Asterixis ("liver flap") is characteristic, but not specific for encephalopathy due to liver failure.
- Spontaneous bacterial peritonitis, comorbid infections such as pneumonia or urinary tract infection, and renal dysfunction are all serious findings that complicate the management of these patients. Acute gastroesophageal bleeding from varices is a catastrophic complication of chronic liver disease discussed in Chap. 41.

DIAGNOSIS AND DIFFERENTIAL

- Laboratory studies for cirrhosis include levels of serum transaminases (GGT, ALT, AST), serum AP, total bilirubin (and its fractions), serum albumin, serum glucose and electrolytes, BUN, creatinine, CBC, and PT. Obtain a serum ammonia if there is suspicion for hepatic encephalopathy.
- Serum transaminases and bilirubin may be mildly elevated or normal in cirrhosis.
- Elevated ammonia level suggests but does not diagnose hepatic encephalopathy, which is a diagnosis of exclusion. A thorough search for other causes of altered mental status (sepsis, meningitis, cerebral hemorrhage, metabolic and toxic derangement) is necessary.
- Spontaneous bacterial peritonitis (SBP) has a yearly incidence of 30% in ascitic patients. SBP should be suspected in any cirrhotic patient with fever, abdominal pain or tenderness, worsening or new ascites, subacute functional decline, or encephalopathy.
- SBP may be confirmed through sampling of ascitic fluid by paracentesis, ideally under ultrasound guidance. Ascitic fluid should be tested for total protein and glucose levels, lactic (acid) dehydrogenase (LDH), Gram's stain, and white blood cell (WBC) count with differential. A total WBC count >1000 per cubic millimeter or neutrophil (PMN) count >250 per cubic millimeter is diagnostic for SBP. Low glucose or high protein values suggest infection.
- Gram's stain and culture results from ascitic fluid are often negative (30-40%), but placing 10 mL of ascitic fluid in a blood culture bottle may improve yield. Gram-negative Enterobacteriaceae (*Escherichia coli*, *Klebsiella*, etc.) account for 63% of SBP, followed

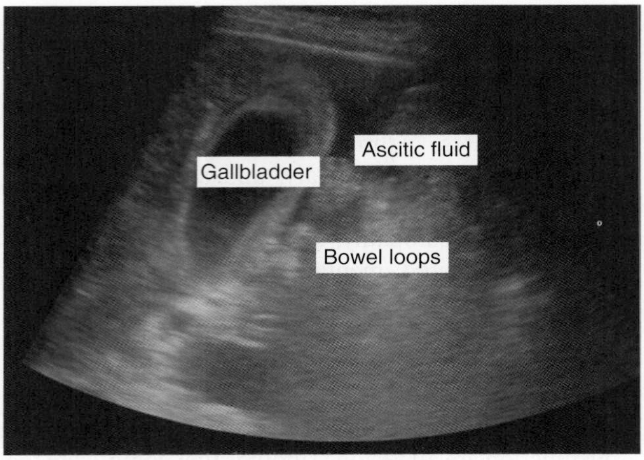

FIG. 50-1. Sonographic image of ascitic fluid showing bowel loops and an edematous gallbladder wall, a common finding in patients with ascites. (Courtesy of and used with permission of MedStar Health and Michael S. Antonis, DO, RDMS, Sonologist.)

by the pneumococcus (15%) and the enterococcus (6-10%). Empirical therapy with antimicrobial agents to cover typical enteric flora should be instituted as soon as SBP is suspected from ascitic fluid analysis.

- Ultrasonography can identify ascites, infectious or mass lesions, cholecystitis, and hepatic and portal vein thrombosis (Fig. 50-1).
- Abdominal CT may help elucidate structural problems. Consider head CT in patients with mental status changes.
- Hepatorenal syndrome is a form of acute renal failure that occurs in cirrhotic patients. It has a poor prognosis and the cause is unknown.
- Gastroesophageal varices form as a result of intrahepatic fibrosis and scarring, leading to portal vein resistance and hypertension, with resulting collateral flow through veins at the gastroesophageal junction. Bleeding may take the form of frank hematemesis, "coffee ground" emesis, with melena, or with massive hemorrhage, hematochezia. Symptoms may be more insidious with light-headedness, generalized weakness, fatigue, or increased confusion being the presenting features.
- Cirrhosis is often caused by ethanol or chronic viral hepatitis; uncommon causes include drugs or toxins, hemochromatosis, Wilson's disease, and primary (idiopathic) biliary cirrhosis.

EMERGENCY DEPARTMENT CARE AND DISPOSITION

- Patients with chronic liver disease can sometimes be managed on an outpatient basis with management and medication changes by the patient's gastroenterologist or primary physician. Abstinence from alcohol and other hepatotoxins is essential for outpatient management.
- Recommended diuretics for management of ascites include **spironolactone**, 50 to 200 milligrams daily, and **amiloride**, 5 to 10 milligrams daily. A protein-restricted diet helps prevent the complication of hepatic encephalopathy.
- Patients with abdominal pain, fever, acidosis, leukocytosis, significant hypo- or hypervolemia, new onset or worsening encephalopathy, coagulopathy with bleeding, or significant electrolyte abnormalities should be admitted to the hospital. Hepatorenal syndrome warrants nephrology consultation.
- Paracentesis is warranted for symptomatic relief of ascites or to diagnose SBP. Paracentesis can be performed in the ED, ideally under ultrasound guidance. Administer **albumin**, 1.5 grams/kg IV before paracentesis. Removal of more than 1 L of ascitic fluid can lead to hypotension, so careful monitoring is required. If performing diagnostic paracentesis, obtain at least 50 mL of ascitic fluid for cell count, Gram's stain, and culture.
- Treatment of SBP involves empiric antibiotic coverage. **Cefotaxime** 2 grams IV every 8 hours (4 grams every 8 hours if life threatening) or **piperacillin-tazobactam** 3.375 grams IV every 6 hours or **ampicillin-sulbactam** 3 grams IV every 6 hours or **ticarcillin-clavulanate** 3.1 grams IV every 6 hours or **ceftriaxone** 2 grams IV every 24 hours are acceptable empiric antimicrobial choices. Give **albumin** 1.5 grams/kg IV if it was not given at the time of paracentesis, as it may reduce the incidence of renal failure and hospital mortality in these patients.
- The mainstay of therapy for hepatic encephalopathy is **lactulose**, 20 grams PO or 300 mL of the syrup diluted with 700 mL of water or normal saline as a 30-minute retention enema. **Flumazenil**, 1 to 4 milligrams IV can cause short-term improvement in symptoms but has no proven long-term effect. Patients should be placed on a protein-restricted diet.
- Suspect gastroesophageal variceal bleeding in any chronic liver patient with hematemesis, melena, or hematochezia. Variceal bleeding is discussed in Chapter 41.
- Elevated PT with signs of bleeding should be treated with **vitamin K**, 10 milligrams PO or IV. Massive or life-threatening bleeding may require fresh frozen plasma transfusion. Decreased or malfunctioning platelets should be repleted with pooled donor platelets.
- Aggressive treatment of comorbidities, including alcohol-related syndromes (withdrawal, ketoacidosis,

Wernicke–Korsakoff syndrome), sepsis, ventilatory and circulatory dysfunction, electrolyte abnormalities, and hypoglycemia, is very important to satisfactory patient outcomes.

- Acute liver failure from any cause (with prolonged PT, hypoglycemia, coagulopathy, encephalopathy, marked jaundice, etc.) should warrant admission to the intensive care unit, aggressive treatment, and consultation with a hepatologist and transplant team, if available.

For further reading in Tintinalli's *Emergency Medicine: A Comprehensive Study Guide,* 7th ed., see Chapter 83, "Hepatic Disorders, Jaundice, and Hepatic Failure," by Susan R. O'Mara and Kulleni Gebreyes.

51 COMPLICATIONS OF GENERAL SURGICAL PROCEDURES

Daniel J. Egan

- Common postoperative disorders seen in the ED include fever, respiratory complications, genitourinary complaints, wound infections, vascular problems, and complications of drug therapy. Specific problems not discussed elsewhere in this book are mentioned here.

CLINICAL FEATURES

FEVER

- The causes of postoperative fever are listed as the five Ws: **W**ind (respiratory), **W**ater (urinary tract infection [UTI]), **W**ound, **W**alking (deep venous thrombosis [DVT]), and **W**onder drugs (pseudomembranous colitis [PMC]).
- Fever in the first 24 hours is usually due to atelectasis, necrotizing fasciitis, or clostridial infections.
- In the first 72 hours, pneumonia, atelectasis, intravenous-catheter-related thrombophlebitis, and infections are the major causes of complications.
- UTIs are seen 3 to 5 days postoperatively.
- DVT does not typically occur until 5 days after a procedure, and wound infections generally appear 7 to 10 days after surgery (see Chapter 27).
- Antibiotic-induced diarrhea (PMC) is seen 6 weeks after surgery.

RESPIRATORY COMPLICATIONS

- Atelectasis develops from postoperative pain, splinting, and inadequate clearance of secretions. Fever, tachypnea, tachycardia, and mild hypoxia may be seen. Pneumonia may develop 24 to 96 hours later (see Chapter 32).
- The diagnosis of pulmonary embolism should be entertained at any point postoperatively. Findings include hypoxia, tachycardia, chest pain, and shortness of breath (see Chapter 27).

GENITOURINARY COMPLICATIONS

- UTIs are more common after instrumentation of the urinary tract.
- Certain patients are at risk of urinary retention following surgical procedures (see Chapter 56).
- Decreased urine output should raise concerns for renal failure resulting from many causes (see Chapter 52).

WOUND COMPLICATIONS

- Hematomas result from inadequate hemostasis and lead to pain and swelling at the surgical site. Careful evaluation and sometimes exploration to rule out infections must be undertaken.
- Seromas are collections of clear fluid under the wound.
- Wound infections present with pain, swelling, erythema, drainage, and tenderness. Extremes of age, diabetes, poor nutrition, necrotic tissue, poor perfusion, foreign bodies, and wound hematomas contribute to the development of wound infections.
- Necrotizing fasciitis should be considered in a patient with a rapidly expanding infection and signs of systemic toxicity (see Chapter 92).
- Wound (superficial or deep fascial) dehiscence can occur due to diabetes, poor nutrition, chronic steroid use, and inadequate or improper closure of the wound.

VASCULAR COMPLICATIONS

- Superficial thrombophlebitis, usually in the upper extremities after intravenous catheter insertion, manifests with erythema, warmth, and fullness of the affected vein.
- DVT commonly occurs in the lower extremities with swelling, pain, and sometimes erythema of the affected limb (see Chapter 27).

DRUG THERAPY COMPLICATIONS

- Many drugs are known to cause fever without any concomitant infection.

- PMC, a dreaded complication, is caused by *Clostridium difficile* toxin. Watery and potentially bloody diarrhea with abdominal cramping are typical features.

DIAGNOSIS AND DIFFERENTIAL

- Patients with a postoperative fever should have an evaluation focusing on the elements above.
- Patient with suspected respiratory complications should have chest radiographs, which may reveal atelectasis, pneumonia, or pneumothorax. Advanced imaging with CT may be required for the evaluation of infection, effusions, or pulmonary embolism.
- Patients with oliguria or anuria should be evaluated for signs of hypovolemia or urinary retention and have laboratory testing of renal function.
- Diagnosis of PMC is established by demonstrating *C. difficile* cytotoxin in the stool. However, the assay is negative in up to 27% of cases.

EMERGENCY DEPARTMENT CARE AND DISPOSITION

- Always discuss patients and proposed treatments with the surgeon who performed the relevant procedure.
- Many patients with atelectasis may be managed as outpatients with pain control and deep breathing exercises or incentive spirometry.
- Postoperative pneumonia may be polymicrobial, and inpatient therapy with antipseudomonal and antistaphylococcal agents is often recommended (see Chapter 32).
- Nontoxic patients with UTI can be managed as outpatients with oral antibiotic therapy. Gram-positive coverage should be considered if instrumentation occurred.
- Wound hematomas may require removal of some sutures and evacuation in consultation with the surgeon. Admission is often unnecessary.
- Seromas can be confirmed and treated with needle aspiration and wound cultures. Admission may not always be necessary.
- Most wound infections can be treated with oral antibiotics unless there is systemic toxicity or significant comorbidities. Perineal infections usually require admission and parenteral antibiotics due to their polymicrobial nature.
- Emergent surgical debridement and parenteral antibiotics are indicated for necrotizing fasciitis. The emergency physicians should initiate broad-spectrum therapy rapidly.
- Most patients with superficial thrombophlebitis can be treated with local heat, NSAIDs, and elevation of the affected area if there is no evidence of cellulitis or lymphangitis. Suppurative thrombophlebitis requires excision of the affected vein.
- Oral **vancomycin** and **metronidazole**, PO or IV, are currently available treatment modalities for drug-induced PMC.

SPECIFIC CONSIDERATIONS

COMPLICATIONS OF BREAST SURGERY

- Wound infections, hematomas, pneumothorax, necrosis of the skin flaps, and lymphedema of the arms after mastectomy are common problems seen after breast surgery.

COMPLICATIONS OF GASTROINTESTINAL SURGERY

- Stimulation of the splanchnic nerves may cause dysmotility and paralytic ileus, which usually resolves within 3 days.
- Prolonged ileus should prompt investigation for non-neuronal causes. Clinical features include nausea, vomiting, obstipation, constipation, abdominal distension, and pain.
- Abdominal radiographs, complete blood count, electrolytes, blood urea nitrogen and creatinine levels, and urinalysis should be obtained.
- Treatment of adynamic ileus consists of nasogastric suction, bowel rest, and hydration.
- Mechanical obstruction is usually due to adhesions and may require surgical intervention if conservative management with nasogastric suction is ineffective.
- Intra-abdominal abscesses are caused by preoperative contamination or postoperative anastomotic leaks. Diagnosis can be confirmed by computed tomography (CT) scan or ultrasonography. Percutaneous drainage or surgical exploration, evacuation, and parenteral antibiotics will be required.
- Pancreatitis may occur after direct manipulation of the pancreatic duct. Patients typically have nausea, vomiting, abdominal pain, and leukocytosis. Serum amylase and lipase levels are usually elevated (although amylase is nonspecific).
- Cholecystitis and biliary colic may occur postoperative. Elderly patients are more prone to develop acalculous cholecystitis.
- Fistulas, either internal or external, may result from technical complications or direct bowel injury and require surgical consultation.
- Anastomotic leaks may occur after esophageal, gastric, or colonic surgery. Esophageal leaks cause significant morbidity and mortality.

- Bariatric surgery procedures are at risk for leak and bleeding. Dumping syndrome can be seen after gastric bypass. Patients are also at risk for mechanical obstruction, ulcers, reflux, and vitamin deficiencies.
- Complications of percutaneous endoscopic gastrostomy (PEG) tubes include infections, hemorrhage, peritonitis, aspiration, wound dehiscence, sepsis, and obstruction of the tube. Tubes may also be dislodged requiring replacement either permanently or temporarily with a Foley catheter.
- Complications arising from stomas are due to technical errors or from underlying disease such as Crohn's disease and cancer. Ischemia, necrosis, bleeding, hernia, and prolapse are sometimes seen.
- The most common colonoscopy complications are hemorrhage (after biopsy procedures) and perforation. Symptoms may be delayed by several hours. Abdominal and upright chest radiographs are necessary to evaluate for free air; however, their limited sensitivity warrants CT imaging if highly suspicious.
- Rectal surgery complications include urinary retention, constipation, prolapse, bleeding, and infections.

For further reading in Tintinalli's *Emergency Medicine: A Comprehensive Study Guide,* 7th ed., see Chapter 90, "Complications of General Surgical Procedures," by Edmond A. Hooker.

Section 8
RENAL AND GENITOURINARY DISORDERS

52 ACUTE RENAL FAILURE

Marc D. Squillante

EPIDEMIOLOGY

- Distinction between community- and hospital-acquired acute renal failure (ARF) is important for differential diagnosis, treatment, and outcome.
- Prerenal ARF is the most common community-acquired cause, accounting for 70% of patients. Majority of cases are due to volume depletion. Up to 90% of patients presenting to an ED have a potentially reversible cause.
- Intrinsic renal causes, particularly acute tubular necrosis (ATN), are the most common etiology for hospital-acquired ARF, accounting for 70% of patients. Common in ICU and multi-organ failure patients.
- Postrenal causes account for 10% of patient in both community- and hospital-acquired ARF.
- Mortality rates depend on severity and cause of renal failure. Most adult ARF deaths are due to sepsis and cardiopulmonary failure. Hospital-acquired ARF has a higher mortality.
- The RIFLE classification has established three grades of renal compromise of increasing severity (Risk, Injury, and Failure), and two outcome measures (Loss, and End-stage renal disease), which correlate with prognosis. Grading renal risk, injury, failure can be accomplished using either serum creatinine/glomerular filtration rate (GFR) criteria, or by urine output criteria over 6 to 24 hours.
- Use of the serum creatinine change from baseline is the most useful for the emergency physician seeing the patient during a small window of time in the ED: renal risk = serum creatinine increased 1.5 times baseline; renal injury = serum creatinine increased 2 times baseline; renal failure = serum creatinine increased 3 times baseline *or* creatinine greater than 4.0 milligrams/dL and acute increase over 0.5 milligram/dL.
- Mortality from ARF has been stable for decades, in spite of use of dialysis.
- Pediatric ARF has a different set of etiologies, and mortality averages 25%.

PATHOPHYSIOLOGY

- Decreases in renal blood flow (RBF) are the final common pathway for most causes of ARF.
- Tubular and glomerular functions are maintained in prerenal failure, but GFR is depressed by compromised renal perfusion.
- Prerenal failure is produced by conditions that decrease renal perfusion (Table 52-1), and is the most common cause of community-acquired ARF (70% of cases). It is a common precursor to ischemic and nephrotoxic causes of intrinsic renal failure as well.
- Ischemic ARF (traditionally known as ATN, but now called *acute kidney injury [AKI]*), is the most common cause of intrinsic renal failure. The renal parenchyma suffers ischemic injury due to significant decreases in renal perfusion. This is the most common cause of hospital-acquired ARF.
- Intrinsic renal failure occurs with diseases of the glomerulus, interstitium, or tubules, associated with the release of renal vasoconstrictors.
- The etiologies of intrinsic renal failure are subdivided anatomically into small-vessel disease, primary glomerular disease, and tubular and interstitial diseases (Table 52-1).
- Nephrotoxins are the second most common cause of ATN, accounting for approximately 25%.
- ARF has a different spectrum in the pediatric population: a higher incidence of intrinsic renal causes for ARF (45%) secondary to diseases such as glomerulonephritis and hemolytic-uremic syndrome.
- Postobstructive ARF increases tubular pressure, which decreases filtration. It has a significantly higher incidence in selected populations (such as elderly men).
- Restoring RBF is key to recovery from ARF.
- Replacement of circulating volume is critical in prerenal ARF.
- Treatment of the underlying cause of intrinsic ARF (toxin clearance, therapy for glomerular diseases) helps restore RBF.
- Vasoconstriction and tubular pressure decrease with relief of postrenal obstruction.

TABLE 52-1 Causes of Renal Failure

PRERENAL	RENAL (INTRINSIC)	POSTRENAL
Hypovolemia GI: decreased intake, vomiting and diarrhea Pharmacologic: diuretics Third spacing Skin losses: fever, burns Miscellaneous: hypoaldosteronism, salt-losing nephropathy, postobstructive diuresis Hypotension Septic vasodilation Hemorrhage Decreased cardiac output: ischemia/infarction, valvulopathy, cardiomyopathy, tamponade Pharmacologic: β-blockers, calcium channel blockers, other antihypertensive medications High-output failure: thyrotoxicosis, thiamine deficiency, Paget's disease, arteriovenous fistula Renal artery and small-vessel disease Embolism: thrombotic, septic, cholesterol Thrombosis: atherosclerosis, vasculitis, sickle cell disease Dissection Pharmacologic: NSAIDs, angiotensin-converting enzyme inhibitors, angiotensin receptor blockers (these act on the microvasculature but have prerenal physiology) Cyclosporine and tacrolimus Microvascular thrombosis: preeclampsia, hemolytic-uremic syndrome, disseminated intravascular coagulation, vasculitis, sickle cell disease Hypercalcemia	Tubular diseases Ischemic acute tubular necrosis: caused by more advanced disease due to the prerenal causes Nephrotoxins: aminoglycosides, radiocontrast agents, cisplatin, amphotericin B, heme pigments (rhabdomyolysis, massive hemolysis) Obstruction: uric acid, calcium oxalate, myeloma light chains, amyloid; pharmacologic: sulfonamide, triamterene, acyclovir, indinavir Interstitial diseases Acute interstitial nephritis: typically a drug reaction (NSAIDs and antibiotics most commonly, but also diuretics, phenytoin, allopurinol, rifampin) Infection: bilateral pyelonephritis, Legionnaire disease, hantavirus infection Infiltrative disease: sarcoidosis, lymphoma Autoimmune diseases: systemic lupus erythematosus Toxicologic: aristolochic acid Glomerular diseases Rapidly progressive glomerulonephritis: Goodpasture syndrome, Wegener granulomatosis, Henoch–Schönlein purpura, membranoproliferative glomerulonephritis Postinfectious glomerulonephritis Small-vessel diseases Microvascular thrombosis: preeclampsia, hemolytic-uremic syndrome, disseminated intravascular coagulation, thrombotic thrombocytopenic purpura, vasculitis Malignant hypertension Scleroderma	All ages Urethra and bladder outlet Phimosis or urethral stricture (male preponderance) Neurogenic bladder: diabetes mellitus, spinal cord disease, multiple sclerosis Parkinson's disease; pharmacologic: anticholinergics, α-adrenergic antagonists, opiates Calculus: in children in Southeast Asia, in adults typically a complication of mechanical intervention Adults Urethra and bladder outlet Benign prostate hypertrophy Cancer of prostate, bladder, cervix, or colon Obstructed catheters Ureter Calculi, uric acid crystals Papillary necrosis: sickle cell disease, diabetes mellitus, pyelonephritis Tumor: carcinoma of ureter, uterus, prostate, bladder, colon, rectum; retroperitoneal lymphoma; uterine leiomyomata Retroperitoneal fibrosis: idiopathic, tuberculosis, sarcoidosis, methylsergide, propranolol Stricture: tuberculosis, radiation, schistosomiasis, NSAIDs Miscellaneous: aortic aneurysm, pregnant uterus, inflammatory bowel disease, blood clot, trauma, accidental surgical ligation Infants and children Urethra and bladder outlet Anatomic malformations such as, anterior and posterior urethral valves (males) Ureter Anatomic malformations such as vesicoureteral reflux (female preponderance)

CLINICAL FEATURES

- Deterioration in renal function leads to excessive accumulation of nitrogenous waste products in the serum. Patients usually have signs and symptoms of their underlying causative disorder but eventually develop stigmata of renal failure.
- Volume overload, hypertension, pulmonary edema, mental status changes or neurologic symptoms, nausea and vomiting, bone and joint problems, anemia, and increased susceptibility to infection (a leading cause of death) can occur as patients develop more chronic uremia.

DIAGNOSIS AND DIFFERENTIAL

- History and physical examination usually provide clues to etiology. Signs and symptoms of the underlying causative disorder (Table 52-1) should be vigorously sought.
- Physical examination should assess vital signs, volume status, establish urinary tract patency and output, and search for signs of chemical intoxication, drug usage, muscle damage, infections, or associated systemic diseases.
- Diagnostic studies include urinalysis (see Table 52-2), blood urea nitrogen and creatinine levels, serum electrolytes, urinary sodium and creatinine, and urinary osmolality. Analysis of these tests allows most patients to be categorized as prerenal, renal, or postrenal. Fractional excretion of sodium can be calculated to help in this categorization (see Table 52-3).
- Normal urinary sediment may be seen in prerenal and postrenal failure, hemolytic-uremic syndrome, and thrombotic thrombocytopenic purpura. The presence of albumin may indicate glomerulonephritis or malignant hypertension.

TABLE 52-2 Urine Findings in Different Types of Renal Failure

CONDITION	MICROSCOPIC ANALYSIS	URINE DIPSTICK RESULTS
Prerenal renal failure	Normal, or a few hyaline casts possible	Normal, or trace proteinuria, specific gravity >1.015
Intrinsic renal failure		
Tubular injury		
Ischemia	Pigmented granular casts, renal tubular epithelial cells	Specific gravity <1.015, mild to moderate proteinuria
Nephrotoxins	Pigmented granular casts	Specific gravity <1.015, mild to moderate proteinuria
Acute interstitial nephritis	White cells, eosinophils, casts, red cells	Mild to moderate proteinuria; hemoglobin, leukocytes
Acute glomerulonephritis	Red cells and red cell casts; red cells can be dysmorphic	Moderate to severe proteinuria; hemoglobin
Postrenal renal failure	Crystals, red cells, and white cells possible	Trace to no proteinuria; hemoglobin and leukocytes possible

- Granular casts are seen in ATN. Albumin and red blood cell casts are found in glomerulonephritis, malignant hypertension, and autoimmune disease. White blood cell casts are seen in interstitial nephritis and pyelonephritis. Crystals can be present with renal calculi and certain drugs (sulfas, ethylene glycol, and radiocontrast agents).
- Renal ultrasound is the radiologic procedure of choice in most patients with ARF when upper tract obstruction and hydronephrosis is suspected. Color flow Doppler can assess renal perfusion and diagnose large vessel causes of renal failure. Bedside sonography can quickly diagnose some treatable causes and give guidance for fluid resuscitation; inspiratory collapse of the intrahepatic IVC can give a good measure of volume status and fluid responsiveness (see Figs. 52-1A and 52-1B, and 52-2A and 52-2B).
- *Prerenal failure* is produced by conditions that decrease renal perfusion (see Table 52-1) and is the most common cause of community-acquired ARF (~70% of cases). It also is a common precursor to ischemic and nephrotoxic causes of intrinsic renal failure.
- *Intrinsic renal failure* has vascular and ischemic etiologies; glomerular and tubulointerstitial diseases are also causative. (Ischemic ARF—traditionally known as ATN—is now called AKI.)
- ATN due to severe and prolonged prerenal etiologies causes most cases of intrinsic renal failure; ATN is also the most common cause of hospital-acquired ARF.
- Nephrotoxins are the second most common cause of ATN.
- *Postrenal azotemia* occurs primarily in elderly men with high-grade prostatic obstruction. Lesions of the external genitalia (ie, strictures) are also common causes. Significant permanent loss of renal function occurs over 10 to 14 days with complete obstruction, and worsens with associated UTI.

TABLE 52-3 Laboratory Studies Aiding in the Differential Diagnosis of Acute Renal Failure

TEST EMPLOYED	PRERENAL	RENAL*	POSTRENAL†
Urine sodium (mEq/L)	<20	>40	>40
FE_{Na} (%)‡	<1	>1	>1
RFI#	<1	>1	>1
Urine osmolality (mOsm/L)	>500	<350	<350
Urine: serum creatinine	>40:1	<20:1	<20:1
Blood urea nitrogen: creatinine	>20:1	10:1	>10:1

*FE_{Na} may be less than 1 in patients with intrinsic renal failure plus glomerulonephritis, hepatorenal syndrome, radiocontrast acute tubular necrosis, myoglobinuric and hemoglobinuric acute renal failure, renal allograft rejection, and certain drugs (angiotensin-converting enzyme inhibitors and nonsteroidal anti-inflammatory agents).
†One can see indices similar to prerenal early in the course of obstruction. With continued obstruction, tubular function is impaired and indices mimic those of renal causes.
‡FE_{Na} = ([urine sodium/serum sodium] ÷ [urine creatinine/serum creatinine]) × 100.
#RFI = (serum sodium ÷ [urine creatinine/serum creatinine]) × 100.
Abbreviation: FE_{Na} = fractional excretion of sodium, RFI = renal failure index.

EMERGENCY DEPARTMENT CARE AND DISPOSITION

- ED goals in the initial care of patients with ARF focus on treating the underlying cause and correcting fluid and electrolyte derangements. Efforts should be made to prevent further renal damage and provide supportive

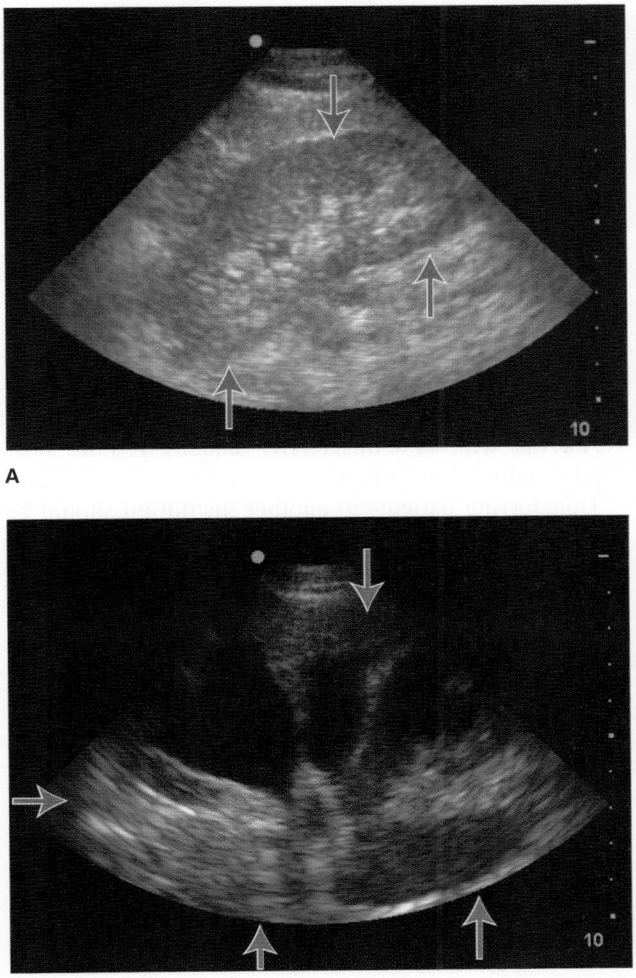

A

B

FIG. 52-1 **A.** US of normal kidney and kidney showing hydronephrosis. Normal kidney, capsule margin at arrows. **B.** Hydronephrosis as would be expected in obstructive uropathy; the dilated kidney fills the majority of the screen, capsule at arrows. (Courtesy of Michael B. Stone, MD, RDMS.)

care until renal function has recovered (see Chap. 6 for treatment of electrolyte and acid-base disorders).

PRERENAL FAILURE

- Effective intravascular volume should be restored with isotonic fluids (normal saline or lactated Ringer solution) at a rapid rate in appropriate patients; volume resuscitation is the first priority.
- If cardiac failure is causing prerenal azotemia, cardiac output should be optimized to improve renal perfusion, and reduction in intravascular volume (ie, with diuretics) may be appropriate.

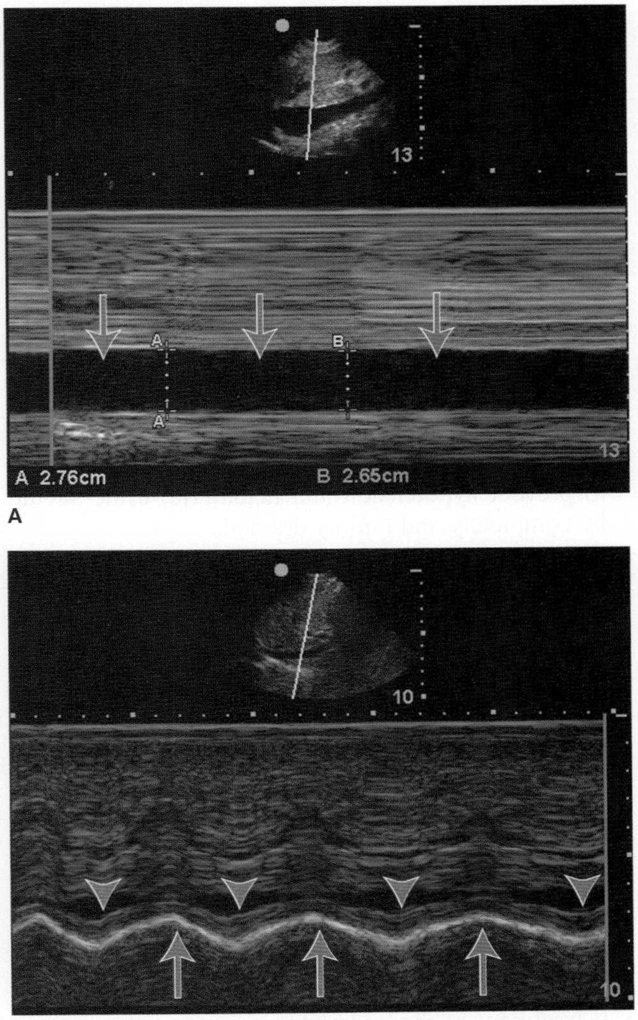

A

B

FIG. 52-2 US of the inferior vena cava. **A.** Plethoric inferior vena cava (arrows) as might be expected in volume overload; there is very little respiratory variation. **B.** An almost fully collapsed inferior vena cava at inspiration (arrows) and expiration (arrowheads) as might be expected in prerenal acute renal failure. (Courtesy of Michael B. Stone, MD, RDMS.)

RENAL FAILURE (INTRINSIC)

- Adequate circulating volume must be restored first; hypovolemia potentiates and exacerbates all forms of ARF.
- Ischemia or nephrotoxic agents are the most common causes of intrinsic ARF. History, physical examination, and baseline laboratory tests should provide clues to the diagnosis. Nephrotoxic agents (drugs and radiocontrast) should be avoided.
- Low-dose dopamine (1-5 micrograms/kg/min) may improve RBF and urine output, but it does not lower mortality rates or improve recovery.

- Renally excreted drugs (digoxin, magnesium, sedatives, and narcotics) should be used with caution because therapeutic doses may accumulate to excess and cause serious side effects. Fluid restriction may be required. Interventions useful in the prevention of radiocontrast nephropathy include acetylcysteine, fenoldopam, and crystalloid infusions.

POSTRENAL FAILURE

- Appropriate urinary drainage should be established; the exact procedure depends on the level of obstruction.
- A Foley catheter should be placed to relieve obstruction caused by prostatic hypertrophy. There is no support for the practice of intermittent catheter clamping to prevent hypotension and hematuria; urine should be completely and rapidly drained.
- Percutaneous nephrostomy may be required for ureteral occlusion until definitive surgery to correct the obstruction can take place once the patient is stabilized.
- For the acutely anuric patient, obstruction is the major consideration. If no urine is obtained on initial bladder catheterization, emergency urologic consultation should be considered.
- With chronic urinary retention, postobstructive diuresis may occur due to osmotic diuresis or tubular dysfunction. Patients may become suddenly hypovolemic and hypotensive. Urine output must be closely monitored, with appropriate fluid replacement.

DIALYSIS

- If treatment of the underlying cause fails to improve renal function, hemodialysis or peritoneal dialysis should be considered. The nephrology consultant usually makes decisions about dialysis (see Table 52-4).

TABLE 52-4 Indications for Emergent Dialysis

Uncontrolled hyperkalemia (K^+ >6.5 mmol/L or rising)
Intractable fluid overload in association with persistent hypoxia, or lack of response to conservative measures
Uremic pericarditis
Progressive uremic/metabolic encephalopathy; asterixis, seizures
Serum sodium level <115 or >165 mEq/L
Severe metabolic acidosis resistant to sodium bicarbonate, or cases in which repeat dosing of sodium bicarbonate is contraindicated
Life-threatening poisoning with a dialyzable drug, such as lithium, aspirin, methanol, ethylene glycol, or theophylline
Bleeding dyscrasia secondary to uremia
Excessive BUN and creatinine levels: trigger levels are arbitrary; it is generally advisable to keep BUN level <100 milligrams/dL, but each patient should be evaluated individually

Abbreviation: BUN = blood urea nitrogen.

- Dialysis often is initiated when the blood urea nitrogen is greater than 100 milligrams/dL or serum creatinine is greater than 10 milligrams/dL.
- Patients with complications of ARF such as cardiac instability (due to metabolic acidosis and hyperkalemia), intractable volume overload, hyperkalemia, and uremia (ie, encephalopathy, pericarditis, and bleeding diathesis) not easily corrected by other measures should be considered for emergency dialysis. However, morality in ARF has changed little since the advent of dialysis.

DISPOSITION

- Patients with new-onset ARF usually require hospital admission, often to an intensive care unit. Transferring patients to another institution should be considered if nephrology consultation and dialysis facilities are not available.

For further reading in Tintinalli's *Emergency Medicine: A Comprehensive Study Guide*, 7th ed., see Chapter 91, "Acute Renal Failure," by Richard Sinert and Peter R. Peacock, Jr.

53 RHABDOMYOLYSIS

Michael Levine

Rhabdomyolysis is a clinical and biochemical syndrome resulting from skeletal muscle necrosis.

EPIDEMIOLOGY

- Conditions associated with rhabdomyolysis are listed in Table 53-1.
- Comatose patients are at risk for rhabdomyolysis due to prolonged immobilization with continual pressure on gravity-dependent parts of the body.

PATHOPHYSIOLOGY

- Skeletal muscle injury results in cellular death with resultant leakage of previously intracellular contents into the vasculature.
- Common cellular agents that leak into the circulation include myoglobin, creatinine kinase, aldolase, lactate dehydrogenase, potassium, and aspartate aminotransferase.

TABLE 53-1 Common Conditions Associated with Rhabdomyolysis in Adults

Trauma	**Immunologic diseases involving muscle**	**Ischemic injury**
Crush injury	Dermatomyositis	Compartment syndrome
Electrical or lightning injury	Polymyositis	Compression
Drugs of abuse	**Bacterial infection**	**Medications**
Amphetamines [including Ecstasy (3,4-methylenedioxymethamphetamine)]	*Clostridium*	Antipsychotics
	Group A β-hemolytic streptococci	*Barbiturates
Caffeine	*Legionella*	*Benzodiazepines
Cocaine	*Salmonella*	*Clofibrate
*Ethanol	*Shigella*	Colchicine
*Heroin	*Staphylococcus aureus*	Corticosteroids
Lysergic acid diethylamide	*Streptococcus pneumoniae*	Diphenhydramine
Methamphetamines	**Viral infection**	Isoniazid
*Opiates	Coxsackievirus	*Lithium
Phencyclidine	Cytomegalovirus	*Monoamine oxidase inhibitors
Environment and excessive muscular activity	Epstein-Barr virus	*Narcotics
Contact sports	Enterovirus	Neuroleptic agents
Delirium tremens	Hepatitis virus	Phenothiazines
Dystonia	Herpes simplex virus	Salicylates
Psychosis	Human immunodeficiency virus	*Selective serotonin reuptake inhibitors
Seizures	Influenza virus (A and B)	Statins
Sports and basic training	Rotavirus	*Theophylline
Heat stroke		*Tricyclic antidepressants
Genetic disorders		Zidovudine
Glycolysis and glycogenolysis disorders		
Fatty acid oxidation disorders		
Mitochondrial and respiratory chain metabolism disorders		

*The marked substances do not cause rhabdomyolysis directly, but may be associated with rhabdomyolysis through predisposition to immobility or compression related muscle injury, or in association with other syndromes (e.g., serotonin syndrome, or neuroleptic malignant syndrome and others).

- Disruption of the sodium/potassium/ATPase and calcium transport results in increased intracellular calcium which, ultimately triggers cellular death.

CLINICAL FEATURES

- A number of clinical histories should raise the clinician's suspicion for this syndrome, the most common of which follow.
- Prolonged immobilization from any cause may lead to rhabdomyolysis, especially in association with drug intoxication such as that caused by narcotics, sedative-hypnotic medications, or ethanol consumption.
- Drug intoxication with sympathomimetics may lead to rhabdomyolysis without immobilization, including cocaine, amphetamine, or phencyclidine (PCP) abuse, or antihistamine use.
- Excessive muscular activity or strenuous exercise may lead to rhabdomyolysis; see Table 53-1 for common causes.
- Injuries that can cause a compartment syndrome or prolonged muscular compression such as crush injuries, heat stroke, and electrical injuries may lead to rhabdomyolysis.
- Certain diseases or disease states are associated with rhabdomyolysis such as polymyositis, dermatomyositis, and neuroleptic malignant syndrome.
- Common complaints include muscle ache/stiffness, malaise, muscle tenderness (especially thigh or calf muscle), and dark-colored urine. However, these signs and symptoms are neither sensitive nor specific.

DIAGNOSIS AND DIFFERENTIAL

- Diagnosis is made by measuring the serum creatinine kinase (CK). An elevation of at least five times the upper limit of normal, with the exclusion of cardiac etiologies is diagnostic of rhabdomyolysis.
- The serum CK rises 2 to 12 hours after the initial injury, and peaks 1 to 3 days after the injury resolves.
- Myoglobinuria can be detected once plasma myoglobin concentration exceeds 1.5 milligrams/dL.
- The presence of heme on the urine dipstick without observing blood cells on microscopy is a diagnostic clue.
- Obtain CK levels and basic metabolic studies for all patients suspected of having rhabdomyolysis.

EMERGENCY DEPARTMENT CARE AND DISPOSITION

- The primary focus is intravenous hydration with crystalloids. Typically, several liters of normal saline are given; use caution in patients who cannot tolerate rapid infusions of fluid.
- Urinary alkalinization is often performed, but has not been clearly demonstrated to improve outcome.
- Electrolytes should be monitored carefully as therapy is given in severe cases.
- Phosphorus and should only be treated when above 7 milligrams/dL or below 1 milligram/dL.
- Hyperkalemia requires aggressive therapy (see Chapter 6); avoid agents that would dehydrate the patient.
- Monitor urine output closely.
- Avoid potentially nephrotoxic drugs, if possible.
- Hydrate patients with mild rhabdomyolysis without comorbidities in the emergency department, after which they may be discharged.
- Admit patients with acute kidney injury, significant comorbid conditions, or marked elevations in the CK.
- Complications include acute kidney injury, hypercalcemia (late), hyperphosphatemia (early), hypophosphatemia (late), hyperkalemia, hyperuricemia, hypocalcemia, and disseminated intravascular coagulation.

For further reading in Tintinalli's *Emergency Medicine: A Comprehensive Study Guide,* 7th ed., see Chapter 92, "Rhabdomyolysis," by Francis L. Counselman and Bruce M. Lo.

54 EMERGENCIES IN RENAL FAILURE AND DIALYSIS PATIENTS

Jonathan A. Maisel

EPIDEMIOLOGY

- End-stage renal disease (ESRD) is primarily a disease of the elderly, with patients over 65 years comprising nearly half of new cases, and over one-third of all living individuals with the disease.
- Diabetes mellitus is the most common disease causing ESRD, followed by hypertension, glomerulonephritis, and cystic kidney disease.
- Cardiac causes account for approximately 50% of all cases of ESRD death. Infectious etiologies account for 10% to 25% of deaths.

PATHOPHYSIOLOGY

- The pathophysiology of renal failure can be categorized by three mechanisms: (1) excretory failure, ie, inability to excrete over 70 chemicals known to accumulate in renal failure, most notably urea; (2) biosynthetic failure, ie, the loss of renal hormones vitamin D and erythropoietin; and (3) regulatory failure, ie, the disruption of normal feedback mechanisms leading to the oversecretion of hormones that exacerbate uremia.
- The diagnosis of uremia is a clinical one, based on a constellation of symptoms. Though a correlation exists between the symptoms of uremia and a low glomerular filtration rate (8-10 mL/min), routine laboratory tests are inaccurate markers of the syndrome. The decision to institute renal replacement therapy (RRT) is a clinical one.
- Patients with ESRD may sustain multiple complications of their disease process and treatment.
- Emergent dialysis is most commonly required for hyperkalemia, severe metabolic acidosis, and pulmonary edema resistant to alternative therapy.

CARDIOVASCULAR COMPLICATIONS

- Creatine phosphokinase (and the MB fraction), troponin I, and troponin T are not significantly elevated in ESRD patients undergoing regular dialysis, and have been shown to be specific markers of myocardial ischemia in these patients.
- *Hypertension* occurs in 80% to 90% of patients starting dialysis. Management includes control of blood volume, followed by use of adrenergic-blocking drugs, angiotensin-converting enzyme inhibitors, or vasodilating agents.
- *Congestive heart failure* (CHF) may be caused by hypertension, coronary ischemia, and valvular disease, as well as uremic cardiomyopathy, fluid overload, and arteriovenous (AV) fistulas (high output failure). Treatment is similar to that in non-ESRD patients.
- Most importantly, preload can be reduced using nitrates, as well as by inducing diarrhea with sorbitol and with phlebotomy (minimum 150 mL). Blood should be collected in a transfusion bag so that it may be transfused back to the patient during subsequent dialysis.
- Diuretics (furosemide 60-100 milligrams) may have a small benefit, even in oliguric patients, as they cause pulmonary vessel vasodilatation.

- Hemodialysis (HD) is the definitive treatment for fluid overload.
- *Pericarditis* in ESRD patients is usually due to worsening uremia. Electrocardiographic (ECG) changes typical of acute pericarditis are not seen. Pericardial friction rubs are louder than in most other forms of pericarditis, often palpable, and frequently persist after the metabolic abnormalities have been corrected. Uremic pericarditis is treated with intensive dialysis.
- *Cardiac tamponade* is the most serious complication of uremic pericarditis. It presents with changes in mental status, hypotension, or dyspnea. An enlarged heart on chest radiograph may suggest the diagnosis, which can be confirmed with echocardiography. Hemodynamically significant pericardial effusions require pericardiocentesis under fluoroscopic or ultrasonographic guidance.

NEUROLOGIC COMPLICATIONS

- *Uremic encephalopathy* presents with cognitive defects, memory loss, slurred speech, and asterixis. The progressive neurologic symptoms of uremia are the most common indications for initiating HD. It should remain a diagnosis of exclusion until structural, vascular, infectious, toxic, and metabolic causes of neurologic dysfunction have been ruled out.
- *Peripheral neuropathy*, manifested by paresthesias, diminished deep tendon reflexes, impaired vibration sense, muscle wasting, and weakness, occurs in 60% to 100% of patients with ESRD.
- *Autonomic dysfunction*, characterized by postural dizziness, gastric fullness, bowel dysfunction, reduced sweating, reduced heart rate variability, and baroreceptor control impairment, is common in ESRD patients, but is not responsible for intradialytic hypotension.
- *Stroke* is seen in 6% of HD patients, with 52% of cases caused by intracranial hemorrhage (subdural hematoma in particular). Stroke may be caused by cerebrovascular disease, head trauma, bleeding dyscrasias, anticoagulation, excessive ultrafiltration, or hypertension. It should be considered in any ESRD patient presenting with a change in mental status.

HEMATOLOGIC COMPLICATIONS

- *Anemia* is caused by decreased erythropoietin, blood loss from dialysis, frequent phlebotomy, and decreased red cell survival.
- *Factitious anemia* reflects changes in plasma volume related to dialysis.
- Abnormal hemostasis in ESRD is multifactorial in origin, resulting in an increased risk of gastrointestinal (GI) tract bleeding, subcapsular liver hematomas, subdural hematomas, and intraocular bleeding.
- *Immunologic compromise*, caused by impaired leukocyte chemotaxis and phagocytosis, leads to high mortality rates from infection. Dialysis does not appear to improve immune system function.

GASTROINTESTINAL COMPLICATIONS

- *Anorexia, nausea*, and *vomiting* are common symptoms of uremia, and are used as an indication to initiate dialysis, and assess its efficacy.
- *Chronic constipation* is common, due to decreased fluid intake, and the use of phosphate-binding gels.

COMPLICATIONS OF HEMODIALYSIS

- *Hypotension* is the most frequent complication of HD. Excessive ultrafiltration from underestimation of the patient's ideal blood volume (dry weight) is the most common cause of intradialytic hypotension.
- Other causes of intradialytic hypotension include myocardial dysfunction from ischemia, hypoxia, arrhythmias, and pericardial tamponade; abnormalities of vascular tone secondary to sepsis, overproduction of nitric oxide, and antihypertensive medications; and volume loss from inadequate oral intake, vomiting, diarrhea, GI bleeding, or blood tubing or filter leaks.
- Treatment consists of Trendelenburg positioning, oral salt solution, or infusion of parenteral normal saline solution. If these interventions fail, excessive ultrafiltration is unlikely, and further evaluation to look for another cause will be required.
- Cardiac compensation for fluid loss may be compromised by diastolic dysfunction common in ESRD patients.
- *Dialysis disequilibrium*, caused by cerebral edema following large solute clearances, is characterized by nausea, vomiting, and hypertension, which can progress to seizures, coma, and death. Treatment consists of terminating dialysis, and administering mannitol intravenously to increase serum osmolarity. This syndrome should be distinguished from other neurologic disorders, such as subdural hematoma, stroke, hypertensive crisis, hypoxia, and seizures.

COMPLICATIONS OF VASCULAR ACCESS

- *Complications of vascular access* account for more inpatient hospital days than any other complication of HD.

- *Thrombosis or stenosis* presents with loss of the bruit and a thrill over the access. These need to be treated within 24 hours with angiographic clot removal, angioplasty, or direct injection of thrombolytic (eg, alteplase 2.2 milligrams) into the access.
- *Vascular access infections* often present with signs of systemic sepsis, including fever, hypotension, and an elevated white blood cell (WBC) count. Classic signs of pain, erythema, swelling, and discharge are often missing. *Staphylococcus aureus* is the most common infecting organism, followed by gram-negative bacteria. Patients usually require hospitalization, and treatment with vancomycin (15 milligrams/kg), and an aminoglycoside (eg, gentamicin 100 milligrams intravenously).
- Potential life-threatening *hemorrhage from a vascular* access may result from a ruptured aneurysm or anastomosis, or over-anticoagulation. Bleeding can often be controlled with 5 to 10 minutes of pressure at the puncture site. If this fails, the addition of an adsorbable gelatin sponge soaked in reconstituted thrombin, or a prothrombotic gauze (eg, HemCon or QuikClot), followed by 10 minutes of direct pressure will be effective. Life-threatening hemorrhage may require placement of a tourniquet proximal to the access, and vascular surgery consultation.
- If the etiology is excessive anticoagulation, the effects of heparin can be reversed with protamine 0.01 milligram/unit heparin dispensed during dialysis (10-20 milligrams protamine if the heparin dose is unknown).
- If a newly inserted vascular access continues to bleed, desmopressin acetate (0.3 micrograms/kg intravenously) can be given as an adjunct to direct pressure.

COMPLICATIONS OF PERITONEAL DIALYSIS

- *Peritonitis* is the most common complication of peritoneal dialysis (PD). Signs and symptoms are similar to those seen in other patients with peritonitis, and include fever, abdominal pain, and rebound tenderness. A cloudy effluent supports the diagnosis.
- Peritoneal fluid should be sent to the lab for cell count, Gram stain, culture, and sensitivity. With peritonitis, cell counts usually reveal >100 leukocytes/mm^3, with >50% neutrophils. Gram stain is positive in only 10% to 40% of culture-proven peritonitis. Organisms isolated include *Staphylococcus epidermidis, S. aureus, Streptococcus* species, and gram-negative bacteria.
- Empiric therapy begins with a few rapid exchanges of dialysate to decrease the number of inflammatory cells within the peritoneum. The addition of heparin (500-1000 units/L dialysate) decreases fibrin clot formation.
- Empiric antibiotics, covering gram-positive organisms (eg, cephalothin or vancomycin 500 milligrams/L dialysate) and gram-negative organisms (eg, gentamicin 100 milligrams/L dialysate), are added to the dialysate.
- Inpatient versus outpatient treatment of PD-related peritonitis should be based on clinical presentation.
- Infections around the PD catheter are characterized by pain, erythema, swelling, and discharge. Causative organisms are *S. aureus* and *Pseudomonas aeruginosa*. Outpatient treatment consists of a first generation cephalosporin or ciprofloxacin.

For further reading in Tintinalli's *Emergency Medicine: A Comprehensive Study Guide,* 7th ed., see Chapter 93, "Emergencies in Renal Failure and Dialysis Patients," by Mark Spektor and Richard Sinert.

55 URINARY TRACT INFECTIONS AND HEMATURIA

David M. Cline

URINARY TRACT INFECTIONS

- Urethritis and cystitis are infections of the lower urinary tract.
- Pyelonephritis is an infection of the upper urinary tract.
- Uncomplicated urinary tract infection (UTI) is defined as UTI without structural or functional abnormalities within the urinary tract or kidney parenchyma, without relevant comorbidities that place the patient at risk for more serious adverse outcome, and not associated with GU tract instrumentation.
- Complicated UTI is defined as infection involving a functional or anatomically abnormal urinary tract, or infection in the presence of comorbidities that place the patient at risk for more serious adverse outcome.

EPIDEMIOLOGY

- UTIs account for up to 3% of emergency department (ED) visits.
- Up to 80% of UTIs are caused by *Escherichia coli*. The remainder of cases are caused by *Klebsiella*, *Proteus*, *Enterobacter*, *Pseudomonas*, group D streptococci, *Chlamydia trachomatis,* and *Staphylococcus saprophyticus.*

- *Chlamydia trachomatis* and *S. saprophyticus* are more commonly associated with the "dysuria-pyuria" syndrome in which sterile or low-colony-count culture results are obtained. *Staphylococcus saprophyticus* may account for up to 15% of acute lower tract infections in young, sexually active females—but rarely progresses to involve the upper tract.
- Adults at risk for UTI include women between 18 and 30 years of age, and the elderly of both sexes.
- Males younger than 50 years of age with symptoms of dysuria or urinary frequency usually have urethritis caused by sexually transmitted infections. UTIs in children are discussed in Chapter 77.
- Table 55-1 lists risk factors for complicated UTIs.

PATHOPHYSIOLOGY

- A thin film of urine remains in the functionally intact bladder after each void. Urinary pathogens, adhering to the uroepithelium with adhesins, fimbriae or pili, are removed from the film by mucosal production of organic acids. Incomplete bladder emptying renders this mechanism ineffective, and is responsible for the increased frequency of UTI in patients with structural or neurogenic bladder outflow abnormalities.
- Ureteral valves restrict the majority of uncomplicated UTIs to the bladder. If ascending infection of the urinary tract occurs, renal defense mechanisms including local antibody secretion and complement activation are induced.
- In uncomplicated UTIs, the most common urinary pathogen is *E. coli*. Up to one-half of women with symptomatic UTI may have low-grade or early infection, usually with 10^2 to 10^4 colony-forming units (CFU) per milliliter of *E. coli*, *S. saprophyticus*, or *C. trachomatis*. In complicated UTIs (ie, in those occurring in patients with underlying urologic or neurologic dysfunction), *Pseudomonas* spp. and enterococci are likely pathogens.
- In young women, the risk of UTI is independently associated with recent sexual intercourse, recent use of a diaphragm with spermicide, and a history of UTI. A "milking action" of the female urethra during intercourse can increase the concentration of bacteria in the bladder by up to a factor of 10. The use of a spermicide enhances vaginal colonization with *E. coli*.

TABLE 55-1 Risk Factors for Complicated Urinary Tract Infection (UTI)

RISK FACTOR	COMMENTS
Male sex	In young males, dysuria is more common secondary to sexually transmitted disease; suspect underlying anatomic abnormality in men with culture-proven UTI.
Anatomic abnormality of the urinary tract or external drainage system	Indwelling urinary catheter, ureteral stent, nephrolithiasis, neurogenic bladder, polycystic renal disease, or recent urinary tract instrumentation.
Recurrent UTI	No universal definition exists. A pragmatic definition is three or more per year.
Advanced age in men	Presence of prostatic hyperplasia, recent instrumentation, recent prostatic biopsy.
Nursing home residency	With or without indwelling bladder catheter.
Neonatal state	See Chap. 77, Urinary Tract Infection in Infants and Children.
Comorbidities	Diabetes mellitus, sickle cell disease, others.
Pregnancy	See Chap. 62, Comorbid Diseases in Pregnancy.
Immunosuppression	Active chemotherapy, acquired immunodeficiency syndrome, immunosuppressive drugs.
Advanced neurologic disease	Stroke with disability, spinal cord injuries, others.
Known or suspected atypical pathogens	Non–*Escherichia coli* infections.
Known or suspected resistance to typical antimicrobial agents for UTI	Resistance to ciprofloxacin predicts multidrug resistance.

CLINICAL FEATURES

- Typical symptoms of lower urinary tract infections are dysuria, frequency, and urgency.
- The addition of flank pain, costovertebral angle (CVA) tenderness, fever, and systemic symptoms, often nausea and vomiting, constitutes pyelonephritis.
- Subclinical pyelonephritis is present in 25% to 30% of patients with cystitis. Atypical symptoms are found in patients at risk for complicated UTI.
- Suspect UTI in elderly or debilitated patients presenting with weakness, general malaise, generalized abdominal pain, or mental status changes.
- Urethral or vaginal discharge is more consistent with urethritis and vaginitis, and the possibility of a sexually transmitted disease.
- Asymptomatic bacteriuria is defined as two positive cultures without symptoms. Since cultures are not available acutely, asymptomatic bacteriuria is diagnosed in the ED when bacteria are found on microscopy in patients with no symptoms.
- Asymptomatic bacteriuria is commonly found in patients with indwelling catheters, up to 30% of pregnant women, and 40% of female nursing home patients.
- Empiric treatment is recommended for asymptomatic bacteriuria during pregnancy.

DIAGNOSIS AND DIFFERENTIAL

- The diagnosis of UTI is based on patient symptoms and signs, with individualized assessment of urine dipstick, urinalysis, and culture in selected patients.
- Typically, urine dipstick and urine microscopy is performed at minimum; woman of child bearing potential should have a pregnancy test.
- Clean catch specimens are adequate for most patients; catheterization should be used in a patient that cannot void spontaneously, is immobilized, or is too ill or obese to be able to provide a clean voided specimen.
- Although the gold standard for the diagnosis is urine culture, it is not required in all cases diagnosed in the ED.
- Uncomplicated lower urinary tract infections (woman with symptoms, such as pyuria, dipstick positive for nitrite, and/or leukocyte esterase) can usually be managed as an outpatient without a culture. Obtain a culture in all other cases.
- *Criteria for complicated UTI* include positive laboratory testing in the setting of prior history of UTI (reoccurrence in <1 month or more than 3 infections per year), which defines recurrent UTI with an atypical organism (non-*E. coli*) or known antibiotic resistance, a functionally or anatomically abnormal urinary tract, comorbidities (metabolic diseases, carcinoma, immune suppression, sickle cell anemia), advanced neurologic disease, advanced age, nursing home residency, indwelling catheter or recent urinary tract instrumentation, pregnancy, or male sex.
- The urine nitrite reaction is greater than 90% specific but only about 50% sensitive in the diagnosis of UTI. A positive result with symptoms and bacteriuria is confirmatory.
- UTI with *Enterococcus*, *Pseudomonas,* or *Acinetobacter* results in a negative nitrite test.
- The leukocyte esterase reaction is more sensitive (77%) but less specific (54%) than the nitrite reaction. If it is positive, it is supportive of UTI.
- In summary, a positive urine dipstick nitrate or leukocyte test result supports the diagnosis of UTI; a negative test result does not exclude it.
- A urine white blood cell per high power field (WBC/HPF) of greater than 2 to 5 in women and 1 to 2 in men, in a patient with appropriate symptoms, is suggestive of a UTI.
- In a symptomatic patient with less than 5 WBC/HPF, one must consider causes of false-negative pyuria. These include dilute urine, systemic leukopenia, partially treated UTI, and obstruction of an infected kidney.
- Any bacteria on an uncentrifuged specimen is abnormal, and more than 1 to 2 bacteria per HPF in a centrifuged specimen is 95% sensitive and more than 60% specific for UTI.
- False-negative results may occur in a low-colony-count infection or in the case of chlamydia. False-positive results may occur due to contamination with fecal or vaginal flora.
- In patients with urinary catheters, the diagnosis of UTI is difficult as both pyuria and asymptomatic bacteriuria are near universal by the fourth week of indwelling.
- Treatment is only recommended in symptomatic patients; see Chapter 59 for detailed criteria of symptomatic catheter-associated infection.
- Renal imaging should be considered acutely in the severely ill, if there is suspicion for a stone associated with infection, and with a poor initial response to therapy.
- Differential diagnostic considerations include upper and lower urinary tract infections, urethritis due to sexually transmitted infections (which are more common than cystitis/pyelonephritis in males younger than 50 years of age), vaginitis (both sexually transmitted and non–sexually transmitted), vulvodynia, prostatitis, epididymitis, and intra-abdominal pathology.

EMERGENCY DEPARTMENT CARE AND DISPOSITION

- Treatment is determined by whether the UTI is complicated or uncomplicated.
- Acute pyelonephritis can be treated as an outpatient if the patient has normal anatomy and is otherwise healthy. Urine culture, larger doses, and longer duration of antibiotics are recommended.
- *Uncomplicated UTI.* **Empiric treatment is best based on local resistance patterns**. For uncomplicated lower urinary tract infections in women, trimethoprim-sulfamethoxazole double strength (TMP-SMX DS) (160/800 milligrams twice a day for 3-5 days) is recommended as first choice **only in areas where** *E. coli* **resistance is less than 20%.** However, 20% to 30% of patients given 3- to 5-day therapy will experience treatment failure or rapid relapse. Alternatives will be determined by local resistance patterns.
- Nitrofurantoin (100 milligrams 4 times a day *or* 100 milligrams extended release twice a day for 5 days) is a first-choice antibiotic with lower resistance. Nitrofurantoin is recommended for asymptomatic bacteriuria during pregnancy.
- *Complicated UTI.* Use fluoroquinolones (ciprofloxacin 500 milligrams twice a day or levofloxacin 500 milligrams once a day), cefpodoxime (200 milligrams twice a day), or fosfomycin (3 grams once) in males, cases where symptoms suggest upper urinary tract involvement or have been present for more than

a week, infection is recurrent, follow-up is unsure, there are complicating factors, or local resistance to TMP-SMX is greater than 20%.

- Duration of therapy should be 10 to 14 days.
- Ciprofloxacin resistance may preclude its effective use in some communities.
- Use caution with nitrofurantoin and the fluoroquinolones in the elderly and in patients with renal insufficiency.
- If there is suspicion for concomitant infection with gonorrhea and/or chlamydia, antibiotic choice is more complex. Consider ofloxacin, 400 milligrams twice a day, and see Chapter 89.
- Consider 1 to 2 days of an oral bladder analgesic such as phenazopyridine 200 milligrams 3 times a day.
- Discharge instructions must include instructions to return for increased pain, fever, vomiting, or intolerance of medications, to take the entire course of antibiotics, and to follow up with primary care provider.
- Encourage fluids (cranberry juice may be helpful), and frequent voiding.
- Admission is indicated for pyelonephritis associated with intractable vomiting and should be considered for complicated UTIs.
- For admitted patients, empiric antibiotic therapy should be initiated in the ED: ciprofloxacin 400 milligrams IV every 12 hours, ceftriaxone 1 gram IV once daily, gentamicin or tobramycin, 3.0 milligrams/kg/d divided every 8 hours ± ampicillin 1 to 2 grams every 4 hours. For patients with unstable vital signs, see Chapter 91.

HEMATURIA

- Hematuria is blood in the urine. It is either visible to the eye, *gross hematuria*, requiring 1 mL of whole blood per liter, or only seen under the microscope, *microscopic hematuria*, defined as greater than 3 to 5 RBCs per high power field (RBC/HPF).

CLINICAL FEATURES

- Gross hematuria suggests a lower urinary tract source, and microscopic hematuria suggests a renal source.
- Asymptomatic hematuria is more often due to neoplasm or vascular causes than infection.
- Asymptomatic hematuria is defined as greater than 3 to 5 RBC/HPF on 2 of 3 properly collected urine specimens in a patient with no symptoms.

DIAGNOSIS AND DIFFERENTIAL

- A urine dipstick is positive with approximately 5 to 20 red blood cells per milliliter of urine.
- All positive dipsticks should be followed by microscopy.
- False-positive results can occur with the presence of myoglobin, porphyrins, free hemoglobin (as opposed to intact RBCs) due to hemolysis, and povidone-iodine.
- Catheterization usually does not cause an abnormal result.
- False-negative results can be seen with very high specific gravity.
- Differential diagnostic considerations are numerous. Consider the patients' age, sex, demographic characteristics, habits, potential risk factors for urologic malignancy, comorbidities, or any history of recent urinary tract instrumentation.
- The most common causes of hematuria are UTI, nephrolithiasis, neoplasms, benign prostatic hypertrophy, glomerulonephritis, and schistosomiasis (most common cause worldwide).
- In the ED consider strenuous exercise, post-streptococcal infection (in younger patients) and life threats including malignant hypertension, eroding abdominal aortic aneurysm, coagulopathy, foreign body, immune-mediated disease (Henoch–Schönlein purpura, pulmonary-renal syndromes), sickle cell disease complications, and renal vein thrombosis.

EMERGENCY DEPARTMENT CARE AND DISPOSITION

- Treatment of hematuria is directed at the cause. ED management consists of the minimization of complications and appropriate referral or admission for further evaluation.
- All hematuria should be followed up by either primary care or urology within 2 weeks.
- Admit patients with infection associated with an obstructive stone, intractable pain, intolerance of medications or oral fluids, newly diagnosed glomerular nephritis, significant anemia, renal insufficiency, significant comorbidity, bladder outlet obstruction, pregnancy with preeclampsia, pyelonephritis, obstructive stone, or any potentially life-threatening causes of hematuria.

For further reading in Tintinalli's *Emergency Medicine: A Comprehensive Study Guide*, 7th ed., see Chapter 94, "Urinary Tract Infections and Hematuria," by David S. Howes and Mark P. Bogner.

56 ACUTE URINARY RETENTION

Casey M. Glass

EPIDEMIOLOGY

- The most common cause of acute urinary retention is benign prostatic hypertrophy. There are a number of other causes of acute urinary retention (Table 56-1) some of which are gender specific (Table 56-2).
- Acute urinary retention is more common in men and is associated with advancing age.
- Precipitated urinary retention referes to retention associated with other causes including recent surgery, medical illness, or drug effect (commonly anticholinergics, antihistamines, anaesthesia agents, cold medications, and α-sympathomimetics).
- Acute urinary retention associated with benign prostatic hypertrophy alone is considered spontaneous urinary retention and is associated with a greater risk of recurrence comapred to precipitated retention (15% vs 9%) and need for surgical intervention (75% vs 26%).

PATHOPHYSIOLOGY

- Acute urinary retention may be secondary to physical obstruction to urine flow or as a result of decreased neurologic control of bladder emptying.
- Sympathetic innervation of the bladder originates from the T10-L2 levels of the spinal cord. Somatic innervation is via the pudendal nerve (S2-4).

TABLE 56-1 Causes of Acute Urinary Retention

CATEGORY	EXAMPLES
Obstruction	Benign prostatic hyperplasia, urethral stricture
Neurogenic dysfunction	Spinal cord injury, cauda equina syndrome, multiple sclerosis, neuropathy associated with diabetes mellitus
Trauma	Spinal cord trauma, trauma to bladder or pelvis
Extraurinary mass	Rectal or retroperitoneal masses, fecal impaction
Psychogenic	Psychosexual stress, acute anxiety
Infection	Cystitis, herpes simplex (genital), prostatitis
Post-operative	General or epidural anesthesia
Congenital abnormality	Posterior urethral valves, urethral atresia
Medication related	Antidepressants, β-adrenergic agents, α-adrenergic agents, antihistamines, antipsychotics, antihypertensives, opiates, anticholinergics

TABLE 56-2 Gender-Specific Causes of Acute Urinary Obstruction

MEN	WOMEN
Obstructive	Obstructive
Benign prostatic hypertrophy*	Cystocele
Prostate cancer	Ovarian tumor
Phimosis	Uterine tumor
Paraphimosis	Operative
Meatal stenosis	Incontinence surgery
Urethral strangulation	Infection
Infection	Pelvic inflammatory disease
Prostatitis	

*Most common cause.

- Progressive obstruction leads to bladder dilation and decreased stream intensity as well as increased frequency of voiding.

CLINICAL FEATURES

- Patients with urinary retention complain of lower abdominal pain and the sensation of needing to void. Chronic retention may present with pain and a history of frequent incomplete voiding (overflow incontinence).
- The history should be directed at identifying the cause of precipitated urinary retention. A history of hematuria may be related to bladder or renal calculi, urinary tract neoplasm, or infection. Patients should be asked about new medications or recent surgical procedures. A comprehensive urologic history including known anatomic abnormalities and recent surgical interventions is vital.
- Prostate examination is necessary to assess for size, consistency, and the possibility of prostatitis. An enlarged, hard, nodular prostate is concerning for malignancy.
- Women with urinary retention should have a pelvic examination to assess for pelvic masses or pelvic inflammatory disease.
- A comprehensive neurologic examination is necessary to exclude a neurogenic cause. The examination should include assessment of rectal tone and perineal sensation.

DIAGNOSIS AND DIFFERENTIAL

- Bedside ultrasound is recommended as an intitial noninvasive test to assess for urinary retention (Fig. 56-1).

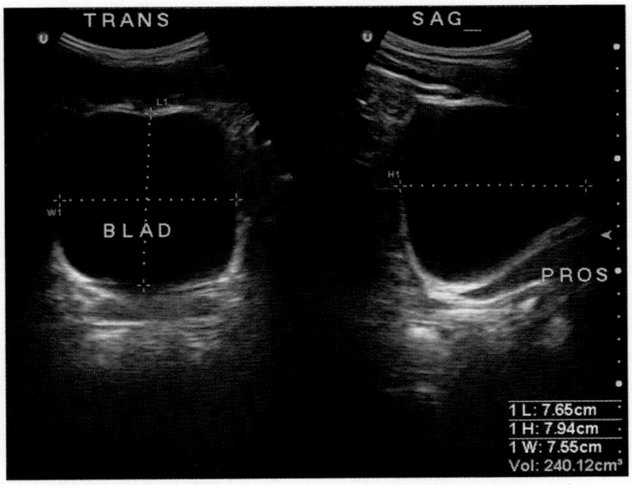

FIG. 56-1. Transverse and sagittal views of the urinary bladder. The prostate is visualized as a medium echogenicity structure posterior and caudal to the bladder. Anterior-posterior, cradio-caudal, and transverse measurements of the bladder are obtained for calculation of the bladder volume. (Reproduced with permission from Casey Glass, MD.)

- When ultrasound is not available, placement of a urethral Foley catheter is both diagnostic and therapeutic.
- Urinary volumes greater than 75 to 150 cc are consistent with retention.
- Urinalysis is necessary to determine the presence or absence of infection.
- CBC is recommended for patients with massive hematuria, suspected infection, and hematologic diseases.
- Serum chemistries are recommended to asses for renal dysfunction.

EMERGENCY DEPARTMENT CARE AND DISPOSITION

- The primary treatment of acute urinary retention is placement of a urethral or suprapubic catheter to allow for bladder drainage.
- Urologist consultation may be necessary if initial attempts at placement of a catheter are unsuccessful.
- Urologist consultation is recommended as the initial intervention when there is a history of a recent urologic procedure or after a traumatic Foley placement attempt with concern for creation of a false passage.
- Chronic obstruction is a risk factor for postobstructive diuresis and renal failure. Patients with chronic obstruction should be observed for 4 hours. Persistent diuresis greater than 200 cc an hour is abnormal. Patients with significant diuresis should be started on IV rehydration. Renal function should be checked regularly.
- Patients with significant hematuria need admission for conintued irrigation as blood clots commonly cause obstruction of the Foley catheter.
- Patients with significant comorbid illness as a cause of their obstruction (eg, cystitis, prostatitis), significant postobstructive diuresis, or abnormal measures of renal function need admission for additional treatment and monitoring.
- Antibiotics are not indicated unless a specific source of infection is noted.
- Men with spontaneous urinary retention can be started on an α-adrenergic blocker (tamsulosin, 0.4 milligram PO daily). They should be warned about the possibility of hypotension related to α-adrenergic blocker use.
- All patients dischared home should be set up with a leg bag for Foley catheter drainage and be instructed in how to care for the catheter and empty the bag.
- Urologist follow up in 4 to 7 days is recommended for discharged patients.
- Patients with precipitated urinary retention may have a trial of voiding in the ED if the precipitating cause is resolved. The bladder is drained and the catheter removed. The patient is observed for a period of time and allowed to attempt to void. Ultrasound can be used to confirm a minimal post-void residual.
- Occasionally medications are needed to manage pain from bladder spasms which are often secondary to irritation from the Foley catheter. The anticholinergic oxybutinin can be tried at a dose of 2.5 milligrams 3 times a day. Consistent with its class, this medication can itself cause urinary retention.

For further reading in Tintinalli's *Emergency Medicine: A Comprehensive Study Guide*, 7th ed., see Chapter 95, "Acute Urinary Retention," by David Hung-Tsang Yen and Chen-Hsen Lee.

57 MALE GENITAL PROBLEMS

Boyd Burns

SCROTUM

- *Scrotal abscesses* may be localized to the scrotal wall or may arise from extensions of infections of scrotal contents (ie, testis, epididymis, and bulbous urethra). A simple hair follicle scrotal wall abscess can be managed by incision and drainage; no antibiotics are required in immunocompetent patients unless signs of cellulitis or systemic involvement are present.

- When a scrotal wall abscess is suspected of arising from an intrascrotal infection, ultrasound and retrograde urethrography may demonstrate pathology in the testis, epididymis, or urethra. Definitive care of any complex abscess calls for a urology consultation.
- *Fournier's gangrene* is a polymicrobial infection of the perineal subcutaneous tissues (see Fig. 57-1). Immunocompromised males, particularly diabetics, are at highest risk.
- Prompt diagnosis is essential to prevent extensive tissue loss. Early surgical consultation is recommended for at-risk patients who present with scrotal, rectal, or genital pain.
- Treatment for Fournier's gangrene begins with aggressive fluid resuscitation (with normal saline). Broad-spectrum antibiotics should cover gram-positive, gram-negative, and anaerobic organisms, such as imipenem 1 gram IV every 24 hours, or meropenem 500 milligrams to 1 gram IV every 8 hours, with vancomycin if methicillin-resistant *Staphylococcus aureus* is suspected; surgical debridement is also necessary.

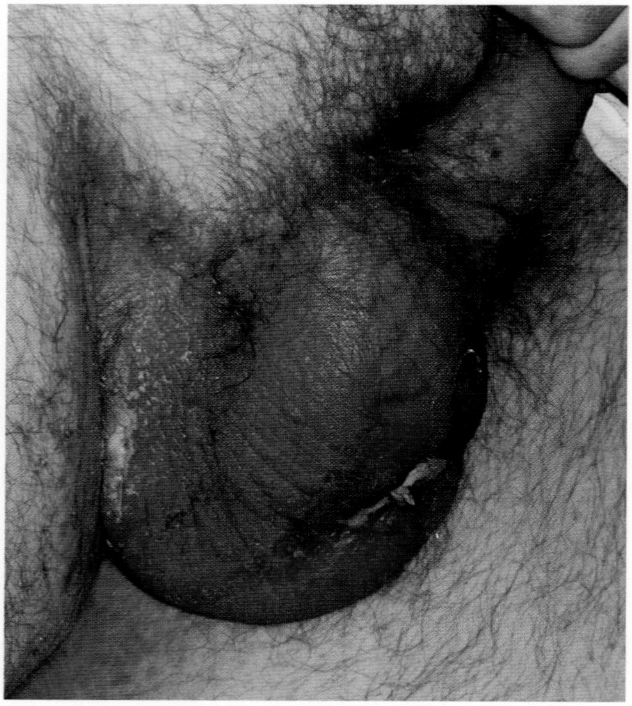

FIG. 57-1. A patient with Fournier's gangrene of the scrotum. Note the sharp demarcation of gangrenous changes and the marked edema of the scrotum and the penis.

PENIS

- *Balanoposthitis* is inflammation of the glans (balanitis) and foreskin (posthitis). Upon foreskin retraction, the glans and prepuce appear purulent, excoriated, malodorous, and tender.
- Treatment of balanoposthitis consists of cleansing with mild soap, assuring adequate dryness, and application of antifungal creams (nystatin qid or clotrimazole bid) and an oral azole (such as fluconazole), with urologic follow-up for possible circumcision. An oral cephalosporin (eg, cephalexin 500 milligrams qid) should be prescribed in cases of secondary bacterial infection. Recurrent balanoposthitis can be the sole presenting sign of diabetes.
- *Phimosis* is the inability to retract the foreskin proximally (see Fig. 57-2). Hemostatic dilation of the preputial ostium relieves the urinary retention until definitive dorsal slit or circumcision can be performed.

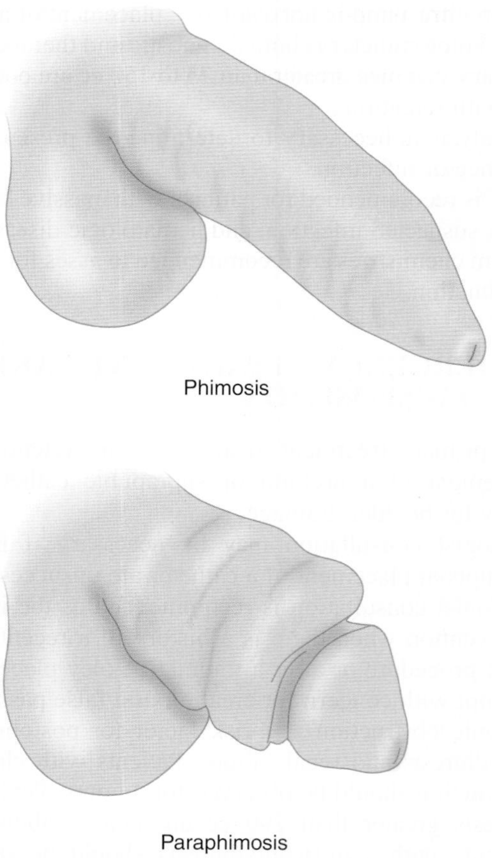

FIG. 57-2. Phimosis and paraphimosis.

- Need for circumcision after phimoisis can often be averted by application of topical steroids (eg, triamcinolone 0.025% bid for 4-6 weeks).
- *Paraphimosis* is the inability to reduce the proximal edematous foreskin distally over the glans (see Fig. 57-2). Paraphimosis is a true urologic emergency because resulting glans edema and venous engorgement can progress to arterial compromise and gangrene.
- If surrounding tissue edema can be successfully compressed, as by wrapping the glans with 2 × 2-in. elastic bandages for 5 minutes, the foreskin may be reduced. Making several puncture wounds with a small (22- to 25-gauge) needle may help with expression of glans edema fluid.
- Local anesthetic block of the penis is helpful for paraphimosis if patients cannot tolerate the discomfort associated with edema compression and removal. If arterial compromise is suspected, local lidocaine (1% without epinephrine) infiltration of the constricting band, followed by superficial vertical incision of the band, will decompress the glans and allow foreskin reduction.
- *Penile entrapment injuries* occur when various objects are wrapped around the penis. Such objects should be removed, and imaging is often necessary to confirm urethral integrity (retrograde urethrogram) and distal penile arterial blood supply (Doppler studies).
- *Penile fracture* occurs when there is an acute tear of the penile tunica albuginea. The penis is acutely swollen, discolored, and tender in a patient with history of intercourse-related trauma accompanied by a snapping sound. Urologic consultation is indicated.
- *Peyronie's disease* presents with patients noting sudden or gradual onset of dorsal penile curvature with erections. Examination reveals a thickened plaque on the dorsal penile shaft. Assurance and urologic follow-up are indicated.
- *Priapism* is a painful pathologic erection, which may be associated with urinary retention. Infection and impotence are other complications. In most cases, the initial therapy for priapism is terbutaline 0.25 to 0.5 milligram (repeated in 20 minutes if needed) injected subcutaneously in the deltoid area.
- Patients with priapism from sickle cell disease are usually treated with simple or exchange transfusion. Corporal aspiration and irrigation with either normal saline solution or an α-adrenergic agonist (ie, phenylephrine) is the next step and may need to be performed by the emergency physician. Even when emergency physicians provide stabilizing care, urologic consultation is indicated in all cases.

TESTICULAR TORSION

CLINICAL FEATURES

- Due to potential for infarction and infertility, testicular torsion must be the primary consideration in any male complaining of testicular pain.
- Though torsion is most common in the peripubertal period (when hormonal stimulation is maximal), this organ-threatening emergency may occur at any age.
- Pain usually occurs suddenly, is severe, and is felt in either the lower abdominal quadrant, the inguinal canal, or the testis.
- The finding with the highest sensitivity (99%) is unilateral absence of the cremasteric reflex.
- Though pain may follow strenuous activity such as athletics, torsion also occurs during sleep (when unilateral cremasteric contraction is the cause). The pain may be constant or intermittent but is not positional, since torsion is primarily an ischemic event.

DIAGNOSIS AND DIFFERENTIAL

- When the diagnosis is obvious, urologic consultation is indicated for exploration, since confirmatory imaging can be too time consuming. With acute torsion, testicular salvage is related to the duration of symptoms before surgical detorsion.
- Excellent salvage rates are expected with detorsion within 6 hours of symptoms, but testicular preservation rates decline rapidly with longer delays to intervention. A rapid evaluation should be performed regardless of the duration of the symptoms. The emergency physician should move as expeditiously as possible in cases of suspected torsion.
- In indeterminate cases, color-flow duplex ultrasound, and less commonly radionuclide imaging, may be helpful. Both techniques are subject to limitations associated with need for timely test availability and image interpretation.
- Compared to radionuclide imaging, ultrasound offers the advantage of providing additional information about scrotal anatomy and differential diagnoses; however, ultrasound is more likely than radionuclide imaging to yield indeterminant results.
- *Torsion of the testicular appendage* is more common than testicular torsion but is not dangerous, since the appendix testis and appendix epididymis have no known function. If the patient is seen early, diagnosis can be supported by the following: pain is most intense near the head of the testis or epididymis; there is an isolated tender nodule; or there is a (pathognomonic) blue-dot appearance of a cyanotic appendage transilluminated through thin prepubertal scrotal skin.

- The differential for testicular torsion also includes epididymitis, inguinal hernia, hydrocele, and scrotal hematoma.

EMERGENCY DEPARTMENT CARE AND DISPOSITION

- The emergency physician can attempt manual detorsion. Most testes twist in a lateral-to-medial direction, so detorsion is performed in a medial-to-lateral direction, similar to the opening of a book (see Fig. 57-3).
- The endpoint for successful detorsion is pain relief; worsening of pain with detorsion may indicate the need for attempts at detorsion by lateral-to-medial rotation.
- Regardless of whether detorsion appears successful, urologic referral is indicated.
- If normal intratesticular blood flow can be demonstrated with color Doppler, immediate surgery is not necessary for torsion of the appendages, since most appendages calcify or degenerate over 10 to 14 days and cause no harm.
- If the diagnosis cannot be ensured, urologic exploration is needed to rule out testicular torsion.

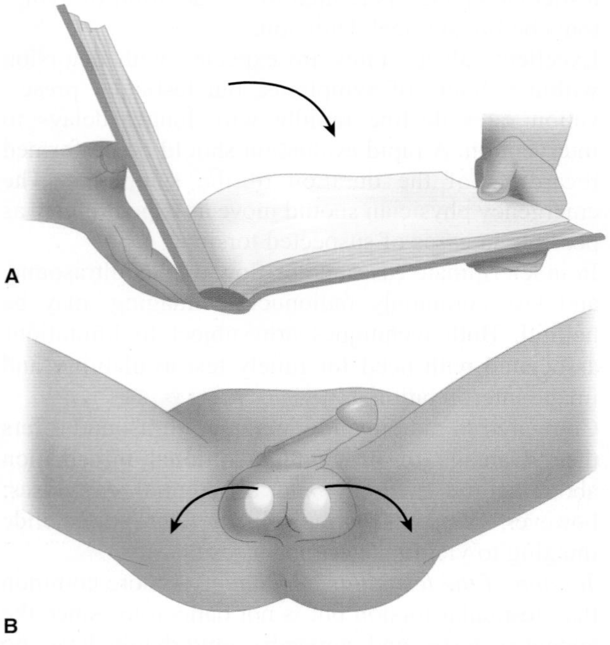

FIG. 57-3. Testicular detorsion. This procedure is best done standing at the foot of or on the right side of the patient's bed. **A.** The torsed testis is detorsed in a fashion similar to opening a book. **B.** The patient's right testis is rotated counterclockwise, and the left testis is rotated clockwise. (Reproduced with permission from Strange GR, Ahrens WR, Schafermeyer RW, et al: Pediatric Emergency Medicine, 3rd ed. © 2009, McGraw-Hill, Inc., New York, NY, p. 679.)

- Consider testicular torsion in the differential of any male presenting with abdominal pain.

EPIDIDYMITIS AND ORCHITIS

CLINICAL FEATURES

- Epididymitis, an inflammatory process, is characterized by gradual onset of pain.
- Bacterial infection is the most common etiology, with infecting agent identity varying with patient age.
- In patients younger than 40 years old, epididymitis is primarily due to sexually transmitted diseases (STDs); culture or DNA probe analysis for gonococci and *Chlamydia* is indicated in patients <40 years old, even in the absence of urethral discharge. In older men (>40 years), common urinary pathogens predominate.
- Epididymitis causes lower abdominal, inguinal canal, scrotal, or testicular pain, alone or in combination. Urinalysis may show pyuria in about half of the patients.
- Due to the inflammatory nature of the pain, patients with epididymitis may note transient pain relief when elevating the scrotal contents while recumbent (positive Prehn's sign).

DIAGNOSIS AND DIFFERENTIAL

- Initially, tenderness is well localized to the epididymis, but progression of inflammation and swelling-mediated obliteration of the sulcus between the epididymis and testis results in the physical examination finding of a single, large testicular mass (epididymoorchitis).
- Orchitis in isolation is rare; it usually occurs with viral or syphilitic disease and is treated with disease-specific therapy, symptomatic support, and urologic follow-up.
- Testicular malignancy should be suspected in patients presenting with asymptomatic testicular mass, firmness, or induration. Ten percent of tumors present with pain due to hemorrhage within the tumor. Urgent urologic follow-up is indicated.

EMERGENCY DEPARTMENT CARE AND DISPOSITION

- If the patient appears toxic, admission for intravenous antibiotics is indicated (treatment is based on the presumed etiology).
- Outpatient treatment is the norm in patients who do not appear toxic; urologic follow-up within a week is indicated.

- In patients age <40, treatment is aimed toward gonorrhea and *Chlamydia* with doxycycline 100 milligrams twice daily for 10 days after IM ceftriaxone while in the ED. In patients age >40 treatment is directed toward gram-negative bacilli with ciprofloxacin 500 milligrams twice daily for 10 to 14 days or levofloxacin 250 milligrams daily for 10 to 14 days
- Additionally, scrotal elevation, ice application, nonsteroidal anti-inflammatory drugs (NSAIDs), opioids for analgesia, and stool softeners are indicated.
- Orchitis is treated with disease-specific therapy, symptomatic support, and urologic follow-up. Patients at risk for syphilitic disease should be treated as directed in Chapter 89, Sexually Transmitted Diseases.

ACUTE PROSTATIS

- Patient complaints may include back pain, perineal, suprapubic, or genital discomfort, urinary obstruction, fever, or chills.
- Diagnosis is clinical as the urinalysis and urine culture may both be negative.
- Initial treatment is fluoroquinolone antimicrobial therapy for 30 days.
- An alternative approach is trimethoprim-sulfamethoxazole double strength (DS), one tablet PO twice daily for 30 days.

URETHRA

URETHRITIS

- Characterized by purulent or mucopurulent urethral discharge. The diagnosis is clinical and most cases are due to *Neisseria gonorrhea* or *Chlamydia trachomatis*; see also Chapter 89.
- Physical examination should exclude other disorders such as epididymitis, disseminated gonococccemia, or Reiter sydrome.
- Treatment is ceftriazone 125 milligrams IM, administered with either azithromycin 1 gram PO × 1 or doxycycline 100 milligrams PO bid for 10 days.

URETHRAL STRICTURE

- Urethral stricture is becoming more common due to the rising incidence of STDs. If a patient's bladder cannot be cannulated with a 14F or 16F Foley or Coudé catheter, the differential diagnosis includes urethral stricture, voluntary external sphincter spasm, bladder neck contracture, or benign prostatic hypertrophy; see also Chapter 56, Acute Unrinary Retension.
- Retrograde urethrography can be performed to delineate the location and extent of urethral stricture. Endoscopy is necessary to confirm bladder neck contracture or define the extent of an obstructing prostate gland.
- Suspected voluntary external sphincter spasm can be overcome by holding the patient's penis upright and encouraging him to relax his perineum and breathe slowly during the procedure.
- After no more than three gentle attempts to pass a 12F Coudé catheter into a urethra prepared with anesthetic lubricant, urology consultation should be obtained.
- In an emergency situation, suprapubic cystostomy can be performed; see Chapter 56.
- Urologic follow-up should occur within 2 to 3 days.

URETHRAL FOREIGN BODIES

- Urethral foreign bodies are associated with bloody urine and slow, painful urination.
- Radiographs of the bladder and urethral areas may disclose a foreign body.
- Removal of the foreign body may be achieved with a gentle milking action; retrograde urethrography or endoscopy is required in such cases to confirm an intact urethra.
- Often, urologic consultation for endoscopy or open cystotomy is required for foreign-body removal.

For further reading in Tintinalli's *Emergency Medicine: A Comprehensive Study Guide,* 7th ed., see Chapter 96, "Male Genital Problems," by Bret A. Nicks and David E. Manthey.

58 UROLOGIC STONE DISEASE

Geetika Gupta

- The acute phenomenon of renal stones migrating down the ureter is referred to as renal colic.

EPIDEMIOLOGY

- Urinary stones are three times more common in males and usually occur in the third to fifth decades.
- Overall incidence is around 12%.

- There is an increased incidence from genetic predisposition and hereditary diseases (eg, renal tubular acidosis, hyperparathyroidism, cystinuria).
- Lifestyle factors augment stone growth. Increasing water intake results in a decreased incidence of calculi. Patients in mountainous, desert, or tropical regions, and those in sedentary jobs suffer a higher frequency of stone disease.
- Medications such as protease inhibitors to treat HIV (indinavir sulfate), laxatives, and diuretics have also shown an increase in prevalence.
- Approximately one-third of the patients suffer recurrences within 1 year and 50% in 5 years.
- Children less than 16 years of age constitute approximately 7% of all cases of renal stones with a 1:1 sex distribution.
- Common etiologies in pediatrics are metabolic abnormality (50%), urologic anomalies (20%), infection (15%), and immobilization syndrome (5%).

PATHOPHYSIOLOGY

- The precise cause of urinary stone formation is unknown. What is known is that it requires three elements: supersaturation, lack of inhibitors, and stasis.
- Approximately 75% of calculi are composed of calcium, occurring in conjunction with oxalate, phosphate, or a combination of both. Calcium excretion is elevated in conditions such as high dietary calcium intake, immobilization syndrome, or hyperparathyroidism. Oxalate excretion is enhanced in patients with inflammatory bowel disease and as a result of small bowel bypass surgery.
- Ten percent to 15% of stones are magnesium-ammonium-phosphate (struvite). These are associated with infection by urea-splitting bacteria and are the most common cause of staghorn calculi. Urea-splitting organisms include *Proteus, Klebsiella, Staphylococcus* species, *Providencia,* and *Corynebacterium*. Antibiotic penetration into these calculi is low and makes patients with stones prone to urosepsis, thus surgical removal of staghorn calculi is recommended.
- Uric acid causes 10% of uroliths, with cystine and other uncommon stones making up the remainder. Twenty-five percent of patients with gout will have a kidney stone.
- The majority (90%) of urinary calculi are radiopaque. Calcium phosphate and calcium oxalate stones have a density similar to bone.
- Common areas of impaction include the ureteropelvic junctions (UPJs), pelvic brim, and ureterovesical junction (UVJ). The UVJ has the smallest diameter of the urinary tract and is the most common location for impacted stones.

CLINICAL FEATURES

- Patients are usually asymptomatic until there is at least a partial obstruction.
- Patients complain of the acute onset of severe pain, which can be associated with diaphoresis, nausea, and emesis. During extreme presentations, the patient is anxious, pacing or writhing, and may be unable to hold still or converse.
- Hematuria is present in 85% of patients.
- Typically pain originates in flank, radiating ipsilaterally and anteroinferiorly around the abdomen and toward the ipsilateral groin. The radiating pattern is the result of autonomic nerve fibers serving both the kidney and respective gonad. Anterior abdominal pain may radiate back toward the flank and is associated with midureteral stones. Stones near the bladder may cause urinary frequency and urgency.
- Young pediatric patients present as nonspecific abdominal pain. Twenty percent to 30% of children diagnosed with ureteral stones may present with painless hematuria.
- During acute obstruction the serum creatinine is unchanged due to the unaffected kidney functions up to 185% of its baseline capacity.
- Stone size determines the likelihood of spontaneous passage. Seventy-five percent of stones <5 mm will pass spontaneously within 4 weeks, 60% of stones 5 to 7 mm, and only 39% of stones >7 mm will pass spontaneously within 4 weeks.
- Irregularly shaped stones with spicules and sharp edges will have a lower passage rate. Rates of passage for stones found in the proximal, middle, and distal ureter are approximately 20%, 50%, and 70%, respectively, regardless of stone size.
- Extracorporeal shock wave lithotripsy (ESWL) is used as an aid to fracture stones into small particles using focused sound waves. The resulting sludge is passed in the urine. When there are large fragments left, an acute episode of renal colic re-occurs. The presentation is identical to the de novo episodes of renal colic.
- Stones with obstruction for >3 weeks will lead to irreversible renal parenchyma damage.

DIAGNOSIS AND DIFFERENTIAL

- All patients with suspected renal colic need a urinalysis to exclude infection. In 11% to 15% of the cases, there is no blood found in the urine. If there is evidence of pyuria, cultures and sensitivities are recommended due to the likelihood of needing prolonged antibiotic therapy. Blood urea nitrogen and creatinine levels should be considered as many patients with stones as they may have a reduced creatinine clearance.

More importantly, 25% of patients with flank pain and hematuria do not have radiographic evidence of nephrolithiasis. As a consequence, other diagnoses must be considered.

- The differential diagnosis in these patients includes a symptomatic abdominal aortic aneurysm, aortic dissection, incarcerated hernia, epididymitis, testicular torsion, ectopic pregnancy, salpingitis, pyelonephritis, papillary necrosis (due to sickle cell disease, diabetes, nonsteroidal analgesic abuse, or infection), renal infarction, appendicitis, diverticulitis, mesenteric ischemia, herpes zoster, drug-seeking behavior, and musculoskeletal strain. A right ureteral stone can also resemble cholecystitis. This list is not exhaustive.
- All female patients of childbearing age should have a pregnancy test.
- Intravenous pyelogram (IVP) yields information regarding renal function as well as anatomy. The first and most reliable indication of the presence of obstruction is a delay in the appearance of the nephrogram. Adjuncts to diagnosis include distension of the renal pelvis, calyceal distortion, dye extravasation, hydronephrosis, and visualization of the entire ureter.
- The sensitivity of an IVP is 64% to 90% and the specificity is 94% to 100%. A falsely negative IVP infrequently occurs when there is a radiolucent, partially obstructing stone.
- Advantages of the IVP are that it provides information on renal function and the degree of obstruction. The major disadvantages are time to perform the examination, contrast allergy, and the risk of nephrotoxicity.
- Noncontrast helical computed tomography (CT) is the diagnostic procedure of choice in the emergency department (ED). This modality should be strongly considered in first time stone presentation. The sensitivity is 95% to 97% and the specificity is 96% to 98%. Advantages of CT include its speed and that it avoids the risk of contrast allergy and can identify other pathologies. The disadvantage is that it doesn't evaluate for renal function and the sensitivity and specificity for other diagnoses is low.
- Positive findings on CT for obstructive stone include ureteral caliber changes, suspicious calcifications, stranding of perinephric fat, increase in renal size, and dilation of the collecting system (see Fig. 58-1).
- Ultrasound (US) is reserved for patients unable to undergo an IVP or CT. US is not a functional test and provides anatomic information only. It is useful in the detection of hydronephrosis and larger stones (>5 mm) in the proximal and distal ureter (see Fig. 58-2).
- The kidney-ureter-bladder (KUB) radiograph's greatest utility is in following the migration of a known stone. Ninety percent ureteral stones are composed of calcium phosphate and calcium oxalate and are radiopaque. Radiopaque stones appear 20% greater than their original size.
- Summary of radiographic imaging is in Table 58-1.

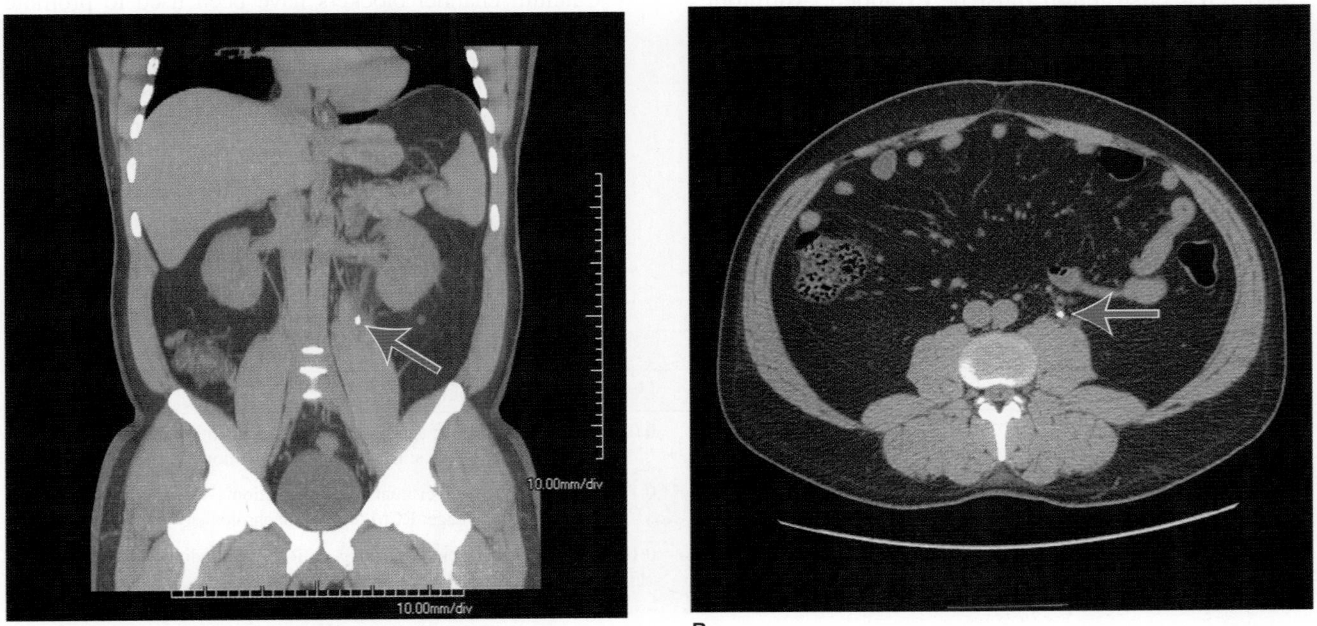

A B

FIG. 58-1. **A.** Red arrow shows 6-mm stone within the proximal third of the left ureter on noncontrast CT reformatted image of upright abdomen. **B.** From same patient as in **A**, note 6-mm stone (*arrow*) within the proximal third of the left ureter on noncontrast CT.

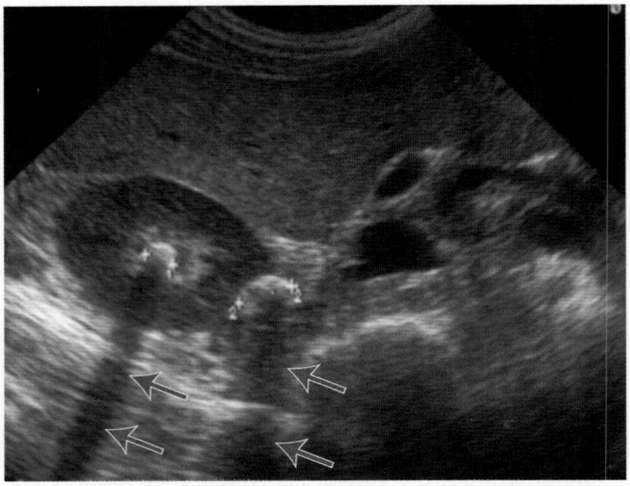

FIG. 58-2. US of renal pelvis showing stones (marked with 1+ and 2+) with shadowing effects (*arrows*).

EMERGENCY DEPARTMENT CARE AND DISPOSITION

- Patients are treated symptomatically. Pain medication including narcotics and nonsteroidal anti-inflammatory drugs should not be delayed pending test results. Intravenous antiemetic should be used. Intravenous fluids have not been shown to promote expulsion of the stone.
- In cases complicated by urinary tract infection (UTI), routine cultures of urine and blood are indicated and renal obstruction must be excluded. Antibiotics should be started promptly while the patient is in the emergency department. Considerations for intravenous (IV) antibiotics include gentamicin or tobramycin, 3.0 milligrams/kg/d divided every 8 hours, plus ampicillin, 1 to 2 grams every 4 hours. One can also consider cefipime, 2 grams IV every 8 hours; ticarcillin-clavulanic acid, 3.1 grams every 6 hours; ciprofloxacin, 400 milligrams every 12 hours; or piperacillin-tazobactam, 3.375 grams IV every 6 hours. Local sensitivites should help guide therapy.
- Hospitalization is required if the patient has an infection with concurrent obstruction, solitary kidney and complete obstruction, hypercalcemic crisis, uncontrolled pain, urosepsis, acute renal failure, or intractable emesis.
- Disposition should be discussed with a urologist in patients with a stone >6 mm, renal insufficiency, severe underlying disease, IVP with extravasation or complete obstruction, or failed outpatient management.
- Discharge is appropriate in patients with rounded stones <4–5 mm, with no significant obstruction, and for whom pain is controlled by oral analgesics. Those patients with infection and no systemic signs of illness may be discharged on ciprofloxacin, 500 milligrams PO bid for 10 to 14 days; levofloxacin, 500 milligrams PO daily for 10 to 14 days; or cefpodoxime, 200 milligrams PO bid 10 to 14 days. The individual should have follow-up with urology in 48 to 72 hours with explicit instructions to return for fever, nausea, or systemic illness.
- Alpha-blockers are associated with increased rate of expulsion, decreased time to expulsion, and decreased pain with a number needed to treat of 3.3 and a 2- to 6-day improvement in time to expulsion. This should be considered in stones in the distal third of the ureter due to theorized increased alpha-receptors in this region. Tamsulosin (0.4 milligram daily), terazosin (5-10 milligrams daily), or doxazosin (4 milligrams daily) can be given daily for up to 4 weeks.
- Calcium channel blockers have been used to promote stone expulsion but have increased adverse effects of hypotension. Nifedipine-XL, 30 milligrams daily up to 8 weeks, has been used. The number needed to treat is 3.9 and time to stone expulsion is reported as <28 days. Steroids are being considered as an adjunct to medical propulsion therapy to improve rates of expulsion.
- Follow-up with a urologist is recommended for those patients with hematuria and no definitive diagnosis.

TABLE 58-1 Ancillary Tests in Urologic Stone Disease

TEST	SENSITIVITY (%)	SPECIFICITY (%)	LR^+	LR^-	COMMENTS
Noncontrast CT	94-97	96-99	24-∞	0.02-0.04	Advantages: speed, no RCM, detects other diagnoses Disadvantages: radiation, no evaluation of renal function
IV urogram	64-90	94-100	15-∞	0.11-0.15	Advantage: evaluates renal function Disadvantage: RCM (allergy, nephrotoxicity, metformin)
US	63-85	79-100	10-∞	0.10-0.34	Advantages: pregnancy, no RCM, no radiation, no known side effects Disadvantages: insensitive in middle third of the ureter, may miss smaller stones (<5 mm)
Plain abdominal radiograph	29-58	69-74	1.9-2.0	0.58-0.64	Advantage: may be used to follow stones Disadvantage: poor sensitivity and specificity

Abbreviation: RCM = radiocontrast media.

• Patients whose stones pass in the emergency department require no further treatment.

For further reading in *Emergency Medicine: A Comprehensive Study Guide*, 7th ed., see Chapter 97, "Urologic Stone Disease," by David E. Manthey and Bret A. Nicks.

59 COMPLICATIONS OF UROLOGIC PROCEDURES AND DEVICES

Roy L. Alson

LITHOTRIPSY

• Hematuria is common complication of extracorporeal shockwave lithotripsy, usually self-limiting and resolves in 1 to 2 days.
• Other post-procedure complications include nausea, vomiting, flank pain and bruising, fever, and renal calculi. All managed with supportive therapy. Monitor creatinine and urine output. Appropriate antibiotics for UTI and fever.
• Steinstrasse (street of stone) is a result of disperals of multiple fragments posttreatment that can obstruct ureters. Symptoms include ureterolithiasis: flank pain and hematuria. Stones may be seen on plain films. Treat like ureterolithiasis. If fully obstructed, repeat lithotripsy or percutaneous nephrostomy.
• Rare injury to viscus or abdominal organs by lithotripsy. Pain with or without signs of peritonitis. CT or US to rule out and surgical or urological consult.

COMPLICATIONS OF URINARY CATHETERS

• Infection is the most common complication of urinary catheters (3%-10% incidence of bacteria per day with 100% by day 30), with females, diabetics, elderly, debility, and BPH increasing risk.
• Presence of catheter interferes wth uriniary clearance of bacteria allowing colonization and/or infection. Longer term catheters are more likely to have polymicrobial infections.
• Antibiotic treatment of asymptomatic bacteriuria in a patient with a short-term catheter is not recommended.
• Pyuria is universal for patients with long-term (1 month) indwelling catheters; pyuria should not be used in the diagnosis of asymptomatic infection. Hematuria is a better indicator of infection.
• Catheter-related UTI in patients with indwelling urethral, indwelling suprapubic, or intermittent catheterization is defined by the presence of symptoms or signs compatible with UTI with no other identified source of infection along with $\geq 10^3$ colony-forming units/mL of ≥ 1 bacterial species in a single catheter urine specimen.
• Signs and symptoms compatible with catheter-related UTI include new onset or worsening of fever, rigors, altered mental status, malaise, or lethargy with no other identified cause; flank pain; costovertebral angle tenderness; acute hematuria; pelvic discomfort; and in those whose catheters have been removed, dysuria, urgent or frequent urination, or suprapubic pain or tenderness.
• In those patients with mild symptoms, treatment is ciprofloxacin 500 milligrams twice a day, or levofloxacin 500 milligrams once a day, or cefpodoxime 200 milligrams twice a day.
• Seven days is the recommended duration of antimicrobial treatment for patients with catheter-related UTI who have prompt resolution of symptoms (A-III), and 10 to 14 days of treatment is recommended for those with a delayed response.
• Pyelonephritis is the most common complication of catheter-related UTI with fever. Admission is frequently required (see Chapter 55, Urinary Tract Infections and Hematuria, for further antibiotic recommendations). Check urine cultures and blood cultures if septic (see Chapter 91 for septic shock). Replace the catheter if it has been in place >7 days.
• Other infectious complications in males include prostatits, urethritis, epididymits, and absecess. See Chapter 57, Male Genital Problems, for diagnosis and treatment.
• Damage to urethra from improper insertion can casue bleeding or creation of false passage. Urethral stricture or prostatic hypertrophy increases risk of injury. Consider use of coude tip catheter.
• Cessation of urine output suggests uretheral disruption or obstruction by clots. Inflation of retention balloon with catheter in urethra may also cause injury.
• Minor traumatic complications of urinary catheters may require no therapy, while major complications (such as bladder perforation or urethral disruption) require consultation with a urologist.

NONDRAINING CATHETER

• Obstruction is suggested if the catheter does not flush easily or if there is no return of the irrigant. Obstruction of the catheter by blood clots often creates a situation in which the catheter is easily flushed, but little or no irrigant is returned.

- If obstruction occurs, the catheter can be replaced with a triple-lumen catheter so that the bladder can be easily irrigated. If after clearing the bladder of all clots evidence of continued bleeding is present, urologic consultation is recommended for possible cystoscopy.
- Some physicians advocate the use of single-lumen catheters to lavage the bladder, as its larger lumen may aid in the evacuation of larger clots.
- Pericatheter leakage may be a result of catheter obstruction by clot or concretions (see bullets immediately above). If not due to obstruction, treat spasm with antispasmodics such as oxybutynin or dicyclomine.
- Make sure after placing catheter that foreskin is returned to normal position to prevent paraphimosis.

NONDEFLATING RETENTION BALLOON

- If the obstruction is distal, the result of a crush or defective valve, the catheter can be cut proximal to the defect. If this does not deflate the balloon, a lubricated guidewire can be introduced into the cut inflation channel in an attempt to clear the obstruction.
- The balloon can be ruptured within the bladder. However, consider urologic consultation prior to rupturing the balloon, as overinflation (using sterile water) often requires 10 to 20 times the normal balloon volume.
- Urologic consultation may be required if simple measures are not successful.

COMPLICATIONS OF PERCUTANEOUS NEPHROSTOMY TUBES

- Percutaneous nephrostomy is a urinary drainage procedure used for supravesical or ureteral obstruction secondary to malignancy, pyonephrosis, genitourinary stones, or ureteral strictures.
- Bleeding may occur, and most episodes can be managed with irrigation to clear the nephrostomy tube of clots. In resistant cases check complete blood count (CBC), renal function, and coagulation studies (as indicated by comorbidities).
- Treat the patient for hemodynamic instability and consult urology.
- Infectious complications of nephrostomy tubes range from simple bacteriuria and pyelonephritis to renal abscess, bacteremia, and urosepsis. Culture any wound drainage, start an antibiotic such as ciprofloxacin 400 milligrams IV, and consult urology.
- Mechanical complications, such as catheter dislodgement and tube blockage, can occur with these devices. The urologist has several techniques available to reestablish access to an obstructed nephrostomy tube.

COMPLICATIONS OF ARTIFICAL URINARY SPHINCTERS

- Artifical sphincter is a device that increases resistance around urethra and provides continence. Several types exist. Basic design is a cuff around urethera with tubing to a pump that moves fluid to cuff, constricting urethra.
- Postoperative complications include hematomas at implantation site. Infections are serious as they are periprosthetic. Appropriate antibiotics need to cover gram negatives and also skin flora. Removal of device is necessary.
- Patients with device in place should receive prophylactic antibiotics when undergoing procedures that may cause hematogenous seeding, such as dental procedures.
- Air in the fluid path of the sphincter may compromise function and pumps or tubes may fail. Urologic evaluation is warranted.
- Never introduce urinary catheter through an artificial sphincter.

COMPLICATIONS OF URETERAL STENTS

- Dysuria, urinary urgency, and frequency, as well as abdominal and flank discomfort, are common complaints in patients with ureteral stents. The baseline discomfort in a functioning, well-positioned stent can range anywhere from minimal to debilitating. However, an abrupt change in the character, location, or intensity of the pain requires further evaluation for stent malposition or malfunction.
- Ureteral stents may remain in place for weeks to months and often function with no complications during the entire period. However, stents can often become encrusted with mineral deposits and may obstruct.
- Complete obstruction of urine flow is possible, although this tends to occur more often in patients with stents in place for long-term use. These patients may require urologic consultation, and in some cases may require stent replacement.

URINARY TRACT INFECTION VERSUS STENT MIGRATION OR MALFUNCTION

- Changing abdominal or flank pain or bladder discomfort may be indicative of stent migration. Radiographic examination is indicated with comparison to a previous film to evaluate stent position, and urologic consultation with further studies to evaluate stent position may eventually be necessary.

- When a urinary tract infection occurs in the presence of a stent, stent removal is not mandatory, because most infections can be managed with outpatient antibiotics. However, if pyelonephritis or systemic infection is evident, then further evaluation and emergent intervention are indicated.
- Plain radiograph examination to check for stent migration, and urologic consultation for evaluation of stent migration and malfunction are indicated, as well as initiation of antibiotic therapy.

URINARY DIVERSION AND ORTHOTOPIC BLADDER SUSBSITUTION

- Ileal conduit most common urinary bladder diversion. Postoperative complications include bowel obstruction, pyelonephritis, renal insufficiency, and stoma breakdown or stenosis. Reflux of urine into implanted ureters is a major cause of these complications.
- Other newer techniques for neobladder construction now exist, with less urine reflux into ureters. Bacturia is common postprocedure.
- Diagnosis of infection should be made based on clinical findings including fever and flank pain or urine culture ($>10^4$ CFU/ML). Consult with urology for treatment recommendations if UTI is found.

For further reading in Tintinalli's *Emergency Medicine: A Comprehensive Study Guide,* 7th ed., see Chapter 98, "Complications of Urologic Procedures and Devices," by Elaine B. Josephson and Moira McCarty.

Section 9
OBSTETRICS AND GYNECOLOGY

60 VAGINAL BLEEDING AND PELVIC PAIN IN THE NONPREGNANT PATIENT

Thomas W. Lukens

VAGINAL BLEEDING

CLINICAL FEATURES

- Patients with the chief complaint of vaginal bleeding are commonly seen in emergency departments (EDs).
- History should include amount, duration, and characteristics of the bleeding along with reproductive and sexual history. Medications, presence of a bleeding diathesis, endocrine disorders, liver disease, and existence of GU and systemic symptoms should also be used in developing the differential diagnosis.
- Assessment of the abdomen and gynecological organs is necessary, as well as a speculum and bimanual examination.
- Conjunctival pallor, skin color, and changes in vital signs can indicate significant anemia.

DIFFERENTIAL DIAGNOSIS

- Sexual assault or genital trauma needs to be excluded in each prepubertal patient.
- Nonspecific vulvovaginitis is the most frequent cause of vaginal bleeding in prepubertal females. Specific etiologies, eg, candidiasis, *Escherichia coli, Shigella*, and pinworms, are less commonly seen.
- Less common causes of bleeding in this age group are precocious puberty and menarche, congenital abnormalities, and tissue sensitivity to soaps and chemicals.
- Bleeding with discharge suggests possible retained foreign body.
- In reproductive age women, abnormal vaginal bleeding may be uterine or cervical in origin.
- Primary coagulation disorders can be found in up to 20% of younger patients with menorrhagia.
- Common causes are anovulation, pregnancy, exogenous hormone use, uterine leiomyomas, pelvic infections, and polyps. Bleeding disorders and thyroid dysfunction are possible etiologies.
- Bleeding in postmenopausal women commonly is associated with exogenous estrogens, atrophic vaginitis, or endometrial lesions or other tumors.
- Dysfunctional uterine bleeding (DUB) is diagnosed only after structural or systemic causes are excluded.
- DUB may be ovulatory or anovulatory, typically anovulatory in perimenarchal and perimenopausal patients.
- Symptoms are prolonged menses, irregular cycles, or intermenstrual bleeding that is usually mild and painless, although severe bleeding may occur.

EMERGENCY DEPARTMENT CARE AND DISPOSITION

- Obtain a pregnancy test in all reproductive age patients to rule out pregnancy-related conditions causing bleeding.
- Other laboratory evaluations are guided by the history and examination.
- Hemoglobin/hematocrit to determine the extent of blood loss, coagulation studies, and thyroid functions, if appropriate.
- If necessary, pelvic ultrasound is the imaging modality of choice and may be obtained as an outpatient in stable patients.
- In those who are hemodynamically stable, no acute intervention is necessary.
- Unstable patients with persistent bleeding need IV resuscitation, consideration of blood products use, and emergent gynecological consultation.
- Estrogens may be used in cases of more severe bleeding; IV and PO have similar efficacy. Hormonal therapy should be deferred, until gynecologic evaluation, if any concern for malignancy.
- Withdrawal bleeding typically begins 3 to 10 days after the hormonal therapy is stopped.
- See Table 60-1 for drug therapy for excessive vaginal bleeding.

TABLE 60-1 Drug Therapy for Excessive Vaginal Bleeding

DRUG	NAME	DOSING
Conjugated estrogen IV	Premarin	25 milligrams every 4-12 hours until bleeding slows
Conjugated estrogen PO		2.5 milligrams every 6 hours for 7-10 days
Ethinyl estradiol + norethindrone PO	Ortho-Novum 1/35	35 micrograms + 1 milligram, 4 tabs daily for 7 days
Medroxyprogesterone PO	Provera	10 milligrams daily, add when bleeding subsides, for 10 days
Tranexamic acid (antifibrinolytic) PO	Lysteda	600-1300 milligrams every 8 hours for 3 days

PELVIC PAIN

- Gynecologic pathology is the usual cause, but referred pain from extrapelvic abdominal conditions needs to be considered. Pregnancy needs to be excluded.

CLINICAL FEATURES

- Differentiate pain as chronic or acute, intermittent or continuous, and determine its characteristics and location to aid diagnosis.
- Ruptured ovarian cysts, torsion, and obstruction typically present as unilateral sudden onset pain. Gradual onset suggests infection or enlarging mass lesion.
- Abdominal and gynecologic assessments, with speculum and bimanual examination, are essential. Other testing is guided by the history and physical examination.

DIAGNOSIS AND DIFFERENTIAL

- Primary dysmenorrhea—excessive pain with menstruation. Pain tapers as bleeding diminishes. Pain can radiate to lower back and thighs, and may be associated with nausea/vomiting.
- Treatment with NSAIDs is usually sufficient, hormonal contraceptives in some cases.
- Mittelschmerz—self-limited unilateral mid-cycle pelvic pain due to leakage of follicular fluid.
- Ovarian cyst—pain from leakage of cyst fluid or pressure on adjacent structures. Sudden onset suggests rupture. Pelvic US is generally diagnostic.
- Cysts less than 5 cm generally involute in 2 to 3 cycles. Follow-up with gynecologic provider recommended.
- Ovarian torsion—a surgical emergency. Sudden onset severe unilateral adnexal pain. Risk factors: pregnancy, large ovarian cysts or tumors, and chemical induction of pregnancy. US with Doppler flow images diagnostic of venous congestion early followed by arterial obstruction.
- Intermittent torsion possible and images during detorsion period can be normal.
- Endometriosis—endometrium-like stroma implanted outside of the uterus, most commonly the ovaries. Recurrent pain associated with menstrual cycle, dysmenorrhea, and dyspareunia are symptoms. Infertility may be associated with endometriosis.
- Nonspecific pelvic pain may be the sole finding on examination and definitive diagnosis usually not made in the ED. Ultrasound may show endometriomas.
- Fibroids (leiomyomas)—benign estrogen-dependent uterine smooth muscle tumors, often multiple, found in the middle or later reproductive years. Symptoms include pain, abnormal vaginal bleeding, bloating, dyspareunia, and possibly urinary complaints. Severe pain can result from torsion of a pedunculated fibroid or ischemia and degeneration of the tumor.
- Bimanual examination often can reveal a mass. Pelvic US is confirmatory. Treatment consists of analgesia and referral to a gynecologist.

EMERGENCY DEPARTMENT CARE AND DISPOSITION

- Most patients with pelvic pain can be discharged from the ED with gynecologic follow-up. Patients need to receive detailed discharge instructions about the signs and symptoms to expect and when to return. Reevaluation in 12 to 24 hours is appropriate if concerns remain.
- Analgesics should be offered and NSAIDs are effective for most conditions. Opioids such as oxycodone/acetaminophen (5 milligrams/325 milligrams) for several days can be used if appropriate.

For further reading in Tintinalli's *Emergency Medicine: A Comprehensive Study Guide*, 7th ed., see Chapter 99, "Vaginal Bleeding in the Nonpregnant Patient," by Laurie J. Morrison and Julie M. Spence and Chapter 100, "Abdominal and Pelvic Pain in the Nonpregnant Female," by Thomas W. Lukens.

61 ECTOPIC PREGNANCY AND EMERGENCIES IN THE FIRST 20 WEEKS OF PREGNANCY

Robert Jones

ECTOPIC PREGNANCY

EPIDEMIOLOGY

- Ectopic pregnancy (EP) occurs in 2% of all pregnancies and is the leading cause of maternal death in the first trimester.
- Twenty percent of EPs are ruptured at the time of presentation.
- Major risk factors include history of pelvic inflammatory disease; surgical procedures on the fallopian tubes, including tubal ligation; previous EP; diethylstilbestrol exposure; intrauterine device use; and assisted reproduction techniques.
- More than 50% of cases of EP occur in patients without recognized risk factors.
- This diagnosis must be considered in every woman of childbearing age presenting with abdominal pain.

PATHOPHYSIOLOGY

- EP is postulated to be caused by (1) mechanical or anatomic alterations in the tubal transport mechanism, or (2) functional/hormonal factors that alter the fertilized ovum.
- Tubal rupture is thought to be spontaneous, but trauma associated with coitus or a bimanual examination may precipitate tubal rupture. Tubal rupture may occur in the early weeks of an EP or as late as 16 weeks estimated gestational age.

CLINICAL FEATURES

- The classic triad of abdominal pain, vaginal bleeding, and amenorrhea used to describe EP may be present, but many cases occur with more subtle findings.
- Presenting signs and symptoms may be different in ruptured versus non-ruptured EP. Ninety percent of women with EP complain of abdominal pain; 80% have vaginal bleeding; and only 70% give a history of amenorrhea.
- The pain may be sudden, lateralized, and extreme, or it may be relatively minor and diffuse.
- The presence of hemoperitoneum causing diaphragmatic irritation may cause pain to be referred to the shoulder or upper abdomen.
- Vaginal bleeding is usually light; heavy bleeding is more commonly seen with threatened abortion or other complications of pregnancy.
- Presenting vital signs may be entirely normal even with a ruptured EP, or may indicate advanced hemorrhagic shock.
- There is poor correlation with the volume of hemoperitoneum and vital signs in EP. Relative bradycardia may be present even in cases with rupture and intraperitoneal hemorrhage.
- Physical examination findings are highly variable. The abdominal examination may show signs of localizing or diffuse tenderness with or without peritoneal signs.
- The pelvic examination findings may be normal, but more often reveal cervical motion tenderness, adnexal tenderness with or without a mass, and possibly an enlarged uterus.
- Fetal heart tones can be auscultated in advanced cases of EP. The presence of fetal heart tones cannot be used to rule out the presence of EP.

DIAGNOSIS AND DIFFERENTIAL

- Urine pregnancy testing (for urinary beta-human chorionic gonadotropin [β-hCG]) should be performed immediately.
- Dilute urine may result in a false-negative result; serum testing will give a more definitive result in such situations.
- The primary goal of ultrasound in suspected EP is to determine if an intrauterine pregnancy (IUP) is present (Fig. 61-1). The presence of a heterotopic pregnancy should be strongly considered in patients who have undergone assisted reproduction.

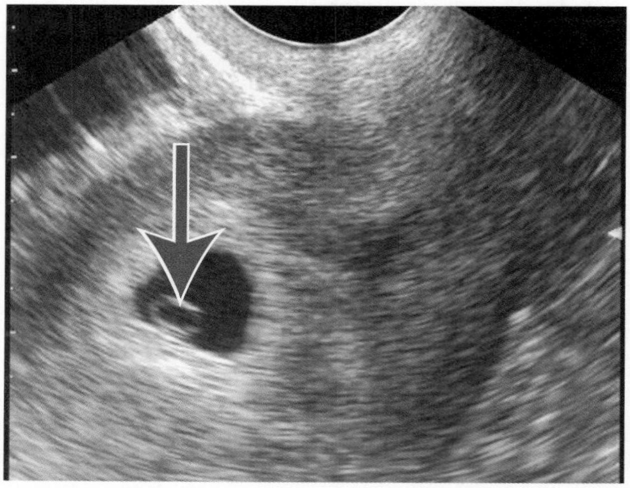

FIG. 61-1. Yolk sac (*arrow*) seen within an intrauterine gestational sac consistent with an early IUP. (Reproduced with permission from Ma OJ, Mateer JR, Blaivas M: *Emergency Ultrasound,* 2nd ed. © 2008, McGraw-Hill Inc., New York.)

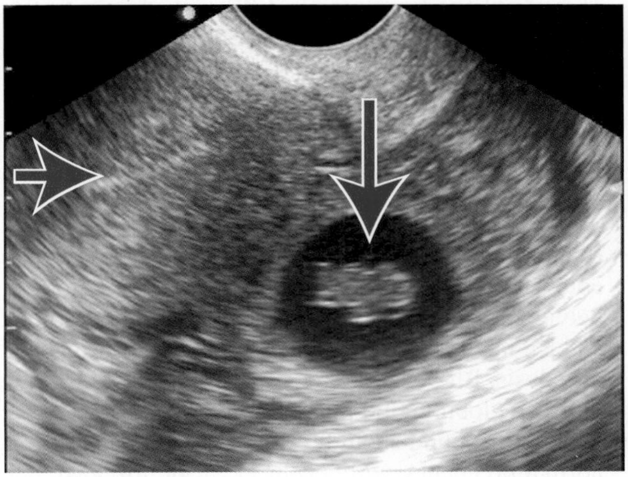

FIG. 61-2. Ectopic pregnancy. A living embryo in the adnexa and empty uterus is seen in this ectopic pregnancy (endometrial echo is visible in the left upper portion of the image). Embryonic cardiac activity was present on real-time imaging. Transvaginal image. *Horizontal arrow* points to empty uterus (uterine stripe) and *vertical arrow* to ectopic pregnancy in the adnexa. (Reproduced with permission from Ma OJ, Mateer JR, Blaivas M: *Emergency Ultrasound*, 2nd ed. © 2008, McGraw-Hill Inc., New York.)

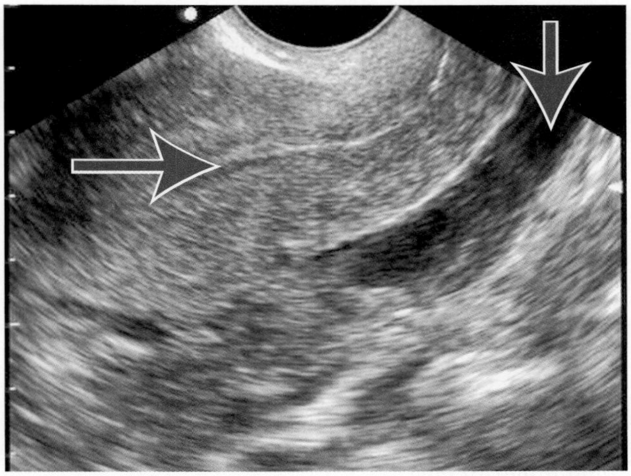

FIG. 61-3. Ectopic pregnancy: empty uterus and free fluid in the posterior cul-de-sac. Transvaginal sagittal image. *Horizontal arrow* points to empty uterus (uterine stripe), and *vertical arrow* points to fluid in the cul-de-sac. (Reproduced with permission from Ma OJ, Mateer JR, Blaivas M: *Emergency Ultrasound*, 2nd ed. © 2008, McGraw-Hill Inc., New York.)

- Transvaginal ultrasound is the test of choice to identify EP and should be performed in cases where transabdominal ultrasound is nondiagnostic.
- Definitive findings of an EP include the presence of an empty uterus along with visualization of extrauterine cardiac activity (Fig. 61-2).
- Findings suggestive of an EP include the presence of an empty uterus and any of the following: adnexal mass (other than a simple cyst) with or without free fluid in the abdomen or moderate/large amount of free pelvic fluid (Fig. 61-3).
- A normal pelvic ultrasound should be considered to be an indeterminate test and should be interpreted in light of the β-hCG levels.
- A β-hCG level above the discriminatory zone (1500 mIU/mL) and an empty uterus suggests EP.
- A β-hCG level below the discriminatory zone (1500 mIU/mL) and an empty uterus is indeterminate.
- A β-hCG level should never be used to determine the need for performing a pelvic ultrasound in the symptomatic patient.
- Failure of the β-hCG level to increase by 53% in 2 days is suggestive of EP or an abnormal IUP. However, an increase of 53% in 2 days does not rule out EP.
- Differential diagnosis in the patient presenting with abdominal pain, vaginal bleeding, and early pregnancy includes threatened, incomplete, or missed abortion; recent elective abortion; or endometritis.

EMERGENCY DEPARTMENT CARE AND DISPOSITION

- Treatment of patients with suspected EP is dependent on the patient's vital signs, physical signs, and symptoms. Close communication with the obstetric-gynecologic consultant is essential.
- For unstable patients, start two large-bore intravenous lines for rapid infusion of crystalloid and/or packed red blood cells to maintain blood pressure.
- Perform a bedside urine pregnancy test.
- Perform a rapid bedside, transabdominal ultrasound in the unstable patient after ABCs have been addressed.
- Notify an obstetric-gynecologic consultant immediately for the unstable patient, even before laboratory and diagnostic tests are complete.
- Draw blood for complete blood count (CBC), blood typing, and Rh (rhesus factor) determination (or crossmatching for the unstable patients), quantitative β-hCG determination (if indicated), and serum electrolyte determination as required.
- If the patient is stable, proceed with diagnostic workup, including transabdominal with or without transvaginal ultrasound. In reliable patients with indeterminate ultrasound results and a β-hCG level below 1000 mIU/mL, discharge with ectopic precautions and arranged follow-up in 2 days for repeat β-hCG determination and obstetric-gynecologic reevaluation is appropriate.

- Definitive treatment, as determined by the obstetric-gynecologic consultant, may include laparoscopy, dilatation and curettage (D&C), or medical management with methotrexate.

EMERGENCIES DURING PREGNANCY AND THE POSTPARTUM PERIOD

- The leading causes of maternal death are pulmonary embolus (see Chapter 27), EP (see Chapter 60), hypertensive disorders of pregnancy, hemorrhage, and infection.
- Risk increases with increased maternal age, increased birth order, lack of prenatal care, unmarried status, and minority race.

EMERGENCIES IN THE FIRST 20 WEEKS

THREATENED ABORTION AND ABORTION

Epidemiology

- Twenty to 40% of pregnancies abort spontaneously.

Pathophysiology

- Chromosomal abnormalities account for most fetal wastage. Risk increases with increasing maternal age and concurrent medical disorders, previous abortion, infections, and anatomic abnormalities.

Clinical Features

- Threatened abortion is defined as vaginal bleeding with a closed cervical os and benign physical examination.
- Inevitable abortion will occur with vaginal bleeding and dilatation of the cervix.
- Incomplete abortion is defined as partial passage of the conceptus and is more likely between 6 and 14 weeks of pregnancy.
- Complete abortion is passage of all fetal tissue before 20 weeks' gestation.
- Missed abortion is fetal death at less than 20 weeks' gestation without passage of fetal tissue for 4 weeks after fetal death.
- Septic abortion implies evidence of infection during any stage of abortion, such as pelvic pain, fever, cervical motion or uterine tenderness, and purulent or foul-smelling discharge.

Diagnosis and Differential

- The differential diagnosis includes EP and gestational trophoblastic disease (GTD). GTD is a neoplastic disease of trophoblastic tissue, and is distinguished from threatened abortion by ultrasound. These patients will have an abnormally large uterus and an abnormally high β-hCG level. It may be noninvasive (hydatidiform mole) or invasive (choriocarcinoma).

Emergency Department Care and Disposition

- Manage hemodynamic instability. Consult a gynecologist emergently in the unstable patient. Perform a pelvic examination, and obtain a CBC, blood typing and Rh factor determination, quantitative β-hCG, and urinalysis. Rh-negative women should receive Rh (D) immune globulin 300 micrograms IM.
- Pelvic ultrasound should reveal a gestational sac in a normal pregnancy with a β-hCG >1500 mIU/Ml, but an IUP cannot be definitively diagnosed until a yolk sac or embryo is visualized. Absence of a gestational sac with a β-hCG >1500 mIU/mL suggests complete abortion or EP. An excessively large uterus in which the placenta has many lucent areas interspersed with brighter areas is seen in GTD.
- Incomplete abortion or GTD requires D&C. GTD patients must receive close follow-up until quantitative β-hCG has returned to zero. Failure of the β-hCG to return to normal could indicate choriocarcinoma.
- Septic abortion requires gynecologic consultation and broad-spectrum antibiotics such as **ampicillin sulbactam** 3.0 grams IV or **clindamycin** 600 milligrams plus **gentamicin** 1 to 2 milligrams/kg IV.
- Patients with threatened abortion or complete abortion may be discharged with close follow-up arranged. Discharge instructions include pelvic rest (no intercourse or tampons) and instructions to return for heavy bleeding, fever, or pain.

NAUSEA AND VOMITING OF PREGNANCY

Epidemiology

- Nausea and vomiting in pregnancy occurs commonly in the first 12 weeks and affects between 60% and 80% of pregnant women.

Pathophysiology

- The pathophysiology is unknown.

Clinical Features

- The physical findings are usually normal in these patients with the exception of volume depletion.
- The presence of abdominal pain is highly unusual and should suggest another diagnosis.

Diagnosis and Differential

- Hyperemesis gravidarum (intractable nausea and vomiting without significant abdominal pain) can cause hypokalemia or ketonemia and may result in a low-birth-weight infant.
- Diagnostic workup should include a CBC, electrolyte panel, and urinalysis.

Emergency Department Care and Disposition

- Treatment consists of rehydration with IV fluid (5% dextrose in normal saline [D5NS] or 5% dextrose in lactated Ringer's [D5LR]), along with antiemetics, until ketonuria clears. Antiemetics that are frequently used are **metoclopramide** 10 milligrams IV, **promethazine** 25 milligrams IV (pregnancy class C, but widely used), or **ondansetron** 4 milligrams IV.
- Patients are candidates for discharge if they have reversal of ketonuria, correction of any electrolyte imbalance, and a successful trial of oral fluids. Patients should be discharged with an antiemetic.
- Patients admitted with intractable hyperemesis gravidarum may be candidates for methylprednisolone. This treatment should be initiated in consultation with the consulting obstetrician.

For further reading in Tintinalli's *Emergency Medicine: A Comprehensive Study Guide*, 7th ed., see Chapter 101, "Ectopic Pregnancy and Emergencies in the First 20 Weeks of Pregnancy," by Richard S. Krause, David M. Janicke, and Rita K. Cydulka.

62 COMORBID DISEASES IN PREGNANCY

Abigail Hankin-Wei

MEDICATION USE DURING PREGNANCY

- Table 62-1 lists recommendations for drug use during pregnancy.

DIABETES

- Diabetes in pregnancy increases patients' risk for complications of both pregnancy and diabetes, including preterm labor, spontaneous abortion, pyelonephritis, fetal demise, hypoglycemia, and diabetic ketoacidosis (DKA).

TABLE 62-1 Use of Medications in Pregnancy*

DRUG	CATEGORY†	COMMENTS
Antibiotic		
Cephalosporins	B	
Penicillins	B	
Erythromycin estolate	B	Maternal hepatotoxicity
Azithromycin	B	
Clarithromycin	C	
Nitrofurantoin	B	
Clindamycin	B	
Metronidazole	B	Fetal facial defects (1st trimester)
Ethambutol	B	
Quinolones	C, D	Toxicity to fetal cartilage
Aminoglycosides	C, D	Some of this class cause ototoxicity
Isoniazid	C	In TB, benefit may outweigh risk
Clavulanate combos	B	
Sulfonamides	C	Kernicterus (near term)
Tetracycline	D	Fetal bone/teeth anomalies
Trimethoprim	C	Folate antagonist (1st trimester)
Antivirals		
Acyclovir	B	
Zidovudine	C	Recommended in HIV+ mothers
Antihypertensives		
α-Methyldopa	B	
β-Blockers	C	
Calcium channel blockers	C	
Hydralazine	C	Frequently used
ACE inhibitors	D, X	Discontinue use at first sign of pregnancy
Anticonvulsants		
Valproic acid	X	Neural tube defects
Phenytoin	C, D	Fetal anomalies (benefit may outweigh risk)
Carbamazepine	C, D	Fetal anomalies
Corticosteroids	C	May exacerbate hyperglycemia
Anticoagulants		
Heparin	C	
Enoxaparin	B	
Warfarin	X	Nasal hypoplasia, optic atrophy

(Continued)

TABLE 62-1 Use of Medications in Pregnancy* (*Continued*)

DRUG	CATEGORY†	COMMENTS
Analgesics		
Acetaminophen	A	
Propoxyphene	C	Avoid close to term, neonatal withdrawal may occur
Opiates	C	
NSAIDs	B, C, D	Should not be used after 32 wk
Sumatriptan	C	
Ergot alkaloids	X	Potential for fetal death and abortion
Antiemetics		
Meclizine	B	
Diphenhydramine	B	
Metoclopramide	B	
Phenothiazine	C	Widely used
Ondansetron	B	
Vaccines		
Live vaccines (measles/mumps/rubella)	X	Potential exists for fetal transmission
Inactivated viral vaccines-rabies, hepatitis B, influenza	C	Commonly given in pregnancy
Pneumococcal vaccine	C	Avoid using in first trimester
Tetanus and diphtheria	C	Commonly given in pregnancy
Tetanus immune globulin	C	Commonly given in pregnancy

*Few studies have been done on pregnant women; therefore, any medication should be used only if clearly necessary. Consult drug reference for more information.

†A = safe, B = presumed safe, C = possible adverse effect, D = unsafe but use may be justifiable in certain circumstances, X = contraindicated.

Abbreviations: ACE = angiotensin-converting enzyme, HIV = human immunodeficiency virus, NSAIDs = nonsteroidal anti-inflammatory drugs, TB = tuberculosis.

- Insulin requirements increase throughout the pregnancy from 0.7 U/kg/d to 1.0 U/kg/d at term.
- Ketosis develops more quickly and at lower glucose levels during pregnancy. Risk factors for DKA include poor compliance, hyperemesis, and use of sympathomimetic tocolytic agents.
- DKA and hypoglycemia are treated the same as in the nonpregnant patient.

HYPERTHYROIDISM

- Hyperthyroidism in pregnancy increases the risk of preeclampsia and neonatal morbidity. Clinical features mimic those of normal pregnancy, and may present as hyperemesis gravidarum. Propylthiouracil (PTU) is the treatment of choice; side effects include rash and agranulocytosis.
- Thyroid storm presents with fever, volume depletion, and cardiac decompensation, and has a high mortality rate. Treat as in nonpregnant patients (see Chapter 133).

DYSRHYTHMIAS

- Pregnancy and labor can precipitate dysrhthmias.
- Supraventricular tachycardias should be treated with vagal maneuvers, then lidocaine, digoxin, procainamide, or verapamil in the usual doses.
- Cardioversion has not been shown to be harmful to the fetus.
- Amiodarone should be used only for life-threatening dysrhythmias not responsive to other measures, as iodine may lead to fetal neurotoxicity.
- Use unfractionated or low-molecular-weight heparin for anticoagulation.

THROMBOEMBOLISM

- Pulmonary embolism (PE) is the most common cause of maternal death in the developed world.
- The incidence of deep venous thrombosis (DVT) ranges between 0.5% and 0.7%.
- Factors associated with increased risk include advanced maternal age, increasing parity, multiple gestation, operative delivery (13- to 16-fold increase), bed rest, obesity, and hypercoagulable states.
- Doppler compression ultrasonography is the preferred test for symptomatic DVTs; some suggest a combination of negative D-dimer and negative doppler compression ultrasound.
- Perform lower extremity compression ultrasound in patients who do not meet low risk criteria. If negative for DVT, perform CT.
- Chest CT exposes the fetus to less radiation than ventilation-perfusion scanning, but exposes maternal breast tissue to a higher dose.
- Treatment of DVT and PE is with heparin or enoxaparin; warfarin is contraindicated.

ASTHMA

- Clinical features, diagnosis, and management are similar in pregnant and nonpregnant patients.
- Acute therapy includes nebulized β_2-agonists such as albuterol. Intravenous methylprednisolone and oral prednisone can be used in pregnancy.
- Supplementary oxygen should be administered to keep O_2 saturation above 95%.

- **Terbutaline** 0.25 milligram SC every 20 minutes can be used if necessary. Epinephrine should be used only in the critically ill patient.
- Criteria for intubation or admission are similar in pregnant and nonpregnant patients; standard agents for rapid-sequence intubation are used.
- Peak expiratory flow rates are unchanged in pregnancy.

URINARY TRACT INFECTIONS

- Urinary tract infection is the most common bacterial infection in pregnancy.
- Simple cystitis may be treated for 3 days with slow release **nitrofurantoin** 100 milligrams PO, or an oral cephalosporin.
- Patients with pyelonephritis should be admitted for IV antibiotics and hydration because of increased risk of preterm labor and sepsis. Antibiotic options include **cefazolin** 1 to 2 grams IV, or **ampicillin** 1 gram IV plus **gentamicin** 1 milligram/kg IV.
- Quinolones are contraindicated during pregnancy. Sulfonamides should be avoided in the third trimester, and trimethoprim should be avoided in the first trimester.

SICKLE-CELL DISEASE

- Women with sickle-cell disease are at higher risk for miscarriage, preterm labor, and vaso-occlusive crises.
- Clinical features, evaluation, and treatment are similar in pregnant and nonpregnant patients. Management includes aggressive hydration and analgesic therapy. Opioids should be used; nonsteroidal anti-inflammatory agents should be avoided after 32 weeks' gestation. Hydroxyurea should be discontinued in pregnancy.
- Parvovirus B19 may precipitate an aplastic crisis and is associated with development of hydrops fetalis.

HEADACHES

- Warning symptoms to suggest a life-threatening etiology of headache include acute onset, postpartum onset, neurological deficits, and papilledema or retinal hemorrhages.
- Migraines should be treated with acetaminophen, antiemetics, and opioids, if needed. Avoid ergot alkaloids and triptans.

SEIZURE DISORDERS

- Altered pharmacokinetics during pregnancy may lead to increased frequency of seizures.
- Management of a pregnant patient with a known seizure disorder is similar to that of a nonpregnant patient.
- Status epilepticus with prolonged maternal hypoxia and acidosis has a high mortality rate for the mother and infant and should be treated aggressively with early intubation and ventilation. Place the patient in the left lateral decubitus position to maximize placental oxygenation.

HIV INFECTION

- All pregnant HIV-infected women beyond 14 weeks' gestation should be on zidovudine therapy to reduce the risk of transmission to the fetus.
- Patients with CD4 counts <200 should be on prophylaxis for *Pneumocystis carinii* pneumonia. Treatment of opportunistic infections is unchanged in pregnancy.

SUBSTANCE ABUSE

- Cocaine use is associated with increased incidence of fetal death in utero, placental abruption, preterm labor, premature rupture of membranes, spontaneous abortion, intrauterine growth restriction, and fetal cerebral infarcts. Treatment of toxicity is unchanged in pregnancy.
- Opiate withdrawal in pregnant women is treated with **methadone** or **clonidine** (0.1-0.2 milligram SL every hour until signs of withdrawal resolve, up to 0.8 milligram total).
- Alcohol use contributes to increased rates of spontaneous abortion, low-birth-weight infants, preterm deliveries, and fetal alcohol syndrome.
- Benzodiazepines, a category D class, are best avoided in early pregnancy, but can be used in the context of a clinically unstable patient in alcohol withdrawal.

DOMESTIC VIOLENCE

- Approximately 4% to 20% of pregnant women are victims of domestic violence. They are at risk for placental abruption, uterine rupture, preterm labor, and fetal fractures. Rh immune globulin (Rhogam 300 micrograms IM) should be considered following blunt abdominal trauma in Rh-negative patients.

DIAGNOSTIC IMAGING IN PREGNANCY

- The risk of radiation exposure varies with gestational age. The second to the eighth week postconception is the period of organogenesis, the most vulnerable

period for birth defects. Mental retardation and other problems may occur after significant radiation exposures between weeks 8 and 25.
- Data suggest that exposures <5 rads do not increase risk of fetal death, or neurological/growth retardation. Total doses from multiple exposures are summative, with a cumulative dose of 10 rads thought to be the threshold for human teratogenesis.
- Ultrasound and magnetic resonance imaging exposures have not shown any teratogenic effects.

HYPERTENSION IN PREGNANCY

- See Chapter 63.

OTHER THROMBOEMBOLIC EVENTS

- See Chapter 27.

For further reading in Tintinalli's *Emergency Medicine: A Comprehensive Study Guide*, 7th ed., see Chapter 102, "Comorbid Diseases in Pregnancy," by Pamela L. Dyne and Matthew A. Waxman.

63 EMERGENCIES DURING THE SECOND HALF OF PREGNANCY

Howard Roemer

For essentially all conditions below, initiate immediate continuous fetal monitoring for a viable fetus.

VAGINAL BLEEDING

- Abruptio placentae, placenta previa, and preterm labor are the most common causes.
- Speculum and digital pelvic examination is contraindicated until ultrasound has been obtained to rule out placenta previa.
- Manage hemodynamic instability with lateral decubitus positioning, IV normal saline (NS), and/or packed RBCs.
- Obtain emergent obstetric consultation, CBC, type- and crossmatching leukoreduced packed cells, disseminated intravascular coagulation (DIC) profile, and electrolyte studies. Administer **Rh (D) immunoglobulin 300 micrograms** to all Rh-negative patients.

ABRUPTIO PLACENTAE

- Abruptio placentae is the premature separation of the placenta from the uterine wall.
- Risk factors include hypertension, advanced maternal age, multiparity, smoking, cocaine use, previous abruption, and abdominal trauma.
- Clinical features include abdominal pain, vaginal bleeding (may be absent), uterine tenderness, or fetal distress; DIC and fetal and/or maternal death may occur. Ultrasound has low sensitivity.
- Management is the same as noted above for vaginal bleeding. Emergency delivery may be needed to save the life of the fetus and/or mother. Avoid tocolytics.

PLACENTA PREVIA

- Placenta previa is the implantation of the placenta over the cervical os.
- Risk factors include multiparity and prior cesarean section.
- Clinical features include painless bright-red vaginal bleeding.
- Diagnosis is made by transabdominal pelvic ultrasound. Transvaginal US and pelvic examinations are contraindicated.

PREMATURE RUPTURE OF MEMBRANES

- Premature rupture of membranes (PROM) is rupture of membranes prior to the onset of labor.
- Clinical presentation is a rush of fluid or continuous leakage of fluid from the vagina.
- Diagnosis is confirmed by finding a pool of fluid with pH >7.0 (dark blue on nitrazine paper) in the posterior fornix, and ferning pattern on smear. Sterile speculum examination may be done; if possible, digital pelvic examination should be deferred or done with sterile gloves.
- Test for the presence of chlamydia, gonorrhea, bacterial vaginosis, and group B streptococci infections. Perform ultrasound to assess fetal age, weight, anatomy, amniotic fluid level.
- Patients with suspected PROM require obstetrics (OB) consultation for admission and possible delivery based on gestational age and possible antibiotics.

PRETERM LABOR

- Preterm labor is defined as labor prior to 37 weeks' gestation. It occurs in 10% of deliveries and is the leading cause of neonatal deaths.
- Risk factors include PROM, abruptio placentae, drug abuse, multiple gestation, polyhydramnios, incompetent cervix, and infection.

- Clinical features include regular uterine contractions with effacement of the cervix. The diagnosis is made by observation, with external fetal monitoring (initiated without delay) and serial sterile speculum examinations.
- Consult an obstetrician for admission and decision regarding tocolytics. If tocolytics are initiated, the mother should receive glucocorticoids to hasten fetal lung maturity (two doses of **betamethasone** 12 milligrams IM 24 hours apart or four doses of **dexamethasone** 6 milligrams IM 12 hours apart). Do not use tocolytics if abruptio placentae is suspected.
- Gestational age less than 34 weeks is associated with poorer outcomes; consider transfer to a tertiary care center with a high-risk intensive care unit if possible.

HYPERTENSION, PREECLAMPSIA, AND RELATED DISORDERS

- Hypertension in pregnancy may be chronic due to preexisting hypertension or gestational (preeclampsia, eclampsia and transient hypertension of pregnancy).
- Complications associated with hypertension in pregnancy include HELLP (hemolysis, elevated liver enzymes, and low platelets) syndrome, abruptio placentae, preterm birth, and low-birth-weight infants.
- Preeclampsia complicates 5% to 10% of pregnancies.
- The following associated findings may or may not be present in patients with preeclampsia:
  - Proteinuria
  - Oliguria
  - Headache or visual disturbances
  - Epigastric, and/or RUQ pain
  - Pulmonary edema or cyanosis
  - Hemolysis
  - Elevated liver enzymes
  - Thrombocytopenia
- HELLP syndrome often presents with abdominal pain; consider it in differential of pregnant women (at >20 weeks' gestation) with abdominal pain. Diagnosis is made by lab tests: schistocytes on peripheral smear, platelet count less than 150,000/mL, and elevated liver function tests. Obtain CBC, urinalysis, electrolyte panel, liver panel, and coagulation profile.
- Consult an obstetrician and initiate immediate continuous fetal monitoring.
- Hypertension treatment usually reserved for patients with BP >160 systolic and >110 diastolic: **labetalol** 20 milligrams IV as the initial bolus, with repeat boluses of 40 to 80 milligrams, if needed, to a maximum of 300 milligrams. A second option is **hydralazine** 5 to 10 milligrams IV initially, followed by 5 to 10 milligrams IV every 10 minutes. Eclampsia is treated with a **magnesium sulfate** loading dose of 4 to 6 grams over 20 minutes, followed by a maintenance infusion of 1 to 2 grams/h to prevent seizure. Serum magnesium and reflexes must be monitored. Definitive treatment requires delivery of the fetus.

EMERGENCIES DURING THE POSTPARTUM PERIOD

- Hemorrhage and infection are the most common postpartum complications presenting to the ED.
- Postpartum preeclampsia or eclampsia, amniotic fluid embolism, and postpartum cardiomyopathy are rare but life-threatening complications.
- Thromboembolic disease is common in the postpartum period.

POSTPARTUM HEMORRHAGE

- The differential diagnosis of postpartum hemorrhage includes uterine atony (most common), uterine rupture, laceration of the lower genital tract, retained placental tissue, uterine inversion, and coagulopathy.
- After the first 24 hours, retained products of conception, uterine polyps or coagulopathy, such as van Willebrand disease are more likely causes.
- The uterus is enlarged and "doughy" with uterine atony. A vaginal mass is suggestive of an inverted uterus. Bleeding in spite of good uterine tone and size may indicate retained products of conception or uterine rupture.
- Manage hemorrhage with crystalloid IV fluids and/or packed red blood cells if needed. Obtain CBC, clotting studies, and type and cross-match.
- Treatment of uterine atony consists of uterine massage, removal of the placental remnants and **oxytocin** 10 units IM or 40 units in 500 mL of IV solution given over 20 to 30 minutes until bleeding is controlled.
- Treatment of retained products of conception requires removing all placental remnants form the uterus. Ultrasound can help identify the retained material.
- When clinically significant bleeding continues despite taking the above measures, consult interventional radiology (if available) to identify and embolize the involved pelvic arteries.
- Minor lacerations may be repaired using local anesthetic. Extensive lacerations, retained products of conception, uterine inversion, or uterine rupture require emergency operative treatment by the obstetrician.

INFECTION

- Postpartum endometritis is usually polymicrobial. Risk factors include cesarean delivery, prolonged ruptured membranes or labor, younger maternal age, and internal fetal monitoring.
- Clinical features include fever, lower abdominal pain, foul-smelling lochia, uterine and cervical motion tenderness, and varying amounts of discharge. Obtain CBC, urinalysis (usually cath), and cervical cultures.
- Admission for antibiotic treatment is indicated for most patients.
- Antibiotic regimens include **gentamicin** 5 miligrams/kg IV plus **clindamycin phosphate** 2700 milligrams IV q 24 hours or **piperacillin/tazobactam**, 3.375 grams IV plus **gentamicin**, 5 milligrams/kg. (French LM, Smaill FM. Antibiotic regimens for endometritis after delivery. Cochrane Database Syst Rev. 2004;4: CD001067.)

AMNIOTIC FLUID EMBOLISM

- Amniotic fluid embolism is a sudden, catastrophic illness with mortality rates of 60% to 80%.
- Clinical features include respiratory distress, altered mental status, profound hypotension, coagulopathy and seizures.
- Intensive management for cardiovascular collapse and DIC is indicated.

MASTITIS

- Mastitis is cellulitis of the periglandular breast tissue.
- Clinical features include swelling, redness, and tender engorgement of the involved portion of the breast. Ultrasound may help differentiate between mastitis and abscess.
- Initiate treatment with **dicloxacillin** 500 milligrams orally four times daily or **cephalexin** 500 milligrams orally four times daily. **Clindamycin** 300 milligrams PO every 6 hours may be used in patients with penicillin allergy or if concerns about MRSA exist.
- Oral analgesics may be needed.
- Patients should continue nursing on the affected breast.

For further reading in Tintinalli's *Emergency Medicine: A Comprehensive Study Guide*, 6th ed., see Chapter 106, "Emergencies During Pregnancy and the Postpartum Period," by Gloria J. Kuhn.

64 EMERGENCY DELIVERY

Stacie Zelman

EPIDEMIOLOGY

- Precipitous delivery in an emergency is a relatively uncommon occurrence. However, when a patient in active labor does present to the ED, careful preparation and education can help avoid serious complications of labor and delivery.

CLINICAL FEATURES

- Any pregnant woman who is beyond 20 weeks' gestation and appears to be in active labor should be evaluated expeditiously. Evaluation includes maternal vital signs, especially blood pressure, and fetal heart monitoring.
- A persistently slow fetal heart rate (<100 beats/min) is an indicator of fetal distress.
- History should include time of onset of contractions, leakage of fluid, vaginal bleeding, and prenatal care.
- A focused physical examination should include an abdominal examination evaluating fundal height, abdominal or uterine tenderness, and fetal position. A bimanual or sterile speculum examination should be performed if no contraindications exist.
- False labor is characterized by irregular, brief contractions usually confined to the lower abdomen. These contractions, commonly called Braxton Hicks contractions, are irregular in intensity and duration.
- True labor is characterized by painful, regular contractions of steadily increasing intensity and duration leading to progressive cervical dilatation. True labor typically begins in the fundal region and upper abdomen and radiates into the pelvis and lower back.

DIAGNOSIS AND DIFFERENTIAL

- Patients without vaginal bleeding should be assessed with a sterile speculum examination and bimanual examination to assess the progression of labor, cervical dilation, and rupture of membranes.
- Patients with active vaginal bleeding require initial evaluation with ultrasound to rule out **placenta previa**.
- **Abruptio placentae** should be considered in patients with a tender, firm uterus and marked bleeding. However, bleeding does not have to be present.
- **Spontaneous rupture of membranes** typically occurs with a gush of clear or blood-tinged fluid. If ruptured membranes are suspected, a sterile speculum examination should be performed and amniotic

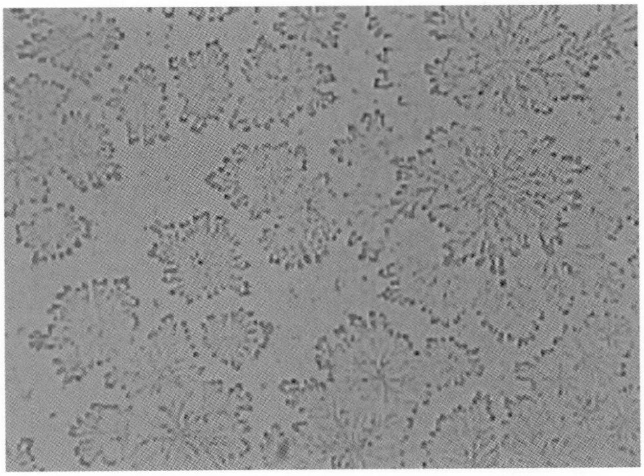

FIG. 64-1. Typical ferning of dried amniotic fluid

fluid obtained from the fornix or vaginal vault. Amniotic fluid is alkaline and will stain nitrazine paper dark blue and will "fern" if dried on a slide (Fig. 64-1). The presence of meconium in amniotic fluid should be noted.

- Avoid digital examinations in the preterm patient in whom prolongation of gestation is desired. Even one examination increases the chance of infection, especially if premature rupture of membranes is suspected.

EMERGENCY DEPARTMENT CARE

- If the cervix is dilated in a woman experiencing active contractions, further transport, even short distances, may be hazardous. Preparations should be made for emergency delivery.
- Assess fetal position by physical examination, and confirm by ultrasound, if possible.
- Place the patient in the dorsal lithotomy position.
- Notify an obstetrician, if one is available.

EMERGENCY DELIVERY PROCEDURE (FIG. 64-2)

1. **Control of the delivery** of the neonate is the major challenge.
   a. As the **infant's head** emerges from the introitus, support the perineum with a sterile towel placed along the inferior portion of the perineum with one hand while supporting the fetal head with the other.
   b. Exert mild counterpressure to prevent the rapid expulsion of the fetal head, which may lead to third- or fourth-degree perineal tears.
   c. As the infant's head presents, use the inferior hand to control the fetal chin while keeping the superior hand on the crown of the head, supporting the delivery.
   d. This controlled extension of the fetal head will aid in the atraumatic delivery.
   e. Ask the mother to breathe through contractions rather than bearing down and attempting to push the baby out rapidly.
2. After delivery of the head, palpate the neck for the presence of a **nuchal cord**.
   a. A nuchal cord is present in up to 35% of all cephalad-presenting deliveries.
   b. If the cord is loose, reduce it over the infant's head; the delivery may then proceed as usual.
   c. If the cord is tightly wound, clamp it in the most accessible area using two clamps in close proximity and cut to allow delivery of the infant.
3. After delivery of the head, the head will restitute or turn to one side or the other.
   a. As the head rotates, place your hands on either side, providing gentle downward traction to deliver the anterior shoulder.
   b. Then guide the fetus upward, delivering the posterior shoulder and allowing the remainder of the infant to be delivered.
4. Place your posterior (left) hand underneath the infant's axilla before delivering the rest of the body. Use the anterior hand to grasp the infant's ankles and ensure a firm grip.
5. Wrap the infant in a towel and stimulate it while drying.
6. Double clamp the umbilical cord and cut with sterile scissors.
7. Finish drying. Place the infant in a warm incubator, where postnatal care may be provided and **Apgar scores** calculated at 1 and 5 minutes after delivery. Scoring includes general color, tone, heart rate, respiratory effort, and reflexes.
8. Use of routine **episiotomy** for a normal spontaneous vaginal delivery is discouraged since it increases the incidence of third- and fourth-degree lacerations at the time of delivery.
9. If an episiotomy is necessary (eg, with a breech presentation), it may be performed as follows:
   a. Inject a solution of 5 to 10 mL of 1% **lidocaine** with a small-gauge needle into the posterior fourchette and perineum.
   b. While protecting the infant's head, make a 2- to 3-cm cut with scissors to extend the vaginal opening.
   c. Support the incision with manual pressure from below, taking care not to allow the incision to extend into the rectum.

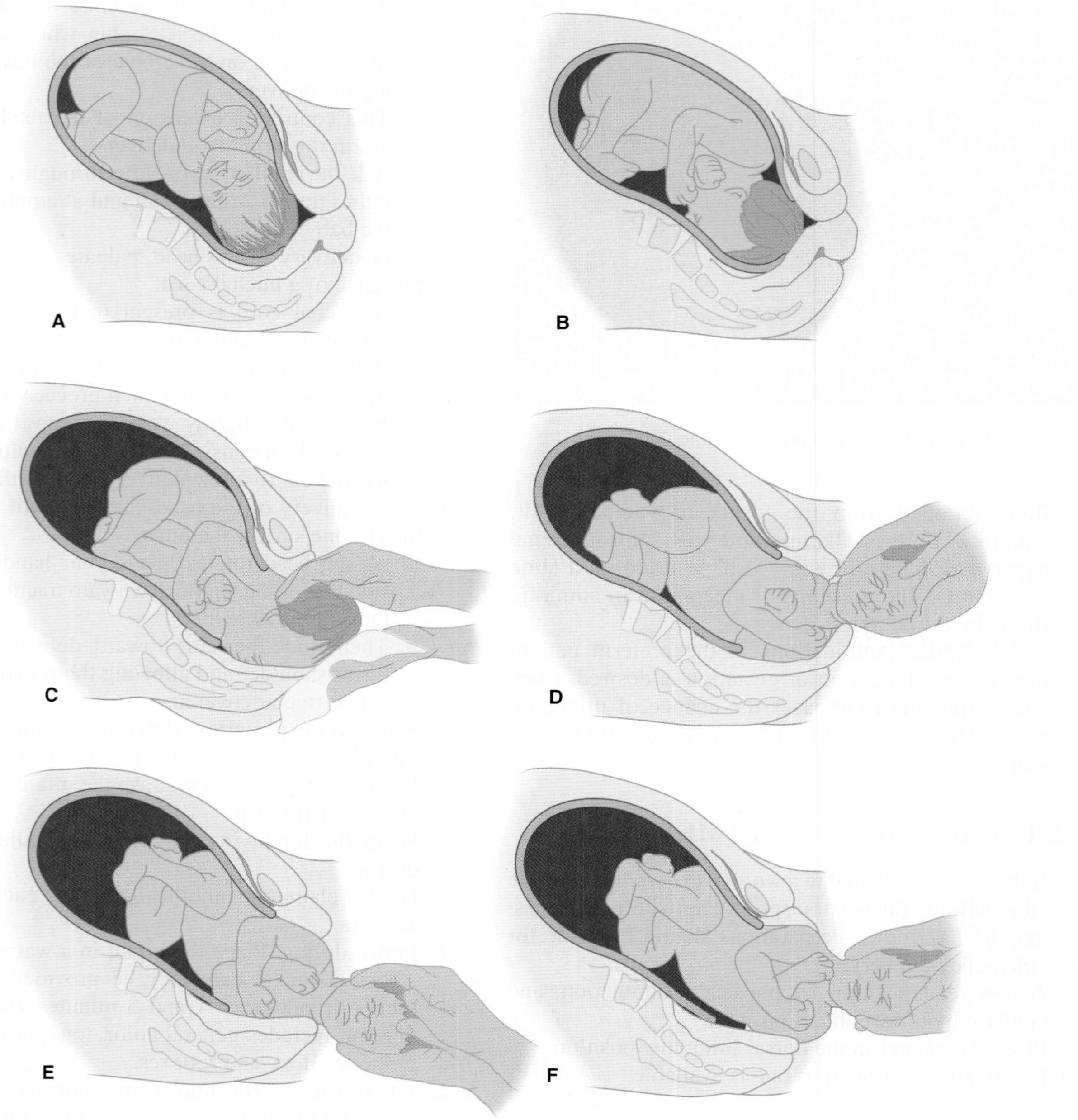

FIG. 64-2. Movements of normal delivery. Mechanism of labor and delivery for vertex presentations. **A.** Engagement, flexion, and descent. **B.** Internal rotation. **C.** Extension and delivery of the head. After delivery of the head, the neck is checked for encirclement by the umbilical cord. **D.** External rotation, bringing the thorax into the anteroposterior diameter of the pelvis. **E.** Delivery of the anterior shoulder. **F.** Delivery of the posterior shoulder. Note that after delivery, the head is supported and used to gently guide delivery of the shoulder. Traction should be minimized.

CORD PROLAPSE

If bimanual examination shows a **palpable, pulsating cord:**

a. Do not remove the examining hand; use the hand to elevate the presenting fetal part to reduce compression of the cord.
b. Immediate obstetric assistance is necessary, as a **cesarean section** is indicated.
c. Keep the examining hand in the vagina while the patient is transported and prepped for surgery to prevent further compression of the cord by the fetal head. Do not attempt to reduce the cord.

SHOULDER DYSTOCIA

- Shoulder dystocia first recognized after the delivery of the fetal head, when routine downward traction is insufficient to deliver the anterior shoulder. The anterior shoulder is trapped behind the pubic symphysis.
- After delivery of the infant's head, the head retracts tightly against the perineum ("Turtle sign").
- Upon recognizing shoulder dystocia, suction the infant's nose and mouth and call for assistance to position the mother in the extreme lithotomy position, with legs sharply flexed up to the abdomen (McRoberts maneuver) and held by the mother or assistant.
- Drain the bladder.
- A generous episiotomy also may facilitate delivery.
- Next, an assistant should apply suprapubic pressure to disimpact the anterior shoulder from the pubic symphysis.
- Do not apply fundal pressure because this will further force the shoulder against the pelvic rim.
- A Woods corkscrew maneuver may be attempted—place a hand behind the posterior shoulder of the infant, and rotate the shoulder girdle 180 degrees.

BREECH PRESENTATION

- The primary concern with breech presentation is head entrapment.
- Breech presentations may be classified as **frank, complete, incomplete**, or **footling.**
- In any breech delivery, immediate obstetric consultation should be requested.
- **Frank and complete breech presentations:**
  a. Serve as a dilating wedge nearly as well as the fetal head, and delivery may proceed in an uncomplicated fashion.
  b. Main point is to allow the delivery to progress spontaneously. This lets the presenting portion of the fetus to dilate the cervix maximally.
  c. Consult obstetrical texts for a detailed description of maneuvers for breech delivery.
- **Footling and incomplete breech positions** are not considered safe for vaginal delivery because of the possibility of cord prolapse or incomplete dilatation of the cervix.

POSTPARTUM CARE

- The placenta should be allowed to separate spontaneously and assisted with gentle traction.
- Aggressive traction on the cord risks uterine inversion, tearing of the cord, or disruption of the placenta, which can result in severe vaginal bleeding.
- After removal of the placenta, gently massage the uterus to promote contraction.
- Infuse **oxytocin** 10 to 40 U/1000 mL NS at a moderate rate to maintain uterine contraction. Oxytocin may also be given as 10 U IM.
- Episiotomy or laceration repair may be delayed until an experienced obstetrician is able to close the laceration and inspect the patient for fourth-degree (rectovaginal) tears.

For further reading in Tintinalli's *Emergency Medicine: A Comprehensive Study Guide*, 7th ed., see Chapter 105, "Emergency Delivery," by Michael J. VanRooyen and Jennifer A. Scott.

65 VULVOVAGINITIS

Stacie Zelman

EPIDEMIOLOGY

- Vulvovaginitis is a common gynecological complaint, affecting females of all ages.
- Bacterial vaginosis (BV) is the most common cause of vaginitis. Up to 50% of women with BV are asymptomatic. BV is associated with preterm labor and premature rupture of membranes (PROM).
- *Candida* is the second most common etiology of vulvovaginitis. Factors associated with increased rates of colonization include pregnancy, oral contraceptives, uncontrolled diabetes mellitus, and frequent visits to STD clinics. Infection is rare in premenarcheal girls and decreases in incidence after menopause unless hormone replacement therapy is used.
- *Trichomonas vaginalis* accounts for up to 20% of cases of vaginitis. The risk of infection increases with increasing numbers of sexual partners, early onset of sexual activity, and lower socioeconomic status. It is associated with preterm delivery, low birthrate, PID, and cervical cancer. *Trichomonas* is also associated with increased transmission of other STDs such as HIV, HSV, and HPV.

PATHOPHYSIOLOGY

- The pathophysiology of vulvovaginitis is related to inflammation of the vulva and vaginal tissues.

Causes include infection, irritants and allergens, foreign bodies, and atrophy.

- In females of childbearing age, estrogen causes the development of a thick vaginal epithelium with glycogen stores that support the normal flora. The glycogen is converted by lactobacilli and acidogenic corynebacteria to lactic acid and acetic acid that forms the acidic environment (pH 3.8-4.5) that discourages the growth of pathogenic bacteria.
- Causes of infectious vulvovaginitis include trichomoniasis, caused by *T. vaginalis*; bacterial vaginosis, caused by replacement of normal flora by overgrowth of both anaerobes and *Gardnerella vaginalis*; and candidiasis, usually caused by *Candida albicans*.
- Contact dermatitis results from exposure of vulvar epithelium and vaginal mucosa to chemical irritants or allergens. Secondary infections can occur.
- Retained foreign bodies can cause severe localized infections from *Escherichia coli*, anaerobes, or overgrowth of other vaginal flora.
- Atrophic vaginitis during menarche, pregnancy, and lactation, and after menopause, results from the lack of estrogen stimulation on the vaginal mucosa. Decreased estrogen results in loss of normal rugae, atrophy of squamous epithelium, and increase in vaginal pH.

CLINICAL FEATURES

- Bacterial vaginosis may present with a malodorous vaginal discharge and pruritus. The associated odor may be described as having a "fishy" smell. Examination findings range from mild vaginal redness to a frothy gray-white discharge.
- *Candida* vaginitis causes vaginal discharge, severe pruritus, dysuria, and dyspareunia. Examination reveals vulvar and vaginal erythema, edema, and thick "cottage cheese" discharge. Odor is an uncommon presenting symptom.
- *Trichomonas vaginalis* causes vaginal discharge, perineal irritation, dysuria, spotting, and pelvic pain. Examination reveals vaginal erythema and a frothy, malodorous discharge.
- Contact vulvovaginitis causes pruritus and a burning sensation. Examination reveals an edematous, erythematous vulvovaginal area.
- Vaginal foreign bodies can cause a bloody or foul-smelling discharge. Examination generally reveals the foreign body.
- Atrophic vaginitis causes vaginal soreness, dyspareunia, and occasional spotting or discharge. Examination reveals a thin, inflamed, and even ulcerated vaginal mucosa.

DIAGNOSIS AND DIFFERENTIAL

- A detailed gynecologic history should be obtained and a gynecologic examination performed.
- Microscopic evaluation of vaginal secretions using normal saline (demonstrating clue cells for BV and motile *T. vaginalis* for trichomoniasis) and 10% potassium hydroxide (KOH) (demonstrating yeast or pseudohyphae for candidiasis and fishy odor for BV) will frequently provide the diagnosis.
- Secretions from the sidewall of the vagina should be tested for pH using nitrazine paper. A pH greater than 4.5 is typical of BV or trichomoniasis. A pH less than 4.5 is typical of physiologic discharge or a candidal infection.
- Historically, bacterial vaginosis is diagnosed according to the Amsel criteria by three of the following four criteria: (1) thin, homogeneous discharge, (2) pH >4.5, (3) fishy odor when 10% KOH is added to the discharge (positive amine test result), and (4) greater than 20% clue cells, which are epithelial cells with clusters of bacilli stuck to the surface, seen on saline wet prep.
- *Candida* vaginitis is diagnosed microscopically by the presence of yeast buds and pseudohyphae. Using a 10% KOH solution will dissolve the epithelial cells, making the findings easier to see. Sensitivity is 80%.
- Trichomoniasis is diagnosed microscopically by the presence of motile, pear-shaped, flagellated trichomonads that are slightly larger than leukocytes. A wet prep for trichomonas may be negative in men.
- Contact vulvovaginitis is diagnosed by ruling out an infectious cause and identifying the offending agent.
- On wet preparation, atrophic vaginitis will show erythrocytes and increased polymorphonuclear leukocytes (PMNs) associated with small, round epithelial cells. These cells are immature squamous cells that have not been exposed to sufficient estrogen.

EMERGENCY DEPARTMENT CARE AND DISPOSITION

- Bacterial vaginosis is treated with **metronidazole** 500 milligrams PO twice daily for 7 days or **clindamycin** 300 milligrams PO twice daily for 7 days. All symptomatic patients should be treated regardless of pregnancy status. Pregnant women, particularly those at high risk for preterm labor, should be considered for treatment even if asymptomatic. The recommended treatment in pregnancy is **metronidazole** 250 milligrams PO three times daily for

7 days, but a single 2-gram PO dose is an alternative regimen. No treatment is necessary for male partners or asymptomatic women. Any patient receiving metronidazole should be counseled to abstain from drinking alcohol during treatment and for the 24 hours following completion of treatment.

- For trichomoniasis, **metronidazole** 2 grams PO in a single dose is the treatment of choice (or alternatively 500 milligrams PO twice daily for 7 days). Metronidazole gel is much less effective, and not recommended. Most infected men are asymptomatic; however, male partners need treatment to avoid retransmission of the disease. Patients should also be counseled to abstaining from sexual activity until the treatment regimen is complete. Any patient receiving metronidazole should be counseled to abstain from drinking alcohol during treatment and for the 24 hours following completion of treatment.
- Uncomplicated *Candida* vaginitis is treated with the topical imidazoles, such as **butoconazole 2% cream**—5 grams daily for 3 days *or* **clotrimazole** 100 milligrams—2 tablets/daily for 3 days *or* **miconazole** 200 milligrams vaginal suppository—1 suppository daily for 3 days. Alternative treatment for uncomplicated or complicated *Candida* is a single dose of **fluconazole** 150 milligrams PO. Treatment of sexual partners is not necessary unless candidal balanitis is present. Pregnant patients should receive topical treatment only.
- Contact vulvovaginitis is treated by removal of the offending agent. Cool sitz baths and wet compresses of dilute boric acid or Burow's solution may provide some relief. Topical corticosteroids can also be used to relieve symptoms and promote healing. Superinfections with *Candida* should be treated as previously discussed.
- Vaginal foreign bodies require removal of the object. No other therapy is necessary, unless superinfection is present.
- Atrophic vaginitis is treated with topical vaginal estrogen cream or tablets. Patients should be warned about possible side effects such as breast or perineal pain, and/or uterine bleeding. Estrogen should not be used if there is a history of cancer of any of the reproductive organs or postmenopausal bleeding. Refer patients to a gynecologist.

For further reading in Tintinalli's *Emergency Medicine: A Comprehensive Study Guide*, 7th ed., see Chapter 106, "Vulvovaginitis," by Gloria J. Kuhn and Robert P. Wall.

66 PELVIC INFLAMMATORY DISEASE

Stacie Zelman

EPIDEMIOLOGY

- Pelvic inflammatory disease (PID) is the most common gynecological complaint presenting to the ED, accounting for over 25,000 visits per year by women aged 15 to 44 years.
- Ten to 20% of untreated gonococcal or chlamydial cervicitis may progress to PID.
- Risk factors include multiple sexual partners, sexual abuse, young age, HIV-1 infection, bacterial vaginosis, history of other STDs, frequent vaginal douching, and use of intrauterine devices (IUDs).
- Risk is reduced with use of barrier contraception and pregnancy; however, PID can occur during the first trimester and may cause fetal loss.
- Bilateral tubal ligation does not confer protection from PID, but disease severity may be less.

PATHOPHYSIOLOGY

- PID represents an ascending infection from the lower genital tract. The spectrum of disease includes salpingitis, endometritis, tubo-ovarian abscess (TOA), and peritonitis.
- *Neisseria gonorrhoeae* and/or *Chlamydia trachomatis* are isolated in many cases, but not all.
- At least 30% to 40% of infections are polymicrobial and include anaerobes, such as *Bacteroides* species, aerobes such as *Gardnerella vaginalis*, enteric gram-negative rods, *Haemophilus influenzae*, and *Streptococcus agalactiae*, and endogenous genital tract mycoplasma such as *Mycoplasma hominis* and *Ureaplasma urealyticum*.
- *Neisseria gonorrhoeae* and *C. trachomatis* may be instrumental in the initial infection of the upper genital tract, whereas other bacterial species and anaerobes are isolated increasingly as inflammation increases and abscesses form.
- Infection may extend beyond the pelvis via direct or lymphatic spread to involve the hepatic capsule, resulting in perihepatitis and focal peritonitis (Fitz-Hugh–Curtis syndrome).

CLINICAL FEATURES

- Lower abdominal pain is the most common presenting complaint.

- Other common symptoms include abnormal vaginal discharge, vaginal bleeding, postcoital bleeding, irritative voiding symptoms, fever, malaise, nausea, and vomiting. However, severity of symptoms varies by individual.
- Physical examination findings include lower abdominal tenderness, mucopurulent cervicitis, cervical motion tenderness, and uterine and/or adnexal tenderness. Peritoneal signs may be present.
- Unilateral adnexal tenderness and palpable fullness or mass may indicate TOA.
- Right upper quadrant tenderness, especially with jaundice, suggests Fitz-Hugh–Curtis syndrome.

DIAGNOSIS AND DIFFERENTIAL

- PID is a clinical diagnosis (Table 66-1).
- Laboratory evaluation should include a pregnancy test, wet prep, and endocervical swabs for gonorrhea and chlamydia. Elevations in white blood cell count, erythrocyte sedimentation rate, and C-reactive protein help support the diagnosis of PID.
- Transvaginal pelvic ultrasound is used to detect TOA, which appears as a complex adnexal mass with multiple internal echoes.
- Procedures such as endometrial biopsy, culdocentesis, and laparoscopy may help to facilitate or confirm the diagnosis; however, their utility in the emergency department setting is limited.
- The differential diagnosis includes cervicitis, ectopic pregnancy, endometriosis, ovarian cyst, ovarian torsion, spontaneous abortion, septic abortion, cholecystitis, gastroenteritis, appendicitis, diverticulitis, pyelonephritis, and renal colic.

TABLE 66-1 Diagnostic Criteria for PID

1. Minimal criteria for diagnosis and empiric treatment:
Lower abdominal or pelvic pain without another identifiable cause
Plus
Uterine tenderness or
Adnexal tenderness or
Cervical motion tenderness
2. Additional criteria improving diagnostic specificity:
Oral temperature >101°F (38.3°C)
Abnormal cervical or vaginal mucopurulent discharge
Abundant numbers of WBC on saline microscopy of vaginal fluid
Elevated erythrocyte sedimentation rate
Elevated C-reactive protein
Laboratory evidence of cervical infection with *Neisseria gonorrhea* or *Chlamydia trachomatis* (ie, culture or DNA probe techniques)
3. Most specific criteria:
Transvaginal ultrasound (or MRI) showing thickened, fluid-filled tubes with or without free pelvic fluid or tuboovarian complex
Laparoscopic confirmation*
Endometrial biopsy showing endometritis*

Abbreviations: MRI = magnetic resonance imaging, PID = pelvic inflammatory disease. *These diagnostic procedures are not usually performed during ED visit.
Source: Centers for Disease Control and Prevention. Sexually Transmitted Diseases Treatment Guidelines, MMWR 2010; 59 (No. RR 12):65.

TABLE 66-2 Parenteral Treatment Regimens for Pelvic Inflammatory Disease

Recommended
1. Cefotetan 2 grams IV every 12 h *or* cefoxitin 2 grams IV every 6 h
Plus
Doxycycline 100 milligrams IV or PO every 12 h
2. Clindamycin 900 milligrams IV every 8 h
Plus
Gentamicin 2 milligrams/kg IV loading dose followed by 1.5 milligrams/kg every 8 h
Alternative
Ampicillin/sulbactam 3 grams IV every 6 h
Plus
Doxycycline 100 milligrams IV/PO every 12 h

Abbreviations: IV = intravenously, PO = orally.
Source: Adapted from Centers for Disease Control and Prevention. Sexually Transmitted Diseases Treatment Guidelines, MMWR 2010; 59 (No. RR 12):65.

EMERGENCY DEPARTMENT CARE AND DISPOSITION

- Analgesia and IV hydration should be provided as needed.
- Immediate initiation of broad-spectrum antibiotics improves long-term outcomes. See Tables 66-2 and 66-3 for treatment options as recommended by the Centers for Disease Control and Prevention.
- Any IUD must be removed after antibiotics are started.
- Sixty percent to 80% of TOAs resolve with antibiotics alone. The remainder requires drainage.

TABLE 66-3 Oral and Outpatient Treatment Regimens for Pelvic Inflammatory Disease

1. Ceftriaxone, 250 milligrams IM once, or cefoxitin, 2 grams IM once, and probenecid, 1 gram PO once
or
Other parenteral third-generation cephalosporin (eg, ceftizoxime or cefotaxime)
plus
Doxycycline, 100 milligrams PO twice a day for 14 d
with or without
Metronidazole, 500 milligrams PO twice a day for 14 d
2. If parenteral cephalosporin therapy is not feasible and community prevalence of fluoroquinolone resistance is low:
Levofloxacin, 500 milligrams PO, *or* ofloxacin, 400 milligrams twice daily every day for 14 d
with or without
Metronidazole, 500 milligrams PO twice a day for 14 d

Note: Other parenteral third-generation cephalosporins can be substituted for ceftriaxone or cefoxitin.
Source: From Updated recommended treatment regimens for gonococcal infections and associated conditions–United States, April 2007. *MMWR Morb Mortal Wkly Rep* 56:332, 2007.

- The decision for hospitalization should be made based on severity of illness, inability to tolerate PO medications/fluids, likelihood of anaerobic infection (IUD use, suspected abscess, recent instrumentation), uncertainty of diagnosis, immunosuppression, pregnancy, patient age, fertility issues, or concerns for compliance.
- Patients started on IV antibiotics may be switched to oral treatment 24 hours after clinical improvement. With outpatient treatment, patients should be followed up within 72 hours to assess substantial response to antibiotic therapy and compliance.
- Patients should be educated regarding prevention, compliance, and the need to have all sexual partners treated. Appropriate referrals for further STD testing including HIV and syphilis should be provided.

For further reading in Tintinalli's *Emergency Medicine: A Comprehensive Study Guide,* 7th ed., see Chapter 107, "Pelvic Inflammatory Disease," by Amy J. Behrman, William H. Shoff, and Suzanne M. Shepherd.

67 COMPLICATIONS OF GYNECOLOGIC PROCEDURES

Anitha Mathew

- The most common reasons for emergency department (ED) visits during the postoperative period following gynecologic procedures are pain, fever, and vaginal bleeding.
- A focused but thorough evaluation should be performed, including a sterile speculum and bimanual examination.
- Consultation with the gynecologist who performed the procedure is typically indicated. (Complications common to gynecologic and general surgery are discussed in Chapter 51.)

COMPLICATIONS OF ENDOSCOPIC PROCEDURES

LAPAROSCOPY

- Major complications associated with laparoscopy are listed in Table 67-1.
- Patients with thermal injury may not develop symptoms for several days to weeks postoperatively and typically present with bilateral lower abdominal pain, fever, elevated white blood cell count, and peritonitis.
- Radiographs can show an ileus or free air under the diaphragm.
- Patients with greater than expected pain after laparoscopy have a bowel injury until proven otherwise; early gynecology consultation should be obtained.

TABLE 67-1 Major Complications Associated with Laparoscopy
Thermal injury of the bowel
Perforation of viscus
Hemorrhage
Vascular injury
Ureteral or bladder injuries
Incisional hernia
Wound dehiscence

HYSTEROSCOPY

- Complications of hysteroscopy include cervical and uterine perforation, postoperative bleeding, fluid overload from absorption of distention media, and infection.
- Consultation with a gynecologist is required.
- Postoperative bleeding is the most likely cause of hospital revisit. After hemodynamic stabilization, the gynecologist may insert a Foley or balloon catheter into the uterus to tamponade the bleeding; vasopressin or misoprostol are alternative treatments.
- Patients with uterine perforation can present with peritoneal signs and require surgical exploration.
- Fluid overload is rare, but affected patients are likely to be hyponatremic.
- Infection as a result of hysteroscopy is uncommon; treat with antibiotics.

COMPLICATIONS RELATED TO MAJOR ABDOMINAL SURGERY

VAGINAL CUFF CELLULITIS

- *Cuff cellulitis*, a common complication after hysterectomy, is an infection of the contiguous retroperitoneal space immediately above the vaginal apex and the surrounding soft tissue.
- Patients typically present between postoperative days 3 and 5 with fever, abdominal pain, pelvic pain, back pain, and abnormal vaginal discharge.
- Cuff tenderness and induration are prominent during the bimanual examination, and a vaginal cuff abscess may be palpable.

- Treat with broad-spectrum antibiotics, such as **ampicillin**, 2 grams IV every 6 hours, plus **gentamicin**, 1 milligram/kg IV every 8 hours, plus **clindamycin**, 900 milligrams IV every 6 hours.
- Admit for continuation of antibiotics and possible abscess drainage.

POSTOPERATIVE OVARIAN ABSCESS

- Patients with ovarian abscesses typically present shortly after hospital discharge with fever and abdominal or pelvic pain.
- A CT scan can help to identify and localize the abscess.
- A sudden increase in pain can signal possible abscess rupture, which requires emergent laparotomy.
- Patients with ovarian abscesses should be admitted for IV antibiotics and possible drainage.

URETERAL INJURY

- Ureteral injury can occur during abdominal hysterectomy, resulting from crushing, transecting, or ligating trauma.
- Patients present soon after surgery with flank pain, fever, and costovertebral angle tenderness.
- Workup includes a urinalysis and either a CT scan with IV contrast or an IVP to evaluate for obstruction.
- Patients should be admitted for ureteral catheterization and possible repair.

OTHER COMPLICATIONS OF GYNECOLOGIC SURGERY

VESICOVAGINAL FISTULA

- Patients typically present 10 to 14 days following abdominal hysterectomy with watery vaginal discharge and should receive prompt gynecologic consultation.
- Patients are treated with Foley catheter drainage after the diagnosis is confirmed.

POSTCONIZATION BLEEDING

- The most common complication associated with loop electrocautery, laser ablation, and cold-knife conization of the cervix is bleeding, which can be rapid and excessive.
- Delayed hemorrhage can occur 1 to 2 weeks postoperatively.
- Directly visualize the bleeding site, then apply Monsel solution, hold direct pressure for 5 minutes with a large cotton swab, or cauterize with silver nitrate.
- If unsuccessful, the bleeding site may be better visualized and treated in the OR.

SEPTIC PELVIC THROMBOPHLEBITIS

- Patients with ovarian vein thrombosis present within a week after delivery or surgery with fever, tachycardia, GI distress, and unilateral abdominal pain.
- Patients with deep septic pelvic thrombophlebitis present a few days after delivery or surgery with spiking fevers that are unresponsive to antibiotics; these patients may also have abdominal pain.
- Ultrasound, CT, and MRI are frequently nondiagnostic, making this a diagnosis of exclusion.
- Patients are admitted for anticoagulation (**heparin or enoxaparin**) and IV antibiotics, such as **ampicillin/sulbactam** 3 grams IV every 6 hours, **piperacillin/tazobactam** 4.5 grams IV every 8 hours, or **ticarcillin/clavulanate** 3.1 grams IV every 4 hours. Monotherapy with a carbapenem, such as **imipenem** 500 milligrams every 6 hours, may be used for patients with beta-lactam intolerance.

INDUCED ABORTION

- Complications associated with induced abortion include uterine perforation, cervical lacerations, retained products of conception, and postabortal endometritis (Table 67-2).
- Patients with retained products of conception usually present with excessive bleeding and abdominal pain.
- Pelvic examination reveals an enlarged and tender uterus with an open cervical os.
- A pelvic ultrasound should be obtained to confirm the diagnosis.

TABLE 67-2 Complications Associated with Induced Abortion

TIMING	COMPLICATION	POSSIBLE ETIOLOGIES
Immediate complications: within 24 h postprocedure	Bleeding, pain	Uterine perforation, cervical lacerations
Delayed complications: between 24 h and 4 wk postprocedure	Bleeding	Retained products of conception, postabortive endometritis
Late complications: >4 wk postprocedure	Amenorrhea, psychological problems, Rh isoimmunization	—

- Treatment is dilatation and curettage.
- Endometritis can occur with or without retained products of conception and is treated with antibiotics, as previously discussed under Vaginal Cuff Cellulitis.
- Women who are Rh negative require **Rh_0 immunoglobulin**, 300 micrograms IM.

ASSISTED REPRODUCTIVE TECHNOLOGY

- Complications related to ultrasound-guided aspiration of oocytes include ovarian hyperstimulation syndrome, pelvic infection, intraperitoneal bleeding, and adnexal torsion.
- Ovarian hyperstimulation syndrome can be a life-threatening complication of assisted reproduction.
- Patients with mild cases present with abdominal distention, ovarian enlargement, and weight gain.
- In severe cases, patients have rapid weight gain, tense ascites from third spacing of fluid into the abdomen, pleural effusions, hemodynamic instability, oliguria, electrolyte abnormalities, and increased coagulability.
- Bimanual pelvic examination is contraindicated to avoid rupturing the ovaries.
- Initiate intravenous volume replacement, obtain CBC, electrolytes, liver function tests and coagulation studies, and consult gynecology for admission.

POSTEMBOLIZATION SYNDROME

- *Postembolization syndrome* consists of postprocedure pelvic pain, nausea, vomiting, and fever lasting 2 to 10 days due to myometrial and fibroid ischemia after fibroid embolization.
- Evaluate patients for other causes of fever, and provide pain control.
- Patients with inadequate pain control or those with infection may require admission.

For further reading in Tintinalli's *Emergency Medicine: A Comprehensive Study Guide*, 7th ed., see Chapter 109, "Complications of Gynecologic Procedures," by Michael A. Silverman.

Section 10
PEDIATRICS

68 FEVER AND SERIOUS BACTERIAL ILLNESS

Milan D. Nadkarni

EPIDEMIOLOGY

- In the pediatric population, fever is the most common chief complaint presenting to an emergency department and accounts for 30% of outpatient visits each year.
- Meningitis risk decreases from about 1% in the first month of life to <0.1% later in infancy while the risk for pyelonephritis remains relatively constant among young girls with fever, and gradually decreases among boys over the first year of life.
- Most studies of febrile infants ≤3 months old cite a bacteremia/sepsis incidence of 2% to 3%. The most common causes of bacteremia and meningitis in this age group are *Escherichia coli*, group B *Streptococcus*, and *Listeria monocytogenes*. Risk factors include premature delivery, ruptured amniotic membranes more than 24 hours prior to delivery, maternal GBS status, and intrapartum fever.
- In older infants and children, *Streptococcus pneumoniae* previously accounted for more than 90% of occult bacteremia with *Neisseria meningitidis*, group A *Streptococcus*, and *Salmonella* responsible for the remainder. *Haemophilus influenzae* type b was a significant cause of bacteremia, but has been nearly eliminated since vaccination against this organism began in the early 1990s.
- Administration of the *H. influenzae* type b vaccine and the heptavalent pneumococcal conjugate vaccine have decreased the occult bacteremia rate of well-appearing, febrile children 3 to 36 months of age from approximately 2% to 3% to 0.5% to 0.7%.

PATHOPHYSIOLOGY

- Fever is the result of the body's thermostat being reset by exogenous pyrogens, such as bacteria, bacterial endotoxins, antigen–antibody complexes, and viruses, which stimulate the production of endogenous pyrogens.
- Infants and young children are thought to be at increased risk for bacteremia due to their immature immune system. The likelihood of various organisms causing bacteremia is age dependent.
- Neonates and young infants demonstrate decreased opsonin activity, decreased macrophage and neutrophil function, and bone marrow exhaustion. Infants and children demonstrate a poor immunoglobulin G antibody response to encapsulated bacteria until 24 months of age.

CLINICAL FEATURES

- In the neonate or infant <2 to 3 months of age, the threshold for concerning fever is 38°C (100.4°F); in infants and children 3 to 36 months old, the threshold is 39°C (102.2°F).
- In general, higher temperatures are associated with a higher incidence of serious bacterial illness.
- Immature development and immature immunity make reliable examination findings difficult. Persistent crying, inability to console, poor feeding, or temperature instability may be the only findings suggestive of a serious bacterial illness.

DIAGNOSIS AND MANAGEMENT BASED ON AGE

INFANTS UP TO 3 MONTHS OLD

- History and physical examination are rarely helpful in diagnosing or excluding serious bacterial illness in this age group as symptoms are typically vague, and physical examination findings are unreliable: meningismus is present in <15% of bacterial meningitis; rales may not be appreciated in the absence of ability to generate negative inspiratory forces; and bacteremia can occur in the well-appearing infant.
- A history of cough, tachypnea, or hypoxia (by pulse oximetry), however, should alert the examiner to a

possible lower respiratory tract infection and prompt chest radiograph.

- **The safest course for 0- to 28-day-old infants is full sepsis testing, admission, and empiric antibiotic treatment.**
- Antibiotic coverage in this age group includes ampicillin for *L. monocytogenes* (see Table 68-1) and either gentamycin or cefotaxime to cover *E. coli*. Sepsis testing includes complete blood count (CBC), blood culture, urinalysis (UA) and urine culture, chest radiograph, and lumbar puncture.
- Criteria used to define infants at low risk for serious bacterial illness in the 31 to 90 days age group include well appearance without a history of prematurity or other comorbidity, and a normal urinalysis.
- Infants with symptoms of lower respiratory tract disease, such as cough, grunting, physical findings such as tachypnea, rales, rhonchi, or low pulse oximeter readings, should have a chest radiograph.
- The Boston, Philadelphia (which include normal CSF, UA, and CBC), and Rochester criteria (which includes normal UA and CBC) should only be applied if the child's presentation warrants the sepsis testing listed above. Obtaining these laboratory tests should be reconsidered for infants in the 31 to 90 days age group because of the lower incidence of bacteremia due to screening and treatment for maternal GBS and declining rates of bacteremia.
- All ill-appearing infants should receive parenteral antibiotic therapy (see Table 68-1) and be admitted to the hospital.
- Management of well-appearing febrile low-risk infants remains a subject of significant debate. Infants older than 28 days at low risk may be managed conservatively as inpatients with **ceftriaxone** (see Table 68-1) pending cultures; as inpatients without antibiotics; as outpatients with **ceftriaxone** 50 milligrams/kg IM; or as outpatients without antibiotics. The key deciding factor should be the physician's comfort level and the ability for close follow-up, typically within 12 hours. **If antibiotics are administered (inpatient or outpatient), CSF and blood cultures should be obtained prior to administration of antibiotics**.
- Most community and academic emergency physicians perform a full septic workup in infants less than 4 weeks of age.
- It is our recommendation to admit all well-appearing febrile infants less than 4 weeks of age. Empiric antibiotics or close observation can be discussed with the hospitalist.
- Infants between the ages of 4 and 12 weeks may be considered for discharge provided a complete workup is negative.
- Well-appearing febrile children between the ages of 29 and 90 days with an identifiable viral source of infection (eg, respiratory syncytial virus [RSV] or influenza) should have urinary tract infection (UTI) ruled out before being discharged from the emergency department, as UTI occurs in 2% to 4% of febrile infants with RSV.

TABLE 68-1 Initial Intravenous Antibiotic Dosages for Bacteremia, Sepsis, and Meningitis

AGE GROUP	BACTEREMIA	SEPSIS*	MENINGITIS
Neonates (age 0-28 d)	Not applicable	Ampicillin, 50-100 milligrams/kg *Plus* cefotaxime, 50 milligrams/kg†	Ampicillin, 100 milligrams/kg *Plus* cefotaxime, 100 milligrams/kg†
Young infants (29-90 d)	Ceftriaxone, 50 milligrams/kg	Ampicillin, 50-100 milligrams/kg *plus* cefotaxime, 50 milligrams/kg *or* ceftriaxone 50 milligrams/kg *plus consider* vancomycin, 15 milligrams/kg‡	Ampicillin, 100 milligrams/kg *plus* cefotaxime, 100 milligrams/kg *or* ceftriaxone, 100 milligrams/kg *plus* vancomycin, 15 milligrams/kg§
Older infants and children (age >90 d)	Ceftriaxone, 50 milligrams/kg#	Cefotaxime, 50 milligrams/kg *or* ceftriaxone, 50 milligrams/kg *plus consider* vancomycin, 15 milligrams/kg§	Cefotaxime, 100 milligrams/kg *or* ceftriaxone, 100 milligrams/kg *plus* vancomycin, 15 milligrams/kg§

*Use meningitis doses if the patient is considered too unstable for lumbar puncture in the emergency department.
†Cefotaxime is used rather than ceftriaxone for neonates ≤28 days old because ceftriaxone can displace bilirubin and worsen hyperbilirubinemia.
‡Consider the addition of vancomycin in sepsis with critical illness, immunocompromised, or indwelling catheters.
§Add vancomycin only if there is evidence of bacterial meningitis in the cerebrospinal fluid.
#May be given IM.

- Chest radiographs are obtained at the discretion of the clinician, but are *not* indicated for infants with clinical bronchiolitis or RSV that is otherwise uncomplicated.
- Lumbar puncture in this group of children may be deferred in those who are well-appearing and test positive for a source of infection.
- For febrile infants less than 3 months of age with an identifiable source of infection requiring antibiotic treatment (eg, otitis media or UTI) blood and CSF cultures should be obtained prior to administration of antibiotics.

INFANTS 3 TO 36 MONTHS OLD

- Physical examination findings become more reliable with increasing age, though meningeal signs remain unreliable in the first year of life. Viral illnesses including pneumonia account for most febrile illnesses in this age group; patients with clinical findings suggesting pneumonia should have a chest radiograph.
- UTI may present with fever and no other symptoms in this age group. UTI is a significant source of bacterial illness in females prior to toilet training, circumcised boys younger than 6 months of age and uncircumcised boys under 1 year of age; these patients should have urinalysis and urine culture (by catheterization) if a source for the fever is not otherwise identified.
- Unless there is an identifiable source of infection through history and physical examination, urinalysis/culture and/or chest radiograph may be the only two tests required for a workup on these febrile infants.
- Infants in this age group who appear ill should receive a full septic workup including lumbar puncture and administration of antibiotics in a timely fashion (see Table 68-1).

OLDER FEBRILE CHILDREN

- The risk for bacteremia in children older than 3 years is <0.2% since the introduction of Prevnar. CBC is no longer predictive of bacteremia and blood cultures are no longer recommended (more likely to yield false positive results) in immunized older children with fever.
- Etiologies to consider in older febrile children include streptococcal pharyngitis, pneumonia, and Epstein–Barr virus infection. Testing is directed by clinical presentation.

EMERGENCY DEPARTMENT CARE AND DISPOSITION

- The management of pneumonia is covered in Chapter 73; UTI is covered in Chapter 77; and infections of the ears, nose, and throat are covered in Chapter 70.
- Table 68-1 lists specific antibiotic recommendations for conditions discussed in this chapter.
- Although fever makes children uncomfortable, it is not harmful to children, though it does lower the seizure threshold. The physician can use several methods to reduce fever:
  1. Remove excessive clothing and blankets to increase heat loss through radiation.
  2. Administer **acetaminophen** 15 milligrams/kg PO/PR every 4 hours (maximum dose, 80 milligrams/kg in 24 hours).
  3. Consider **ibuprofen** 10 milligrams/kg PO in children older than 1 year of age; the dose can be repeated every 6 hours (maximum of 40 milligrams/kg in 24 hours), and can be given concurrently with acetaminophen.

SEPSIS

EPIDEMIOLOGY

- Sepsis is an infectious inflammatory syndrome with clinical evidence of infection that may include focal infections and meningitis. Multiorgan failure and death can rapidly develop. The clinical situations in which sepsis may develop or be suspected are quite varied and therefore the true incidence in children is not well described.

PATHOPHYSIOLOGY

- The progression from bacteremia to sepsis begins with colonization with a bacterial pathogen (usually nasopharyngeal), and progresses to invasion of the blood by encapsulated organisms, the release of inflammatory mediators, and failure of host defenses.
- Risk factors include impaired immunity, prematurity, recent invasive procedures, and indwelling foreign objects such as catheters, splenic function, congenital metabolic disease, and the presence of and obstruction to drainage of a body cavity.
- Age-dependent etiologies of sepsis are listed in Table 68-2.

CLINICAL FEATURES

- Clinical signs may be vague and subtle in the young infant, and include lethargy, poor feeding, vomiting, irritability, or hypotonia.
- Fever is common; however, very young infants with sepsis may be hypothermic. Tachypnea and tachycardia are usually present as a result of fever but also may be secondary to hypoxia and metabolic acidosis.

TABLE 68-2 Common Organisms Causing Sepsis and Meningitis

AGE	ORGANISMS
0-2 mo	Group B *Streptococcus* *Escherichia coli* *Listeria monocytogenes*
2 mo to 5 y	*Streptococcus pneumoniae* *Neisseria meningitidis* β-Hemolytic *Streptococcus* *Haemophilus influenzae* b* *Salmonella* sp (gastroenteritis) *E. coli* (pyelonephritis) *Rickettsia rickettsii*†

*Marked decline in cases since the introduction of the *Haemophilus influenzae* vaccine; consider in the unimmunized.
†Etiologic agent for Rocky Mountain spotted fever; seen in endemic areas after tick bites, with summer or fall predominance.

- Sepsis can rapidly progress to shock manifest as prolonged capillary refill, decreased peripheral pulses, altered mental status, and decreased urinary output. Hypotension is usually a very late sign of septic shock in children and, and, in conjunction with respiratory failure and bradycardia, indicates a grave prognosis.

DIAGNOSIS AND DIFFERENTIAL

- Diagnosis is based on clinical findings and confirmed by positive blood culture results.
- Though international criteria for sepsis have been published, all infants who appear toxic should be considered septic. The laboratory evaluation of a child with presumed sepsis includes a CBC, blood culture, complete metabolic panel, catheterized urinalysis with culture and sensitivities, chest radiograph, lumbar puncture, and stool studies in the presence of diarrhea.
- A serum glucose level should be performed on any critically ill child with altered mental status or cardiorespiratory instability. Serum lactate may be useful for predicting severity of the clinical course, but rarely changes the emergency department management.

EMERGENCY DEPARTMENT CARE AND DISPOSITION

- Administer high-flow oxygen, institute cardiac monitoring, and secure IV or IO access immediately. Endotracheal intubation should be performed in the presence of respiratory failure.
- Treat shock with 20-mL/kg boluses of **normal saline** solution. Repeat boluses until vital signs, perfusion, and mental status and urine output improve, up to 100 mL/kg total volume.
- Treat hypoglycemia with 4 to 5 mL/kg D10 in neonates and young infants and 2 mL/kg D25 in older infants and children.
- Initiate antibiotic therapy promptly, as soon as IV access is achieved. Do not delay due to difficulty with procedures such as lumbar puncture. Empiric antibiotic choices are listed in Table 68-1.
- Treat volume-refractory shock with **dopamine** 5 to 20 micrograms/kg/min or **norepinephrine** 0.1 to 0.2 micrograms/kg/min.
- Consider the presence of drug-resistant organisms or immunoincompetence and infection with unusual or opportunistic organisms.

MENINGITIS

EPIDEMIOLOGY

- Since the advent of the *H. influenzae* type b (Hib) vaccine, the epidemiology of pediatric meningitis in the United States has changed dramatically. In 1986, the median age for all patients with meningitis was 15 months; in 1995 the median age for meningitis was 25 years. Meningitis has shifted from being predominantly a disease of infants and young children to a disease predominantly of adults.

PATHOPHYSIOLOGY

- Typically, meningitis is a complication of primary bacteremia. It is thought that the products of bacterial multiplication alter the permeability of the blood-brain barrier and extend the infection to the brain and surrounding cerebrospinal fluid spaces.
- Less commonly, meningitis may result from hematogenous spread from a distant primary focal infection, direct extension from adjacent infection, or following cribriform plate or sinus fracture.
- The neurologic damage that sometimes follows meningitis is thought to result from direct inflammatory effects, brain edema, increased intracranial pressure, decreased cerebral blood flow, and vascular thrombosis.
- Impaired splenic function and immunosuppression or immunodeficiency is associated with a relatively increased risk of meningitis.
- Bacterial agents responsible for meningitis vary with age. Group B streptococci, *E. coli*, and *L. monocytogenes* predominate in neonates. *Streptococcus pneumoniae* and *N. meningitidis* are most common in older infants and children.

CLINICAL FEATURES

- Meningitis may present with the subtle signs that accompany less serious infections, such as otitis media or sinusitis. Irritability, inconsolability, hypotonia, and lethargy are most common in infants.
- Older children may complain of headache, photophobia, nausea, and vomiting and exhibit the classic signs of meningismus with complaints of neck pain and stiffness.
- Occasionally, meningitis presents as a rapidly progressive, fulminant disease characterized by shock, seizures, or coma, or with febrile status epilepticus. In infants presenting with hypothermia a full septic workup should be initiated to rule out meningitis.

DIAGNOSIS AND DIFFERENTIAL

- Diagnosis is made by lumbar puncture and analysis of the cerebrospinal fluid (CSF). The CSF should be examined for white blood cells, glucose, and protein and undergo Gram stain and culture.
- Herpes encephalitis should be considered in the seizing neonate and any child with CSF pleocytosis.
- In the presence of immunoincompetence, infections with opportunistic or unusual viral organisms should be considered.
- Cranial computed tomography should be performed before lumbar puncture in the presence of focal neurologic signs or increased intracranial pressure.

EMERGENCY DEPARTMENT CARE AND DISPOSITION

- Treatment should always begin with the ABCs and restoration of oxygenation and perfusion (see specific treatment recommendations under Sepsis, above).
- Empiric antibiotic therapy is based on the patient's age and listed in Table 68-1.
- Antibiotics should not be deferred or delayed when meningitis is strongly suspected.
- Strongly consider the addition of acyclovir 10 milligrams/kg/dose in neonates with seizures, or ill-appearing neonates and in neonates with vesicular lesions.
- The role of steroids in the management of meningitis in children is controversial. If given, the dose should ideally be administered before antibiotics.
- For any patient suspected of having meningitis for whom efforts at lumbar puncture fail, the patient should be admitted, hydrated, given meningitis doses of antibiotics, and blood and urine cultures obtained. Lumbar puncture may be successful after hydration.

POSITIVE BLOOD CULTURES

- Recall all children with positive blood cultures.
- In the case of positive *S. pneumoniae* cultures:
  1. If the child is receiving appropriate antibiotics, is clinically well, and afebrile, the child should complete the course of therapy.
  2. If afebrile and clinically well but not receiving antibiotics, opinions differ regarding the need for additional blood cultures and antibiotic therapy. Most physicians would treat this group of infants with antibiotics and repeat a blood culture 24 to 48 hours after initiation of antibiotics. These children can be managed on an outpatient basis.
  3. The febrile child who appears ill should receive a complete sepsis evaluation (CBC, urinalysis, CSF indices, and blood, urine, and CSF cell count and cultures).
- For the persistently febrile patient who is well appearing and has a normal evaluation, admission is usual, although empiric treatment with ceftriaxone and follow-up as an outpatient may be considered.
- For any patient who is ill appearing, complete a sepsis evaluation and admit for parenteral antibiotics.
- Children with cultures positive for *N. meningitidis*, methicillin-resistant *Staphylococcus aureus* or gram-negative organisms should be admitted for parenteral antibiotic therapy.
- Children who are thought to be at risk for a serious bacterial illness and do not have reliable follow-up or the ability to return to the hospital should also be admitted for inpatient management.

For further reading in Tintinalli's *Emergency Medicine: A Comprehensive Study Guide*, 7th ed., see Chapter 113, "Fever and Serious Bacterial Illness," by Vincent J. Wang.

69 NEONATE EMERGENCIES AND COMMON NEONATAL PROBLEMS

Shad Baab

- This chapter covers common neonatal problems that my present to the emergency department (ED). For discussion of fever and/or sepsis in the neonate, see Chapter 68.
- In general, the signs and symptoms of illness are vague and nonspecific in neonates (ie, infants in the first month of life).

- Improved survival of premature infants has increased the number of infants whose corrected gestational age (chronological age since birth in weeks minus number of weeks of prematurity) makes them similar to neonates. Some of these children have multiple medical problems and may present frequently to the ED.
- Common neonatal ED complaints ranging from benign to critical are summarized in Table 69-1.

NORMAL VEGETATIVE FUNCTIONS

- Bottle-fed infants generally feed 6 to 9 times per 24-hour period, with a relatively stable pattern developing by the end of the first month of life. Breast-fed infants typically feed every 1 to 3 hours.
- Infants lose 5% to 10% of their birth weight during the first 3 to 7 days of life. After this time, they are expected to gain about 1 ounce per day (20 to 30 grams) for the first 3 months of life.
- The number, color, and consistency of stools vary from day to day. Normal breast-fed infants may go 5 to 7 days without stooling or have up to 9 stools per day. Color has no significance unless blood is present or stools are acholic (white). Typical neonatal stool is yellow with a mustard-seed appearance.
- Respiratory rates in newborns vary, with normal ranges from 30 to 60 breaths per minute. Periodic breathing (brief pauses in respiration from 3 to 10 seconds alternating with short periods of tachypnea) is normal but may be frightening to parents.
- Normal newborns awaken at variable intervals that can range from every 20 minutes to 6 hours. Neonates and young infants tend to have no day–night differentiation until about 3 months of age.

ACUTE, UNEXPLAINED, EXCESSIVE CRYING (INCONSOLABILITY)

- There are multiple causes of prolonged crying in infants (Table 69-2), which range from benign to life threatening. Acute onset of inconsolable crying represents a serious condition in the majority of infants and requires careful evaluation.
- Neonates and infants who present with excessive crying but have a normal head-to-toe physical examination, normal temperature and vital signs, and return to baseline in the ED can safely be discharged without further invasive testing.

INTESTINAL COLIC

- Intestinal colic is defined as crying for 3 hours or more per day for 3 or more days per week over a

TABLE 69-1 Common Pediatric Emergency Presenting Complaints

COMPLAINT CATEGORIES (PROPORTION OF INFANT VISITS)	SUBCATEGORIES
Respiratory symptoms (27.5%)	Viral upper respiratory infection (54.5%) Bronchiolitis (35%) Apparent life-threatening event (8%) Pneumonia (1%) Congenital (eg, laryngotracheomalacia) (1.5%)
GI and GU complaints (21%)	Vomiting (37%) Scrotal swelling (15%) Constipation (11%) Vomiting and diarrhea (10%) Blood in emesis or stools (8%) Diarrhea (8%) Feeding tube problems (3%) Oral thrush (3%) Renal and urinary concerns (2%) Congenital anomalies (2%) Vaginal discharge (1%)
Normal infant queries (18%)	Crying/colic (21%) Miscellaneous variant of normal infants (79%) Feeding patterns and weight gain Periodic breathing Diaper rash Umbilical cord questions Postimmunization reaction Infantile breast tissue Sleep pattern Normal newborn temperature
Fever, rule out sepsis (11%)	Fever without focus, for septic workup (64.5%) Urinary tract infection (33%) Respiratory symptoms (2%) CNS symptoms (<1%)
Jaundice (8%)	—
Skin lesions (5.5%)	Erythema toxicum, seborrhea, atopic dermatitis Perianal abscesses Birth marks
CNS (3%)	Head injuries Seizures Myoclonus Lethargy
Eye complaints (2%)	Eye discharge, including nasolacrimal duct obstruction Conjunctivitis
Cardiac (2%)	Tachyarrhythmia Heart murmurs Symptoms of known congenital malformation
Musculoskeletal (1.5%)	Injuries (falls, nonaccidental trauma) Hair tourniquets to digits
Hematology (0.5%)	Anemia (hemolysis, surgery-related blood loss)
Sudden infant death syndrome (one case seen)	—

Abbreviation: CNS = central nervous system.

TABLE 69-2 Conditions Associated with Uncontrollable Crying, Irritability, and/or Lethargy in Neonates

SYSTEM	EMERGENT	NONEMERGENT
Central nervous system	Intracranial hemorrhage (neonatal alloimmune thrombocytopenia, birth trauma, vitamin K deficiency) Meningitis Elevated intracranial pressure	—
Eye, ear, nose, throat	Nasal obstruction (choanal atresia or stenosis)	Corneal abrasion, ocular foreign body Otitis media Nasal congestion (upper respiratory infection) Oral thrush Stomatitis
Pulmonary	Pneumonia	—
Cardiac	Supraventricular tachycardia Heart failure	—
GI	Volvulus Intussusception Incarcerated hernia	Gastroesophageal reflux disease (reflux) Gastroenteritis Anal fissure Colic
GU	Testicular torsion Penile hair tourniquets Paraphimosis	Urinary tract infection Diaper rash
Musculoskeletal	Hair tourniquet of finger/toe Nonaccidental trauma	Injuries (diaper pin, sharp or irritating objects from clothing)
Infectious	Sepsis Pneumonia Meningitis	Upper respiratory infection
Metabolic	Inborn errors of metabolism Hypoglycemia Congenital adrenal hyperplasia	—

3-week period. It is the most common cause of excessive (but not inconsolable) crying.

- The cause of colic is unknown and the incidence is about 13% of all neonates. Colic seldom lasts beyond 3 to 4 months of age but can produce significant stress in caregivers and is a risk factor for nonaccidental trauma. Colic is benign and reassurance is usually all that is required.

NONACCIDENTAL TRAUMA (CHILD ABUSE)

- A battered child may present with unexplained bruises at varying ages, skull fractures, intracranial injuries, extremity and/or rib fractures, cigarette burns, retinal hemorrhages, or unexplained irritability, lethargy, or coma (see Chapter 189 for detailed discussion).

GASTROINTESTINAL SYMPTOMS

SURGICAL CONDITIONS

- Surgically treated abdominal emergencies in neonates are uncommon, but may present with nonspecific symptomatology, and when suspected require prompt consultation with an experienced pediatric surgeon.
- The most common signs and symptoms are nonspecific and include irritability and crying, poor feeding, vomiting, constipation, and abdominal distention. **Bilious vomiting is suggestive of malrotation with midgut volvulus and requires emergent surgical consultation and radiologic evaluation (upper GI contrast study) prior to ED discharge**. A groin or scrotal mass may represent an incarcerated hernia or testicular torsion, and should be evaluated with ultrasound.

FEEDING DIFFICULTIES

- Parents may present to the ED with the perception of inadequate oral intake. If the patient's weight gain is appropriate and the infant appears satisfied after feeding, simple reassurance is appropriate. A successful trial of feeding in the ED can reassure parents, ED nurses, and physicians alike.
- Anatomic abnormalities interfering with feeding or swallowing (eg, esophageal stenosis, esophageal stricture, laryngeal clefts, and compression of the esophagus or trachea by a double aortic arch) typically present with difficulty feeding from birth, choking or gagging with feeds, failure to thrive, and dehydration.
- Infants with a recent and actual decrease in intake usually have acute disease, most commonly infection, and warrant further evaluation.

GASTROINTESTINAL REFLUX

- Gastroesophageal reflux in neonates and infants is universal, although variable in severity, and caused by reduced lower esophageal sphincter pressure and relatively increased intragastric pressure.
- Reflux of a small amount of feedings regurgitated through the mouth or nose is typically a self-limited condition; in the well-appearing and growing infant, reassurance alone is appropriate.
- Although rare, reflux associated with poor weight gain, respiratory symptoms, fussiness, or feeding aversion requires a more thorough evaluation. If dehydration or persistent respiratory symptoms are present, inpatient evaluation should be considered.

VOMITING

- Vomiting is differentiated from regurgitation by forceful contraction of the diaphragm and abdominal muscles. Vomiting has a variety of causes and is rarely an isolated symptom.
- Vomiting from birth is usually due to an anatomic anomaly (eg, tracheoesophageal fistula, duodenal atresia, midgut malrotation) and often diagnosed prior to discharge from the nursery.
- Vomiting is a nonspecific but serious symptom in neonates. Diverse etiologies include increased intracranial pressure (eg, shaken-baby syndrome), infections (eg, urinary tract infections [UTIs], sepsis, gastroenteritis, meningitis), hepatobiliary disease (usually accompanied by jaundice), and inborn errors of metabolism (usually accompanied by hypoglycemia or metabolic acidosis).
- Pyloric stenosis most commonly presents between 6 weeks and 6 months of age with nonbilious, projectile vomiting after feeding in the hungry infant. Classically an olive-shaped mass can be palpated on abdominal examination, and measurement of electrolytes may reveal hypochloremic alkalosis, but these signs are present in less than 10% of cases in neonates at the time of diagnosis. Diagnosis is made with pyloric ultrasound or upper GI radiography. Treatment is surgical after correction of electrolyte abnormalities.
- **Bilious vomiting in a neonate should be considered a surgical emergency until proven otherwise**.

DIARRHEA

- The most common causes of blood in the stool in infants less than 6 months of age are cow's milk intolerance and anal fissures. Breast-fed infants may have heme-positive stool from swallowed maternal blood due to bleeding nipples. Although bacterial enteritis is a cause of bloody diarrhea, it is rare in neonates.
- Oral rehydration should be attempted if the patient is less than 5% dehydrated (see Chapter 75 for detailed discussion of dehydration in infants) with a total intake goal of 150 cc/kg/d.
- Dehydrated neonates (and neonates with impending dehydration from rotavirus) should be admitted for rehydration. Although routine electrolyte measurement is not helpful in older children, infants <6 months of age have a higher incidence of sodium abnormalities and serum electrolytes may help guide therapy.
- Necrotizing enterocolitis may present with bloody diarrhea, although usually with accompanying signs of serious illness (eg, jaundice, lethargy, fever, poor feeding, and abdominal distention). Abdominal radiography may demonstrate pneumatosis intestinalis, hepatic portal air, or free air. Treatment includes bowel rest and broad-spectrum antibiotics (clindamycin, cefotaxime, and ampicillin) and pediatric surgery consultation.

ABDOMINAL DISTENTION

- Relatively large abdominal girth can be normal in the neonate and is usually due to lax abdominal muscles and relatively large intra-abdominal organs. In general, if the neonate appears comfortable and is feeding well, and the abdomen is soft, there is no need for concern.

CONSTIPATION

- Infrequent bowel movements in neonates do not necessarily mean that the infant is constipated. Stool

patterns are variable, with normal ranging from multiple bowel movements per day to intervals of up to a week. Painful, hard, or pencil-shaped infrequent stools, by contrast, are more likely to signal underlying abnormalities.
- Normal newborns pass meconium in the first 24 hours of life; failure to stool in the first 2 days of life may be associated with intestinal stenosis or atresias, Hirschsprung's disease, and meconium ileus or plug associated with cystic fibrosis. A perinatal stooling history should be obtained in all patients presenting to the ED for evaluation of constipation.

CARDIORESPIRATORY SYMPTOMS

BREATHING AND STRIDOR

- Noisy breathing in a neonate is usually benign. Infectious causes of stridor seen commonly in older infants and young children (eg, croup) are rare in neonates.
- Stridor in a neonate is often due to a congenital anomaly, most commonly laryngomalacia. Other causes include webs, cysts, atresias, stenoses, clefts, and hemangiomas.
- Neonates are obligate nasal breathers and feed for relatively prolonged times, breathing only through their noses (having the bottle or breast occlude the mouth). Nasal congestion from upper respiratory tract infections can cause significant respiratory distress. The use of saline drops and frequent nasal bulb suctioning is often effective.

APNEA AND PERIODIC BREATHING

- Periodic breathing is normal in neonates.
- Apnea is the cessation of respiration for 20 seconds, or less when accompanied by bradycardia, cyanosis, or change in muscle tone. Apnea generally signifies critical illness or injury, and further investigation and admission for monitoring should be considered (see Apparent Life-Threatening Event below).
- Apnea may be the first sign of bronchiolitis with respiratory syncytial virus (RSV) in neonates and often occurs before wheezing. Neonates and young infants with documented apnea and clinical bronchiolitis require admission to the hospital, even when other signs of disease are mild. Apnea is also associated with pertussis and chlamydia infections in young infants.

CYANOSIS AND BLUE SPELLS

- Many disorders can present with cyanosis, and differentiating among them can be a challenge. However, some symptom patterns are helpful.
- Rapid, unlabored respirations and cyanosis suggest cyanotic heart disease with right-to-left shunting (see Chapter 74, Pediatric Heart Disease).
- Irregular, shallow breathing and cyanosis suggests sepsis, meningitis, cerebral edema, or intracranial hemorrhage.
- Labored breathing with grunting and retractions is suggestive of pulmonary disease such as pneumonia, aspiration, or bronchiolitis.
- All cyanotic neonates should be admitted to the hospital for monitoring, therapy, and further investigation.

BRONCHOPULMONARY DYSPLASIA

- Premature infants who required prolonged mechanical ventilation in the neonatal intensive care unit (NICU) may have residual lung injury and bronchopulmonary dysplasia (BPD). Young infants with BPD may be on home oxygen, diuretics, bronchodilators, or steroids.
- Infants with BPD can have respiratory deterioration due to acute illnesses, including bronchiolitis, pneumonia, dehydration, sepsis, gastroesophageal reflux with aspiration, and congestive heart failure.
- The most common cause of acute respiratory deterioration in an infant with BPD is a lower respiratory tract infection. RSV infections are particularly common and may be quite severe.
- Basic treatment for BPD exacerbations includes oxygenation and bronchodilators. Antibiotics, admission, and mechanical ventilation may be required based on the clinical presentation.

JAUNDICE

- There are multiple causes of jaundice, and the likelihood of each is based on the age at which the patient first develops signs.
- Jaundice that occurs within the first 24 hours of life is pathologic. The most likely causes include ABO or Rh incompatibility, congenital or acquired infections, or birth trauma that produces severe bruising or cephalohematoma.
- Jaundice that develops during the second or third day of life is usually physiologic. Classically the bilirubin rise is slow with a peak less than 6 milligrams/dL. It is more common in breast-fed infants and rarely requires treatment.
- Jaundice that develops after the third day of life is usually pathologic. Causes include sepsis, congenital or acquired infections (eg, UTI), congenital hemolytic anemias, breast-milk jaundice, hypothyroidism, and hepatobiliary disease.

TABLE 69-3 Reported Final Diagnoses for Patients Presenting with Apparent Life-Threatening Event

COMMON DIAGNOSES	LESS COMMON DIAGNOSES	RARE REPORTED DIAGNOSES
Seizure/febrile seizure	Pertussis	Arrhythmia or other cardiac process
Gastroesophageal reflux	Inflicted injury	Anemia
Respiratory tract infection (upper or lower tract)	Poisoning	Breath-holding spell
Misinterpretation of benign process such as periodic breathing	Serious bacterial infection	Metabolic disease
Vomiting/choking episode	Electrolyte abnormality (including glucose)	Anatomic maxillofacial obstruction

- Diagnostic evaluation includes direct and indirect bilirubin levels in well-appearing infants with suspected benign causes of jaundice. If other pathologic conditions are suspected, evaluation is guided by the suspected differential (septic workup, including a lumbar puncture, a peripheral blood smear and reticulocyte count, liver function tests). Empiric antibiotics should also be administered when sepsis is suspected.
- Phototherapy and exchange transfusion treatment thresholds for hyperbilirubinemia are guided by nomograms from the AAP, which can be found online at http://aappolicy.aappublications.org/cgi/content/full/pediatrics;114/1/297.

ORAL THRUSH

- Oral thrush may prompt a visit to the ED because the parent notices something white in the mouth or because the discomfort from extensive lesions interferes with feeding. Intraoral lesions due to candida are white, adherent, and may be noted on the tongue, lips, or buccal mucosa.
- Treatment consists of the topical application of oral nystatin suspension.

APPARENT LIFE-THREATENING EVENTS

- An apparent life-threatening event (ALTE) is defined as an episode that is frightening to the observer and involves any combination of apnea, color change (pallor, plethora, or cyanosis), change in muscle tone (limp or stiff), choking, or gagging.
- An ALTE is a symptom (or constellation of symptoms) for which the emergency physician must look for an underlying diagnosis. Many of the symptoms in an ALTE can represent normal or expected infant phenomena (eg, periodic breathing, reflux, acrocyanosis), but perilous etiologies are also possible.
- A careful history and physical examination will help differentiate between benign and serious events. Particular attention should be paid to past history of prematurity, respiratory or feeding difficulties, infant siblings with unexplained death, stillbirths or miscarriage, as well as the duration of event, contemporaneous events (feeding, sleeping, vomiting, etc.), changes in color or motor tone, and infectious exposures.
- The differential diagnosis for an ALTE is broad and listed in Table 69-3.
- Gastroesophageal reflux disease (GERD) is ubiquitous in infancy and usually represents a benign physiologic process in which gastric contents are regurgitated into the esophagus. In pathological cases, complications including severe discomfort, failure to thrive, and aspiration can occur. GERD is problematic in the evaluation of ALTE because it can produce symptoms that trigger an ED visit in both physiological and pathological forms.
- The evaluation for an ALTE depends on the history of the event and the patient's condition in the ED.
- Stable patients with clear diagnoses (eg, witnessed seizure in ED that is identical to episode that prompted visit) can be managed according to etiology.
- Unstable patients should be resuscitated according to Pediatric Advanced Life Support (PALS) guidelines and have a differential diagnosis and diagnostic workup similar to stable patients without a clear diagnosis (by far the largest group of patients).
- Stable patients without a clear diagnosis are the largest group; screening labs (ABG, CBC, BMP, glucose, EKG, head CT, and fundoscopic examination) are directed by the history and physical examination, and can often be deferred to the inpatient team.
- Admission is usually required for any infants less than 2 months of age. Infants greater than 2 months with a clear and benign diagnosis (eg, reflux with choking episode), strong social support, reliable parents, and close primary care follow-up can be considered for discharge if both the physician and the family are confident in the diagnosis and its benign nature.
- Home apnea monitors have not been shown to affect outcomes and are not recommended.

SUDDEN INFANT DEATH SYNDROME

- Sudden infant death syndrome (SIDS) is the unexpected death of an infant under 1 year of age for which no cause can be determined by history, physical examination, postmortem examination, or scene investigation.
- Patients should be resuscitated per PALS guidelines with the exception of patients with rigor mortis, dependent livedo, initial serum pH <6, or significant hypothermia without explanatory environmental exposure.
- If resuscitation is unsuccessful, the treating physician must report the death to the medical examiner, but should not sign the death certificate as the medical examiner will complete the certificate after autopsy. The physician should also strongly consider involving the primary care physician, chaplain, and social worker (after discussion with the family).

For further reading in Tintinalli's *Emergency Medicine: A Comprehensive Study Guide,* 7th ed., see Chapter 111, "Neonatal Emergencies and Common Neonatal Problems," by Quynh H. Doan and Niranjan Kisson.

70 COMMON INFECTIONS OF THE EARS, NOSE, NECK, AND THROAT

David M. Spiro

ACUTE OTITIS MEDIA

EPIDEMIOLOGY

- Acute otitis media (AOM) accounts for 13% of emergency departments visits.
- The incidence is higher in males, children who attend day care, children exposed to smoke, and those with a family history of AOM.
- The most common pathogens are *Streptococcus pneumoniae* (31%) and non-typeable *Haemophilus influenzae* (56%).

PATHOPHYSIOLOGY

- Abnormal function of the eustachian tube appears to be the dominant factor in the pathogenesis of middle ear disease.

CLINICAL FEATURES

- The peak age is 6 to 36 months.
- Symptoms include fever, poor feeding, irritability, vomiting, otalgia, and otorrhea.

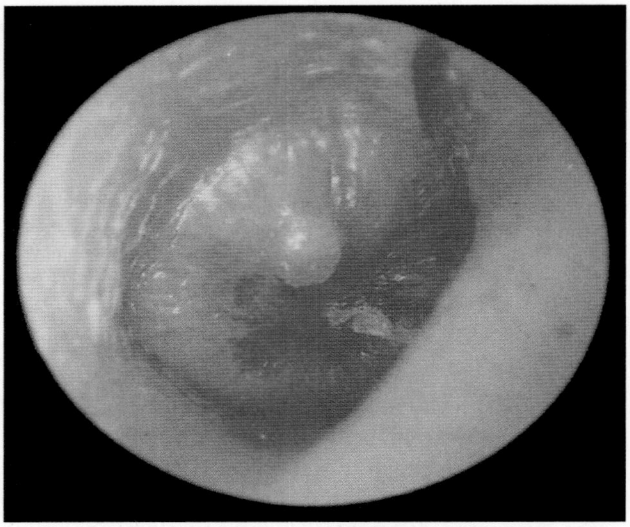

FIG. 70-1. Acute otitis media in a 3-year-old child with an outward bulge of the tympanic membrane and an exudative process in the middle ear space. (Courtesy of Dr. Shelagh Cofer, Department of Otolaryngology, Mayo Clinic.)

- Signs include bulging pus behind the tympanic membrane (TM) (Fig. 70-1), an immobile TM, loss of visualization of bony landmarks within the middle ear, and bullae on the TM (bullous myringitis).

DIAGNOSIS AND DIFFERENTIAL

- Making an accurate diagnosis is the most important first step.
- The definition of acute otitis media requires (A) acute onset (<48 hours) of signs and symptoms, (B) middle ear effusion (Fig. 70-1), and (C) signs and symptoms of middle ear inflammation. A red TM alone does not indicate the presence of an ear infection. Fever, prolonged crying, and viral infections can cause hyperemia of the TM. The normal TM is translucent and pearly grey (see Fig. 70-2).
- The most common causes of acute otalgia include AOM, otitis media with effusion, foreign body in the external ear canal, and otitis externa.

EMERGENCY DEPARTMENT CARE AND DISPOSITION

- *Treatment of pain is essential for all children diagnosed with AOM.* Topical analgesics such as benzocaine-antipyrene are recommended for routine use, unless there is a known perforation of the TM. Ibuprofen 10 milligrams/kg/dose is the preferred oral analgesic for AOM.

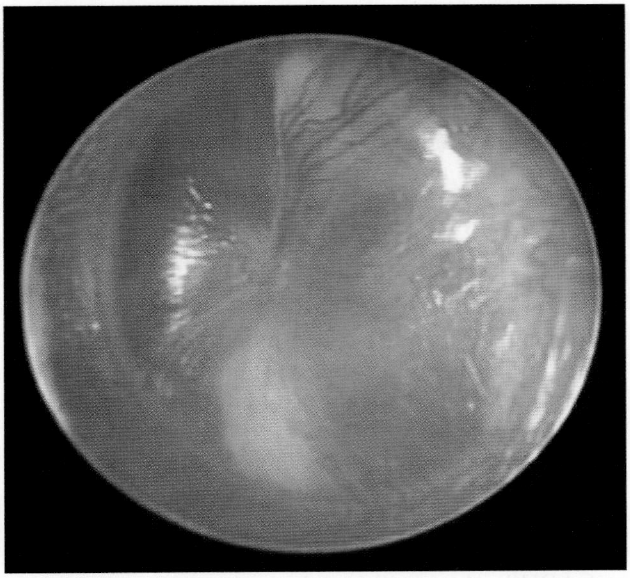

FIG. 70-2. Normal right tympanic membrane in 6-year-old child. (Courtesy of Dr. Shelagh Cofer, Department of Otolaryngology, Mayo Clinic.)

- Consider use of a "wait-and-see" prescription for the treatment of uncomplicated AOM. Parents are given a prescription and told to wait and see for 48 hours, and if the child is not better to fill the prescription. Treat AOM with immediate antibiotics with any of the following: age <6 months, an immunocompromised state, ill-appearance, recent use of antibiotics, or the diagnosis of another bacterial infection.
- Amoxicillin 40 to 50 milligrams/kg/dose PO twice daily remains the first drug of choice for uncomplicated AOM.
- Second-line antibiotics include amoxicillin/clavulanate 40 to 50 milligrams/kg/dose twice daily, cefpodoxime 5 milligrams/kg/dose PO twice daily, cefuroxime axetil 15 milligrams/kg/dose PO twice daily, cefdinir 7 milligrams/kg/dose PO twice daily, and ceftriaxone 50 milligrams/kg/d IM for three doses are alternatives. For patients allergic to the previously mentioned antibiotics, azithromycin 10 milligrams/kg/single dose PO on the first day followed by 5 milligrams/kg/single dose PO for 4 more days can be used.
- Infants less than 30 days of age with AOM are at risk for infection with group B *Streptococcus*, *Staphylococcus aureus*, and gram-negative bacilli and should undergo evaluation and treatment for presumed sepsis.
- In uncomplicated AOM, symptoms resolve within 48 to 72 hours; however, the middle ear effusion may persist as long as 8 to 12 weeks. Routine follow-up is not necessary unless the symptoms persist or worsen.
- Mastoiditis is the most common, serious complication of AOM. If mastoiditis is suspected, obtain a CT scan of the mastoid. If the diagnosis is confirmed, obtain consultation with an otolaryngologist and start IV antibiotics.

OTITIS EXTERNA

EPIDEMIOLOGY

- Otitis externa (OE) is an inflammatory process involving the auricle, external auditory canal (EAC), and surface of the TM. It is commonly caused by *Pseudomonas aeruginosa, Staphylococcus epidermidis*, and *Staph. aureus,* which often coexist.

PATHOPHYSIOLOGY

- OE occurs when protective features are compromised, often due to hyperhydration and maceration of the epithelial tissue, such as when a child is submerged during swimming.

CLINICAL FEATURES

- Peak seasons for OE are spring and summer, and the peak age is 9 to 19 years.
- Symptoms include earache, itching, and fever.
- Signs include erythema, edema of the EAC, white exudate in the EAC, pain with motion of tragus or auricle, and periauricular or cervical adenopathy.

DIAGNOSIS AND DIFFERENTIAL

- Diagnosis of OE is based on clinical signs and symptoms. A foreign body within the external canal should be excluded by carefully removing any debris that may be present.

EMERGENCY DEPARTMENT CARE AND DISPOSITION

- Cleaning the ear canal with a small tuft of cotton attached to a wire applicator is the first step. Place a wick in the canal if significant edema obstructs the EAC.
- Mild OE may be treated with acidifying agents alone, such as 2% acetic acid.
- Consider oral analgesics, such as ibuprofen at 10 milligrams/kg/dose every 6 hours as needed.
- Fluoroquinolone otic drops are now considered the preferred agents over neomycin-containing drops. Ciprofloxacin with hydrocortisone, 0.2% and 1% suspension (Cipro HC), three drops twice daily or

ofloxacin 0.3% solution 10 drops twice daily can be used. Ofloxacin is used when TM rupture is found or suspected.
- Oral antibiotics are indicated if auricular cellulitis is present.
- Follow-up should be advised if improvement does not occur within 48 hours; otherwise routine follow-up is not recommended.

ACUTE BACETRIAL SINUSITIS

EPIDEMIOLOGY

- Sinusitis is an inflammatory process that may be secondary to infection or allergy and may be acute, subacute, or chronic.
- Approxiamately 8% of upper respiratory infections (URIs) develop into acute sinusitis.

PATHOPHYSIOLOGY

- Blockage of the ostia by mucous and inflammation predisposes to acute sinusitis.
- The major pathogens in childhood are *Strep. pneumoniae, Moraxella catarrhalis,* and nontypeable *H. influenzae.*

CLINICAL FEATURES

- Acute sinusitis is associated with persistant (nasal drainage for 10-30 days) and severe symptoms (fever >39°C, purulent drainage, headaches, and localized swelling and tenderness or erythema over the sinuses).
- Reproducible, unilateral tenderness to percussion or direct pressure over the frontal or maxillary sinuses may indicate acute infection.

DIAGNOSIS AND DIFFERENTIAL

- The diagnosis is made on clinical grounds without routine use of imaging studies.
- Nasal congestion or colored drainage from the nose lasting up to 7 days often indicates a viral URI and should not be diagnosed as acute sinusitis and does not need treatment with antibiotics.

EMERGENCY DEPARTMENT CARE AND DISPOSITION

- For children with mild to moderate sinusitis, treat with high-dose amoxicillin (40-45 milligrams/kg/dose PO twice daily) for 10 to 14 days.
- For children who present with severe symptoms, are in day care, or have recently been treated with antibiotics, prescribe cephalosporins such as cefprozil (7.5-15 milligrams/kg/dose PO twice daily), cefuroxime (15 milligrams/kg/dose PO twice daily), and cefpodoxime (5 milligrams/kg PO twice daily).
- Intranasal steroids have shown modest benefits and are recommended if antibiotics do not result in improvement in the first 3 to 4 days of treatment.

STOMATITIS AND PHARYNGITIS

EPIDEMIOLOGY

- Herpangina, hand-foot-and-mouth disease (HFM), and herpes simplex gingivostomatitis are the primary infections that cause stomatitis and are all viral etiologies.
- The vast majority of pharyngitis is caused by viral infections (~85%) including Epstein–Barr virus (EBV) pharngitis.
- Peak seasons for group A β-hemolytic *Streptococcus* (GABHS) pharyngitis are late winter or early spring, the peak age is 5 to 15 years, and it is *rare before the age of two*.

PATHOPHYSIOLOGY

- GABHS and *Neisseria gonorrhoeae* are bacterial etiologies that require accurate diagnosis.
- The identification and treatment of GABHS pharyngitis is important in order to prevent the suppurative complications and the sequelae of acute rheumatic fever.

CLINICAL FEATURES

- Herpangina causes a vesicular enanthem of the tonsils and soft palate. The vesicles are painful and can be associated with fever and dysphagia.
- HFM disease usually begins as macules which progress to vesicles of the palate, buccal mucosa, gingiva, and tongue. Similar lesions may present on the palms of hands, soles of feet, and buttocks.
- Herpes simplex gingivostomatitis often presents with abrupt onset of fever, irritability, and decreased oral intake with edematous and friable gingival. Vesicular lesions, often with ulcerations, are seen in the anterior oral cavity.
- Symptoms of GABHS pharyngitis include sore throat, fever, headache, abdominal pain, enlarged anterior cervical nodes, palatal petechiae, and hypertrophy of the tonsils. With GABHS pharyngitis, there is usually an absence of cough, coryza, laryngitis, stridor, conjunctivitis, and diarrhea.
- EBV often presents much like streptococcal pharyngitis. Common symptoms are fever, sore throat, and malaise. Cervical adenopathy may be prominent and hepatosplenomegaly may be present.

DIAGNOSIS AND DIFFERENTIAL

- The diagnoses of herpangina, HFM, and herpes simplex gingivostomatitis are based on clinical findings.
- To diagnose GABHS, current guidelines recommend the use of **Centor criteria**: (a) tonsillar exudates, (b) tender anterior cervical lymphadenopathy, (c) absence of cough, and (d) history of fever. With two or more criteria, testing should be performed with a rapid antigen detection test and/or culture. If the rapid antigen test is negative, a confirmatory throat culture is recommended.
- Diagnosis of EBV is often clinical. The monospot test can aid in the diagnosis. The monospot may be insensitive in children <2 years of age and is often negative in the first week of illness. If obtained, the white blood cell count may show a lymphocytosis with a preponderance of atypical lymphocytes.

EMERGENCY DEPARTMENT CARE AND DISPOSITION

- Treatment of herpangina, HFM, and herpes simplex gingivostomatitis is primarily supportive. Systemic analgesics such as the combination of ibuprofen and tylenol should be considered. Occasionally oral narcotics may be required. IV hydration may be necessary if the child cannot tolerate oral fluids.
- Antibiotics for the treatment of GABHS pharyngitis are reserved for patients with a positive rapid antigen test or culture. Antibiotic choices for GABHS include penicillin (PCN) V 250 milligrams PO twice daily for children, 500 milligrams PO twice daily for adolescent/adults, benzathine PCN G 1.2 million U IM (600,000 units IM for patients weighing less than 27 kilograms), or erythromycin ethylsuccinate 10 to 20 milligrams/kg/dose PO twice daily for 10 days. *Antipyretics and analgesics should be routinely prescribed until symptoms resolve.*
- EBV is usually self-limited and requires only supportive treatment of antipyretics, fluids, and bedrest. A dose of dexamethasone 0.5 milligrams/kg PO to a maximum of 10 milligrams daily may be prescribed for more severe disease.

CERVICAL LYMPHADENITIS

EPIDEMIOLOGY

- Acute, unilateral cervical lymphadenitis is commonly caused by *Staph. aureus* or *Streptococcus pyogenes*.
- Bilateral cervical lymphadenitis is often caused by viral entities such as EBV and adenovirus.
- Chronic cervical lymphadenitis is less common but may be caused by *Bartonella henselae* (also called occuloglandular fever) or *Mycobacterium* species.

PATHOPHYSIOLOGY

- Infectious agents are transported by afferent lymph vessels to lymph nodes.
- The lymph nodes filter infectious and antigenic materials from the lymphatic fluid, lymphocytes, then proliferate, causing subsequent nodal enlargement.

CLINICAL FEATURES

- Acute cervical lymphadenitis presents with tender nodules often with overlying erythema.
- Bilateral cervical lymphadenitis presents with small, rubbery lymph nodes and usually self-resolves after 3 to 5 days of symptoms.
- *Bartonella henselae* results from a kitten scratch with ipsilateral cervical lymphadenitis and sometimes associated conjunctivitis and fever ("occuloglandular fever").

DIAGNOSIS AND DIFFERENTIAL

- Most cases are diagnosed clinically. Differential may also include sialoadenitis (infection of the salivary glands), which is usually caused by *Staph. aureus* or *Strep. pyogenes*. Malignancy and deep neck infections are additional considerations—the former are typically firm, immobile, and nontender; the latter are often associated with systemic signs such as fever and torticollis.

EMERGENCY DEPARTMENT CARE AND DISPOSITION

- For the treatment of acute cervical lymphadenitis, either amoxicillin plus clavulanic acid 15 to 20 milligrams/kg/dose twice daily or clindamycin 10 to 13 milligrams/kg/dose three times daily.
- The presence of a fluctuant mass may require incision and drainage in addition to antimicrobial therapy.
- Most cases of acute bilateral cervical lymphadenitis resolve without antibiotics, as they often represent viral infection or reactive enlargement.
- Chronic cases of lymphadenitis are often treated surgically, with directed antimicrobial therapy.

For further reading in Tintinalli's *Emergency Medicine: A Comprehensive Study Guide*, 7th ed., see Chapter 114, "Ear and Mastoid Disorders in Infants and Children," by David M. Spiro and Donald H. Arnold, and Chapter 118, "Neck Masses in Children," by Osama Y. Kentab and Nadeemuddin Qureshi.

71 STRIDOR AND DROOLING

Kathleen M. Adelgais

UPPER AIRWAY OBSTRUCTION

EPIDEMIOLOGY

- Diseases that cause upper respiratory tract (URT) obstruction account for a significant number of pediatric emergency department visits. While some diseases of the URT are common and benign, others, although rare, can be life threatening.
- Most causes of stridor among children younger than 6 months of age are a result of congenital abnormalities while stridor in older children is typically caused by acquired illnesses. Table 71-1 lists the common acquired causes of stridor.

PATHOPHYSIOLOGY

- Stridor is the physical sign common to all causes of URT obstruction and can be inspiratory, expiratory, or mixed.
- Stridor results from Venturi effects created by airflow through a narrow semicollapsible airway. With inhalation, the relative pressure in the center of the tube becomes greater than at the edges; the pressure differential leads to collapse of airway walls, obstruction, and turbulent airflow creating the sound of stridor.

TABLE 71-1 Common Acquired Causes of Stridor

	VIRAL CROUP	BACTERIAL TRACHEITIS	EPIGLOTTITIS	PERITONSILLAR ABSCESS	RETROPHARYNGEAL ABSCESS	FOREIGN BODY ASPIRATION
Etiology	Parainfluenza viruses (occasionally respiratory syncytial virus and rhinovirus)	*Staphylococcus aureus* (most) *S. pneumoniae* *Haemophilus influenzae*	*Streptococcus pneumoniae* *S. aureus* *H. influenzae*	Polymicrobial *S. pyogenes* *S. aureus* Oral anaerobes	Polymicrobial *S. pyogenes* *S. aureus* Gram-negative rods Oral anaerobes	Variable Foods Peanuts Sunflower seed Balloons/other toys
Age	6 mo-3 y old Peak 1-2 y old	3 mo-13 y old Mean, 5-8 y old	All ages Classically 1-7 y old	10-18 y old (most) 6 mo-5 y old (rare)	6 mo-4 y old Rare >4 years	Any 6 mo-5 y old most common 80% <3 years
Onset	1-3 d	2-7 d viral upper respiratory infection Suddenly worse over 8-12 h	Rapid, hours	Antecedent pharyngitis	Insidious over 2-3 d after an upper respiratory infection or local trauma	Immediate or delayed possible
Effect of positioning on symptoms	None	None	Worse supine prefer erect, chin forward	Worse supine	Neck stiffness and hyperextension	Usually none Location-dependent
Stridor	Inspiratory and expiratory	Inspiratory and expiratory	Inspiratory	Uncommon	Inspiratory when severe	Location-dependent
Cough	Seal-like bark	Usually Possible thick sputum	No	No	No	Often transient or positional
Voice	Hoarse Not muffled	Usually normal Possibly raspy	Muffled "Hot potato"	Muffled "Hot potato"	Often muffled "Hot potato"	Location-dependent Primarily if at or above glottis
Drooling	No	Rare	Yes	Often	Yes	Rare—often if esophageal
Dysphagia	Occasional	No	Yes	Yes	Yes	Rare—typically if esophageal
Radiologic appearance	Subglottic narrowing "steeple"	Subglottic narrowing Irregular tracheal margins	Enlarged epiglottis Thickened aryepiglottic folds	May see enlarged tonsillar soft tissue	Thickened bulging retropharyngeal soft tissue	Often normal Possible radiopaque density Ball-valve effect Segmented atelectasis

- Resistance is inversely proportion to the fourth power of the airway radius during laminar gas flow and the fifth power during turbulent flow. In the normal pediatric subglottis, 1 mm of edema will reduce its cross-sectional area by 50%.
- As air progresses from the supraglottic to the glottic and subglottic areas and finally the trachea, there is an increase in physiologic support structure that decreases the amount of collapse that occurs during inspiration. These structures (eg, tracheal rings) are less developed in young infants.
- Expiratory stridor, or wheeze, is common in distal airways since intrathoracic pressure may become much greater than atmospheric pressure during expiration. The pressure differential creates high relative laminar flow through semicollapsible bronchi, resulting in wheezes.

CLINICAL FEATURES

- Inspiratory stridor indicates obstruction at or above the larynx (ie, supraglottic). There is often marked inspiratory and expiratory variation.
- Glottic and subglottic obstructions commonly cause both inspiratory and expiratory stridor of lesser magnitudes. Obstruction at the level of the trachea and primary bronchi may be associated with inspiratory or expiratory stridor, but usually to a much lesser degree.
- Expiratory stridor usually implies obstruction below the carina.
- Hypoxia may be present with or without cyanosis, which depends on the hemoglobin level and peripheral circulation. Cyanosis in upper airway obstruction is an ominous sign.
- Tachypnea, retractions (subcostal, intercostal, supraclavicular), and nasal flaring or head bobbing, are signs of labored respirations.
- Grunting is a valuable diagnostic sign as it localizes disease to the lower respiratory tract and correlates with disease severity.

DIAGNOSIS AND DIFFERENTIAL

- The diagnosis of upper airway obstruction is clinical through observation of signs of increased work of breathing and stridor.
- The differential diagnosis is aided by considering the age of the patient and duration of symptoms.
- Children less than 6 months old with a long duration of symptoms characteristically have a congenital cause of stridor. Common congenital causes of stridor include laryngomalacia, tracheomalacia, vocal cord paralysis, and subglottic stenosis. Less common, but important causes include airway hemangiomas, vascular rings, and slings.
- Patients over 6 months of age with a short duration of symptoms characteristically have an acquired cause of stridor such as viral croup, epiglottitis, foreign body aspiration, peritonsillar abscess, or retropharyngeal abscess.
- The differential diagnosis and disease severity determine further diagnostic testing, which may include imaging (eg, soft-tissue neck and chest radiography or CT, barium swallow), blood work (eg, CBC, blood cultures), or endoscopy.

■ STRIDOR IN NEONATES

EPIDEMIOLOGY

- Laryngomalacia accounts for 60% of all neonatal laryngeal problems.
- After tracheomalacia, vocal cord paralysis is the most common causes of neonatal stridor.

PATHOPHYSIOLOGY

- Laryngomalacia is caused by a developmentally weak larynx, which results in airway collapse at the epiglottis, aryepiglottic folds, and arytenoids during inspiration.
- Vocal cord paralysis may be congenital or acquired. There may be a history of birth trauma, shoulder dystocia, macrosomia, forceps delivery, or other intrathoracic anomaly.

CLINICAL FEATURES

- Stridor from laryngomalacia worsens with crying or agitation and improves with neck extension or when prone.
- Laryngomalacia is usually a self-limited disorder that resolves in 90% of cases by 18 months of age.
- Stridor from vocal cord paralysis is typically chronic and may worsen with agitation or secondary viral infection; signs of respiratory distress or cyanosis may be present.

DIAGNOSIS AND DIFFERENTIAL

- A presumptive diagnosis can be made clinically, though definitive diagnosis is made by fiberscopic laryngeal examination.
- The differential diagnosis includes tracheomalacia, vascular anomalies, foreign body, and infectious causes of stridor.

EMERGENCY DEPARTMENT CARE AND DISPOSITION

- Laryngomalacia is usually a self-limiting disease and is only rarely associated with respiratory failure, failure to thrive, apnea, or feeding problems.
- Patients with respiratory failure and vocal cord paralysis require cautious airway management: endotracheal intubation can be quite difficult in a child with bilateral cord paralysis. Placing the bevel of the tube parallel to the small remaining glottic opening and rotating the tube one-quarter turn with gentle pressure may facilitate passing the tube. Force should never be applied since this may cause damage to laryngeal structures.
- Minimally symptomatic patients with lifelong stridor and no signs of distress or hypoxia can be referred to outpatient pediatric otolaryngology for definitive diagnosis.
- Patients with signs of respiratory distress or hypoxia should be admitted to the hospital.

VIRAL CROUP (LARYNGOTRACHEOBRONCHITIS)

EPIDEMIOLOGY

- Viral croup is responsible for most cases of stridor after the neonatal period, and is usually a benign, self-limited disease, though it can rarely cause life-threatening airway obstruction.
- Children ages 6 months to 3 years are most commonly affected, with a peak at age 12 to 24 months. Croup is rare after 6 years of age but can occur as late as 12 to 15 years of age.
- Croup is seasonal and occurs mainly in late fall and early winter in North America.

PATHOPHYSIOLOGY

- Croup is caused by a number of viral infections, parainfluenza (I, II, and III) being the most common; influenza, respiratory syncytial virus (RSV), adenovirus, enterovirus, rhinovirus, and metapneumovirus can also cause croup.
- Transmission is usually airborne with infection entering the nose and pharynx and spreading to the larynx and trachea.
- Inflammation and edema result from viral invasion and cytotoxicity, particularly in the subglottic larynx and trachea around the cricoid cartilage, leading to upper airway obstruction.
- Spasmodic croup results from subglottic edema that may be related to allergy or viral infection.

CLINICAL FEATURES

- Croup typically begins with a 1- to 5-day prodrome of cough and coryza, which is followed by a 3- to 4-day period of classic barking cough, stridor, and hoarseness. Symptoms peak on days 3 to 4 and then wane.
- Spasmodic croup is typically sudden in onset and occurs at night without antecedent symptoms of infection; it may be recurrent.
- Croup represents a spectrum of illness from barking cough to stridor at rest with associated labored breathing and hypoxia.

DIAGNOSIS AND DIFFERENTIAL

- The diagnosis of croup is clinical.
- Physical examination classically reveals a barking cough with or without stridor, which is classically inspiratory but can be biphasic. Stridor may occur with crying or at rest, and may be associated with signs of increased work of breathing.
- Laboratory and radiographic studies are not necessary for typical croup, though may aid in the differential diagnosis, which includes epiglottitis, bacterial tracheitis, or foreign body aspiration.
- If obtained, a lateral neck and chest radiograph may demonstrate that the normally squared shoulders of the subglottic tracheal air shadow are shaped like a pencil tip, hourglass, or steeple. This "steeple sign" is neither sensitive nor specific for croup.

EMERGENCY DEPARTMENT CARE AND DISPOSITION

- Place patients on pulse oximetry and administer oxygen for hypoxia.
- Give dexamethasone 0.15 to 0.6 milligram/kg (10 milligrams max) PO or IM. The IV form of dexamethasone may be given orally, is concentrated and thus smaller volume, and is well tolerated. Nebulized budesonide (2 milligrams) may be clinically useful in moderate to severe cases. Even patients with mild croup have been shown to benefit from steroids.
- Administer nebulized racemic epinephrine, 0.05 mL/kg/dose up to 0.5 mL of 2.25% solution, for patients with stridor at rest and signs of respiratory distress. Alternatively L-epineprhine (1:1000) 0.5 mL/kg (max 5 mL) can be used. Children with stridor associated only with agitation do not need epinephrine.
- Helium plus oxygen (Heliox) in a 70:30 mixture may prevent the need for intubation in children with severe croup. Heliox is only effective to a maximum concentration of oxygen of 40%, and is therefore not useful in patients requiring additional oxygen for hypoxia.

TABLE 71-2	Criteria for Discharge from ED in Patients with Croup
3 h since last epinephrine	
Nontoxic appearance	
Able to take fluids well	
Caretaker able to recognize change in child's condition and has adequate transportation to return if necessary	
Parents have a phone and no social issues for concern	

- Although intubation should be performed whenever clinically indicated, when treated aggressively, less than 1% of admitted patients require intubation. When necessary, consider using smaller endotracheal tubes than recommended to avoid trauma to inflamed mucosa.
- Most patients can be safely discharged to home if they meet criteria listed in Table 71-2.
- Children with persistent stridor at rest, tachypnea, retractions, and hypoxia or those who require more than two treatments of epinephrine should be admitted to the hospital.

EPIGLOTTITIS

EPIDEMIOLOGY

- Epiglottitis is life threatening and can occur at any age. Since the introduction of *Haemophilus influenzae* vaccine the incidence and demographics have changed remarkably, with less than 25% of cases caused by *Haemophilus*, and a median age of presentation shifting to older children and adults.
- In immunized children, most cases are caused by gram-positive organisms, including *Streptococcus pyogenes*, *Staphylococcus aureus*, and *Streptococcus pneumoniae*.
- In immunocompromised children, herpes, *Candida*, and varicella can cause epiglottitis.

CLINICAL FEATURES

- Classically there is abrupt onset of high fever, sore throat, and drooling. Symptoms may rapidly progress to stridor and respiratory distress. Cough may be absent.
- Patients usually appear toxic and may assume a tripod or sniffing position to maintain their airway.
- Symptoms in older children and adults may be subtle; severe sore throat, with or without stridor may be the primary complaint.

DIAGNOSIS AND DIFFERENTIAL

- The diagnosis is clinical and suggested by severe sore throat, a normal-appearing oropharynx, and tenderness with gentle movement of the hyoid.
- Radiographs are usually unnecessary in patients with a classic presentation.
- When the diagnosis is uncertain, lateral neck radiographs should be obtained with the neck extended during inspiration. The normal epiglottis is tall and thin, but appears swollen, squat, and flat like a thumbprint when inflamed (Fig. 71-1).
- False-negative radiographs can occur, and if clinical suspicion exists, direct visualization of the epiglottis, preferably in the operating room with anesthesiology and otolaryngology present.
- Blood cultures are positive in up to 90% of patients, while cultures from the epiglottis are less sensitive.
- A CBC may reveal leukocytosis and left shift.

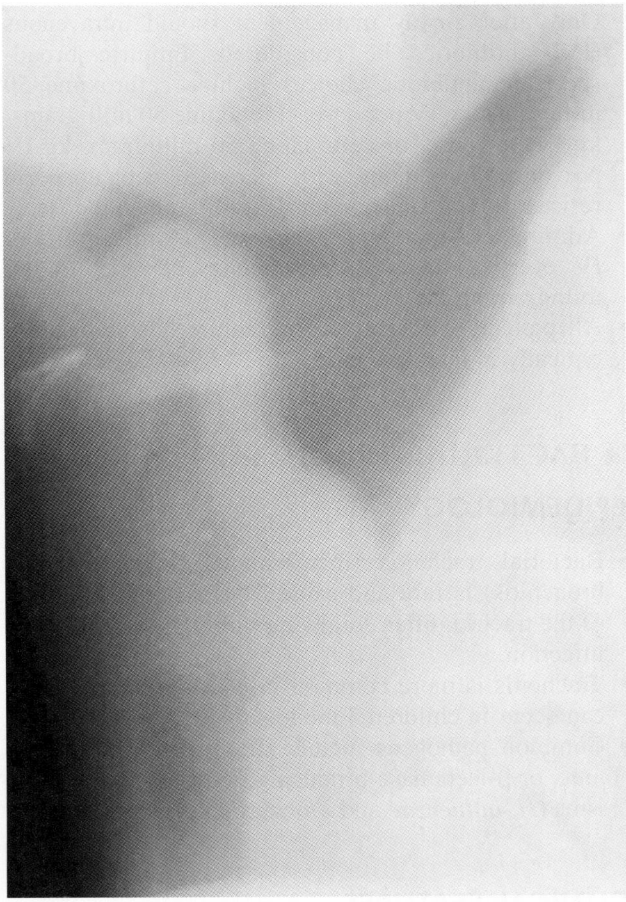

FIG. 71-1. Lateral neck view of a child with epiglottitis. (Courtesy of W. McAlister, MD, Washington University School of Medicine, St. Louis, MO.)

EMERGENCY DEPARTMENT CARE AND DISPOSITION

- Anticipation of airway loss is of primary importance in epiglottitis, and preparation for emergent advanced airway management (medical and surgical) should take place early; patients should be accompanied by a physician if moved to a radiograph suite.
- Keep patients seated and upright. Provide oxygen and administer nebulized racemic or L-epinephrine. Consider heliox if available.
- If total airway obstruction or apnea occurs, children with epiglottitis sometimes can be effectively ventilated with a bag-valve-mask device.
- The most experienced individual should perform intubation as soon as the diagnosis is made. Ensure that multiple endotracheal tube sizes are immediately available. Use of paralytics in the patient who is able to maintain their airway must be accompanied by the certainty that intubation will be successful or that a surgical airway can immediately be performed if unsuccessful.
- Only after airway management should intravenous (IV) antibiotics be considered. Empiric broad-spectrum antibiotic choices include cefuroxime 50 milligrams/kg IV per dose, cefotaxime 50 milligrams/kg IV per dose, or ceftriaxone 50 milligrams/kg IV per dose. In regions with increased cephalosporin resistance, add vancomycin 10 milligrams/kg/dose.
- Administer methylprednisolone 1 milligram/kg IV every 6 hours or dexamethasone 0.15 to 0.6 milligram/kg IV.
- All patients with epiglottitis require hospitalization, typically in intensive care.

BACTERIAL TRACHEITIS

EPIDEMIOLOGY

- Bacterial tracheitis (membranous laryngotracheobronchitis) is rare and caused by bacterial infection of the trachea, often following viral upper respiratory infection.
- Tracheitis is more common in children under 3, but can occur in children 3 months to 13 years of age.
- Common pathogens include *S. aureus*, *S. pneumoniae*, or β-lactamase-producing gram-negative organisms (*H. influenzae* and *Moraxella catarrhalis*).

CLINICAL FEATURES

- Symptoms of tracheitis resemble severe croup or epiglottitis.
- Patients often appear toxic, and may have cough, stridor (inspiratory and expiratory), hoarseness, and occasionally thick sputum production.
- Dysphagia is uncommon with tracheitis.

DIAGNOSIS AND DIFFERENTIAL

- Radiographs of the lateral neck and chest usually demonstrate subglottic narrowing of the trachea, and an irregular "shaggy" boarder (Fig. 71-2).
- Bacterial cultures of tracheal secretions and blood may identify a pathogen and antibiotic sensitivities; a CBC may reveal leukocytosis.

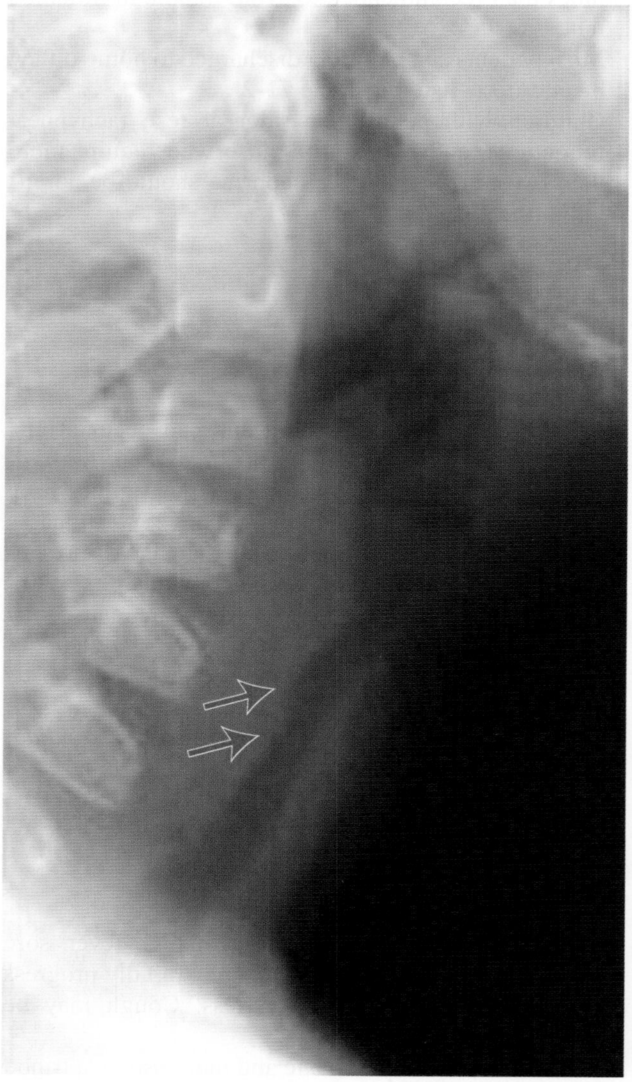

FIG. 71-2. Lateral neck view of patient with bacterial tracheitis. Note presence of irregular tracheal margins (*arrows*). (Courtesy of W. McAlister, MD, Washington University School of Medicine, St. Louis, MO.)

EMERGENCY DEPARTMENT CARE AND DISPOSITION

- Management is similar to that of epiglottitis, with primary attention to airway and anticipation of airway loss. Greater than 85% of patients ultimately require intubation. As with epiglottitis, ideal intubating conditions include an operating room for sedation, paralysis, intubation, and bronchoscopy. The emergency department physician must be prepared to perform emergent intubation and should prepare multiple endotracheal tube sizes.
- Initial antibiotic choices include ampicillin/sulbactam 50 milligrams/kg/dose IV, or the combination of a third-generation cephalosporin such as **ceftriaxone** 50 milligrams/kg IV per dose and clindamycin 10 milligrams/kg/dose. In areas with increasing *S. aureus* resistance, consider **vancomycin** 10 milligrams/kg IV every 6 hours.

RETROPHARYNGEAL ABSCESS

EPIDEMIOLOGY

- Retropharyngeal abscesses, although rare, are the second most common deep neck infection, usually occurring in children aged 6 months to 6 years of age.
- Infection in the retropharyngeal space can be caused by aerobic organisms (eg, β-hemolytic streptococci and *S. aureus*) anaerobes (eg, *Bacteroides*), and gram-negative organisms (eg, *Haemophilus*).
- The incidence of retropharyngeal abscess appears to be increasing in the United States in recent years.

CLINICAL FEATURES

- Patients usually present with fever, sore throat, neck pain, drooling, dysphagia/odynophagia. Dysphagia and refusal to feed occur before significant respiratory distress.
- Patients typically appear toxic and neck swelling or torticollis may be noted on examination along with drooling.
- Rapidly fatal airway obstruction from sudden rupture of the abscess pocket can occur.
- Aspiration pneumonia, empyema, mediastinitis, and erosion into the jugular vein and carotid artery have been reported.

DIAGNOSIS AND DIFFERENTIAL

- Physical examination of the pharynx may demonstrate posterior pharyngeal fullness. Additional examination findings include nuchal rigidity or torticollis, cervical adenopathy, drooling, and fever.
- Plain radiographs of the lateral neck during inspiration may show a widened retropharyngeal space; the diagnosis is suggested when the retropharyngeal space at C2 is twice the diameter of the vertebral body or greater than one-half the width of C4.
- CT of the neck with IV contrast is thought to be near 100% sensitive and is the diagnostic study of choice.
- Blood tests are rarely helpful for diagnosis or acute management.

EMERGENCY DEPARTMENT CARE AND DISPOSITION

- Immediate airway stabilization is the first priority. Unstable patients should be intubated before performing imaging.
- Empiric antibiotic choice is controversial since most retropharyngeal abscesses contain mixed flora. Consider broad-spectrum coverage with ampicillin-sulbactam, 200 milligrams/kg/d divided every 6 hours, and/or clindamycin 25 to 40 milligrams/kg IV divided every 6 hours. In penicillin-allergic patients, clindamycin and a third-generation cephalosporin are recommended.
- Steroids may reduce airway inflammation and prevent progression of cellulitis to abscess.
- Consult otolaryngology for operative incision and drainage; although cellulitis and some very small abscesses may improve with antibiotics alone, most require surgery.

PERITONSILLAR ABSCESS

EPIDEMIOLOGY

- Peritonsillar abscesses occur most frequently in adolescents and young adults.
- Most are unilateral, with <10% becoming bilateral.

CLINICAL FEATURES

- Symptoms include fever, sore throat (often unilateral), dysphagia, odynophagia, and neck pain.
- Patients usually appear acutely ill with fever, and may have trismus, drooling, and a muffled "hot potato" voice. The uvula is displaced away from the affected side. As a rule the affected tonsil is anteriorly and medially displaced.

DIAGNOSIS AND DIFFERENTIAL

- Careful visualization of the oral cavity can reliably confirm or exclude peritonsillar abscess in most cases.

The presence of uvular deviation, soft palate displacement, trismus, airway compromise, or localized areas of fluctuance are sufficient for diagnosis and no imaging is required.
- For ambiguous cases computed tomography (CT) or ultrasound (US) of the neck may be helpful.

EMERGENCY DEPARTMENT CARE AND DISPOSITION

- The majority of cases can be safely treated in the ED with needle drainage followed by outpatient antibiotics and analgesics.
- Formal incision and drainage in the operating room is sometimes necessary, especially in young or uncooperative patients.
- Parenteral antibiotic choices include clindamycin 10 milligrams/kg IV or ampicillin-sulbactam 50 milligrams/kg; oral options include **amoxicillin/clavulanate** 45 milligrams/kg/d divided twice a day or clindamycin 10 to 20 milligrams/kg/d divided every 6 to 8 hours.
- Close outpatient follow-up is essential for all discharged patients.

FOREIGN BODY ASPIRATION

EPIDEMIOLOGY

- Foreign body (FB) aspirations cause over 3000 deaths each year, and have a peak incidence between ages 1 and 3 years. In children under 6 months of age, the cause is usually secondary to a feeding by a well-meaning sibling.
- Commonly aspirated foreign bodies include foods and toys.

CLINICAL PRESENTATION

- Clinical symptoms and signs depend on the size and location of the aspirated foreign body and range from mild coughing to acute airway obstruction and respiratory failure. Many patients are completely asymptomatic.
- Classic teaching is that an FB in the laryngotracheal area causes stridor, whereas a bronchial FB causes wheezing. There is significant overlap in symptoms, however, and wheeze is present in 30% of laryngotracheal FB aspirations, and stridor in up to 10% of bronchial aspirations.

DIAGNOSIS AND DIFFERENTIAL

- A high index of suspicion is required to diagnose FB aspiration. Since as many as one-third of the aspirations are not witnessed or remembered by the parent, FB aspirations should be considered in all children with unilateral wheezing or persistent symptoms that do not respond to standard bronchodilator therapy.
- Plain chest radiograph can be normal: >50% of tracheal FB, 25% of bronchial FB, and more than 75% of FB in children < 3 years of age are radiolucent. In cases of complete obstruction, atelectasis may be found. In partial obstructions, air trapping with asymmetric hyperinflation of the obstructed lung may occasionally be seen. There is little additional value to expiratory or decubitus views.
- Definitive diagnosis requires laryngoscopy or bronchoscopy in the operating room, which should be considered in any patient with a history of choking, asymmetric breath sounds, or suggestive findings on chest radiograph.
- The differential diagnosis of upper airway foreign body includes esophageal foreign body: radiographically, flat foreign bodies such as coins are usually oriented in the sagittal plane when located in the trachea (ie, appears as a thick line in an antero-posterior chest radiograph) and in the coronal plane when in the esophagus (ie, appears round on an anteroposterior chest radiograph).

EMERGENCY DEPARTMENT CARE AND DISPOSITION

- If FB aspiration or airway obstruction is clearly present, BLS procedures to relieve airway obstruction should be implemented immediately.
- If BLS maneuvers fail, perform direct laryngoscopy and attempt to remove the FB with Magill forceps. If the FB cannot be seen, orotracheal intubation with distal displacement of the FB into a bronchus may be lifesaving.
- Consider racemic epinephrine or Heliox for patients with stridor and respiratory distress as a temporizing measure.
- Definitive treatment usually requires rigid laryngoscopy or bronchoscopy under general anesthesia.
- Foreign bodies in the proximal airways require immediate treatment while distal foreign bodies may be removed in the outpatient setting after consultation with subspecialists when reliable follow-up can be ensured.

For further reading in Tintinalli's *Emergency Medicine: A Comprehensive Study Guide*, 7th ed., see Chapter 119, "Stridor and Drooling," by Joseph D. Gunn III.

72 WHEEZING IN INFANTS AND CHILDREN

Donald H. Arnold

WHEEZING

EPIDEMIOLOGY

- Eighty percent of wheezing in patients <1 year is due to viral bronchiolitis and resolves by 3 years.

PATHOPHYSIOLOGY

- Wheezing implies diffuse or focal obstructive lower airway disease.
- Dynamic airway compression results in auto-PEEP with increased work of breathing and V/Q mismatch.
- V/Q mismatch results in mild hypoxemia (>92%) that responds to minimal oxygen supplementation. If more severe hypoxemia, consider pneumonia or pneumothorax.

CLINICAL FEATURES

- Wheezing may diminish as air entry becomes more compromised.
- Air entry and accessory muscle use are the most valid bedside measures of severity but may diminish if the patient becomes fatigued.
- Retractions progress in a rostral-caudal direction with subcostal, intercostal, and supraclavicular accessory muscle use.

DIAGNOSIS AND DIFFERENTIAL

- Asthma and bronchiolitis account for most episodes of wheezing, but other causes should always be considered (Table 72-1).

EMERGENCY DEPARTMENT CARE AND DISPOSITION

- Determine precipitating events and whether wheezing is diffuse or localized.

TABLE 72-1 Differential Diagnosis of Wheezing According to Presenting Signs and Symptoms

SIGNS, SYMPTOMS, AND CONTEXT	POSSIBLE DIAGNOSES	ANCILLARY TESTING
Feeding-related cough, gagging, or emesis; present from birth	Gastroesophageal reflux Tracheoesophageal fistula	Esophageal pH probe Barium swallow
Multiple lower respiratory tract illnesses or infections; failure to thrive; present from birth	Cystic fibrosis Ciliary dyskinesia Immunodeficiency	Sweat chloride concentration Ciliary biopsy Immunoglobulin assays
Diffuse rales; tachycardia; hepatomegaly; cardiac murmur	Congenital heart disease with left-to-right shunt and congestive heart failure Myocarditis	CXR; ECG; echocardiography
Associated stridor; positional changes with neck flexion, extension, or rotation	Vascular ring or other great vessel malformation; airway polyp or hemangioma	CXR; CT angiography; barium swallow; bronchoscopy
Stridor with high fever; ill appearance; drooling	Epiglottitis	Soft tissue radiographs of neck
Abrupt-onset stridor and/or wheezing; history of choking episode	Foreign-body aspiration Vocal cord dysfunction (paradoxical vocal cord motion)	CXR Bronchoscopy Flexible fiberoptic laryngoscopy
Stridor and/or wheezing that changes with position, or is exacerbated during feeding or upper respiratory illness and present from birth	Tracheomalacia Laryngomalacia	Observation Bronchoscopy
Tachypnea; fever; rales; grunting	Pneumonia	CXR
URI symptoms; seasonal outbreaks; nasal flaring	Bronchiolitis	Viral antigen testing
Episodic exacerbations with wheezing and/or cough; seasonal or after exposure to allergens; responds to bronchodilators	Asthma	Pulmonary function testing; trial of albuterol; allergy testing

Abbreviations: CHF = congestive heart failure, CXR = chest radiograph, URI = upper respiratory infection.

- Quickly evaluate for adequacy of air entry, work of breathing, and oxygenation.
- Use standardized respiratory distress score to establish baseline severity and response to treatment.
- Fatigue, drowsiness, and altered mental status are signs of respiratory failure.

ASTHMA

EPIDEMIOLOGY

- Asthma is the most common chronic disease of childhood and most frequent reason for pediatric hospitalizations in North America.
- Exacerbations occur in 57% of children with asthma and account for 640,000 ED visits each year.
- Rhinovirus wheezing illnesses in early childhood are the strongest predictor of asthma at 6 years of age. Other risk factors include second-hand smoke exposure, urban household (cockroach) exposure, family history, and race (non-Hispanic black children).
- Near-fatal or fatal asthma may occur even in patients with previously mild episodes. Risk factors include massive allergen exposure, emotional distress, obesity, limited access to health care, improper medication administration, history of prior respiratory failure, African-American race, and impaired perception of dyspnea.

PATHOPHYSIOLOGY

- The primary pathophysiologic event is airway inflammation, leading to airway hyperresponsiveness and obstruction. Each of these three components must be treated.
- The most common triggers are allergens, irritants, and viral respiratory infections.
- Bronchospasm, mucosal edema, and mucous plugging cause variable and reversible airflow obstruction, dynamic airway compression, and V/Q mismatch. Airway obstruction may become nonreversible over time.
- During early stages of exacerbation, mild hypoxemia and hypocapnia with respiratory alkalosis are observed. With decreasing alveolar ventilation, increased work of breathing and tissue hypoxia, $Paco_2$ increases and metabolic acidosis may predominate over respiratory alkalosis. Thus, rising $Paco_2$ may be an ominous indicator of respiratory failure.

CLINICAL FEATURES

- Acute asthma exacerbations comprise progressively worsening wheezing, cough, shortness of breath, and/or chest tightness. Any exacerbation may progress to unresponsive asthma (status asthmaticus), respiratory failure, and fatal asthma.
- Wheezing, cough, dyspnea, and fever (due to viral illness as precipitant) are the most common manifestations of an acute asthma exacerbation.
- The quiet chest is an ominous sign of severely compromised ventilation and indicates airflow insufficient to generate wheezing.
- Critical elements of physical assessment include mental status, accessory muscle use, respiratory rate, and air entry by auscultation.
- Hypoxia may result in agitation, whereas somnolence may result from hypercarbia and indicate respiratory failure and impending arrest.
- End-tidal CO_2 monitoring may be useful but may not be sensitive to rising $Paco_2$ if alveolar emptying is impaired.
- Pulsus paradoxus and PEF or FEV measurement are recommended by NHLBI guidelines but accurate measurement is difficult in the ED environment.

DIAGNOSIS AND DIFFERENTIAL

- Essential diagnostic questions are (1) Does this patient have asthma? (2) What is the severity of airway obstruction? (3) Is there a treatable condition that precipitated the exacerbation?
- Most children <3 years with wheezing do not have asthma. Children >3 years with wheezing, dyspnea, or cough that responds to albuterol may be given a provisional diagnosis of asthma. Spirometry for FEV is the criterion standard for airway obstruction but is generally not possible in children <6 years and in those in respiratory distress.
- Indications for chest radiograph in asthma include a first episode of wheezing, localized findings (dullness or rales) that do not resolve with bronchodilator treatment (possible foreign body or pneumonia), significant chest pain (possible pneumothorax), or respiratory distress out of proportion to the degree of airflow limitation. Viral infections are the most common precipitant, and thus many patients present with fever. Presence of fever alone is *not* an indication for chest radiograph. Chest radiograph findings include hyperinflation and atelectasis.

EMERGENCY DEPARTMENT CARE AND DISPOSITION

- Quickly identify the patient experiencing an acute severe exacerbation and escalate therapy as appropriate to prevent respiratory failure.

- Oxygen should be administered if saturation is <95%. Titrated oxygen to maintain saturation 95% to 98% may result in more rapid resolution of V/Q mismatch.
- Albuterol is the mainstay of treatment and can be administered by Metered Dose Inhaler (MDI) with expansion chamber (4-8 puffs every 20 minutes × 3 doses then Q 1-4 hours); by intermittent nebulization (0.15 milligram/kg, or 2.5 milligrams, every 20 minutes × 3 doses, then 0.15-0.3 milligram/kg up to 10 milligrams every 1-4 hours); or by continuous nebulization (0.5 milligram/kg/h).
- Ipratropium should be administered with nebulized albuterol (0.25-0.5 milligram Q 20 minutes × 3 doses).
- Systemic β-agonists have no advantage over inhaled albuterol except in the patient with minimal ventilation. Terbutaline can be administered SQ (0.01 milligram/kg, max 0.4 milligram, Q 20 minutes × 3 doses) or IV (0.01 milligram/kg load over 5-10 minutes then 0.001-0.01 milligram/kg/min). Epinephrine has β- and α-agonist activity that may shrink edematous mucosa (SQ: 0.01 milligram/kg, max 0.5 milligram, Q 15 minutes).
- Systemic corticosteroids (CCS) should be considered in all but the mildest cases that respond immediately to albuterol. CCS decrease airway inflammation and increase the effectiveness of β_2-agonists. Early administration decreases hospital admission rates. Prednisone (2 milligrams/kg/d, maximum 60 milligrams/d) as a 3 to 5 day course is usually sufficient and does not require tapering. Dexamethasone, 0.6 milligram/kg administered orally (IV formulation) or IM as a single dose may be as effective as a 3 to 5 day course and better tolerated (less vomiting). These medications are generally contraindicated in varicella-susceptible patients who have or might have exposure to varicella.
- Magnesium sulfate (50-75 milligrams/kg, maximum 2 grams, IV over 10-20 minutes) may provide rapid bronchodilation in the patient who is not ventilating sufficiently for nebulized albuterol delivery to peripheral airways.
- Ketamine (2 milligrams/kg IV followed by 2-3 milligrams/kg/h) is an effective bronchodilator and may delay or prevent respiratory failure and the need for assisted ventilation in the patient with severe status asthmaticus.
- Helium-oxygen (Heliox) as a 60:40 or 70:30 (helium:oxygen) mix may restore laminar airflow and improve alveolar ventilation. Nebulized albuterol may be administered with this treatment.
- IV fluids should be considered for the patient in status asthmaticus who has decreased oral intake or who is NPO due to the severity of the episode.
- Aminophylline is no longer recommended by the NHLBI guidelines.
- Respiratory failure may be avoided by rapid escalation of the above treatments. However, patient fatigue or persistent bronchospasm may nonetheless occur, and for this reason the need for endotracheal intubation and mechanical ventilation should be anticipated and planned. Laryngoscopy may precipitate severe laryngo- or bronchospasm; the decision to intubate should be carefully considered. Rapid-sequence intubation may include premedication with atropine (0.02 milligram/kg, minimum 0.5 milligram; maximum 1 milligram) and lidocaine (1.5 milligrams/kg) and sedation with ketamine (2 milligrams/kg), followed by paralysis using succinylcholine (2 milligrams/kg) or rocuronium (1 milligram/kg) to provide optimal intubating conditions.

Disposition

- Hospital admission is necessary for children who do not respond adequately to treatment (eg, persistent hypoxemia or failure to normalize aeration over 2-4 hours) or whose caretaker may not be able to provide necessary ongoing care.
- Discharge planning should include an "action plan" (available at http://www.nhlbi.nih.gov/health/public/lung/asthma/actionplan_text.htm), albuterol as MDI or nebulizer, oral CCS, and follow-up with the primary care provider.
- Inhaled corticosteroids should be prescribed for all patients with persistent asthma (as defined by NHLBI at Web site above).

BRONCHIOLITIS

EPIDEMIOLOGY

- Bronchiolitis affects 20% to 30% of all infants and is most frequent lower respiratory infection in first 2 years of life.
- Respiratory syncytial virus (RSV) and rhinovirus are the most common viruses associated with this illness, with RSV predominating during winter and rhinovirus in fall and spring.
- Peak bronchiolitis season is November to March but may occur throughout the year.
- Infants less than 2 years old are most commonly affected. The peak incidence in urban populations is 2 months of age.
- Young infants and those with history of prematurity, bronchopulmonary dysplasia, congenital heart disease, or immunosuppression are at increased risk of complicated courses of disease.

- Infection is highly contagious and is transmitted by direct contact with secretions and self-inoculation by contaminated hands via the eyes and nose. Infection does not confer immunity, and infants may develop multiple episodes.

PATHOPHYSIOLOGY

- There is acute airway inflammation and edema, small airway epithelial cell necrosis and sloughing, increased mucus production and mucus plugging, and bronchospasm, all of which vary considerably between patients and over the course of the illness.
- Nasal passages account for 50% total airway resistance and thus suctioning is usually beneficial. Increased overall airway resistance and decreased compliance result in increased work of breathing.
- Sustained immunity does not reliably occur, and reinfection with recurrence of illness is common.

CLINICAL FEATURES

- Clinical features indicate severity of illness and include dyspnea, coryza, cough, wheezing, variable hypoxemia, use of accessory muscles, nasal flaring, and poor feeding.
- Severity increases over the first 3 to 5 days with a total duration of illness of 7 to 14 days.
- Apnea (see below), cyanosis, or altered mental status or fatigue are ominous signs and may portend respiratory failure.
- Somnolence or apparent fatigue (including an inability to take fluids) or significant hypoxia or cyanosis signify more severe illness and warrant greater intensity of observation or intervention.
- Infants at risk of apnea include those who were born at <37 weeks gestation and are <12 weeks of age or postconception age <48 weeks; born at term but <4 weeks of age; have had witnessed apnea; have hemodynamically significant congenital heart disease (CHF, moderate to severe pulmonary hypertension, cyanotic lesions); have chronic lung disease (BPD, congenital malformations, CF); or are immunocompromised.

DIAGNOSIS AND DIFFERENTIAL

- Diagnosis is clinical and should not routinely involve laboratory or radiologic studies. Routine chest radiograph is not indicated for mild and typical episodes without focal chest findings.
- Patients with severe disease, possible respiratory failure, and/or apnea should be identified early.
- Testing for RSV or other pathogens and other lab studies is not routinely indicated.
- Serial assessment and oximetry is a key component for disposition decisions.

EMERGENCY DEPARTMENT CARE AND DISPOSITION

- Nasal suctioning and saline drops: nasal airflow resistance is 50% of total airways resistance and suctioning of the nasal passages after saline instillation alone may substantially decrease work of breathing, correct hypoxemia, and enable the patient to feed normally. Nasal vasoconstrictors are not indicated and have resulted in tachydysrrythmia.
- Oxygen saturation should be maintained >92%. Hypoxemia may result from V/Q mismatch and require minimal supplemental oxygen, or may result from significant airspace (alveolar) disease and require more intensive treatment.
- Nebulized α- and β-agonists should not be routinely used. However, use of a β_2-agonist (albuterol) might be considered, particularly if there is a personal or family history of asthma.
- Epinephrine (0.5 mL of 1:1000 in 2.5 mL saline) may be beneficial due to α-agonist mediated mucosal vasoconstriction with reduction of edema. If these medications are used, an objective measure (eg, respiratory rate or bronchiolitis score) should be used to assess response.
- Nebulized hypertonic saline (3% or 5%, 3-5 mL by nebulizer) may decrease mucus production and viscidity and, if beneficial, may be administered every 4 hours.
- Hydration should be assessed and managed with IV fluids if necessary. Patients with bronchiolitis may not be able to feed normally, and respiratory rates >60/minute increase the risk of aspiration.
- Helium-oxygen (heliox) may delay or prevent respiratory failure and need for intubation.
- Noninvasive ventilation (CPAP or BiPAP) may improve oxygenation and ventilation, decrease work of breathing, and delay or obviate the need for endotracheal intubation. Additionally, application of CPAP may prevent further apnea in affected infants.
- CCS should not be used routinely for patients with bronchiolitis. A single study suggests potential synergy when high-dose CCSs are coadministered with racemic epinephrine.
- Disposition decision making must consider the timepoint of disease progression (severity increases over the first 3-5 days of illness), the ability of caretakers to manage the illness, the availability of follow up,

and whether risk factors for apnea and/or severe disease are present.

- Indications for hospitalization include persistent hypoxia, tachypnea, increased work of breathing, and inability to feed or maintain hydration. Discharged patients should have follow-up with their primary care provider within 24 hours.

For further reading in Tintinalli's *Emergency Medicine: A Comprehensive Study Guide*, 7th ed., see Chapter 120, "Wheezing in Infants and Children," by Donald H. Arnold, David M. Spiro, and Melissa L. Langhan.

73 PNEUMONIA IN INFANTS AND CHILDREN

Chad D. McCalla

EPIDEMIOLOGY

- Pneumonia is more common in early childhood than at any other age and the incidence decreases with age (eg, 40 per 1000 in preschool children, 9 per 1000 in 10-year olds in North America).
- Viruses or bacteria usually cause pediatric pneumonia, though in most cases, the causative organism is unknown due to difficulties obtaining appropriate specimens, and age is the best predictor of etiology.
- Infants less than 4 months of age are at risk for *Chlamydia trachomatis*, RSV, other respiratory viruses, and *Bordetella pertussis*.
- In the 1 to 24 months age group, mild to moderate pneumonia can be caused by respiratory viruses as well as *Streptococcus pneumoniae*, *Haemophilus influenzae* (less commonly), and *Mycoplasma pneumoniae*.
- Although viral pathogens dominate during years 2 to 5, the above bacterial pathogens are common. By the sixth year through 18 years of age, influenza virus A or B and adenovirus are common.
- At any age, severe pneumonia may be caused by *Staphylococcus aureus*, *Strep. pneumoniae, M. pneumoniae*, *H. influenzae* B, and group A streptococci.
- Special consideration to unusual organisms must be given to children with immunosuppression (*Pneumocystis jiroveci*, CMV, fungi), cystic fibrosis (*Staph. aureus*, *Pseudomonas*), and sickle cell disease (encapsulated organisms).
- Risk factors for pneumonia and disease severity include prematurity, malnutrition, low socioeconomic status, passive exposure to smoke, and day care attendance.
- Although the mortality rate is less than 1% in industrialized nations, 5 million children less than 5 years of age in developing countries die each year from pneumonia.

PATHOPHYSIOLOGY

- Most cases of pneumonia develop after aspiration of infectious viruses or bacteria into the lower respiratory tract.
- Protective mechanisms include nasal entrapment of aerosolized particles, mucus and ciliary movement in the upper respiratory tract, laryngeal reflexes and coughing, alveolar macrophages, activation of complement and antibodies, and lymphatic drainage.
- Children who are at a higher risk for pneumonia include those with anatomic abnormalities of the airways, immune deficiencies, neuromuscular weakness, and abnormal mucus production.

CLINICAL FEATURES

- Clinical features of pneumonia vary with patient age and underlying health as well as infectious etiology.
- Neonates and young infants with pneumonia typically present with a sepsis syndrome. Signs and symptoms are nonspecific and include fever or hypothermia, tachycardia, or bradycardia, tachypnea or apnea, hypoxemia, poor feeding, lethargy or irritability, grunting, vomiting, and shock.
- Tachypnea is the most common physical sign in children with pneumonia. In an otherwise well-appearing child, the absence of tachypnea suggests another diagnosis, especially in the absence of respiratory distress, rales, or abnormal breath sounds.
- Signs and symptoms of pneumonia in older children include fever, cough, pleuritic chest pain, tachypnea, and abnormal lung examination. Associated signs and symptoms may include malaise, headache, rhinitis, conjunctivitis, pharyngitis, wheezing, and rash.
- Occasionally, abdominal pain is the primary complaint of a child with lower lobe pneumonia and respiratory symptoms may be omitted during the history.
- The clinical manifestations of bacterial and viral pneumonias overlap, making the clinical distinction between them problematic; no single physical examination finding is diagnostic, though combinations of signs and symptoms have better predictive value: the combination of fever, plus either tachypnea, decreased breath sounds or fine crackles predict radiograph positivity with a sensitivity of 93% to 96%.

DIAGNOSIS AND DIFFERENTIAL

- As discussed above, individual clinical signs and symptoms cannot reliably distinguish bacterial from viral pneumonia, and chest radiographs are commonly used for this purpose as consolidation is considered a reliable sign of pneumonia.
- Though radiologic distinction among viral, atypical, and bacterial pneumonias is not perfect, viral infections typically reveal diffuse interstitial infiltrates with hyperinflation, peribronchial thickening or cuffing, and areas of atelectasis. Bacterial infections tend to produce focal lobar or segmental infiltrates. Care must be taken to distinguish a normal pediatric thymus from focal consolidation (Figs. 73-1 and 73-2).
- Indications for chest radiography include (1) age 0 to 3 months as part of a "rule out sepsis" evaluation; (2) age <5 years with temperature >39°C (102.2°F), WBC count >20,000/mm^3, and no other source of infection; (3) ambiguous clinical findings; (4) suspicion for pulmonary complications (eg, pleural effusion or pneumothorax); (5) pneumonia that is prolonged or unresponsive to treatment; (6) suspicion of foreign body aspiration; suspected congenital lung malformations; (7) follow-up of "round pneumonia."
- Sputum cultures are generally unhelpful as they are difficult to obtain in young children, though they may be helpful for older children with cystic fibrosis or children with tracheostomies.
- Rapid viral antigen tests are available for RSV and influenza, and may be useful in reducing the inappropriate use of antibiotics or unnecessary invasive testing of infants and young children with fever.
- A CBC may reveal leukocytosis; a left shift is typical for bacterial pneumonia, or atypical, or cleft lymphocytes may be seen in children with viral infection or pertussis.

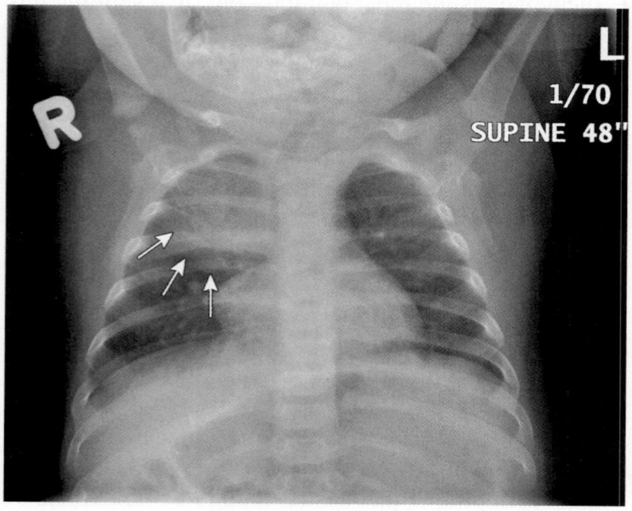

FIG. 73-1. Arrows indicate a normal thymus. Rotation, apparent from the location of the heart, trachea, and clavicles, makes this thymus appear to be far right of midline. (Courtesy of BC Children's Hospital, Vancouver, BC, Canada.)

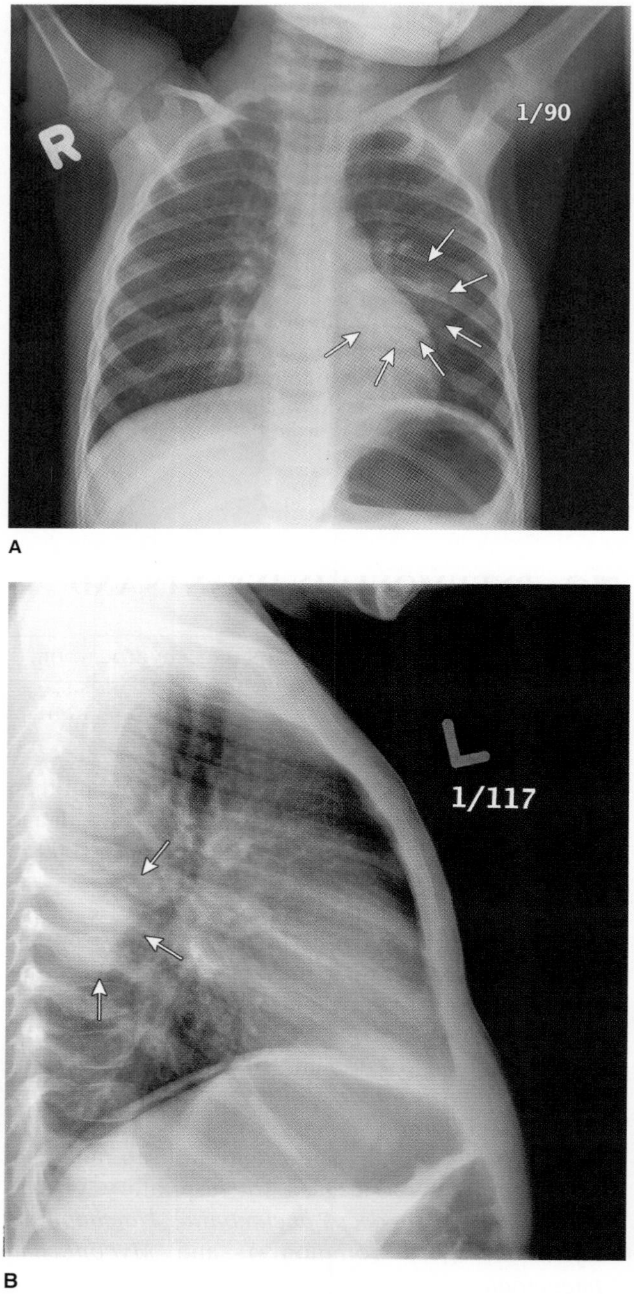

FIG. 73-2. Anterior-posterior (**A**) and lateral views (**B**) shows lower lobe consolidation (*arrows*). (Courtesy of BC Children's Hospital, Vancouver, BC, Canada.)

TABLE 73-1 Empiric Treatment for Pneumonia in Healthy Children

AGE GROUP	INPATIENT TREATMENT	OUTPATIENT TREATMENT
Neonates	Ampicillin 50 milligrams/kg IV *and* cefotaxime 50 milligrams/kg IV *or* gentamicin 2.5-5.0 milligrams/kg IV	Not recommended
1-3 months	Afebrile: erythromycin 10 milligrams/kg IV Febrile pneumonia: cefuroxime 50 milligrams/kg IV ± erythromycin IV	Not recommended
3 months-5 years	Ampicillin 50 milligrams/kg IV *or* cefuroxime 50 milligrams/kg IV ± erythromycin IV	Amoxicillin 40-50 milligrams/kg/dose twice daily *or* amoxicillin-clavulanate 22.5 milligrams/kg/dose twice daily *or* cefuroxime axetil 15 milligrams/kg/dose twice daily
5-18 years	Ampicillin 50 milligrams/kg IV *and* erythromycin 10 milligrams/kg IV Alternative: cefuroxime 50 milligrams/kg IV ± erythromycin	Azithromycin 10 milligrams/kg × 1 on day 1 then 5 milligrams/kg daily for 4 days *or* amoxicillin-clavulanate as above *or* cefuroxime axetil as above

- Blood cultures are positive <10% of the time in children with proven bacterial pneumonia and are not routinely recommended.
- The differential diagnosis for pneumonia in children includes congestive heart failure, atelectasis, tumors, congenital pulmonary anomalies, aspiration pneumonitis, chemical pneumonitis (eg, hydrocarbons), foreign body aspiration, diabetic ketoacidosis, GI emergencies (eg, appendicitis), and chronic pulmonary diseases.

EMERGENCY DEPARTMENT CARE AND DISPOSITION

- Treat hypoxia with supplemental oxygen.
- Consider positive pressure support (eg, continuous positive airway pressure) for severe respiratory distress and endotracheal intubation for respiratory failure.
- Administer isotonic crystalloid for dehydration caused by increased insensible losses and inability to tolerate oral intake (eg, young infants with significant tachypnea, children with vomiting).
- Treat bronchospasm with β-agonists.
- Treat bacterial pneumonia with empiric antibiotics selected by likely etiologic agent and whether treatment is inpatient or outpatient (Table 73-1).
- Most children with pneumonia can be treated as outpatients. Indications for admission include age <3 months, a history of apnea or cyanosis, toxic appearance, severe respiratory distress, pulmonary complications (eg, empyema), vomiting with inability to tolerate oral intake or medication, an unreliable home caretaker, and hypoxemia.
- The exact pulse oximetry threshold at which an otherwise well-appearing young child with pneumonia should be admitted to the hospital is unknown, however, POX <90% on room air correlates with an increased risk of amoxicillin treatment failure.

For further reading in Tintinalli's *Emergency Medicine: A Comprehensive Study Guide*, 7th ed., see Chapter 121, "Pneumonia in Infants and Children," by Joseph E. Copeland.

74 PEDIATRIC HEART DISEASE

Garth D. Meckler

- This chapter covers common presentations of congenital heart disease as they present to the emergency department (ED): cyanosis, shock, and congestive heart failure.
- Other cardiovascular topics such as dysrhythmias (Chapter 4), syncope and sudden death (Chap. 80), myocarditis, pericarditis, and cardiomyopathies (Chapter 26), endocarditis (Chapter 95) and Kawasaki's disease (Chapter 85) are discussed elsewhere.
- There are six common clinical presentations of pediatric heart disease: cyanosis, shock, congestive heart failure (CHF), pathologic murmur in an asymptomatic patient, hypertension, and syncope or palpitations. Table 74-1 lists the most common lesions in each category.
- The evaluation of an asymptomatic murmur is a nonemergent diagnostic workup that can be done on an outpatient basis. Innocent murmurs, often described as flow murmurs, are of low intensity, are brief, and occur during systole. In general, common pathologic murmurs in children are typically harsh, holosystolic, continuous, or diastolic in timing and often radiate. They may be associated with abnormal pulses or symptoms such as syncope or CHF. Common benign pediatric murmurs are listed in Table 74-2.

TABLE 74-1	Clinical Presentation of Pediatric Heart Disease
Cyanosis	TGA, TOF, TA, Tat, TAPVR
Shock	Coarctation, HPLHS
Congestive heart failure	Coarctation, PDA, ASD, VSD (see Table 74-4 for other causes)
Murmur/symptomatic patient	Shunts: VSD, PDA, ASD
	Obstructions (eg, valvular stenosis)
	Valvular incompetence
Hypertension	Coarctation
Syncope	
Cyanotic	TOF
Acyanotic	Critical AS

Abbreviations: AI = aortic insufficiency, AS = aortic stenosis, ASD = atrial septal defect, HPLHS = hypoplastic left heart syndrome, PDA = patent ductus arteriosus, TA = truncus arteriosus, TAPVR = total anomalous pulmonary venous return, Tat = tricuspid atresia, TGA = transposition of the great arteries, TOF = tetralogy of Fallot, VSD = ventricular septal defect.

EPIDEMIOLOGY

- Pediatric cardiac conditions are relatively rare. Congenital heart disease is a broad term encompassing a multitude of anatomic abnormalities. Congenital heart disease is the most common form of pediatric heart disease and is present in only 8 cases per 1000 live births in all forms.
- Ventricular septal defects (VSDs) are the most common congenital heart defect, comprising 25% of all such lesions. Transposition of the great arteries (TGA) and tetralogy of Fallot (TOF) are the most common cyanotic lesions presenting in the neonatal and post-infancy period, respectively.
- Acquired heart disease is less common and includes complications secondary to rheumatic fever (now quite uncommon), Kawasaki's disease, cardiomyopathies, severe chronic anemia, myocarditis, pericarditis, and endocarditis.

CYANOSIS

PATHOPHYSIOLOGY

- Cyanosis results from deoxygenation of hemoglobin.
- Congenital heart lesions produce cyanosis through one of three mechanisms: decreased pulmonary blood flow, mixing or shunting of deoxygenated blood (ie, right-to-left shunts), or poor cardiac output causing deoxygenation in peripheral capillary beds.

CLINICAL FEATURES

- Central cyanosis (a blue discoloration of the skin and mucus membranes) is the cardinal sign of cyanotic congenital heart disease (Fig. 74-1A), and may be associated with a murmur. Acral cyanosis (limited to the distal extremities, Fig. 74-1B) can be a normal finding in neonates.
- Cyanosis may present in the immediate neonatal period (eg, transposition of the great arteries, critical pulmonary stenosis, TOF) or later in infancy (eg, total anomalies venous return, TOF, Eisenmenger complex).
- Hypercyanotic episodes associated with TOF ("tet spells") typically present with an inconsolable infant with deep central cyanosis.
- Effortless tachypnea may be associated with cyanotic congenital heart disease.

TABLE 74-2 Benign Pediatric Murmurs

MURMUR	AGE	CHARACTER/LOCATION	VARIATION
Still's vibratory murmur	Infancy through childhood	1-3/6 vibratory, early systolic murmur at left lower sternal border to apex	Louder supine
Pulmonary flow murmur	Childhood to young adult	2-3/6 crescendo-decrescendo, early systolic at left upper sternal border, 2nd intercostal space	Louder supine and on full expiration
Peripheral pulmonic stenosis murmur	First year of life	1-2/6 low pitched, early to midsystolic in pulmonic area radiating to the back	Increased with slower heart rate, decreased with tachycardia
Supraclavicular or brachiocephalic murmur	Childhood to young adult	Crescendo-decrescendo, systolic, short, low pitched above clavicles radiating to neck	Decreases with hyperextension of shoulders or reclining
Venous hum	Childhood	1-6 continuous, humming, low anterior neck to lateral SCM muscle to anterior chest below clavicle	Louder sitting, head away from murmur. Softer lying with head toward murmur

Abbreviation: SCM = sternocleidomastoid.

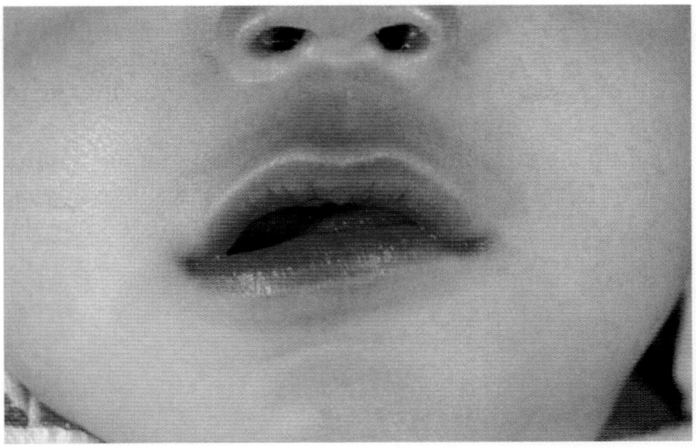

A

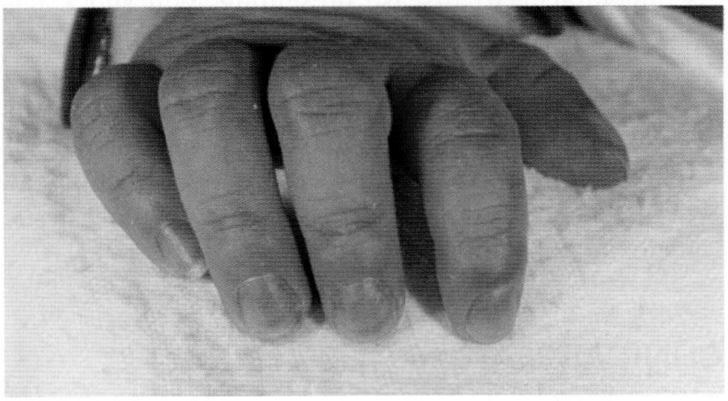

B

FIG. 74-1. Cyanosis of the mucous membranes (**A**) and nail beds (**B**). [Reproduced with permission from Shah BR, Lucchesi M (eds): *Atlas of Pediatric Emergency Medicine.* New York, NY, McGraw-Hill, 2006.]

DIAGNOSIS AND DIFFERENTIAL

- The most common congenital heart lesions causing cyanosis are transposition of the great arteries (TGA), TOF, tricuspid atresia, truncus arteriosus, and total anomalous venous return ("the five Ts").
- Cyanosis in the neonate or infant resulting from congenital heart disease must be differentiated from that caused by noncardiac causes such as lung disease and sepsis.
- A full set of vital signs including four-extremity blood pressure, and oxygen saturations measured in both the right arm (pre-ductal) and left arm (post-ductal) is essential.
- The "hyperoxia test" may help distinguish cyanotic heart disease from noncardiac causes of cyanosis: administer 100% oxygen; infants with cyanotic heart disease will not increase their $Pa{O_2}$ by more than 20 mm Hg.
- A chest radiograph should be obtained in all cyanotic neonates and infants, both to exclude pulmonary causes, and to evaluate the size and shape of the heart as well as pulmonary blood flow, which may provide clues to the diagnosis.
- An ECG should also be obtained. The typical ECG and chest radiograph findings associated with various cyanotic heart lesions are described in Table 74-3.
- Echocardiography and occasionally cardiac catheterization provide definitive diagnosis of cyanotic congenital heart disease, but are rarely performed in the ED and require pediatric sonographers and cardiologists.
- Transposition of the great vessels represents the most common cyanotic defect presenting with symptoms during the first week of life. This entity is easily missed due to the absence of cardiomegaly or murmur. Symptoms (prior to shock) include dusky lips, increased respiratory rate, and/or feeding difficulty. ECG may show right-sided-force dominance.
- TOF produces the following features: a holosystolic murmur of a VSD, a diamond-shaped murmur of pulmonary stenosis, and cyanosis. Chest radiograph may reveal a boot-shaped heart with decreased pulmonary vascular markings or a right-sided aortic arch (Fig. 74-2). The ECG may reveal right ventricular hypertrophy and right axis deviation.

TABLE 74-3 Cyanotic Congenital Cardiac Lesions: Typical Chest Radiograph and ECG Findings

CARDIAC LESION	CHEST RADIOGRAPH	ECG
Tetralogy of Fallot	Boot-shaped heart, normal-sized heart, decreased pulmonary vascular markings	Right axis deviation, right ventricular hypertrophy
Transposition of the great arteries	Egg-shaped heart, narrow mediastinum, increased pulmonary vascular marking	Right axis deviation, right ventricular hypertrophy
Total anomalous pulmonary venous return	Snowman sign, significant cardiomegaly, increased pulmonary vascular markings	Right axis deviation, right ventricular hypertrophy, right atrial enlargement
Tricuspid atresia	Heart of normal to slightly increased size, decreased pulmonary vascular markings	Superior QRS axis with right atrial hypertrophy, left atrial hypertrophy, left ventricular hypertrophy
Truncus arteriosus	Cardiomegaly, increased pulmonary vascular markings	Biventricular hypertrophy

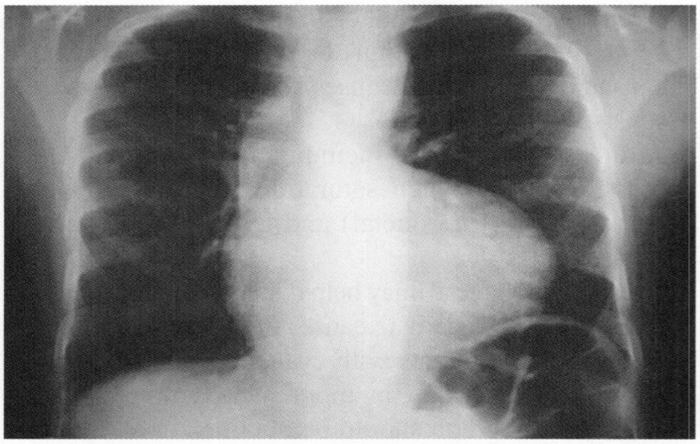

FIG. 74-2. Chest radiograph revealing the classic "boot-shaped heart" of tetralogy of Fallot. [Reproduced with permission from Shah BR, Lucchesi M (eds): *Atlas of Pediatric Emergency Medicine*. New York, NY, McGraw-Hill, 2006.]

- Hypercyanotic episodes, or "tet spells," may bring children with TOF to the ED with dramatic presentations. Symptoms include paroxysmal dyspnea, labored respiration, increased cyanosis, and possibly syncope. These episodes frequently follow exertion due to feeding, crying, or straining at stool, and last from minutes to hours.

EMERGENCY DEPARTMENT CARE AND DISPOSITION

- The ED management is primarily focused on stabilization, and definitive diagnosis (if not known); most cyanotic congenital defects are treated surgically.
- Though high-flow oxygen should be placed initially and maintained until noncardiac causes of cyanosis such as pneumonia or sepsis have been excluded, it is important to remember that neonates have significant amounts of oxygen-avid fetal hemoglobin and tolerate saturations in the 70s without tissue hypoxia. Oxygen is a potent pulmonary vasodilator and may lead to pulmonary over circulation in some lesions, and should be reserved for those with signs of inadequate tissue perfusion.
- Noncardiac causes should be considered and treated appropriately including a fluid challenge (10 mL/kg in neonates, 20 mL/kg in infants) and antibiotics if indicated.
- Management of hypercyanotic spells from TOF include placing the patient in the knee-chest position, administration of high-flow oxygen, and calming the infant; if these measures fail, morphine sulfate (0.2 milligram/kg SC or IM) may be given and refractory cases can be treated with IV phenylephrine or propranolol.
- Immediate consultation with a pediatric cardiologist and intensivist should be obtained for neonates and infants with suspected undiagnosed cyanotic heart disease or hemodynamic instability.
- While new diagnoses and unstable patients require hospitalization (usually to intensive care), hypercyanotic spells that have been successfully treated may be discharged safely.

SHOCK

PATHOPHYSIOLOGY

- Congenital heart disease presenting with shock has two main causes: inadequate left-ventricular outflow (eg, critical aortic stenosis, hypoplastic left heart syndrome) or closure of a patent ductus arteriosus upon which systemic circulation depends (eg, coarctation of the aorta). Both of these mechanisms lead to inadequate systemic perfusion with resultant tissue hypoxia and acidosis.

CLINICAL FEATURES

- The presentation of congenital heart defects resulting in shock is usually quite dramatic and infants may arrive in the ED in extremis. Most patients present in the first or second week of life as the ductus arteriosus closes.
- Early symptoms include poor feeding or sweating with feeds, vomiting, and parents may note rapid breathing, irritability, or lethargy.
- Tachycardia, tachypnea, pallor, mottling of skin, and sometimes cyanosis (from inadequate tissue perfusion) are typically noted on presentation to the ED.
- Mental status changes including profound lethargy are common with severe shock.

DIAGNOSIS AND DIFFERENTIAL

- The congenital heart defects most commonly associated with shock in the neonate are hypoplastic left heart syndrome, coarctation of the aorta, and interrupted aortic arch.
- Noncardiac causes of shock such as sepsis, inborn errors of metabolism, abdominal catastrophes, nonaccidental trauma, and congenital adrenal hyperplasia must be considered.
- A full set of vital signs including four-extremity blood pressures should be obtained. Extreme tachycardia, tachypnea, and differential upper extremity and lower extremity blood pressures with delayed or absent

femoral pulses strongly suggest ductal dependent congenital heart disease.

- A chest radiograph and ECG may help exclude noncardiac causes of shock such as pneumonia with sepsis and suggest a cardiac lesion.
- Routine blood tests are not helpful to diagnose ductal dependent heart lesions, but may be useful to guide management and exclude other causes and may include a complete blood count (for infectious causes), electrolytes (for metabolic and endocrine disease), venous blood gas, and lactate. Cultures may be helpful to exclude infection.
- Echocardiography and occasionally cardiac catheterization provide definitive diagnosis of congenital heart disease, but are rarely performed in the ED and require pediatric sonographers and cardiologists.

EMERGENCY DEPARTMENT CARE AND DISPOSITION

- Neonates presenting with shock from congenital heart disease require urgent resuscitation, continuous monitoring, and pharmacologic treatment.
- Provide high-flow oxygen to improve delivery to tissues, though recognize that oxygen may hasten closure of the ductus arteriosus or cause pulmonary steal of systemic blood flow through dilation of pulmonary vasculature.
- Obtain vascular or osseous access and administer normal saline in 10 to 20 mL/kg boluses repeated as necessary.
- Begin infusion of prostaglandin E1 in all patients suspected of ductal dependent congenital heart disease, as this may be lifesaving: start at 0.1 microgram/kg/min and gradually decrease to the lowest effective dose.
- Consider epinephrine for further treatment of hypotension (0.05-0.5 microgram/kg/min).
- Obtain immediate consultation with a pediatric cardiologist and intensivist.
- By definition, these patients require admission to intensive care.

CONGESTIVE HEART FAILURE

PATHOPHYSIOLOGY

- Congestive heart failure in infants and children develops because of one of two mechanisms (sometimes a combination of both): poor ventricular outflow or pulmonary vascular over-circulation.
- Poor ventricular outflow may be structural (eg, hypoplastic left ventricle, coarctation of the aorta) or functional (eg, cardiomyopathy, severe anemia, sustained tachydysrhythmia).
- Pulmonary vascular over-circulation is typically the result of left-to-right shunting, which can occur through a patent ductus arteriosus or a septal defect.

CLINICAL FEATURES

- Feeding difficulties (slow feeding, sweating with feeds) are often the first symptoms of congenital heart disease causing congestive heart failure (CHF).
- Respiratory symptoms develop as pulmonary edema progresses resulting in tachypnea (usually effortless initially, later with signs of distress), nasal flaring, and grunting. Rales can sometimes be heard on auscultation.
- Hepatomegaly and dependent edema (back, scalp, scrotum) can sometimes develop.
- The timing and age at which CHF develops may be helpful in determining the likely cause (see Diagnosis and Differential below).

DIAGNOSIS AND DIFFERENTIAL

- Diagnosis is made through a combination of physical examination and radiologic findings. Tachypnea, tachycardia, decreased breath sounds, or rales may be the only signs in left-sided CHF, while hepatomegaly and peripheral edema suggest right-sided failure.
- Chest radiograph reveals cardiomegaly and pulmonary vascular congestion (see Fig. 74-3), sometimes with an effusion.
- The rapidity and age of onset of CHF help determine the differential diagnosis (Table 74-4).
- Onset of CHF after the first 6 months of life usually signifies acquired heart disease such as cardiomyopathy, myocarditis, or pericarditis, though acute

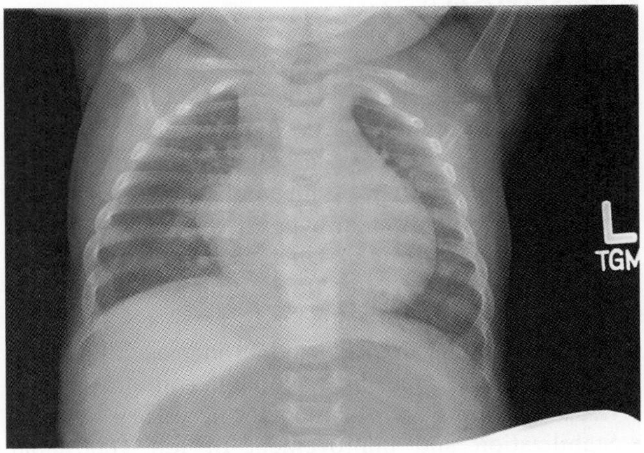

FIG. 74-3. Cardiomegaly and pulmonary edema in a 74-day-old infant.

TABLE 74-4 Differential Diagnosis of Congestive Heart Failure Based on Age at Presentation

AGE	SPECTRUM	
1 min	Noncardiac origin: anemia (isoimmunization), meconium aspiration, acidosis, asphyxia, hypoglycemia, supraventricular tachycardia (intra-uterine)	Congenital or acquired
1 h	Hypocalcemia, sepsis	
1 d	PDA in premature infants	Congenital
1 wk	HPLHS	
2 wk	Coarctation of the aorta	
1 mo	Ventricular septal defect	
3 mo	Large atrial septal defect, supraventricular tachycardia	
1 y	Myocarditis	Acquired
	Cardiomyopathy	
	Severe anemia	
10 y	Rheumatic fever	

Abbreviations: HPLHS = hypoplastic left heart syndrome, PDA = patent ductus arteriosus.

respiratory infection can precipitate CHF in the setting of underlying structural disease.

- Myocarditis is often preceded by a viral respiratory illness and may be difficult to distinguish from pneumonia, though patients with myocarditis may show ECG changes such as ST segment elevations, dysrhythmias, or ectopy.
- Pericarditis may be associated with muffled heart sounds and a friction rub and a pericardial effusion may be noted on bedside ultrasound.
- Cardiomyopathy is usually more insidious in onset with malaise, gradual progression of respiratory distress, signs of CHF accompanied by weak peripheral pulses, cardiomegaly on chest radiograph, and often chamber enlargement on ECG.
- Once CHF is diagnosed, echocardiography is indicated to define anatomy and cardiac function.

EMERGENCY DEPARTMENT CARE AND DISPOSITION

- The infant who presents with mild tachypnea, hepatomegaly, and cardiomegaly should be seated upright in a comfortable position, oxygen should be given, and the child should be kept in a neutral thermal environment to avoid metabolic stresses imposed by either hypothermia or hyperthermia.
- If the work of breathing is increased or CHF is apparent on chest radiograph, 1 to 2 milligrams/kg of furosemide parenterally is indicated.
- Fluid restriction, diuresis, and an increased FiO_2 can usually correct hypoxemia, although continuous positive airway pressure is sometimes necessary.
- Stabilization and improvement of left ventricular function can often first be accomplished with inotropic agents. Digoxin is used in milder forms of CHF. The appropriate loading/digitalizing dose to be given in the ED is 0.02 milligram/kg.
- At some point, CHF progresses to cardiogenic shock, in which distal pulses are absent and end-organ perfusion is threatened. In such situations, continuous infusions of inotropic agents, such as dopamine or dobutamine, are indicated instead of digoxin. The initial starting range is 2 to 10 micrograms/kg/min.
- Aggressive management is often necessary for secondary derangements, including respiratory insufficiency, acute renal failure, lactic acidosis, disseminated intravascular coagulation, hypoglycemia, and hypocalcemia.
- For definitive diagnosis and treatment of congenital lesions presenting in CHF, cardiac catheterization followed by surgical intervention is often necessary. See the previous section for recommendations regarding administration of prostaglandin E1 as a temporizing measure prior to surgery.

For further reading in Tintinalli's *Emergency Medicine: A Comprehensive Study Guide,* 7th ed., see Chapters 122A, "Congenital Heart Defects," and 122B, "Acquired Heart Disease," by Linton L. Yee and Garth D. Meckler.

75 VOMITING AND DIARRHEA IN INFANTS AND CHILDREN

Stephen B. Freedman

EPIDEMIOLOGY

- Acute viral gastroenteritis is the most common cause of vomiting and diarrhea in children. Clinical diagnosis requires the presence of diarrhea.

- Acute vomiting is usually caused by a self-limited viral illness. Nonetheless, more serious diagnoses must be considered.
- Acute gastroenteritis is defined by the presence of three or more diarrheal stools in a 24-hour period. An increase in stooling frequency and/or change in consistency in infants is consistent with diarrhea. Recognition is important, as young infants can develop gastroenteritis and, given their small size and limited fluid reserves, are at high risk for developing dehydration and hypoglycemia.
- Most enteric infections are self-limited, but excessive water and electrolyte loss resulting in clinical dehydration may occur in 10% and is life threatening in 1%.
- Pathogenic viruses, bacteria, or parasites may be isolated from nearly 50% of children with diarrhea. Viral infection is the most common, but bacterial pathogens are isolated in 1% to 4% of cases.
- The major bacterial enteropathogens in the United States are *Campylobacter jejuni*, *Shigella* species, *Salmonella* species, *Yersinia enterocolitica*, *Clostridium difficile*, and *Escherichia coli*. *Escherichia coli* has three pathogenic varieties, including enterohemorrhagic (serotype O157:H7), which is associated with hemolytic-uremic syndrome.
- *Giardia lamblia* is a parasitic infection and a common cause of diarrhea in infants and young children in day care centers.

PATHOPHYSIOLOGY

- Viral, parasitic, and bacterial pathogens cause disease by tissue invasion and alteration of intestinal absorption of water and electrolytes.
- Some bacterial pathogens such as *E. coli*, *Vibrio cholerae*, and *Shigella* cause diarrhea through production of enterotoxins and cytotoxins and invasion of the mucosal absorptive surface.
- The small bowel absorbs the vast majority of water in the gastrointestinal tract. Pathogens that interfere with water absorption in this area tend to produce voluminous diarrhea. By contrast, disease processes that affect the colon, such as dysentery, produce frequent, small-volume, often bloody stools.
- Fasting, which frequently occurs with gastroenteritis, worsens the capacity of the bowel to absorb fluids. Continued feeding not only slows progression of dehydration by increasing the volume of fluid available to the intravascular space, but the presence of nutrients in the bowel lumen promotes mucosal recovery and improves fluid absorption.

CLINICAL FEATURES

- Evaluation of a child's state of hydration is most important. If possible, it is best to determine the degree of fluid loss by comparing the child's current weight to a recent previous weight. A history of normal fluid intake and normal urine output drastically reduce the likelihood of significant dehydration.
- When objective measurements such as pre- and post-illness weights are not available, the state of hydration can be assessed by physical examination (Table 75-1).

DIAGNOSIS AND DIFFERENTIAL

- History and physical examination are the most important tools in diagnosis. Most children with acute vomiting and diarrhea have self-limited viral illness.
- Specific clinical findings, such as bilious or bloody vomitus, hematochezia, or abdominal pain, should trigger concerns of a disease process other than simple viral gastroenteritis (Table 75-2), or a potential complication of gastroenteritis.
- Check a bedside glucose on all patients with vomiting or diarrhea and altered mental status and in infants and toddlers with protracted symptoms, which may cause hypoglycemia.
- Serum electrolytes are usually not necessary because dehydration caused by diarrhea is usually isotonic and laboratory parameters are subject to inaccuracy. They should, however, be performed in moderately dehydrated children whose history and physical examination findings are inconsistent with acute gastroenteritis, severely dehydrated children, and all children requiring intravenous rehydration, or those with potential hyper- or hyponatremia (see Chapter 83).
- Obtain stool cultures in children with the following high-risk features: >10 stools in the previous 24 hours, travel to high-risk area, fever, older age, and blood or mucus in the stool. In the context of an outbreak of hemolytic uremic syndrome or a positive blood culture for *E. coli* O157:H7, further testing to rule out evidence of renal failure, thrombocytopenia, and hemolytic anemia should be performed.
- Special attention should be given to those children who have chronic debilitating illnesses, high-risk social situations, or malnutrition, since they are at particular risk for rapid decompensation.
- Bilious vomiting should always raise suspicion for an obstructive lesion distal to the ampulla of Vater.
- The differential diagnosis of vomiting is age specific, and serious diagnoses that need to be considered include metabolic (eg, inborn errors of metabolism, congenital

TABLE 75-1 Clinical Signs in Dehydration

SIGN	NONE–MINIMAL DEHYDRATION (<3% LOSS OF BODY WEIGHT)	MILD–MODERATE DEHYDRATION (3%-9% LOSS OF BODY WEIGHT)	SEVERE DEHYDRATION (>9% LOSS OF BODY WEIGHT)
Mental status	Well, alert	Fatigued, restless, irritable	Apathetic, lethargic, unconscious
Thirst	Normal, slight increase, or refusing	Increased, eager to drink	Very thirsty or too lethargic to indicate
Heart rate	Normal	Normal to increased	Tachycardic with bradycardia in severe cases
Blood pressure	Normal	Normal	Normal to reduced
Pulse quality	Normal	Normal to reduced	Weak, thready
Breathing	Normal	Normal to tachypneic	Deep
Eyes	Normal	Slightly sunken orbits	Deeply sunken orbits
Tears	Present	Decreased	Absent
Mucous membranes	Moist	Dry	Parched
Anterior fontanelle	Normal	Sunken	Sunken
Skin turgor	Instant recoil	Recoil in <2 s	Recoil in >2 s
Capillary refill	Normal	Prolonged 1-2 s	Prolonged >2 s
Extremities	Warm	Cool	Cold, mottled, cyanotic
Urine output	Normal to decreased	Decreased (<1 mL/kg/h)	Minimal (<0.5 mL/kg/h)

adrenal hyperplasia, diabetes mellitus), neurologic (eg, intracranial hemorrhage, hydrocephalus, cerebral edema), surgical/gastrointestinal (eg, esophageal or intestinal stenosis/atresia, pyloric stenosis, malrotation ± volvulus, incarcerated hernia, Hirschsprung disease, intussusception, foreign body, Meckel's diverticulum), renal (eg, urinary tract infection, obstructive uropathy, renal insufficiency), infectious (eg, gastroenteritis, meningitis, sepsis, pneumonia), and other disease states (eg, gastroesophageal reflux, necrotizing enterocolitis, milk allergy, appendicitis, pregnancy, cyclic vomiting syndrome).

- The differential diagnosis of diarrhea includes infection (eg, viral, bacterial, parasitic), dietary disturbances (eg, food allergy, starvation stools), anatomic abnormalities (eg, Hirschsprung disease, partial obstruction, appendicitis), inflammatory bowel disease, malabsorptive or secretory diseases (eg, cystic fibrosis, celiac disease), systemic diseases (eg, immunodeficiency, endocrinopathy), and other causes (eg, antibiotic associated diarrhea, secondary lactase deficiency).
- Causes of diarrhea that may result in significant morbidity include infection (eg, *Salmonella* gastroenteritis with bacteremia, *Shigella*, *C. difficile*), anatomic abnormalities (eg, intussusception, toxic megacolon, appendicitis), inflammatory bowel disease, and hemolytic uremic syndrome. Appendicitis may cause diarrhea, particularly after the appendix has perforated.

EMERGENCY DEPARTMENT CARE AND DISPOSITION

Therapy is determined by the severity of dehydration:

- Mild: Continue with the child's preferred, usual, and age-appropriate diet.
- Moderate: Administer oral rehydration therapy. Aim for 25 to 50 mL/kg over 1 to 2 hours. Reassess in 1 hour. If sufficient intake and clinically less dehydrated, then continue age-appropriate diet at home. If no improvement, options include continuing oral rehydration for 1 additional hour, nasogastric rehydration, or intravenous rehydration.
- Severe: Treat emergently as indicated for hypovolemic shock with isotonic crystalloids administered as 20 mL/kg boluses and repeated until clinical improvement is noted (see Chapter 83).

If vomiting is the prominent symptom:

- Treat with oral rehydration with a glucose-electrolyte oral rehydration solution (ORS) using frequent, small volumes. Aim for 1 ounce (30 mL) of ORS/kg/h. Avoid other beverages (eg, tea, juice, sports drinks),

TABLE 75-2 Etiologies of Vomiting That May Result in Significant Morbidity, Categorized by Age

Newborn Period (birth-2 wk)	
Obstructive intestinal anomaly	Esophageal or intestinal stenosis/atresia, bowel malrotation ± midgut volvulus, meconium ileus/plug, Hirschsprung disease, imperforate anus, enteric duplications
Other GI disease processes	Necrotizing enterocolitis, perforation with secondary peritonitis
Neurologic	Mass lesion, hydrocephalus, cerebral edema, kernicterus
Renal	Obstructive anomaly, uremia
Infectious	Sepsis, meningitis
Metabolic	Inborn errors of metabolism, congenital adrenal hyperplasia
Infant (2 wk-12 mo)	
Acquired esophageal disorders	Foreign body, retropharyngeal abscess
GI obstruction	Bezoar, foreign body, pyloric stenosis, malrotation ± volvulus, enteric duplications, complications of Meckel diverticulum, intussusception, incarcerated hernia, Hirschsprung disease
Other GI disease processes	Gastroenteritis with dehydration, peritonitis
Neurologic	Mass lesion, hydrocephalus
Renal	Obstruction, uremia
Infectious	Sepsis, meningitis, pertussis
Metabolic	Inborn errors of metabolism
Toxic ingestions	—
Child (>12 mo)	
GI obstruction	Bezoar, foreign body, posttraumatic intramural hematoma, malrotation ± volvulus, complications of Meckel diverticulum, intussusception, incarcerated hernia, Hirschsprung disease
Other GI disease processes	Appendicitis, peptic ulcer disease, pancreatitis, peritonitis
Neurologic	Mass lesions
Renal	Uremia
Infectious	Sepsis, meningitis
Metabolic	Diabetic ketoacidosis, adrenal insufficiency, inborn errors of metabolism
Toxic ingestion	—

which are deficient in sodium and provide excess sugar, resulting in amplified losses.

- Consider intravenous rehydration with isotonic crystalloid administered via IV, IO, or NG routes in children with severe dehydration, with hemodynamic compromise, or when altered mental status precludes safe oral fluid administration.
- A single dose of ondansetron, a 5-hydroxytryptamine receptor antagonist, may be used as an adjunct to ORT in children with persistent vomiting at a dose of 0.15 mg/kg PO or 0.1 mg/kg IV.
- **Dopamine receptor antagonists should not be used to treat vomiting in children because of the potential for serious side effects and lack of evidence of efficacy.**

If diarrhea is the prominent symptom:

- Children with mild diarrhea who are not dehydrated should continue routine feedings.
- Children with moderate to severe dehydration should first receive adequate rehydration before resuming routine feedings. Food should be reinstated after the rehydration phase is completed and never delayed more than 4 hours. There is no need to dilute formula, or recommendation of a lactose-free milk or the bananas, rice, applesauce, and toast (BRAT) diet.
- Dietary recommendations include a diet high in complex carbohydrates, lean meats, vegetables, fruits, and yogurt. Fatty foods and foods high in simple sugars should be avoided.
- **Antidiarrheal medications are not recommended in children due to safety concerns and a lack of effectiveness data. Antimotility agents, which can reduce diarrhea, have potential serious adverse effects (eg, lethargy, paralytic ileus, death), and are contraindicated in children.**
- Bismuth, which can reduce the severity of diarrhea, can cause salicylate poisoning, and is not recommended in children <12 years of age.
- Antibiotics are unnecessary for the vast majority of children with acute gastroenteritis and are only indicated for specific pathogens or clinical settings (Table 75-3).
- Admit all infants and children who appear toxic or have high-risk social situations, significant dehydration, intractable vomiting, altered mental status, an inability to drink, or laboratory evidence of hemolytic anemia, thrombocytopenia, or elevated creatinine levels.
- Families of discharged patients should be given instructions to return or seek care with their primary physician if the child has increased emesis, bilious vomiting, or signs of dehydration such as decreased activity level, or urination.

TABLE 75-3 Clinical Features and Treatment of Etiologic Agents of Bacterial Gastroenteritis

ORGANISM	CLINICAL FEATURES	RISK FACTORS	COMPLICATIONS	ANTIMICROBIAL THERAPY
Shigella	Mild: watery stools without constitutional symptoms Severe: fever, abdominal pain, tenesmus, mucoid stools, hematochezia	Poor sanitation, crowded living, day care	Bacteremia, Reiter syndrome, hemolytic uremic syndrome, toxic encephalopathy, seizures, dehydration, toxic megacolon ± perforation	Typically self-limited (48-72 h) Treat if: immunocompromised, severe disease, dysentery, or systemic symptoms Options: azithromycin, trimethoprim-sulfamethoxazole, ceftriaxone, ciprofloxacin
Salmonella	Mild: watery diarrhea, mild fever, abdominal cramps Typhoid fever: high fever, constitutional symptoms, abdominal pain, hepatosplenomegaly, rose spots, altered mental status	Direct contact with animals: poultry, livestock, reptiles, pets Contact/ingestion of contaminated food: beef, poultry, eggs, dairy, water	Meningitis, osteomyelitis, bacteremia, dehydration, endocarditis, typhoid fever	Typically self-limited Treat if: <3 mo of age, hemoglobinopathy, immunodeficiency, chronic GI tract disease, malignancy, severe colitis, bacteremia, sepsis Gastroenteritis: ampicillin, amoxicillin, trimethoprim-sulfamethoxazole, cefotaxime, ceftriaxone, fluoroquinolone Invasive disease: cefotaxime, ceftriaxone
Campylobacter	Diarrhea, abdominal pain, fever, malaise Often hematochezia in infants	Improperly cooked poultry, untreated water, unpasteurized milk, pets (dogs, cats, hamsters, birds)	Acute: dehydration, bacteremia, focal infections Convalescence: reactive arthritis, Reiter syndrome, erythema nodosum, idiopathic polyneuritis, Miller Fisher syndrome	Typically self-limited; 20% have relapse or prolonged symptoms Treat if: moderate-severe symptoms, relapse, immunocompromised, day care, and institutions Options: erythromycin, azithromycin, ciprofloxacin
Yersinia	Bloody diarrhea with mucus, fever, abdominal pain Pseudoappendicitis syndrome: fever, right lower quadrant pain, leukocytosis	Contaminated food: improperly cooked pork, unpasteurized milk, untreated water	Acute: bacteremia, pharyngitis, meningitis, osteomyelitis, pyomyositis, conjunctivitis, pneumonia, empyema, endocarditis, acute peritonitis, liver/spleen abscess Convalescence: erythema nodosum, glomerulonephritis, reactive arthritis	Typically self-limited Treat if: sepsis, non-GI infections, immunocompromised, excess iron storage condition (desferrioxamine use, sickle cell anemia, thalassemia) Options: trimethoprim-sulfamethoxazole, aminoglycosides, cefotaxime, fluoroquinolones, tetracycline, doxycycline, chloramphenicol
Escherichia coli–Shiga toxin producing	Bloody or nonbloody diarrhea, severe abdominal pain	Food or water contaminated with feces, undercooked beef, unpasteurized milk	Hemorrhagic colitis, hemolytic uremic syndrome, thrombotic thrombocytopenic purpura	None indicated; debated risk of increased incidence of hemolytic uremic syndrome with treatment
E. coli–enteropathogenic	Severe watery diarrhea	Food or water contaminated with feces	Dehydration	Options: trimethoprim-sulfamethoxazole, azithromycin, ciprofloxacin
E. coli–enterotoxigenic	Moderate watery diarrhea, abdominal cramps	Food or water contaminated with feces	Dehydration	Treat if severe Options: trimethoprim-sulfamethoxazole, azithromycin, ciprofloxacin
E. coli–enteroinvasive	Fever, bloody, or nonbloody dysentery	Food or water contaminated with feces	Dehydration	Treat if dysentery Options: trimethoprim-sulfamethoxazole, azithromycin, ciprofloxacin
E. coli–enteroaggregative	Watery, occasionally bloody diarrhea	Food or water contaminated with feces	Dehydration	Options: trimethoprim-sulfamethoxazole, azithromycin, ciprofloxacin

For further reading in Tintinalli's *Emergency Medicine: A Comprehensive Study Guide*, 7th ed., see Chapter 123, "Vomiting, Diarrhea, and Dehydration in Children," by Stephen Freedman and Jennifer Thull-Freedman.

76 PEDIATRIC ABDOMINAL EMERGENCIES

David I. Magilner

EPIDEMIOLOGY

- The causes of abdominal pain and gastrointestinal (GI) bleeding vary by age and are listed in Tables 76-1 and 76-2.

TABLE 76-1 Classification of Abdominal Pain by Age Group

AGE	EMERGENT	NONEMERGENT
0-3 mo old	Necrotizing enterocolitis Volvulus Testicular torsion Incarcerated hernia Trauma Toxic megacolon Tumor	Colic Acute gastroenteritis Constipation
3 mo-3 y old	Intussusception Testicular torsion Trauma Volvulus Appendicitis Toxic megacolon Vaso-occlusive crisis	Acute gastroenteritis Constipation Urinary tract infections HSP
3 y old-adolescence	Appendicitis Diabetic ketoacidosis Vaso-occlusive crisis Toxic ingestion Testicular torsion Ovarian torsion Ectopic pregnancy Trauma Toxic megacolon Tumor	Constipation Acute gastroenteritis Nonspecific viral syndromes *Streptococcus* pharyngitis Urinary tract infections Pneumonia Pancreatitis Cholecystitis Renal stones HSP Inflammatory bowel disease Gastric ulcer disease/gastritis Ovarian cyst Pregnancy

Abbreviation: HSP = Henoch–Schönlein purpura.

TABLE 76-2 Age-Based Causes of Upper and Lower GI Bleeding

UPPER GI BLEEDING		
<2 MO	2 MO-2 Y	>2 Y
Swallowed maternal blood Stress ulcer Vascular malformation Hemorrhagic disease of newborn (vitamin K deficiency) Coagulopathy/bleeding diathesis	Gastroenteritis Toxic ingestion Mallory–Weiss tear Vascular malformation Esophagitis Stress ulcer Bleeding diathesis GI duplication Foreign body	Gastroenteritis Mallory–Weiss tear Peptic ulcer disease Toxic ingestion Vascular malformation Gastritis Varices Hematobilia Foreign body
LOWER GI BLEEDING		
<2 MO	2 MO-2 Y	>2 Y
Swallowed maternal blood Milk allergy Infectious colitis Intussusception Volvulus Meckel's diverticulum Necrotizing enterocolitis Vascular malformation Hemorrhagic disease of newborn Hirschsprung's disease Congenital duplications	Anal fissure Gastroenteritis Milk allergy Intussusception Volvulus Meckel's diverticulum Hemolytic uremic syndrome Henoch–Schönlein purpura Polyps; benign, familial Inflammatory bowel disease GI duplication Dieulafoy lesion	Anal fissure Gastroenteritis Hemorrhoids Polyps Colitis (infectious, ischemic) Meckel's diverticulum Intussusception Hemolytic uremic syndrome Henoch-Schönlein purpura Inflammatory bowel disease Angiodysplasia Celiac disease Dieulafoy lesion Rectal ulcer syndrome Peptic ulcer disease

PATHOPHYSIOLOGY

- Abdominal pain can be caused by infection, inflammation, or obstruction of any of the GI or genitourinary (GU) organs. In addition, abdominal pain may be caused by a systemic illness, pregnancy, or its complications, or may be referred from an extra-abdominal site. See Chapter 38 for further discussion on the pathophysiology of abdominal pain.
- GI bleeding can occur anywhere along the GI tract from the esophagus to the anus, or be swallowed from bleeding in the nose or mouth. Bleeding can be caused by mucosal injury from a localized process; by infection, food allergy, and ingestion of a toxin or foreign body; or by a condition that increases bleeding.

CLINICAL FEATURES

- Pain: The quality, timing, location, and exacerbating factors of abdominal pain provide clues to diagnosis. The two main types of abdominal pain in emergent conditions are peritoneal and obstructive: peritoneal pain is exacerbation by motion, while obstructive pain is spasmodic, and usually causes restlessness.
- Associated symptoms and exposure to ill close contacts may also provide clues to etiology. In children less than 2 years of age, abdominal pain may be nonspecific and manifest as fussiness or lethargy.
- Bleeding: The volume and quality of bleeding, along with associated symptoms, helps identify the cause of GI bleeding.
- Associated symptoms: In addition to pain and bleeding, patients with abdominal emergencies may have associated symptoms such as vomiting, diarrhea, constipation, fever, anorexia, or jaundice. Jaundice often indicates a serious condition. **Bilious vomiting in the first year of life should always be considered a symptom of obstruction and a true surgical emergency.**
- Physical examination in the child with abdominal pain or GI bleeding must first identify the need for resuscitation by assessment of general appearance, vital signs, perfusion, mental status, and hydration status. Abdominal examination may reveal distension, masses, localized tenderness, or peritoneal signs such as guarding, rebound pain, and "shake" or "hop" tenderness. A rectal examination should be considered to test for blood.
- Non-GI sources of abdominal pain, such as pharyngitis, pneumonia, and testicular torsion, should be sought and all patients examined for hernias. A pelvic examination should be considered in any female patient who is post-menarchal.

DIAGNOSIS AND DIFFERENTIAL

- The specific diagnosis for abdominal emergencies can be narrowed by the patient's age. Tables 76-1 and 76-2 list the age-based causes of abdominal pain and GI bleeding. The most important diagnoses and some of their key characteristics are discussed below.
  - *Intussusception* may occur at any age, but has a peak incidence of 3 months to 2 years. Key features may include colicky abdominal pain, vomiting, "currant jelly" stool, and listlessness between episodes of pain. A sausage-like mass may be felt in the right abdomen. Diagnosis can be suggested by abdominal radiographs, but ultrasound has a higher sensitivity and specificity, and air contrast enema provides definitive diagnosis and potential treatment. Ultrasound may show a classic "target sign" (Fig. 76-1). A surgeon should be consulted prior to enema in case of failure or perforation.
  - *Malrotation* and *volvulus* can also occur at any age, but the vast majority of patients present in the first year of life. Volvulus occurs when a malrotated gut twists, compromising perfusion and leading to bowel ischemia and necrosis. Key features may include sudden abdominal pain and distension, bilious emesis, irritability, and eventually peritonitis and shock. If the diagnosis is in question and the patient is stable, radiographs including plain films and an upper GI series may aid in diagnosis, but surgical consultation should never be delayed.

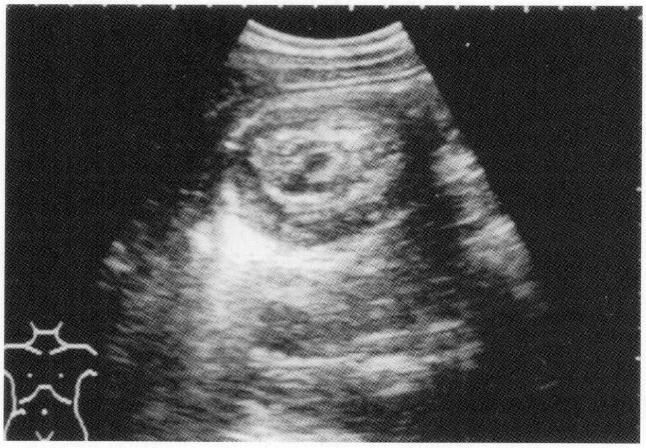

A

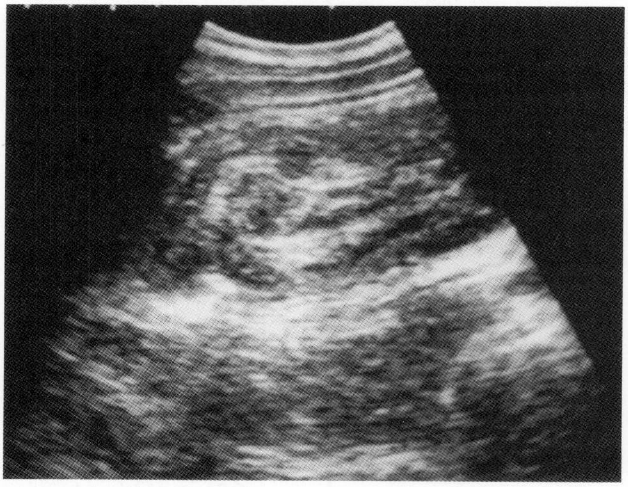

B

FIG. 76-1. **A** and **B**. US image of intussusception showing the classic target appearance of bowel within bowel. (Reprinted with permission from Reardon RF, Joing SA: Cardiac, in Ma OJ, Mateer JR, Blaivas M (eds): *Emergency Ultrasound,* 2nd ed. © 2008, The McGraw-Hill Companies, All rights reserved, New York. Figure 9-15A&B.)

- *Incarcerated hernia* can present at any time in life, and the diagnosis is made by the presence of an inguinal or scrotal mass. Additional symptoms may include poor feeding, irritability, or vomiting. See Chapter 45 for further discussion on hernias.
- *Appendicitis* can occur at any age, but peak incidence is between 9 and 12 years. Patients under 5 years of age are at high risk of perforation because of atypical symptoms and delayed diagnosis. Key features include periumbilical pain that migrates to the right lower abdomen, anorexia, nausea, vomiting, and fever; diarrhea may occur. However, this constellation of symptoms is present in <50% of cases. Studies that may aid in the diagnosis include the white blood cell (WBC) count, which if normal or low makes appendicitis less likely, and ultrasound (US) or CT imaging. Both ultrasound and CT are highly sensitive and specific (around 90%), but US is operator dependent. If a CT is performed, it should be done with IV (and possibly PO or rectal) contrast.
- *Necrotizing enterocolitis (NEC)* is more common in low-birth-weight and premature infants, but 10% to 15% of cases occur in term infants. Most cases present in the first week of life. Key features include poor feeding, lethargy, and abdominal distension, and peritonitis and shock can result from intestinal perforation. Stool may test positive for occult blood, and plain films of the abdomen show air bubbles in the wall of the bowel (pneumatosis coli), which is diagnostic of NEC, and possibly portal venous or free air.
- *Nonspecific (or functional) abdominal pain* is a diagnosis of exclusion. It is the most common diagnosis in children who present to the emergency department with abdominal pain, and may be considered a provisional diagnosis if the history, physical examination, and laboratory and radiologic studies (if needed) are normal. Most children have vague, periumbilical, or lower abdominal pain, which can be associated with nausea. All children discharged with this diagnosis should follow up with a physician within 24 hours if pain is not resolved.
- *Constipation* is a clinical diagnosis, defined by either infrequent and hard stools or pain with defecation. Most cases are functional or related to diet, but constipation may be indicative of a more serious condition such as Hirschsprung's disease or cystic fibrosis. Physical examination should include examination of the spine for signs of dysraphism (dimples, clefts, tufts of hair) and possibly rectal examination to assess sphincter tone and the presence or absence of stool in the vault.
- *Henoch–Schönlein purpura (HSP)*, also known as anaphylactoid purpura, is a vasculitis that affects vessels in the skin, intestine, kidneys, and joints. The rash is purpuric and palpable, and typically presents on the lower extremities and buttocks first. Arthritis and arthralgia are migratory and usually involve the ankles and knees. Renal involvement may manifest as hematuria or hypertension (see Chapter 28). Abdominal pain is present in 60% to 80% of cases, and is usually diffuse and colicky. It may be accompanied by vomiting and/or GI bleeding. In most cases, the pain is a direct result of intestinal vasculitis, but in about 5% of patients an intussusception will develop secondary to the vasculitis.
- *Pyloric stenosis* presents with projectile non-bilious vomiting that occurs after feeds, and may present anytime from 2 to 12 weeks of life. The diagnosis may be suggested by palpation of an "olive" in the left upper abdomen, confirmed by ultrasound. Laboratory evaluation may show a hypokalemic, hypochloremic metabolic alkalosis, but this is a late finding.
- *Meckel's diverticulum* most commonly causes painless hematochezia, but may act as a lead point for volvulus or intussusception.

- Other causes of GI bleeding are listed in Table 76-2. In most cases, the responsibility of the emergency room caregiver is to ensure that the patient is stable by assessing vital signs, hydration status, and presence or absence of anemia. Most entities will require either emergent or non-emergent referral to a pediatric gastroenterologist or surgeon for definitive diagnosis (eg, endoscopy or biopsy) and management.
- Systemic infectious and noninfectious diseases that may cause abdominal pain are discussed elsewhere, but include streptococcal pharyngitis, pneumonia, diabetic ketocidosis, urinary tract infection, and sickle-cell disease.
- Other important causes of abdominal pain discussed elsewhere include colic (Chapter 69), gastroenteritis (Chapter 75), cholesystitis (Chapter 44), pancreatitis (Chapter 44), renal stones (Chapter 58), and inflammatory bowel disease (Chapter 39).

EMERGENCY DEPARTMENT CARE AND DISPOSITION

- In all cases the first responsibility is to assess whether the patient is stable. This includes an assessment of general appearance, vital signs, perfusion, mental status, and hydration. Standard resuscitation efforts should begin immediately when necessary.

- Treat shock from abdominal emergencies with aggressive isotonic crystalloid boluses: 20 mL/kg of normal saline or lactated Ringer's solution should be administered and repeated until clinical improvement is noted.
- Consider administration of blood products (eg, packed red blood cells, fresh frozen plasma—see Chapter 87) for patients with life-threatening and ongoing GI bleeding.
- Treat significant pain with parenteral narcotics such as morphine 0.1 milligram/kg IV; **administration of narcotics does not alter the reliability of the physical examination to detect peritoneal signs and should not be withheld**.
- Obtain laboratory and radiographic studies as directed by the presentation and suspected etiology.
- Obtain surgical or GI consultation as indicated, and consider rapid transfer to a pediatric facility after initial resuscitation for patients with a suspected surgical process.

For further reading in Tintinalli's *Emergency Medicine: A Comprehensive Study Guide*, 7th ed., see Chapter 124, "Acute Abdominal Pain in Children," by Anupam B. Kharbanda and Rasha D. Sawaya, and Chapter 125, "Gastrointestinal Bleeding in Children," by Robert W. Schafermeyer and Emily MacNeill.

77 URINARY TRACT INFECTION IN INFANTS AND CHILDREN

Justin W. Sales

EPIDEMIOLOGY

- Pediatric urinary tract infections (UTIs) are now the most common serious bacterial infection in children following the introduction of successful immunizations.
- Pediatric UTI occurs in up to 8% of febrile children presenting to the ED with no obvious source of infection.
- Two percent of boys and up to 8% of girls have a UTI during the first 8 years of life, with the highest incidence during the first year of life in both sexes.
- Prevalence of UTI is three times higher in females; amongst males, uncircumcised infant boys have a 10 times higher risk than circumcised boys.

PATHOPHYSIOLOGY

- UTIs typically occur from retrograde contamination of the lower urinary tract with organisms from the perineum and periurethral area. In neonates, however, UTIs typically develop after seeding of the renal parenchyma from hematogenous spread.
- *Escherichia coli* is the most common cause of UTI in children. Additional pathogens include *Klebsiella, Proteus,* and *Enterobacter* species.
- Enterococcus species, *Staphylococcus aureus,* and group B streptococci are the most common gram-positive organisms and are more common in neonates. *Chlamydia trachomatis* may be present in adolescents with urinary tract symptoms and microhematuria. Adenovirus may cause culture-negative acute cystitis in young boys.
- Factors influencing the development of UTI include virulence of the pathogen, congenital urinary tract abnormalities, vesicoureteral reflux, urolithiasis, poor hygiene, voluntary urinary retention, circumcision, and constipation.

CLINICAL FEATURES

- Clinical features vary markedly by age as described below.
- Neonatal UTI may present with a septic-like appearance. Features may include fever, jaundice, poor feeding, irritability, and lethargy.
- Infants and young children typically present with gastrointestinal complaints, which may include fever, abdominal pain, vomiting, and change in appetite.
- In school-aged children and adolescents, cystitis and urethritis (lower tract disease) typically present with urinary frequency, urgency, hesitancy, and dysuria. Pyelonephritis (upper tract disease) typically presents with fever, chills, back or flank pain, vomiting, and dehydration.

DIAGNOSIS AND DIFFERENTIAL

- The American Acadamy of Pediatrics clinical practice guideline from 2011 proposes criteria for UTI in infants and young children 2 to 24 months of age to include evidence of pyuria in addition to positive culture results.
- For infants less than 2 months of age, urine culture remains the gold standard for this age group.
- A positive urine culture is defined as $\geq 5 \times 10^4$ colony-forming units (CFU)/mL of a single urinary pathogen. Growth of a urinary pathogen in any number from a suprapubic aspiration is considered a positive culture.

TABLE 77-1 Treatment of UTI in Infants and Children

AGE	DISPOSITION CONSIDERATIONS	ANTIMICROBIAL CHOICES AND DOSES
≥1 mo old	Hospital admission and IV antibiotics	Ampicillin (50 milligrams/kg/dose) + Cefotaxime (50 milligrams/kg/dose) or Gentamicin (2.5 milligrams/kg/dose)
>1 mo-2 y old	Toxic—admit to hospital and IV antibiotics	Ceftriaxone (50 milligrams/kg/dose) or Cefotaxime (50 milligrams/kg/dose)
	Non-toxic, able to tolerate PO: outpatient treatment	Consider ceftriaxone (50 milligrams/kg/dose) IV/IM, then choice of oral treatments below
> 2 y old	Select oral antibiotic therapy based on local resistance patterns Adolescent girls (>13 y old), option to treat for 3 d	Cefixime 8 milligrams/kg/d in two doses Cefprozil 30 milligrams/kg/d in two doses Cephalexin 75 milligrams/kg/d in three doses Cefdinir 14 milligrams/kg/d in two doses

- Urine culture results are not available to the emergency physician during the initial visit; therefore, urine chemical test strips that can detect leukocyte esterase and urinary nitrites in conjunction with microscopic urinalysis are employed to help predict the results of the urine culture and initiate treatment.
- In infants and children who are not able to void on command, bladder catheterization is the preferred method for urine collection. Suprapubic aspiration, although invasive, is also an acceptable means of obtaining a cultured specimen. High false-positive results and low specificity seriously limit the use of perineal bag specimens.
- Urinary nitrites and leukocyte esterase alone are not sensitive markers for children who empty their bladders frequently. Urinary nitrites are highly specific and therefore helpful when positive.
- Pyuria alone does not confirm a UTI. Causes of culture-negative pyuria include urethritis from kawasaki disease, pelvic abscess or infections (appendicitis, pelvic inflammatory disease, colitis), or sexually transmitted diseases.
- Causes of culture-negative dysuria include viral urethritis/cystitis, balanitis, and irritant urethritis from poor hygiene or clothing.

EMERGENCY DEPARTMENT CARE AND DISPOSITION

- Treatment and disposition depends on the age of the patient and severity of the illness.
- Physicians should be familiar with the local susceptibilities of the common urinary pathogens in their geographic region. Medications listed in Table 77-1 are generally acceptable, but emerging resistance is a continuing problem.
- Neonates (under 1 month of age) with fever and UTI should be hospitalized and given intravenous antibiotics.
- Children over 1 month of age with fever and uncomplicated UTI may be appropriate for outpatient care with oral antibiotics if they appear well, can tolerate oral medication, are not dehydrated, and are not immunocompromised. They may receive a single dose of intramuscular or intravenous ceftriaxone (50 milligrams/kg) in the emergency department and start on outpatient oral antibiotics with close primary care follow-up.
- Older infants and children with fever and UTI complicated by vomiting, dehydration, any suspicion of sepsis, or inability to take oral antibiotics are hospitalized for intravenous antibiotics until they are afebrile and able to take oral medications.
- Length of antimicrobial therapy should be 7 to 14 days.
- Adolescent girls (>13 years old) with UTI may be treated like adults with option for 3-day oral antibiotic regimen.
- Febrile infants with UTIs should undergo renal and bladder ultrasonography. The necessity of routine voiding cystourethrogram after the first febrile UTI has recently been challenged unless ultrasonography reveals high-grade or obstructive uropathy. This testing is arranged as an outpatient or performed during hospitalization and is not typically facilitated from the emergency department.

For further reading in Tintinalli's *Emergency Medicine: A Comprehensive Study Guide,* 7th ed., see Chapter 126, "Urinary Tract Infection in Infants and Children," by Julie S. Byerley and Michael J. Steiner.

78 SEIZURES AND STATUS EPILEPTICUS IN CHILDREN

James C. O'Neill

- Unusual movements and changes in behavior in children often lead to an ED visit. Although seizures account for many of these events, as many as 30% or more of paroxysmal events may be misdiagnosed as seizures.
- Most seizure activity stops before the child is seen in an ED. Therefore, history is key to making the correct diagnosis.
- There are many different causes of pediatric seizures. The goal is to identify and treat the underlying cause. Some seizures require emergency management and extensive evaluation (eg, neonatal seizures); others are very common and benign and need little evaluation (eg, febrile seizures).

EPIDEMIOLOGY

- Approximately 1% to 2% of the U.S. population has epilepsy, although the lifetime likelihood of at least one seizure is nearly 9%.
- Simple febrile seizures constitute a separate category, with an incidence of 3% to 5% in children.

PATHOPHYSIOLOGY

- Seizures represent synchronous firing of neurons in the brain leading to paroxysmal involuntary motor activity and/or changes in behavior or consciousness. The release of glutamate from a firing neuron activates *N*-methyl-d-aspartic acid receptors that subsequently initiate and propagate seizure activity.
- Seizures are inhibited by γ-aminobutyric acid (GABA), and failure of this inhibition facilitates seizure spread.

CLINICAL FEATURES

- Seizures can be generalized (involving both hemispheres with alteration in consciousness) or partial (involving a limited area of the brain), although partial seizures can become generalized and vice versa.
- A *convulsive* generalized seizure involves both hemispheres of the brain and rhythmic motor stiffening and/or shaking affects both sides of the body.
- A *nonconvulsive* generalized seizure also involves both hemispheres of the brain but manifests no motor activity—seizure activity is recognizable only on EEG and as altered level of consciousness.
- During both convulsive and nonconvulsive generalized seizures, the patient loses consciousness and a postictal period follows.
- An ***absence seizure*** manifests as a brief episode of staring without a postictal state.
- In ***atonic seizures*** a patient suddenly loses muscle tone and drops to the ground.
- Myoclonic seizures occur when a patient has a sudden, brief, total body jerking movement.
- Partial seizures are focal, involving only part of the brain, with manifestations correlating with the affected area. In a ***simple partial seizure***, the patient is awake.
- ***Complex partial seizures*** are focal but involve loss of consciousness.
- ***Status epilepticus*** is a "prolonged seizure" or recurrent seizures lasting >5 minutes without the patient's regaining consciousness. Rapid cessation of status epilepticus is important to prevent irreversible neuronal damage.

DIAGNOSIS AND DIFFERENTIAL

- The diagnosis of seizure disorder is based primarily on history and physical examination, with laboratory studies (other than a bedside glucose) obtained in a problem-focused manner.
- True seizures must be distinguished from mimics that include breath-holding spells, vasovagal events, hypoglycemia, acute life-threatening event (ALTE), benign sleep myoclonus, movement disorders, night terrors, Sandifer syndrome (gastroesophageal reflux disease), and nonepileptic paroxysmal event (pseudoseizures).
- Unlike adults, routine laboratory testing and neuroimaging are not recommended for most pediatric seizures including simple febrile seizures, complex febrile seizures with return to baseline, or new-onset afebrile seizures. ED investigations are helpful in some specific circumstances, however.
- Serum drug level determinations are useful for phenobarbital, phenytoin, valproic acid, and carbamazepine in patients with known epilepsy and breakthrough seizures or status epilepticus, whereas levels of the newer agents may not be immediately available or useful in guiding therapy.
- Serum chemistry studies (ie, electrolytes, magnesium, calcium, creatinine, and blood urea nitrogen levels) are usually not indicated except in neonatal seizures, infantile spasms, and status epilepticus, or suspected metabolic or gastrointestinal disorders.
- Serum ammonia, TORCH (toxoplasmosis, rubella, cytomegalovirus, and herpes) titers, and urine and

serum amino acid screening may be useful in evaluating neonatal seizures.

- Blood gas analysis is indicated in neonatal seizures and status epilepticus.
- ECG is useful to assess the PR and QT intervals and the possibility of cardiac dysrhythmia as the precipitant of seizure.
- Toxicology screening may be useful in adolescents suspected of recreational drug use (eg, cocaine).
- Magnetic resonance imaging is the preferred neuroimaging procedure for most cases of new-onset seizures, but can usually be performed as an outpatient. Noncontrast computed tomography is indicated in cases of suspected head trauma, afebrile status epilepticus, and focal seizures or focal neurologic signs.
- Lumbar puncture should be performed in patients with neonatal seizure, infantile spasms, and febrile status epilepticus as well as patients with meningeal signs, or persistent alteration in consciousness.

EMERGENCY DEPARTMENT CARE AND DISPOSITION

STATUS EPILEPTICUS

- Most seizures stop within 5 minutes and do not require medical treatment. Status epilepticus (seizure activity lasting for >5 minutes or multiple seizures over a period of >5 minutes) is more responsive to medications when treated early, and medical treatment becomes less effective with time.
- Pediatric Advanced Life Support (PALS)® guidelines should be implemented in patients who present in status epilepticus. IV access is essential, but other routes of medication delivery can be used (IO, IM, intranasal, PR, or buccal) so as not to delay treatment.
- Benzodiazepines are first-line therapy in the seizing patient and are summarized in Table 78-1.
- Figure 78-1 outlines the initial and subsequent management of refractory status epilepticus including second-line pharmacologic options for patients unresponsive to benzodiazepines.
- Rapid bedside testing for electrolytes and glucose levels (glucose, sodium, and calcium) is recommended in status epilepticus when available. Order a complete blood count (CBC), full chemistry panel, hepatic and renal studies, and anticonvulsant levels, if appropriate, when an IV or IO is placed. Other studies may be needed depending upon the suspected underlying cause of seizures. Consider CNS infection and lumbar puncture in the child with febrile status epilepticus. The decision to intubate is clinical, the most common causes being apnea and hypoxia.
- The use of a paralytic with intubation will obscure the ability to assess ongoing seizure activity, and continuous EEG monitoring should be arranged for intubated patients with status epilepticus.
- All patients with status epilepticus require hospitalization and those with persistent seizure activity require admission to intensive care.

FEBRILE SEIZURES

- Simple febrile seizures are defined as generalized tonic-clonic, lasting <15 minutes, with a fever ≥38°C (≥100.4°F) in a child 6 months to 5 years of age that occurs only once in a 24-hour period.
- Identification and treatment of the cause of fever is the primary goal of therapy for febrile seizures, and specific laboratory and radiologic evaluation is otherwise not needed.

TABLE 78-1 Benzodiazepines for Initial Treatment of Status Epilepticus

DRUG	ROUTE	DOSE*	MAXIMUM	ONSET OF ACTION	DURATION OF ACTION
Lorazepam	IV, IO, IN†	0.1 milligram/kg	4 milligrams	1-5 min	12-24 h
	IM	0.1 milligram/kg	4 milligrams	15-30 min	12-24 h
Diazepam	IV, IO	0.1-0.3 milligram/kg	10 milligrams	1-5 min	15-60 min
	PR	0.5 milligram/kg	20 milligrams	3-5 min	15-60 min
Midazolam	IV, IO	0.1-0.2 milligram/kg	4 milligrams	1-5 min	1-6 h
	IM	0.2 milligram/kg	10 milligrams	5-15 min	1-6 h
	IN	0.2 milligram/ kg	10 milligrams	1-5 min	1-6 h
	Buccal†	0.5 milligram/kg	10 milligrams	3-5 min	1-6 h

Abbreviation: IN = intranasal.
*Repeat *dose* is the same.
†Not widely studied.

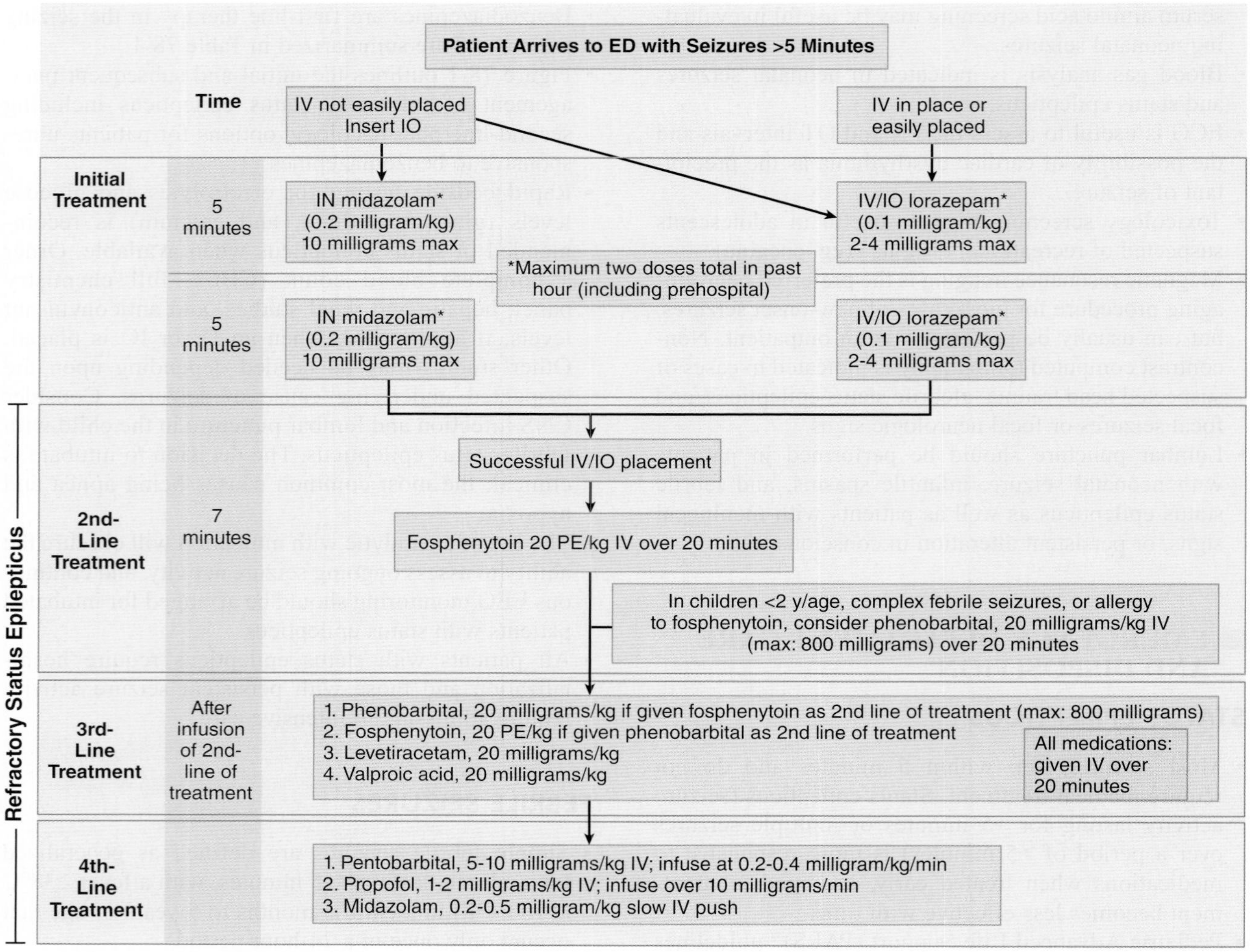
Patient Arrives to ED with Seizures >5 Minutes
Time
IV not easily placed Insert IO
IV in place or easily placed
Initial Treatment
5 minutes
IN midazolam* (0.2 milligram/kg) 10 milligrams max
IV/IO lorazepam* (0.1 milligram/kg) 2-4 milligrams max
*Maximum two doses total in past hour (including prehospital)
5 minutes
IN midazolam* (0.2 milligram/kg) 10 milligrams max
IV/IO lorazepam* (0.1 milligram/kg) 2-4 milligrams max
Refractory Status Epilepticus
Successful IV/IO placement
2nd-Line Treatment
7 minutes
Fosphenytoin 20 PE/kg IV over 20 minutes
In children <2 y/age, complex febrile seizures, or allergy to fosphenytoin, consider phenobarbital, 20 milligrams/kg IV (max: 800 milligrams) over 20 minutes
3rd-Line Treatment
After infusion of 2nd-line of treatment
1. Phenobarbital, 20 milligrams/kg if given fosphenytoin as 2nd line of treatment (max: 800 milligrams)
2. Fosphenytoin, 20 PE/kg if given phenobarbital as 2nd line of treatment
3. Levetiracetam, 20 milligrams/kg
4. Valproic acid, 20 milligrams/kg
All medications: given IV over 20 minutes
4th-Line Treatment
1. Pentobarbital, 5-10 milligrams/kg IV; infuse at 0.2-0.4 milligram/kg/min
2. Propofol, 1-2 milligrams/kg IV; infuse over 10 milligrams/min
3. Midazolam, 0.2-0.5 milligram/kg slow IV push

FIG. 78-1. Treatment of status epilepticus. IN = intranasal; PE = phenytoin sodium equivalents.

- Complex febrile seizures are defined as seizures with fever that last >15 minutes, recur within a 24-hour period, are focal, or occur in children <6 months or >5 years of age without signs of serious infection. Recent guidelines recommend against routine lumbar puncture or neuroimaging in patients who return to baseline and have a normal examination in the ED. All patients with persistent focal deficits or meningeal signs, however, require further ED evaluation and testing.
- Anticonvulsant therapy is not recommended for simple febrile seizures. Although antipyretics are indicated in children with fever, there is no evidence that antipyretics can prevent subsequent febrile seizures.

NEONATAL SEIZURES

- Neonates (<1 month of age) do not have a fully developed neurologic system. Seizures occurring in this age group can be subtle, are more likely to be focal, and often carry a poor prognosis.
- Regardless of fever history, neonates with seizures need a full evaluation for sepsis (blood, urine, and CSF) and IV antibiotics. Neonatal seizures may be caused by herpes simplex encephalitis regardless of the maternal history. Blood and CSF testing for herpes simplex virus and treatment with acyclovir are indicated.
- A toxicologic evaluation may provide the physician with evidence of withdrawal or overdose of abused substances. Neonates with seizures are more likely to have electrolyte abnormalities than older children. Head CT evaluates for concerns of nonaccidental trauma, intracranial hemorrhage, infarction, or mass.
- If inborn errors of metabolism are suspected, levels of lactate, ammonia, and serum amino and urine organic acids should be obtained.

HYPONATREMIA

- Excessive water drinking can lead to hyponatremia (<135 mEq/L). Hyponatremia is most commonly seen in infants <6 months of age and sometimes in athletes. Babies who drink several bottles of water a day or who drink dilute infant formula are at risk for hyponatremia. Athletes can also suffer from water intoxication.
- Hyponatremia can cause seizures, especially if the sodium level is <120 mEq/L. The goal of therapy is to correct the level to >120 mEq/L quickly to treat or prevent further seizure activity, and then correct the sodium to normal levels over the next 24 hours.
- If a patient is actively experiencing seizure, the treatment of choice is 3% NaCl. An infusion of 20 mL/kg of 0.9% NaCl should be started immediately for patients in status epilepticus if delivery of 3% NaCl is delayed.

HYPOGLYCEMIA

- Hypoglycemia is defined as a glucose level of <50 milligrams/dL regardless of whether symptoms exist. Seizures can occur with hypoglycemia, so glucose levels should be measured in all patients presenting with seizures.
- If hypoglycemia is present, patients should be treated with a rapid infusion of 4 mL/kg of 10% dextrose in water (2 mL/kg D25 in older children).

HYPOCALCEMIA

- Hypocalcemia is caused by abnormal calcium absorption, excretion, or distribution and can also cause seizures. Hypocalcemia is more common in neonates and young infants and may be associated with congenital anomalies such as DiGeorge syndrome.
- Treat with 10% calcium gluconate (0.3 mL/kg administered slowly over 5-10 minutes).

SEIZURES IN CHILDREN WITH EPILEPSY

- Epilepsy is defined as two or more unprovoked seizures (eg, no fever or trauma). Diagnosing the type of seizure and determining the best treatment can be complex.
- Parents, old records, and pediatric neurologists can be very helpful in identifying past causes of seizures, successful treatment, and other issues that can help direct care.
- When children with epilepsy who are taking anticonvulsant medications are brought to the ED with seizure, drug levels should be checked if the corresponding assays are available.
- Children with epilepsy may have a lower seizure threshold with febrile illness, even with therapeutic anticonvulsant levels.

SEIZURES IN CHILDREN WITH A VENTRICULOPERITONEAL SHUNT

- Many children with ventriculoperitoneal (VP) shunts also have a medical history of seizures. Considerations include underlying epilepsy, shunt malfunction, and CNS infection.
- The standard approach to the evaluation for a shunt malfunction consists of a radiographic VP shunt series and a head CT or "quick brain MRI" (fast spin echo T2-weighted images performed rapidly typically without sedation) to evaluate for increased ventricular size. If a CNS infection is a concern, a pediatric neurosurgeon should be consulted to consider tapping the shunt for CSF analysis.

SEIZURES IN CHILDREN WITH HEAD TRAUMA

- Children with acute trauma who have seizures may have experienced intracranial injury.
- Those with obvious significant trauma should undergo imaging. "Impact seizures" (seizures that occur within minutes of head trauma) are not associated with severe head injuries. However, seizures that occur in a delayed fashion following injury are more likely to be indicative of severe intracranial injuries.

FIRST-TIME AFEBRILE SEIZURES

- The overall risk of recurrence after a single afebrile seizure is roughly 40%.
- Most neurologists do not recommend daily administration of anticonvulsant medications after a first seizure.
- Only patients with prolonged or repetitive witnessed seizures, especially with concomitant neurologic deficit, are started on antiepileptic drugs. The choice of antiepileptic drug is based on seizure type, side-effect profile, and ease of administration, and should usually be discussed with the primary physician or neurologist.

For further reading in Tintinalli's *Emergency Medicine: A Comprehensive Study Guide*, 7th ed., see Chapter 129, "Seizures and Status Epilepticus in Children," by Maija Holsti.

79 ALTERED MENTAL STATUS AND HEADACHE IN CHILDREN

Kathleen M. Adelgais

ALTERED MENTAL STATUS

EPIDEMIOLOGY

- Altered mental status (AMS) in children is defined as failure to respond to verbal or physical stimulation in a manner appropriate for the child's developmental level.
- The incidence and etiologies of AMS in children are quite varied, and depend on the type of institution and specific definition of AMS used.
- Aggressive resuscitation, stabilization, diagnosis, and treatment must occur simultaneously to prevent morbidity and death in children with AMS.

PATHOPHYSIOLOGY

- Alterations in mental status result from either depression of both cerebral cortices or localized abnormalities of the reticular activating system in the brain stem and midbrain, and range from confusion or delirium to lethargy, stupor, and coma.
- Pathologic conditions that result in AMS can be divided into three broad categories: supratentorial mass lesions, subtentorial mass lesions, and metabolic encephalopathy.
- Supratentorial mass lesions cause AMS by compressing the brain stem and/or diencephalon. Focal motor abnormalities are often present from the onset of alteration in consciousness. Neurologic dysfunction progresses from rostral to caudal, with sequential failure of midbrain, pontine, and medullary function. Supratentorial lesions cause slow nystagmus toward, and fast nystagmus away from a cold stimulus during caloric testing.
- Subtentorial lesions produce rapid loss of consciousness (due to dysfunction of the reticular activating system), cranial nerve abnormalities, abnormal breathing patterns (eg, Cheyne–Stokes respirations, neurogenic hyperventilation, ataxic breathing), and asymmetric or fixed pupils.
- Metabolic encephalopathy produces decreased level of consciousness before exhibiting motor signs, which are symmetrical when present. Pupillary reflexes are intact except with profound anoxia, opiates, barbiturates, and anticholinergics. Respiratory changes are common and are often due to associated acid–base disturbances.

CLINICAL FEATURES

- Historical data should focus on prodromal events, such as recent illnesses, infectious exposures, toxic exposures, and the possibility of trauma or abuse. Ask about antecedent fever, headaches, head tilt, abdominal pain, vomiting, diarrhea, gait disturbance, seizures, drug ingestion, palpitations, weakness, hematuria, weight loss, and rash; review developmental milestones, past medical history, immunization history, and family history.
- Focus the physical examination on signs of infection, trauma, toxidromes, or metabolic disease.
- The neurologic examination includes the child's response to sensory input, motor activity, pupillary reactivity, oculovestibular reflexes, and respiratory pattern, as well as the child's performance on the AVPU (alert, response to verbal stimuli, response to painful stimuli, unresponsive) or pediatric Glasgow coma score.

DIAGNOSIS AND DIFFERENTIAL

- The differential diagnosis for AMS in children is diverse and differs slightly from that for adults. The familiar mnemonic AEIOU TIPS remains a useful tool in organizing diagnostic possibilities (Table 79-1).
- Diagnostic adjuncts are guided by the clinical presentation and may include analysis of blood, gastric fluid, urine, stool, cerebrospinal fluid (CSF), electrocardiography, or selected radiographic studies. Obtain a rapid bedside glucose in all patients with AMS.
- For suspected meningitis or encephalitis, obtain a lumbar puncture for CSF analysis as rapidly as possible after initial resuscitation and stabilization.
- Capnometry may be useful for rapid assessment of acid–base status.
- Obtain 12-lead ECG if pathologic auscultatory findings or rhythm disturbances are noted.
- Consider blood ammonia level, serum osmolality, blood alcohol level, thyroid function tests, blood lead level, and skeletal survey and head CT for concerns of trauma or abuse.
- A portable electroencephalograph may diagnose nonconvulsive status epilepticus.

EMERGENCY DEPARTMENT CARE AND DISPOSITION

- Initial treatment priorities are airway, breathing, and circulation.
- Immobilize cervical spine for suspected trauma.
- Initiate continuous pulse oximetry and consider capnometry; administer oxygen.

TABLE 79-1 AEIOU TIPS Mnemonic for Diagnosing Altered Mental Status (AMS)

A	**Alcohol.** Changes in mental status can occur with serum levels <100 milligrams/dL. Concurrent hypoglycemia is common. **Acid–base and metabolic.** Hypotonic and hypertonic dehydration. Hepatic dysfunction, inborn errors of metabolism, diabetic ketoacidosis, primary lung disease, and neurologic dysfunction causing hypercapnia. **Arrhythmia/cardiogenic.** Stokes–Adams, supraventricular tachycardia, aortic stenosis, heart block, ventricular fibrillation, pericardial tamponade
E	**Encephalopathy.** Hypertensive encephalopathy can occur with diastolic pressures of 100-110 mm Hg. Reye's syndrome. HIV. Post-immunization encephalopathy. Encephalomyelitis. **Endocrinopathy.** AMS is rare as a presentation in this category. Addison's disease can present with AMS or psychosis. Thyrotoxicosis can present with ventricular dysrhythmias. Pheochromocytoma can present with hypertensive encephalopathy. **Electrolytes.** Hyponatremia becomes symptomatic around 120 mEq/L. Hypernatremia and disorders of calcium, magnesium, and phosphorus can produce AMS.
I	**Insulin.** AMS from hyperglycemia is rare in children, but diabetic ketoacidosis is the most common cause. Hypoglycemia can be the result of many disorders. Irritability, confusion, seizures, and coma can occur with blood glucose levels <40 milligrams/dL. **Intussusception.** AMS may be the initial presenting symptom.
O	**Opiates.** Common household exposures are to Lomotil®, loperamide, diphenoxylate, and dextromethorphan. Clonidine, an α-agonist, can also produce similar symptoms.
U	**Uremia.** Encephalopathy occurs in over one-third of patients with chronic renal failure. Hemolytic-uremic syndrome can also produce AMS in addition to abdominal pain. Thrombocytopenic purpura and hemolytic anemia can also cause AMS.
T	**Trauma.** Children with blunt trauma are more likely to develop cerebral edema than adults. The child should be examined for signs of abuse, particularly shaken baby syndrome with retinal hemorrhages. **Tumor.** Primary, metastatic, or meningeal leukemic infiltration. **Thermal.** Hypo- or hyperthermia.
I	**Infection**. One of the most common causes of AMS in children. Meningitis should be high on the differential list, particularly among febrile children. **Intracerebral vascular disorders.** Subarachnoid, intracerebral, or intraventricular hemorrhages can be seen with trauma, ruptured aneurysm, or arteriovenous malformations. Venous thrombosis can follow severe dehydration or pyogenic infection of the mastoid, orbit, middle ear, or sinuses.
P	**Psychogenic.** Rare in the pediatric age group, characterized by decreased responsiveness with normal neurologic examination including oculovestibular reflexes. **Poisoning**. Drugs or toxins can be ingested by accident, through neglect or abuse, or in a suicide gesture.
S	**Seizure**. Generalized motor seizures are often associated with prolonged unresponsiveness in children. Seizure in a young febrile patient suggests intracranial infection. Shunt malfunction should be considered among patients with a ventriculo-peritoneal shunt for hydrocephalus.

Abbreviations: AMS = altered mental status, HIV = human immunodeficiency virus.

- Provide fluid resuscitation (20 mL/kg three times as needed) for signs of shock.
- Perform bedside glucose determination and treat hypoglycemia with 4 mL/kg of D10 in infants or 2 mL/kg of D25 in children.
- Treat hypothermia or hyperthermia.
- Control seizures with benzodiazepines (eg, lorazepam, 0.1 milligram/kg IV/IO).
- Give naloxone for suspected opiate or clonidine overdose, 0.01 to 0.1 milligram/kg IV/IO every 2 minutes as needed.
- Give flumazenil for suspected pure benzodiazepine overdose, 0.01 milligram/kg IV/IO.
- Avoid sodium bicarbonate except as specifically indicated for select toxic ingestions or serum pH <7.0.
- Administer empiric broad-spectrum antibiotics as quickly as possible, before lumbar puncture if unstable, to all patients with suspected sepsis or meningitis.
- Most infants and children with AMS require admission to an intensive care unit, although benign and transient causes of AMS may be treated and monitored in the ED with discharge after observation.

HEADACHE

EPIDEMIOLOGY

- Headaches comprise up to 1% of pediatric ED visits.
- The vast majority of headaches in children have a benign etiology. Occipital location of the headache and the inability of the child to describe the quality of the head pain are associated with potentially serious underlying causes.
- Emergent neurosurgical conditions presenting with headache are usually associated with neurologic signs.

PATHOPHYSIOLOGY

- The pathogenesis of headache is complex and varies by cause. The brain, the cranium, and most of the overlying meninges lack pain receptors. Pain is perceived from structures between the epidermis of the scalp and periosteum of the skull.
- Extracranial pain can arise from cervical nerve roots, cranial nerves, or extracranial arteries traversing muscles, leading to pain within specific areas of the head and neck region.
- Intracranial pain can arise from venous sinuses, dural veins or arteries, and arteries around the base of the brain. Posterior fossa pain can be referred to the occiput, ear, or throat, secondary to nociceptors from the vagus and glossopharyngeal nerves.

CLINICAL FEATURES

- Headaches can be classified as either primary or secondary: primary headaches are physiologic (migraine, tension), while secondary headaches have an anatomic basis (vascular malformation, tumor, or infectious). Table 79-2 outlines elements of the history and physical examination that aid in the differentiation between primary and secondary headaches.
- Secondary headache is suggested by acute onset; morning vomiting; behavioral changes; AMS; worst headache ever; awakening from sleep; association with fever, trauma, or toxic exposure; or aggravation by coughing, valsalva, or position.

TABLE 79-2 Features Suggesting Secondary Headache

HISTORICAL DESCRIPTION	PHYSICAL FINDINGS
• Abrupt onset	• Altered mental status
• First or worst ever	• Septic or toxic appearance
• Posttraumatic	• External evidence of head trauma
• Present with fever or stiff neck	• Bradycardia, hypertension, or irregular respirations
• Aggravated by sneezing, coughing, lying down	• Diaphoresis
• Vomiting or worsening pain in morning	• Petechiae
• Altered mental status or focal neurologic findings	• Café au lait or ash-leaf spots
• Change in behavior	• Asymmetry of papillary response
• Change in pattern or worsening over time	• Ptosis
• Toxic exposure	• Visual field defects
• Family history of subarachnoid hemorrhage	• Retinal hemorrhage or optic disc distortion
• Abrupt onset	• Asymmetry of motor or sensory responses
• First or worst ever	• Thyromegaly
	• Nuchal rigidity
	• Head tilt

- Benign headaches are more likely to occur in school-aged children and are often described as pulsating. They tend to be unilateral/bilateral, frontal or temporal in location, and vary from mild to intense without associated neurologic symptoms or signs.
- Life-threatening headaches are more likely in preschool-aged children. The pain may be occipital and constrictive in nature if described. Pain is usually intense, and the headache is often associated with neurologic changes such as focal deficits, papilledema, ataxia, and AMS.
- Physical findings suggestive of a secondary headache include blood pressure abnormalities, nuchal rigidity, head tilt, ptosis, retinal hemorrhage or optic nerve distortion, visual field defects, gait disturbances, or focal motor or sensory deficits (Table 79-3).

DIAGNOSIS AND DIFFERENTIAL

- There are no evidence-based studies to guide the diagnostic work-up of headache in children. The selection of studies should be guided by the history and physical examination.
- Practice guidelines state that routine imaging is not indicated in children with recurrent headaches and a normal neurologic examination. Neuroimaging (computed tomography or magnetic resonance imaging) may be indicated in trauma or when history or physical examination suggests a secondary type of headaches.
- Perform a lumbar puncture if infection or subarachnoid hemorrhage is suspected.

EMERGENCY DEPARTMENT CARE AND DISPOSITION

- Obtain a throughout history and physical examination to distinguish primary from secondary headache.
- For secondary headaches, treat the underlying cause and manage pain. Narcotics can be used for pain related to secondary headaches but have no role in the management of primary headaches. For secondary headaches, consider morphine 0.1 milligram/kg IV, or hydrocodone with acetaminophen (0.1 milligram/kg of hydrocodone component, PO).
- For primary headaches, treat based on type of headache diagnosed by historical features. Most primary headaches can be treated with first-line oral therapy, typically ibuprofen 10 milligrams/kg PO or acetaminophen 15 milligrams/kg PO/PR.
- For migraines, consider prochlorperazine 0.15 milligram/kg IV with diphenhydramine 1 milligram/kg IV to prevent dystonic reactions or use of a triptan (see cluster headache below). Dihydroergotamine 0.1 milligram/kg (ages 6-9 years), 0.15 milligram/kg (ages

TABLE 79-3 Physical Examination Findings Associated with Potential Secondary Causes of Headache

EXAMINATION COMPONENT	FINDING	POTENTIAL CAUSES
Growth parameters	Abnormal height, weight, head circumference	Failure to thrive suggests systemic disease; enlarged head circumference suggests increased intracranial pressure
Vital signs	Abnormal heart rate, blood pressure, respiratory rate, temperature	Bradycardia, hypertension, and irregular respirations indicate intracranial hypertension; sever hypertension may be associated with hypertensive crisis; tachypnea suggests metabolic acidosis; fever suggests CNS or systemic infection
Head and neck	Cranial or carotid bruits Signs of trauma	Arteriovenous malformation Accidental or nonaccidental trauma
Eyes	Papilledema Unilateral conjunctival injection, tearing, eyelid edema Retinal hemorrhage Bilateral periorbital edema, facial tenderness, nasal discharge	Increased intracranial pressure Cluster headache Nonaccidental trauma Sinusitis
Ear, nose, throat	Signs of infection Malocclusion, TMJ tenderness	Otitis media, mastoiditis, sinusitis, pharyngitis, dental abscess or caries TMJ dysfunction
Heart	Murmurs	Potential shunting with risk of embolic event or cerebral abscess
Skin	Café au lait spots, ash-leaf spots, vascular malformations	Neurofibromatosis, tuberous sclerosis, congenital vascular malformations

Abbreviation: TMJ = temporomandibular joint.

9-12 years), or 0.2 milligram/kg (ages 12-16 years) is an alternative, but is contraindicated in patients with complex migraine.

- Cluster and tension headaches are managed much the same way as migraines. Sumatriptan 10 milligrams (20-39 kg) or 20 milligrams (>40 kg) intranasal or 0.06 milligram/kg subcutaneously and high-flow oxygen (7 L/minute via non-rebreather mask) may be effective for cluster headaches. Tension headaches usually respond to first-line oral therapy such as ibuprofen 10 milligrams/kg.
- Address potential precipitating factors to avoid reoccurrence of the headache. Consider prophylactic regimens such as β-blockers for migraines, usually in consultation with neurology.
- In general, most patients with primary headache can be discharged after relief of symptoms. Those with intractable pain may require inpatient management.
- Patients with secondary headache of emergent origin (eg, meningitis, tumor, severe hypertension, or hemorrhage) require inpatient treatment for definitive care.

For further reading in Tintinalli's *Emergency Medicine: A Comprehensive Study Guide*, 7th ed., see Chapter 130, "Headaches in Children," by Brian R. E. Schultz and Charles G. Macias and Chapter 131, "Altered Mental Status in Children," by Jonathan I. Singer.

80 SYNCOPE AND SUDDEN DEATH IN CHILDREN

Derya Caglar

EPIDEMIOLOGY

- Syncope is common in adolescents and less common in younger children. Between 20% and 50% of adolescents experience at least one episode of syncope. This condition is transient and usually self-limited.
- The most common type of benign syncope is neurally mediated (vasovagal) syncope.
- Twenty percent of children referred to a cardiologist or neurologist for evaluation are diagnosed with a serious illness.
- The rate of sudden unexpected death in children is 2.3% of all pediatric deaths. Sudden cardiac death makes up about one-third of these cases.
- Except for trauma, sudden cardiac death is the most common cause of sports-related deaths, more commonly associated with basketball, football, and track.
- The two most common causes of sudden cardiac death in adolescent athletes without known cardiac disease are hypertrophic cardiomyopathy and aberrant coronary arteries.
- Other causes of sudden cardiac death in children are myocarditis, cardiomyopathy, congenital heart disease, and conduction disturbances.

PATHOPHYSIOLOGY

- Syncope is the temporary loss of consciousness from reversible disruption of cerebral functioning, and is usually caused by inadequate cardiac output causing cerebral hypoperfusion.
- Vascular syncope occurs when venous pooling occurs in the legs, leading to a decrease in ventricular preload with a compensatory increase in heart rate and myocardial contractility.
- Neurally mediated syncope (NMS), or reflex syncope, occurs when receptors in the atria, ventricles, and pulmonary arteries sense a decrease in venous return, and an efferent brain stem response via the vagal nerve causes bradycardia, hypotension, or both. Types of NMS include vasovagal, orthostatic, situational (urination, coughing), and familial. NMS is usually preceded by sensations of nausea, warmth, or lightheadedness, with a gradual visual grayout.
- Cardiac syncope occurs when there is an interruption of cardiac output from an intrinsic cardiac problem. These causes are divided into tachydysrhythmias, bradydysrhythmias, outflow obstruction, and myocardial dysfunction. Syncope resulting from these causes usually begins and ends abruptly and may be exercise induced.
- Long QT syndrome may be inherited or acquired, is associated with hypertrophic cardiomyopathy, and accounts for half of the cases of sudden cardiac death. Patients with long QT syndrome have a QTc >0.44 seconds on ECG. Drugs that prolong the QT interval include antibiotics, tricyclic antidepressants (TCAs), antipsychotics, antifungals, GI motility and antinausea agents, antihistamines, antiarrhythmics, and appetite suppressants.
- Other known causes of syncope include breath holding, hyperventilation, hypoglycemia, hysteria, and atypical migraines.
- Any event that causes sufficient cerebral hypoperfusion can lead to sudden death.

CLINICAL FEATURES

- Syncope is the sudden onset of falling, accompanied by a brief episode of loss of consciousness.
- Involuntary motor movements may occur with all types of syncopal episodes, but are most common with seizures.
- Two-thirds of children experience lightheadedness or dizziness prior to the episode.
- Table 80-1 lists the most common causes of syncope by category.
- Structural cardiac disease, cardiac dysfunction, rhythm disturbances, and systemic disease are predisposing factors for sudden cardiac death.

TABLE 80-1 Causes of Syncope in Children and Adolescents

Neurally mediated: most common cause of syncope in children Orthostatic: lightheadedness with standing Situational: urination, defecation, coughing, and swallowing Familial dysautonomia
Cardiac dysrhythmias: events that usually start and end abruptly Prolonged QT syndrome Wolff–Parkinson–White syndrome Sick sinus syndrome: associated with prior heart surgery Supraventricular tachycardia Atrioventricular block: most common in children with congenital heart disease Pacemaker malfunction
Structural cardiac disease Hypertrophic cardiomyopathy: exertional syncope most common presentation; but infants can present with congestive heart failure and cyanosis; echocardiography necessary to confirm Dilated cardiomyopathy: may be idiopathic, post-myocarditis, or congenital
Congenital heart disease Valvular diseases: aortic stenosis is usually congenital, Ebstein's malformation, or mitral valve prolapse (which is not associated with increased risk of sudden death) Dysrhythmogenic right ventricular dysplasia Pulmonary hypertension: dyspnea on exertion, exercise intolerance, shortness of breath Coronary artery abnormalities: aberrant left main artery causing external compression during physical exercise
Endocrine abnormalities: hyperthyroid, hyperglycemia, adrenal insufficiency
Medications and drugs: antihypertensives, tricyclic antidepressants, cocaine, diuretics, antidysrhythmics
Gastrointestinal disorders: reflux

- Risk factors associated with serious causes of syncope include exertion preceding the event, a personal or family history of cardiac disease or dysfunction, recurrent episodes, associated chest pain or palpitations, or prolonged loss of consciousness (see Table 80-2).
- Events easily mistaken for syncope are presented in Table 80-3 along with common associated symptoms.

TABLE 80-2 Risk Factors for Serious Causes of Syncope

Exertion preceding the event
History of cardiac disease in patient
Recurrent episodes
Recumbent episode
Family history of sudden death, cardiac disease, deafness
Chest pain, palpitations
Prolonged loss of consciousness
Medications that affect cardiac conduction

TABLE 80-3 Events Mistaken for Syncope

Basilar migraine: headache, loss of consciousness, neurologic symptoms
Seizure: loss of consciousness, simultaneous motor movements, prolonged recovery
Vertigo: no loss of consciousness, spinning or rotating sensation
Hysteria: no loss of consciousness, indifference to the event
Hypoglycemia: confusion, gradual onset associated with diaphoresis
Breath-holding spell: crying prior to the event, age 6-18 months
Hyperventilation: severe hypocapnia can cause syncope

DIAGNOSIS AND DIFFERENTIAL

- No specific historical or clinical features reliably distinguish between vasovagal syncope and other causes. However, a thorough history and physical examination, with particular focus on the cardiac examination, can help to arouse suspicion for serious causes.
- The most important step in evaluation of children with syncope is a detailed history, including medications, drugs, intake, and food.
- Syncope during exercise suggests a more serious cause. Many of the diseases that cause syncope also cause sudden death in children. Approximately 25% of children who suffer sudden death have a history of syncope. However, syncope is a very common event, and a syncopal episode by itself is not associated with an increased risk of sudden death.
- If witnesses note that the patient appeared dead or cardiopulmonary resuscitation was performed, a search for a serious pathologic condition must be undertaken.
- Cardiac dysrhythmia should be suspected if syncope is associated with fright, anger, surprise, or physical exertion.
- The physical examination should include a complete cardiovascular, neurologic, and pulmonary examination. Any abnormalities noted in the cardiovascular examination require additional work-up.

EMERGENCY DEPARTMENT CARE AND DISPOSITION

- Routine laboratory studies are not needed if vasovagal syncope is clearly identified from the history. Laboratory assessment is guided by the history, physical examination, and clinical suspicion. In patients with atypical presentation or worrisome symptoms, one might consider serum chemistry, hematocrit, thyroid function tests, a chest radiograph, and a urine drug screen.
- An ECG should be done on all patients except those with a clear vasovagal episode. The QT interval should be assessed. Patients with hypertrophic cardiomyopathy, prolonged QT interval, or other cardiac dysrhythmias should be managed in consultation with a cardiologist.
- An echocardiogram is recommended for patients with known or suspected cardiac disease.
- Patients resuscitated from sudden death must have a complete evaluation including a creatinine phosphokinase level (CPK-MB) and troponin I unless a clear cause of the arrest is apparent. One should be alert for complications resulting from the arrest. All such patients should be admitted to a pediatric intensive care unit.
- If no clear cause is found for the syncopal episode, the child may be discharged to be further evaluated and followed by the primary care physician, unless there are cardiac risk factors or exercise-induced symptoms, in which case referral to a cardiologist is warranted, and further participation in sports should be prohibited until cleared by cardiology.
- Children with documented dysrhythmias should be admitted with continuous cardiac monitoring. Patients with a normal ECG but a history suggesting a dysrhythmic event are candidates for outpatient monitoring and cardiac work-up.

For further reading in Tintinalli's *Emergency Medicine: A Comprehensive Study Guide*, 7th ed., see Chapter 140, "Syncope and Sudden Death in Children," by William E. Hauda II and Maybelle Kou.

81 HYPOGLYCEMIA AND METABOLIC EMERGENCIES IN INFANTS AND CHILDREN

Matthew Hansen

EPIDEMIOLOGY

- Hypoglycemia is more common in neonates and infants than older children. Conditions associated with hypoglycemia in infants and children are listed in Table 81-1.
- Congenital adrenal hyperplasia occurs in about 1:10,000 live births. Seventy-five percent of affected newborns exhibit the classic salt wasting, virulizing variant.
- Inborn errors of metabolism encompass a diverse group of rare disorders, and many are included on state newborn screening exams in the United States, although disorders screened vary by state.

TABLE 81-1 Conditions Associated with Hypoglycemia in Infants and Children

PERINATAL PERIOD	INFANCY AND CHILDHOOD
Infant of a diabetic mother	Idopathic ketotic hypoglycemia/ starvation
Congenital heart disease	Diabetes mellitus/endocrine disorder
Infection/sepsis	Infection/sepsis
Adrenal hemorrhage	Inborn errors of metabolism
Hypothermia	Hypothermia
Hypoglycemia-inducing drug use by mother	Drug induced (salicylates, etc.) Hyperinsulinism
Maternal eclampsia	Idiopathic
Fetal alcohol syndrome	
Hypopituitarism	

PATHOPHYSIOLOGY

- Young children are predisposed to hypoglycemia because of a higher basal metabolic rate and lesser glycogen stores.
- For children younger than 2 years who are fasting, nearly all endogenously produced glucose is required and used by the brain.
- As glucose levels fall, counterregulatory hormones including glucagon, cortisol, growth hormone, and epinephrine are released, stimulating gluconeogenesis. The clinical effects of epinephrine release are called the adrenergic response.
- Congenital adrenal hyperplasia is caused by a deficiency of one of several enzymes in the cortisol production pathway.
- Inborn errors of metabolism result from abnormal metabolism of fat, carbohydrates, or protein; symptoms are caused by the accumulation of toxic substrates resulting from the metabolic derangement.

CLINICAL FEATURES

- Hypoglycemic patients present with either neuroglycopenic or adrenergic signs and symptoms.
- Neurologic symptoms associated with hypoglycemia include altered level of consciousness, focal neurologic deficits, and seizures in young infants, as well as confusion, ataxia, and blurred vision in older children.
- Adrenergic symptoms associated with hypoglycemia include anxiety, tachycardia, perspiration, tremors, pallor, weakness, abdominal pain, and irritability; these symptoms may be absent in young infants.
- Hypoglycemia in neonates and infants are usually nonspecific and include poor feeding, jitteriness, emesis, ravenous hunger, lethargy, altered personality, repetitive colic-like symptoms, hypotonia, and hypothermia.
- Hypoglycemia often accompanies a critical illness (eg, sepsis) and the features of that illness may dominate the clinical picture.
- Congenital adrenal hyperplasia most frequently presents within the second week of life with vague symptoms such as lethargy, poor feeding, irritability, vomiting, or shock. Female infants will frequently have virulized genitalia (ie, cliteromegally).
- Inborn errors of metabolism present with nonspecific symptoms similar to those of sepsis, congenital adrenal hyperplasia, or hypoglycemia. Seizures may occur.

DIAGNOSIS AND DIFFERENTIAL

- Plasma glucose concentration <45 milligrams/dL constitutes hypoglycemia in any symptomatic patient and <35 milligrams/dL in any asymptomatic patient. *Bedside glucose should be checked immediately in any critically ill child.*
- The differential diagnosis of hypoglycemia differs by age, and may accompany many systemic disorders, illnesses, and ingestions, but is commonly associated with critical illness from any cause including sepsis, congenital heart disease, and inborn errors of metabolism.
- The classic electrolyte abnormalities seen in congenital adrenal hyperplasia are hyponatremia and hyperkalemia. The differential diagnosis includes sepsis, congenital heart disease, and metabolic diseases.
- Diagnosis of specific metabolic disorders is beyond the scope of ED care and not important for initial stabilization. Key labs include glucose, urine ketones, plasma ammonia, complete metabolic screen, blood gas analysis, and lactate.
- Figure 81-1 outlines disorders associated with specific patterns of lab abnormalities.

EMERGENCY DEPARTMENT CARE AND DISPOSITION

HYPOGLYCEMIA

- The dose of dextrose is 0.5 to 1 gram/kg for any age patient, which can be given via IV, IO, NG, or PO route. Table 81-2 outlines the age-based ED management of hypoglycemia.

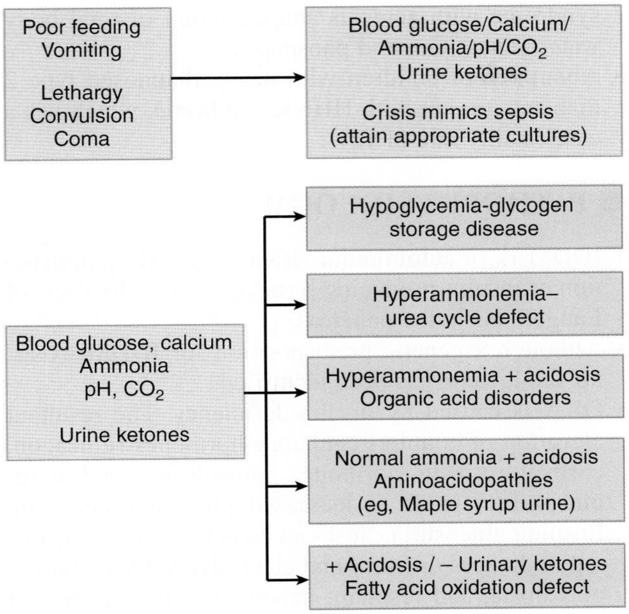

FIG. 81-1. Approach to suspected metabolic disorders.

- Administration of D25W and D50W is not recommended for younger patients since both are hyperosmolar and increase the risk in smaller veins for phlebitis, extravasation, and surrounding tissue necrosis, and potentially intracranial hemorrhage in neonates.
- Consider glucagon, 0.3 milligram/kg IM when IV or IO access is unavailable. Glucagon only works in patients with intact glycogen stores, and may be ineffective in those with severe systemic or metabolic disease.

CONGENITAL ADRENAL HYPERPLASIA OR ADRENAL INSUFFICIENCY

- Administer hydrocortisone empirically when standard resuscitation efforts fail to improve the clinical condition, especially when considering adrenal insufficiency as a cause. The dose is 25 milligrams for neonates and infants, 50 milligrams for children, and 100 milligrams for adolescents. Hydrocortisone can be given IV, IO, or IM in all age groups.
- Treat patients with congenital adrenal hyperplasia and hyperkalemia associated with ECG changes or arrhythmias with IV calcium gluconate 100 milligrams/kg. *Do not give insulin and glucose to neonates* as this may cause profound hypoglycemia. Asymptomatic hyperkalemia will correct with hydrocortisone treatment.

INBORN ERRORS OF METABOLISM

- Initial stabilization of children with inborn errors of metabolism focuses on restoring circulatory volume with normal saline boluses of 10 to 20 mL/kg, providing glucose to stop catabolism and further production of toxic metabolites, and enhancing elimination of toxic metabolites.
- Stabilize and support airway and breathing, but exercise caution with paralysis and mechanical ventilation as severe metabolic acidosis may be worsened by a relative respiratory acidosis from inadequate ventilatory rate.
- Treatment for hypoglycemia is listed in Table 81-2.
- Make patients NPO and begin D10 infusion at twice normal maintenance rate (see Chapter 83 for maintenance fluid calculations).

TABLE 81-2 Emergency Department Treatment of Hypoglycemia

PATIENT AGE	DEXTROSE BOLUS DOSE	DEXTROSE MAINTENANCE DOSAGE	OTHER TREATMENTS TO CONSIDER
Neonate	D10 5 mL/kg PO/NG/IV/IO	6 mL/kg/h D10	Glucagon, 0.3 milligram/kg IM Hydrocortisone, 25 grams PO/IM/IV/IO
Infant	D10 5 mL/kg PO/NG/IV/IO *or* D25 2 mL/kg	6 mL/kg/h D10	Glucagon, 0.3 milligram/kg IM Hydrocortisone, 25 grams PO/IM/IV/IO
Child	D25 2 mL/kg PO/NG/IV/IO	6 mL/kg/h D10 for the first 10 kg + 3 mL/kg/h for 11-20 kg + 1.5 mL/kg/h for each additional kg >20 kg	Glucagon, 0.3 milligram/kg/IM Hydrocortisone, 50 grams PO/IM/IV/IO
Adolescent	D50 one ampule	6 mL/kg/h D10 for the first 10 kg + 3 mL/kg/h for 11-20 kg + 1.5 mL/kg/h for each additional kg >20 kg	Glucagon, 0.3 milligram/kg IM Hydrocortisone, 100 grams PO/IM/IV/IO

Abbreviations: D10 = 10% dextrose; D25 = 25% dextrose; NG = (via) nasogastric tube.

- Treat hyperammonemia with sodium benzoate, 250 milligrams/kg IV or IO as a continuous infusion over 24 hours and arginine 210 milligrams/kg IV or IO over 90 minutes. Consider hemodialysis for serum ammonia levels >300 milligrams/dL.
- Consider carnitine, 400 milligrams IV, IO, or PO for patients with known organic acidemias.
- In children with known or suspected metabolic disorders, discharge criteria include stable vital signs, ability to tolerate PO, normal electrolytes, normal pH, normal ammonia level, and overall well appearance on examination. Prior to disposition from the ED, care of children with known or suspected metabolic disorders should ideally be discussed with a local metabolic specialist. There should be a low threshold for admission or transfer of these patients to a children's hospital.

For further reading in Tintinalli's *Emergency Medicine: A Comprehensive Study Guide*, 7th ed., see Chapter 137, "Hypoglycemia and Metabolic Emergencies in Infants and Children," by Nadeemuddin Qureshi, Mohammed Al-Mogbil, and Osama Y. Kentab.

82 THE CHILD WITH DIABETES

Adam Vella

EPIDEMIOLOGY

- Insulin-dependent diabetes mellitus (IDDM) is the most common endocrine disorder of childhood, with an estimated prevalence of 1 in 400.
- As many as 27% to 40% of new-onset diabetics present with diabetic ketoacidosis (DKA).
- In known diabetics, DKA is much less common and tends to be clustered in a small subset of patients, with 5% of diabetic children accounting for nearly 60% of DKA episodes.
- DKA is the most common cause of death in diabetic patients under 24 years of age, and cerebral edema is the leading cause of mortality in DKA.
- Mortality rates for children who develop cerebral edema are 40% to 90%, and only 14% to 57% of those children affected recover neurologically normal.
- DKA is much more common in patients with type 1 diabetes, but patients with type 2 diabetes can develop hyperglycemic, hyperosmolar nonketotic (HHNK) syndrome with acidosis and depletion of total body water, potassium, and phosphorus.
- About 4% of children with newly diagnosed type 2 diabetes present with HHNK syndrome, which has a case fatality rate of 12%.

PATHOPHYSIOLOGY

- IDDM is an autoimmune disease caused by destruction of insulin-producing β (beta) cells of the islets of Langerhans in the pancreas.
- Although a genetic predisposition for IDDM exists, no single gene has been identified.
- DKA is caused by insulin-deficiency. The resultant elevation of counter-regulatory hormones (glucagon, cortisol, growth hormone, epinephrine, and norepinephrine) leads to increased glucose production. Ensuing glucosuria causes an osmotic diuresis, resulting in the loss of fluids and electrolytes. Dehydration, polydipsia, and resultant hyperosmolality occur as a result of fluid losses.
- Lack of insulin and excess glucagon result in the production of ketone bodies from free fatty acids. Production of ketones, primarily β-hydroxybutyrate and acetoacetate, exceeds the capacity for peripheral utilization, contributing to metabolic acidosis and compensatory respiratory alkalosis. The presence of increased ketones and acidemia manifest as the classic fruity breath odor of ketosis.

CLINICAL FEATURES

- Classic symptoms of IDDM include polyuria, polydipsia, and polyphagia; however, other common complaints include weight loss, secondary enuresis, anorexia, abdominal discomfort, visual changes, headache, and genital candidiasis in a toilet-trained child.
- Physical examination may reveal signs of dehydration, abdominal tenderness, Kussmaul's respirations, decreased level of consciousness, or coma.
- DKA should be considered in patients with hyperventilation, fruity breath odor of ketosis, dehydration, lethargy, altered mental status, hyperglycemia, vomiting, abdominal pain, or polyuria.
- Cerebral edema is the most dreaded complication of DKA and should be suspected in all comatose patients. Premonitory symptoms of cerebral edema occur in as few as 50% and include severe headache, declining mental status, seizures, and papilledema.

DIAGNOSIS AND DIFFERENTIAL

- DKA is defined by hyperglycemia (blood glucose >250 milligrams/dL), ketonemia, and metabolic acidosis (pH <7.2 and plasma bicarbonate level <15 mEq/L), associated with glucosuria and ketonuria.

- Laboratory tests required to diagnose and manage DKA include serum electrolytes, urinalysis, and venous blood gas analysis.
- Cerebral edema in DKA is a clinical diagnosis based on altered mental status not attributed to hypovolemia, and treatment should begin prior to neuroimaging when suspected. CT can confirm the diagnosis, and intracranial pressure monitoring may be indicated.
- Sepsis should be considered in the setting of fever when the cause of DKA is not apparent, and a complete blood count, a chest radiograph, and appropriate cultures should be obtained as clinically directed.
- Other causative factors include trauma, vomiting, noncompliance, and stress.
- The abdominal pain associated with DKA can mimic acute appendicitis or other surgical abdominal emergencies, which must be considered in the differential diagnosis.

EMERGENCY DEPARTMENT CARE AND DISPOSITION

- The treatment of DKA consists of judicious fluid resuscitation, insulin therapy, correction of electrolyte abnormalities, and close monitoring.
- Patients should have continuous monitoring of cardiorespiratory status, and vascular access should be established.
- Initially, hourly monitoring of electrolytes and pH is necessary.
- Administer 10 to 20 mL/kg NS boluses until hemodynamically stable. Give an initial 20 mL/kg bolus of NS if the child is in shock and repeat if needed. Once vital signs have stabilized, resist the desire to correct the fluid deficit too rapidly, especially if there is a high calculated serum osmolarity (ie, >340 mOsm/L).
- Begin regular insulin at 0.05 to 0.1 units/kg/h after the initial IV fluid bolus (if given). Adjust the rate to maintain correction of serum glucose of 50 to 100 milligrams/dL/h. **Do not decrease insulin infusion below 0.05 unit/kg/h until ketonuria has resolved**; dextrose may be added to the IVF when the serum glucose approaches 200 milligrams/dL if ketonuria persists. **High-dose insulin therapy and insulin boluses increase the risk of complications and are not recommended**.
- Correction of serum sodium is accomplished by administration of NS and treatment of hyperglycemia. Patients with DKA typically have sodium deficits of 5 to 10 mEq/kg, although initial hyponatremia may be overestimated due to effects of hyperglycemia and hyperlipidemia on reported sodium levels. Monitor serum sodium closely, since a slower than expected increase in serum sodium is a risk factor for developing cerebral edema.
- Patients with DKA have total body deficits of potassium that require careful management. Extracellular shifts of potassium occur with metabolic acidosis and initial serum potassium levels do not reflect total body stores. If the pH is 7.10 or less and the K^+ level is normal or low, begin replacement therapy immediately: for initial [K^+] 3.5 to 5.5 mEq/L with adequate urine output, add 30 to 40 mEq potassium per liter (half as KCl and half as potassium phosphate); for initial [K^+] of 2.5 to 3.5 mEq/L, add 40 mEq [K^+] per liter; consider adding more if the [K^+] is <2.5 mEq/L. If the K^+ level is elevated (>6.0 mEq/L) consider withholding K^+ therapy until adequate urine output is achieved and monitor serum K^+ closely.
- **The use of bicarbonate in the treatment of DKA is not recommended**, as it does not improve outcome and it has been associated with a fourfold increase in the development of cerebral edema. Bicarbonate should be used only in life-threatening situations in which other therapy has failed (including adequate ventilation), such as cardiac dysrhythmias or dysfunction.
- Add dextrose to IV fluids when blood glucose is <200 to 250 milligrams/dL. *Serum glucose corrects faster than ketoacidosis, so insulin must be continued with supplemental glucose until ketoacidosis has resolved.*
- Measure serum electrolyte levels and glucose hourly initially, then electrolyte monitoring can be spaced to every 2 hours as the patient stabilizes.
- Cerebral edema is a potentially fatal complication of DKA and typically occurs 6 to 10 hours after initiating therapy; it presents with mental status changes progressing to coma. Although the etiology of this complication is unknown, it is felt that several factors may contribute, including overly aggressive fluid therapy, rapid correction of blood glucose levels, bicarbonate therapy, and failure of the serum sodium level to increase with therapy.
- **Management of cerebral edema:** patients with DKA and altered mental status suggestive of cerebral edema should be treated empirically with mannitol 0.5 to 1 gram/kg or 3% hypertonic saline, 10 mL/kg over 20 to 30 minutes. Restrict additional IV fluids to a minimum required to maintain IV access. Use caution if endotracheal intubation is required and *avoid eucapnea*, as severe metabolic acidosis requires compensatory respiratory alkalosis and a rise in CO_2 may worsen systemic and intracellular acidosis.
- Most patients with DKA require admission to the intensive care unit, even when stable, because of intensive monitoring needs. Furthermore, many hospitals

restrict the use of insulin infusions to intensive care settings. Patients with cerebral edema require ICU admission and possible intracranial pressure monitoring. Consultation with the patient's primary care physician and a pediatric endocrinologist should be made early in the course of therapy.

For further reading in Tintinalli's *Emergency Medicine: A Comprehensive Study Guide*, 7th ed., see Chapter 139, "The Child with Diabetes," by Adam Vella.

83 FLUID AND ELECTROLYTE THERAPY IN INFANTS AND CHILDREN

Jennifer R. Reid

EPIDEMIOLOGY

- While the incidence of dehydration and electrolyte abnormalities in children is unknown, they account for more than 3 million physician visits, 220,000 hospitalizations, and hundreds of deaths annually in the United States. Worldwide, dehydration and electrolyte abnormalities, primarily from gastrointestinal illness, are a leading cause of death among children.
- The most common cause of fluid and electrolyte disturbances in infants and children presenting to the emergency department is acute gastroenteritis (see Chapter 75).
- Inappropriate home remedies for gastrointestinal illness may contribute to electrolyte abnormalities, especially in children <6 months of age.

■ DEHYDRATION

PATHOPHYSIOLOGY

- During the first 2 years of life, infants and children have tremendous caloric and water maintenance requirements as a result of rapid growth and metabolism. The relative daily free water turnover is three to four times that of an adult.
- Factors contributing to increased fluid requirements in children include high metabolic rate, large relative body surface area, increased insensible losses from the skin and respiratory tract (especially with fever), a relative inability to concentrate urine, and a relatively large percentage of total body water in the extracellular space.
- Causes of dehydration include decreased intake, due to voluntary or involuntary causes such as anatomic or pathologic disease (eg, pharyngitis, stomatitis, cleft lip/palate or GI obstruction), neurologic disease (eg, meningitis, brain tumor, seizures), or febrile illness.
- Another cause of dehydration is increased output due to insensible losses (eg, fever, heat, respiratory illness, diaphoresis, thyroid disease, cystic fibrosis), GI losses (vomiting, diarrhea), renal losses (eg, osmotic, such as diabetic ketoacidosis or nonosmotic such as renal disease or diabetes insipidus), or sodium losing conditions (eg, adrenal disease or diuretic use).
- Systemic disorders such as burns, secondary ascites, respiratory disease, peritonitis, or anaphylaxis may also cause dehydration.
- Dehydration can be classified as isotonic, hyponatremic, and hypernatremic, depending on the relative loss of free water and electrolytes.
- Isotonic dehydration (serum sodium 130-150 mEq/L) is most common and results from a proportionately equal loss of sodium and water.
- Hyponatremic dehydration (serum sodium <130 mEq/L) develops when acute fluid losses are replaced with free water (eg, tea, diluted formula). Hyponatremia may also occur in the setting of increased total body water relative to sodium (eg, syndrome of inappropriate secretion of antidiuretic hormone, and edema-forming states, such as nephrotic syndrome, cirrhosis, psychogenic or infantile water intoxication).
- Hypernatremic dehydration (serum sodium >150 mEq/L) develops when there is a relatively greater loss of free water than sodium. This typically occurs when a young patient is fed salt-rich solutions (eg, inappropriately mixed formula, boiled skim milk, chicken broth).

CLINICAL FEATURES

- The clinical appearance of patients depends on the degree of dehydration, the rate of fluid loss, and the age of the patient.
- Older children may tolerate gradual loss of as much as 40% of intracellular volume without decompensation.
- Rapid loss of large volumes in young infants can cause hypovolemic shock with cardiovascular collapse.

DIAGNOSIS AND DIFFERENTIAL

- The gold standard for assessing dehydration is comparison of a pre-illness weight with post-illness weight where 1 L water = 1 kg. Based on weight lost, the fluid deficit (as a percentage of body weight) can be calculated. Dehydration is then classified as mild (<5%), moderate (5%-10%), or severe (>10%). Unfortunately, accurate pre-illness weights are rarely available in the emergency department.

TABLE 83-1 Clinical Estimate of Pediatric Dehydration

CLINICAL CHARACTERISTIC	NONE TO MILD DEHYDRATION	MODERATE DEHYDRATION	SEVERE DEHYDRATION
Percent dehydrated*	<5%	5%-10%	>10%
Overall appearance	Active and playful	Restless and fussy	Limp and sleepy
Eyes	Not sunken	Somewhat sunken	Clearly sunken
Tears	Present when cries	May be absent when cries	Absent when cries
Mouth	Moist mucous membranes	Somewhat dry mucous membranes	Dry mucous membranes
Thirst	Not particularly thirsty	Drinks eagerly	Too sick to drink
Skin pinch	Returns immediately	Returns somewhat slow	Returns slowly

*The number used to calculate the fluid deficit.

- In lieu of accurate weights, clinical features have been shown to provide a reliable estimation of the degree of dehydration (Table 83-1). Hypernatremic dehydration, however, may present with vital signs and skin turgor that can underestimate the total fluid losses since intravascular volume is relatively preserved.
- In general, routine laboratory studies are not helpful in children older than 6 months of age unless the history or examination suggests underlying electrolyte abnormalities (see Electrolyte Disorders below).
- In severe dehydration or suspected underlying systemic disease, a comprehensive metabolic panel may help classify the type of dehydration (ie, isotonic, hyponatremic, hypernatremic) and identify related problems (eg, renal failure, hypoglycemia, ketoacidosis).
- Other laboratory investigations are directed by the clinical picture and aimed at diagnosis of underlying causes of dehydration (eg, infectious enteritis, metabolic disease, toxic ingestions).

EMERGENCY DEPARTMENT CARE AND DISPOSITION

- The management of fluid and electrolyte disturbances in infants and young children revolves around a few basic principles: (1) identify and treat shock; (2) identify and treat underlying causes if possible (eg, diabetic ketoacidosis, pyloric stenosis, respiratory distress); (3) administer appropriate fluids to replace fluids already lost, maintenance fluids, and ongoing fluid losses.
- Treat hypovolemic shock with prompt isotonic crystalloid: administer 20 mL/kg of normal saline or lactated Ringer's solution by rapid IV or IO bolus and repeat until vital signs, peripheral perfusion, and mental status improve. A minimum of 60 mL/kg or more in the first hour should be given, unless contraindicated based on the patient's underlying disease (eg, diabetic ketoacidosis).
- Treat children with mild to moderate dehydration with oral rehydration therapy (ORT). See Chapter 76 for a detailed discussion of ORT in the setting of vomiting and diarrhea.
- Administer ondansetron 0.15 milligram/kg PO or 0.1 milligrams/kg IV for children in whom vomiting prevents adequate oral rehydration.
- Consider nasogastric rehydration with isotonic crystalloids or oral rehydration solution as an alternative to oral or parenteral rehydration.
- Maintenance fluids are calculated as follows: for children ≤10 kg administer 100 mL/kg/d over 24 hours (4 mL/kg/h); for children 11 to 20 kg administer 1000 mL + 50 mL/kg for each kg >10 over 24 hours; for children >20 kg administer 1500 mL + 20 mL/kg for each kg >20 over 24 hours.
- Fluid deficit is determined from the estimated percentage of dehydration (see Table 83-1). The calculations are performed in the following manner: If the patient weighs 15 kg on presentation and is estimated to be 10% dehydrated, then the estimated fluid loss is 15 kg × 10% = 1.5 kg = 1.5 L.
- Administer half of the total fluid deficit over the first 8 hours and the remaining half over the following 16 hours. The hourly IV fluid rate is determined by the sum of maintenance and deficit fluid requirements for the patient.

ELECTROLYTE DISORDERS

PATHOPHYSIOLOGY

- The most common electrolyte abnormalities in children involve sodium. Hyponatremia, defined as a serum sodium <130 mEq/L, is most commonly caused by GI losses or water intoxication (eg, ingestion of hypotonic replacement fluids, such as water, especially during infancy).

- Hypernatremia, defined as serum sodium >150 mEq/L, is most commonly associated with diarrhea, as well as renal disease and diabetes insipidus.
- Hypokalemia, serum potassium <3.4 mEq/L, is usually due to profuse vomiting ± diarrhea, or loop diuretics. In diabetic ketoacidosis, total body potassium stores may be significantly depleted due to osmotic diuresis, while serum levels remain normal or falsely elevated. Uncommon causes of hypokalemia include renal tubular acidosis and familial hypokalemia-induced paralysis.
- Hyperkalemia, potassium >5.5 mEq/L, is usually due to hemolysis artifact during blood draws. True hyperkalemia can be caused by renal failure, rhabdomyolysis, and adrenal corticoid insufficiency.
- Disorders of calcium are relatively uncommon in children. Hypocalcemia may be caused by hyperparathyroidism, end organ resistance to parathyroid hormone associated with vitamin D deficiency, young infant's ingestion of cow's milk, hyperventilation or chronic renal failure.
- Hypercalcemia, serum level >11 milligrams/dL most often results from increased bone absorption.
- Magnesium disorders are defined by serum levels outside of the normal range of 1.5 to 2.2 mEq/L.
- Causes of hypomagnesemia include diarrhea, malabsorption, short gut, fistulas, and renal loss (osmotic diuretics, chemotherapeutics).

CLINICAL FEATURES

- Signs and symptoms of various electrolyte abnormalities, as well as their causes and treatment are listed in Table 83-2.

DIAGNOSIS AND DIFFERENTIAL

- The diagnosis is made through a careful history, physical examination, and measurement of serum electrolytes.
- Rapid bedside glucose should be obtained in all patients presenting with signs of dehydration and altered mental status.
- Additional laboratory studies are directed by the initial electrolyte abnormalities and the clinical picture.

TABLE 83-2 Causes, Symptoms, and Treatment of Electrolyte Disorders in Infants and Children

ELECTROLYTE DISORDER	COMMON CAUSES	SYMPTOMS AND SIGNS	INITIAL TREATMENT RECOMMENDATIONS
Hyponatremia	Vomiting, diarrhea, excess free water intake	Mental status changes, seizures, hyporeflexia	IV normal saline starting with a 20 mL/kg bolus For seizures: 4 mL/kg of 3% saline over 30 minutes
Hypernatremia	Vomiting, diarrhea, insensible losses, diabetes insipidus, renal disease	Diarrhea, mental status changes, ataxia, doughy skin, seizures, hyperreflexia	IV normal saline starting with a 20 mL/kg bolus Further correction to take place slowly over 48 hours
Hypokalemia	Vomiting, DKA	Muscle weakness, ileus	Generally tolerated well, replace orally over several days If severe: IV 0.2-0.3 mEq/kg/h of KCl
Hyperkalemia*	Cortical adrenal hyperplasia (neonates), renal failure. May be due to hemolysis of blood sample	ECG changes: peaked T waves, prolonged PR interval, widening of QRS	Insulin 0.1 unit/kg *plus* 25% glucose, 0.5 gram/kg IV Calcium gluconate 10%, 1 mL/kg IV, no faster than 1 mL/min Albuterol, 0.5% solution, 2.5 milligrams via nebulization
Hypocalcemia	Dietary or, vitamin D deficiency, hypoparathyroid and chronic renal failure	Vomiting, irritability, muscle weakness, tetany, seizures	Calcium gluconate 10%, 1 mL/kg IV, no faster than 1 mL/min
Hypercalcemia	Malignancy, hypervitaminosis D or A	Fatigue, irritability, anorexia, vomiting, constipation	IV normal saline starting at 20 mL/kg Bisphosphonates if admission required
Hypomagnesemia	Diarrhea, short gut, diuretics, chemotherapy	Muscle spasms, weakness, ataxia, nystagmus, seizures ECG changes: prolonged PR and QTc, torsades de pointes	For seizures or arrhythmia: IV magnesium sulfate 1 mEq/kg slowly over 4 hours Asymptomatic patients can be treated with oral supplements
Hypermagnesemia	Ingestion of antacids or renal dysfunction	Hypotension, respiratory failure, loss of deep tendon reflexes ECG changes: widening of QRS, PR, QTc	Remove exogenous source of magnesium If severe: calcium gluconate 10% 1 mL/kg IV, no faster than 1 mL/min

*Mild hyperkalemia usually well tolerated in neonates.

- Consider toxic ingestions and occult injury in children with vomiting and altered mental status.

EMERGENCY DEPARTMENT CARE AND DISPOSITION

- Treat hypovolemic shock and dehydration as above (see dehydration).
- Specific therapy for various electrolyte abnormalities is presented in Table 83-2.
- Avoid rapid correction of sodium abnormalities, which can cause cerebral edema or central pontine myelinolysis.
- Electrolyte requirements remain constant throughout childhood. The daily requirement for sodium is 2 to 3 mEq/kg/d and for potassium is 2 mEq/kg/d. All infant formulas contain sufficient electrolytes.

For further reading in Tintinalli's *Emergency Medicine: A Comprehensive Study Guide,* 7th ed., see Chapter 142, "Fluid and Electrolyte Therapy in Infants and Children," by Alan Nager.

84 MUSCULOSKELETAL DISORDERS IN CHILDREN

Mark X. Cicero

PATHOPHYSIOLOGY

- The long bones of children are generally less dense and more porous than the long bones of adults. The resulting increased compliance contributes to the tendency of children's long bones to respond to mechanical stress by bowing and buckling, rather than fracturing through and through.
- The periosteum of the diaphysis and the metaphysis is thicker in children and is continuous from the metaphysis to the epiphysis, surrounding and protecting the mechanically weaker physis.
- The blood supply to the physis arises from the epiphysis, so separation of the physis from the epiphysis may be disastrous for future growth.
- The ligaments of children are stronger and more compliant than those of adults, and sprains are less common than fractures in young children.

CHILDHOOD PATTERNS OF INJURY

- The growth plate (physis) is the weakest point in children's long bones and the frequent site of fractures. The ligaments and periosteum are stronger than the physis, tolerating mechanical forces at the expense of physeal injury.
- The Salter–Harris classification is widely used to describe fractures involving the growth plate.

TYPE I PHYSEAL FRACTURE

- Type I physeal fractures involve injury through the growth plate alone: the epiphysis separates from the metaphysis. The reproductive cells of the physis stay with the epiphysis. There are no bony fragments. Bone growth is undisturbed.
- Diagnosis of this injury is suspected clinically in children with point tenderness over a growth plate. On radiograph, the only abnormality may be an associated joint effusion. There may be epiphyseal displacement from the metaphysis.
- Treatment consists of splint immobilization, ice, and elevation. Type I fractures of the distal fibula and radius are common, benign, and do not require orthopedic referral.

TYPE II PHYSEAL FRACTURE

- Type II physeal fracture is the most common (75%) physeal fracture.
- The fracture extends through the physis and metaphysis (Fig. 84-1). The periosteum remains intact over

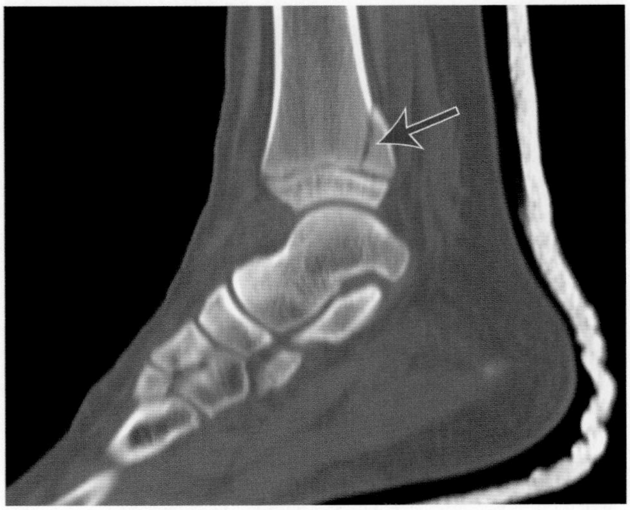

FIG. 84-1. Salter–Harris type II fracture of distal tibia. CT image illustrating fracture extending through physeal growth plate and metaphysis (*arrow*). (Courtesy of Wake Medical Center, Raleigh, NC)

the metaphyseal fragment, but is torn on the opposite side. Growth is preserved since the physis remains with the epiphysis.
- Treatment is closed reduction with analgesia and sedation followed by cast immobilization.

TYPE III PHYSEAL FRACTURE

- The hallmark of type III physeal fracture is an intraarticular fracture of the epiphysis with the cleavage plane continuing along the physis. This injury usually involves the proximal or distal tibia (Fig. 84-2).
- The prognosis for bone growth depends on the circulation to the epiphyseal bone fragment and is usually favorable.
- Reduction of the unstable fragment with anatomic alignment of the articular surface is critical. Open reduction is often required.

TYPE IV PHYSEAL FRACTURE

- The fracture line of type IV physeal fractures begins at the articular surface and extends through the epiphysis, physis, and metaphysis (Fig. 84-3).
- This most often involves the distal humerus.

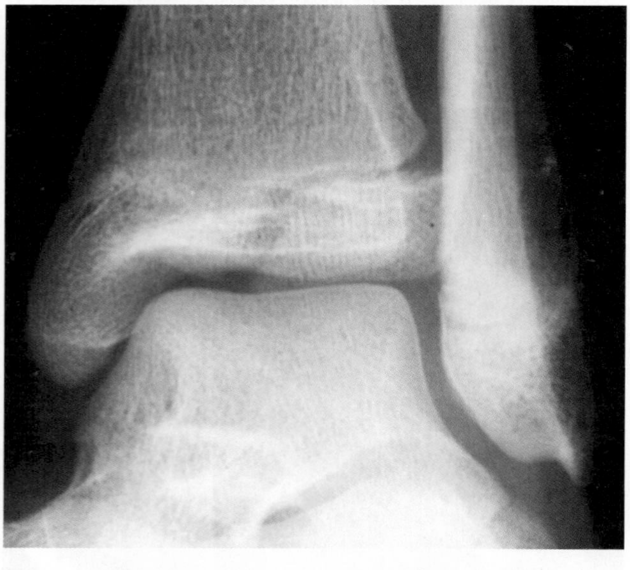

FIG. 84-2. A radiograph of a Salter–Harris type III fracture of the lateral portion of the distal tibia. Note the intra-articular component extending through the growth plate and the medial epiphysis of the tibia. (Reproduced with permission from Shah BR, Lucchesi M: *Atlas of Pediatric Emergency Medicine,* © 2006, McGraw-Hill, New York.)

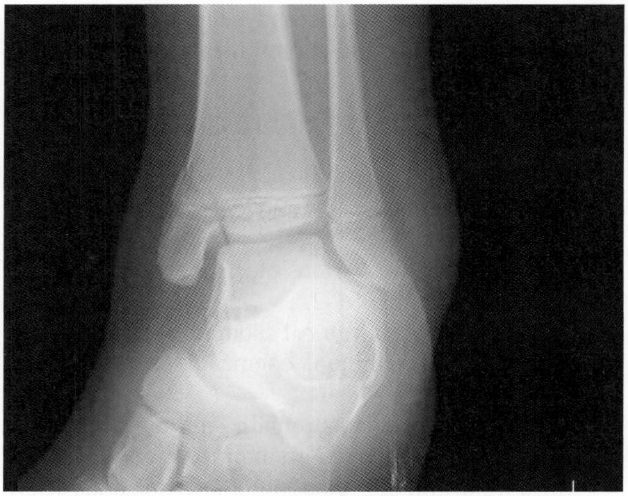

FIG. 84-3. Radiograph of a Salter–Harris type IV fracture of the medial malleolus. (Reproduced with permission from Shah BR, Lucchesi M: *Atlas of Pediatric Emergency Medicine,* © 2006, McGraw-Hill, New York.)

- Open reduction is required to reduce the risk of premature bone growth arrest.

TYPE V PHYSEAL FRACTURE

- Type V physeal fracture is rare and usually involves the knee or ankle. The physis is crushed by severe compressive forces. There is no epiphyseal displacement.
- The diagnosis is often difficult: initial diagnosis of sprain or type I injury may prove incorrect when later growth arrest occurs. Radiographs may look normal or demonstrate focal narrowing of the epiphyseal plate. There is usually an associated joint effusion.
- Treatment consists of cast immobilization, nonweight bearing, and close orthopedic follow-up in anticipation of focal bone growth arrest.

TORUS FRACTURES

- Children's long bones are more compliant than those of adults and tend to bow and bend under forces where an adult's might fracture. Torus (also called cortical or buckle) fractures involve a bulging or buckling of the bony cortex, usually at the metaphysis.
- Patients have soft tissue swelling and point tenderness over the fracture site. Radiographs may be subtle but show cortical disruption.

- Torus fractures are not typically angulated, rotated, or displaced, so reduction is rarely necessary. Splinting or casting in a position of function for 3 to 4 weeks with orthopedic follow-up is recommended.

GREENSTICK FRACTURES

- In greenstick fracture, the cortex and periosteum are disrupted on one side of the bone, but intact on the other.
- Treatment is closed reduction and immobilization.

PLASTIC DEFORMITIES

- Plastic deformities are seen in the forearm and lower leg in combination with a completed fracture in the companion bone. The diaphyseal cortex is deformed, but the periosteum is intact.
- Prompt orthopedic consultation is required for any plastic deformities, as proper reduction and realignment is essential.

FRACTURES ASSOCIATED WITH CHILD ABUSE

See Chapter 189, "Child and Elder Abuse."

SELECTED PEDIATRIC INJURIES

CLAVICLE FRACTURE

- A clavicle fracture is the most common fracture in children.
- Fractures may occur in the newborn during a difficult delivery. Neonates may demonstrate nonuse of the arm. If the fracture was not initially appreciated, parents may notice a bony callus at 2 to 3 weeks of age.
- In older infants and children, the usual mechanism is a fall onto the outstretched arm or shoulder.
- Care of the patient with a clavicle fracture is directed toward pain control. Even if anatomic alignment is not achieved in the emergency department (ED), displaced fractures usually heal well, although there may be a residual bump at the fracture site.
- Figure-of-eight shoulder abduction restraints have been the traditional treatment, but many patients have more pain with this device. A simple sling or shoulder immobilizer are equally effective and less painful. Orthopedic follow-up can be arranged in the next week.
- Orthopedic consultation in the ED is required for an open fracture (which also requires antibiotics), anterior or posterior displacement of the medial clavicle, or a skin-tenting fracture fragment that has the potential to convert to an open fracture.

SUPRACONDYLAR FRACTURES

- The most common elbow fracture in children is a supracondylar fracture of the distal humerus. The usual mechanism is a fall on an outstretched arm.
- The close proximity of the brachial artery to the fracture predisposes the arterial injury. Subsequent arterial spasm or compression by casts may further compromise distal circulation. Forearm compartment syndrome, known as Volkmann's ischemic contracture, may occur.
- Symptoms include pain in the proximal forearm upon passive finger extension, stocking-glove anesthesia of the hand, and hard forearm swelling. Children complain of pain on passive elbow flexion and maintain the forearm pronated.
- Pulses may remain palpable at the wrist despite serious vascular impairment.
- Injuries to the ulnar, median, and radial nerves are common too, occurring in 5% to 10% of all supracondylar fractures.
- Radiographs show the injury, but the findings may be subtle. A posterior fat pad sign is indicative of intra-articular effusion and thus fracture. The anterior humeral line should be assessed (Fig. 84-4). In subtle supracondylar fractures, the line often lies more anteriorly.
- Supracondylar fractures are often classified as types I-III: type I fractures are subtle and may only be detected on radiograph through a fat-pad sign (Fig. 84-5); type II fractures reveal angulation but the posterior cortex is usually displaced; type III fractures disrupt both cortices with displacement of the distal fracture fragment.
- In cases of neurovascular compromise, immediate fracture reduction is indicated. If an ischemic forearm compartment is suspected after reduction, surgical decompression or arterial exploration may be indicated.
- Type I supracondylar fractures can usually be splinted (posterior long-arm splint with the elbow at 90 degrees flexion and the wrist in neutral position, or a double sugar-tong splint) and referred for outpatient follow-up.
- Types II and III supracondylar fractures typically require surgical pinning.
- Admission is recommended for patients with displaced fractures or significant soft tissue swelling. Open reduction is often required.
- Lateral and medial condylar fractures and intercondylar and transcondylar fractures carry risks of neurovascular compromise, especially to the ulnar nerve.

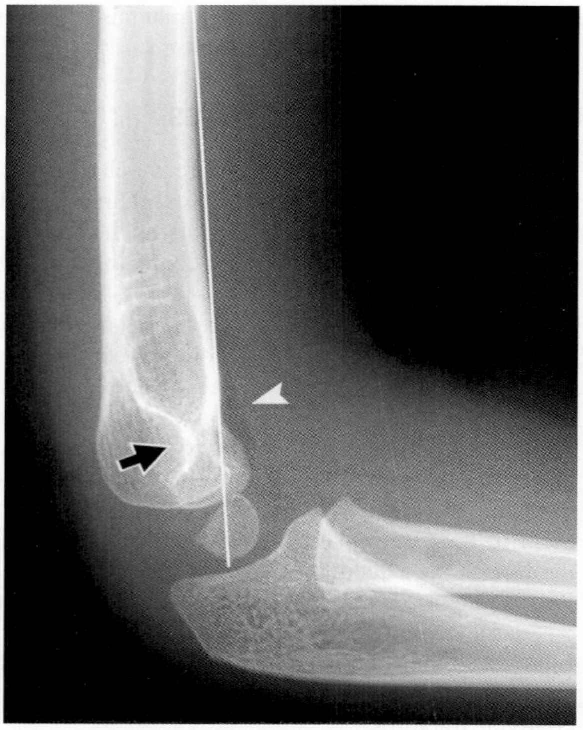

FIG. 84-4. Anterior humeral line. A line drawn along the anterior cortex of the humeral shaft normally intersects the middle third of the capitellum. A normal radiographic teardrop is seen where the cortices of the olecranon and coronoid fossae come together (*black arrow*). A small normal anterior fat pad is visible (*arrowhead*). (Reproduced with permission from Schwartz D: *Emergency Radiology Case Studies*, ©2008, McGraw-Hill, New York.)

These patients have soft tissue swelling and tenderness, maintaining the arm in flexion. Most patients require open reduction.

RADIAL HEAD SUBLUXATION ("NURSEMAID'S ELBOW")

- Radial head subluxation is a very common injury that is seen most often in children between the ages of 1 and 4 years. The typical history is that the child was lifted up by an adult pulling on the hand or wrist. Sometimes there is a history of trauma, and sometimes there is no memorable event at all, but the child refuses to use the arm.
- The arm is held close to the body, flexed at the elbow with the forearm pronated. Gentle examination reveals no tenderness to direct palpation, but any attempts to supinate the forearm or move the elbow cause pain.

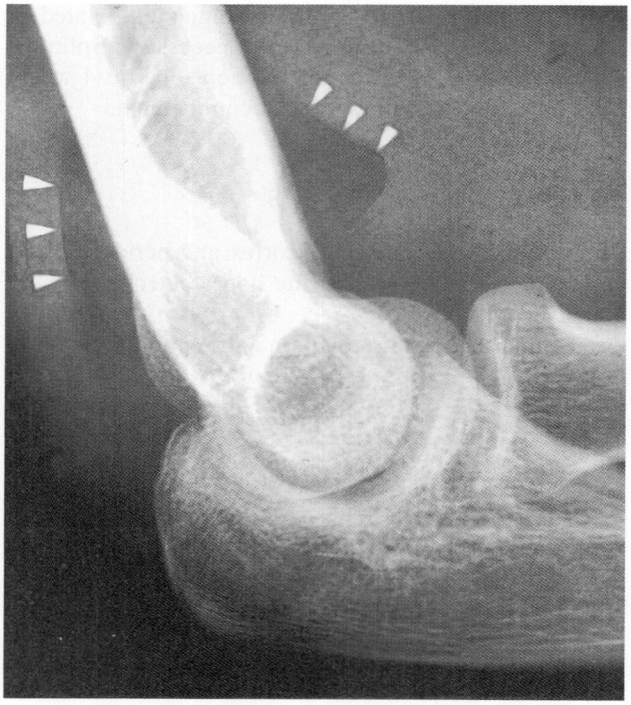

FIG. 84-5. Type I supracondylar fracture: Note the anterior and posterior fat pad signs suggestive of fracture without displacement of the distal fragment.

- If the history and examination are classic, radiographs are not needed, but if the history is atypical or there is point tenderness or signs of trauma, radiographs should be obtained.
- There are two maneuvers for reduction. The supination-flexion technique (Fig. 84-6) is performed by holding the patient's elbow at 90 degrees with one hand, then

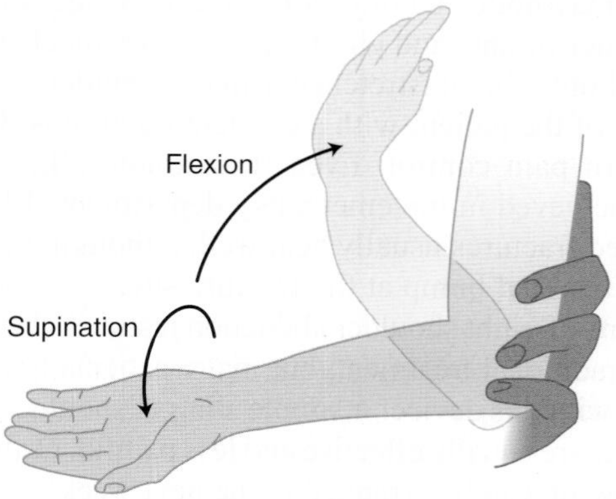

FIG. 84-6. Supination-flexion technique. Hold the elbow at 90 degrees; then firmly supinate the wrist and the forearm toward the ipsilateral shoulder.

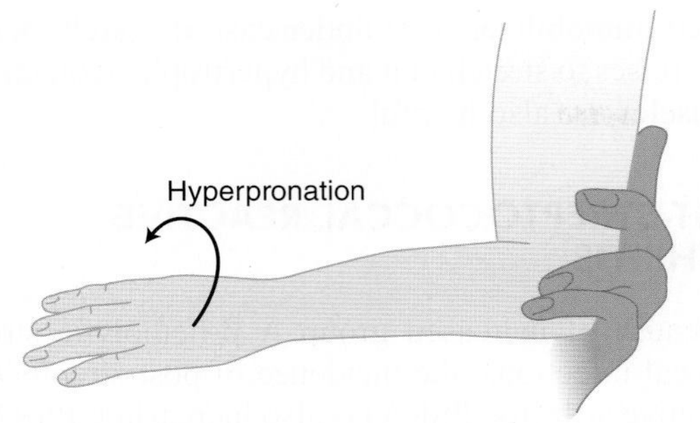

FIG. 84-7. Hyperpronation. Hold the elbow at 90 degrees; then firmly pronate the wrist.

firmly supinating the wrist and simultaneously flexing the elbow so the wrist is directed to the ipsilateral shoulder. There may be a "click" with reduction and the child may transiently cry and resist.

- The hyperpronation technique (Fig. 84-7) is reported to be more successful, less painful, and can be used primarily, or as a back-up if supination fails. The hyperpronation technique is performed by holding the child's elbow at 90 degrees or in full extension in one hand, then firmly pronating the wrist. Usually the child will resume normal activity in 15 to 30 minutes if reduction is achieved. If the child is not better after a second reduction attempt, alternate diagnoses and radiographs should be considered. No specific therapy is needed after successful reduction. Parents should be reminded to avoid linear traction on the arm, as there is an increased risk of recurrence.

SLIPPED CAPITAL FEMORAL EPIPHYSIS

- Slipped capital femoral epiphysis (SCFE) is more common in boys, with peak incidence between ages 12 and 15 years, and in girls between ages 10 and 13 years.
- With a chronic SCFE, children complain of dull pain in the groin, anteromedial thigh, or knee, which becomes worse with activity. With walking, the leg is externally rotated and the gait is antalgic. Hip flexion and rotation are restricted and painful.
- Acute presentation of SCFE is usually due to trauma or may occur in a patient with preexisting chronic SCFE. Patients present in great pain, with marked external rotation of the thigh and leg shortening. The hip should not be forced through full range of motion, as this may displace the epiphysis further.
- The differential includes septic arthritis, toxic synovitis, Legg–Calvé–Perthes' disease, and other hip fractures.
- Children with SCFE are not febrile or toxic and have normal white blood cell counts (WBCs) and erythrocyte sedimentation rates (ESRs) which are not needed unless the patient is febrile.
- On radiograph, medial displacement of the femoral epiphysis will be seen on anteroposterior (AP) views, while frog-leg views detect posterior displacement. In the AP view, a line along the superior femoral neck should transect the lateral quarter of the femoral epiphysis in normal children.
- Management of SCFE is operative. Patients should be made non-weight bearing and NPO and admitted to the hospital. The main long-term complication is avascular necrosis of the femoral head.

SELECTED NONTRAUMATIC MUSCULOSKELETAL DISORDERS OF CHILDHOOD

- Kawasaki's disease is discussed in Chapter 84.
- Acute supperative arthritis is discussed in Chapter 180.

JUVENILE IMMUNE ARTHRITIS

- The group of diseases comprising juvenile immune arthritis (JIA; formerly juvenile rheumatoid arthritis) share the findings of chronic noninfectious synovitis and arthritis, with varying systemic manifestations.
- Pauciarticular disease is the most common form, usually involving a single large joint such as the knee. Permanent joint damage occurs infrequently.
- Polyarticular disease occurs in one-third of cases; both large and small joints are affected, and there may be progressive joint damage.
- Systemic JIA occurs in 20% of patients. This form is associated with high fevers and chills. Extra-articular manifestations are common, including a red macular coalescent rash, hepatosplenomegaly, and serositis.
- The diagnosis of JIA will likely not be made in the ED, as it requires 6 weeks of persistent joint swelling. Lab tests focus mostly on excluding other diagnoses. Complete blood count (CBC), ESR, and C-reactive protein (CRP) may be normal. Arthrocentesis may be necessary to exclude septic arthritis, particularly in pauciarticular disease.
- Radiographs initially show joint effusions but are nonspecific.
- Initial therapy for patients with an established diagnosis includes nonsteroidal anti-inflammatory drugs (NSAIDs). Glucocorticoids are occasionally used, for example, for unresponsive uveitis or decompensated pericarditis or myocarditis. Systemic immunosuppressents are often prescribed by rheumatologists for severe disease.

LEGG-CALVÉ-PERTHES' DISEASE

- Legg-Calvé-Perthes' disease is avascular necrosis of the femoral head with subchondral stress fracture. Collapse and flattening of the femoral head ensues, with potential subluxation.
- The hip is painful with limited range of motion, muscle spasm, and soft tissue contractures. Onset of symptoms occurs between 4 and 9 years of age, with boys outnumbering girls 4:1. The disease is bilateral in 10% of patients. Children present with limp and chronic dull pain in the groin, thigh, or knee, which becomes worse with activity. Systemic symptoms are absent.
- Hip motion is restricted; there may be a flexion-abduction contracture and thigh muscle atrophy.
- Initial radiographs (in the first 1-3 months) show widening of the cartilage space in the affected hip and diminished ossific nucleus of the femoral head. The second sign is subchondral stress fracture of the femoral head. The third finding is increased femoral head opacification. Finally, deformity of the femoral head occurs, with subluxation and protrusion of the femoral head from the acetabulum.
- Bone scan and magnetic resonance imaging are helpful in making this diagnosis, showing bone abnormalities well before plain films.
- The differential diagnosis includes toxic tenosynovitis, tuberculous arthritis, tumors, and bone dyscrasias.
- In the ED, the most important thing is to consider this chronic but potentially crippling condition. Nearly all children are hospitalized initially for traction.

OSGOOD-SCHLATTER DISEASE

- Osgood-Schlatter disease is a common apophysitis that affects preteen boys more than girls. Repetitive stress on the tibial tuberosity by the quadriceps muscle initiates inflammation of the tibial tuberosity, without necrosis.
- Children present with pain and tenderness over the anterior knee, which becomes worse with flexion and better with rest.
- The patellar tendon is thick and tender, with the tibial tuberosity enlarged and inflammed.
- Radiographs show soft-tissue swelling over the tuberosity and patellar tendon thickening without knee effusion. Normally, the ossification site at the tubercle at this age will be irregular, but the prominence of the tubercle is characteristic of Osgood-Schlatter disease.
- The disorder is self-limited. Acute symptoms improve after restriction of physical activities, ice, and NSAIDs. Crutches may be necessary, although a knee immobilizer or cylinder cast are rarely needed. Exercises to stretch taut and hypertrophied quadriceps muscles are also helpful.

POST-STREPTOCOCCAL REACTIVE ARTHRITIS

- Because of increased group A β-hemolytic streptococcal infections, the incidence of post-streptococcal reactive arthritis (PSRA) is also increasing. PSRA is a sterile, inflammatory, nonmigratory mono- or oligoarthritis occurring in the setting of antecedent infection at a distant site with β-hemolytic streptococci and also *Staphylococcus* and *Salmonella* species.
- Unlike acute rheumatic fever, PSRA is not associated with carditis, and in general is a milder illness. However, the arthritis in PSRA is more severe and prolonged compared to acute rheumatic fever, and may be resistant to NSAIDs.
- To establish the diagnosis of PSRA, antecedent infection with group A streptococci must be established, either with throat culture or a fourfold rise in antistreptolysin O (ASO) or anti-DNase B titer.
- PSRA is responsive to NSAIDs. The issue of penicillin prophylaxis, a mainstay of therapy in acute rheumatic fever, is controversial in PSRA. However, if group A *Streptococcus* is recovered from the throat, an acute course of treatment with penicillin or erythromycin should be instituted.

ACUTE RHEUMATIC FEVER

- Acute rheumatic fever (ARF) is an acute inflammatory multisystem illness affecting primarily school-age children. It is not common in the United States, although occasional epidemics have been described and sporadic cases occur.
- ARF follows infection with certain strains of group A β-hemolytic *Streptococcus*, which stimulates antibody production that cross-react with host tissues. Children develop ARF 2 to 6 weeks after symptomatic or asymptomatic streptococcal pharyngitis.
- Arthritis, which occurs in most initial attacks, is migratory and polyarticular, primarily affecting large joints.
- Carditis occurs in one-third of patients, and can affect valves, muscle, and pericardium. Carditis confers greatest mortality and morbidity.
- Sydenham's chorea occurs in 10% of patients and may occur months after the initial infection. Manifestations include sudden, aimless, irregular movements and muscle weakness, and may be the sole clinical manifestation of ARF.
- The classic rash of ARF, erythema marginatum, is fleeting, faint, and serpiginous, usually accompanying

carditis. Subcutaneous nodules, found on the extensor surfaces of extremities, are quite rare.

- Laboratory tests are used to confirm prior streptococcal infection (throat culture and streptococcal serology) or to assess carditis (electrocardiogram, chest radiograph, and echocardiogram).
- The differential diagnosis includes JIA, septic arthritis, Kawasaki's disease, leukemia, and other cardiomyopathies and vasculitides.
- Significant carditis is managed with prednisone 1 to 2 milligrams/kg/dose given daily. Arthritis is initially treated with high-dose aspirin (75-100 milligrams/kg/d).
- All children with ARF are treated with penicillin (PCN): benzathine PCN 1.2 million U intramuscularly, procaine PCN G 600,000 U intramuscularly daily for 10 days, or oral PCN VK 6.25 to 12.5 milligrams/kg/dose four times a day for 10 days. Use erythromycin if the patient is PCN allergic.
- Long-term prophylaxis is indicated for patients with ARF, and lifelong prophylaxis is recommended for patients with carditis.

TRANSIENT TENOSYNOVITIS OF THE HIP

- Transient tenosynovitis is the most common cause of hip pain in children less than age 10 years of age. The peak age is 3 to 6 years, and boys are affected more than girls. The cause is unknown.
- Symptoms may be acute or gradual: patients have pain in the hip, thigh, or knee, and an antalgic gait (or refusal to bear weight). Pain limits the hip's range of motion. There may be a low-grade fever or history of recent upper respiratory infection, although patients do not appear toxic.
- The WBC and ESR are usually normal. Radiographs of the hip are normal or show a mild-to-moderate effusion. The main ED task is differentiation from septic arthritis, particularly if the patient is febrile, with elevation of WBC or ESR and effusion.
- Diagnostic arthrocentesis is required, either with fluoroscopic or ultrasound guidance or in the operating room, in ambiguous cases. The fluid in transient tenosynovitis is a sterile clear transudate.
- Once septic arthritis and hip fracture have been ruled out, patients can be treated with anti-inflammatory agents such as ibuprofen 10 milligrams/kg, and close follow-up.

For further reading in Tintinalli's *Emergency Medicine: A Comprehensive Study Guide,* 7th ed., see Chapter 133, "Musculoskeletal Disorders in Children," by Courney Hopkins-Mann, Damilola Ogunnaike-Joseph, and Donna Moro-Sutherland.

85 RASHES IN INFANTS AND CHILDREN

Kim Askew

- Rashes in children are typically benign and self-limited with only a handful of serious or potentially life-threatening rashes that require intervention, though they are commonly of great concern to parents and may prompt ED visit.
- Essential information for accurate diagnosis includes associated signs and symptoms, immunization history, human and animal contacts, and environmental and medication exposures.
- An exanthem is a rash involving the skin, and may have an infectious and noninfectious cause; an enanthem involves the mucus membranes.
- Pediatric exanthems can be broadly classified as viral, bacterial, rickettsial, and those of unclear etiology. Rickettsial disease is covered in Chapter 99, and cutaneous anthrax is discussed in Chapter 100.

VIRAL INFECTIONS

ENTEROVIRUSES

- Enteroviruses are small, single-stranded RNA viruses that include coxsackieviruses and echoviruses that commonly cause human disease and produce a wide range of clinical symptoms, typically in the summer and early fall.
- Clinically enteroviral infection can cause a wide range of disease including nonspecific febrile illness, upper respiratory tract infections (common cold, croup, pneumonia), conjunctivitis, parotitis, gastroenteritis (vomiting, diarrhea, abdominal pain), hepatitis, pancreatitis, pericarditis, myocarditis, orchitis, nephritis, arthritis, meningitis, and encephalitis.
- The rashes of enteroviral infections are also varied and include macular eruptions, morbilliform erythema, vesicular lesions, petechial and puerperal eruptions, rubelliform rash, roseola-like rash, and scarlatiniform eruptions.
- One of the enterovirus infections that is common and has distinctive features is hand-foot-and-mouth disease. At the outset, patients typically have fever, anorexia, malaise, and mouth pain. Oral lesions appear on day 2 or 3 of illness, followed by skin lesions. The oral lesions start as painful vesicles on an erythematous base that subsequently ulcerate. The typical location is on the buccal mucosa, tongue, soft palate, and gingiva. Skin lesions start as red papules that change to gray vesicles that heal in 7 to 10 days; the distribution of lesions includes the palms, soles, and buttocks.

- Differentiation between enteroviral viruses is difficult. Because there is no specific therapy, it is more important to consider and exclude bacterial diseases in the differential diagnosis.
- Management is symptomatic: provide analgesia (topical or systemic, including narcotics), and ensuring adequate hydration; antipyretics may also be given.

MEASLES

- Due to widespread immunizations, measles is no longer common in North America, though local epidemics do occur in unvaccinated communities. This myxovirus infection typically occurs in the winter and spring.
- The incubation period is 10 days, followed by a 3-day prodrome of upper respiratory symptoms, then malaise, fever, coryza, conjunctivitis, photophobia, and cough. Patients typically appear ill.
- The exanthem develops 14 days after exposure. Initially a red, blanching, maculopapular rash develops, progressing from the head to the feet and rapidly coalescing on the face. As the rash resolves over about 1 week, a coppery brown discoloration may be seen and desquamation may occur.
- Koplik's spots, tiny white to bluish-white spots on the buccal mucosa, may be seen just before the exanthem appears, and are pathognomonic for measles.
- Measles is self-limited and treatment is supportive.

RUBELLA

- Now quite rare due to immunizations, rubella (German measles) can occur in teenagers, typically in the spring. The incubation period is 12 to 25 days with a 1 to 5 day prodrome of fever, malaise, headache, and sore throat.
- The exanthem develops as fine, irregular pink macules and papules on the face, which then spread to the neck, trunk, and arms in a centrifugal progression. The rash coalesces on the face as the eruption reaches the lower extremities and then clears in the same order as it appeared.
- Lymphadenopathy typically involves the suboccipital and posterior auricular nodes. Treatment is supportive.

ERYTHEMA INFECTIOSUM

- Erythema infectiosum (fifth disease) is a febrile illness, typically occurring in the spring, caused by infection with parvovirus. School-aged children 5 to 15 years old are most commonly affected.

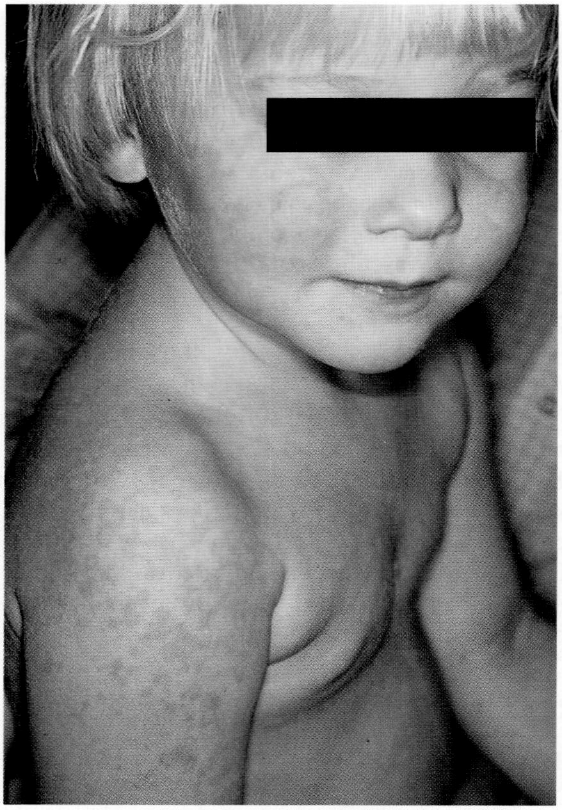

FIG. 85-1. Erythema infectiosum (fifth disease). Toddler with the classic slapped cheek appearance of fifth disease. (Photo contributed by Anne W. Lucky, MD. Reproduced with permission from Knoop K, Stack L, Storrow A, Thurman RJ: *Atlas of Emergency Medicine*, 3rd ed. © 2010, McGraw-Hill, New York.)

- The rash typically starts abruptly as bright red discoloration of the cheeks, giving the so-called "slapped-cheek" appearance (Fig. 85-1). The lesions are closely grouped tiny papules on an erythematous base with slightly raised edges. The eyelids and chin are characteristically spared and circumoral pallor is typical. This rash fades after 4 to 5 days.
- As the illness progresses, and 1 to 2 days after the facial rash appears, a nonpruritic erythematous macular or maculopapular rash appears on the trunk and limbs. This rash may last for 1 week and is not pruritic. As it fades, central clearing of the lesions yields a lacy appearance. Palms and soles are rarely affected.
- The rash may recur intermittently in the weeks following the onset of illness and may be exacerbated by sun exposure or hot baths.
- Associated symptoms include fever, malaise, headache, sore throat, cough, coryza, nausea, vomiting, diarrhea, and myalgias. Treatment is symptomatic.

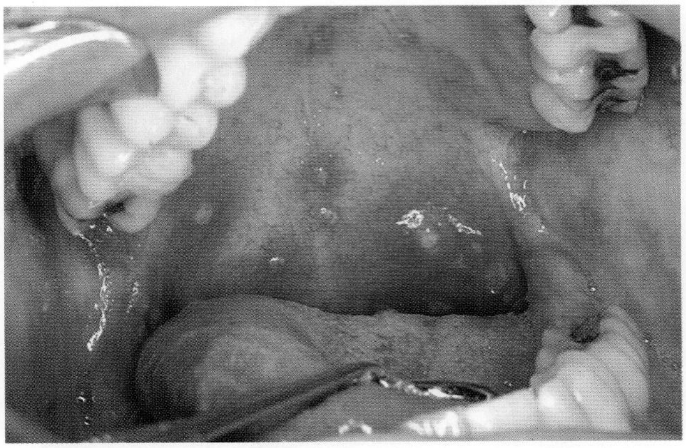

FIG. 85-2. Gingivostomatitis caused by herpes simplex virus. (Courtesy of the Centers for Disease Control and Prevention.)

- Fetal injury may occur with acute infection in pregnant women, and those who have been exposed should receive appropriate counseling.

HERPES VIRUS

- *Herpes labialis* ("cold sores") and *gingivostomatitis* (Fig. 85-2) are two common mucocutaneous presentations of herpes virus infection in children and young adults. Lesions may be single or clustered with herpes labialis; in gingivostomatitis, they are often distributed diffusely throughout the oral cavity including the gingiva, tongue, buccal mucosa, and palate.
- Most herpetic infections are vesicular and extremely painful; lesions eventually unroof and crust over. Herpes labialis is typically localized to the vermillion border.
- Treatment for oral lesions is symptomatic with antipyretics and analgesics. Narcotics may be needed to ensure adequate pain control to maintain oral intake.
- For herpes labialis, oral antivirals may shorten the course of an acute outbreak and viral shedding when provided early in the disease. Topical acyclovir is ineffective. The dosing of oral acyclovir is variable based on age and location of the lesions, but is typically 25 milligrams/kg/dose every 8 hours for 5 days.
- Children with an oral infection can inoculate the distal fingers, causing *herpetic whitlow*.
- In children with existing eczema, a rare life-threatening viral infection can arise: *eczema herpeticum*. Herpes simplex virus is the most common etiologic agent but bacterial superinfection with staphylococci or streptococci is almost universal.

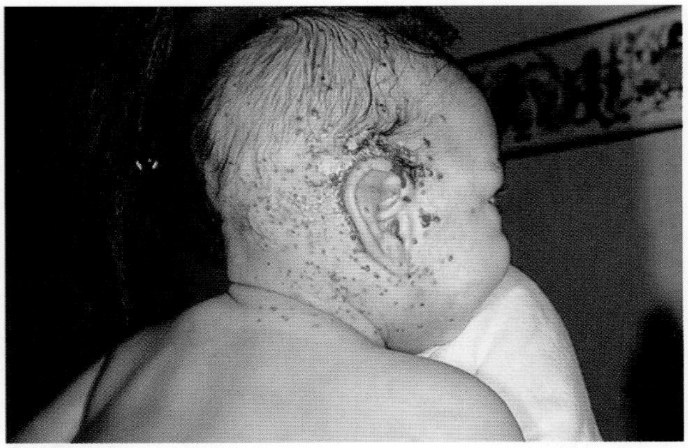

A

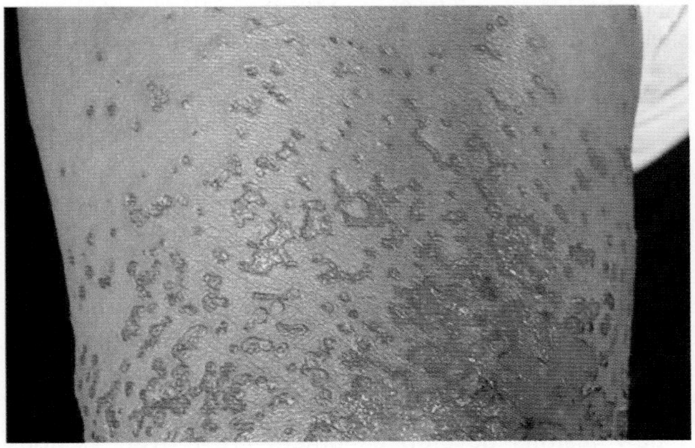

B

FIG. 85-3. **A** and **B.** Typical appearance of eczema herpeticum. (Reproduced with permission from Shah BR, Lucchesi M: *Atlas of Pediatric Emergency Medicine*, © 2006, McGraw-Hill, New York.)

- Clinical manifestations of eczema herpeticum include fever and vesicular eruptions in areas of skin contemporaneously affected by eczematous lesions (Fig. 85-3). Treatment includes acyclovir (25 milligrams/kg/dose PO every 8 hours) and either trimethoprim-sulfamethoxazole (5-10 milligrams/kg/dose twice daily) or clindamycin (5-7.5 milligrams/kg/dose three times daily) for 10 days. Inpatient treatment is recommended.

VARICELLA (CHICKENPOX)

- Due to immunizations, the incidence of varicella has declined dramatically. Varicella-zoster virus (VZV) is a herpes virus.
- Infection typically occurs in children younger than 10 years, but it can occur at any age in susceptible individuals. Varicella occurs most often in the late winter and early spring.

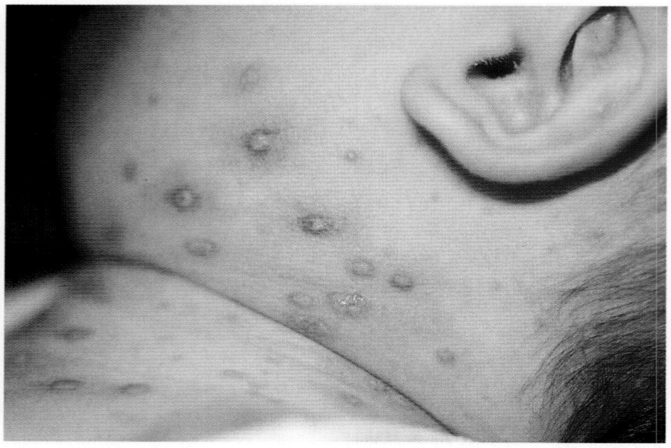

FIG. 85-4. Typical rash of varicella (chicken pox). (Photo contributed by Lawrence B. Stack, MD. Reproduced with permission from Knoop K, Stack L, Storrow A, Thurman RJ: *Atlas of Emergency Medicine*, 3rd ed. © 2010, McGraw-Hill, New York.)

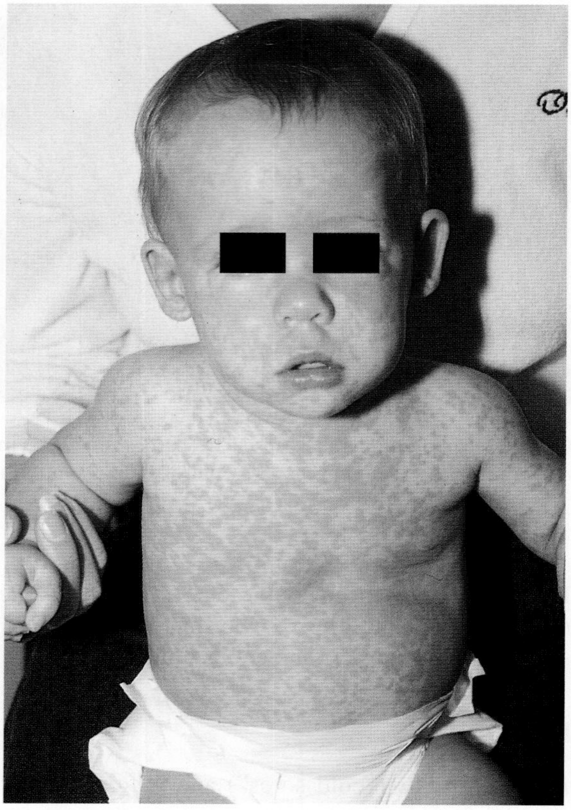

FIG. 85-5. An infant with roseola infantum. (Photo contributed by Raymond C. Baker, MD. Reproduced with permission from Knoop K, Stack L, Storrow A, Thurman RJ: *Atlas of Emergency Medicine*, 3rd ed. © 2010, McGraw-Hill, New York.)

- Patients are highly contagious from the prodrome phase of the illness until all cutaneous lesions are crusted.
- The exanthem starts as faint red macules on the scalp or trunk. Within the first day, lesions vesiculate and develop a red base, giving the characteristic appearance (Fig. 85-4). Over the next few days, crops of new lesions develop as others crust over. Lesions are usually intensely pruritic and spread is typically centrifugal (outward from the center). The palms and soles are often spared.
- Low-grade fever, malaise, and headache are frequently seen but are typically mild.
- Immunized children may present with atypical or limited skin involvement without systemic signs of illness when infected with VZV.
- Treatment is symptomatic including antipyretics and antipruritic medication. *Aspirin should be avoided* as it has been associated with Reye syndrome in patients with VZV infection. Although not needed in previously healthy children, varicella-zoster immune globulin and acyclovir may be indicated for immunocompromised children.

ROSEOLA INFANTUM (EXANTHEM SUBITUM)

- Roseola is a common acute febrile illness in young children, usually between 6 months and 3 years of age and is thought to be most commonly caused by human herpesvirus 6 (HHV6).
- Roseola starts with the abrupt onset of high fevers for 3 to 5 days; associated symptoms are typically mild and may include irritability, cough, coryza, anorexia, and abdominal discomfort. Febrile seizures may occur. The exanthem of roseola appears as the fever abates, which is characteristic and diagnostic for this exanthem. The lesions are discrete, blanching, macular or maculopapular, rose-colored or pink and typically involve the neck, trunk, and buttocks, but may also include the face and proximal extremities (Fig. 85-5); mucous membranes are spared. The rash lasts 1 to 2 days and rapidly fades. Treatment is symptomatic.

FUNGAL INFECTIONS

- Tinea infections are common in infants and children and named for the body parts affected: tinea capitis (scalp), corporis (skin), pedis (foot), and cruris (groin). Tinea infections typically manifest as scaly patches, usually circular with central clearing, and with pruritus of varying intensity (intense with cruris, barely present with corporis).

- Successful treatment for all but tinea capitis is usually accomplished with topical antifungal creams including those available over-the-counter (clotrimazole, miconazole, tolnaftate) or by prescription (ketoconazole, oxiconazole, ciclopirox, terbinafine) and should be continued for 7 to 10 days after resolution of the lesions, which may take 2 to 3 weeks to fade.
- Tinea capitis ranges from mild scalp lesions with patchy alopecia, to a painful, boggy mass known as *kerion*. Tinea capitis is treated with oral griseofulvin (ultramicrosize 15 milligrams/kg/dose once daily) and selenium sulfide shampoo. Treatment is usually continued for at least 8 weeks and close follow up to monitor response and liver function is important. Consider adding a 10-day course of cephalexin (8.3-16.7 milligrams/kg/dose given every 8 hours) for painful kerions that appear secondarily infected. The role of steroids is controversial.

BACTERIAL INFECTIONS

IMPETIGO

- This superficial infectious exanthem is typically caused by group A β-hemolytic streptococci or *Staphylococcus aureus* and commonly affects young children. Outbreaks in daycare or school settings can occur.
- Lesions can occur in areas of minor trauma or insect bites, but there may be no apparent preceding injury. The lesions start as red macules and papules that subsequently form vesicles and pustules. Rupture of the vesicles results in the formation of a characteristic golden crust and lesions may become confluent. The most common sites include the face, neck, and extremities.
- With the exception of lymphadenopathy, fever and systemic signs are rare with impetigo. Diagnosis is based on the clinical appearance of the rash (Fig. 85-6).
- Localized areas of infection can be treated with topical mupirocin. Larger areas usually require oral antibiotics; appropriate choices include cephalexin, erythromycin, clindamycin, amoxicillin-clavulanate, and dicloxacillin.

BULLOUS IMPETIGO AND STAPHYLOCOCCAL SCALDED SKIN SYNDROME (SSSS)

- Bullous impetigo occurs primarily in newborns and young children, while SSSS predominantly occurs in children <6 years of age, with most cases in children <2 years of age. Both are toxin-mediated erythrodermas, caused by toxin serotypes A and B produced by *Staphylococcus*.

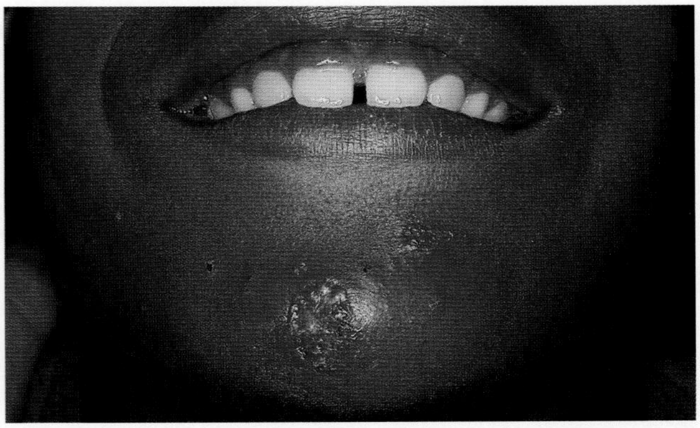

FIG. 85-6. A young girl with crusting impetiginous lesions on her chin. (Photo contributed by Michael J. Nowicki, MD. Reproduced with permission from Knoop K, Stack L, Storrow A, Thurman RJ: *Atlas of Emergency Medicine*, 3rd ed. © 2010, McGraw-Hill, New York.)

- In bullous impetigo, lesions are superficial, thin-walled bullae filled with clear fluid that characteristically occur on the extremities, rupture easily, leave a denuded base, dry to a shiny coating, and contain fluid, which harbors staphylococci.
- Diagnosis is usually made by the appearance of characteristic bullae (Fig. 85-7).
- Treatment includes local wound care and oral antistaphylococcal agents such as cephalexin, and topical agents such as mupirocin. Coverage for community acquired methicillin resistant *Staphylococcus aureus* (CA-MRSA) may be indicated in certain communities.
- In SSSS, the rash progresses from erythroderma to extensive areas of exfoliation, and Nikolsky sign is usually present. Symptoms such as fever, malaise, irritability, and tenderness of the skin are often present.
- Patients with diffuse SSSS often require admission for IV fluids and parenteral antibiotics, with treatment in a burn unit sometimes required. Antibiotics such as nafcillin, penicillin G, amoxicillin-clavulanate, and cephalexin are acceptable therapies; vancomycin should be used when CA-MRSA is suspected.

SCARLET FEVER

- Scarlet fever typically occurs in school-aged children and is diagnosed by the presence of exudative pharyngitis, fever, and a characteristic rash. Associated symptoms include sore throat, fever, headache, vomiting, and abdominal pain.
- Scarlet fever is usually caused by group A β-hemolytic streptococci (recently group C streptococci have been implicated as well).

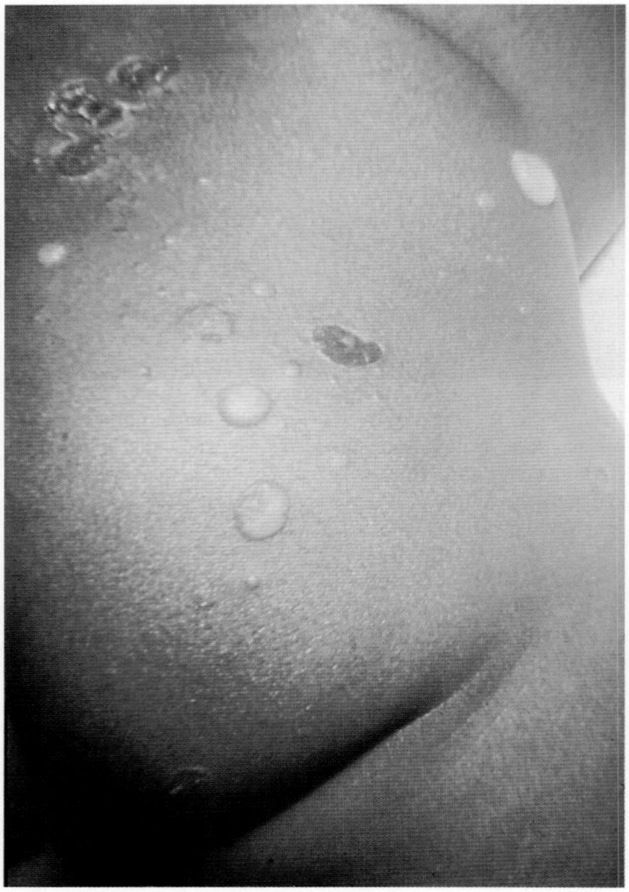

FIG. 85-7. A child with bullous impetigo. (Courtesy of the Centers for Disease Control and Prevention.)

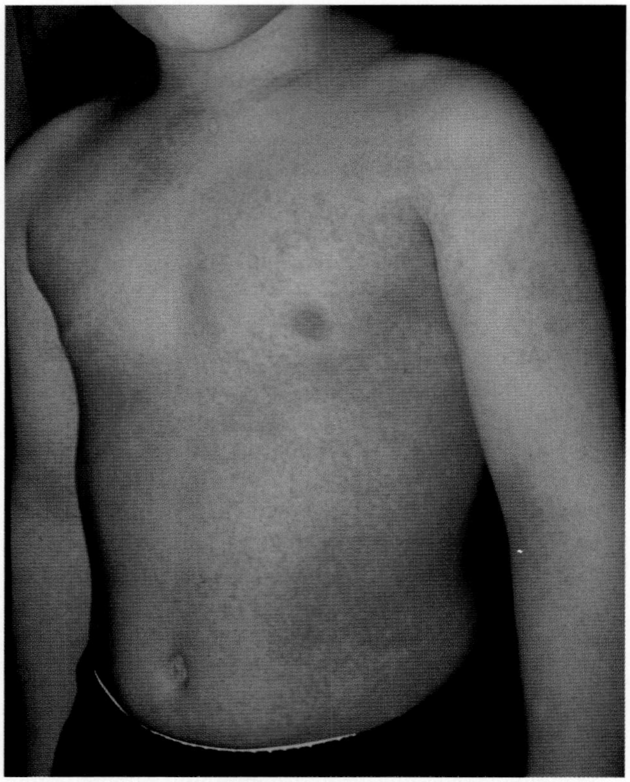

FIG. 85-8. Scarlatiniform rash of scarlet fever; texture is typically sandpaper-like. (Photo contributed by Lawrence B. Stack, MD. Reproduced with permission from Knoop K, Stack L, Storrow A, Thurman RJ: *Atlas of Emergency Medicine*, 3rd ed. © 2010, McGraw-Hill, New York.)

- The characteristic rash typically starts in the neck, groin, and axillae, with accentuation in flexural creases (Pastia's lines). The rash is red and punctate, blanches with pressure, and has a rough sandpaper feel (Fig. 85-8). Early in the course of illness, the tongue has a white coating through which hypertrophic, red papillae project (the "white strawberry tongue"); hemorrhagic spots may be seen on the soft palate. The exanthem typically develops 1 to 2 days after the onset of illness and facial flushing and circumoral pallor are characteristic. Desquamation usually occurs with healing in about 2 weeks.
- The diagnosis is generally made on clinical grounds, though throat culture, if obtained, reveals group A β-hemolytic streptococci or group C streptococci.
- Treatment is penicillin (azithromycin in the penicillin-allergic patient) which shortens the course of the illness and reduces the incidence of rheumatic fever and nephritis.

ERYSIPELAS AND CELLULITIS

- Erysipelas is a cellulitis and lymphangitis of the skin caused by group A β-hemolytic streptococci. Fever, chills, malaise, headache, and vomiting are common.
- The face is the most common site, and the lesion typically forms in an area of prior injury or inflammation. The rash begins as a red plaque that rapidly enlarges. Increased warmth, swelling, and a raised, sharply demarcated, indurated border are characteristic (Fig. 85-9). Diagnosis is clinical.
- Initial parenteral treatment with penicillin G procaine (300,000 U/d IM for <30 kg, 600,00-1 million U/d IM >30 kg) is usually warranted (erythromycin, clarithromycin, or clindamycin in the penicillin-allergic patient). Outpatient treatment includes cephalexin (6.25-12.5 milligrams/kg/dose four times daily), erythromycin (10-15 milligrams/kg/dose three times daily), or clindamycin (5-7.5 milligrams/kg/dose three times daily). Rapid clinical improvement is expected with treatment.

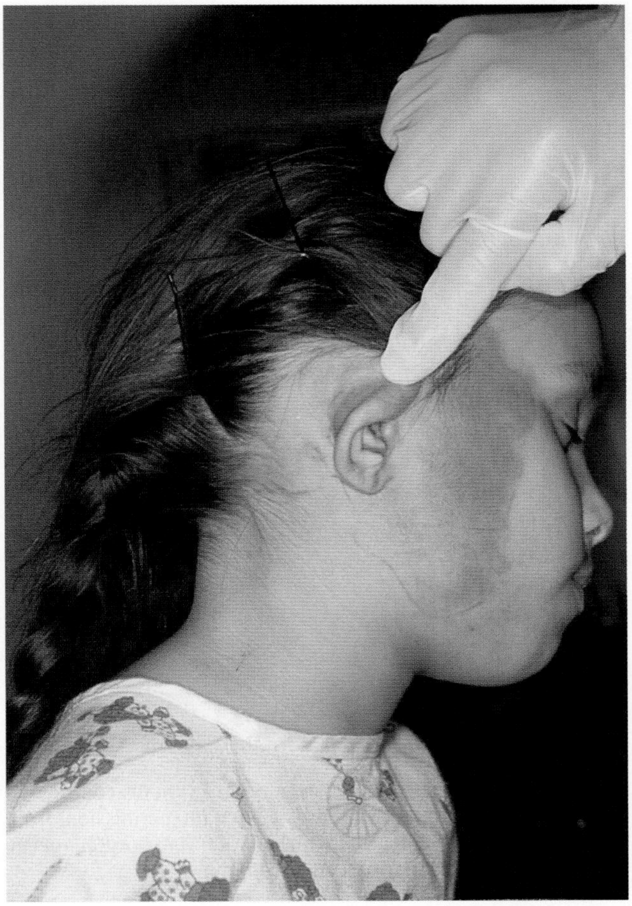

FIG. 85-9. Erysipelas. (Reproduced with permission from Shah BR, Lucchesi M: *Atlas of Pediatric Emergency Medicine*. © 2006, McGraw-Hill, New York.)

- Other forms of cellulitis are treated similarly, however, CA-MRSA is an increasingly common cause of cellulitis in children, and treatment should be based on local sensitivities.
- Traditionally, oral cephalexin (8.3-16.7 milligrams/kg/dose three times daily) has been the antibiotic of choice. With the rise of CA-MRSA, clindamycin (5-7.5 milligrams/kg/dose three times daily) or trimethoprim-sulfamethoxazole (5-10 milligrams of trimethoprim component/kg/dose twice daily) are more common choices.

INFESTATIONS

- Scabies and lice infestations are covered in Chapter 157.

COMMON NEONATAL RASHES

- *Erythema toxicum is* a benign, self-limited rash that occurs in up to 50% of newborns in the first and sometimes second week of life. Characteristic erythematous macules on the trunk, face, and extremities with central pustules suggest the diagnosis. No treatment is needed and lesions resolve in about a week.
- *Neonatal acne* typically appears around the third week of life and affects boys more commonly than girls. Erythematous papules and pustules on the face and trunk suggest the diagnosis in the older neonate, and reassurance of spontaneous clearing is all that is needed.
- *Seborrheic dermatitis* affects neonates and infants and is thought to be the result of genetic and environmental factors. In newborns, greasy yellow or red scales on the scalp, around the ears, eyebrows, and cheeks develop in the second to sixth week of life and are treated with topical application of oils and removal of scales with a fine comb.
- *Atopic dermatitis* is a chronic, recurrent inflammatory disorder with a strong genetic predisposition. Characteristic dry skin and erythematous papular or papulovesicular lesions and plaques appear in the second to sixth months of life (later than seborrheic dermatitis), are usually pruritic, and may become weeping. The typical flexural distribution seen in older children may not be seen in young infants. Therapy is aimed at reducing drying of the skin, application of emollients, and treatment of inflammation with topical steroid ointments.

DIAPER RASH

- A complaint specific to neonates and infants, there are two common forms of diaper rash: contact (irritation from reducing substances in stool and irritants in urine) and candidal dermatitis.
- Contact diaper dermatitis is an erythematous, macular or maculopapular rash with well-demarcated borders that spares skin folds. Treatment includes good hygiene, air-drying, and use of barrier creams/ointments such as zinc oxide.
- Candidal diaper dermatitis is characterized by erythematous papules and pustules with scaling margins and associated small pustules beyond the margins of the main rash known as *satellite lesions*. Diagnosis is clinical and treatment involves antifungal agents, such as nystatin (100,000 U/gram as cream, ointment, or powder applied 3-4 times daily for 10-14 days). Barrier creams (zinc oxide after nystatin application) can be useful. Topical steroids (1%-2% hydrocortisone cream) may be useful if severely inflamed. Oral thrush may be associated with candidal diaper dermatitis and should be treated with oral nystatin.

EXANTHEMS OF UNKNOWN ETIOLOGY

- Erythema multiforme, Stevens–Johnson syndrome, and toxic epidermal necrolysis are covered in Chapter 156, Dermatologic Emergencies.

KAWASAKI'S DISEASE

- Kawasaki's disease (KD), or mucocutaneous lymph node syndrome, is a generalized vasculitis of unknown etiology that peaks around 18 to 24 months of age, and rarely occurs <4 months or >5 years.
- Children may present with classic (complete) findings or incomplete findings; younger children and infants are more likely to have atypical or incomplete features and are at higher risk for complications, which include coronary artery aneurysms and sudden cardiac death.
- **Classic KD** is diagnosed in patients who have fever for at least 5 days and at least four of the following clinical features: (1) bilateral non-exudative conjunctivitis; (2) rash (variable in nature); (3) cervical lymphadenopathy >1.5 cm; (4) mucous membrane changes, including injection of the pharynx and lips with prominent papillae of the tongue (strawberry tongue); and (5) erythema or edema of the extremities, with peeling in the convalescent stage.
- The rash of KD is variable, and may be erythematous, morbilliform, urticarial, scarlatiniform, or erythema multiforme–like. Perineal rash is common.
- **Incomplete KD** is defined by fever for 5 days, *plus* at least two of the classic clinical symptoms listed above, plus a CRP >3.0 milligrams/L and or ESR >40 mm/h *plus* three or more of the following laboratory findings: (1) albumin <3 grams/dL; (2) anemia for age; (3) elevated ALT; (4) sterile pyuria (obtained by clean catch or bag rather than catheterization); (5) WBC >12,000/mm^3; (6) platelets >450,000/mm^3 after 7 days of fever onset.
- Patients with either classic or incomplete KD are often irritable, and may have associated arthralgias, refusal to bear weight, and desquamation.
- If complete or incomplete KD is suspected, admission and specialty referral is indicated. Treatment consists of intravenous gamma globulin (IVIG) and aspirin. The use of steroids is typically not indicated unless patients do not improve with IVIG.

HENOCH–SCHÖNLEIN PURPURA

- Henoch–Schönlein purpura (HSP) is the most common vasculitis in childhood.
- There are four main clinical features to HSP: palpable purpura ranging in size from 2 to 10 mm primarily involving the buttocks, thighs, legs, and arms; gastrointestinal symptoms including vomiting, diarrhea, abdominal pain, and GI bleeding; polyarthralgias; and hematuria and proteinuria (nephritis).

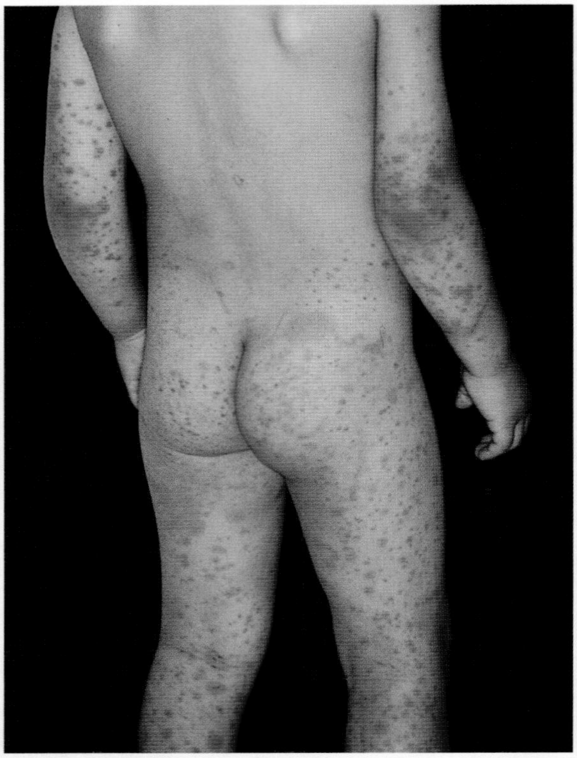

FIG. 85-10. Henoch–Schönlein purpura. (Photo contributed by Kevin J. Knoop, MD. Reproduced with permission from Knoop K, Stack L, Storrow A, Thurman RJ: *Atlas of Emergency Medicine*, 3rd ed. © 2010, McGraw-Hill, New York.)

- Children with HSP are generally well appearing and afebrile. Diagnosis can be made clinically in the presence of the characteristic rash (Fig. 85-10) and requires no laboratory evaluation other than urinalysis to assess for hematuria (if present, renal function tests are indicated).
- Treatment is symptomatic for arthralgias or arthritis with analgesics (typically NSAIDs), though prednisone (1 milligram/kg/dose PO) for 2 weeks followed by a 2-week taper may reduce severe joint and gastrointestinal symptoms.
- HSP is usually self-limited, but may be recurrent. Follow-up for repeat urine testing should be assured in patients with nephritis.

PITYRIASIS ROSEA

- Pityriasis rosea is characteristically seen in older school-aged children and young adults in the spring and fall. It is not contagious and does not appear to occur in epidemics.

- The rash evolves over weeks: it begins with a "herald patch," one red lesion with a raised border, typically on the trunk, which may not be noted by parents; 1 to 2 weeks later, a widespread eruption of pink maculopapular oval patches erupts on the trunk in a pattern following the ribs (the so-called "Christmas tree distribution"). Lesions may be pruritic. There may be mucous membrane involvement.
- Pityriasis rosea typically lasts 3 to 8 weeks. In adolescents, the differential diagnosis includes secondary syphilis, which has a similar appearance.
- Treatment is symptomatic and includes antihistamines for itching.

For further reading in Tintinalli's *Emergency Medicine: A Comprehensive Study Guide*, 7th ed., see Chapter 134, "Rashes in Infants and Children," by Gary Bonfante and Alexander M. Rosenau.

86 SICKLE CELL DISEASE

Ilene Claudius

- Sickle cell anemia–related emergencies in children include vaso-occlusive crises, hematologic crises, and infections. All children with sickle cell anemia presenting with fever, pain, respiratory distress, or a change in neurologic function require a rapid and thorough emergency department (ED) evaluation.

EPIDEMIOLOGY

- In the United States about 8% of the African-American population carries the hemoglobin (HbS) gene and about 0.15% are homozygous (HbSS).
- While vaso-occlusive crises are most common, infection is the leading cause of death.
- Symptoms are rarely seen before 4 months of age due to the predominance of fetal hemoglobin.

PATHOPHYSIOLOGY

- When deoxygenated, HbS polymerizes abnormally, creating chains that distort the red blood cell membrane into the characteristic sickle shape, impeding blood flow. The resultant tissue hypoxia and acidosis encourages further sickling.
- Decline in splenic function from infarction begins at 4 months of age and results in susceptibility to overwhelming infection with encapsulated organisms.

VASO-OCLUSIVE CRISES

- Vaso-occlusive episodes represent tissue ischemia and infarction from intravascular sickling. Bones, soft tissue, viscera, and the central nervous system can all be affected.

PAIN CRISES

Clinical Features

- The classic pain crisis is usually typical (ie, similar to prior episodes) in body location, character, and severity for each individual patient. Long bones and the lower back are common sites of pain.
- Crises can be triggered by stress, cold, dehydration, hypoxia, anemia, or infection, but most often occur without a specific cause.
- Often there are no physical findings, although pain, local tenderness, swelling, and warmth may occur.
- Dactylitis (painful swelling of hands or feet) due to ischemia of the metatarsal/metacarpal nutrient vessels may be the initial presenting manifestation of sickle cell anemia in infants. A low-grade temperature elevation can accompany dactylitis.
- Abdominal pain crises from mesenteric, hepatic, or splenic ischemia commonly present as recurrent episodes of abrupt-onset poorly localized pain and tenderness without rebound or rigidity.

Diagnosis and Differential

- Pain crises can be associated with low-grade fever and leukocytosis.
- Temperatures >38.3°C (101°F) or a left shift in the leukocyte distribution likely indicate an infectious cause (eg, osteomyelitis, septic arthritis).
- Consider avascular necrosis of the femoral head in patients with hip pain (see Fig. 86-1).
- With abdominal pain, cholelithiasis, splenic sequestration, and non-sickle cell anemia–related causes should be considered as well.

Emergency Department Care and Disposition

- Hydrate with oral or IV fluids (D5.45 normal saline) at a rate 1½ times maintenance. IV boluses of normal saline are indicated in the dehydrated or hypotensive patient (20 mL/kg), with careful attention to avoid fluid overload.

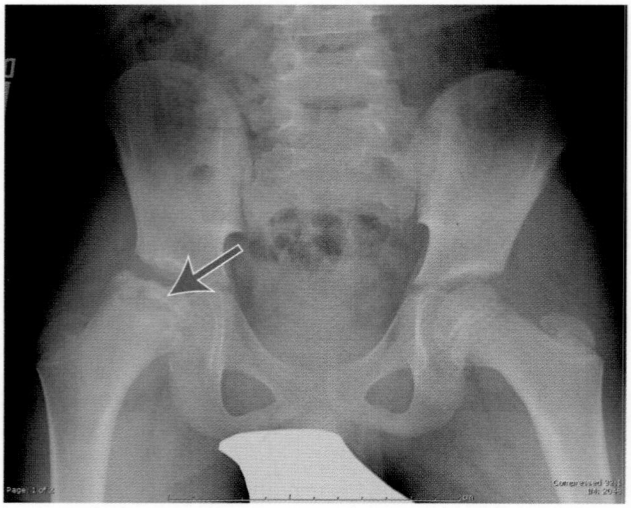

FIG. 86-1. Avascular necrosis of the femoral head. (Courtesy of Hollie Jackson, MD.)

- Mild to moderate pain can often be managed with oral hydration and analgesics, such as narcotics and nonsteroidal anti-inflammatory drugs (NSAIDs).
- Parenteral, long-acting narcotics (morphine 0.1-0.15 milligram/kg IV/IM or hydromorphone 0.015 milligram/kg IV/IM) and NSAIDs (ketorolac 0.5 milligram/kg) are indicated if oral regimens are inadequate.
- Oxygen is rarely useful in a patient without hypoxemia.
- Consider transfusion for acute drop in hemoglobin from baseline, or Hb <5 grams/dL.
- Admission is warranted for poor pain control or inadequate oral fluid intake.

ACUTE CHEST SYNDROME

- Acute chest syndrome, due to ischemia and infarction, is frequently a complication of pneumonia in children.

Clinical Features

- Acute chest syndrome should be considered in all patients with sickle cell disease (SCD) who present with complaints of chest pain. Signs and symptoms include pleuritic chest pain, cough, fever, dyspnea, hypoxia, tachypnea, rhonchi, or rales. Patients can deteriorate rapidly.
- Common concurrent infections include *Chlamydia*, *Mycoplasma*, viral, *Streptococcus pneumoniae*, *Staphylococcus aureus*, and *Haemophilus influenzae*.

Diagnosis and Differential

- Chest radiographs should be obtained, but may be normal initially (see Fig. 86-2).

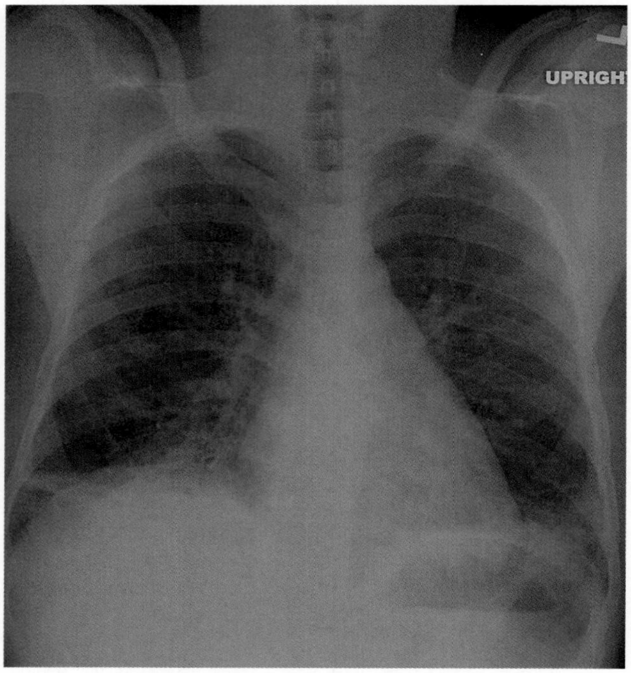

FIG. 86-2. Acute chest crisis. (Courtesy of Hollie Jackson, MD.)

- A complete blood count (CBC) typically indicates a leukocytosis in pneumonia or acute chest crisis. Low Hb may indicate need for transfusion. Low platelets predict poor outcome.
- Asthma, pulmonary hypertension, and fat embolus (from bony infarct) are other complications of sickle cell anemia to consider in the patient with respiratory distress.

Emergency Department Care and Disposition

- Monitor pulse oximetry and work of breathing.
- Supplemental oxygen should be provided if respiratory distress is present or if oxygen saturation is persistently less than or equal to 94%.
- Adequate analgesia for chest pain should be provided (see above), as well as IV hydration with D5.45NS at 1 to 1½ times maintenance.
- Treat underlying bacterial pneumonia with empiric antibiotic therapy such as ceftriaxone 50 milligrams/kg and a macrolide.
- Consider transfusion, in consultation with a pediatric hematologist, for persistent $Pao_2 < 70$ mm Hg or oxygen saturation drop of 10% from baseline. Packed red blood cell (PRBC) transfusions are indicated for Hb levels <10 grams/dL and exchange transfusions are indicated for patients with Hb levels ≥10 grams/dL in these circumstances.
- All children with suspected acute chest syndrome warrant hospital admission.

ACUTE CENTRAL NERVOUS SYSTEM EVENTS

CLINICAL FEATURES

- Ischemic strokes are not uncommon in children with sickle cell anemia and can present with transient or persistent ischemic symptoms, seizure, altered mental status, or coma. Sickle cell anemia patients are also at increased risk of aneurysmal subarachnoid hemorrhage, although this rarely presents before adolescence.

DIAGNOSIS AND DIFFERENTIAL

- Computed tomography (CT) scan should be obtained to assess for acute hemorrhage.
- Magnetic resonance imaging (MRI) scan of the brain may be useful to confirm the diagnosis of ischemic stroke, although should not delay treatment.
- A lumbar puncture may be necessary to exclude subarachnoid hemorrhage or meningitis if symptoms are suggestive.
- A CBC, reticulocyte count, and type and screen should be obtained.

EMERGENCY DEPARTMENT CARE AND DISPOSITION

- Transfuse or exchange transfuse to reduce the percentage of HbS <30%.
- Minimize secondary injury by correcting hypoglycemia, hypovolemia, and hyperpyrexia.
- Thrombolysis is not recommended for acute ischemic stroke in this setting.
- There is no consensus on blood pressure management.
- Coordinate care with pediatric hematology and neurology or neurosurgery, depending on type of stroke. All children with diagnosed or suspected CNS event should be admitted to the pediatric intensive care unit for close monitoring and further care.

PRIAPISM

- Priapism, a painful sustained erection in the absence of sexual stimulation, occurs when sickled cells accumulate in the corpora cavernosa. It can affect all males with SCD regardless of age, and severe prolonged attacks can cause impotence.
- Patients with priapism should receive IV hydration with D5.45NS at 1½ times maintenance, appropriate analgesia, and bladder catheterization if the patient is unable to void spontaneously.
- Treatment options include oral α-adrenergic agonists (eg, terbutaline), needle aspiration of the corpora cavernosa, or intrapenile injection of dilute epinephrine.
- Transfusion or exchange transfusion to decrease the percentage of HbS may be necessary.
- Management and admission decisions should be made promptly in consultation with a urologist and pediatric hematologist.

HEMATOLOGICAL CRISES

ACUTE SPLENIC SEQUESTRATION CRISES

Clinical Features

- The spleen of a young child with sickle cell anemia can enlarge, trapping much of the circulating blood volume. This condition can quickly progress to hypotension, shock, and death.
- Classically, children present with sudden-onset left upper quadrant pain, pallor, and lethargy and have a markedly enlarged, tender, and firm spleen on abdominal examination.
- Minor episodes can occur with insidious onset of abdominal pain, slowly progressive splenomegaly, and a more minor fall in hemoglobin level (Hb >6 grams/dL).
- Because of splenic infarction, this rarely occurs after age 5 years in children with HbSS, but can occur later in patients with HbSC or HbS/β-thalassemia.
- Less commonly, sequestration can occur in the liver. Clinical features include an enlarged and tender liver with associated hyperbilirubinemia, severe anemia, and elevated reticulocyte count. Cardiovascular collapse is rare in this condition.

Diagnosis and Differential

- A CBC reveals a profound anemia with normal to elevated reticulocyte count.

Emergency Department Care and Disposition

- Transfusion with PRBCs is often required. Profoundly anemic children require more gentle transfusions, with the following amounts given over 3 to 4 hours: 3 mL/kg for pre-transfusion Hb <4 milligrams/dL, 5 mL/kg for pre-transfusion Hb 4 to 6 milligrams/dL, 10 mL/kg for pre-transfusion Hb >6 milligrams/dL.

APLASTIC EPISODES

- Potentially life threatening, aplastic episodes are precipitated primarily by viral infections (classically, parvovirus B19), but can also be caused by bacterial infections, folic acid deficiency, or bone-marrow-suppressive drugs.
- Patients present with gradual onset of pallor without pain or jaundice.
- A CBC reveals unusually low hemoglobin with decreased or absent reticulocytosis.

- Blood transfusion may be required for severe anemia or symptoms (see guideline below). Hb <6 grams/dL or a drop of 3 grams/dL or symptoms are considered criteria for transfusion.

HEMOLYTIC CRISES

- Bacterial and viral infections in children with SCD can also precipitate an increasing degree of active hemolysis.
- Onset is usually sudden. A CBC reveals a hemoglobin level decreased from baseline, with markedly increased reticulocytosis. Increased jaundice and pallor are noticed on physical examination.
- Specific therapy is rarely required. Hematologic values return to normal as the infectious process resolves. Care should be directed toward treating the underlying infection. Close follow-up to monitor hemoglobin and reticulocyte count should be arranged at discharge.

INFECTIONS

CLINICAL FEATURES

- Due to functional asplenia, deficient antibody production, and impaired phagocytosis, bacterial infections, especially with encapsulated organisms, pose a serious and potentially fatal threat to young children with SCD and require aggressive management.
- Sickle cell anemia patients should receive penicillin prophylaxis until 5 years of age as well as routine vaccinations, including pneumococcus.

DIAGNOSIS AND DIFFERENTIAL

- A CBC, reticulocyte count, and blood cultures should be obtained for all children with SCD and fever or history of fever. Clinical signs and symptoms should direct the remainder of the workup, including lumbar puncture as indicated.

EMERGENCY DEPARTMENT CARE AND DISPOSITION

- Ill-appearing children or those <1 year of age should be treated empirically with an antibiotic active against *S. pneumoniae* and *H. influenzae* (eg, ceftriaxone 50 milligrams/kg).
- Well-appearing children over 1 year of age with temperature <40°C, WBC between 5,000 and 30,000 cells/mm^3, platelets >100,000/mcL, Hb>5 grams/dL, no infiltrate on CXR, and no history of pneumococcal sepsis can be discharged after a single dose of ceftriaxone and a 4-hour period of observation with follow-up in 24 hours. Children not meeting these criteria should be admitted for parenteral antibiotics and observation.

DISPOSITION GUIDELINES

- Hospital admission is warranted for the following:
  - Febrile children not meeting discharge criteria listed earlier
  - Acute chest crisis
  - Splenic sequestration
  - Any new CNS findings or presentations
  - Prolonged priapism
  - Any vaso-occlusive crises not responsive to analgesia and hydration (usually after 4-6 hours of therapy)
  - Inability to maintain adequate hydration
  - Inadequate assurance of follow-up

VARIANTS OF SICKLE CELL DISEASE

- Sickle cell trait is the carrier state of SCD and the most common variant. These patients are typically asymptomatic. They have vaso-occlusive complications only in the presence of extreme hypoxia or high altitude. They have minimal complications, the most common being hematuria (1%), most likely due to papillary necrosis in the renal medullary tissue.
- Sickle cell-Hemoglobin C disease is a heterozygous condition characterized by mild to moderate anemia and mild reticulocytosis. The smear reveals abundant target cells and few sickled cells. Many adults have splenomegaly, and these patients are at risk for pain crisis and organ infarcts. Most patients, however, have few clinical complications.
- Sickle cell–β-thalassemia disease is a heterozygous condition with varying degrees of severity of symptoms, dependent on the amount of normal β-hemoglobin chains that are produced. The severity can range from mild symptoms to a syndrome similar to SCD.

For further reading in Tintinalli's *Emergency Medicine: A Comprehensive Study Guide,* 7th ed., see Chapter 135, "Sickle Cell Disease," by Ilene Claudius.

87 ONCOLOGIC AND HEMATOLOGY EMERGENCIES IN CHILDREN

Ilene Claudius

- Childhood leukemia, the most common childhood malignancy, will be covered in detail in this chapter. Most complications can be extrapolated to other malignancies as well.
- Please refer to Chapters 137, Hemophilias and von Willebrand Disease, and 141, Emergent Complications of Malignancy, for more information on those entities.

CHILDHOOD LEUKEMIA

EPIDEMIOLOGY

- Acute lymphoblastic leukemia (ALL) accounts for three-fourths of pediatric leukemia.
- Peak incidence is 3 to 5 years of age.
- Five-year survival is 75% to 80%.

PATHOPHYSIOLOGY

- Certain chromosomal abnormalities (eg, Philadelphia translocation), radiation exposure, and chemotherapy treatment for prior malignancy are risk factors for leukemia.

CLINICAL FEATURES

- Leukemia can present with symptoms of direct infiltration of bone marrow and suppression of cell lines, including pallor, fatigue, easy bruising, fever, or bone pain.
- Two-thirds of patients have hepatomegaly or splenomegaly at diagnosis.
- Several findings are classically associated with particular subtypes of acute myelogenous leukemia (AML), including gingival hyperplasia and subcutaneous masses (chloromas).

DIAGNOSIS AND DIFFERENTIAL

- CBC often shows abnormalities of two or more cell lines, although can be normal early in the course.
- Obtain electrolytes, creatinine, uric acid, phosphate, and calcium to assess for tumor lysis; a disseminated intravascular coagulation (DIC) panel, liver function tests (LFTs), and lactate dehydrogenase (LDH); blood and urine cultures if febrile; and a type and screen if anemic.
- Obtain CXR to assess for mediastinal mass.
- Viral syndromes and rheumatologic diseases can present similarly.

EMERGENCY DEPARTMENT CARE AND DISPOSITION

- Anemia: For hemorrhage or significant symptoms, transfuse 10 mL/kg irradiated, leukodepleted packed red blood cells (PRBCs) (caution in hyperviscosity syndrome). In the absence of these indications, transfusions are done non-emergently for Hb <8 grams/dL.
- Thrombocytopenia: For bleeding with platelets <50,000 to 100,000/mL^3 or procedure with platelets <50,000/mL^3, give 10 mL/kg or 0.1 random donor unit/kg of platelets. In the absence of these indications, platelets are given non-emergently when <10,000/mL^3.
- Infection: In newly presenting patients or known patients returning with neutropenia (absolute neutrophil count <1000/mL^3), antibiotics with coverage for pseudomonas (eg, cefepime 50 milligrams/kg) should be given empirically with addition of gentamycin (2.5 milligrams/kg) and vancomycin (15 milligrams/kg) for patients who are ill appearing or suspected to have gram-positive infections. Attention should be paid to the possibility of typhlitis, inflammation of the terminal ileum, and anaerobic coverage added if suspected (see Table 87-1).

TABLE 87-1 Management of Neutropenic Fever

Definition of neutropenia
Absolute neutrophil count (segs + bands) <500/mL^3
Absolute neutrophil count <1000/mL^3 and expected to fall*
Definition of fever†
Temperature ≥38.3°C (100.9°F) orally once
or
Temperature 38°C-38.3°C (100.4°F-100.9°F) persisting for 1 h
or
Age <12 mo old with temperature ≥38°C (100.4°F)
Caveats
Some add 0.5°C (1.0°F) to axillary temperatures for oral equivalent
Confirm with oral temperature when possible
Avoid rectal measurements
Parental history of objective fever is sufficient
Cultures‡
One culture from each central line lumen (label appropriately)
Peripheral culture only in absence of central line
Urine culture (clean catch or bagged)
Antibiotics¶
Well-appearing**
Broad-spectrum antipseudomonal monotherapy
Cefepime, 50 milligrams/kg to maximum dose 2 grams, or ceftazidime, 50 milligrams/kg to maximum dose of 2 grams††
Ill-appearing (ie, septic)
Cefepime, 50 milligrams/kg (or ceftazidime, 50 milligrams/kg) + gentamicin, 2.5 milligrams/kg + vancomycin, 15 milligrams/kg up to 1 gram
Abdominal/perirectal pain
Cefepime, 50 milligrams/kg (or ceftazidime, 50 milligrams/kg) + metronidazole, 7.5 milligrams/kg to 1 gram maximum (± vancomycin 15 milligrams/kg up to 1 gram maximum)

*Based on serial measurements or history of chemotherapy in the previous 5-10 days.
† Definitions will vary by institution.
‡ Most patients will only require aerobic cultures. Consider anaerobic cultures if significant GI symptoms or visible mucositis.
¶ Do not wait for absolute neutrophil count results if patients is expected to be neutropenic to administer antibiotics.
**Indications for the addition of vancomycin include: high-dose cytarabine, acute myelogenous leukemia patients, significant mucositis, evidence of skin or soft tissue or line infections, presence of orthopedic appliances.
†† Vancomycin + aztreonam for cephalosporin-allergic patients.

- Tumor lysis syndrome describes the release of intracellular potassium, phosphate, and uric acid and the subsequent decline in calcium. It occurs with cell lysis, which can precede the initiation of chemotherapy in patients with a high WBC count. Hyperkalemia is managed in the standard fashion, and uric acid elevations can be emergently managed with IV fluids and rasburicase.
- Hyperleukocytosis can cause microvascular obstruction with injury particularly to the lungs or CNS. Patients with symptoms or asymptomatic patients with WBC counts >200,000/mL^3 should be aggressively hydrated. If hydration is ineffective, the patient will require emergent leukapheresis.

LYMPHOMA

- Hodgkin's lymphoma is a lymphoid neoplasm that typically presents as non-tender, non-erythematous cervical or supraclavicular lymph nodes in adolescence. About one-third of patients have systemic symptoms ("B-symptoms") such as fever, weight loss, or night sweats.
- Non-Hodgkin's lymphoma (NHL) occurs in older children, particularly those with immunosuppression, and can occur anywhere in the body. The location typically drives the presenting manifestations.
- Initial workup of lymphoma requires a CXR to assess for mediastinal mass, CBC for bone marrow involvement, electrolytes, uric acid, phosphate, and creatinine to assess for tumor lysis syndrome (more likely with NHL).
- ED care is supportive, with steroids being reserved for situations where a mass causes life- or limb-threatening compression.

CENTRAL NERVOUS SYSTEM TUMORS

- Brain tumors are the most common solid tumors in pediatrics, and most present with signs of increased intracranial pressure. Sleep-related headache is the strongest predictor, with vomiting, ataxia, cranial nerve palsies, and vague neurologic symptoms being common in older children and bulging fontanel, increasing head circumference, and sunsetting (upward gaze paresis) being common in infants. The notable exception is primary brain stem tumors (eg, brain stem glioma), which may present initially with cranial nerve findings without signs of increased intracranial pressure.
- CT and MRI are appropriate studies in the emergency department.
- Seizures, if present, are treated in the standard fashion. Dexamethasone should typically be given to reduce vasogenic edema unless CNS lymphoma is likely (dose: 1 milligram/year of life to a maximum of 10 milligrams).

NEUROBLASTOMA

- Neuroblastoma is a primitive ganglion tumor that can occur in the adrenal, abdomen, chest, or neck.
- Typically, neuroblastoma presents as a painless mass, but can cause compressive symptoms as well. If retrobulbar, raccoon eyes and proptosis can occur and, if located in the superior cervical ganglion, can cause Horner's syndrome and tracheal compression. Paraneoplastic symptoms include hypertension, watery diarrhea, and opsoclonus-myoclonus syndrome (rapid, multidirectional eye movements and jerking of the extremities).
- Chest radiographs should be obtained to assess for mediastinal mass and CBC to assess for bone marrow infiltration. CT can assist in diagnosis and staging.

WILMS TUMOR

- Wilms tumor, or nephroblastoma, arises from embryonal renal cells, typically in children <10 years of age.
- Typically, children present with a painless mass, but may have hematuria, hypertension, or signs of compression of abdominal organs.
- Abdominal CT and chest radiograph can assist in diagnosis and staging. Recommended laboratories include CBC, liver and coagulation profiles, serum chemistries, and urinalysis.

RETINOBLASTOMA

- Retinoblastoma is a white-gray intraocular malignancy arising from the retina caused by an inherited or spontaneous mutation inactivating the RB1 tumor suppressor gene. It is typically diagnosed prior to age 2 years.
- Patients frequently have leukocoria (see Fig. 87-1), or loss of the normal red reflex due to the gray-white intraocular tumor mass. Other possible presentations include strabismus, unilateral fixed pupil, or a painful, red eye (possibly associated with glaucoma). One-quarter of lesions are bilateral.
- Diagnosis is by CT scan and ophthalmology consultation.

BONE AND TISSUE SARCOMAS

- Rhabdomyosarcoma presents as a painless tissue mass, and can be further elucidated on CT scan.
- Osteosarcoma is a bony tumor that primarily affects adolescents. Common sites are proximal humerus and

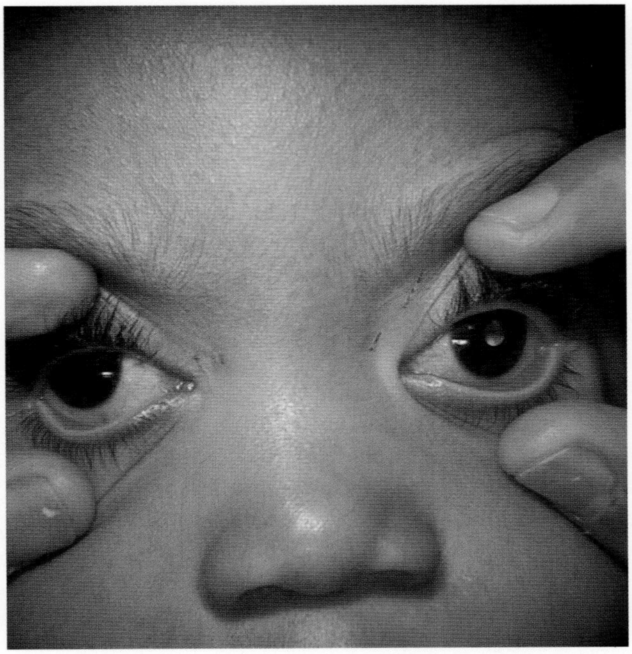

FIG. 87-1. Leukocoria in retinoblastoma. An 18-month-old child presenting with white pupil. (Reproduced with permission from Shah BR, Lucchesi M: *Atlas of Pediatric Emergency Medicine,* © 2006, McGraw-Hill, New York.)

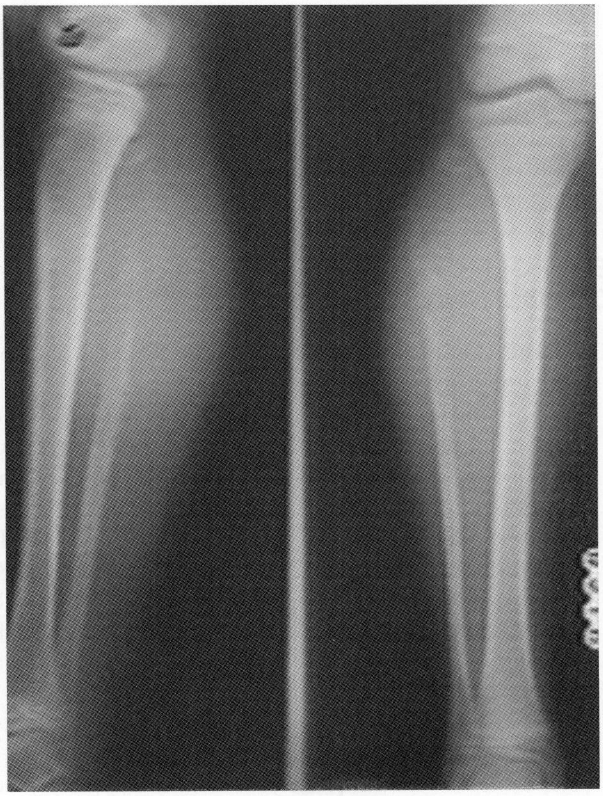

FIG. 87-2. Ewing sarcoma of the fibula.

distal femur, with tumors in the pelvis or mandible occurring rarely. Patients experience a dull ache in the affected area, particularly at night, and may have a palpable mass on examination. Systemic symptoms are rare, and typically indicate metastatic disease.

- Ewing sarcoma is also a painful bony tumor. It presents in the long bones (femur, tibia, humerus) or axial skeleton (pelvis, ribs, or spine). Presentation can be insidious, with weeks of localized pain, or as a mass and discomfort first noted after a minor trauma.
- Radiograph demonstrates a destructive moth-eaten tumor displacing the native cortex outward and creating and onion-peel appearance (see Fig. 87-2).

ANEMIA

EPIDEMIOLOGY

- Iron deficiency anemia from ingestion of cow's milk is common from 6 months to 3 years. Beyond that, or without an appropriate clinical history, gastrointestinal bleeding should be considered.

PATHOPHYSIOLOGY

- Iron deficiency anemia in infants and toddlers is frequently secondary to excessive milk intake (>32 ounces/d) causing poor dietary intake of iron and blood loss through colitis.
- Autoimmune hemolytic anemia due to the production of autoantibodies is typically primary in infants and small children, and in adolescents, secondary to malignancy, rheumatologic disease, or HIV.

CLINICAL FEATURES

- Children with anemia can present with pallor and fatigue. Occasionally, severe anemia can present with congestive heart failure.

DIAGNOSIS AND DIFFERENTIAL

- A CBC, reticulocyte count, and peripheral smear should be obtained. In severe cases, type and screen may be necessary. If hemolysis is suspected, a peripheral smear, bilirubin, and LDH may be helpful. If iron deficiency anemia is suspected outside of the toddler age group, a stool hemocult should be obtained.
- In iron deficiency anemia, there is isolated low hemoglobin with a decreased reticulocyte count and mean corpuscular volume (MCV). Involvement of additional

cell lines should prompt investigation for a hematologic malignancy.
- In autoimmune hemolytic anemia, the low hemoglobin is accompanied by a high MCV and an elevated indirect bilirubin. A direct Coomb's test is positive, and a peripheral smear will show spherocytes and schistocytes.

EMERGENCY DEPARTMENT CARE AND DISPOSITION

- Children with anemia from nontraumatic causes rarely require transfusion in the ED.
- Transfusion can be considered for a symptomatic patient with Hb <6 to 8 milligrams/dL. Typically, the dose is based on the pre-transfusion hemoglobin, and is given over 3 to 4 hours. Patients with Hb <4 grams/dL receive 3 mL/kg, Hb 4 to 6 grams/dL receive 5 mL/kg, and Hb >6 grams/dL receive 10 mL/kg of PRBCs. Transfusion of patients with autoimmune hemolytic anemia is not without risk and should be performed after consultation with a hematologist.
- Corticosteroids are appropriate treatment for patients with autoimmune hemolytic anemia.
- Patients with iron deficiency anemia can typically be discharged from the emergency department. If the etiology is thought to be over-ingestion of cow's milk, reduction of intake to <24 ounces/day is recommended. They should be started on iron therapy at a dose 1 to 2 milligrams/kg/dose of elemental iron three times daily.

THROMBOCYTOPENIA

EPIDEMIOLOGY

- Idiopathic thrombocytopenic purpura (ITP) occurs as an isolated disorder in the preschool-aged child, and is often a feature of systemic infections (HIV, hepatitis) or rheumatologic disorders in the adolescent.

PATHOPHYSIOLOGY

- ITP is an autoimmune disorder in which macrophages of the reticuloendothelial system destroy antibody-coated platelets.

CLINICAL FEATURES

- Patients present with signs of thrombocytopenia such as diffuse petechiae, bruising, and bleeding (mainly epistaxis and mucus membrane) days to weeks after a viral upper respiratory infection. Systemic symptoms should not occur.

DIAGNOSIS AND DIFFERENTIAL

- CBC will reveal significant thrombocytopenia without abnormalities in the other cell lines. Platelet volume is large. Blood type should also be sent if anti-Rh immunoglobulin is planned therapy.

EMERGENCY DEPARTMENT CARE AND DISPOSITION

- The three primary treatments for ITP are prednisone 1 to 2 milligrams/kg/d, IVIG 1 gram/kg, and anti-Rh immunoglobulin (WinRho®). Steroids should not be given unless the possibility of hematologic malignancy has been excluded. Anti-Rh immunoglobulin will typically cause some hemolysis, lowering the patient's hemoglobin by 1 gram/dL in the days following treatment. However, several cases of severe and fatal intravascular hemolysis have been reported, and this should only be given in conjunction with a hematologist comfortable with the contraindications to anti-Rh immunoglobulin.
- Although platelet transfusions are not usually effective, for life-threatening bleeds, a transfusion of two to three times the normal dose of platelets can be useful. Methylprednisolone (30 milligrams/kg) and IVIG (1 gram/kg) should be given as well.
- Admission decisions should be made in conjunction with pediatric hematology.

NEUTROPENIA

EPIDEMIOLOGY

- Multiple disorders can cause an isolated transient neutropenia in children, including benign transient neutropenia from viral infections or medications, autoimmune neutropenia, and cyclic neutropenia. More serious forms are chronic and persistent, such as congenital agranulocytosis or chemotherapy induced.

PATHOPHYSIOLOGY

- Absolute neutrophil counts below $1000/mL^3$ increase the risk for bacterial infection; however, this is rarely true in the transient types of neutropenia.

CLINICAL FEATURES

- Neutropenia may be asymptomatic and incidentally noted on a CBC obtained for other reasons or may be associated with systemic infections and fever.

DIAGNOSIS AND DIFFERENTIAL

- CBC and blood cultures should be sent for a febrile patient in whom neutropenia is suspected.
- Children with neutropenia who are ill appearing should be presumed to have a significant infection.

EMERGENCY DEPARTMENT CARE AND DISPOSITION

- Patients with benign forms of neutropenia and evidence of infection can typically be discharged home, although consultation with the patient's hematologist and a single dose of ceftriaxone (50 milligrams/kg IV/IM) may be considered.
- Ill-appearing patients and those with a fever and a more serious persistent type of neutropenia should be admitted on broad-spectrum antibiotics, such as cefepime (50 milligrams/kg IV).

For further reading in Tintinalli's *Emergency Medicine: A Comprehensive Study Guide,* 7th ed., see Chapter 136, "Oncology and Hematology Emergencies in Children," by Rick Place, Anne Marie T. Lagoc, Thomas A. Mayer, and Christopher J. Lawlor.

88 RENAL EMERGENCIES IN INFANTS AND CHILDREN

Deborah R. Liu

- Renal emergencies in children represent a large and varied group of disease processes. This chapter covers common renal emergencies, including acute renal failure (ARF) in children, acute glomerulonephritis, and nephrotic syndrome.
- For discussion of other renal emergencies, see the following topics and chapters: end-stage renal disease (Chapter 54, Emergencies in Renal Failure and Dialysis Patients), urolithiasis (Chapter 56, Urologic Stone Disease), hypertension (Chapter 28, Hypertension), Henoch–Schönlein Purpura (Chapter 76, Pediatric Abdominal Emergencies), hemolytic uremic syndrome (Chapter 135, Evaluation of Anemia and the Bleeding Patient), and hematuria (Chapter 55, Urinary Tract Infections and Hematuria).

■ ACUTE RENAL FAILURE

- ARF is the abrupt loss of renal function such that body fluid homeostasis is no longer maintained.
- Mortality among children with ARF ranges from 8% to 89% and varies by cause.
- Common causes of ARF in children include severe dehydration, sepsis, pyelonephritis, hemolytic uremic syndrome, acute glomerulonephritis, postoperative complications, and posterior urethral valves in boys.

CLINICAL FEATURES

- Patients present with symptoms of the underlying cause (eg, bloody diarrhea and abdominal pain in hemolytic uremic syndrome; or fever, hypotension, and petechiae in sepsis).
- Ultimately, the patient manifests symptoms and signs of renal failure: nausea and anorexia due to uremia, headache from hypertension, edema (periorbital, scrotal or labial, dependent, or generalized), weight gain, and decreased urine output.

DIAGNOSIS AND DIFFERENTIAL

- ARF may be anatomically categorized as prerenal, renal, or postrenal in etiology. Table 88-1 lists common causes of renal failure in infants and children.
- Urinalysis helps distinguish among the three forms of ARF and should be obtained along with microscopic evaluation. Children who are not toilet trained or in those with significantly decreased urine output require catheterization to obtain urine.
- Prerenal causes of ARF are associated with little blood or protein on urinalysis, but typically manifest high urine specific gravity (≥1.025).
- Children with acute tubular necrosis typically have granular casts on urinalysis but usually have a normal specific gravity.
- Glomerulonephritis and other glomerular disease are characterized by hematuria and proteinuria.
- A positive urine dipstick test for blood without red blood cells on microscopy suggests hemoglobinuria or myoglobinuria.
- Basic blood tests such as serum electrolytes, BUN and creatinine, as well as a complete blood count (CBC) should be obtained in all cases of ARF to help identify the cause and guide management. Additional blood tests may be indicated depending on the clinical scenario.

EMERGENCY DEPARTMENT CARE AND DISPOSITION

- The goals of treatment for ARF are to identify the underlying cause of renal failure and to correct fluid and electrolyte imbalances.

TABLE 88-1 Causes of Renal Failure in Infants and Children

PRERENAL OR INADEQUATE RENAL PERFUSION	RENAL OR INTRINSIC RENAL INJURY OR DISEASE	POSTRENAL OR OBSTRUCTION
Dehydration from GI losses	Tubular diseases (tubular necrosis; effects of contrast agents, chemotherapy)	Solitary kidney
Blood loss from trauma	Myoglobinuria, hemoglobinuria, tumor lysis syndrome	Urethral obstruction (posterior urethral valves, uteropelvic junction obstruction)
Capillary leakage in burns, sepsis, third spacing	Glomerular diseases (Henoch–Schönlein purpura, glomerulonephritis, nephrotic syndrome)	Pelvic mass (lymphoma, rhabdomyosarcoma)
Limited cardiac output in congenital heart disease, myocarditis, cardiogenic shock	Interstitial lesions from medications (antibiotics, antifungals, NSAIDs)	Nephrolithiasis

- Address life-threatening complications, such as severe hyperkalemia (see Chaps. 6 and 83) or hypertensive emergency (see Chapter 28) immediately.
- Consult a pediatric nephrologist for most cases of ARF as many cases require inpatient admission.
- Treatment recommendations for prerenal ARF, intrinsic renal failure, and postrenal failure are listed in Table 88-2.
- Treat hypertension with antihypertensive agents as described in Chapter 28.
- For postrenal (obstructive) ARF, insert a Foley catheter to relieve the obstruction (see also Table 88-2).
- When conservative measures fail, acute renal replacement therapy (dialysis) should be considered.
- Indications for dialysis include severe electrolyte abnormalities, fluid overload not relieved by administration of loop diuretics, and intractable metabolic acidosis not responding to bicarbonate therapy.
- Peritoneal dialysis is the preferred method of acute dialysis for children, because it is inexpensive and requires less expertise to perform than hemodialysis.

ACUTE GLOMERULONEPHRITIS

- Glomerulonephritis is an inflammatory process affecting the glomerulus.
- Acute glomerulonephritis is characterized by hematuria and proteinuria. There are many causes of acute glomerulonephritis, including postinfectious etiologies, the most common of which follows infection with group A β-hemolytic streptococcus. Other less frequent causes include Henoch–Schönlein purpura, hemolytic uremic syndrome, systemic lupus erythematosus, IgA nephropathy, and Goodpasture's syndrome.

CLINICAL FEATURES

- Patients typically present with sudden onset of brown, tea-colored, or grossly bloody urine. Patients may also note foamy urine due to proteinuria.
- Other symptoms include decreased urine output, headaches due to hypertension, or peripheral edema.

TABLE 88-2 Emergency Management of Children with Acute Renal Failure

PRERENAL	RENAL	POSTRENAL
Dehydration with hypovolemic shock Crystalloid bolus of normal saline 10-20 mL/kg; do not add potassium to fluids	Depending on the clinical state, treat oliguria with fluid restriction and limit replacement to insensible water loss and previous 24-h loss.	Depending on the clinical state, treat oliguria with fluid restriction and limit replacement to insensible water loss and previous 24-h loss.
Furosemide, 2 milligrams/kg IV after adequate IV fluid if no urine output	Measure baseline weight and strictly monitor input and output.	Measure baseline weight and monitor input and output.
Hemorrhagic shock Crystalloid bolus as above until blood products are available Transfusion of packed red blood cells 10-15 mL/kg + fresh frozen plasma	Offending medications should be discontinued or adjusted based on glomerular filtration rate. Administer antihypertensive agents and diuretics to control blood pressure (avoid ACE inhibitors).	Offending medications should be discontinued or adjusted based on glomerular filtration rate. Administer antihypertensive agents and diuretics to control blood pressure (avoid ACE inhibitors). Insert Foley catheter to relieve obstruction.
Monitoring of blood pressure and heart rate		

Abbreviation: ACE = angiotensin-converting enzyme.

- In post-streptococcal glomerulonephritis, there may be a history of sore throat 1 to 2 weeks preceding urinary symptoms.
- The physical examination can be completely normal, or may demonstrate hypertension, edema, or signs of congestive heart failure.

DIAGNOSIS AND DIFFERENTIAL

- The diagnosis of glomerulonephritis is made by examination of the urine. The urinalysis shows hematuria and proteinuria (usually at least 2+ protein [100 milligrams/dL] on the urine dipstick). Red blood cell casts are seen on microscopy.
- Additional laboratory testing should include a CBC, electrolytes, BUN and creatinine, and urine culture (infection may present as hematuria with proteinuria).
- Further evaluation for post-streptococcal glomerulonephritis includes antistreptolysin O titers and C3 and C4 complement levels.
- Serum albumin, triglycerides, and cholesterol should be obtained to help differentiate acute glomerulonephritis from nephrotic syndrome.

EMERGENCY DEPARTMENT CARE AND DISPOSITION

- The treatment of glomerulonephritis is determined by the underlying cause.
- Address hypertensive emergencies first.
- Patients with new-onset glomerulonephritis and oliguria or hypertension usually require admission.
- Patients with mild disease may be discharged home on a low-sodium diet with monitoring of fluid intake and with close follow-up with a pediatric nephrologist.

NEPHROTIC SYNDROME

- Nephrotic syndrome is a chronic disease in children characterized by increased permeability of the glomerular capillary wall, with resulting urinary loss of protein.
- Nephrotic syndrome is characterized by significant proteinuria, hypoproteinemia, edema, and hyperlipidemia.
- Nephrotic syndrome can be divided into primary (only affecting the kidney) or secondary (multisystem disease with kidney involvement) nephrotic syndrome.
- The most common form of primary nephrotic syndrome is minimal change disease.
- Other causes include focal glomerulosclerosis, mesangial proliferative glomerulonephritis, and membranoproliferative glomerulonephritis.
- Secondary forms of nephrotic syndrome include lupus, Henoch–Schönlein purpura, sickle-cell disease, and drug or toxin exposure (eg, heavy metals).

CLINICAL FEATURES

- Patients typically present with edema, which may involve the face, abdomen, scrotum or labia, or extremities.
- Because facial swelling or puffy eyes are not specific symptoms, patients are easily misdiagnosed as having an allergic reaction.
- The patient or parent may note foamy urine (proteinuria) or dark urine (hematuria).
- Extreme hypoproteinemia can cause pleural effusions with associated shortness of breath or orthopnea; abdominal ascites can cause pain, nausea, vomiting, or anorexia.

DIAGNOSIS AND DIFFERENTIAL

- Diagnostic criteria include edema, heavy proteinuria (usually 3+ [300 milligrams/dL] or 4+ [2000 milligrams/dL] on urine dipstick testing), and hypoproteinemia (serum albumin <3.0 grams/dL). Hypercholesterolemia (>200 milligrams/dL) is classically seen with nephrotic syndrome, although an inconsistent finding.
- Further testing is useful to distinguish primary from secondary nephrotic syndrome, and may include serum antinuclear antibody, serum immunoglobulins, screening for sickle-cell disease, or serum complement levels.

EMERGENCY DEPARTMENT CARE AND DISPOSITION

- Fluid management in the nephrotic patient can be challenging. Patients may be intravascularly depleted but have signs of fluid overload (edema).
- Mild cases of nephrotic syndrome do not require fluid resuscitation. Treatment of most cases of nephrotic syndrome should be performed in consultation with a pediatric nephrologist.
- Treat hypovolemic shock with 20 mL/kg normal saline, even in the setting of severe edema.
- Treat mild to moderate dehydration with small but frequent amounts of a low-sodium oral solution.
- Treat volume overload and edema with furosemide 1 milligram/kg/dose. If the serum albumin is extremely low, administer 25% albumin (0.5-1 g/kg) over 4 hours followed by furosemide 1 to 2 milligrams/kg IV (higher dose of furosemide may be needed in this setting).

- Definitive treatment of nephrotic syndrome often includes oral corticosteroids; however, this should be initiated only after consultation with a pediatric nephrologist.
- Many patients with nephrotic syndrome can safely be discharged home on a low-salt diet with close follow-up.
- Indications for admission include severe edema (eg, pulmonary effusion or ascites causing respiratory symptoms), symptomatic hypertension, suspected bacterial infection (eg, spontaneous bacterial peritonitis with ascites), significant intravascular dehydration, and renal insufficiency.

For further reading in Tintinalli's *Emergency Medicine: A Comprehensive Study Guide,* 7th ed., see Chapter 128, "Renal Emergencies in Infants and Children," by Christine E. Koerner.

Section 11
INFECTIOUS DISEASES

89 SEXUALLY TRANSMITTED DISEASES

David M. Cline

- This chapter covers the major sexually transmitted diseases (STDs) in the United States, with the exception of human immunodeficiency virus (HIV), which is discussed in Chapter 94. Vaginitis and pelvic inflammatory disease (PID) are covered separately in Chapters 65 and 66, respectively.

GENERAL RECOMMENDATIONS

- Multiple STD infections frequently occur concurrently, compliance and follow-up are often limited or unreliable, and infertility and other long-term morbidities may result from lack of treatment.
- When an STD is suspected, treat with single-dose regimens whenever possible.
- Ascertain pregnancy status and consider an obstetrics consultation if the patient is pregnant.
- Screen for other STDs (HIV infection, syphilis, and hepatitis) in the ED or through follow-up.
- Provide counseling for STD prevention in the ED and assure HIV testing in the ED or through follow-up as indicated.
- Advise that the partner(s) seek treatment and counsel on the appropriate time to reengage in sexual relations.
- Arrange follow-up as local resources allow.

CHLAMYDIAL INFECTIONS

CLINICAL FEATURES

CHLAMYDIA TRACHOMATIS

- *Chlamydia trachomatis* is an obligate intracellular bacteria that causes urethritis, epididymitis, orchitis, proctitis, or Reiter syndrome (nongonococcal urethritis, conjunctivitis, and rash) in men and urethritis, cervicitis, PID, and infertility in women.
- In both sexes, asymptomatic infection is common. There is a high incidence of coinfection with *Neisseria gonorrhoeae.*
- The incubation period is 1 to 3 weeks, with symptoms varying from mild dysuria with purulent or mucoid urethral discharge to sterile pyuria and frequency (urethritis).
- Women may present with mild cervicitis or with abdominal pain, findings of PID, or peritonitis. Men may present with a tender swollen epididymis or testicle.

DIAGNOSIS AND DIFFERENTIAL

- Diagnosis is best made with indirect detection methods—such as enzyme-linked immunosorbent assay or DNA probes, which have a sensitivity of 75% to 90%.
- The Centers for Disease Control and Prevention (CDC) recommends a nucleic acid amplification test to be used as screening tests for *Chlamydia.* Culture is possible but difficult and produces a low yield.

EMERGENCY DEPARTMENT CARE AND DISPOSITION

- Azithromycin 1 gram PO as a single dose, or doxycycline 100 milligrams PO twice daily for 7 days, is the treatment of choice for uncomplicated urethritis or cervicitis.
- Alternatives include 7-day treatment with erythromycin base 500 milligrams PO four times a day, ofloxacin 300 milligrams twice daily, or levofloxacin 500 milligrams PO daily.
- For pregnant patients, the CDC recommends azithromycin 1 gram PO as a single dose, amoxicillin 500 milligrams PO three times daily for 7 days, or erythromycin base 500 milligrams PO four times a day for 7 days.

GONOCOCCAL INFECTIONS

CLINICAL FEATURES

- *Neisseria gonorrhoeae* (GC) is a gram-negative diplococcus that causes urethritis, epididymitis, orchitis, and prostatitis in men and urethritis, cervicitis, PID, and infertility in women.

- Rectal infection and proctitis with mucopurulent anal discharge and pain can occur in both sexes.
- The incubation period ranges from 3 to 14 days.
- Women tend to present with nonspecific lower abdominal pain and mucopurulent vaginal discharge with findings of cervicitis and possibly PID.
- Eighty percent to 90% of men develop symptoms of urethritis: dysuria and purulent penile discharge within 2 weeks. Men also may present with acute epididymitis and orchitis or prostatitis.
- Occasionally, GC can be isolated from the throat, but it rarely causes symptomatic pharyngitis.
- Disseminated GC is a systemic infection that occurs in 2% of untreated patients with GC, most often women, and is the most common cause of infectious arthritis in young adults. An initial febrile bacteremic stage includes skin lesions (tender pustules on a red base, usually on the extremities, and may include palms and soles), tenosynovitis, and myalgias. Over the next week, these symptoms subside, followed by mono- or oligoarticular arthritis with purulent joint fluid.

DIAGNOSIS AND DIFFERENTIAL

- For uncomplicated GC, urethral or cervical cultures are the standard diagnostic tests.
- A Gram stain of urethral discharge showing intracellular gram-negative diplococci is very useful in men; cervical smears are unreliable in women.
- Diagnosis of disseminated GC is primarily clinical because results of culture of blood, skin lesions, and joint fluid are positive in only 20% to 50% of patients. Culturing the cervix, rectum, and pharynx may improve the yield. A positive GC culture result from a partner supports the diagnosis.

EMERGENCY DEPARTMENT CARE AND DISPOSITION

- Effective therapy for uncomplicated gonorrhea (not PID) includes single-dose regimens of cefixime 400 milligrams PO, or ceftriaxone 250 milligrams IM.
- Alternatives include single-dose regimens of ceftizoxime, 500 milligrams IM single dose, or cefoxitin, 2 grams IM single dose, plus probenecid, 1 gram PO single dose, or cefotaxime, 500 milligrams IM single dose, or spectinomycin 2 grams IM (may not be available in the United States).
- Disseminated gonorrhea is treated initially with parenteral ceftriaxone 1 gram daily IM/IV until 24 to 48 hours after there is clinical improvement; then the patient can be switched to oral cefixime 400 milligrams daily for 7 to 10 total antibiotic therapy days.
- Treatment for possible coinfection with *Chlamydia* also should be given.

■ TRICHOMONAS INFECTIONS

CLINICAL FEATURES

- *Trichomonas vaginalis* is a flagellated protozoan that causes vaginitis with malodorous yellow-green discharge and urethritis. Abdominal pain also may be present.
- Trichomoniasis in pregnancy has been associated with premature rupture of membranes, preterm delivery, and low birth weight.
- In men, infection is often asymptomatic (90%-95%), but urethritis may be present. The incubation period varies from 3 to 28 days.

DIAGNOSIS AND DIFFERENTIAL

Diagnosis is based on finding the motile, flagellated organism on a saline wet preparation of vaginal discharge or in a spun urine specimen.

EMERGENCY DEPARTMENT CARE AND DISPOSITION

- Metronidazole 2 grams PO in a single dose is the treatment of choice (alternatively, 500 milligrams PO twice daily for 7 days).
- Alternatively tinidazole 2 grams PO may be given as a single dose.
- Metronidazole is a pregnancy category B drug, and it is the drug of choice for treating symptomatic pregnant patients. The CDC guidelines state that pregnant women may be treated with a single 2-gram dose of metronidazole.

■ SYPHILIS

CLINICAL FEATURES

- *Treponema pallidum,* a spirochete, causes syphilis. It enters the body through mucous membranes and nonintact skin.
- Syphilis occurs in three stages.
- The primary stage is characterized by the chancre (see Fig. 89-1), a single painless ulcer with indurated borders that develops after an incubation period of 21 days on the penis, vulva, or other areas of sexual

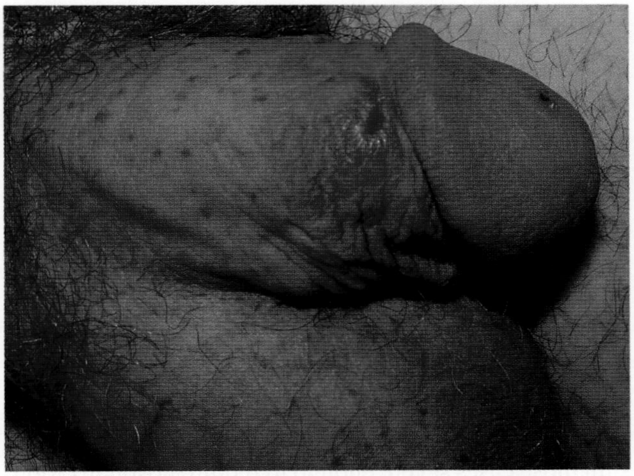

FIG. 89-1. Syphilis chancre in a male. A painless ulcer caused by syphilis is seen on the distal penile shaft with a smaller erosion on the glans. The ulcer is quite firm on palpation. (Reproduced with permission from Wolff K, Johnson RA: *Fitzpatrick's Color Atlas and Synopsis of Clinical Dermatology*, 6th ed. © 2009 by McGraw-Hill, Inc., New York.)

contact (including the vagina or cervix). The primary chancre heals and disappears after 3 to 6 weeks.

- The secondary stage occurs several weeks after the chancre disappears. Rash and lymphadenopathy are the most common symptoms. The rash starts on the trunk, spreads to the palms and soles, and is polymorphous, most often dull red and papular (similar to that of *Pityriasis rosacea*), but it may also take on other forms such as psoriatic or pustular lesions. The rash is not pruritic.
- Constitutional symptoms are common in the secondary stage, including fever, malaise, headache, and sore throat. Mucous membrane involvement ("mucous patches") includes oral or vaginal lesions, and condyloma lata, which are flat, moist, wartlike growths, may occur at the perineum, anogenital region, or adjacent areas (thighs). This stage also resolves spontaneously.
- *Latency* refers to the period between stages during which a patient is asymptomatic.
- Any patient with secondary or latent syphilis who presents with neurologic symptoms or findings should have a lumbar puncture and cerebrospinal fluid testing for neurosyphilis.
- Late- stage or tertiary syphilis, which is much less common (classically found in 33% of untreated patients), occurs years after the initial infection and affects primarily the cardiovascular and neurologic systems.
- Specific manifestations include neuropathy (tabes dorsalis), meningitis, dementia, and aortitis with aortic insufficiency and thoracic aneurysm formation.

DIAGNOSIS AND DIFFERENTIAL

- Syphilis may be diagnosed in the early stages with dark-field microscopic identification of the treponemes from the primary chancre or secondary condyloma or oral lesions.
- Serologic tests include nontreponemal (VDRL and rapid plasma reagin) and treponemal (fluorescent treponemal antibody absorption test).
- Nontreponemal test results are positive about 14 days after the appearance of the chancre. There is a false-positive rate of approximately 1% to 2% of the population.
- Treponemal tests are more sensitive and specific but harder to perform.

EMERGENCY DEPARTMENT CARE AND DISPOSITION

- Syphilis in all stages remains sensitive to penicillin, which is the drug of choice: benzathine penicillin G 2.4 million units IM as a single dose. Latent or tertiary syphilis is treated as above with 3-weekly IM injections.
- Doxycycline, 100 milligrams PO twice daily for 14 days, or Tetracycline, 500 milligrams four times daily for 14 days.
- Intravenous high-dose penicillin is the only treatment with proven benefit for neurosyphilis (tertiary).

HERPES SIMPLEX INFECTIONS

CLINICAL FEATURES

- Herpes simplex virus type 2 and, less often, type 1 cause genital herpes by invading mucosal surfaces or nonintact skin.
- In primary infections, clusters of painful pustules or vesicles on an erythematous base occur 7 to 10 days after contact with an infected person (see Fig. 89-2). These lesions ulcerate and may coalesce over the next 3 to 5 days, and in women a profuse watery vaginal discharge may develop.
- Tender inguinal adenopathy is usually present. Dysuria is common and may lead to frank urinary retention due to severe pain.
- Systemic symptoms are common in first infections and include fever, chills, headache, and myalgias.

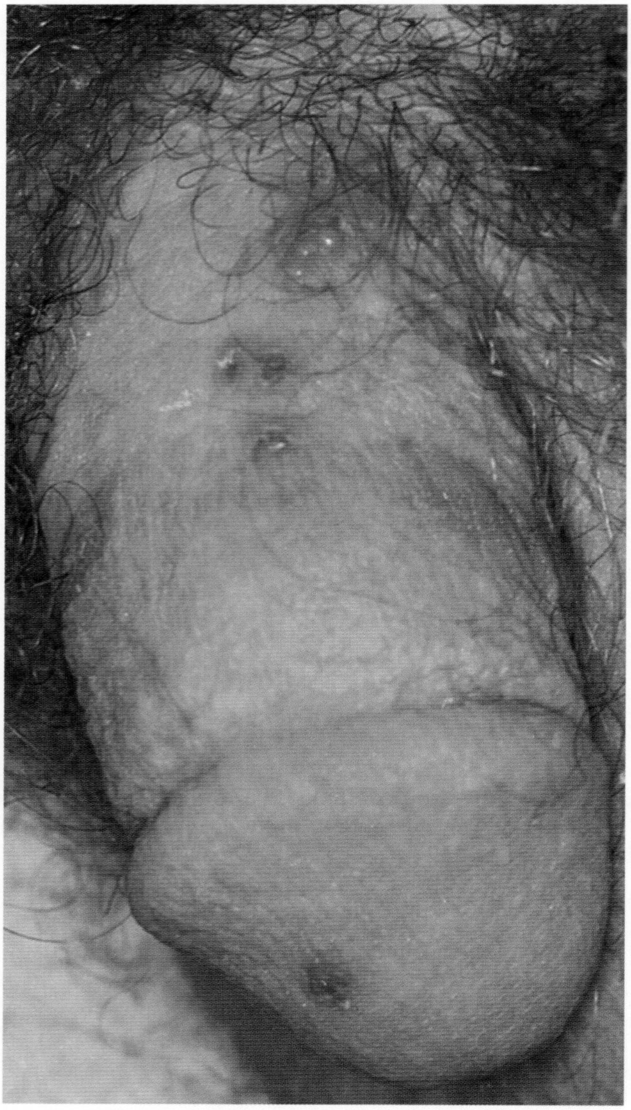

FIG. 89-2. Genital herpes in a male. Classic vesicles are shown proximally on the penis; several formerly vesicular lesions have crusted over. (Reproduced with permission from Wolff K, Goldsmith LA, Katz SI, et al: *Fitzpatrick's Dermatology in General Medicine*, 7th ed. © 2008 by McGraw-Hill, Inc., New York.)

The untreated illness lasts 2 to 3 weeks and then heals without scarring.

- The virus remains latent in the body, however, and continues to be shed in urogenital secretions of asymptomatic patients, making transmission to partners possible.
- Recurrences occur in most patients (60%-90%) but are usually briefer and milder without systemic symptoms.

DIAGNOSIS AND DIFFERENTIAL

- The diagnosis is usually clinical, based on the characteristic appearance.
- Viral cultures for herpes simplex virus taken from vesicles or early ulcers are more reliable than the Tzanck smear for intranuclear inclusions.

EMERGENCY DEPARTMENT CARE AND DISPOSITION

- Treatment of choice for primary genital herpes is a 7- to 10-day course of acyclovir 400 milligrams PO three times daily, valacyclovir 1 gram PO twice daily, or famciclovir 250 milligrams PO three times daily.
- In those cases severe enough to require hospitalization, treatment with intravenous acyclovir 5 to 10 milligrams/kg body weight every 8 hours IV may be given.
- Treatment for episodes of recurrent genital herpes consist of a 5-day course of acyclovir 400 milligrams PO three times daily, valacyclovir 500 milligrams twice daily or 1 gram PO once daily, or famciclovir 125 milligrams PO twice daily.
- If started at the onset of symptoms, antiviral therapy may reduce the severity and duration of the episode.

CHANCROID

CLINICAL FEATURES

- Caused by *Haemophilus ducreyi,* a pleomorphic gram-negative bacillus, chancroid is more common in the tropics, but in recent years there has been a rise in cases in the United States, with epidemic outbreaks.
- Incubation is 4 to 10 days.
- A tender papule on an erythematous base appears on the external genitalia and then over 1 to 2 days erodes to become a painful purulent or pustular ulcer with irregular edges (see Fig. 89-3).
- Multiple ulcers may be present. The ulcers are usually 1 to 2 cm in diameter with sharp, undermined margins and are very painful. "Kissing lesions" may occur due to autoinoculation of adjacent skin.
- Tender inguinal adenopathy, usually unilateral, follows in 50% of untreated patients within 1 to 2 weeks, and these nodes may mat together to form a mass (bubo) that becomes necrotic, suppurates, and drains. Constitutional symptoms are rare.

DIAGNOSIS AND DIFFERENTIAL

- Diagnosis is usually clinical, with care to exclude syphilis. Sometimes the organism may be cultured from a swab of the ulcer or pus from a bubo, but special media are required.

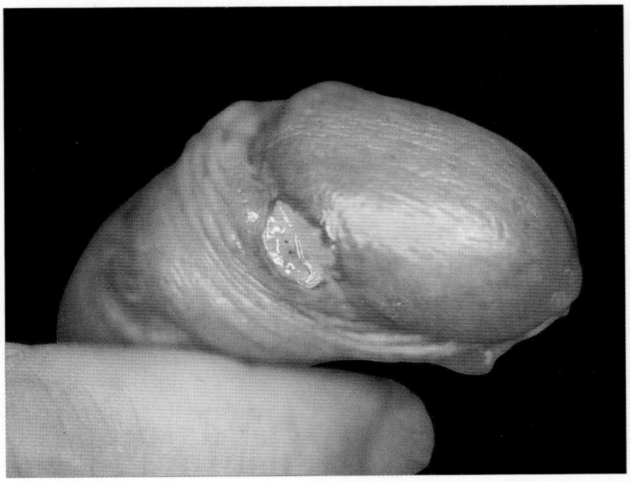

FIG. 89-3. Chancroid ulcer in a male. The lesion is very painful. The friable base of the ulcer is covered with yellow-gray necrotic exudates. (Reproduced with permission from Wolff K, Goldsmith LA, Katz SI, et al: *Fitzpatrick's Dermatology in General Medicine*, 7th ed. © 2008 by McGraw-Hill, Inc., New York.)

EMERGENCY DEPARTMENT CARE AND DISPOSITION

- Treatment regimens include azithromycin 1 gram PO as a single dose, ceftriaxone 250 milligrams IM as a single dose, erythromycin 500 milligrams PO three times a day for 7 days, or ciprofloxacin 500 milligrams PO twice daily for 3 days.
- Symptoms usually improve within 3 days, but large ulcers may require 2 to 3 weeks to heal.
- Buboes may be aspirated to relieve pain from swelling but should not be excised.

LYMPHOGRANULOMA VENEREUM

CLINICAL FEATURES

- Three serotypes of *C. trachomatis* are associated with lymphogranuloma venereum (LGV), which is endemic in other parts of the world but uncommon in the United States.
- The primary lesion, usually occurring 5 to 21 days after exposure, is a painless, small papule or vesicle (see Fig. 89-4) that may go unnoticed and heals spontaneously in 2 to 3 days.
- After anal intercourse, primary LGV may present as painful mucopurulent or bloody proctitis.
- Several weeks to months after the primary lesion, painful inguinal adenopathy (unilateral in 60%) occurs. The nodes mat together to form a bubo (often with a purplish hue to the overlying skin) and often suppurate and form fistulae.
- "Groove sign," an indentation across the bubo that parallels the inguinal ligament, may be seen. Systemic symptoms may include fever, chills, arthralgias, erythema nodosum, and, rarely, meningoencephalitis. Late sequelae include scarring; urethral, vaginal, and anal strictures; and occasionally lymphatic obstruction.

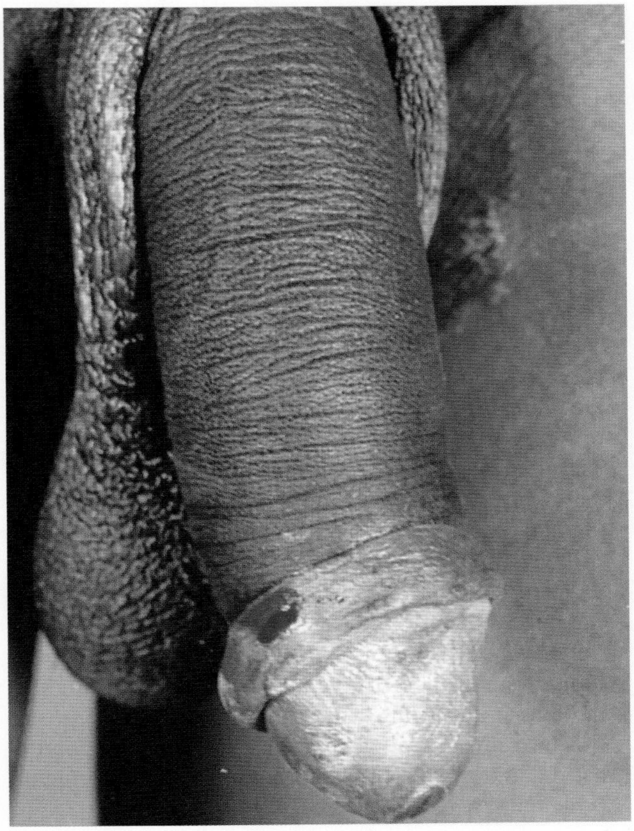

FIG. 89-4. Lymphogranuloma venereum chancre. This ulceration was painless to the patient. (Reproduced with permission from Wolff K, Goldsmith LA, Katz SI, et al: *Fitzpatrick's Dermatology in General Medicine*, 7th ed. © 2008 by McGraw-Hill, Inc., New York.)

DIAGNOSIS AND DIFFERENTIAL

- Diagnosis is through serologic testing and culture of LGV from a lesion. A complement fixation titer for LGV greater than 1:64 is consistent with infection.

EMERGENCY DEPARTMENT CARE AND DISPOSITION

- Doxycycline 100 milligrams PO twice daily for 21 days is the treatment of choice.
- An alternative is erythromycin 500 milligrams PO four times daily for 21 days.

■ GENITAL WARTS

CLINICAL FEATURES

- Human papillomaviruses (HPV) are DNA viruses that are transmitted by direct contact and cause venereal or anogenital warts.
- The incubation period from contact to appearance of warts varies from 1 to 8 months.
- Genital warts begin as flesh-colored papules or cauliflower-like projections that may eventually coalesce to form condyloma acuminata. They may take on a flat appearance on the cervix.
- Venereal warts commonly occur at the urethra, frenulum, coronal sulcus of the penis, and perianal regions in men, and in women they are common at the posterior introitus and adjacent labia, in the vagina, on the cervix, and often spread to other parts of the perineum (vulva and anus).

DIAGNOSIS AND DIFFERENTIAL

- Diagnosis is often clinical, but may be confirmed by skin biopsy and histologic methods or by soaking the suspected skin with dilute acetic acid for 3 minutes; normal skin remains shiny white in color, while areas of wart-neoplasia become dull gray-white in color.

EMERGENCY DEPARTMENT CARE AND DISPOSITION

- One treatment option is podofilox, 0.5% solution or gel, applied with a cotton swab or a finger to the visible warts twice a day for 3 days, followed by 4 days of no therapy, with the cycle repeated up to four times.
- Also recommended is imiquimod, 5% cream, applied at bedtime three times a week for up to 16 weeks. The treatment area should be washed 6 to 10 hours after treatment with imiquimod.
- Most patients experience a local inflammatory reaction after treatment.
- Many patients prefer treatment by a dermatologist using cryotherapy or trichloroacetic acid, and referral is needed for large accumulations of warts.
- Refer patients to a dermatologist, urologist, or ob-gyn specialist.

For further reading in Tintinalli's *Emergency Medicine: A Comprehensive Study Guide,* 7th ed., see Chapter 141, "Sexually Transmitted Diseases," by Joel Kravitz and Susan B. Promes.

90 TOXIC SHOCK SYNDROME AND STREPTOCOCCAL TOXIC SHOCK SYNDROME

Manoj Pariyadath

■ TOXIC SHOCK SYNDROME

EPIDEMIOLOGY

- Toxic shock syndrome (TSS) is a severe, toxin-mediated, life-threatening syndrome that initially was associated with the use of tampons by menstruating women, although most cases are no longer related to these factors.
- Risk factors for TSS include current menstruation, cutaneous lesions including burns, recent surgical procedures, postpartum/postabortion status, use of vaginally inserted devices such as sponges or diaphragms, and nasal packing. Other less common associations include sinusitis, pharyngitis, intrauterine device use, and body art such as tattoos or piercings.
- Risk factors in children <2 years of age include nonsurgical skin and soft tissue lesions and infections.
- One-tenth of the TSS cases are seen in men, with a mortality rate 3.3 times that of menstruating women.

PATHOPHYSIOLOGY

- The majority of TSS cases have been directly associated with colonization or infection with *Staphylococcus aureus*. Production of toxic shock syndrome toxin-1 (TSST-1) is responsible for the clinical manifestation of most cases of menstruation-related TSS via direct toxic effects or through release of secondary mediators. Biochemically similar toxins have been identified in non-menstruation-related TSS.
- TSS-1 production is enhanced by certain vaginal conditions including temperature of 39°C to 40°C, neutral pH, partial pressure of oxygen >5%, and supplemental carbon dioxide. These conditions can be met during menses and with the introduction of tampons or intravaginal devices.
- Marked vasodilatation, movement of serum proteins and fluids from the intravascular to the extravascular space, depressed cardiac function, and total body

water deficits result in hypotension. Subsequent multisystem organ failure may reflect either a direct effect of the toxin on tissues or the rapid onset of hypotension and decreased perfusion.

CLINICAL FEATURES

- TSS is characterized by high fever, profound hypotension, diffuse erythrodermatous rash, mucous membrane hyperemia, diffuse myalgias, headache, sore throat, vomiting, diarrhea, and constitutional symptoms that rapidly progress to multisystem dysfunction.
- Patients are ill appearing. Other features include tender painful genitalia with vaginal hyperemia, nonpitting edema, rhabdomyolysis, and non-focal neurologic abnormalities without signs of meningeal irritation.
- Women with menstruation-related TSS typically present between the third and fifth day of menses. Postoperative patients develop symptoms in 2 days.
- The rash associated with TSS is a diffuse, blanchable erythroderma, often described as a "painless sunburn." Generalized desquamation with notable peeling over the palms and soles occurs on day 6 to 10 of illness.

DIAGNOSIS AND DIFFERENTIAL

- Diagnostic criteria are listed in Table 90-1.
- TSS should be considered in any acute febrile illness associated with erythroderma, hypotension, and multiorgan involvement and should be considered before all diagnostic criteria are met.
- Lab values involved in the diagnostic criteria of TSS and that should be included in the workup are complete blood cell count, serum creatinine and blood urea nitrogen (BUN), urine analysis, liver function tests, and blood cultures. Throat cultures, cerebrospinal fluid cultures, and titers for disease processes such as Rocky Mountain spotted fever should be obtained if indicated.
- Other syndromes to consider in the differential diagnosis of TSS include streptococcal TSS, Kawasaki's disease, staphylococcal scalded skin syndrome, Rocky Mountain spotted fever, and septic shock.

EMERGENCY DEPARTMENT CARE AND DISPOSITION

- The treatment of TSS consists of airway management, aggressive management of circulatory shock, continuous monitoring of vital signs and urinary output, use of antistaphylococcal antimicrobial agents with β-lactamase stability, and the search for a focus of infection.
- Crystalloid IV fluids should be used initially for hypotension and fluid resuscitation. A central venous pressure (CVP) or Swan–Ganz catheter may be necessary for patient monitoring if there is an inadequate response to initial fluid resuscitation. Large volumes of fluid (up to 20 L) may be required over the first 24 hours.

TABLE 90-1 Diagnostic Criteria for Toxic Shock Syndrome

Fever	Temperature ≥ 38.9°C (102°F)	
Skin findings	Rash: diffuse macular edema Desquamation: 1-2 weeks after onset of illness	
Hypotension	Systolic BP <90 mm Hg for adults or less than fifth percentile by age for children	
Multisystem involvement	Three or more of the following:	
	Gastrointestinal	Vomiting or diarrhea at onset of illness
	Hepatic	Total bilirubin, alanine aminotransferase enzyme, or aspartate aminotransferase enzyme levels at least twice the upper limit of normal for laboratory
	Hematologic	Platelets <100,000/mL
	Mucous membranes	Vaginal, oropharyngeal, or conjunctival hyperemia
	Central nervous system	Disorientation or alterations in consciousness
	Muscular	Severe myalgias or creatinine phosphokinase elevation twice normal
	Renal	Blood urea nitrogen or creatinine at least twice the upper limit of normal or laboratory or urinary sediment with pyuria (≥5 leukocytes per high-power field) in the absence of urinary tract infection
Lab findings	Negative cultures and titers for alternative organisms	

Case is considered probable when five of these six criteria are met and confirmed when all six are present unless mortality occurs before desquamation.

- Patients with evidence of bleeding and abnormal coagulation profiles or thrombocytopenia may require blood products.
- Culture all potentially infected sites, including blood, prior to initiating antibiotic therapy.
- Tampons or nasal packing should be removed, if present.
- A dopamine or norepinephrine infusion may be necessary to augment fluid resuscitation for refractory hypotension.
- Initiate antistaphylococcal antimicrobial therapy with β-lactamase stability. Nafcillin or oxacillin in doses of 2 grams IV every 4 hours, or a cephalosporin such as cefazolin given 2 grams every 6 hours, provides adequate coverage. Some authors recommend clindamycin, 600 to 900 milligrams IV every 8 hours, or linezolid, 600 milligrams IV every 12 hours because of evidence that these antibiotics may decrease toxin production. Vancomycin, 1 gram every 12 hours, should be used if methicillin-resistant strains of staphlococci are suspected. In penicillin-allergic patients, clindamycin, vancomycin, or potentially cephalosporins may be used.
- Administration of methylprednisolone and intravenous immunoglobulin (IVIG) may result in clinical improvement. IVIG, 1 to 2 grams/kg, should be considered if there is no clinical improvement after 6 hours of aggressive supportive care.
- Patients are typically admitted to the ICU.
- Recurrence of TSS can be seen in patients not treated with β-lactamase–stable antibiotics.

STREPTOCOCCAL TOXIC SHOCK SYNDROME

EPIDEMIOLOGY

- Streptococcal TSS is defined as any group A streptococcal infection associated with invasive soft tissue infection, early onset of shock, and organ failure. Streptococcal toxic shock is very similar to staphylococcal TSS; however, streptococcal toxic shock is associated with a soft tissue infection that is culture positive for *Streptococcus pyogenes*.
- Streptococcal toxic shock commonly affects individuals between the ages of 20 and 50 years who may be without predisposing illness.
- Risk factors for group A streptococcal infections include extremes of age, diabetes, alcohol or drug abuse, treatment with NSAIDs, and immunodeficiency.

PATHOPHYSIOLOGY

- Virulent streptococcal pyogenic exotoxins are produced by 90% of group A streptococcal isolates and are felt to be accountable for the multisystem failure seen with streptococcal toxic shock.
- The portals of entry of streptococci include the pharynx, vagina, mucosa, and skin in 50% of streptococcal toxic shock cases, but the source cannot be identified in most cases.
- Infection may begin with minor local trauma, although disruption of the skin is not required.

CLINICAL FEATURES

- Pain is the most common presenting symptom, and is often out of proportion to physical findings and abrupt in onset.
- Disease may be heralded by a prodromal episode of fever, chills, myalgias, and diarrhea.
- The development of vesicles and bullae at the site of soft tissue infection, which progresses to violaceous or blue discoloration, is considered an ominous sign of necrotizing fasciitis or myositis.
- Adult respiratory distress syndrome develops in 55% of patients, usually following the onset of hypotension.
- Patients are usually febrile, hypotensive, and confused, and develop multisystem organ dysfunction.

DIAGNOSIS AND DIFFERENTIAL

- Diagnostic criteria are listed in Table 90-2.
- When considering streptococcal toxic shock, look for soft tissue infection and culture the site. Laboratory evaluation includes CBC, arterial blood gas (ABG), liver function tests, serum creatinine and BUN, serum electrolytes including magnesium and calcium, coagulation profile, blood cultures, CXR, ECG, and urinalysis (UA).
- Consider TSS, invasive infections caused by group A streptococci, serious infections caused by other bacteria including *Clostridium perfringens*, Kawasaki's disease, Rocky Mountain spotted fever, and septic shock.

EMERGENCY DEPARTMENT CARE AND DISPOSITION

- Treatment is similar to that for TSS, with airway management and aggressive fluid resuscitation with vasopressors as needed.
- Begin antistreptococcal antimicrobial therapy with IV penicillin G, 24 million U/d in divided doses; IV clindamycin, 900 milligrams every 8 hours; or IV linezolid, 600 milligrams IV every 12 hours. In penicillin-allergic patients substitute ceftriaxone 2 grams IV q24h (at the discretion of the treating physician) and clindamycin 900 milligrams IV q8h.

TABLE 90-2 Diagnostic Criteria for Streptococcal Toxic Shock Syndrome

Skin findings	Generalized erythematous macular rash that may desquamate	
Hypotension	Systolic BP <90 mm Hg for adults or less than fifth percentile by age for children	
Multisystem involvement	Two or more of the following:	
	Respiratory	Acute respiratory distress syndrome
	Hepatic	Enzyme or bilirubin level twice normal
	Hematologic	Platelet count <100,00 or DIC
	Soft tissue	Necrosis, including necrotizing fasciitis or myositis, or gangrene
	Renal	Creatinine level twice normal
Lab findings	Negative cultures and titers for alternative organisms	

Case is considered probable if all criteria are met and group A streptococcus cultured from nonsterile side and confirmed if all criteria are met and group A streptococcus cultured from a site normally considered sterile.

- Obtain immediate surgical consultation, as most patients with streptococcal toxic shock require debridement, fasciotomy, or amputation.
- IVIG may be considered.
- All patients suspected of having streptococcal toxic shock require admission to the ICU.

For further reading in Tintinalli's *Emergency Medicine: A Comprehensive Study Guide*, 7th ed., see Chapter 145, "Toxic Shock Syndrome and Streptococcal Toxic Shock Syndrome," by Shawna J. Perry and Reneé D. Reid.

91 SEPTIC SHOCK

John Gough

EPIDEMIOLOGY

- The majority of sepsis is caused by gram-negative and gram-positive bacteria; however, sepsis can be caused by any class of microorganism including fungi, mycobacteria, viruses, rickettsiae, and protozoa.
- Predisposing factors for gram-negative bacterial sepsis include diabetes mellitus, lymphoproliferative diseases, cirrhosis, burns, invasive procedures, and chemotherapy.
- Risk factors for gram-positive sepsis include vascular catheters, burns, indwelling mechanical devices, and injection drug use.
- Nonbacterial sepsis is more commonly seen in immunocompromised individuals.

DEFINITIONS

- **SIRS (systemic inflammatory response syndrome):** Not synonymous with sepsis. SIRS is a means of stratifying patients with an inflammatory response and is defined by identifying at least two of the following criteria:
  A. Core temperature—>38.3°C (100.9°F) (>38.5°C [101.3°F] in children), or <36°C (96.8°F)
  B. Tachycardia—>90 bpm (>2 SD [standard deviations] above normal for children, or in <1 year bradycardia [10th percentile for age] in absence of external stimuli, long-term use of drugs, or pain)
  C. Mean respiratory rate—>20 breaths/min (>2 SD above normal for age in children) or $Paco_2$ <32
  D. Leukocyte count—>12,000/mm^3, or <4000/mm^3, or >10% bands (in children elevated or depressed for age)
- **Sepsis:** A systemic response to infection, manifested by two or more of the SIRS criteria
- **Severe sepsis:** Sepsis plus either cardiovascular organ dysfunction or acute respiratory distress syndrome (ARDS), or two other organ dysfunctions
- **Septic shock:** Acute circulatory failure characterized by persistent arterial hypotension

CLINICAL FEATURES

- Hyperthermia or hypothermia may be seen with sepsis.
- The most frequent mental status change is obtundation. Neurologic findings are nonfocal and range from mild disorientation to confusion, lethargy, agitation, and coma.

- Cardiovascular manifestations in the early stages commonly include tachycardia, wide pulse pressure, and vasodilation. Cardiac output (CO) and stroke volume are usually initially maintained. As sepsis progresses, hypotension is common.
- Respiratory manifestations—tachypnea and hypoxemia—are common. Sepsis is the most common condition associated with acute lung injury and ARDS.
- Renal manifestations include acute renal failure with azotemia, oliguria, and active urinary sediment. Factors associated with the development of renal failure in septic shock include hypotension, dehydration, aminoglycoside administration, and pigmenturia.
- The most frequent hepatic abnormality is cholestatic jaundice. Concentrations of transaminase, alkaline phosphatase, and bilirubin increase. Red blood cell hemolysis causes jaundice.
- Major blood loss secondary to upper GI bleeding occurs in only a small percentage of patients with sepsis. However, minor blood loss may be seen within 24 hours.
- The most frequent hematologic changes are neutropenia or neutrophilia, thrombocytopenia, and disseminated intravascular coagulation (DIC). Neutrophilic leukocytosis with a "left shift" is common. Neutropenia, occurring rarely, is associated with an increase in mortality.
- Thrombocytopenia frequently arises as a consequence of DIC, although isolated thrombocytopenia is present in >30% of cases of sepsis. Thrombocytopenia may be an early clue to bacteremia, and serial platelet measurements may be useful in evaluating the patient's response to therapy.
- DIC is a frequent finding in patients with septic shock. Gram-negative infections precipitate DIC more readily than do gram-positive infections. Laboratory studies suggesting the presence of DIC include thrombocytopenia, prolonged prothrombin and activated partial thromboplastin values, decreased fibrinogen and antithrombin III levels, and increased fibrin monomer, fibrin split products, and D-dimer levels.
- Hyperglycemia can develop, even without a history of diabetes. Uncontrolled hyperglycemia is a significant risk for adverse outcome. Hypoglycemia is reported but uncommon.
- Blood gas analysis performed early in the course of septic shock usually demonstrates respiratory alkalosis. As perfusion worsens and continues, tissue hypoxia generates more lactic acid and metabolic acidosis worsens.
- Cutaneous lesions that occur as a result of sepsis can be divided into five categories: direct bacterial involvement of the skin and underlying soft tissues (cellulitis, erysipelas, and fasciitis); lesions from hematogenous seeding of the skin or the underlying tissue (petechiae, pustules, cellulitis, ecthyma gangrenosum); lesions resulting from hypotension and/or DIC (acrocyanosis and necrosis of peripheral tissues); lesions secondary to intravascular infections (microemboli and/or immune complex vasculitis); and lesions caused by toxins (toxic shock syndrome).

DIAGNOSIS AND DIFFERENTIAL

- Septic shock should be suspected in any patient with a temperature of >38.3°C (>100.9°F) (>38.5°C [101.3°F] in children) or <36°C (<96.8°F) and a systolic blood pressure of <90 mm Hg (or 2 SD below normal for age in children) with evidence of inadequate organ perfusion. The hypotension of septic shock does not typically reverse with rapid volume replacement.
- Other common features of sepsis include obtundation; hyperventilation; hot, flushed skin; and a widened pulse pressure.
- In elderly, very young, or immunocompromised patients, the clinical presentation may be atypical, with no fever or localized source of infection.
- The differential diagnosis of septic shock includes the other nonseptic causes of shock such as cardiogenic, hypovolemic, anaphylactic, neurogenic, obstructive (pulmonary embolism, tamponade), and endocrine (adrenal insufficiency, thyroid storm) causes.
- There is no specific laboratory test for the diagnosis of septic shock. Basic laboratory studies should include a complete blood count and platelet count; DIC panel; levels of serum electrolytes; liver function panel; renal function panel; arterial blood gas analysis and lactic acid level; and urinalysis. Blood should be typed and crossmatched if low hematocrit is suspected.
- A chest radiograph (CXR) should be part of the basic evaluation. Flat and upright abdominal views are helpful in patients in whom perforation is suspected as a potential source of abdomen-related sepsis. Use of CT scanning and US should be obtained when appropriate.
- Perform lumbar puncture in any patient with a clinical presentation compatible with meningitis. In individuals with papilledema, focal neurologic deficits, or the potential for brain abscess or epidural or subdural empyema, defer lumbar puncture until an imaging study is performed. If meningitis is an important consideration, however, give an empiric antimicrobial prior to the imaging study.
- Obtain at least two separate sets of specimens for blood cultures. Perform gram staining and culture of secretions from any potential site of infection.

- C-reactive protein (CRP) levels are elevated in sepsis. Procalcitonin level has greater sensitivity, specificity, and overall accuracy, and better predictive power in sepsis and septic shock than does CRP level.
- Serum lactate acid level can help in determining prognosis. Patients with higher early clearance of lactic acid have improved outcomes; those with intermediate to high lactate levels have a higher mortality.

EMERGENCY DEPARTMENT CARE AND DISPOSITION

EARLY GOAL-DIRECTED THERAPY

- (1) Optimization of oxygenation, ventilation, and circulation; (2) initiation of drug therapy, including antibiotics; and (3) control of the source of sepsis. Studies have demonstrated that mortality rates for goal-directed therapy are lower than with usual care.
- The ABCs of resuscitation should be addressed. Aggressive airway management with high-flow oxygen (keeping oxygen saturation greater than 90%) through endotracheal intubation may be necessary.
- Hemodynamic stabilization: rapid infusion of crystalloid IV fluid (LR or NS) at 500 mL (20 mL/kg in children) every 5 to 10 minutes should be accomplished. Often, 4 to 6 L (60 mL/kg in children) is necessary.
- In the early goal-directed therapy guidelines, early invasive monitoring (central venous pressure and, in appropriate cases, monitoring via arterial catheter) is recommended. Current recommendations are to maintain central venous pressures between 8 and 12 mm Hg, mean arterial pressure >65 mm Hg, and venous oxygenation saturation level >70%. Keep the patient's hematocrit at >30%.
- If there is no hemodynamic response after administration of 3 to 4 L of fluid, or if there are signs of fluid overload, an infusion of dopamine or norepinephrine can be started. The dopamine dose ranges from 5 to 20 micrograms/kg/min. If there is no response to an infusion of 20 micrograms/kg/min, start norepinephrine to keep the mean arterial pressure at least at 65 mm Hg. Usual doses of norepinephrine range from 2.5 to 20 micrograms/kg/min. Once the blood pressure and perfusion have been stabilized by norepinephrine, use the lowest dose that maintains blood pressure to minimize vasoconstriction.
- Pediatric septic shock requires a different approach to inotropic support. Low cardiac output is associated with mortality. Oxygen delivery, not oxygen extraction, is the major determinant of oxygen consumption. Infants <6 months of age are insensitive to dopamine and dobutamine. Pediatric dopamine-resistant shock commonly responds to norepinephrine or epinephrine.
- The source of infection must be removed (eg, removal of indwelling catheters and incision and drainage of abscesses).
- Empiric antibiotic therapy is ideally begun after obtaining cultures, but administration should not be delayed. Dosages should be the maximum allowed and given intravenously. A partial list of initial doses is listed below.

ADULTS (NON-NEUTROPENIC)

- When the source is unknown, therapy should be effective against gram-positive and gram-negative organisms. In adults imipenem 500 milligrams IV every 6 hours can be used.
- Alternatives include ertapenem, 1 gram IV every 24 hours, plus vancomycin, 15 milligrams/kg every 6 hours or 1 gram IV every 12 hours.
- If pneumonia is a suspected source: ceftriaxone, 1 to 2 grams IV every 12 hours, plus azithromycin, 500 milligrams IV, then 250 milligrams IV every 24 hours, or levofloxacin, 750 milligrams IV every 24 hours, or moxifloxacin, 400 milligrams IV every 24 hours, plus vancomycin, 15 milligrams/kg IV every 6 hours, or 1 gram IV every 12 hours.
- If a biliary source is suspected: ampicillin/sulbactam, 3 grams IV every 6 hours, or piperacillin/tazobactam, 4.5 grams IV every 6 hours, or ticarcillin/clavulanate, 3.1 grams IV every 4 hours.
- When an intra-abdominal source is suspected: imipenem, 500 milligrams IV every 6 hours to 1 gram IV q8 hours, or meropenem, 1 gram IV 8 hours, or doripenem, 500 milligrams IV every 8 hours, or ertapenem, 1 gram IV every 24 hours, or ampicillin/sulbactam, 3 grams IV every 6 hours, or piperacillin/tazobactam, 4.5 grams IV every 6 hours.
- If a urinary source: piperacillin/tazobactam, 4.5 grams IV every 6 hours, or ampicillin, 1 to 2 grams IV every 4 to 6 hours, plus gentamicin, 1.0 to 1.5 milligrams/kg every 8 hours.
- With IV drug use or indwelling devices, there is a high probability of gram-positive etiology; vancomycin 15 milligrams/kg IV every 6 hours or 1 gram IV every 12 hours is recommended.

CHILDREN (NON-NEUTROPENIC)

- Neonates <1 week of age: ampicillin, 25 milligrams/kg IV every 8 hours, plus cefotaxime, 50 milligrams/kg IV every 12 hours.
- Neonates 1 to 4 weeks: ampicillin, 25 milligrams/kg IV every 6 hours, plus cefotaxime, 50 milligrams/kg IV every 8 hours.

- Infants over 3 months: ceftriaxone, 75 milligrams/kg IV every 24 hours, or cefotaxime, 50 milligrams/kg IV every 8 hours.
- Children over 3 months: ceftriaxone, 75 to 100 milligrams/kg every 24 hours, or cefotaxime, 50 milligrams/kg IV every 8 hours. Consider vancomycin, 15 milligrams/kg IV every 6 hours, or 1 gram IV every 12 hours.

NEUTROPENIC CHILDREN AND ADULTS

- Ceftazidime, 2 grams IV every 8 hours; for children, 50 milligrams/kg IV every 8 hours up to adult dosage *or* imipenem, 500 milligrams IV every 6 hours to 1 gram IV every 8 hours; for children: age >3 months, 15 to 25 milligrams/kg IV every 6 hours; age 1 to 3 months, 25 milligrams/kg IV every 6 hours; age 1 to 4 weeks, 25 milligrams/kg IV every 8 hours; age <1 week, 25 milligrams/kg IV every 12 hours, *select one agent above plus* vancomycin, 15 milligrams/kg IV 6 hours.
- DIC should be treated with fresh-frozen plasma, 15 to 20 mL/kg initially, to keep PT at 1.5 to 2 times normal, and treated with a platelet infusion of 6 U, to maintain a serum concentration of at least 50,000/μL.
- Corticosteroids are not recommended for septic patients who are not in shock. Dosages of hydrocortisone should be ≤300 milligrams/d. An adrenocorticotropic hormone stimulation test is not recommended, and hydrocortisone is preferred over dexamethasone.
- Current international guidelines recommend "judicious glycemic control" to keep glucose levels <150 milligrams/dL in patients with septic shock.

For further reading in Tintinalli's *Emergency Medicine: A Comprehensive Study Guide,* 7th ed., see Chapter 146, "Septic Shock," by Jonathan Jui.

92 SOFT TISSUE INFECTIONS

David M. Cline

- The management of soft tissue infections in the ED involves an understanding of appropriate antibiotic treatment, outpatient or inpatient treatment options, and an understanding of when surgical intervention is necessary.

METHICILLIN-RESISTANT *STAPHYLOCOCCUS AUREUS*

- Community-acquired methicillin-resistant *Staphylococcus aureus* (MRSA) is epidemic across all populations.
- A significant majority of soft tissue infections in adults and children are caused by community-acquired MRSA.
- Understanding the treatment of community-acquired MRSA is vital for those managing soft tissue infections in the ED.

CLINICAL FEATURES

- Lesions are typically warm, red, and tender, and may be draining a purulent fluid.
- MRSA lesions are frequently mistaken as spider bites by patients as well as clinicians.

DIAGNOSIS AND DIFFERENTIAL

- The diagnosis of MRSA is largely clinical.
- Community-acquired MRSA should be considered in any infection where *S. aureus* or *Streptococcus* is typically considered the etiologic agent. This includes skin and soft tissue infections as well as sepsis and pneumonia.
- Bedside ultrasound is helpful to identify abscess collections in equivocal cases (see Fig. 92-1).

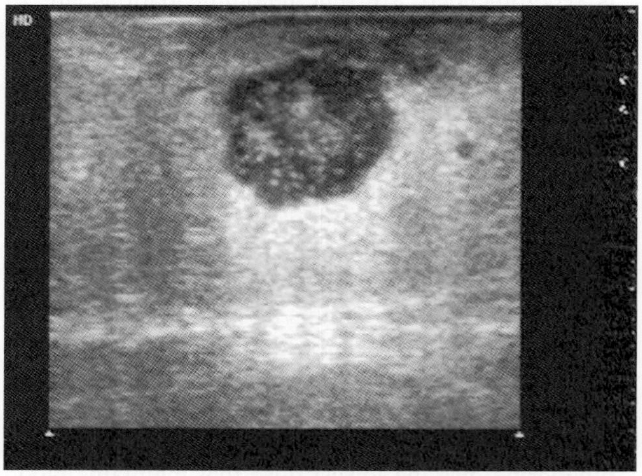

FIG. 92-1. Typical appearance of a subcutaneous abscess on a thigh. The abscess cavity is rounded and hypoechoic with mixed internal echogenicity. There is posterior acoustic enhancement that reflects the liquid nature of the abscess contents. The surrounding skin is hyperechoic because of adjacent tissue edema and possibly cellulitis. (Reproduced with permission from Ma OJ, Mateer JR, Blaivas M: *Emergency Ultrasound*, 2nd ed. Copyright © The McGraw-Hill Companies, 2008. All rights reserved. Figure 16-89.)

EMERGENCY DEPARTMENT CARE AND DISPOSITION

- For many community-acquired MRSA cutaneous infections, adequate incision and drainage is adequate to manage these infections. Suggested criteria for withholding antibiotics include abscesses that are small <5 cm, abscesses in immunocompetent patients, and abscesses without accompanying cellulitis.
- If local epidemiology supports MRSA as the likely etiology of cellulitis, antibiotics effective against MRSA should be given. These include clindamycin 300 milligrams PO four times daily or trimethoprim/sulfamethoxazole double-strength 1 to 2 tablets twice a day for 7 to 10 days.
- Consider adding cephalexin 500 milligrams four times daily to a regimen with trimethoprim/sulfamethoxazole to cover *Streptococcus*. If the infection is severe, vancomycin 1 gram every 12 hours should be used, and inpatient therapy is indicated.
- Patients who are at the extremes of age and have fever, significant comorbidities, or a large number of lesions may require admission for parenteral antibiotics.

NECROTIZING SOFT TISSUE INFECTIONS

- Necrotizing soft tissue infections are a spectrum of conditions that may be polymicrobial or monomicrobial.
- Group A *Streptococcus* and *S. aureus* are often the etiologic agents in monomicrobial infections.
- Clostridial infections are now uncommon due to improved hygiene and sanitation.

CLINICAL FEATURES

- Patients present with pain out of proportion to physical findings and a sense of heaviness in the affected part.
- Physical findings typically include a combination of edema, brownish skin discoloration, bullae, malodorous serosanguineous discharge, and crepitance.
- The patient frequently has a low-grade fever and tachycardia out of proportion to the fever.
- Mental status changes, including delirium and irritability, may accompany necrotizing soft tissue infections.

DIAGNOSIS AND DIFFERENTIAL

- Familiarity with the disease and an appreciation of the subtle physical findings are the most important factors in making the diagnosis of necrotizing soft tissue infections.
- Additional findings that may confirm the clinical suspicion include gas within soft tissue on plain radiographs, metabolic acidosis, coagulopathy, hyponatremia, leukocytosis, anemia, thrombocytopenia, myoglobinuria, and renal or hepatic dysfunction.

EMERGENCY DEPARTMENT CARE AND DISPOSITION

- The patient with necrotizing soft tissue infections should be adequately resuscitated with crystalloid intravenous (IV) fluids and packed red blood cells if there is significant hemolysis with anemia.
- Urine output and central venous pressure readings should be used to assess volume status.
- Vasoconstrictors should be avoided in these patients because of compromised perfusion in the affected extremity.
- IV antibiotics should be administered, including vancomycin 1 gram IV every 12 hours *plus* meropenem 500 to 1000 milligrams IV every 8 hours. Alternatively, piperacillin/tazobactam 4.5 grams IV every 6 hours may be used. The use of clindamycin should also be considered as it inhibits toxin synthesis.
- Tetanus prophylaxis should be administered as indicated.
- Surgical consultation for debridement should be obtained immediately and may include fasciotomy or amputation.
- Hyperbaric oxygen therapy and IV immunoglobulin therapy are controversial and typically the decision of the treating surgeon.

CELLULITIS

- Cellulitis is a local soft tissue inflammatory response secondary to bacterial invasion of the skin.
- Cellulitis is more common in the elderly, immunocompromised patients, and patients with peripheral vascular disease.

CLINICAL FEATURES

- Cellulitis presents as localized tenderness, erythema, and induration.
- Lymphangitis and lymphadenitis may accompany cellulitis and indicate a more severe infection.
- Patients may have fever and chills but are infrequently bacteremic.

DIAGNOSIS AND DIFFERENTIAL

- The clinical presentation is usually sufficient for diagnosis.

- Obtaining a white cell count or blood cultures rarely changes management of otherwise healthy patients with simple cellulitis.
- The differential diagnosis includes any erythematous skin condition. Cellulitis of the lower extremity is sometimes complicated by deep venous thrombosis and may require venogram or Doppler studies for a complete evaluation.
- In patients with systemic toxicity (fever and leukocytosis), cultures of pus, bullae, or blood should be obtained.

EMERGENCY DEPARTMENT CARE AND DISPOSITION

- Simple cellulitis in which MRSA is not suspected can be treated in an outpatient setting using cephalexin 500 milligrams PO four times daily, dicloxacillin 500 milligrams PO four times daily, or clindamycin 300 milligrams four time daily.
- If local epidemiology supports a high likelihood of MRSA in patients with soft tissue infections, antibiotics effective against MRSA should be given. In these cases clindamycin, trimethoprim/sulfamethoxazole, or doxycycline ± cephalexin should be given (see treatment of MRSA in the first section of this chapter).
- All patients discharged should have close follow-up within 2 to 3 days to evaluate the cellulitis and response to therapy.
- Skin markers may be helpful to mark the extent of cellulitis in patients discharged from the ED.
- All patients with systemic toxicity or evidence of bacteremia should be admitted to the hospital. Patients with diabetes mellitus, alcoholism, or other immunosuppressive disorders should be considered for admission for IV antibiotics.
- IV antibiotics, such as clindamycin, vancomycin, or linezolid, should be used in patients requiring hospital admission.

ERYSIPELAS

- Erysipelas is a superficial cellulitis with lymphatic involvement caused primarily by group A *Streptococcus*. Infection is usually through a portal of entry in the skin.

CLINICAL FEATURES

- Onset is acute, with sudden high fever, chills, malaise, and nausea.
- Over the next 1 to 2 days, a small area of erythema with a burning sensation develops.

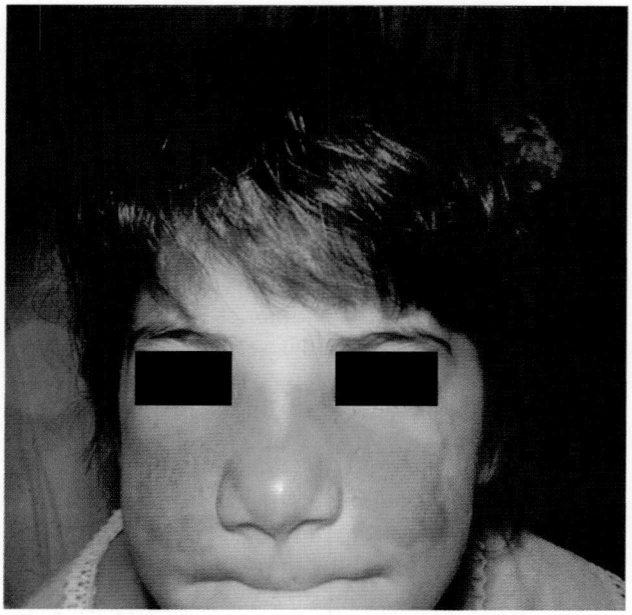

FIG. 92-2. Butterfly rash of erysipelas. The sharp demarcation between the salmon-red erythema and the normal surrounding skin is evident. (Reproduced with permission from Shah BR, Lucchesi M: *Atlas of Pediatric Emergency Medicine*, © 2006, McGraw-Hill, New York.)

- The erythema is sharply demarcated from the surrounding skin and is tense and painful (see Fig. 92-2).
- Lymphangitis and lymphadenitis are common.
- Purpura, bullae, and necrosis may accompany the erythema.
- It is primarily an infection of the lower extremities.

DIAGNOSIS AND DIFFERENTIAL

- The diagnosis is based primarily on physical findings.
- Leukocytosis is common.
- Cultures, Antistreptolysin O (ASO) titers, and anti-DNAase B titers are of little use in the ED. Differential diagnosis includes other forms of local cellulitis.
- Some believe necrotizing fasciitis is a complication of erysipelas and should be considered in all cases.

EMERGENCY DEPARTMENT CARE AND DISPOSITION

- Treatment is with parenteral antibiotics active against streptococci, including ceftriaxone 1 gram every 24 hours or cefazolin 1 to 2 grams every 8 hours.
- If it is difficult to distinguish between cellulitis and erysipelas, cover for *S. aureus* as well as streptococci (see above).

- If the disease is severe, treat for MRSA with vancomycin, clindamycin, or linezolid and admit to the hospital.
- Patients with mild disease may be treated with an initial dose of parenteral antibiotics and discharged on penicillin 500 milligrams PO every 6 hours.
- If the patient is allergic to penicillin, a macrolide or cephalosporin may be used.
- Duration of treatment is 5 to 10 days, and these patients should be re-evaluated in 2 days for follow-up.

CUTANEOUS ABSCESSES

- Cutaneous abscesses are the result of a breakdown in the cutaneous barrier, with subsequent contamination with resident bacterial flora. Incision and drainage is usually the only necessary treatment.

CLINICAL FEATURES AND DIAGNOSIS

- Patients present with an area of swelling, tenderness, and overlying erythema.
- The area of swelling is frequently fluctuant.
- Cutaneous abscesses are usually localized, although they may cause systemic toxicity in the immunosuppressed.
- Cutaneous abscesses should be inspected closely for predisposing injury and foreign bodies.
- Radiography may be indicated if foreign body is suspected.
- Needle aspiration or ultrasound may aid in the diagnosis when it is unclear whether the patient has an abscess or cellulitis (see Fig. 92-1).

EMERGENCY DEPARTMENT CARE AND DISPOSITION

- See Chapter 9 for information on procedural sedation.

Bartholin gland abscess

- Bartholin gland abscess presents as unilateral painful swelling of the labia with a fluctuant 1- to 2-cm mass.
- These infections are typically polymicrobial but may contain *Neisseria gonorrhoeae* and *Chlamydia trachomatis*.
- Routine antimicrobial treatment is not necessary unless there is a suspicion of sexually transmitted disease.
- Treatment involves incision and drainage along the vaginal mucosal surface of the abscess, generally followed by the insertion of a Word catheter.
- The Word catheter can be left in place for up to 4 weeks. Sitz baths are recommended after 2 days.
- Follow-up with gynecology is recommended within 2 days in patients with severe symptoms and within 1 week in patients with mild symptoms.

Hidradenitis suppurativa

- Hidradenitis suppurativa is a recurrent chronic infection involving the apocrine sweat glands.
- These abscesses tend to occur in the axilla and in the groin. The causative organism is usually *Staphylococcus*, although *Streptococcus* also may be present.
- The abscesses are typically multiple and in different stages of progression.
- ED treatment involves incision and drainage of any acute abscess, treating with antibiotics for any cellulitis that may be present, and referral to a surgeon for definitive treatment.

Infected sebaceous cysts

- Infected sebaceous cysts may develop in the sebaceous glands, which occur diffusely throughout the skin.
- Cysts present with an erythematous, tender, cutaneous mass that is often fluctuant.
- Incision and drainage is the appropriate ED treatment, with wound rechecks in 2 to 3 days in the ED or physician's office.
- The cyst contains a capsule that must be removed to prevent recurrence. This capsule can sometimes be grasped at the time of the initial incision and drainage; however, this is typically done at a later follow-up visit.

Pilonidal abscess

- Pilonidal abscess presents as a tender, swollen, and fluctuant mass along the superior gluteal fold.
- Treatment includes incision and drainage followed by iodoform gauze packing.
- The patient should be rechecked in 2 to 3 days, and the wound should be repacked.
- Surgical referral is usually necessary for definitive treatment.
- Antibiotics are not necessary unless there is an accompanying cellulitis.

Folliculitis and Carbuncles

- Staphylococcal soft tissue infection may cause folliculitis; the inflammation of a hair follicle is caused by bacterial invasion, and is usually treated with warm compresses.
- When deeper invasion occurs, the soft tissue surrounding the hair follicle becomes infected, and a furuncle (boil) is formed.

- Warm compresses are usually adequate to promote spontaneous drainage.
- If several furuncles coalesce, they may form a large area of interconnected sinus tracts and abscesses called a *carbuncle.*
- Carbuncles usually require surgical referral for wide excision.
- In the healthy, immunocompetent patient, routine use of antibiotics following abscess incision and drainage is not indicated unless there is a secondary infection.
- In the potentially immunocompromised patient, the threshold for antibiotic use should be lowered.
- Patients presenting with secondary cellulitis or systemic symptoms should be considered for antibiotic therapy.
- Abscesses involving the hands and face also should be treated more aggressively with antibiotics.
- Prophylaxis for endocarditis in patients with structural cardiac abnormalities should be considered (see Chapter 95 for information on those at risk).

SPOROTRICHOSIS

- Sporotrichosis is caused by traumatic inoculation of the fungus *Sporothrix schenckii,* which is found on plants and in the soil.

CLINICAL FEATURES

- After a 3-week incubation period, three types of infection may occur.
- The fixed cutaneous type occurs at the site of inoculation and looks like a crusted ulcer or verrucous plaque.
- The local cutaneous type also remains at the site of inoculation but presents as a subcutaneous nodule or pustule. The surrounding skin may become erythematous.
- The lymphocutaneous type is the most common of the three. It presents as a painless nodule at the site of inoculation that develops subcutaneous nodules that migrate along lymphatic channels.

DIAGNOSIS AND DIFFERENTIAL

- The diagnosis is based on the history and physical examination.
- Tissue biopsy cultures are often diagnostic but of limited use in the ED.
- The differential diagnosis includes tuberculosis, tularemia, cat-scratch disease, leishmaniasis, nocardiosis, and staphylococcal lymphangitis.

EMERGENCY DEPARTMENT CARE AND DISPOSITION

- Itraconazole 100 to 200 milligrams/d PO for 3 to 6 months is highly effective when treating sporotrichosis.
- If disseminated, sporotrichosis may be treated with IV amphotericin B 0.5 milligram/kg/d (after test doses to determine tolerability).
- Most cases of cutaneous sporotrichosis can be treated on an outpatient basis.
- Those patients who have systemic symptoms or who are acutely ill should be admitted for possible treatment with amphotericin B.

For further reading in Tintinalli's *Emergency Medicine: A Comprehensive Study Guide*, 7th ed., see Chapter 147, "Soft Tissue Infections," by Elizabeth W. Kelly and David Magilner.

93 DISSEMINATED VIRAL INFECTIONS

Matthew J. Scholer

- Viral illnesses are among the most common reasons that people come to an emergency department.
- This chapter focuses on some of the more serious viral infections that may cause disseminated illness or have a predilection for the central nervous system (CNS). Treatment of human immunodeficiency virus (HIV) is covered in Chapter 94, and cytomegalovirus (CMV) in Chapter 101. Viral encephalitis is covered in more detail in Chapter 150.

HERPES SIMPLEX VIRUS 1

EPIDEMIOLOGY

- Herpes labialis, or HSV-1, is usually acquired during childhood through nonsexual contact, and more than 85% of the world's population is thought to be seropositive.
- Encephalitis due to herpes labialis occurs most commonly in patients <20 and >50 years of age and is one of the most common causes of viral encephalitis in the United States.
- Encephalitis in neonates is most often caused by herpes simplex virus-2 (HSV-2), which is acquired from the maternal genital tract at the time of delivery (HSV-2 is covered in Chapter 89, Sexually Transmitted Diseases).

PATHOPHYSIOLOGY

- Transmission of HSV is via contact of infected fluids (saliva, vesicle fluid, semen, and cervical fluid) with mucous membranes or with open skin.
- After exposure, the virus replicates locally in the epithelial cells, causing lysis of the infected cells and producing an inflammatory response that results in the characteristic rash of HSV.
- Following primary infection, the virus becomes latent in a sensory nerve ganglion (trigeminal ganglia for herpes labialis, sacral ganglia for genital herpes).
- Reactivated virus may travel to the cutaneous surface and cause localized vesicular eruptions resulting in periodic outbreaks of herpes labialis or genital herpes.

CLINICAL FEATURES

- Herpes labialis primarily causes oral lesions, but may cause genital infection. The primary infection of herpes labialis may be mild or even asymptomatic.
- Symptomatic infection typically produces more extensive orofacial lesions involving both mucosal and extramucosal sites.
- The lesions consist of small, thin-walled vesicles on an erythematous base, although they do not always become vesicular. These primary lesions generally last 1 to 2 weeks.
- In children under age 5 years, herpes labialis infection may present as a pharyngitis or gingivostomatitis associated with fever and cervical lymphadenopathy.
- Less common skin manifestations include herpetic whitlow (finger) and herpes gladiatorum (commonly seen in wrestlers and other athletes involved in close contact sports).
- Eczema herpeticum can occur in patients with atopic dermatitis.
- Recurrent oral lesions occur in 60% to 90% of infected individuals, are usually milder, and generally occur on the lower lip at the outer vermilion border. Recurrences are often triggered by local trauma, sunburn, or stress. The patient may have pain or tingling prior to developing lesions, which begin as erythematous papules and then become vesicular.
- HSV encephalitis typically presents with the acute onset of fever and neurologic symptoms including focal motor or cranial nerve deficits, ataxia, seizures, and altered mental status or behavioral abnormalities.
- HSV infections in immunocompromised hosts can lead to widespread dissemination with multiorgan involvement (Fig. 93-1).

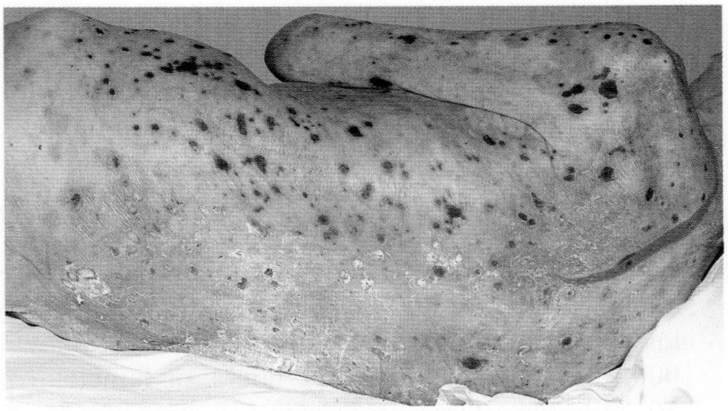

FIG. 93-1. Disseminated herpes simplex in an immunocompromised host. The rash of disseminated herpes simplex begins as vesicular lesions on an erythematous base, which may umbilicate and may blister and crust over as seen here. (Reproduced with permission from Wolff K, Johnson RA: *Fitzpatrick's Color Atlas and Synopsis of Clinical Dermatology*, 5th ed. © 2005 by McGraw-Hill, Inc., New York.)

DIAGNOSIS AND DIFFERENTIAL

- The diagnosis of mucocutaneous HSV lesions is largely clinical. If desired, confirmation can be obtained via HSV polymerase chain reaction (PCR) or direct fluorescent antibody testing performed on swabbed tissue.
- Viral culture from the fluid of an unroofed vesicle may be obtained but takes days to weeks to be performed. A Tzanck test is generally not useful.
- Temporal lobe lesions on CT scan or MRI are strongly suggestive of HSV encephalitis.
- CSF analysis shows a lymphocytic pleocytosis in most cases. CSF erythrocytosis is not a common finding. PCR testing of the CSF is the testing modality of choice for confirming HSV meningoencephalitis, but treatment should not be delayed while these results return are pending.

EMERGENCY DEPARTMENT CARE AND DISPOSITION

- Because CNS herpes virus infections can be difficult to distinguish from other types of meningoencephalitis, empiric treatment should be considered in patients being treated for suspected bacterial meningitis, especially those with increased severity of illness, associated neuropsychiatric symptoms or encephalopathy, history of herpes virus exposure or infection, concomitant mucocutaneous lesions concerning for HSV, negative Gram stain, or immunocompromised state.
- Herpes simplex infections are treatable with antiviral drugs, so early recognition of serious infection is important.

- Severe disease, including suspected or confirmed CNS infection or disseminated disease, should be treated with IV acyclovir 10 to 15 milligrams/kg every 8 hours (based on ideal body weight). Immunocompromised patients with severe mucocutaneous involvement may be treated with IV acyclovir 5 milligrams/kg every 8 hours.
- Immunocompetent adult patients with primary herpes simplex virus infection can be treated orally with acyclovir 400 milligrams three times daily, valacyclovir 1000 milligrams PO every 12 hours, or famciclovir 250 milligrams three times daily. Treatment is most effective if initiated within 48 to 72 hours of symptom onset and should be continued for 7 to 10 days.
- Recurrent herpes simplex virus may be treated orally with acyclovir 400 milligrams PO three times daily × 5 days, valacyclovir 2000 milligrams PO every 12 hours × 1 day (labialis) or 500 milligrams PO every 12 hours × 3 days (genital), or famciclovir 1500 milligrams PO × 1 dose (orolabial) or 1000 milligrams PO every 12 hours for 1 day (genital). Less severe outbreaks may be treated with topical acyclovir 5% ointment applied six times a day for 7 days. Treatment should be started as soon as is possible after symptom onset.

VARICELLA AND HERPES ZOSTER

EPIDEMIOLOGY

- The introduction of the varicella vaccine to routine childhood immunizations in 1995 has dramatically reduced the clinical burden of the disease.
- Herpes zoster can occur once immune response against the virus wanes, with the majority of cases occurring in the elderly. Other risk factors include HIV infection, lymphoproliferative disorders, and iatrogenic immunosuppression. Lifetime incidence is almost 20%.

PATHOPHYSIOLOGY

- Herpes zoster spreads to the respiratory mucosa of a susceptible host via aerosolized droplets of respiratory secretions from patients with chickenpox or direct contact with vesicle fluid in herpes zoster.
- After the initial infection resolves, the virus remains latent in the dorsal root ganglion and can later reactivate along dermatomes, resulting in herpes zoster.

CLINICAL FEATURES

- Varicella is a febrile illness with a characteristic vesicular rash that is superficial, is concentrated more on the torso and face, and typically has lesions at varying stages, including papules, vesicles, and crusted lesions (Fig. 93-2). Nonspecific symptoms of headache, malaise, and loss of appetite are often present.
- Zoster begins with a prodrome of pain in the affected area for 1 to 3 days, followed by the outbreak of a maculopapular rash that quickly progresses to a vesicular rash. The lesions of shingles are identical to those of chickenpox and HSV, but are limited to a unilateral dermatomal in distribution, with trigeminal (face) and thoracic dermatomes being most common (Fig. 93-3).
- The course of the disease is usually around 2 weeks, but may persist for a full month. Rash involving more than three dermatomes or crossing the midline should

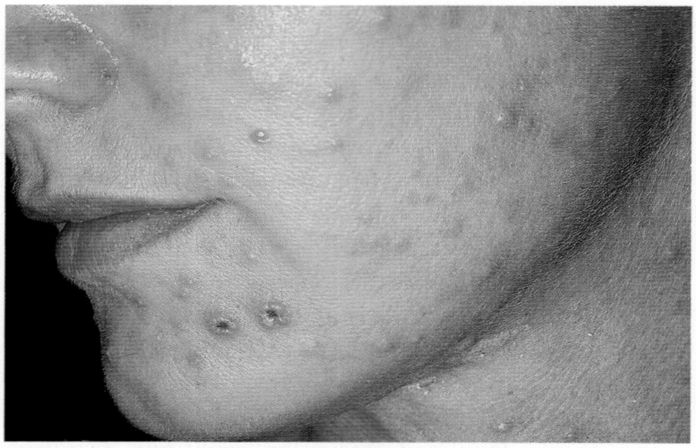

FIG. 93-2. Rash of primary varicella (chickenpox), demonstrating lesions of multiple stages, including papules, vesicles, and crusted lesions. (Reproduced with permission from Wolff K, Johnson RA: *Fitzpatrick's Color Atlas and Synopsis of Clinical Dermatology*, 6th ed. © 2009 by McGraw-Hill, Inc., New York.)

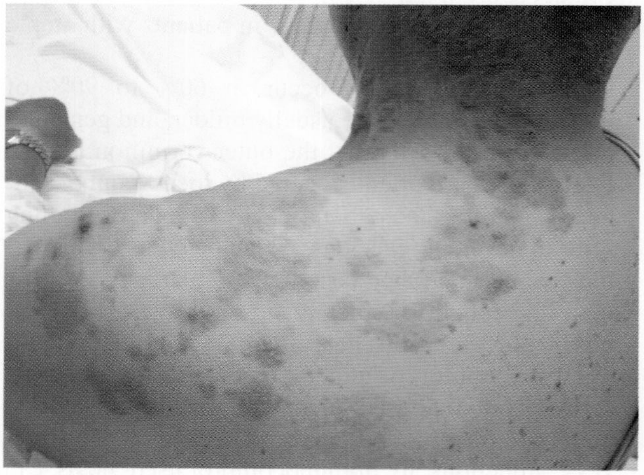

FIG. 93-3. Dermatome distribution of the classic rash of herpes zoster (shingles). (Courtesy of Gregory Moran, MD.)

raise the suspicion of disseminated disease, which can occur in immunocompromised patients.

- Ocular involvement (herpes zoster ophthalmicus) may occur due to involvement of the ocular branch of the trigeminal nerve (see Chapter 151, Ocular Emergencies). Involvement of the geniculate ganglion on CN VII may result in Ramsay Hunt syndrome, which presents clinically as an auricular lesion with associated facial nerve palsy resembling Bell's palsy.
- Bacterial superinfections of herpes zoster skin lesions, most often with group A streptococci, can cause serious illness including necrotizing fasciitis. CNS complications such as cerebellar ataxia, meningitis, and meningoencephalitis are well described.
- Pain that continues beyond 30 days is termed postherpetic neuralgia, occurs more often with advancing age, and may last for months to years. Postherpetic neuralgia occurs in 10% to 20% of all patients after an episode of acute zoster, but in up to 70% of patients aged 70 years or older.

DIAGNOSIS AND DIFFERENTIAL

- Clinical diagnosis is sufficient in most cases. Confirmation can be obtained via herpes zoster PCR or direct fluorescent antibody testing performed on swabbed tissue or by viral culture from the fluid of an unroofed vesicle. CT or MRI of the brain with lumbar puncture and PCR testing of CSF for herpes zoster are appropriate for suspected central neurologic involvement.
- Smallpox is distinguished from varicella by larger lesions that are distributed more on the extremities and are all at the same stage of development.

EMERGENCY DEPARTMENT CARE AND DISPOSITION

- Healthy children need only supportive care for chickenpox. Acyclovir 20 milligrams/kg (max 800 milligrams) PO qid × 5 days is appropriate for high-risk patients including children >12 years of age, adults, those with chronic skin or pulmonary disorders, those receiving long-term salicylate therapy, and immunocompromised patients.
- The primary goal in the treatment of herpes zoster is to reduce the severity of postherpetic neuralgia. Start antiviral medication within 72 hours of the onset of rash, and consider treatment at >72 hours if new vesicles are still present or developing. Treat immunocompromised patients regardless of the time since rash onset.
- For zoster, a 7- to 10-day course of acyclovir 800 milligrams PO five times daily, valacyclovir 1 gram PO three times daily, or famciclovir 500 milligrams PO three times daily may be used.
- Herpes zoster can be extremely painful and may require narcotic analgesia acutely. Corticosteroids in combination with antivirals do not decrease the incidence of postherpetic neuralgia but may provide a modest decrease in acute pain and should be considered in older individuals with severe pain who do not have contraindications to their use.

EPSTEIN–BARR VIRUS INFECTION

- Epstein–Barr virus (EBV) is implicated in a variety of human illnesses. It is the causative agent of heterophile-positive **infectious mononucleosis**.
- There are two age-related peaks of infection: early childhood and young adulthood.
- In developing countries, EBV infection is widespread in early childhood and is often asymptomatic.
- College students and military recruits experience the highest morbidity.

PATHOPHYSIOLOGY

- EBV is transmitted via salivary secretions. After infecting the oropharyngeal epithelium, it disseminates through the blood stream.
- The virus infects B lymphocytes and causes an increase in T lymphocytes, which results in enlargement of lymphoid tissue.

CLINICAL FEATURES

- Infections in infants and young children are often asymptomatic or consist of mild pharyngitis.
- Teenagers and young adults can develop infectious mononucleosis, which presents as fever, lymphadenopathy, and pharyngitis.
- Tonsillar exudates are frequent and often extensive or even necrotic appearing.
- Splenomegaly occurs in more than half of patients.
- Symptoms generally resolve over 2 to 3 weeks, and most patients recover uneventfully. Severe fatigue is a prominent feature and can persist for months.
- Patients treated with ampicillin or amoxicillin for suspected streptococcal pharyngitis often develop a morbilliform rash if they have infection with EBV.
- EBV can affect nearly all organ systems. Neurologic complications such as encephalitis, meningitis, and Guillain–Barré syndrome have been described. Hepatitis, myocarditis, and hematologic disorders are also known complications.

DIAGNOSIS AND DIFFERENTIAL

- If infectious mononucleosis is suspected based on the history and physical examination, a complete blood count and a monospot test can provide confirmation.
- Typically there is lymphocytosis with >50% lymphocytes, and atypical lymphocytes are found on examination of the smear.
- These are reactive cytotoxic T cells that can also be found in other illnesses, including CMV infection, HIV infection, and viral hepatitis.
- The monospot test identifies heterophile antibodies that agglutinate animal erythrocytes, and a positive result is considered diagnostic of EBV infection in the right clinical setting.
- The monospot test result may be negative early in the course of disease, and the test may need to be repeated.
- The sensitivity of the test is also decreased in infants and the elderly. Testing is particularly important in pregnant patients, because some other causes of heterophile-negative mononucleosis can be teratogenic.

EMERGENCY DEPARTMENT CARE AND DISPOSITION

- Most cases are self-limited and do not require specific therapy.
- Use of corticosteroids is associated with increased complications and is recommended only for patients with severe disease, such as upper airway obstruction, neurologic disease, or hemolytic anemia.
- Advise patients to avoid all contact sports for a minimum of 4 weeks after illness onset to avoid splenic injury.

ARBOVIRAL INFECTIONS

EPIDEMIOLOGY

- Arboviral infections are infections spread by biting mosquitoes, ticks, and flies. Infections tend to be seasonal with increased incidence in warmer months due to the breeding patterns of the arthropod vectors.
- West Nile virus and the viruses that cause La Cross encephalitis, St. Louis encephalitis, eastern equine encephalitis, and western equine encephalitis are found in North America and are reviewed in this chapter. Viral encephalitis is covered in more detail in Chapter 150, CNS and Spinal Infections.

PATHOPHYSIOLOGY

- After inoculation by an infected arthropod, the virus enters the reticuloendothelial system and then disseminates, often causing a low-grade viremia. If the host is unable to clear the virus via the production of immunoglobulin M (IgM) neutralizing antibodies, encephalitis may occur.

CLINICAL FEATURES

- Most arbovirus infections are asymptomatic or cause a nonspecific mild viral syndrome.
- The classic presentation of viral encephalitis is fever, headache, and altered level of consciousness. Patients can be lethargic and confused, and occasionally present with seizures.

DIAGNOSIS AND DIFFERENTIAL

- Arboviral infection should be considered based on clinical presentation combined with knowledge of local epidemiologic patterns, suspicious travel, or exposure history.

EMERGENCY DEPARTMENT CARE AND DISPOSITION

- Supportive and symptomatic therapy is the mainstay of management. Specific antiviral drugs, interferon, and steroids are not useful.
- The decision whether or not to admit to the hospital should be based on severity of symptoms, clinical assessment, and level of suspicion for other serious etiologies.
- When CNS infection is suspected, empiric treatment with antibiotics and acyclovir is appropriate until bacterial meningitis and HSV encephalitis are ruled out.
- Cerebrospinal fluid typically shows a lymphocytic pleocytosis and a slightly elevated protein level, although these findings are nonspecific.
- If arboviral infection without encephalitis is suspected and the patient presents with a mild, nonspecific viral illness, discharge with strict return precautions for any signs or symptoms of encephalitis may be appropriate.

INFLUENZAE A AND B

EPIDEMIOLOGY

- In the United States, influenza generally occurs from November to April.
- Transmission is via respiratory droplets, commonly generated by coughing or sneezing.
- During epidemics, attack rates are in the 20% to 30% range, and may be as high as 50% during pandemics.
- After exposure, the incubation period is usually about 2 days. Viral shedding (contagiousness) starts approximately 24 hours before the onset of symptoms, rises to peak levels within 48 hours, and then declines over the next 3 to 7 days.

PATHOPHYSIOLOGY

- Influenza viruses are single-stranded RNA viruses of the orthomyxovirus family.
- Following exposure, the virus enters the columnar cells of the respiratory tract epithelium. The invaded epithelial cells release large numbers of virions before cell death, which are then available for spread in respiratory droplets.
- Antigenic drift caused by minor mutations in the RNA genome results in a change in antigenicity that facilitates annual epidemics.
- Antigenic shift occurs by genetic reassortment and is responsible for flu pandemics.

CLINICAL FEATURES

- Classic flu symptoms include fever of 38.6 to 39.8°C (101-103°F), with chills or rigor, headache, myalgia, and generalized malaise.
- Respiratory symptoms include dry cough, rhinorrhea, and sore throat, frequently with bilateral tender, enlarged cervical lymph nodes.
- The elderly do not usually have classical symptoms and may present only with fever, malaise, confusion, and nasal congestion.
- Almost half of affected children have gastrointestinal symptoms, but these are unusual in adults.
- The fever generally lasts 2 to 4 days, followed by rapid recovery from most of the systemic symptoms. Cough and fatigue may persist for several weeks.

DIAGNOSIS AND DIFFERENTIAL

- A clinical diagnosis of influenza during a known outbreak is highly accurate. Although rapid diagnostic tests are available for influenza, the performance characteristics of these tests vary and results should be interpreted in the context of the clinical and epidemiologic information available.
- Common respiratory complications of acute influenza infection include primary influenza pneumonitis, secondary bacterial pneumonia, croup, and exacerbation of chronic obstructive pulmonary disease. The presence of hypoxia should raise the suspicion for pulmonary involvement.

EMERGENCY DEPARTMENT CARE AND DISPOSITION

- Four antiviral agents (amantadine, rimantadine, oseltamivir, and zanamivir) are approved for preventing or treating influenza.
- Zanamivir is an inhaled medication and may cause bronchospasm. It should be avoided in patients with underlying pulmonary disease.
- When started within 48 hours of symptom onset, these medications can reduce the duration of uncomplicated influenza illness by approximately 1 day.
- Dosage recommendations and duration of administration vary by age group and medical conditions.
- In general, treatment is recommended for any patient with confirmed or suspected influenza who is hospitalized, has severe, complicated, or progressive illness, or is at higher risk for influenza complications. Specific recommendations for use of individual drugs vary by susceptibility and resistance patterns. Up-to-date CDC guidelines can be accessed at their influenza Web site: www.cdc.gov/flu.

For further reading in *Emergency Medicine: A Comprehensive Study Guide*, 7th ed., see Chapter 148, "Disseminated Viral Infections," by Sukhjit S. Takhar and Gregory J. Moran.

94 HUMAN IMMUNODEFICIENCY VIRUS INFECTION AND ACQUIRED IMMUNODEFICIENCY SYNDROME

David M. Cline

- Risk factors for HIV infection include unprotected sexual activity, injection drug use, blood transfusion before 1985, and maternal–neonatal transmission.

EPIDEMIOLOGY

- Increasing use of ED services by HIV-infected persons is due in part to changes in the demographic distribution of HIV cases and acquired immunodeficiency syndrome (AIDS)–related illnesses.
- Seroprevalence studies in one inner-city ED reflect these trends, with rates of HIV infection among unselected adult patients rising from 6% to 11.4% over a 4- year period.
- The range of seroprevalence across the United States is 2% to 14% among adult ED patients.

PATHOPHYSIOLOGY

- HIV is a cytopathic retrovirus that kills infected cells. The viral genes are carried as a single-stranded RNA molecule within the viral particle. Following infection, the virus selectively attacks host cells involved in immune function, primarily CD4 T lymphocytes.

- As a result of infection, immunologic abnormalities eventually occur, including lymphopenia, qualitative CD4 T-lymphocyte function defects, and autoimmune phenomena. Profound defects in cellular immunity ultimately result in a variety of opportunistic infections and neoplasms.
- Transmission of HIV has been shown to occur via semen, vaginal secretions, blood or blood products, breast milk, and transplacental transmission in utero.

CLINICAL FEATURES

- Acute HIV infection, essentially indistinguishable from a "flulike" illness, usually goes unrecognized but is reported to occur in 50% to 90% of patients.
- The time from exposure to onset of symptoms is usually 2 to 4 weeks, and the most common symptoms include fever (>90%), fatigue (70%-90%), sore throat (>70%), rash (40%-80%), headache (30%-80%), and lymphadenopathy (40%-70%).
- Other reported symptoms include myalgias, diarrhea, and weight loss. Seroconversion, reflecting detectable antibody response to HIV, usually occurs 3 to 8 weeks after infection.
- This is followed by a long period of asymptomatic infection except for possible persistent generalized lymphadenopathy.
- Early symptomatic infection is characterized by conditions that are more common and more severe in the presence of HIV infection but, by definition, are not AIDS indicator conditions.
- Examples include thrush, persistent vulvovaginal candidiasis, peripheral neuropathy, cervical dysplasia, recurrent herpes zoster infection, and idiopathic thrombocytopenic purpura. At this time CD4 counts are 200 to 500 cells/mm^3. As the CD4 count drops below 200 cells/mm^3, the frequency of opportunistic infections dramatically increases.
- AIDS is defined by the appearance of any indicator condition (Table 94-1) including a CD4 count lower than 200 cells/mm^3.
- Late symptomatic or advanced HIV infection exists in patients with a CD4 count lower than 50 cells/mm^3 or clinical evidence of end-stage disease, including disseminated *Mycobacterium avium* complex or disseminated cytomegalovirus.
- In today's era of highly active antiretroviral therapy (HAART), longevity is more dependent on age and other comorbidities than HIV status, provided the patient adheres to HAART and the therapy is effective in suppressing viral load and maintaining normal CD4 counts.

TABLE 94-1 Indicator Conditions for Case Definitions of Acquired Immunodeficiency Syndrome
Esophageal candidiasis
Cryptococcosis
Cryptosporidiosis
Cytomegalovirus retinitis
Herpes simplex virus
Kaposi sarcoma
Brain lymphoma
Mycobacterium avium complex infection
Pneumocystis jiroveci (*P. carinii*) pneumonia
Progressive multifocal leukoencephalopathy
Brain toxoplasmosis
HIV encephalopathy
HIV wasting syndrome
Disseminated histoplasmosis
Isosporiasis
Disseminated *Mycobacterium tuberculosis* disease
Recurrent Salmonella septicemia
Added in 1993:
CD4+ T-cell count of <200 cells/mm^3
Pulmonary tuberculosis
Recurrent bacterial pneumonia
Invasive cervical cancer

Abbreviation: HIV = human immunodeficiency virus.

CONSTITUTIONAL SYMPTOMS AND FEBRILE ILLNESSES

- Systemic symptoms, such as fever, weight loss, and malaise, are common in HIV-infected patients and account for most HIV-related ED presentations.
- Appropriate laboratory investigation includes electrolytes, complete blood count, blood cultures, urinalysis and culture, liver function tests, chest radiographs, and in selected patients, serologic testing for syphilis, cryptococcosis, toxoplasmosis, cytomegalovirus, and coccidioidomycosis.
- Lumbar puncture should be considered if there are neurologic signs or symptoms or unexplained fever.
- In HIV patients without obvious focalizing signs or symptoms, sources of fever vary by stage of disease.
- Patients with CD4 counts higher than 500 cells/mm^3 generally have sources of fever similar to those in nonimmunocompromised patients.
- Those with CD4 counts between 200 and 500 cells/mm^3 are most likely to have early bacterial respiratory infections.
- For patients with CD4 counts lower than 200 cells/mm^3, likely infections include *Pneumocystis* pneumonia (PCP; actually *P. jiroveci*), central-line infection, *M. avium* complex (MAC), *Mycobacterium tuberculosis,* cytomegalovirus, drug fever, and sinusitis.
- Disseminated MAC occurs predominately in patients with CD4 counts below 100 cells/mm^3. Persistent fever and night sweats are typical.

- Associated symptoms of disseminated MAC include weight loss, diarrhea, malaise, and anorexia.
- Diagnosis is made with acid-fast stain of stool or other body fluids or culture.
- A more focal and invasive form of MAC has emerged, called *immune reconstitution illness to MAC,* which presents with lymphadenitis and follows weeks to months after starting HAART.
- Cytomegalovirus is the most common cause of serious opportunistic viral disease in HIV-infected patients. Disseminated disease commonly involves the gastrointestinal or pulmonary system.
- The most important manifestation is cytomegalovirus retinitis.
- Infective endocarditis is a concern especially in intravenous (IV) drug users (see Chapter 95).
- Non-Hodgkin lymphoma is the most commonly occurring neoplasm in HIV patients and typically presents as a high-grade, rapidly growing mass lesion.

PULMONARY COMPLICATIONS

- Pulmonary presentations are among the most common reasons for ED visits by HIV-infected patients.
- The most common causes of pulmonary abnormalities in HIV-infected patients include community-acquired bacterial pneumonia, PCP, *M. tuberculosis,* cytomegalovirus, *Cryptococcus neoformans, Histoplasma capsulatum,* and neoplasms.
- Nonopportunistic bacterial pneumonias outnumber atypical infections including *Streptococcus pneumoniae* (most common), *Haemophilus influenzae,* and *Staphylococcus aureus.*
- Productive cough, leukocytosis, and the presence of a focal infiltrate suggest bacterial pneumonia, especially in those with earlier-stage disease.
- Evaluation should include pulse oximetry, arterial blood gas analysis, sputum culture and Gram stain, acid-fast stain, blood cultures, and chest radiograph.
- The classic presenting symptoms of PCP are fever, cough (typically nonproductive), and shortness of breath (progressing from being present only with exertion to being present at rest).
- Negative radiographs are reported in 15% to 20% of patients. Hypoxia or increased alveolar–arterial oxygen gradient identifies patients at risk.
- Classic pulmonary manifestations of tuberculosis (TB) include cough with hemoptysis, night sweats, prolonged fevers, weight loss, and anorexia.
- TB is common in patients with CD4 counts between 200 and 500 cells/mm^3. Classic upper lobe involvement and cavitary lesions are less common, particularly among late-stage AIDS patients.
- False-negative purified protein derivative TB test results are frequent among AIDS patients due to immunosuppression.
- There is a high index of suspicion for TB in HIV patients with pulmonary symptoms due to high rates of person-to-person transmission.
- Consider disseminated fungal infection in the severely immunosuppressed.

NEUROLOGIC COMPLICATIONS

- Central nervous system (CNS) disease occurs in 90% of patients with AIDS, and 10% to 20% of HIV-infected patients initially present with CNS symptoms.
- ED evaluation includes neuro examination, computed tomography, and lumbar puncture.
- Cerebrospinal fluid studies should include pressures; complete cell count; glucose; protein; Gram stain; India ink stain; bacterial, viral, and fungal cultures; toxoplasmosis; and *Cryptococcus* antigen and coccidioidomycosis titer.
- Common causes of neurologic symptoms include AIDS dementia, *Toxoplasma gondii,* and *C. neoformans.*
- Symptoms may include headache, focal neurologic deficits, altered mental status, or seizures.
- AIDS dementia complex (also referred to as HIV encephalopathy or subacute encephalitis) is a progressive process commonly heralded by subtle impairment of recent memory and other cognitive deficits caused by direct HIV infection.
- Other, less common CNS infections that should be considered in the presence of neurologic symptoms include bacterial meningitis, histoplasmosis (usually disseminated), cytomegalovirus, progressive multifocal leukoencephalopathy, herpes simplex virus, neurosyphilis, and TB.
- HIV patients may experience HIV neuropathy characterized by painful sensory symptoms of the feet.

GASTROINTESTINAL COMPLICATIONS

- The most frequent presenting symptoms include odynophagia, abdominal pain, bleeding, and diarrhea.
- ED evaluation includes stool for leukocytes, ova, parasites, acid-fast staining, and culture.
- Diarrhea is the most frequent gastrointestinal complaint and is estimated to occur in 50% to 90% of AIDS patients. Common causes include bacterial organisms, such as *Shigella, Salmonella,* enteroadherent *Escherichia coli,* and *Campylobacter;* parasitic organisms; viruses; fungi; and antiviral therapy.

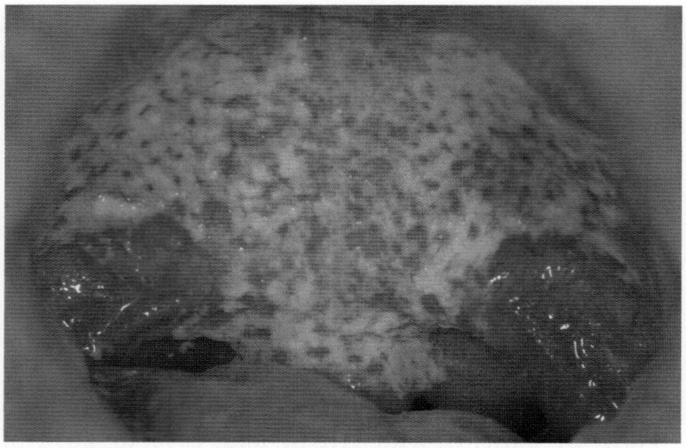

FIG. 94-1. Oral candidiasis (thrush). Extensive thrush is seen on the hard and soft palate of this immunocompromised patient. (Photograph contributed by Lawrence B. Stack. Reproduced with permission from Knoop KJ, Stack LB, Storrow AB, Thurman RJ: *The Atlas of Emergency Medicine*, 3rd ed. © 2009, McGraw-Hill Inc., New York.)

- Oral candidiasis, or thrush, affects more than 80% of AIDS patients.
- The tongue and buccal mucosa are commonly involved, and the plaques characteristically can be easily scraped from an erythematous base (see Fig. 94-1). Esophageal involvement may occur with *Candida,* herpes simplex, and cytomegalovirus. Complaints of odynophagia or dysphagia are usually indicative of esophagitis and may be extremely debilitating.
- Hepatomegaly occurs in approximately 50% of AIDS patients. Elevation of alkaline phosphatase levels is frequently seen. Jaundice is rare. Coinfection with hepatitis B and hepatitis C is common, especially among IV drug users.
- Anorectal disease is common in AIDS patients. Proctitis is characterized by painful defecation, rectal discharge, and tenesmus.
- Common causative organisms include *Neisseria gonorrhoeae, Chlamydia trachomatis,* syphilis, and herpes simplex.

CUTANEOUS MANIFESTATIONS

- Generalized conditions such as xerosis, seborrheic eczema, and pruritus are common.
- Kaposi sarcoma appears more often in homosexual men than in other risk groups.
- Clinically, it consists of painless, raised brown-black or purple papules and nodules that do not blanch.
- Common sites are the face, chest, genitals, and oral cavity.
- Reactivation of varicella zoster virus is more common in patients with HIV infection and AIDS than in the general population.
- Herpes simplex virus infections are common. HIV patients may develop bullous impetigo and *Pseudomonas*-associated chronic ulcerations. MRSA infection, scabies, human papillomavirus, and hypersensitivity reactions to medications are common.

OPHTHALMOLOGIC MANIFESTATIONS

- Seventy-five percent of patients with AIDS develop ocular complications.
- Cytomegalovirus retinitis is the most frequent and serious ocular opportunistic infection and the leading cause of blindness in AIDS patients.
- The presentation of cytomegalovirus retinitis is variable. It may be asymptomatic early on but later causes changes in visual acuity, visual field cuts, photophobia, scotoma, or eye redness or pain.
- Herpes zoster ophthalmicus is another diagnosis to consider and is recognized by the typical zoster rash in the distribution of cranial nerve VI.

DIAGNOSIS AND DIFFERENTIAL

- Benefits of early HIV diagnosis include early and aggressive antiretroviral therapy that can lead to immune reconstitution, prevention of viral mutation and drug resistance, slowing of disease progression, and improved long-term prognosis.
- The most common assay used to detect viral antibody is a screening enzyme-linked immunoassay (ELISA) followed by a confirming Western blot test on ELISA-positive specimens.
- ELISA is approximately 99% specific and 98.5% sensitive; the Western blot test is nearly 100% sensitive and specific if performed under ideal laboratory circumstances.
- Diagnosis of acute-stage HIV infection is not possible with standard serologic tests because seroconversion has not yet occurred.
- Methods for earlier detection of HIV-1 include techniques to detect DNA, RNA, or HIV antigens.
- The single-use diagnostic system is used to screen rapidly for antibodies to HIV-1 in serum or plasma. Rapid tests are available in many EDs nationwide but must be confirmed with Western blot testing.
- Knowledge of current or recent CD4 counts and a HIV viremia load will help in the management of HIV patients.
- CD4 counts below 200 cells/mm^3 and viral load greater than 50,000 copies/mL is associated with increased risk of progression to AIDS-defining illness.

- When these levels are unavailable, a total lymphocyte count of <1200 cells/mm^3 combined with clinical symptoms is strongly predictive of a positive CD4 count of <200 cells/mm^3.

EMERGENCY DEPARTMENT CARE AND DISPOSITION

- The initial evaluation of HIV-infected and AIDS patients begins with a heightened awareness of the need for universal precautions. Respiratory isolation should be instituted for patients with suspected TB.
- All unstable patients should have airway management as indicated, oxygen, pulse oximetry, cardiac monitoring, and IV access.
- Seizures, altered mental status, gastrointestinal bleeding, and coma should be managed with standard protocols.
- Suspected bacterial sepsis and focal bacterial infections should be treated with standard antibiotics (see Chapter 91).
- Systemic *M. avium* should be treated with clarithromycin 500 milligrams PO twice daily plus ethambutol 15 milligrams/kg PO daily plus rifabutin 300 milligrams PO daily.
- Treatment of immune reconstitution illness to MAC should include continuation of HAART, antimicrobials as above, and possibly steroids.
- Systemic cytomegalovirus should be treated with ganciclovir 5 milligrams/kg IV every 12 hours or foscarnet 90 milligrams/kg IV every 12 hours.
- Ophthalmologic cytomegalovirus is treated with a ganciclovir implant plus ganciclovir 1.0 to 1.5 grams PO three times daily or 5 milligrams/kg IV twice daily for 14 to 21 days.
- Pulmonary PCP should be treated with trimethoprim-sulfamethoxazole (TMP-SMX), with TMP 15 to 20 milligrams/kg/d IV or PO divided three times daily, for 3 weeks. The typical oral dose is two tablets of TMP-SMX double strength three times daily. An alternative is pentamidine 4 milligrams/kg/d IV or IM for 3 weeks.
- Oral steroids should be given if hypoxic: prednisone 40 milligrams twice daily for 5 days, then 40 milligrams daily for 5 days, and then 20 milligrams daily for 11 more days.
- Pulmonary TB may be treated with INH 5 milligrams/kg/d PO plus rifabutin 10 milligrams/kg/d PO or rifampin 10 milligrams/kg/d PO plus pyrazinamide 15 to 30 milligrams/kg/d PO plus ethambutol 15 to 20 milligrams/kg/d PO daily.
- CNS toxoplasmosis can be treated with pyrimethamine 200 milligrams initially and then 50 to 75 milligrams daily PO plus sulfadiazine 4 to 6 grams daily PO plus folinic acid 10 milligrams daily PO for 6 to 8 weeks, plus/minus leucovorin 10 to 25 milligrams daily.
- CNS cryptococcosis can be treated with amphotericin B 0.7 milligrams/kg/dose daily IV and flucytosine 25 milligrams/kg IV four times daily for 2 weeks. When improved, fluconazole 400 milligrams PO daily for 8 to 10 weeks can be used.
- Candidiasis (thrush) can be treated with clotrimazole 10-milligram troches five times per day or nystatin 500,000 units/mL gargle with 5 mL five times per day.
- Esophagitis can be treated with fluconazole 100 to 400 milligrams daily PO.
- Salmonellosis can be treated with ciprofloxacin 500 milligrams PO twice daily for 2 to 4 weeks.
- Cutaneous herpes simplex can be treated with acyclovir 200 milligrams PO five times daily for 7 days or famciclovir 125 milligrams PO twice daily for 7 days or valacyclovir 1 gram PO BID for 7 days or acyclovir 5 to 10 milligrams/kg IV every 8 hours for 7 days for severe illness.
- Cutaneous herpes zoster can be treated with acyclovir 800 milligrams PO five times daily, or valacyclovir 1 gram PO three times daily, or famciclovir 500 milligrams PO three times daily.
- Herpes zoster ophthalmicus should be treated with acyclovir 800 milligrams PO five times daily for 7 to 10 days.
- *Candida* or *Trichophyton* should be treated with topical clotrimazole or miconazole or ketoconazole three times daily for 3 weeks.
- Although rarely started in the ED, antiretroviral therapy is started for CD4 counts below 350 cells/mm^3 or history of AIDS-defining illness (see Table 94-1) or pregnancy, HIV-associated neuropathy, and hepatitis B confection regardless of the CD4 count.
- New protocols recommending treatment upon initial HIV-positive testing may be forthcoming, but are not currently available. Initial treatment includes two nucleoside reverse transcriptase inhibitors plus one or two protease inhibitors or one non-nucleoside reverse transcriptase inhibitor drug. See the Centers for Disease Control and Prevention Web site: http://www.cdc.gov/hiv/.
- The decision to admit an AIDS patient should be based on severity of illness, with attention to new presentation of fever of unknown origin, hypoxia worse than baseline, or Pao_2 below 60 mm Hg, suspected PCP, suspected TB, new CNS symptoms, intractable diarrhea, suspected cytomegalovirus retinitis, herpes zoster ophthalmicus, or a patient unable to perform self-care.
- Post-exposure prophylaxis should be initiated as quickly as possible, preferably within 1 to 2 hours.

Risks for seroconversion include (1) deep injury, (2) visible blood on the injuring device, (3) needle placement in a vein or an artery of the source patient, and (4) a source patient with late-stage HIV infection. Treatment regimes vary by type of exposure.

- CDC guidelines recommend two general alternatives: a basic regimen, which consists of two-drug therapy, often consisting of azidothymidine and lamivudine, and an expanded regimen, which adds a third drug, such as indinavir or nelfinavir.

For further reading in Tintinalli's *Emergency Medicine: A Comprehensive Study Guide*, 7th ed., see Chapter 149, "Human Immunodeficiency Virus Infection and Acquired Immunodeficiency Syndrome," by Richard E. Rothman, Catherine A. Marco, and Samuel Yang.

95 INFECTIVE ENDOCARDITIS

John C. Nalagan

EPIDEMIOLOGY

- In infective endocarditis (IE), the mitral valve is the most affected valve, followed by the aortic, tricuspid, and pulmonic valve.
- Most cases occur in patients with an identifiable cardiac structural abnormality or a recognized risk factor for the disease.
- In native valve endocarditis, rheumatic heart disease is the leading risk factor and mitral valve prolapse is a common predisposing cardiac lesion.
- Endocarditis in injection drug users has a predilection for the tricuspid valve. It is also associated with a 40% recurrence rate and high mortality in patients with AIDS.
- Early prosthetic valve endocarditis (cases within 60 days post-surgery) is usually acquired in the hospital, whereas late prosthetic valve endocarditis (>60 days) is community acquired.

PATHOPHYSIOLOGY

- Normal endothelium is typically resistant to infection and thrombus unless injured by abnormal hemodynamic states such as valvular or congenital cardiac defects. The turbulent flow then leads to denuding of the endothelium.
- In injection drug use, endothelial damage occurs from damage from particulate matter present in the injected substance, or from vasospasm from the drug itself.
- Endothelial damage results in deposition of platelets and fibrin, resulting in the formation of sterile vegetations (nonbacterial thrombotic endocarditis).
- Transient bacteremia may result in colonization of vegetations and conversion of nonbacterial thrombotic endocarditis to IE.
- The infecting bacteria must be able to adhere to the thrombus to result in IE. Different organisms vary in this ability. Certain pathogens (eg, *Staphylococcus aureus* in injection drug users) are so invasive that nonbacterial thrombus on the endothelium does not need to be present to induce IE.

CLINICAL FEATURES

- Fever is the most common manifestation (80%) followed by chills, weakness, and dyspnea (40% each).
- Cardiac manifestations such as heart murmurs are present in up to 85% of cases.
- Dyspnea is common and often due to acute or progressive CHF (70% of cases).
- Embolic phenomenon occurs about 50% of the time and is due to the embolization of friable vegetation fragments. Findings include strokes (most common), chest and abdominal pain, flank pain with hematuria, and acute limb ischemia.
- Cutaneous findings occur in 18% to 50% of patients and include petichiae, splinter/subungual hemorrhages, Osler nodes (tender subcutaneous nodules on finger/toe pads), and Janeway lesions (hemorrhagic plaques on the palms or soles).

DIAGNOSIS AND DIFFERENTIAL

- Hospitalize all patients at risk for IE. This includes patients with unexplained fever and risk factors for the disease, patients with prosthetic valves, and those with new or changing murmurs and evidence of arterial emboli.
- The necessary components for diagnosis are blood cultures, echocardiogram, and clinical observation. Blood cultures should be drawn prior to administration of antibiotics and from three separate sites, with an hour elapsing between the first and last set of cultures.
- Echocardiography should be performed as soon as possible.

EMERGENCY DEPARTMENT CARE AND DISPOSITION

- Patients may present with respiratory compromise and require emergent airway stabilization.
- Intra-aortic balloon counterpulsion is indicated for mitral valve rupture but contraindicated for aortic valve rupture.
- Patients with native valve endocarditis do not require anticoagulation. Patients with prosthetic valves already on anticoagulation should continue their current regimen unless requested otherwise by the consultant.
- Antibiotics should be initiated in patients with suspected endocarditis after appropriate cultures are obtained. Table 95-1 lists empiric treatment regimens. Definitive therapy is based on culture and sensitivity results and typically requires 4 to 6 weeks of antibiotics.
- Prophylactic antibiotics before procedures should be administered for patients only with the highest risk factors (eg, prior history of IE, patients with prosthetic heart valve, unrepaired congenital heart disease, or a cardiac transplant recipient with valve regurgitation).

TABLE 95-1 Empiric Therapy of Suspected Bacterial Endocarditis*

PATIENT CHARACTERISTICS	RECOMMENDED AGENTS, INITIAL DOSE
Uncomplicated history	Ceftriaxone, 1-2 grams IV *or* Nafcillin, 2 grams IV *or* Oxacillin, 2 grams IV *or* Vancomycin, 15 milligrams/kg *plus* Gentamicin, 1-3 milligrams/kg IV *or* Tobramycin, 1 milligram/kg IV
Injection drug use, congenital heart disease, hospital-acquired, suspected methicillin-resistant *Staphylococcus aureus*, or already on oral antibiotics	Nafcillin, 2 grams IV *plus* Gentamicin, 1-3 milligrams/kg IV *plus* Vancomycin, 15 milligrams/kg IV
Prosthetic heart valve	Vancomycin, 15 milligrams/kg IV *plus* Gentamicin, 1-3 milligrams/kg IV *plus* Rifampin, 300 milligrams PO

*Because of controversy in the literature regarding the optimal regimen for empiric treatment, antibiotic selection should be based on patient characteristics, local resistance patterns, and current authoritative recommendations.

- The only ED procedures where prophylactic antibiotics should be considered are procedures on known infected skin, such as abscess drainage. Agents suggested are dicloxacillin 2 grams PO, cephalexin 2 grams PO, clindamycin 600 milligrams IM or IV, or vancomycin 1 gram IV, 30 to 60 minutes before procedure. Antibiotic prophylaxis is *not* indicated for common emergency department procedures.

For further reading in Tintinalli's *Emergency Medicine: A Comprehensive Study Guide*, 7th ed., see Chapter 150, "Infective Endocarditis," by Richard E. Rothman, Samuel Yang, and Catherine A. Marco.

96 TETANUS AND RABIES

Vincent Nacouzi

TETANUS

EPIDEMIOLOGY

- The reported cases of tetanus worldwide are about a million cases per year. The mortality is close to 30% mostly in Africa and Asia. In the United States, tetanus is uncommon and mostly seen in temperate areas. Texas, California, and Florida report most cases annually.
- Intravenous drug user has a disproportionate risk of contracting tetanus.
- Only 30% of elderly Americans over the age of 70 years have adequate immunization; they also have the highest incidence of death from the disease.

PATHOPHYSIOLOGY

- Tetanus is caused by *Clostridium tetani*, a gram-positive rod. The wound is often contaminated by the spore-forming organism. Later when oxygen tension decreases in the wound, as seen in crushed, devitalized tissue, the toxin-producing *C. tetani* develops.
- *Clostridium tetani* produces two exotoxins: tetanospasmin, the most potent of both neurotoxins, is responsible for the clinical manifestations of tetanus. Incubation varies from 24 hours to over 30 days. Dissemination is initially hematogenous then via the nervous system.
- Tetanospasmin acts on the motor endplates of skeletal muscle, in the spinal cord, in the brain, and in

the sympathetic nervous system. This prevents the release of the inhibitory neurotransmitters glycine and gamma-amino butyric acid (GABA), resulting in loss of normal inhibitory control.

CLINICAL FEATURES

- The clinical manifestations of tetanus are neuromuscular irritability, muscular rigidity, violent contractions, and instability of the autonomic nervous system.
- Wounds that become infected with toxin-producing *C. tetani* are most often puncture wounds, but can vary in severity from lacerations to minor corneal abrasion.
- Local tetanus is manifested by rigidity of the muscles in proximity to the site of the wound and usually resolves after weeks without squeal. It may progress to generalized tetanus.
- Generalized tetanus is the most common form of the disease.
- The most frequent presenting complaints are pain and stiffness in the masseter muscles (lockjaw).
- Nerves with short axons are affected initially; therefore, symptoms appear first in the facial muscles, with progression to the neck, trunk, and extremities.
- Trismus manifest as a sardonic smile, hence the term "rhesus sardonicus." Dysphagia, opisthotonus, and extension of lower extremities are also seen, but of importance, the mental status remains normal. This helps differentiate other pathologies.
- Instability of the autonomic nervous system, mostly a hyper sympathetic state, typically occurs in the second week of clinical tetanus and presents as tachycardia, hypertension, diaphoresis, and fever.
- Cephalic tetanus follows injuries to the head, and some cases of chronic otitis, resulting in dysfunction of the cranial nerves, most commonly the seventh. The prognosis is poor.
- Neonatal tetanus occurs only if the mother is inadequately immunized. Most cases of neonatal tetanus arise from unsterile handling of the umbilical cord at the time of birth or the umbilical stump after birth. The infant is weak, irritable, and unable to suck.

DIAGNOSIS AND DIFFERENTIAL

- Tetanus is a clinical diagnosis. There is no laboratory test to diagnose it.
- Strychnine poisoning most closely mimics the clinical picture of generalized tetanus.
- The differential diagnosis includes strychnine poisoning, serotonin syndrome, peritonitis, and malignant neuroleptic syndrome, dystonic reactions to the phenothiazines, hypocalcemic tetany, rabies, and temporomandibular joint disease.

EMERGENCY DEPARTMENT CARE AND DISPOSITION

- Patients with tetanus should be managed in an intensive care unit due to the potential for respiratory compromise. Minimize stimuli to prevent reflex convulsive spasms. Debridement of the inciting wound, if present, is necessary to minimize further toxin production.
- Tetanus immune globulin (TIG), 3000 to 6000 U intramuscularly in a single injection, should be given. TIG neutralizes circulating toxin but not toxin already fixed to the nervous system. Always give away from the tetanus vaccine site, and do not use the same syringe for both vaccine and immunoglobulin.
- Always give before any wound debridement, because more exotoxin may be released during wound manipulation.
- Antibiotics are of questionable value in the treatment of tetanus. If warranted, parenteral metronidazole (500 milligrams intravenously every 6 hours) is the antibiotic of choice. Do not use penicillin as it may potentiate the effects of tetanospasmin.
- Midazolam (5-15 milligrams IV as a continuous drip to effect) is best to use and results in sedation as well as amnesia. Lorazepam can be used but should be avoided in prolonged and repeated doses since the diluent, glycol, can cause acidosis.
- Neuromuscular blockade is often required to control ventilation and muscular spasm and to prevent fractures and rhabdomyolysis. Vecuronium, the agent of choice, is given (6-8 milligrams/h intravenously) because of its minimal cardiovascular side effects. Sedation during neuromuscular blockade is of primary importance.
- The combined α- and β-adrenergic blocking agent labetalol (0.25-1 milligram/min continuous intravenous infusion, 0.3 to 1 milligrams/kg/h in children) has been used to treat the manifestation of sympathetic hyperactivity.
- Propranolol is contraindicated because of its unopposed beta effects with sudden death cases reported.
- Magnesium sulfate (70 milligrams/kg loading dose, then 1-4 grams/h intravenously) has been advocated as a treatment for this condition as well.
- Morphine sulfate (0.5-1 milligram/kg/h) is also useful and provides sympathetic control without compromising cardiac output. Clonidine may be helpful in the management of cardiovascular instability.
- Patients that recover from clinical tetanus must undergo active immunization (see Chapter 18, and Table 18-1,

Recommendations for Tetanus Prophylaxis, for the treatment schedule).

RABIES

EPIDEMIOLOGY

- Rabies, primarily a disease of animals, claims over 60,000 deaths annually, worldwide.
- Ninety percent of transmission is due to dogs and where there is no canine control, wild animals accounted for almost 94% of the reported cases in decreasing order: raccoons; skunks; bats; foxes; and other wild animals, including rodents and lagomorphs. Rabid domestic animals included cats; cattle; dogs; horses and mules; sheep and goats; and other animals such as ferrets.
- Bat exposure even without a documented bite may require rabies prophylaxis. Such exposure maybe as simple as awakening in a room with a bat, or witnessing a bat in a room with a mentally disabled person, a child, or an intoxicated person; all those may require prophylaxis.
- In the United States most reports of rabies in wildlife far exceed those in domestic animals. Most other cases of human rabies diagnosed in the United States are attributable to infections acquired in areas of enzootic canine rabies outside of the United States; most persons with a case of rabies that originated in the United States have no history of an animal bite.
- The following animals are almost never found to be rabid: rodents (squirrels, chipmunks, rats, mice, etc.) and lagomorphs (rabbits, hares, and gophers); therefore, postexposure prophylaxis may not be needed. Do contact the health officials for management.

PATHOPHYSIOLOGY

- The rabies virus resides in the infected salivary glands of the animal. Once introduced, the incubation is 20 to 90 days where the virus remains close to the inoculation site.
- Subsequently the virus spreads across the motor endplate, and ascends and replicates along peripheral nervous system to the spinal cord and central nervous system (CNS). Following CNS replication, the virus spreads outward by peripheral nerves to most tissues and organ systems.

CLINICAL FEATURES

- Fever, malaise, headache, anorexia, nausea, sore throat, cough, and pain or paresthesia at the bite site (80%) are initial symptoms of human rabies and last 1 to 4 days.
- Later, CNS involvement leads to restlessness and agitation, altered mental status, painful bulbar and peripheral muscular spasms, opisthotonos, and motor paresis.

DIAGNOSIS AND DIFFERENTIAL

- Rabies is diagnosed clinically; there is no laboratory test for rabies. It should be suspected in any case of encephalitis.
- Most confirmatory diagnoses are made by postmortem analysis of brain tissue. Cerebrospinal fluid (CSF) and serum antibody titers should be sent to laboratories skilled in rabies identification. Elevated CSF protein and a mononuclear pleocytosis are also seen.
- The differential diagnosis includes other infectious encephalitis, polio, viral process, meningitis, brain abscess, cavernous sinus thrombosis, cholinergic poisoning, Guillain–Barre syndrome, and tetanus (normal mentation and normal CSF).

EMERGENCY DEPARTMENT CARE AND DISPOSITION

- When rabies exposure is suspected: If the person is bitten, scratched, or exposed to saliva of a possible rabid animal, treatment begins with the assessment of true risk for rabies, notification of public health and animal control, and if at risk, the administration of postexposure prophylaxis.
- Local wound care and debridement of devitalized tissue, if any, is important in reducing the viral inoculum and increasing oxygen tension in the tissue. Do not suture wounds of special concern, as this promotes rabies virus replication. Recall that the depth of the wound, the number of wounds, and their location increase the risk of developing the disease. Tetanus prophylaxis when needed should also be administered.
- Awakening in a room with a bat has been associated with the development of rabies. For this reason, the CDC recommends rabies postexposure prophylaxis for all persons who have been exposed to a bat unless the bat is available for testing and is negative for evidence of rabies.
- The CDC recommends that a healthy dog, cat, or ferret that bites a person should be confined and observed for 10 days.
- Human rabies immune globulin (HRIG) is administered only once at the outset of therapy. The dose is 20 IU/kg, with half the dose (based upon tissue volume constraints) infiltrated locally at the exposure site and the remainder administered intramuscularly.
- Human diploid cell vaccine (HDCV) for active immunization is available in two formulations of the same vaccine. The HDCV can be administered intramuscularly

or intradermal in five 1-mL doses on days 0, 3, 7, and 14. Day 28 is no longer recommended by the Advisory Committee on Immunization Practices (ACIP).
- Use only the regimens recommended by the US ACIP, from the CDC, because of their proven efficacy.
- Preexposure prophylaxis does not eliminate the need for prophylaxis after a rabies exposure, but it does simplify it by reducing the number of doses needed.
- The recommendations for postexposure prophylaxis should be followed *exactly* as given in the package insert. While there have been no failures in the United States, failures in other countries have been due to alterations in the method of administration or dosing interval.
- Healthcare workers with mucous or non-intact skin exposed to a patient with suspected rabies should receive postexposure prophylaxis for rabies.
- Ordinarily, dogs and cats involved in an attack on someone are quarantined for 10 days. If no signs become apparent within that period, the animal can be considered nonrabid.
- State or local officials should be consulted regarding the risk of rabies in local animal populations before initiating rabies prophylaxis. This action may not be possible before the first treatment, but may affect subsequent treatments. Animal bites should be reported to the local animal control unit so that animals can be captured or quarantined for observation in a timely fashion.
- The Centers for Disease Control and state and county health departments can provide assistance in the management of rabies complications. The rabies home page, which is produced and updated regularly by the Centers for Disease Control at www.cdc.gov/ncidod/dvrd/rabies, offers good update resources.

For further reading in Tintinalli's *Emergency Medicine: A Comprehensive Study Guide,* 7th ed., see Chapter 151, "Tetanus," by Joel L. Moll and Donna L. Carden, and Chapter 152, "Rabies," by David J. Weber, David A. Wohl, and William A. Rutala.

97 MALARIA

David M. Cline

- Malaria must be considered in any person who has traveled to the tropics (even months later) and presents with an unexplained febrile illness.

EPIDEMIOLOGY

- Five species of the protozoan *Plasmodium* infect humans: *Plasmodium falciparum, Plasmodium vivax, Plasmodium ovale, Plasmodium malariae,* and *Plasmodium knowlesi.*
- Malaria transmission occurs in large areas of Central and South America, the Caribbean, sub-Saharan Africa, the Indian subcontinent, Southeast Asia, the Middle East, and Oceania (New Guinea, Solomon Islands, etc.). More than 50% of all US cases of malaria, including most cases due to *P. falciparum,* arise from travel to sub-Saharan Africa. Resistance of *P. falciparum* to chloroquine and other drugs continues to spread (see Table 97-1). Strains of *P. vivax* with chloroquine resistance have been identified. The Centers for Disease Control and Prevention (CDC) has a malaria hotline: 770-488-7788 M-F, 8 a.m. to 4:30 p.m. EST, and 770-488-7100 after-hours, weekends and holidays. Alternatively, the CDC Web site can be accessed at http://www.cdc.gov/malaria/ for information on resistance patterns in various countries and information on malaria prophylaxis and treatment. When in doubt, chloroquine resistance for initial treatment should be assumed.

PATHOPHYSIOLOGY

- Transmitted by blood transfusion or passed transplacentally from mother to fetus.
- Plasmodial sporozoites are injected into a host's bloodstream during the feeding of the female anopheline mosquito, and travel directly to the liver where they invade hepatic parenchymal cells (exoerythrocytic stage). In the liver the parasites undergo asexual reproduction, forming thousands of daughter merozoites, which after an incubation period of one to several weeks rupture their host hepatic cells and are released into the peripheral circulation.
- The merozoites then rapidly invade circulating erythrocytes, where they mature and take on various morphologic forms—early ring forms, trophozoites, and schizonts, which are a mass of new merozoites (erythrocytic stage).
- Eventually the target red blood cell (RBC) lyses, releasing the merozoites to invade additional erythrocytes, continuing the infection. RBC lysis then often recurs at regular 2- to 3-day intervals, corresponding with the classic periodicity of symptoms. This cyclical feature may be absent in *P. falciparum* infection.
- With *P. vivax* or *P. ovale* infection, portions of the intrahepatic forms are not released, remain dormant for months, and can later activate, resulting in a clinical relapse.

TABLE 97-1 Geographic Distribution of Malaria, Including Resistant Strains

GEOGRAPHIC REGION	AREAS WITH MALARIA	COUNTRIES WITH CHLOROQUINE-RESISTANT *PLASMODIUM FALCIPARUM*
Central America	All countries	Areas east of the Panama Canal
Caribbean	Dominican Republic and Haiti	None
South America		
Temperate	Argentina	None
Tropical	Most countries	All countries except Paraguay
East Asia	China	China
Eastern South Asia	All countries except Brunei and Singapore	All infected areas
Middle South Asia	All countries	All countries
Western South Asia and Middle East	Iraq, Oman, Saudi Arabia, Syria, Turkey, and United Arab Emirates	All countries except Syria and Turkey
Northern Africa	All countries except Tunisia	None
Sub-Saharan Africa	All countries except Reunion and Seychelles	Widespread
Southern Africa	All countries except Lesotho and Saint Helena	Widespread
Oceania	Limited to Papua New Guinea, Solomon Islands, and Vanuatu (small foci elsewhere)	Widespread

- *Plasmodium* infection may also be acquired via transplacental transmission, via infected blood during transfusion, or by sharing of IV needles among drug abusers.
- The classic febrile paroxysm of malaria results from hemolysis of infected RBCs and the resulting release of antigenic agents that activate macrophages and produce cytokines.
- Infected RBCs lose their flexibility and thus are prone to cause congestion and obstruction of the capillary microcirculation of various organs, resulting in sequestration of blood in the spleen and anoxic injury to the lungs, kidneys, brain, and other vital organs.
- Hemolysis is often high with *P. falciparum* infection because of its predilection for erythrocytes of all ages (while the other three *Plasmodium* species target young or old RBCs). RBC sequestration accounts for the paucity of observed mature parasites sometimes seen on the peripheral blood smear in *P. falciparum* infection.
- Immunologic sequelae such as glomerulonephritis, nephrotic syndrome, thrombocytopenia, and polyclonal antibody stimulation may occur. Hypersplenism with subsequent pancytopenia may occur, especially with prolonged untreated malaria.

CLINICAL FEATURES

- The incubation period ranges from 1 to 4 weeks. Partial chemoprophylaxis or incomplete immunity can prolong the incubation period to months or even years.
- Initially malaria manifests with nonspecific fever and malaise, and then progresses to chills and high-grade fevers; frequent symptoms include headache, myalgia, arthralgia, cough, abdominal pain, nausea, and diarrhea.
- The patient may have tachycardia, orthostatic dizziness, and extreme weakness.
- Classically, cycles of fever and chills followed by profuse diaphoresis and exhaustion occur at regular intervals, reflecting hemolysis of infected erythrocytes.
- Physical examination findings are typically nonspecific. During a febrile paroxysm, most patients appear acutely ill, with high fever, tachycardia, and tachypnea.
- Splenomegaly is common. In *P. falciparum* infections, hepatomegaly, edema, and icterus often occur.
- Laboratory features include normocytic normochromic anemia with evidence of hemolysis and thrombocytopenia. The white blood cell count is normal or low.
- Complications of malaria can occur rapidly, particularly with *P. falciparum.*
- All forms cause hemolysis and splenomegaly, and splenic rupture may occur. Hypersplenism with subsequent pancytopenia may be seen in advanced cases.
- Glomerulonephritis, most often in *P. malariae* infections, and nephrotic syndrome may occur.
- Cerebral malaria, characterized by somnolence, coma, delirium, and seizures, has a mortality rate greater than 20%.

- Other life-threatening complications associated with *P. falciparum* include noncardiogenic pulmonary edema and metabolic abnormalities, including lactic acidosis and profound hypoglycemia.
- Blackwater fever is a severe complication seen almost exclusively in *P. falciparum* infections, with massive intravascular hemolysis, jaundice, hemoglobinuria (dark urine), and acute renal failure.

DIAGNOSIS AND DIFFERENTIAL

- The definitive diagnosis is established by identification of the parasite on Giemsa-stained thin and thick smears of peripheral blood.
- In early infection, especially with *P. falciparum,* parasitemia may be undetectable initially due to intraorgan sequestration.
- Parasite load in the peripheral circulation fluctuates over time and is highest during an acute rising fever with chills.
- Therapy should *not* be withheld if malaria is suspected, even though the parasite is not detected on initial blood smears.
- If plasmodia are not visualized, repeated smears should be taken at least twice daily (preferably during febrile episodes) for 3 days to fully exclude malaria.
- Once plasmodia are identified, the smear is also evaluated for the degree of parasitemia (percentage of red blood cells infected—which correlates with prognosis), and species type (in particular *P. falciparum*) is present.
- Antigen-detecting rapid diagnostic tests are available in certain areas, and are recommended by the World Health Organization (WHO), provided quality control measures are in place.
- Further, the WHO recommends parasite-based diagnosis except for young children in areas of high transmission when testing availability is limited; in these situations, clinically based diagnoses and treatment are recommended, with monitoring for clinical improvement.

EMERGENCY DEPARTMENT CARE AND DISPOSITION

- Unless it is certain that a patient could *not* have a chloroquine-resistant case, based on history of geographic exposure, the infection must be assumed to be resistant and treated with one of the chloroquine-resistant regimens listed immediately below.
- Patients with uncomplicated infection with chloroquine-resistant *P. falciparum* can be treated with one of several regimens.
- *Option 1* is artemether/lumefantrine, dose twice daily for 3 days, a total of six doses. For adults, 20 milligrams/ 120 milligrams tablets, 4 tablets initially, 4 tablets in 8 hours, then 4 tablets every 12 hours × 2 days. For children, 5 to 15 kg, one tablet initially, one tablet in 8 hours, then one tablet every 12 hours × 2 days; 15 to 25 kg, 2 tablets initially, 2 tablets in 8 hours, then 2 tablets every 12 hours × 2 days; 25 to 35 kg, 3 tablets initially, 3 tablets in 8 hours, then 3 tablets every 12 hours × 2 days; >35 kg, follow adult dosing.
- *Option 2* is atovaquone-proguanil. For adults, give four adult strength (250 milligrams/100 milligrams) tablets daily × 3 days. For children >41 kg, give adult dose; 31 to 40 kg, three adult tablets × 3 days; 21 to 30 kg, two adult tablets × 3 days; 11 to 20 kg, one adult tablet × 3 days; 9 to 10 kg, three pediatric tablets × 3 days; 5 to 8 kg, two pediatric tablets × 3 days.
- *Option 3* is quinine sulfate 542 milligrams base (= 650 milligrams salt) PO three times daily (10 milligrams salt/kg/dose maximum) for 3 to 7 days plus doxycycline 100 milligrams PO twice daily for 7 days. Options 1 and 2 are preferred for children.
- A final option is mefloquine plus doxycycline, but mefloquine has an increased frequency of neuropsychiatric reactions, making it the least favored choice.
- If *P. falciparum* can be excluded (travelers returning from Central America west of the Panama Canal, Haiti, the Dominican Republic, and most of the Middle East), patients with adequate home care and oral hydration can be treated as outpatients with close follow-up, including repeated blood smears to assess treatment response.
- Recommended treatment for uncomplicated malaria infection due to *P. vivax, P. ovale, P. malariae,* and *P. knowlesi* is chloroquine plus primaquine phosphate.
- For adults: chloroquine 600 milligrams base (= 1 gram salt), then 300 milligrams base (= 500 milligrams salt) in 6 hours, then 300 milligrams base per day for 2 days (total dose 1550 milligrams base), plus primaquine phosphate 30 milligrams base per day for 14 days on completion of chloroquine therapy.
- For children: chloroquine 10 milligrams/kg base to maximum of 600 milligrams load, then 5 milligrams/kg base in 6 hours and 5 milligrams/kg base per day for 2 days, *plus* primaquine phosphate 0.5 milligram/kg base for 14 days on completion of chloroquine therapy.
- Chloroquine has no effect on the exoerythrocytic forms of *P. vivax* and *P. ovale,* which remain dormant in the liver.
- Unless treated with primaquine, relapse will occur. Primaquine should be avoided in patients with glucose-6-phosphate dehydrogenase deficiency because of hemolysis.

- Patients with significant hemolysis or with comorbid conditions that can be aggravated by high fevers or hemolysis are best hospitalized, as are infants and pregnant women.
- *Plasmodium falciparum* infections are best managed in the hospital, as are patients with more than 3% parasitemia (typical in the USA and developed countries).
- Patients with complications due to *P. falciparum* or with high parasitemia but unable to tolerate oral medication should receive intravenous treatment.
- For severe malaria, with chloroquine-resistant *P. falciparum*, there are two recommended treatments.
- *Option 1* is quinidine, 6.25 milligrams base (= 10 milligrams salt)/kg IV load over 2 hours (maximum, 600 milligrams), then 0.0125 milligram base (= 0.02 milligram salt)/kg/min continuous infusion until patient is stabilized and able to tolerate PO therapy (see above). Parenteral quinidine and quinine can cause severe hypoglycemia. They are also myocardial depressants and are contraindicated in patients with heart disease. Cardiac monitoring is required during administration.
- *Option 2* is artesunate, which is available from the CDC quarantine station, follow artesunate with atovaquone-proguanil plus doxycycline as above. The dose of artesunate is 2.4 milligrams/kg IV at 0, 12, and 24 hours, and then 2.4 milligrams/kg once daily for 3 days.
- Aggressive supportive care should be provided to all hospitalized ill patients, including judicious fluid replacement, correction of metabolic derangements, and advanced support (dialysis, mechanical ventilation, etc.).

For further reading in Tintinalli's *Emergency Medicine: A Comprehensive Study Guide,* 7th ed., see Chapter 153, "Malaria," by John J. Szela, Josiah J. Tayali, and Jeffrey D. Band.

98 FOODBORNE AND WATERBORNE DISEASES

David M. Cline

EPIDEMIOLOGY

- Foodborne disease is an illness that occurs in two or more people after the consumption of common food source. Contamination can come from bacteria, viruses, or protozoans.
- Viruses are the most common source, including Norwalk-type (58% overall, United States), astrovirus, rotaviruses, and enteric adenoviruses.
- Bacterial sources include nontyphoidal *Salmonella* (11% overall, most common cause for hospitalization and associated death in the United States), *Clostridium perfringens*, *Campylobacter* spp., *Listeria monocytogenes*, *Shigella* spp., Shiga toxin–producing *Escherichia coli* (STEC), and *Staphylococcus aureus*.
- Parasitic causes include *Giardia lamblia*, *Toxoplasma gondii, Entamoeba histolytica,* and *Cryptosporidium.*
- The most common associated foods are poultry, leafy vegetables, and fruits/nuts.
- In addition, after eating reef fish that feed on certain dinoflagellates (algae), patients may experience scombroid or ciguatera poisoning, which is a toxin-induced syndrome.
- Waterborne diseases occur from ingestion of or contact with contaminated water from swimming pools, hot tubs, spas, or naturally occurring fresh or salt water.
- Symptoms of waterborne diseases can be either GI or dermatologic. Common organisms include the majority of those associated with foodborne illness plus *Vibrio* species, *Aeromonas* species, *Pseudomonas aeruginosa*, *Yersinia* species, hepatitis A, nontuberculous *Mycobacterium,* and less frequent organisms.

PATHOPHYSIOLOGY

- Foodborne pathogens are responsible for >200 known diseases and can cause illnesses through a variety of mechanisms.
- Some pathogens, such as *S. aureus*, *Bacillus cereus*, and *Clostridium botulinum* (botulism), produce toxins capable of causing illness.
- Preformed toxins are present in the food before ingestion and result in the rapid onset (1-6 hours) of vomiting.
- Other pathogens, such as *Vibrio*, *Shigella*, and STEC, produce toxins after ingestion, causing diarrhea and lower GI symptoms (cramping and sometimes bloody diarrhea) with onset at approximately 24 hours.
- Some of the most common pathogens, such as the enteric viruses, *Salmonella*, *Campylobacter*, and *Shigella*, directly invade the intestinal epithelial barrier. These pathogens often cause systemic symptoms such as fever and upper and lower GI symptoms lasting from 24 hours to weeks.
- Alteration of the gastrointestinal tract's protective mechanisms by medications, chronic systemic diseases, surgery, age, or the pathogen itself can increase susceptibility to foodborne disease.

- Proton pump inhibitors, histamine-2 (H2) blockers, and antacids reduce gastric pH.
- Recent antibiotic use, chemo- or radiation therapy, and recent surgery alter the intestinal flora.
- Decreased intestinal motility from narcotics, antiperistaltic drugs, and surgery may encourage pathogen growth and migration.

CLINICAL FEATURES

- Symptoms of both foodborne and waterborne illness include vomiting, diarrhea, abdominal cramping, fever, dehydration, malaise, and in some, bloody stool.
- Physical examination may be remarkable for features of dehydration, and in some, stool positive for frank or occult blood.
- Prolonged illness beyond 2 weeks suggests protozoan parasites. STEC may be complicated by hemolytic uremic syndrome (decreased urine output, symptoms of anemia), especially after antibiotic treatment.
- STEC classically presents with vomiting, moderate to marked stomach cramps, diarrhea (often bloody), and mild fever, not over 101°F/38.5°C.
- Patients with scombroid fish poisoning or ciguatera poisoning have symptoms similar to foodborne illness described immediately above, 1 to 24 hours after ingestion of reef fish. In addition, patients with scombroid poisoning frequently have flushing and headache due to histamine reaction.
- Those with ciguatera poisoning may have headaches, muscle aches, paresthesias, or a burning sensation on contact with cold, due to sodium channel–mediated nerve depolarizations.
- Neurologic symptoms may be prolonged beyond the ED visit.
- The skin manifestations of waterborne illness vary from simple cellulitis, the painful indurated plaque of *Mycobacterium marinum*, to necrotizing infections, which may include hemorrhagic bulla with *Vibrio vulnificus*.
- Patients with *Aeromonas hydrophila* skin infections often have a history of trauma associated with freshwater exposure, and may have foul-smelling wounds.

DIAGNOSIS AND DIFFERENTIAL

- Bedside testing for fecal occult blood is the most commonly indicated test; otherwise most patients need no laboratory testing, unless significantly dehydrated or other significant diagnoses are being considered.
- For those more acutely ill, consider fecal leukocytes, the neurophil marker lactoferrin, electrolytes, and complete blood count.
- Stool Gram stain may reveal *Campylobacter*. Stool cultures are more likely to be positive in those with positive fecal leukocytes or lactoferrin.
- STEC and *Vibrio* cultures require specific procedures (check local laboratory guidelines).
- Reserve ova and parasite testing for those patients with chronic symptoms, immunocompromised, or patients with a confirmed source of parasite.
- Other considerations include Rotavirus antigen testing in children from daycare settings, daycare workers, or older adults.
- *Clostridium difficile* antigen testing may be indicated in those with prolonged symptoms, recent antibiotic use, significant comorbidities, or extremes of age.

EMERGENCY DEPARTMENT CARE AND DISPOSITION

- Most cases are self-limited and improve with nonspecific treatment.
- Initiate oral rehydration fluids initially if tolerated. Intravenous rehydration with normal saline will benefit those significantly dehydrated, or those with continued vomiting.
- Antiemetics, such as metoclopramide 10 milligrams PO or IV, or ondansetron 4 milligrams PO or IV may facilitate oral rehydration.
- Antihistamines, such as diphenhydramine 25 milligrams PO or IV, may improve the symptoms of scombroid fish poisoning.
- Loperamide 4 milligrams initially and then 2 milligrams after every unformed stool up to a maximum of 16 milligrams/d is indicated in mild to moderate, non-bloody diarrhea in adults without fever (do not use in patients with STEC).
- Antibiotics are favored only in those patients with an increasing number of the following features: significant abdominal pain, bloody diarrhea, fever over 101°F/38.5°C, symptom duration >48 hours, impaired host, positive fecal leukocytes, or lactoferrin; however, **antibiotics are contraindicated in patients with STEC**.
- When treatment is indicated, recommended agents include ciprofloxacin 500 milligrams PO twice per day, or trimethoprim-sulfamethoxazole double-strength twice daily, for 3 to 5 days.
- Organism-specific antibiotic recommendations can be found in the parent text cited at the end of this chapter.
- *Vibrio vulnificus* skin infections are treated with doxycycline 100 milligrams IV or PO twice daily, plus ceftazidime 2 grams IV every 8 hours.
- *Aeromonas* skin infections are treated with ciprofloxacin 500 milligrams twice daily (mild cases) or with piperacillin-tazobactam 3.375 grams IV every 6 hours in severe cases.

- Necrotizing infections require emergent surgical debridement.
- Most patients can be treated as outpatients, and admission is indicated in those appearing toxic, those in whom vomiting cannot be controlled, the immunocompromised, or those at the extremes of age with significant symptoms.

For further reading in Tintinalli's *Emergency Medicine: A Comprehensive Study Guide,* 7th ed., see Chapter 154, "Foodborne and Waterborne Diseases," by Patrick L. McGauly and Simon A. Mahler.

99 ZOONOTIC INFECTIONS

Christopher R. Tainter

- Zoonoses are diseases transmitted between vertebrate animals and humans. They remain common and often underestimated in prevalence in North America.
- Infection may occur by direct contact, ingestion of contaminated water or food, inhalation, or through arthropod vectors.
- Most zoonoses in the United States have the highest incidence in the spring and summer. These diseases are easily mistaken for other nonspecific self-limited diseases, and many patients at risk fail to volunteer their exposure history (eg, cannot recall a tick bite). Rabies and West Nile virus are discussed separately.

■ ROCKY MOUNTAIN SPOTTED FEVER

EPIDEMIOLOGY

- Transmission of Rocky Mountain spotted fever (RMSF) to humans via tick bite occurs primarily between April and September, with the highest incidence in the mid-Atlantic states (although cases have been reported in most of the continental United States). Two-thirds of all cases are reported in children <15 years old.

PATHOPHYSIOLOGY

- RMSF is caused by *Rickettsia rickettsii*, a pleomorphic, obligate intracellular organism, carried by *Dermacentor* ticks. Deer, rodents, horses, cattle, cats, and dogs are the usual animal reservoir hosts.

CLINICAL FEATURES

- RMSF is classically defined by a triad of fever, rash, and history of tick exposure. Unfortunately, only about 50% of afflicted patients can recall a tick bite, and rash may be absent in up to 20% ("spotless RMSF," which is usually seen in African Americans, in the elderly, and in severe, fatal cases).
- The incubation period following a tick bite is usually 4 to 10 days and is followed by onset of nonspecific symptoms such as fever, malaise, severe headache, myalgias, nausea and vomiting, diarrhea, anorexia, abdominal pain, and photophobia.
- Additional signs and symptoms may include lymphadenopathy, hepatosplenomegaly, conjunctivitis, confusion, meningismus, renal or respiratory failure, and myocarditis.
- A rash usually begins 2 to 4 days after the onset of fever. It is generally maculopapular, typically begins on the extremities around the wrists and ankles (often involving the palms and soles), and spreads centripetally to the trunk, usually sparing the face (it may become petechial or purpuric later).

DIAGNOSIS AND DIFFERENTIAL

- Lab findings are usually nonspecific, but the combination of neutropenia, thrombocytopenia, hyponatremia, and elevated liver function tests (LFTs) suggests RMSF.
- The mortality rate for RMSF is between 5% and 10%. The clinical diagnosis must be presumed in order to start therapy early, since serology to confirm a rise in antibody titer is not reliably positive until 6 to 10 days after onset of symptoms (diagnosis may also be confirmed by skin rash biopsy with immunofluorescent testing).
- Differential diagnosis includes viral illness, ehrlichiosis, disseminated gonorrhea, meningococcemia, secondary syphilis, scarlet fever, leptospirosis, typhoid, gastroenteritis, pneumonia, and toxic shock syndrome.

EMERGENCY DEPARTMENT CARE AND DISPOSITION

- Treatment for adults includes doxycycline 100 milligrams PO or IV twice daily for 5 to 10 days. Alternatives include tetracycline 500 milligrams PO four times daily, or chloramphenicol 12.5 to 18.75 milligrams/kg/dose IV every 6 hours.
- Treatment for children <45 kg includes doxycycline 2.2 milligrams/kg twice daily. Tetracycline and IV chloramphenicol are alternatives, although chloramphenicol is contraindicated in children less than 2 years old.

- Doxycycline is the first-line therapy for rickettsial diseases recommended in all ages by the Centers for Disease Control and Prevention and the American Academy of Pediatrics.

LYME DISEASE

EPIDEMIOLOGY

- Lyme disease remains the most common vector-borne zoonosis in the United States, and is most prevalent in the north-central, northeastern, and mid-Atlantic states, but has been reported in all 48 contiguous states.

PATHOPHYSIOLOGY

- *Borrelia burgdorferi*, a spirochete, is the responsible organism and is transmitted to humans by *Ixodes* species (black-legged) ticks, with rabbits, rodents, and deer serving as host reservoir animals. The overall risk of contracting Lyme disease after a deer tick bite is relatively low, about 3% in highly endemic areas, and proportional to the length of tick attachment. There is almost no risk when the duration of attachment is less than 24 hours.

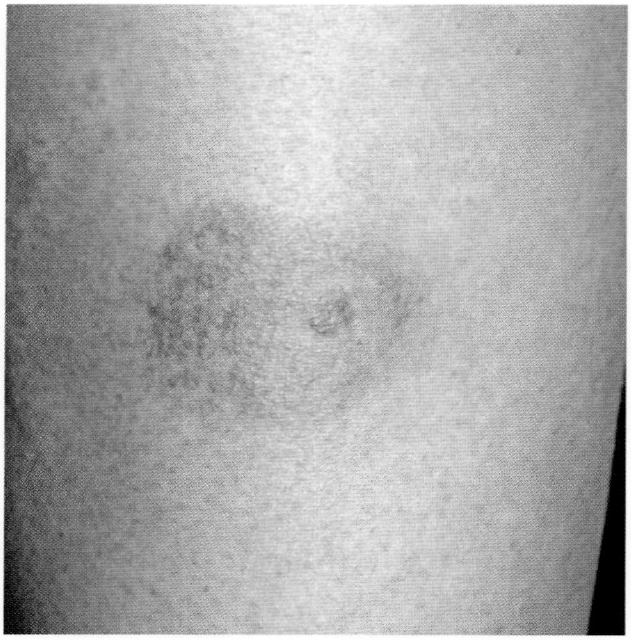

FIG. 99-1. Erythema chronicum migrans. This pathognomonic eruption of Lyme disease forms at the site of the tick bite. The initial papule forms into a slowly enlarging oval area of erythema while clearing centrally. Reproduced with permission from Knoop K, Stack L, Storrow A: Atlas of Emergency Medicine, 3rd ed. © 2010 McGraw-Hill, New York. (Photo contributed by David Effron, MD.)

CLINICAL FEATURES

- Lyme disease is divided into three distinct stages, but not all patients suffer all stages; stages may overlap and remissions between stages may occur.
- *Stage I* is characterized by the erythema chronicum migrans (ECM) skin lesion, which occurs in 60% to 80% of cases. It consists of an annular, erythematous skin plaque with central clearing (see Fig. 99-1), which develops 2 to 20 days after a tick bite at the inoculation site, as a result of a vasculitis. It resolves after 3 to 4 weeks, and may recur during the second stage.
- *Stage II* corresponds to dissemination of the spirochete, resulting in multiple secondary annular skin lesions (ECM), fever, adenopathy, splenomegaly, and flulike constitutional symptoms. Neurologic symptoms may occur during stage II, most often cranial neuritis (especially uni- or bilateral facial nerve palsy), but may also include headache, neck stiffness, cerebellar ataxia, or encephalitis. Asymmetric oligoarticular arthritis (usually in large joints, especially knees) may develop as well. Cardiac abnormalities occur in approximately 8% of patients and typically present as first-, second-, or third-degree atrioventricular nodal heart block or myocarditis.
- *Stage III* represents chronic persistent infection, and occurs years after the initial infection. It may include chronic intermittent migratory arthritis, myocarditis, encephalopathy, and axonal polyneuropathy.

DIAGNOSIS AND DIFFERENTIAL

- Diagnosis is made clinically, and may be confirmed by polymerase chain reaction (PCR), polyvalent fluorescence immunoassay, or Western immunoblot testing.
- The differential diagnosis depends on clinical manifestation of the disease stage, and may include cellulitis, erythema multiforme, tinea corporis, viral/bacterial meningitis/encephalitis, rheumatic fever, septic arthritis, endocarditis, and other inflammatory/autoimmune and viral syndromes.

EMERGENCY DEPARTMENT CARE AND DISPOSITION

- The treatment of choice for early Lyme disease is oral doxycycline 100 milligrams PO twice daily for 14 to 21 days for primary stage infection (28 days if treating secondary stage, and 28 to 60 days for tertiary stage).

Acceptable alternatives include amoxicillin, cefuroxime, ceftriaxone, or erythromycin.

- A single dose of doxycycline 200 milligrams given within 72 hours of the deer tick bite can prevent Lyme disease, but this is not routinely suggested due to the low transmission rate, the potential to depress the immune response to the disease, and the high incidence of gastrointestinal side effects from high-dose oral doxycycline.

EHRLICHIOSIS

EPIDEMIOLOGY

- A zoonotic disease with two clinical subtypes (*human granulocytic* and *human monocytic*). The *human monocytic* form (*Ehrlichia chaffeensis*) predominates in the United States.

PATHOPHYSIOLGY

- Caused by *Ehrlichia* species, small gram-negative coccobacilli that infect circulating leukocytes. Transmission occurs via bite or exposure to *Amblyomma americanum* (lone star tick) and *Dermacentor variabilis*. The major animal reservoir in North America is the white-tailed deer in the southeastern United States.

CLINICAL FEATURES

- Symptoms usually develop within 10 to 14 days of tick bite, and may include fever, headache, malaise, nausea, vomiting, diarrhea, abdominal pain, and arthralgias.
- More serious complications of renal or respiratory failure and encephalitis occur in a minority of patients.
- The acute phase of illness lasts less than 4 weeks, with most patients recovering and proceeding to a convalescent phase.

DIAGNOSIS AND DIFFERENTIAL

- Diagnosis is made clinically, but can be confirmed by a rise in antibody titer between the acute and convalescent phase.
- Laboratory findings may include leukocytopenia, thrombocytopenia, and elevated serum hepatic enzymes.
- The differential diagnosis includes cholecystitis/cholangitis, Lyme disease, babesiosis, malaria, meningitis, RMSF, and typhoid.

EMERGENCY DEPARTMENT CARE AND DISPOSITION

- The treatment of choice for both adults and children is doxycycline 100 milligrams PO twice daily for 7 to 14 days (for children, 2.2 milligrams/kg PO twice daily).

COLORADO TICK FEVER

EPIDEMIOLOGY

- Colorado tick fever is endemic to the western mountainous regions of the United States, at elevations above 4000 ft. Only about 300 cases are reported annually.

PATHOPHYSIOLOGY

- An acute viral illness caused by an RNA virus of the genus *Coltivirus*, transmitted to humans primarily via *Dermacentor andersoni* (wood tick). Animal reservoirs are deer, marmots, and porcupines.

CLINICAL FEATURES

- Symptoms begin suddenly 3 to 6 days following tick bite and include fever, chills, headache, myalgias, and photophobia. There may be a macular or petechial rash. Complications are rare.

DIAGNOSIS AND DIFFERENTIAL

- Diagnosis is based on clinical findings and geography.
- Differential diagnosis includes meningitis (bacterial or viral), and other tick-borne illnesses (especially RMSF).

EMERGENCY DEPARTMENT CARE AND DISPOSITION

- No specific therapy exists, and supportive care is usually sufficient.

TULAREMIA

EPIDEMIOLOGY

- Tularemia has been widely reported in the continental United States, with the highest incidence in Arkansas, Missouri, and Oklahoma. Incidence is highest in early winter (adults) and early summer (children).

PATHOPHYSIOLOGY

- Tularemia is caused by *Francisella tularensis*, a nonmotile, gram-negative coccobacillus carried by *Dermacentor* and *Amblyomma* ticks. The principal animal reservoirs are rabbits, hares, cats, and deer.
- Transmission occurs via arthropod bite or direct innoculation from an infected host.

CLINICAL FEATURES

- There are several distinct clinical syndromes, depending on the route of inoculation: *ulceroglandular, glandular, typhoidal, pneumonic,* and *oropharyngeal.*
- The *ulceroglandular* form is the most common, characterized by an ulcer at the site of the tick bite, and painful regional adenopathy. *Glandular* tularemia consists of tender regional adenopathy without a skin lesion.
- *Typhoidal* tularemia (any form of transmission) is associated with fever, chills, cephalgia, and abdominal pain. *Ocular-oropharyngeal* and *pneumonic* forms are the result of deposition of the bacterium in the eyes, or inhalation.

DIAGNOSIS AND DIFFERENTIAL

- Clinical diagnosis can be confirmed by culture and enzyme-linked immunosorbent assay (ELISA). Other laboratory findings are nonspecific.
- The multiple clinical variations of tularemia lead to a broad differential diagnosis that should include pyogenic bacterial infection, syphilis, anthrax, plague, Q fever, psittacosis, typhoid, brucellosis, and rickettsial infection.

EMERGENCY DEPARTMENT CARE AND DISPOSITION

- Treatment is with streptomycin 1 gram IM twice daily or IM or IV (pediatric dose is 15 milligrams/kg IM twice daily, max 2 grams/d), or gentamicin 5 milligrams/kg IM or IV once daily. Other alternatives include doxycycline, chloramphenicol, and ciprofloxacin. Therapy is given for 10 to 14 days.

HANTAVIRUS

EPIDEMIOLOGY

- Hantavirus infection is a viral zoonosis identified in 1977. In North America the etiologic agent is the Sin Nombre virus (a member of Bunyaviridae family), and to date at least 10 distinct serotypes have been identified, each with a specific rodent vector, geographic distribution, and clinical manifestation.

PATHOPHYSIOLOGY

- In the southwestern United States, *Peromyscus maniculatus* (deer mouse) is the primary vector, with transmission to humans accomplished via inhalation of dried particulate feces, contact with urine, or by rodent bite.

CLINICAL FEATURES

- Worldwide the majority of hantavirus serotypes have a predilection for the kidney, with a clinical presentation of acute renal failure, thrombocytopenia, ocular abnormalities, and flulike symptoms.
- In the United States, the most common presentation is hantavirus pulmonary syndrome: a flulike prodrome for 3 to 4 days, followed by pulmonary edema, hypoxia, hypotension, tachycardia, and metabolic acidosis. The presence of dizziness, nausea and vomiting, and thrombocytopenia and the absence of a cough may help with clinical diagnosis.

DIAGNOSIS AND DIFFERENTIAL

- Diagnosis relies on clinical features and a history of exposure, but may be confirmed by an immunofluorescent or immunoblot assay. Differential diagnosis includes bacterial pneumonia, acute respiratory distress syndrome (ARDS), and influenza pneumonia.

EMERGENCY DEPARTMENT CARE AND DISPOSITION

- Hantavirus pulmonary syndrome has reported a mortality rate of 50% to 70%. Treatment is primarily with supportive care (especially oxygenation and ventilation) and possibly inhaled ribavirin.

ANTHRAX

EPIDEMIOLOGY

- Anthrax infection is very rare in North America, but remains a concern in part because of its potential use as an agent of biological warfare or terrorism.

PATHOPHYSIOLOGY

- Anthrax is an acute bacterial infection caused by *Bacillus anthracis*, an aerobic gram-positive rod that forms central oval spores.

- In nature, the disease is most commonly seen in domestic herbivores (cattle, sheep, horses, and goats) and wild herbivores. Human infection can result from inhalation of spores, inoculation of broken skin, arthropod bite (fleas), or ingestion of inadequately cooked infected meat.

CLINICAL FEATURES

- Inhalational anthrax is a mediastinitis without alveolar involvement, and therefore not a true pneumonia. Initially patients suffer a flulike illness that progresses over 3 to 4 days to respiratory failure, and is generally fatal.
- Cutaneous anthrax (woolsorter's disease) accounts for 95% of infections. Spores are deposited in a wound (usually on the hands or fingers), and in 1 to 5 days progresses to a pruritis macule.
- The lesion then becomes an ulcer with multiple sero-sanguinous vesicles containing the bacilli, and are infectious. The ulcer eventually becomes a black eschar and falls off within 2 weeks.

DIAGNOSIS AND DIFFERENTIAL

- Diagnosis may be established via Gram's stain, direct fluorescent antibody stain, or culture of skin lesions or vesicular fluid.
- The differential diagnosis depends on the type of exposure. For inhalational anthrax, it may include influenza, tuberculosis, and other causes of mediastinitis (bacterial, viral, parasitic, sarcoidosis). With cutaneous anthrax, warfarin necrosis, calciphylaxis, ischemic necrosis, tularemia, plague, spider/insect bite, mycobacterial infection, ecthyma gangrenosum, and aspergillosis/mucormycosis should be considered.

EMERGENCY DEPARTMENT CARE AND DISPOSITION

- Treatment for both inhalational and cutaneous anthrax is ciprofloxacin 400 milligrams (10-15 milligrams/kg for children) IV every 12 hours or doxycycline 100 milligrams (2.2 milligrams/kg for children) IV every 12 hours, plus either clindamycin or rifampin. Extended treatment for adults is ciprofloxacin 500 milligrams PO every 12 hours or doxycycline 100 milligrams PO every 12 hours for 60 days.
- A vaccine is available for high-risk populations (military personnel and laboratory technicians).
- Prophylaxis for exposed individuals can be done with either ciprofloxacin 500 milligrams PO twice per day or doxycycline 100 milligrams PO twice per day for 60 days in combination with a three-dose vaccination course.

PLAGUE (YERSINIA)

EPIDEMIOLOGY

- Plague is endemic to the United States, most often found in the Southwest, but may also be carried by cats and dogs.

PATHOPHYSIOLOGY

- *Yersinia pestis* is a gram-negative bacillus of the Enterobacteriaceae family. Rock squirrels and ground rodents are the animal reservoir, and the rodent flea is the primary vector.
- Transmission to humans occurs via the bite of a flea from an infected animal host or through handling or ingestion of infected rodents.

CLINICAL FEATURES

- There are three clinical forms of human disease: bubonic or suppurative (most common), which may progress to the pneumonic or septicemic forms.
- The incubation period ranges from 2 to 7 days following exposure. Frequently an eschar develops at the bite site, followed by a painful, sometimes suppurative bubo (enlarged regional lymph nodes), often at the groin. Associated symptoms may include fever, headache, malaise, abdominal pain, nausea and vomiting, and bloody diarrhea.
- The pulmonary form is highly contagious and can be transmitted from person to person via aerosolized respiratory secretions (respiratory isolation is required). It is rapidly fatal if not aggressively treated.

DIAGNOSIS AND DIFFERENTIAL

- Diagnosis must be made on clinical findings in a patient with possible contact with a vector or animal host. Blood culture or culture of suspected sites may reveal organisms, but treatment should be initiated in suspected cases without awaiting these results.
- The differential diagnosis includes lymphogranuloma venereum, syphilis, staphylococcal or streptococcal lymphadenitis, other causes of pneumonia, or tularemia.

EMERGENCY DEPARTMENT CARE AND DISPOSITION

- Therapy should begin immediately for any suspected case with gentamicin 2.0 milligrams/kg IV loading dose, then 1.7 milligrams/kg IV every 8 hours (2-2.5 milligrams/kg/dose for children), or streptomycin

15 milligrams/kg or 1 gram IV or IM every 12 hours. Therapy is continued for 10 to 14 days. Alternatives include doxycycline or ciprofloxacin.

For further reading in Tintinalli's *Emergency Medicine: A Comprehensive Study Guide*, 7th ed., see Chapter 155, "Zoonotic Infections," by John T. Meredith.

100 WORLD TRAVELERS

David M. Cline

EPIDEMIOLOGY

- Fever and other symptoms of infection are the most common complaints for returning travelers (see Table 100-1).
- The evaluation of infectious disease in the returning traveler requires an understanding of the geographical distribution of infections (see Table 100-2), risk factors, incubation periods, clinical manifestations, and appropriate laboratory investigations.
- See Centers for Disease Control and Prevention (CDC) Web site for further information: http://wwwnc.cdc.gov/travel/destinations/list.aspx.
- Traveler's diarrhea, enteroviral infections, gastroenteritis, giardiasis, salmonellosis, and shigellosis are discussed in Chapter 98, Foodborne and Waterborne Diseases, as well as in Chapter 39, Diseases Presenting Primarily with Diarrhea; malaria is discussed in Chapter 97, Malaria; upper respiratory infection and pertussis are discussed in Chapter 32, Pneumonia, Bronchitis, and Upper Respiratory Tract Infection; STDs are discussed in Chapter 89, Sexually Transmitted Diseases; hepatitis A and B are discussed in Chapter 50, Hepatic Disorders, Jaundice, and Hepatic Failure; HIV (human immunodeficiency virus) infections and acquired immune deficiency syndrome are discussed in Chapter 94; anthrax and plague are discussed in Chapter 99, Zoonotic Diseases.
- This chapter covers the most common infectious disease presentations in returning travelers; the reader is referred to the source material, cited at the end of the chapter, for further information, and discussion of less common diseases.

TABLE 100-2 Common Regional Tropical Illness

Africa	Malaria, human immunodeficiency virus, TB, hookworm, tapeworm, roundworm, brucellosis, yellow fever (and other hemorrhagic fevers), relapsing fever, schistosomiasis, tick typhus
Central and South America	Malaria, relapsing fever, dengue fever, filariasis, TB, schistosomiasis, Chagas disease, louse-borne typhus
Mexico, Caribbean	Dengue fever, hookworm, malaria, cysticercosis, amebiasis, louse-borne typhus
Australia	Dengue fever
Middle East	Malaria, hookworm, anthrax, brucellosis
China and East Asia	Dengue fever, hookworm, malaria, strongyloidiasis, hemorrhagic fever, scrub typhus

CLINICAL FEATURES

- The incubation period for disease is most commonly longer than a traveler's foreign stay, and therefore, travelers commonly become febrile/symptomatic upon return.

TABLE 100-1 Traveler Risk of Exposure to Infectious Agents

RISK (FREQUENCY)	DISEASES/SYNDROMES (# REFERENCES TO OTHER JUST THE FACTS CHAPTERS)
High risk (1 in 10)	Traveler's diarrhea (98), upper respiratory illness (32)
Moderate risk (1 in 200)	Chikungunya, dengue fever, enteroviral infection (98), gastroenteritis (98), giardiasis, hepatitis A (50), malaria (97), salmonellosis (98), sexually transmitted diseases (89), shigellosis
Low risk (1 in 1000)	Amebiasis, ascariasis (roundworm), enterobiasis (pinworm), hepatitis B (50), scabies (157), tuberculosis (33), typhoid/paratyphoid
Very low risk (1 in >1000)	Anthrax (99), brucellosis, Chagas disease, cysticercosis, hemorrhagic fevers (including yellow fever), human immunodeficiency virus (94), hookworm, leishmaniasis, leptospirosis, pertussis (32), plague (99), schistosomiasis/Katayama syndrome, typhus/rickettsial disease, trypanosomiasis

- Travel history should include query concerning visits to game parks, farms, caves, health facilities, consumption of exotic foods, activities involving fresh- or saltwater exposure, insect exposure, sexual activities, epidemics in the area visited, contact with ill people, as well as pre-trip immunizations, and prophylactic antibiotics taken.
- A history of chronological disease presentation should be taken including height, quality, and duration of fever and chills.
- Examination findings such as current temperature, rash, eschar, hepatosplenomegaly, lymphadenopathy, jaundice, and other skin findings should be documented.

DIAGNOSIS AND DIFFERENTIAL

- General laboratory assessment includes malaria smear (and dipstick antigen test if available) for all febrile travelers returning from locations with endemic malaria.
- Complete blood count: look for lymphopenia (dengue, HIV, and typhoid) or eosinophilia (parasites, fungal disease) and thrombocytopenia (malaria, dengue, acute HIV, typhoid).
- Urinalysis may show proteinuria and hematuria in cases of leptospirosis. Blood cultures should be obtained prior to antibiotics.
- Liver function tests are indicated if patient is jaundiced. Consider specific testing for diseases suspected by symptoms and risk of exposure.
- Obtain a chest radiograph for respiratory symptoms, and consider a liver ultrasound if amebic liver abscess is suspected.

ASSESSMENT, EMERGENCY DEPARTMENT CARE, AND DISPOSITION FOR SPECIFIC DISEASES

- Malaria is the most important disease to rule out in returning travelers (discussed in Chapter 97, Malaria).
- The other most common diseases in returning travelers (see also references at the beginning of this chapter) are discussed below.

DENGUE FEVER

- Dengue fever is spread by the day-biting *Aedes aegypti* mosquito. Incubation is 4 to 7 days.
- Symptoms of classic dengue are high fever, headache, nausea, vomiting, myalgias, and rash (late), lasting several days.
- Dengue fever acquired in Southeast Asia typically is accompanied by hemorrhagic symptoms and often shock; in this form abdominal pain may be marked.
- Diagnosis is by polymerase chain reaction (PCR) (1-8 days post symptom onset) or IgM ELISA, after 4 days of symptoms.
- Daily blood counts are recommended.
- Outpatient treatment is recommended in mild cases, with oral hydration as tolerated and close follow-up for blood work. Avoid aspirin and NSAIDs.
- Inpatient treatment for supportive care is recommended if there is a drop in hematocrit or platelets, hemorrhagic symptoms, or abnormal vital signs.

CHIKUNGUNYA

- Chikungunya is the second most common arbovirus infection in returning travelers, after dengue fever.
- Also spread by day-biting mosquitos, chikungunya presents very much like classic dengue fever but additionally with generalized arthralgia.
- From 5% to 30% of patients will go on to have chronic arthropathy.
- Diagnosis is by PCR (1-4 days post symptom onset) or IgM, after 5 days of symptoms.
- Treatment is supportive; chloroquine may reduce long-term arthralgias but is not standard therapy. NSAIDs are helpful, but should be avoided until dengue fever has been ruled out.

TYPHOID FEVER

- Typhoid fever, or enteric fever, is caused by *Salmonella typhi* and *Salmonella paratyphi*.
- Transmission is from contaminated food or water, after contact with the infected urine or feces of symptomatic individuals, or asymptomatic carriers.
- After malaria is ruled out (by lack of potential exposure or by testing), typhoid fever is the most common febrile disease lasting more than 10 days in returning travelers.
- Incubation is 1 to 3 weeks.
- Symptoms include fever with headache initially, then high fever with chills, headache, cough, abdominal distention, myalgias, constipation (most common, but some have diarrhea), and prostration.
- A classic presentation is bradycardia relative to the height of fever, but is often absent.
- After several days, a pale red macular rash appears on the trunk, "rose spots."
- Complications include small-bowel ulceration, anemia, disseminated intravascular coagulopathy (DIC), pneumonia, meningitis, myocarditis, and renal failure.

- Remarkable lab findings may include leukopenia and elevated liver enzymes, however not typical.
- Diagnosis is clinical, and confirmation is by stool culture. After initiation of supportive care with fluids and fever control, treatment is ceftriaxone, 2 grams IV/IM for 14 days, or ciprofloxacin 500 to 750 milligrams PO twice daily for 14 days.
- For severe typhoid fever complicated by delirium, coma, shock, or DIC, administer dexamethasone, 3 milligrams/kg IV load.
- Blood transfusion may be required in severe cases.

BRUCELLOSIS

- Brucellosis is caused by the bacterium *Brucella*, most commonly following contact with cattle, goats, camels, dogs, or pigs, or after ingestion of unpasteurized milk or cheese.
- Symptoms include fever, abdominal pain, back pain, fatigue, headache, joint pain, and loss of appetite.
- Common history is relapsing fever, but can be chronic low-grade fever. Examination findings include lymphadenopathy, hepatomegaly, as well as splenomegaly, and may include septic arthritis.
- Diagnosis is by blood culture, or serology.
- Consult infectious disease for treatment with doxycycline, rifampicin, and an aminoglycoside, streptomycin, or gentamicin for 2 weeks.

RICKETTSIAL SPOTTED FEVERS INCLUDING SCRUB TYPHUS

- Rickettsial spotted fevers are transmitted by the bite, body fluid, or feces of ixodid arthropod ticks.
- Mortality without treatment approaches 25%. Scrub typhus (*Rickettsia orientalis*) and African tick typhus (*Rickettsia conorii*) are the most common forms in travelers returning from the Southeast Asia and Africa, respectively.
- Incubation is 3 to 14 days.
- Symptoms are fever, malaise, myalgias, severe headache, rash (may be absent), nausea, and vomiting followed by lymphadenopathy and splenomegaly.
- The skin lesion in scrub typhus starts as a papule at the bite site, which becomes necrotic and forms a crusted black eschar.
- African scrub typhus is, in general, less severe.
- Diagnosis is clinical; serologic tests confirm the diagnosis after empiric treatment with doxycycline 100 milligrams twice daily for 7 to 10 days; chloramphenicol is an alternative.

TYPHUS EPIDEMIC LOUSE-BORNE TYPHUS

- Epidemic louse-borne typhus, common in Mexico, Guatemala, Ethiopia, and the Himalayas, is caused by *Rickettsia prowazekii* and should not be confused with the disease caused by *S. typhi*.
- Incubation is 8 to 12 days. Patients may or may not be aware of the louse. Symptoms include high fevers, severe headache, and a maculopapular rash between 4 and 7 days.
- Diagnosis is clinical; serologic tests confirm the diagnosis after empiric treatment with doxycycline 100 milligrams twice daily for 7 to 10 days; chloramphenicol is an alternative.

LEPTOSPIROSIS (WEIL DISEASE)

- Leptospirosis occurs after freshwater exposure to *Leptospira interrogans* or after exposure to infected dogs.
- Incubation is 2 to 20 days.
- Symptoms include high fever, severe headache, chills, myalgias, hepatitis with or without jaundice, and conjunctival injection without purulent discharge.
- Diagnosis requires serology. Mild disease (within 3 days of symptoms) is treated with amoxicillin 500 milligrams three times daily, or doxycycline 100 milligrams twice daily.
- More severe cases should be treated with penicillin G, 5 million units every 6 hours IV, or ceftriaxone 1 gram IV/IM daily.
- Treatment duration is 7 to 14 days.

CRIMEAN–CONGO HEMORRHAGIC FEVER

- Crimean–Congo hemorrhagic fever is a tick-borne viral disease that is rising in frequency in Africa, Asia, Eastern Europe, and the Middle East.
- Agricultural workers are at the greatest risk, but it can be acquired from contact with the blood of patients.
- Symptoms include sudden onset of fever, headache, myalgia, dizziness, and possibly mental confusion.
- The hemorrhagic period is short (2-3 days), starts the third to fifth day of illness, and may manifest with epistaxis, hemoptysis, GI bleeding, vaginal bleeding, or hematuria.
- Patients may have thrombocytopenia, elevated liver enzymes, and creatinine, Prothrombin time and activated partial thromboplastin time may be prolonged.
- Diagnosis is clinical with confirmation by serology. Treatment is supportive, and may require transfusions and/or respiratory support.

- Ribavirin is used in moderate to severe cases, 30 milligrams/kg load, then 15 milligrams/kg every 6 hours for 4 days, and then 7.5 milligrams/kg for 6 days.

YELLOW FEVER

- Yellow fever is caused by a flavivirus, transmitted by a day-biting mosquito, occurring along a broad equatorial belt in South and Central America and Africa.
- Symptoms range from a mild flulike illness to hemorrhagic fever with 20% mortality.
- After an incubation period of 3 to 6 days, typical early symptoms include fever, headache, myalgias, conjunctival injection, abdominal pain, prostration, facial flushing, and relative bradycardia; subsequently the classic jaundice, black emesis, and albuminuria are found.
- Symptoms may progress to shock, multiorgan failure, and bleeding diathesis.
- Treatment is supportive, including transfusion as needed.

CYSTICERCOSIS

- Cysticercosis is the systemic illness caused by dissemination of the larval form of the pork tapeworm.
- Humans become infected by ingesting the contaminated food (undercooked pork), or inadvertent contact with contaminated soil.
- Involvement of almost any tissue can occur.
- CNS infection is known as neurocysticercosis, and is the most important cause of seizures worldwide.
- Additional symptoms of neurocysticercosis include headache, visual or mental status changes, stroke, meningoencephalitis, and obstructive hydrocephalus.
- Noncontrast CT shows calcifications of inactive disease, and may reveal hydrocephalus.
- Therapy is praziquantel, 17 milligrams/kg/dose three times daily (albendazole also used).
- Steroids are recommended for those with encephalitis, hydrocephalus, or vasculitis.

AFRICAN TRYPANOSOMIASIS (AFRICAN SLEEPING SICKNESS)

- Sleeping sickness is transmitted by the aggressive tsetse fly.
- After a bite, a localized inflammatory reaction occurs followed in 2 to 3 days by a painless chancre that increases in size for 2 to 3 weeks, and then gradually regresses.
- Intermittent fevers follow the skin lesion, with malaise, rash, and eventual CNS involvement, causing behavioral and neurologic changes, encephalitis, coma, and death.
- Other complications include hemolysis, anemia, pancarditis, and meningoencephalitis.
- Diagnosis is made by rapid evaluation of blood smears for the mobile parasite.
- Consult infectious disease expert for diagnosis and treatment with suramin and other agents.

CHAGAS DISEASE (AMERICAN TRYPANOSOMIASIS)

- The protozoan *Trypanosoma cruzi* is endemic in regions of Latin America and is reported as far north as Texas.
- It is spread by the reduviid "kissing bug " or "assassin" bug.
- The bug typically bites nocturnally after emerging from rural adobe walls or thatched roofs.
- Symptoms of the acute phase are unilateral periorbital edema (Romaña sign) or painful cutaneous edema at the site of skin penetration (chagoma) followed by a toxemic phase with parasitemia causing lymphadenopathy and hepatosplenomegaly.
- The acute phase diagnosis is made by examination of peripheral blood smears demonstrating motile parasites, or by blood culture. In the chronic phase, serologic tests or tissue biopsies are useful.
- Recommended treatment is nifurtimox (consult infections disease).

LEISHMANIASIS (VISCERAL)

- *Leishmania* is an intracellular protozoan transmitted by *Lutzomyia* or *Phlebotomus* sandflies.
- Leishmaniasis should be suspected in the military and their families living proximal to jungles, adventure travelers, field biologists, and emigrants from endemic zones.
- The disease has a variety of syndromic presentations, the most important of which is visceral leishmaniasis, or kala-azar, or black fever.
- It is typified by a pentad of fever, weight loss, hepatosplenomegaly, pancytopenia, and hypergammaglobulinemia.
- Treat visceral disease with pentavalent antimonials, either sodium stibogluconate (available through the CDC) or meglumine antimonate, available in some European countries.

SCHISTOSOMIASIS (SNAIL FEVER)

- Schistosomiasis should be suspected in travelers presenting with GI symptoms exposed to freshwater.

- The larvae are released into freshwater by snails. Soon after exposure, "swimmer's itch" occurs with a macular-papular pruritic dermatitis over the lower legs, which can last for days.
- Four to eight weeks later, fever occurs, with headache, cough, urticaria, diarrhea, hepatosplenomegaly, and hypereosinophilia (Katayama fever).
- Worms mature in the venous blood, and (if untreated) deposit eggs in the bladder, GI tract, brain, skin, and liver.
- Diagnosis is suspected from eosinophilia, and microscopic identification of eggs in mid-day urines, or stools.
- Treatment is with praziquantel, 20 milligrams/kg two doses in a single day, except with GI involvement, where three doses in a single day are suggested.

AMEBIASIS

- Pathogenic species such as *Entamoeba histolytica* are endemic to Asia, Africa, and Latin America.
- Amebiasis is typically spread by asymptomatic carriers whose excrement contains encysted organisms.
- Incubation is 1 to 3 weeks for colitis, and weeks to months for liver abscess.
- Symptoms include alternating constipation with diarrhea, over weeks, to abdominal pain, fever, dehydration, and weight loss.
- Complication such as liver abscess cause fever, right upper quadrant pain, chronic vague abdominal pain, and weight loss.
- Stool for ova and parasites is diagnostic (specimen should be examined within 30 minutes of collection).
- Ultrasound should identify liver abscess. Most common treatment is with metronidazole, 500 to 750 milligrams three times daily for 10 days.

ASCARIASIS

- Infection with *Ascaris lumbricoides* should be suspected following ingestion of street vendor foods or vegetables fertilized by "night soil" (human feces) or animal feces.
- Symptoms may include a dry cough or pneumonia as young worms are expectorated and migrate from the lungs to the esophagus and gut.
- A large worm burden can lead to malnutrition and weakness, and a mass of worms may lead to bowel obstruction.
- Diagnosis is with stool examination, and serology. Treatment is with mebendazole, 100 milligrams daily for 3 days, or albendazole, 400 milligrams twice a day for 3 days or 500 milligrams single dose, or ivermectin, 150 to 200 micrograms/kg single dose.
- The single dose regimens are used, but have a lower cure rate.

ENTEROBIASIS (SEATWORM OR PINWORM)

- Infection is typically from fecal-oral contact from contaminated objects.
- Presentation is intense perianal itching.
- Diagnosis is with cellophane tape swab of anus to look for worms.
- Treatment is with mebendazole, 100 milligrams single dose and repeat in 2 weeks, or albendazole, 400 milligrams single dose and repeat in 2 weeks, or pyrantel pamoate, 11 milligrams/kg (up to 1 gram) single dose and repeat in 2 weeks.

ANCYLOSTOMA DUODENALE AND *NECATOR AMERICANUS* (HOOKWORM)

- Infection follows exposure to contaminated soil; larvae penetrate skin.
- Worms may migrate to the lungs, may be coughed up, and access the GI tract after being swallowed.
- Symptoms include abdominal pain, severe anemia, and cutaneous larva migrans, red, wormlike burrows visible underneath the skin.
- Treatment is with albendazole 400 milligrams single dose (preferred), or mebendazole 100 milligrams twice daily for 3 days, or pyrantel pamoate 11 milligrams/kg (maximum, 1 gram) daily for 3 days.

TAENIA SOLIUM (PORK TAPEWORM), *TAENIA SAGINATA* (BEEF TAPEWORM), *DIPHYLLOBOTHRIUM LATUM* (FISH TAPEWORM)

- Infection follows ingestion of undercooked pork, beef, or fish.
- Symptoms include diarrhea, abdominal pain, bowel obstruction, taenia cysts in eye, heart, and brain (see cysticercosis above).
- Diagnosis is by stool examination or serology (may be negative if cysts are calcified). Treatment is with praziquantel, 5 to 10 milligrams/kg single dose.

For discussion of other diseases that may be acquired during travel, or other parasites, see the chapter referenced immediately below.

For further reading in Tintinalli's *Emergency Medicine: A Comprehensive Study Guide*, 7th ed., see Chapter 156, "World Travelers," by Michael J. VanRooyen and Raghu Venugopal.

101 THE TRANSPLANT PATIENT

David M. Cline

- Management of the transplant patient in the emergency department can be divided into three general areas: disorders specific to the transplanted organ, disorders common to all transplant patients due to their immunosuppressed state or antirejection medication, and disorders unrelated to their transplant; yet special care is required due to their medications or altered physiology.
- Disorders specific to the transplanted organ are manifestations of acute rejection, surgical complications specific to the procedure performed, and altered physiology (most important in cardiac transplantation).
- The most common presentations of transplant patients to the emergency are infection (39%) followed by noninfectious GI/GU pathology (15%), dehydration (15%), electrolyte disturbances (10%), cardiopulmonary pathology (10%) or injury (8%), and rejection in 6%.
- Before prescribing any new drug for a transplant recipient, the treatment plan should be discussed with a representative from the transplant team.

POSTTRANSPLANT INFECTIOUS COMPLICATIONS

- Predisposing factors to infections posttransplant include ongoing immunosuppression in all patients and the presence of diabetes mellitus, advanced age, obesity, and other host factors. Table 101-1 lists the broad array of potential infections and the time after transplant they are most likely to occur.

CLINICAL FEATURES

- The initial presentation of a potentially life-threatening infectious illness may be quite subtle in transplant recipients.
- As many as 50% of transplant patients with serious infections will not have fever.
- A nonproductive cough with little or no findings on physical examination may be the only clue to emerging *Pneumocystis jiroveci* pneumonia or cytomegalovirus (CMV) pneumonia.
- Urinary tract infections are a very common cause of fever in this group of patients.

TABLE 101-1 Infections in Transplant Patients Stratified by Posttransplant Period

First month posttransplant
Wound infection/anastomotic leaks: MRSA, gram-negative bacteria
Pneumonia: *Pseudomonas, Klebsiella, Legionella, Aspergillus*
UTI: Gram-negative bacteria, *Enterococcus, Candida*
Line-related sepsis: *S. aureus, S. epidermidis*, gram-negative bacteria, *Candida*
Abdomen: VRE, *Clostridium difficile*, intra-abdominal infections (liver transplant)
Viral: Disseminated/local, HSV, RSV (HSCT patients)
Febrile neutropenia: *Streptococcus viridans* (HSCT patients)
Oral: Candidal pharyngitis, esophagitis
Second to 6 months posttransplant
Pneumonia: CAP, *Nocardia*, CMV, *Aspergillus*, TB, *Pneumocystis, Listeria*
Meningitis: *Listeria, Cryptococcus*
UTI/cystitis/nephritis: Common pathogens, polyomavirus BK
Abdominal colitis: *C. difficile*, visceral leishmaniasis
Oral: Candidal pharyngitis, esophagitis
Viral: CMV, EBV, HSV, VZV, adenovirus, influenza, hepatitis A, B, C
Fever: Toxoplasmosis, common presentation of most listed pathogens
Beyond sixth months posttransplant
Pneumonia: CAP, *Aspergillus*, CMV, *Pneumocystis, Listeria, Nocardia*
UTI/cystitis: Common pathogens, Polyomavirus BK
Meningitis: *Listeria, Cryptococcus*
Oral: Candidal pharyngitis, esophagitis
Viral: CMV (chorioretinitis, colitis), VZV, HSV, hepatitis C, B, West Nile

Abbreviations: CAP = community-acquired pneumonia, CMV = cytomegalovirus, EBV = Epstein–Barr virus, HBV = hepatitis B virus, HCV = hepatitis C virus, HSCT = hematopoietic stem cell transplant, HSV = herpes simplex virus, MRSA = methicillin-resistant *Staphylococcus aureus*, PTLD = posttransplantation lymphoproliferative disorder, RSV = respiratory syncytial virus, TB = tuberculosis, UTI = urinary tract infection, VRE= vancomycin-resistant *Enterococcus faecalis*, VZV = varicella-zoster virus.

DIAGNOSIS AND DIFFERENTIAL

- Blood counts, inflammatory markers, and baseline tests of renal and liver function may be helpful in this group of complex patients.
- The threshold for obtaining chest radiographs for these patients should be low.
- Cultures of all appropriate fluids, including blood, are essential before (or simultaneous with) initiating antimicrobial therapy.
- Central nervous system infections such as meningitis (*Listeria monocytogenes* and cryptococci) should be considered.
- Complaints of recurrent headaches, therefore, with or without fever, should be investigated vigorously, first with a structural study to exclude a mass lesion (central nervous system lymphomas occur with increased frequency, too) and then with a lumbar puncture.

- Liver transplant patients are especially susceptible to intra-abdominal infections during the first postoperative month.
- Lung transplant patients are especially prone to pneumonia.
- Cardiac transplant patients may develop mediastinitis during the first postoperative month.

EMERGENCY DEPARTMENT CARE AND DISPOSITION

- Drug choice, dose, and ultimate management should be accomplished in consultation with the transplant team.
- The following recommended drugs are listed for the event of urgent patient need due to instability or delay in reaching the transplant team.
- For skin and superficial wounds, a broad-spectrum antibiotic plus an agent specific to MRSA is recommended. Therefore, imipenem 500 milligrams IV every 6 hours, *or* meropenem 1 gram IV every 8 hours, *or* piperacillin/tazobactam 3.375 IV every 6 hours can be initiated, *plus* vancomycin 1 gram IV every 12 hours *or* linezolid 600 milligrams IV every 12 hours is recommended.
- Pneumonia may be caused by a wide variety of organisms from common to atypical to opportunistic.
- Treatment options for pneumonia include imipenem 500 milligrams IV every 6 hours, meropenem 1 gram IV every 8 hours, cefotaxime 1 to 2 grams IV every 6 to 8 hours plus gentamicin 1 to 2 milligrams/kg IV every 8 hours, or piperacillin/tazobactam 3.375 grams IV every 6 hours. Add MRSA specific therapy, listed above, and fungal therapy, listed below, if suspected.
- Intra-abdominal infection may be due to enteric gram-negative aerobic, obligate anaerobic bacilli and facultative bacilli, and enteric gram-positive streptococci.
- Recommended coverage for intra-abdominal infection is to combine metronidazole 500 milligrams IV every 12 hours *plus* one of the following agents: imipenem 500 milligrams IV every 6 hours, meropenem 1 gram IV every 8 hours, doripenem 500 milligrams IV every 8 hours, piperacillin/tazobactam 3.375 grams IV every 6 hours. Ampicillin-sulbactam is not recommended for use because of high rates of resistance to this agent among community-acquired *Escherichia coli*.
- Meningitis is frequently due to *L. monocytogenes*, and patients with suspected meningitis should be treated cefotaxime 2 grams IV every 4 to 6 hours plus vancomycin 1 gram IV every 12 hours. The addition of vancomycin should be considered.
- The initial treatment of suspected fungal disease is fluconazole 400 milligrams daily IV; amphotericin B 0.7 milligram/kg/d IV has been a mainstay of treatment, but has more toxicity than fluconazole. Oral or esophageal candidiasis is treated with fluconazole 200 milligrams on day 1, and then 100 milligrams PO daily.
- Suspected CMV disease is treated with ganciclovir, with a dose of 5 milligrams/kg IV twice daily; in bone marrow transplant patients, add immunoglobulin.
- Varicella and herpes simplex virus are typically treated with acyclovir 800 milligrams IV five times a day for dissemination or ocular involvement. Acyclovir has renal excretion, and the dose must be adjusted for renal insufficiency. Alternatives include valacyclovir 1000 milligrams every 8 hours and famciclovir 500 milligrams every 8 hours.
- Epstein–Barr virus is typically treated with a reduction in the immunosuppression regimen. Both acyclovir and ganciclovir have also been used, but not routinely.
- Treatment of choice for *P. jiroveci* pneumonia starts with prednisone 80 milligrams per day followed immediately by antimicrobial therapy. First choice is trimethoprim/sulfamethoxazole (TMP-SMX), TMP 15 milligrams/kg/d IV divided every 8 hours while critically ill. Oral therapy is TMP-SMX double strength (DS) 2 tablets PO every 8 hours for 3 weeks of total therapy. Pentamidine 4 milligrams/kg/d IV or IM for 3 weeks and clindamycin 600 milligrams IV *plus* primaquine 30 milligrams orally daily are reserved as alternative therapies if TMP-SMX is not tolerated.
- Toxoplasmosis can be treated initially with pyrimethamine 200 milligrams PO initially and then 50 to 75 milligrams PO daily plus sulfadiazine 1 to 4 grams PO daily plus folinic acid 10 milligrams PO daily.
- Urinary tract infections (see Chapter 55), invasive gastroenteritis (due to *Salmonella, Campylobacter,* and *Listeria*; see Chapters 39 and 98), and diverticulitis (see Chapter 46) can be treated with the usual antimicrobial agents.

COMPLICATIONS OF IMMUNOSUPPRESSIVE AGENTS

- Therapeutic immunosuppression is accompanied by a number of adverse effects and complications.
- These adverse effects are typically gradual in onset, but may be life threatening, such as pancreatitis, bleeding, hypoglycemia or hyperglycemia, bradycardia or tachycardia, hyperkalemia, hypertension or

hypotension, cardiotoxicity, pulmonary edema, seizures, thromboembolic events, and thrombocytopenia.

- Side effects such as fever or rigors may also be confused for life-threatening infections.
- A headache syndrome often indistinguishable from migraine is common in transplant recipients and usually develops within the first 2 months of immunosuppression.
- An important differential must include infectious causes and malignancy when headache first presents and usually requires computed tomography of the head with subsequent biochemical analysis of cerebrospinal fluid.
- As the number of immunosuppressive drugs has increased dramatically, a complete listing of adverse effects is beyond the scope of this review book.
- The reader is referred to the parent textbook, referenced at the end of this manual chapter, or to Web resources, or a personal digital assistant, for a more complete listing of side effects of these medications.
- Any illness that prevents transplant patients from taking or retaining their immunosuppressive therapy warrants hospital admission for IV therapy, preferably at a transplant center.
- Starting even simple medications can precipitate complications. For example, nonsteroidal anti-inflammatory drugs may increase nephrotoxicity.
- In general, any new medications should be discussed with a representative of the patient's transplant team.

CARDIAC TRANSPLANTATION

- Transplantation results in a denervated heart that does not respond with centrally medicated tachycardia in response to stress or exercise but does respond to circulating catecholamines and increased preload.
- Patients may complain of fatigue or shortness of breath with the onset of exercise, which resolves with continued exertion as an appropriate tachycardia develops.
- The donor heart is implanted with its sinus node intact to preserve normal atrioventricular conduction. The normal heart rate for a transplanted heart is 90 to 100 beats/min.
- The technique of cardiac transplantation also results in the preservation of the recipient's sinus node at the superior cavoatrial junction.
- The atrial suture line renders the two sinus nodes electrically isolated from each other.
- Thus, electrocardiograms frequently will have two distinct P waves.
- The sinus node of the donor heart is easily identified by its constant 1:1 relation to the QRS complex, whereas the native P wave marches independently through the donor heart rhythm.

CLINICAL FEATURES

- Because the heart is denervated, myocardial ischemia does not present with angina.
- Instead, recipients present with heart failure secondary to silent myocardial infarctions or with sudden death.
- Transplant recipients who have new-onset shortness of breath, chest fullness, or symptoms of congestive heart failure should be evaluated, in routine fashion with an electrocardiogram and serial cardiac enzymes levels, for the presence of myocardial ischemia or infarction.
- Although most episodes of acute rejection are asymptomatic, symptoms can occur. The most common presenting symptoms are dysrhythmias and generalized fatigue.
- The development of atrial or ventricular dysrhythmia in a cardiac transplant recipient (or congestive heart failure) must be assumed to be due to acute rejection until proven otherwise.
- In children, rejection may present with low-grade fever, fussiness, and poor feeding.

EMERGENCY DEPARTMENT CARE

- Rejection: Management of acute rejection is methylprednisolone 1 gram IV after consultation with a representative from the transplant center.
- Treatment for rejection without biopsy confirmation is contraindicated except when patients are hemodynamically unstable.
- Dysrhythmias: If patients are hemodynamically compromised by dysrhythmias, empiric therapy for rejection with methylprednisolone 1 gram IV may be given after consultation.
- Atropine has no effect on the denervated heart; isoproterenol is the drug of choice for bradydysrhythmia in these patients.
- Patients who present in extremis should be treated with standard cardiopulmonary resuscitation measures.
- Hypotension: Low-output syndrome, or hypotension, should be treated with inotropic agents such as dopamine or dobutamine when specific treatment for rejection is instituted.
- Hospitalization: Transplant patients suspected of having rejection or acute illness should be hospitalized, preferably at the transplant center, if stable for transfer.

LUNG TRANSPLANTATION

CLINICAL FEATURES

- Clinically, the patient suffering rejection may have a cough, chest tightness, fatigue, and fever (>0.5°C above baseline).
- Acute rejection may manifest with frightening rapidity, causing a severe decline in patient status in only 1 day.
- Isolated fever may be the only finding. Spirometry may show a 15% drop in forced expiratory volume in 1 second, the patient may be newly hypoxic, and examination may show rales and adventitious sounds.
- Chest radiograph may demonstrate bilateral interstitial infiltrates or effusions but may be normal when rejection occurs late in the course.
- The longer a patient is from transplant, the less classic a chest radiograph may appear for acute rejection.
- Infection, such as interstitial pneumonia, may present with a clinical picture similar to acute rejection.
- Diagnostically, bronchoscopy with transbronchial biopsy is usually needed not only to confirm rejection but also to exclude infection.
- Two late complications of lung transplant are obliterative bronchiolitis and posttransplant lymphoproliferative disease (PTLD).
- Obliterative bronchiolitis presents with episodes of recurrent bronchitis, small airway obliteration, wheezing, and eventually respiratory failure.
- PTLD is associated with Epstein–Barr virus and presents with painful lymphadenopathy and otitis media (due to tonsillar involvement) or may present with malaise, fever, and myalgia.

DIAGNOSIS AND DIFFERENTIAL

- Evaluation of the lung transplant patient should include chest radiograph, pulse oximetry, arterial blood gas analysis (if CO_2 retention is suspected), spirometry, complete blood cell count, serum electrolytes, creatinine and magnesium levels, and appropriate drug levels.

EMERGENCY DEPARTMENT CARE AND DISPOSITION

- Rejection: After consultation with the transplant center representative, and infection is excluded, methylprednisolone 500 to 1000 milligrams IV should be given for acute rejection.
- Patients who have a history of seizures associated with the administration of high-dose glucocorticoids also will need concurrent benzodiazepines to prevent further seizure episodes.
- Late complications: Obliterative bronchiolitis is treated with increased immunosuppression including high-dose steroids, whereas PTLD is treated with reduced immunosuppression and other therapy such as rituximab.
- These decisions should be made in consultation with specialists from the transplant center.

RENAL TRANSPLANT

CLINICAL FEATURES

- Diagnosis and treatment of acute rejection is most critical.
- Without timely recognition and intervention, allograft function may deteriorate irreversibly in a few days.
- Renal transplant recipients, when symptomatic from acute rejection, complain of vague tenderness over the allograft (in the left or right iliac fossa).
- Patients also may describe decreased urine output, rapid weight gain (from fluid retention), low-grade fever, and generalized malaise.
- Physical examination may disclose worsening hypertension, allograft tenderness, and peripheral edema.
- The absence of these symptoms and signs, however, does not exclude the possibility of acute rejection.
- With improved methods of maintenance immunosuppression, the only clue may be an asymptomatic decline in renal function.

DIAGNOSIS AND DIFFERENTIAL

- Even a change in creatinine levels from 1.0 milligram/dL to 1.2 or 1.3 milligrams/dL may be important.
- When such changes in creatinine levels are reproducible, a careful workup consists of complete urinalysis, possibly renal ultrasonography, and levels of immunosuppressive drugs if available, in addition to a careful history and examination.
- It is critical to interpret changes in renal function in the context of prior data (eg, trends of recent serum creatinine levels, recent history of rejection, or other causes of allograft dysfunction).
- Evaluation should consider the multiple etiologies of decreased renal function in the renal transplant recipient.
- The two most common causes, apart from acute rejection causing an increase in creatinine, are volume contraction and cyclosporine-induced nephrotoxicity.

EMERGENCY DEPARTMENT CARE AND DISPOSITION

- Rejection: After consultation with the transplant center representative, treatment of allograft rejection consists of high-dose glucocorticoids, typically methylprednisolone 500 milligrams IV.

LIVER TRANSPLANT

CLINICAL FEATURES

- Although frequently subtle in presentation, a syndrome of acute rejection includes fever, liver tenderness, lymphocytosis, eosinophilia, liver enzyme elevation, and a change in bile color or production.
- In the perioperative period, the differential diagnosis must include infection, acute biliary obstruction, or vascular insufficiency.
- Diagnosis can be made with certainty only by hepatic ultrasound and biopsy, which usually requires referral back to the transplant center for management and follow-up.
- Two possible surgical complications in liver transplant patients are biliary obstruction or leakage and hepatic artery thrombosis.
- Biliary obstruction follows three typical presentations. The most common is intermittent episodes of fever and fluctuating liver function tests.
- The second is a gradual worsening of liver function tests without symptoms.
- Third, obstruction may present as acute bacterial cholangitis with fever, chills, abdominal pain, jaundice, and bacteremia.
- It can be difficult to distinguish clinically from rejection, hepatic artery thrombosis, CMV infection, or a recurrence of a preexisting disease, especially hepatitis.
- If a biliary complication is suspected, all patients should have a complete blood count; serum chemistry levels; liver function tests; basic coagulation studies; and lipase levels; cultures of blood, urine, bile, and ascites, if present; chest radiograph; and abdominal ultrasound.
- Ultrasound looks for the presence of fluid collections, screens for the presence of thrombosis of the hepatic artery or portal vein, and identifies any dilatation of the biliary tree. Alternatively, abdominal computed tomography can be used.
- Biliary leakage is associated with 50% mortality. It occurs most frequently in the third or fourth postoperative week.
- The high mortality may be related to a high incidence of concomitant hepatic artery thrombosis, infection of leaked bile, or difficult bile repair when the tissue is inflamed.
- Patients most often have peritoneal signs and fever, but these signs may be masked by concomitant use of steroids and immunosuppressive agents.
- Presentation is signaled by elevated prothrombin time and transaminase levels and little or no bile production, but this complication also may present as acute graft failure, liver abscess, unexplained sepsis, or a biliary tract problem (leak, obstruction, abscess, or breakdown of the anastomosis).

EMERGENCY DEPARTMENT CARE AND DISPOSITION

- Rejection: After consultation with the transplant center representative, acute rejection is managed with a high-dose glucocorticoid bolus of methylprednisolone 500 to 1000 milligrams IV.
- Surgical complications are best managed at the transplant center. Biliary obstruction is managed with balloon dilatation, and all patients should receive broad-spectrum antibiotics against gram-negative and gram-positive enteric organisms, such as metronidazole 500 milligrams IV every 12 hours *plus* one of the following agents: imipenem 500 milligrams IV every 6 hours, or piperacillin/tazobactam 3.375 grams IV every 6 hours. Biliary leakage is treated with reoperation, and hepatic artery thrombosis is treated with retransplantation.

HEMATOPOIETIC STEM CELL TRANSPLANT

- Hematopoietic stem cell transplant (HSCT) is performed for a variety of conditions, including hematopoietic malignancies, severe anemia, and other conditions.
- The most common complication of HSCT is graft-versus-host disease, affecting approximately 50% of HSCT patients.

CLINICAL PRESENTATION (GRAFT-VERSUS-HOST DISEASE)

- A HSCT recipient presenting to the ED with nonspecific rash (see Fig. 101-1) should be suspected of having graft-versus-host disease.
- The rash may be pruritic or painful, frequently demonstrating a brownish hue and slight scaling. The distribution varies greatly but often affects palms and soles initially, and later progresses to cheeks, ears, neck, trunk, chest, and upper back. In the more severe

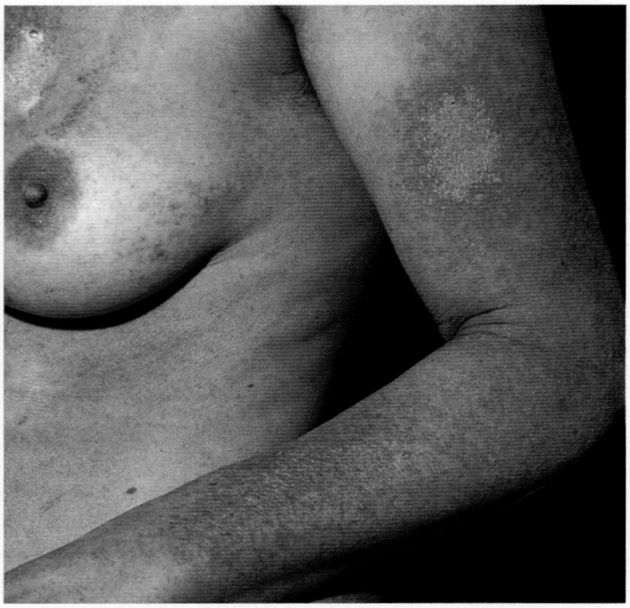

FIG. 101-1. Rash of acute cutaneous graft-versus-host disease. The maculopapular lesions have acquired a brownish hue and there is slight scaling. (Reproduced with permission from Wolff KL, Johnson R, Suurmond R: *Fitzpatrick's Color Atlas & Synopsis of Clinical Dermatology*, 6th ed. © 2009, McGraw-Hill, New York.)

forms, skin involvement is erythrodermic or may show bullae formation.

- Mucositis has been reported to occur in 35% to 70% of patients.
- As many as 90% of patients undergoing combined chemotherapy and radiotherapy develop severe skin disease.
- The second most common presentation is gastrointestinal with diarrhea.
- Upper GI symptoms such as anorexia, nausea, and emesis are common.
- The patient may develop painful cramping, ileus, and, sometimes, life-threatening hemorrhage from the colon.

DIAGNOSIS AND DIFFERENTIAL (GRAFT-VERSUS-HOST DISEASE)

- The diagnosis of graft-versus-host disease is made on clinical grounds initially.
- The patient with serious GI hemorrhage in the early post-transplant period may have coagulation deficits, especially thrombocytopenia.
- The differential diagnosis of GI bleeding in this setting includes all the usual causes of GI bleeding in addition to infection (viral, fungal, or bacterial).
- Liver involvement presents with hyperbilirubinemia and increases in alkaline phosphatase and transaminase levels.

EMERGENCY DEPARTMENT CARE AND DISPOSITION

- Most patients with graft-versus-host disease will need supportive care in consultation with the patient's transplant team for management including possible admission or transfer to the transplant center.
- Initiation of prednisone 60 milligrams PO daily or methylprednisolone 1 to 2 milligrams/kg IV daily until clinical improvement is seen is the usual management.
- If other immunosuppressants have recently been tapered or discontinued, generally these are increased or reinstituted.

For further reading in Tintinalli's *Emergency Medicine: A Comprehensive Study Guide,* 7th ed., see Chapter 295, "The Transplant Patient," by Raymond M. Fish and Malek G. Massad.

Section 12
TOXICOLOGY

102 GENERAL MANAGEMENT OF POISONED PATIENTS

L. Keith French

EPIDEMIOLOGY

- In 2008, nearly 2.5 million toxic exposures were reported to poison centers in the United States, resulting in 1315 deaths.
- Over half of all reported poisonings occur in children <12 years of age.
- Most accidental poisonings are preventable through increased educational efforts and public awareness.

PATHOPHYSIOLOGY

- All substances have dose-dependent toxic potential.
- Poisons cause harm through various mechanisms including alteration or inhibition of cellular function(s); disruption of cellular uptake or transportation of substances within the body; or interference with utilization of essential substrates from the environment.
- Although ingestion is the most common route of poisoning, toxins can enter the body via inhalation, injection, transdermal or ocular absorption, or insufflation.

CLINICAL FEATURES

- A detailed history is paramount for proper management of the poisoned patient; however, a complete assessment may be difficult to obtain due to alteration in cognition or secondary motives.
- Every attempt should be made to ascertain the type(s), amount, timing, and route of exposure(s) as well as the number of persons involved. Corroboration may be needed from bystanders, family, hospital records, EMS personnel, or paraphernalia in the patient's possession.
- A thorough physical examination is essential and special emphasis should focus on assessment of mental status, pupil size and reactivity, skin temperature and the presence or absence of sweat, muscular tone, gastrointestinal motility, and mucous membrane moisture.

DIAGNOSIS AND DIFFERENTIAL

- Recognition of a toxidrome can help narrow the differential diagnosis in the situation of an unknown or suspected poisoning (Table 102-1).
- In the emergency setting, toxicologic screening tests of blood and/or urine do not contribute significantly to the evaluation, management, or outcome for most patients.
- There are, however, instances where knowledge of serum concentrations of certain drugs can help guide or change management (Table 102-2).
- Caution should be used when interpreting urine drug screens as false-positive or negative results can be misleading.
- Acetaminophen and aspirin are common and treatable coingestants and should be screened for in any suspected intentional ingestion, unknown poisoning, or patient who presents with altered mental status of unknown etiology.
- Other helpful studies to consider include serum glucose, electrocardiography, arterial blood gas, serum electrolytes, complete blood count, liver function tests, pregnancy screening, and blood ethanol concentration.

EMERGENCY DEPARTMENT CARE AND DISPOSITION

- Except in rare circumstances, resuscitation of the poisoned patient begins with assessment and stabilization of the airway, breathing, and circulation rather than administration of a specific antidote (Table 102-3).
- For patients externally contaminated, removal of clothing and copious irrigation of the skin is a priority and should occur as soon as possible, before entry into the hospital. Rescue and hospital personnel

TABLE 102-1 Common Toxidromes

TOXIDROME	REPRESENTATIVE AGENT(S)	MOST COMMON FINDINGS	ADDITIONAL SIGNS AND SYMPTOMS	POTENTIAL INTERVENTIONS
Opioid	Heroin Morphine Oxycodone	Central nervous system depression, miosis, respiratory depression	Hypothermia, bradycardia Death may result from respiratory arrest, acute lung injury	Ventilation or naloxone
Sympathomimetic	Cocaine Amphetamine	Psychomotor agitation, mydriasis, diaphoresis, tachycardia, hypertension, hyperthermia	Seizures, rhabdomyolysis, myocardial infarction Death may result from seizures, cardiac arrest, hyperthermia	Cooling, sedation with benzodiazepines, hydration
Cholinergic	Organophosphate insecticides Carbamate insecticides	Muscarinic effects (salivation, lacrimation, diaphoresis, nausea, vomiting, urination, defecation, bronchorrhea) Nicotinic effects (muscle fasciculations and weakness)	Bradycardia, miosis/mydriasis, seizures, respiratory failure, paralysis Death may result from respiratory arrest from paralysis, bronchorrhea, or seizures	Airway protection and ventilation, atropine, pralidoxime
Anticholinergic	Scopolamine Atropine	Altered mental status, mydriasis, dry flushed skin, urinary retention, decreased bowel sounds, hyperthermia, dry mucous membranes	Seizures, dysrhythmias, rhabdomyolysis Death may result from hyperthermia and dysrhythmias	Physostigmine (if appropriate), sedation with benzodiazepines, cooling, supportive management
Salicylates	Aspirin Oil of wintergreen	Altered mental status, respiratory alkalosis, metabolic acidosis, tinnitus, hyperpnea, tachycardia, diaphoresis, nausea, vomiting	Low-grade fever, ketonuria Death may result from acute lung injury or cerebral edema	Multidose activated charcoal, alkalinization of urine with potassium repletion, hemodialysis
Sedative-hypnotic	Barbiturates Benzodiazepines	Depressed level of consciousness, slurred speech, ataxia	Stupor to coma, depressed respirations, apnea, bradycardia	Ventilatory support
Hypoglycemic	Sulfonylureas Insulin	Altered mental status, diaphoresis, tachycardia, hypertension	Paralysis, slurring of speech, bizarre behavior, seizures Death may result from seizures, altered behavior	Glucose-containing solution IV and oral feedings if possible, frequent glucose measurement, octreotide
Hallucinogenic	Phencyclidine Lysergic acid diethylamide Psilocybin Mescaline	Hallucinations, dysphoria, anxiety	Hyperthermia, mydriasis, nausea, sympathomimetic symptoms	Generally supportive
Serotonin	SSRIs Meperidine A variety of drug interactions with dextromethorphan, monoamine oxidase inhibitors, tricyclic antidepressants, other SSRIs, and amphetamines	Altered mental status, increased muscle tone, hyperreflexia, hyperthermia	Intermittent whole-body tremor Death may result from hyperthermia	Cooling, sedation with benzodiazepines, supportive management, theoretical benefit of cyproheptadine
Extrapyramidal	Haloperidol Phenothiazines Risperidone Olanzapine	Dystonia, torticollis, tremor, muscle rigidity	Choreoathetosis, hyperreflexia, seizures	Diphenhydramine Benztropine Benzodiazepines

Abbreviation: SSRI = selective serotonin reuptake inhibitor.

TABLE 102-2 Substances for Which Serum Level May Affect Therapy
Acetaminophen
Salicylate
Lithium
Digoxin
Valproate
Phenytoin
Carbamazepine
Theophylline
Carbon monoxide
Methemoglobin
Methanol
Ethylene glycol
Iron
Paraquat

should always wear personal protective gear, which may include gowns, eye protection, and masks.

- Patients presenting with sedation, obtundation, or coma, should receive empiric treatment with naloxone (0.2-2.0 milligram IV), glucose (50 mL 50% dextrose IV), and thiamine (100 milligrams IV), which are reasonable and generally accepted as safe. Empiric use of flumazenil, a benzodiazepine antagonist, is generally not recommended for adults, although may be helpful in children.
- Hypotension is first managed with fluid resuscitation; vasopressors should be considered only when blood pressure is refractory to fluid administration. Ventricular dysrhythmias are treated according to standard Advanced Cardiac Life Support (ACLS) measures unless treatment of a specific toxin dictates alternative therapy.
- Benzodiazepines are first-line therapy for seizures following exposure to most toxins.

TABLE 102-3 Common Antidotes: Initial Dosages and Indications

ANTIDOTE	DOSE: PEDIATRIC	DOSE: ADULT	INDICATION
Acetylcysteine	140 milligrams/kg PO load, followed by 70 milligrams/kg PO every 4 h for 17 total doses or 150 milligrams/kg IV load over 60 min, followed by 50 milligrams/kg IV over 4 h and then 100 milligrams/kg IV over 16 h		Acetaminophen
Activated charcoal	1 gram/kg PO	50-100 grams	Most ingested poisons
Antivenom Fab	4-6 vials IV initially over 1 h, may be repeated to gain control of progressive symptoms		Envenomation by Crotalidae
Calcium chloride 10% (27.2 milligrams/mL elemental calcium)	0.2-0.25 mL/kg IV	10 mL IV	Calcium channel antagonists
Calcium gluconate 10% (9 milligrams/mL elemental calcium)	0.6-0.8 mL/kg IV	10-30 mL IV	Hypermagnesemia Hypocalcemia
Cyanide antidote kit			
Amyl nitrite	Not typically used	1 ampule in oxygen chamber of ventilation bag 30 s on/30 s off	Cyanide Hydrogen sulfide (use only sodium nitrite)
Sodium nitrite (3% solution)	0.33 mL/kg IV	10 mL IV	—
Sodium thiosulfate (25% solution)	1.65 mL/kg IV	50 mL IV	—
Deferoxamine	90 milligrams/kg IM (1 gram maximum) or 15 milligrams/kg/h IV (maximum dose, 1 gram/d)	2 grams IM or 15 milligrams/kg/h IV (maximum dose, 6-8 grams/d)	Iron

(Continued)

TABLE 102-3 Common Antidotes: Initial Dosages and Indications (Continued)

ANTIDOTE	DOSE: PEDIATRIC	DOSE: ADULT	INDICATION
Dextrose (glucose)	0.5 gram/kg IV	1 gram/kg IV	Insulin Oral hypoglycemics
Digoxin Fab			
Acute	1-2 vials IV	5-10 vials	Digoxin and other cardioactive steroids
Chronic	1-2 vials IV	3-6 vials IV	Cardioactive steroids
Ethanol (10% for IV administration)	10 mL/kg IV over 30 min, then 1.2 mL/kg/h*	10 mL/kg IV over 30 min, then 1.2 mL/kg/h*	Ethylene glycol Methanol
Folic acid/leucovorin	1-2 milligrams/kg IV every 4-6 h	1-2 milligrams/kg IV every 4-6 h	Methotrexate (only leucovorin)
Fomepizole	15 milligrams/kg IV, then 10 milligrams/kg every 12 h	15 milligrams/kg IV, then 10 millgrams/kg every 12 h	Methanol Ethylene glycol Disulfiram-ethanol interaction
Flumazenil	0.01 milligram/kg IV	0.2 milligram IV	Benzodiazepines
Glucagon	50-150 micrograms/kg IV	3-10 milligrams IV	Calcium channel antagonists β-Blockers
Hydroxocobalamin	70 milligrams/kg IV (not to exceed 5 grams) over 30 min; can be repeated up to three times Administered in combination with sodium thiosulfate		Cyanide Nitroprusside
IV lipid emulsion 20%	1.5 mL/kg IV bolus over 1 min (may be repeated two times at 5-min intervals), followed by 0.25 mL/kg/min IV	100 mL IV bolus over 1 min, followed by 400 mL IV over 20 min	IV bupivacaine Rescue therapy for calcium channel antagonists and β-blockers
Methylene blue	1-2 milligrams/kg IV Neonates: 0.3-1.0 milligram/kg	1-2 milligrams/kg IV	Oxidizing chemicals (eg, nitrites, benzocaine, sulfonamides)
Octreotide	1 microgram/kg SC every 6 h	50-100 micrograms SC every 6 h	Refractory hypoglycemia after oral hypoglycemic agent ingestion
Naloxone	As much as is needed Typical starting dose is 0.01 milligram IV	As much as needed Typical starting dose is 0.4-2.0 milligrams IV	Opioid Clonidine
Physostigmine	0.02 milligram/kg IV	0.5-2.0 milligrams slow IV over 2-5 min	Anticholinergic agents (not cyclic antidepressants)
Pralidoxime (2-PAM)	20-40 milligrams/kg IV over 5-10 min, followed by 20 milligrams/kg/h infusion	1-2 grams IV over 5-10 min, followed by 500 milligrams/h infusion	Cholinergic agents
Protamine	1 milligram neutralizes 100 units of unfractionated heparin, administered over 15 min 0.6 milligram/kg IV (empiric dose)	25-50 milligrams IV (empiric dose)	Heparin
Pyridoxine	Gram for gram of ingestion if amount of isoniazid is known 70 milligrams/kg (maximum 5 grams) IV	5 grams IV	Isoniazid *Gyromitra esculenta* Hydrazine
Sodium bicarbonate	1-2 mEq/kg IV bolus followed by 2 mEq/kg/h IV infusion	1-2 mEq/kg IV bolus followed by 2 mEq/kg/h IV infusion	Sodium channel blockers For urinary alkalinization

(Continued)

TABLE 102-3 Common Antidotes: Initial Dosages and Indications (Continued)

	DOSE		
ANTIDOTE	PEDIATRIC	ADULT	INDICATION
Thiamine	5-10 milligrams IV	100 milligrams IV	Wernicke syndrome Wet beri-beri
Vitamin K_1	1-5 milligrams/d PO	20 milligrams/d PO	Anticoagulant rodenticides

*This is an approximation. Dose should be titrated to level (see Chapter 106, Alcohols).

- Ocular exposures are treated with copious irrigation using isotonic crystalloid. Administration of an ocular anesthetic can facilitate decontamination.
- The three general methods of GI decontamination involve removing toxin(s) from the gut, binding toxin(s) in the stomach, and enhancing transit through the intestines.
- Syrup of ipecac is no longer routinely recommended and should only be used in rare circumstances under the direction of a poison center.
- Orogastric lavage is reserved for potentially lethal poisonings (determined by the toxin and dose). Efficacy is increased when performed in a timely manner, generally within an hour of ingestion. Contraindications include an unprotected airway, caustic or hydrocarbon ingestion, or ingestion of pills that are known to be too large to fit through the side ports of the orogastric tube (OG tube).
- Activated charcoal (1 gram/kg or in a 10:1 AC to drug ratio, whichever is larger) is the agent most commonly used to decontaminate the GI tract and works by adsorbing substances in the gut lumen. Activated charcoal will bind to most organic and some inorganic substances.
- Benefit of activated charcoal is generally greater when administered soon after drug ingestion (up to an hour), although benefit outside this time frame cannot necessarily be excluded.
- Awake and cooperative patients can drink activated charcoal; alternatively, it can be instilled through an NG tube. If orogastric lavage is utilized, a dose of activated charcoal should be given before the OG tube is removed.
- Activated charcoal should not be used if the ingested substance is known not to bind to charcoal, for caustic or volatile substances, if the airway is not protected, or if the patient is actively vomiting.
- Multidose activated charcoal may improve the clearance of theophylline, carbamazepine, phenobarbital, quinine, and dapsone.
- Osmotic cathartics (1 gram/kg or 70% sorbitol or 4 milligrams/kg of 10% magnesium citrate) may be given with the first dose of activated charcoal, although evidence is lacking to support improved outcomes when compared to use of AC alone. Contraindications to cathartic use include age <5 years, caustic ingestions, bowel obstructions, renal failure, and poisonings by substances known to cause significant diarrhea.
- Whole bowel irrigation may enhance elimination of sustained-released products, heavy metals, drugs carried by body stuffers/packers, or agents known to form bezoars. Instill polyethylene glycol via an NG tube (1.5-2.0 L/h in adults, 1.0-1.5 L/h in children 6-12 years of age, and 0.5 L/h in children <6 years of age) until rectal effluent is clear.
- Along with, or subsequent to decontamination, specific techniques to enhance elimination, such as urinary alkalinization and hemodialysis, may be indicated.
- The duration of observation for asymptomatic patients following poisonings or potentially toxic exposures is variable and toxin specific. Consultation with a regional poison center or medical toxicologist may be warranted for expert opinion or assistance with management.
- All patients with intentional poisonings should be referred for psychiatric evaluation once medically stable. Pediatric poisonings may require social work evaluation.

For further reading in Tintinalli's *Emergency Medicine: A Comprehensive Guide*, 7th ed., see Chapter 170, "General Management of the Poisoned Patient," by Jason B. Hack and Robert S. Hoffman.

103 ANTICHOLINERGICS

O. John Ma

EPIDEMIOLOGY

- Anticholinergic toxicity is encountered because of the common use of phenothiazines, mydriatics, skeletal muscle relaxants, antihistamines (particularly diphenhydramine), antidepressants, antispasmotics, and antiparkinsonian drugs.
- Jimsonweed is a plant associated with anticholinergic toxicity.

PATHOPHYSIOLOGY

- The mechanism of action involves cholinergic blockade of muscarinic receptors (primarily in the brain), nicotinic receptors, or both. The clinical effects of these agents result from disturbances in the parasympathetic nervous system (peripheral effects) and the brain (central effects).
- Drug absorption can occur after ingestion, smoking, or ocular use.
- Table 103-1 describes muscarinic and antimuscarinic effects.

CLINICAL EFFECTS

- Clinical findings include mydriasis, hypoactive or absent bowel sounds, tachycardia, flushed skin, disorientation, urinary retention, hyperthermia, dry skin and mucus membranes, dysarthria, confusion, agitation, and auditory or visual hallucinations.
- Clinical findings can be remembered as: Dry as a Bone, Red as a Beet, Hot as a Hare, Blind as a Bat, Mad as a Hatter, and Stuffed as a Pipe.
- The most common ECG finding is sinus tachycardia. Wide-complex tachydysrhythmias and QT-interval prolongation can also be seen.

DIAGNOSIS AND DIFFERENTIAL

- Diagnosis is primarily clinical. In isolated anticholinergic toxicity, routine laboratory studies should be normal. Nonetheless, obtain electrolytes, glucose level, toxicology screening, and pulse oximetry in the presence of altered mental status.
- In contrast, sympathomimetic toxicity and delirium tremens present with moist skin and active bowel sounds. Acute psychiatric disorders may have tachycardia and tachypnea, but the physical examination is otherwise unremarkable.

TABLE 103-1 Muscarinic and Antimuscarinic Effects

ORGAN	STIMULATION OR MUSCARINIC EFFECT	ANTAGONISM OR ANTIMUSCARINIC EFFECT
Brain	Complex interactions, possible improvement in memory	Complex interactions, impairs memory, produces agitation, delirium, hallucinations, and fever
Eye	Constricts pupil (miosis), decreases intraocular pressure, increases tear production	Dilates pupil (mydriasis), loss of accommodation (blurred vision), increases intraocular pressure
Mouth	Increases saliva production	Decreases saliva production, dry mucous membranes
Lungs	Bronchospasm, increases bronchial secretions	Bronchodilation
Heart	Bradycardia, slows atrioventricular condition	Tachycardia, enhances atrioventricular conduction
Peripheral vasculature	Vasodilation (modest)	Vasoconstriction (very modest)
GI	Increases motility, increases gastric acid production, produces emesis	Decreases motility, decreases gastric acid production
Urinary	Stimulates bladder contraction and expulsion of urine	Decreases bladder activity, promotes urinary retention
Skin	Increases sweat production	Decreases sweat production (dry skin), cutaneous vasodilation (flushed appearance)

- The differential diagnosis includes viral encephalitis, Reye's syndrome, head trauma, other intoxications, neuroleptic malignant syndrome, alcohol withdrawal, delirium tremens, acute psychiatric disorders, and sympathomimetic toxicity.

EMERGENCY DEPARTMENT CARE AND DISPOSITION

- Treatment is primarily supportive. Place the patient on a cardiac monitor and secure intravenous access.
- GI decontamination with activated charcoal may be useful even outside the 1-hour window of ingestion because of diminished GI motility.
- Treat hyperthermia and seizures with conventional measures.
- Standard antiarrhythmics are usually effective, but class Ia medications should be avoided. Treat wide

complex tachydysrhythmias with intravenous sodium bicarbonate.
- Treat agitation with benzodiazepines, such as lorazepam. Phenothiazines should be avoided.
- Physostigmine treatment is controversial. Consider its use if conventional therapy fails to control agitation and delirium. The initial dose is 0.5 to 2 milligrams IV, administered slowly over 5 minutes. When effective, a significant decrease in agitation may be apparent within 15 to 20 minutes.
- Physostigmine may lead to severe bradycardia and asystole. It is contraindicated in patients with asthma, intestinal or bladder obstruction, or heart block.
- Discharge patients with mild anticholinergic toxicity after 6 hours of observation if their symptoms have resolved. Admit more symptomatic patients for 24 hours of observation. Patients receiving physostigmine usually require at least a 24-hour admission.

For further reading in Tintinalli's *Emergency Medicine: A Comprehensive Study Guide*, 7th ed., see Chapter 196, "Anticholinergics," by Paul M. Wax and Amy C. Young.

104 PSYCHOPHARMACOLOGIC AGENTS

C. Crawford Mechem

CYCLIC ANTIDEPRESSANTS

EPIDEMIOLOGY

- Cyclic antidepressants are the most common antidepressants to cause overdose-related deaths. In 2008, 11,000 exposures were reported to US poison control centers.

PATHOPHYSIOLOGY

- Cyclic antidepressants are first-generation antidepressants. They have a low therapeutic index, troublesome side effects, and the potential to produce severe toxicity in overdose.
- Pharmacologic effects include antagonism of histamine and α-adrenergic receptors, inhibition of norepinephrine and serotonin reuptake, and inhibition of sodium and potassium channels.

CLINICAL FEATURES

- Toxicity can occur both at therapeutic doses and in overdose. Manifestations range from mild antimuscarinic symptoms (dry mouth, sinus tachycardia) to severe cardiotoxicity.
- Altered mental status is the most common symptom of toxicity.
- Sinus tachycardia is the most frequent dysrhythmia.
- Serious toxicity is almost always seen within 6 hours of ingestion and consists of coma, cardiac conduction delays, supraventricular tachycardia, hypotension, respiratory depression, premature ventricular beats, ventricular tachycardia, and seizures.

DIAGNOSIS AND DIFFERENTIAL

- ECG abnormalities develop within 6 hours of ingestion and identify patients at increased risk for seizures and ventricular dysrhythmias. However, life-threatening complications can occur in the absence of significant ECG abnormalities.
- Classic findings are sinus tachycardia, right axis deviation of the terminal 40 milliseconds (positive terminal R wave in aVR, negative S wave in lead I), and prolongation of the PR, QRS, and QT intervals. Less common findings are right-bundle branch block and the Brugada pattern.

EMERGENCY DEPARTMENT CARE AND DISPOSITION

- Obtain IV or IO access, initiate continuous cardiac monitoring, and perform an ECG on all patients.
- Suggested laboratory studies include serum electrolytes, creatinine, glucose, an ABG, and quantitative serum acetaminophen and aspirin levels.
- Patients may require urinary catheterization, and an NG tube may be needed to relieve urinary retention and ileus.
- Administer 1 gram/kg of activated charcoal PO/NG. Consider gastric lavage followed by activated charcoal in patients presenting within an hour of ingestion.
- Treat hypotension with IV/IO isotonic crystalloids in increments of 20 mL/kg. Administer sodium bicarbonate if no response. Treat persistent hypotension with an infusion of norepinephrine starting at 1 microgram/min, and titrating to effect, up to 30 micrograms/min.
- Administer sodium bicarbonate to patients with hypotension refractory to IV fluids, cardiac conduction abnormalities (prolonged QRS duration or Brugada pattern), and ventricular dysrhythmias. Give an initial IV bolus of 1 to 2 mEq/kg, and repeat until the patient improves

or blood pH equals 7.50 to 7.55; after the bolus, begin a continuous infusion (150 mEq added to 1 L of 5% dextrose in water, or 100 mEq added to 5% dextrose in 0.45% saline) at 2 to 3 mL/kg/h, to maintain alkalemia. Anticipate and treat associated hypokalemia as needed.

- Treat agitation with reassurance, a quiet environment, and benzodiazepines.
- Treat seizures with lorazepam or diazepam, followed by IV phenobarbital, 15 milligrams/kg in refractory cases. Anticipate hypotension. Consider paralysis with a neuromuscular blocking agent followed by continued anticonvulsant therapy for refractory seizures; ongoing electroencephalographic monitoring is required in these cases.
- No therapy is required for asymptomatic patients with sinus tachycardia, isolated PR prolongation, or first-degree AV block; however, consider sodium bicarbonate in asymptomatic or minimally toxic patients if the QRS duration is >100 milliseconds.
- Treat ventricular dysrhythmias with sodium bicarbonate. Lidocaine is a second-line agent. Synchronized cardioversion is appropriate for unstable tachydysrhythmias.
- Treat torsades de pointes with 2 grams (50 milligrams/kg in children) of IV magnesium sulfate.
- Patients who remain asymptomatic after 6 hours of observation do not require hospital admission for toxicologic reasons. Admit all symptomatic patients to a monitored bed, and those with signs of moderate to severe toxicity to the ICU.

ATYPICAL ANTIDEPRESSANTS, SEROTONIN REUPTAKE INHIBITORS, AND SEROTONIN SYNDROME

EPIDEMIOLOGY

- These newer antidepressants comprise a heterogeneous group that are more selective in their pharmacologic activity and have a different presentation in overdose than monoamine oxidase inhibitors (MAOIs) and cyclic antidepressants. They are associated with less toxicity and fewer fatalities.

PATHOPHYSIOLOGY

- The mechanism of action of atypical antidepressants most likely involves inhibition of neurotransmitter reuptake or interruption of negative feedback loops.
- Almost all agents have serotoninergic activity and can produce serotonin syndrome, particularly when combined with other serotoninergic drugs (Table 104-1).
- Atypical antidepressants are less likely to cause the ECG conduction abnormalities and cardiotoxicity seen with cyclic antidepressants.

TABLE 104-1 Serotoninergic Drugs

Antidepressants	
Monoamine oxidase inhibitors: phenelzine, tranylcypromine, isocarboxazid, pargyline, rasagiline, and selegiline	
Selective serotonin reuptake inhibitors: fluoxetine, sertraline, paroxetine, fluvoxamine, citalopram, and escitalopram	
Serotonin/norepinephrine reuptake inhibitors: venlafaxine, desvenlafaxine, and duloxetine	
Cyclic antidepressants: amitriptyline, clomipramine, desipramine, doxepin, imipramine, nortriptyline, protriptyline, and trimipramine	
Miscellaneous: trazodone (moderate potency), bupropion (low potency)	
Other Agents	
Amantadine (low potency)	L-tryptophan and 5-hydroxytryptophan (high potency)
Amphetamines (moderate potency)	Lysergic acid diethylamide (moderate potency)
Bromocriptine (low potency)	
Buspirone (moderate potency)	Meperidine (high potency)
Carbamazepine (low potency)	Mescaline (moderate potency)
Cocaine (moderate potency)	Metoclopramide (low potency)
Codeine (low potency)	Pentazocine (low potency)
Dextromethorphan (high potency)	Pergolide (low potency)
	Reserpine (low potency)
Fentanyl (moderate potency)	St. John's wort (moderate potency)
Levodopa (moderate potency)	Sumatriptan and related triptans (high potency)
Linezolid (high potency)	
Lithium (high potency)	Tramadol (high potency)

- Newer antidepressants (except bupropion) have a higher safety margin than the MAOIs and cyclic antidepressants. However, they can still cause fatalities.

TRAZODONE

CLINICAL FEATURES

- Adverse effects include orthostatic hypotension, sedation, priapism, and liver toxicity.
- Cardiac dysrhythmias include sinus arrest, sinus bradycardia, AV blocks, complete heart block, atrial fibrillation, premature ventricular beats, and torsades de pointes.
- ECG findings include sinus bradycardia and tachycardia and QT prolongation.
- Serious toxicity in an average adult is not expected with acute, isolated ingestions of <2 grams.
- Following acute ingestion, the most common symptom is CNS depression. Other neurologic symptoms include ataxia, dizziness, coma, and seizures.

- Commonly reported GI complaints include nausea, vomiting, and nonspecific abdominal pain.

EMERGENCY DEPARTMENT CARE AND DISPOSITION

- Obtain a 12-lead ECG and initiate cardiac monitoring for all patients.
- Administer single-dose activated charcoal. Consider gastric lavage followed by activated charcoal in patients presenting within 1 hour of ingesting >2 grams of trazodone or those with toxic coingestions.
- Treat hypotension with isotonic IV fluids, followed by norepinephrine for refractory shock.
- Treat torsades de pointes with IV magnesium sulfate or defibrillation.
- Patients who remain asymptomatic for 6 hours can be discharged, provided that any necessary psychiatric evaluation has been completed.
- Admit patients with neurologic and/or cardiac symptoms persisting >6 hours after ingestion to a monitored bed.

BUPROPION

CLINICAL FEATURES

- Adverse effects include dry mouth, dizziness, agitation, nausea, headache, constipation, tremor, anxiety, confusion, blurred vision, and increased motor activity. Abrupt discontinuation may pose a theoretical risk of precipitating neuroleptic malignant syndrome.
- Bupropion has a low therapeutic index, and toxicity can occur at dosages equal to or just slightly greater than the maximum therapeutic dose of 450 milligrams/d.
- The most common symptoms in overdose are agitation, dizziness, tremor, nausea, vomiting, drowsiness, tachycardia, and hyperthermia.
- Sinus tachycardia is the most common ECG finding.
- Hypotension may develop in mixed overdoses, and hypertension may also occur.
- Coma and cardiac arrest can occur with severe overdoses.
- Seizures are more common than with other atypical antidepressants and can develop in otherwise asymptomatic patients.
- Laboratory studies are usually normal except for occasional hypokalemia.

EMERGENCY DEPARTMENT CARE AND DISPOSITION

- Anticipate generalized seizures in all cases.
- Obtain IV access and initiate cardiac rhythm monitoring.
- Perform GI decontamination if it can be done within 1 hour of ingestion. Whole-bowel irrigation is helpful in overdoses of sustained-release products.
- Treat seizures with benzodiazepines and phenobarbital (15 milligrams/kg) if needed.
- Admit all patients with seizures, persistent sinus tachycardia, or lethargy. Asymptomatic patients who have ingested regular-release bupropion should be observed for 8 hours before discharge. Adult patients ingesting >450 milligrams of sustained-release bupropion require monitoring for longer periods up to 24 hours.

MIRTAZAPINE

CLINICAL FEATURES

- Mirtazapine has limited toxicity in overdose. Signs and symptoms include sedation, confusion, sinus tachycardia, and mild hypertension.
- The risk of coma and respiratory depression is greatest at larger doses or when mirtazapine is combined with other sedative drugs.

EMERGENCY DEPARTMENT CARE AND DISPOSITION

- Isolated mirtazapine overdoses are generally managed with supportive care.
- Administer activated charcoal, 1 gram/kg, and consider gastric lavage if performed early after large overdoses or with significant coingestions.
- Admit symptomatic patients to a monitored bed, although life-threatening cardiac toxicity is rare. Asymptomatic patients can be discharged after 8 hours of observation.

SELECTIVE SEROTONIN REUPTAKE INHIBITORS

EPIDEMIOLOGY

- Selective serotonin reuptake inhibitors (SSRIs) currently available in the United States are fluoxetine, sertraline, paroxetine, fluvoxamine, citalopram, and escitalopram, which, as a group, have a high therapeutic-to-toxic ratio.

CLINICAL FEATURES

- The most serious adverse effect is serotonin syndrome.
- Other adverse effects include headache, sedation, insomnia, dizziness, weakness or fatigue, tremor, nervousness, nausea, vomiting, diarrhea, constipation, and anorexia. Dystonic reactions, akathisia, dyskinesia, hypokinesia, and parkinsonian symptoms can develop.

- Most patients remain asymptomatic following overdose, but may develop nausea, vomiting, sedation, tremor, and sinus tachycardia. Sinus bradycardia is more commonly observed with fluvoxamine overdoses. QRS and QT prolongation have been reported with citalopram ingestions. In most cases, ECG abnormalities gradually resolve over 24 hours.
- Life-threatening complications are uncommon. Patients at higher risk include those with underlying seizure disorders, symptoms of serotonin syndrome, or mixed-drug overdoses.

EMERGENCY DEPARTMENT CARE AND DISPOSITION

- Supportive care is generally all that is required for SSRI overdoses.
- For symptomatic patients, obtain vascular access and initiate cardiac monitoring.
- Administer single-dose activated charcoal for most ingestions.
- Treat seizures with benzodiazepines.
- Observe patients for at least 6 hours. Patients with persistent tachycardia or lethargy and those with ECG conduction abnormalities 6 hours after ingestion require admission.

SEROTONIN/NOREPINEPHRINE REUPTAKE INHIBITORS

EPIDEMIOLOGY

- Serotonin/norepinephrine reuptake inhibitors available in the United States include venlafaxine, desvenlafaxine, and duloxetine. Adverse effects are similar to those of the SSRIs.

CLINICAL FEATURES

- Venlafaxine can produce hypertension. Duloxetine may cause nausea, dizziness, and vomiting.
- In acute overdose, all three medications can cause tachycardia, hypertension, diaphoresis, tremor, and mydriasis. Altered mental status is common. Generalized seizures are more frequent in overdose with these medications than with SSRIs and can occur shortly after ingestion.
- ECG abnormalities include sinus tachycardia, QRS widening, and QT prolongation.

EMERGENCY DEPARTMENT CARE AND DISPOSITION

- Experience with overdoses of these agents is limited. Toxic effects may appear precipitously.
- Obtain vascular access and initiate cardiac monitoring.
- Administer single-dose activated charcoal and consider gastric lavage with early presentation after large ingestions. Consider whole-bowel irrigation in the case of a massive ingestion of sustained-release preparations.
- Treat seizures with benzodiazepines.
- Treat hypotension with isotonic crystalloid and direct-acting α-agonists for refractory cases.
- Observe all patients for at least 6 hours and longer for those with extended-release ingestions. Admit all symptomatic patients to a monitored bed.

SEROTONIN SYNDROME

PATHOPHYSIOLOGY

- Serotonin syndrome is a potentially fatal adverse drug reaction to serotoninergic medications, characterized by cognitive impairment and autonomic and neuromuscular dysfunction.
- Serotonin syndrome can be caused by any drug or combination of drugs that increase serotonin transmission.

CLINICAL FEATURES

- Cognitive and behavioral findings include confusion, agitation, coma, anxiety, hypomania, lethargy, seizures, insomnia, hallucinations, and dizziness.
- Autonomic signs include hyperthermia, diaphoresis, sinus tachycardia, hypertension or hypotension, tachypnea, dilated or unreactive pupils, flushed skin, diarrhea, and salivation.
- Neuromuscular findings include myoclonus, hyperreflexia, muscle rigidity, tremor, hyperactivity, ataxia, shivering, Babinski sign, nystagmus, opisthotonus, and trismus.

DIAGNOSIS AND DIFFERENTIAL

- The diagnosis is made on clinical grounds after exclusion of other psychiatric and medical conditions. There are no confirmatory laboratory tests.

EMERGENCY DEPARTMENT CARE AND DISPOSITION

- Therapy involves discontinuing all serotoninergic agents and providing supportive care.
- Consider administration of antiserotonergic agents such as cyproheptadine, 4 to 12 milligrams PO, repeated in 2 hours if no response, to a maximum of 32 milligrams. Patients who respond are

given 4 milligrams PO every 6 hours for 48 hours. Chlorpromazine may also be used.
- Administer benzodiazepines to relieve muscle rigidity and discomfort.
- Monitor all patients with muscle rigidity, seizures, or hyperthermia for development of rhabdomyolysis and/or metabolic acidosis.
- Admit all patients with serotonin syndrome to the hospital.

MONOAMINE OXIDASE INHIBITORS

EPIDEMIOLOGY

- Monoamine oxidase inhibitors (MAOIs) were the first class of antidepressants. Their use is now limited to treating atypical and refractory cases of depression, and some cases of Parkinson's disease.
- MAOIs have a low therapeutic index, and can cause tyramine reactions, serotonin syndrome, and potentially fatal drug interactions.

PATHOPHYSIOLOGY

- Monoamine oxidase is an intracellular enzyme that inactivates norepinephrine, dopamine, serotonin, and tyramine.
- Inhibition leads to accumulation of neurotransmitters in presynaptic nerve terminals and increased systemic availability of dietary amines.
- Toxicity results from ingestion of foods containing tyramine, drug interactions, or overdose.

CLINICAL FEATURES

- Tyramine reactions develop within 15 to 90 minutes of ingestion of dietary tyramine, which is found in foods such as aged meats and cheeses. Symptoms include severe headache, hypertension, diaphoresis, mydriasis, neck stiffness, pallor, neuromuscular excitation, palpitations, and chest pain. Fatalities have been reported.
- Drug interactions involving MAOIs can result in a hyperadrenergic state or the serotonin syndrome. Physicians should exercise caution when administering medications to patients who have taken MAOIs within the past 2 weeks.
- Appearance of toxicity is often delayed 6 to 12 hours after ingestion, and as long as 24 hours.
- Initial symptoms of overdose include headache, agitation, irritability, nausea, palpitations, and tremor.
- Signs of toxicity include sinus tachycardia, hyperreflexia, hyperactivity, fasciculations, mydriasis, hyperventilation, nystagmus, and generalized flushing.
- In more severe cases, muscle rigidity, diaphoresis, chest pain, hypertension, diarrhea, hallucinations, combativeness, confusion, hyperthermia, and trismus may be noted.
- Severe toxicity is accompanied by coma, seizures, bradycardia, hypoxia, worsening hyperthermia, and hypotension. Death usually results from multiorgan failure.

DIAGNOSIS AND DIFFERENTIAL

- MAOI overdose is diagnosed clinically.
- Laboratory tests can assist in the differential diagnosis and identify possible complications, including hypoxia, rhabdomyolysis, renal failure, hyperkalemia, metabolic acidosis, hemolysis, and disseminated intravascular coagulation. Leukocytosis and thrombocytopenia are common.
- The most common ECG abnormality is sinus tachycardia; T-wave changes may also be seen.
- The differential includes other causes of a hyperadrenergic state, altered mental status, or muscle rigidity (Table 104-2).

TABLE 104-2 Differential Diagnosis of Monoamine Oxidase Inhibitor Overdose

Intoxications	Medical conditions	Adverse drug reactions
Amphetamines	Heat stroke	Dystonic reactions
Antimuscarinics	Hypoglycemia	Malignant hyperthermia
Cathinone	Hyperthyroidism	Serotonin syndrome
Cocaine	Pheochromocytoma	Tyramine reaction
Methylphenidate	**Infectious diseases**	Spontaneous hypertensive crisis
MDMA (3,4-methylenedioxy-methamphetamine)	Encephalitis	Neuroleptic malignant syndrome
Phencyclidine	Meningitis	**Psychiatric condition**
Phenylpropanolamine	Rabies	Lethal catatonia
Strychnine	Sepsis	
Theophylline	Tetanus	
Tricyclic antidepressants (early)		
Withdrawal states		
Ethanol (delirium tremens)		
Sedative-hypnotics		
Clonidine		
β-Blockers		

EMERGENCY DEPARTMENT CARE AND DISPOSITION

- ED management consists of supportive care and treatment of complications.
- Obtain IV/IO access, initiate cardiac monitoring, and provide supplemental oxygen.
- Gastric lavage is recommended for all significant exposures if it can be performed within 1 hour of ingestion. After gastric lavage, or if presentation is delayed for >1 hour, administer a single dose of activated charcoal.
- Treat hypertension with short-acting parenteral antihypertensive agents because of the potential for precipitous hypotension: consider phentolamine in 2.5- to 5.0 milligram IV boluses every 10 to 15 minutes until hypertension is controlled. Nitroprusside may be given as an alternative as a continuous infusion starting at a rate of 0.25-1.0 micrograms/kg/min, titrated to effect.
- Give nitroglycerin for relief of anginal chest pain and in patients with signs of myocardial ischemia.
- Treat hypotension with isotonic crystalloid boluses, followed by norepinephrine.
- Treat ventricular dysrhythmias with lidocaine or procainamide.
- Give atropine, isoproterenol, or dobutamine for bradycardia and consider cardiac pacing.
- Treat seizures with lorazepam or diazepam. Phenobarbital is effective but can cause hypotension. General anesthesia and muscle paralysis with a *nondepolarizing neuromuscular agent* such as vecuronium may be necessary for status epilepticus. Paralyzed patients require electroencephalographic monitoring.
- Treat hyperthermia with benzodiazepines to reduce muscle hyperactivity and evaporative cooling methods or ice baths. Consider muscle paralysis for diffuse rigidity refractory to benzodiazepines. Dantrolene may be considered for hyperthermia resistant to other measures: the dose is 0.5 to 2.5 milligrams/kg IV every 6 hours.
- Admit all patients with intentional overdoses or accidental exposures of >1 milligram/kg to an ICU. Admit patients with accidental exposures of <1 milligram/kg to a monitored bed. Asymptomatic patients should be monitored for at least 24 hours.

■ ANTIPSYCHOTICS

EPIDEMIOLOGY

- Antipsychotics are a group of medications used to treat symptoms of psychosis, as well as nausea and vomiting, various types of headaches, hiccups, and involuntary motor disorders.
- Isolated overdose is rarely fatal, and most patients develop mild to moderate symptoms.

PATHOPHYSIOLOGY

- All antipsychotics bind to and inhibit CNS dopamine receptors. This results in decreased dopamine production and release, along with dopamine receptor blockade.
- Some antipsychotics bind to histamine, muscarinic, α-adrenergic, and serotonin receptors.

CLINICAL FEATURES

- Adverse effects can develop at therapeutic doses and include acute dystonia, akathisia, parkinsonism, tardive dyskinesia, and neuroleptic malignant syndrome.
- Acute dystonia is characterized by intermittent, uncoordinated, involuntary contractions of the muscles of the face, tongue, neck, trunk, or extremities.
- Akathisia is a subjective sensation of motor restlessness that typically occurs within minutes to days of initiating or increasing the dose of an antipsychotic.
- Parkinsonism is a delayed effect and is characterized by cogwheel-type muscle rigidity, pill-rolling tremor, mask facies, shuffling gait, bradykinesia or akinesia, and cognitive impairment.
- Tardive dyskinesia is a late-onset, often irreversible, extrapyramidal syndrome and is characterized by painless, stereotyped, repetitive movements of the face.
- Neuroleptic malignant syndrome is a rare but potentially fatal complication that most often occurs shortly after the start of therapy or after a dosage adjustment. It is characterized by fever, muscular rigidity, autonomic dysfunction, and altered mental status.
- CNS depression is common and may range from lethargy, ataxia, dysarthria, and confusion to coma. Respiratory depression is more common in multidrug overdoses.
- Paradoxical agitation and delirium may occur in mixed overdoses.
- Seizures occur in 1% of overdoses and are more common with loxapine and clozapine.
- Patients may manifest anticholinergic toxicity, including tachycardia, dry mucous membranes and skin, mydriasis, decreased bowel sounds, urinary retention, delirium, and hyperthermia.
- Cardiovascular manifestations include sinus tachycardia and orthostatic hypotension.
- ECG changes include PR, QRS, and QT prolongation, ST depression, T-wave flattening, and a rightward shift of the terminal 40 milliseconds of the QRS frontal plane axis.

DIAGNOSIS AND DIFFERENTIAL

- In neuroleptic malignant syndrome, laboratory abnormalities include elevated creatine kinase, leukocytosis, elevated liver transaminases, hypernatremia or hyponatremia, metabolic acidosis, myoglobinuria, elevated BUN and creatinine, and decreased serum iron level.
- Obtain a CBC for any patient presenting with a fever while taking clozapine or chlorpromazine because of the possibility of associated leukopenia and agranulocytosis.
- In acute overdose, routine laboratory analysis should include a CBC, basic chemistry tests, acetaminophen and aspirin levels, and a pregnancy test for women of childbearing age.

EMERGENCY DEPARTMENT CARE AND DISPOSITION

- Treat acute akathisia and acute dystonia with diphenhydramine, 25 to 50 milligrams, or benztropine, 1 to 2 milligrams, IM or IV.
- Treat drug-induced parkinsonism by lowering the dosage, changing to a different agent, adding diphenhydramine or benztropine, or adding amantadine.
- Treatment of neuroleptic malignant syndrome is primarily supportive. Patients with airway compromise, acidosis, hypoxia, or severe fever and rigidity should be intubated using a nondepolarizing agent for rapid sequence induction and benzodiazepines for sedation. Consider dantrolene (1.0-2.5 milligrams/kg IV load, followed by 1 milligram/kg IV every 6 hours) in severe cases.
- Following acute overdose, management is supportive.
- Obtain vascular access, initiate cardiac rhythm monitoring, and provide oxygen.
- Consider naloxone and thiamine, and serum glucose determination, for patients with altered mental status.
- Treat seizures with benzodiazepines.
- Treat hypotension with fluid resuscitation, followed by phenylephrine or norepinephrine.
- Patients with a QTc interval of >500 milliseconds are at risk for torsades de pointes and should receive magnesium sulfate, 2 to 4 grams IV over 10 minutes.
- Treat patients with QRS prolongation or ventricular arrhythmias with sodium bicarbonate, 1 to 2 mEq/kg IV bolus, followed by intermittent boluses or a continuous infusion.
- Observe patients for at least 6 hours. Patients with no mental status changes, pulse and blood pressure abnormalities, orthostatic hypotension, and normal ECG 6 hours from the time of ingestion are candidates for discharge.
- Monitor patients with thioridazine or mesoridazine ingestion for 24 hours.
- Patients with sinus tachycardia, QT prolongation, seizure, respiratory depression, hypotension, or acidosis require admission to a monitored bed; those with altered mental status, cardiotoxicity, or suspected neuroleptic malignant syndrome should be admitted to an ICU bed.

LITHIUM

EPIDEMIOLOGY

- Lithium is used for treatment of bipolar disorder and acute mania.
- Toxicity most often results from accidental or intentional overdose or from an alteration in clearance secondary to renal impairment.
- Up to 75% to 90% of patients on long-term lithium therapy will develop toxicity.

PATHOPHYSIOLOGY

- Lithium competes with sodium, potassium, magnesium, and calcium, displacing them from intracellular and extracellular sites.
- Lithium inhibits adenylate cyclase, decreasing cAMP and possibly cGMP.
- Lithium interferes with the release and reuptake of norepinephrine at nerve terminals.
- Lithium enhances serotonin release from the hippocampus.
- Acute toxicity may result from overdose or develop in those on long-term therapy. Decreased renal clearance and intravascular volume depletion are the most common causes.
- Most often, toxicity involves a drug–drug interaction. An important potential interaction is that the effect of neuromuscular blocking agents such as succinylcholine and vecuronium may be prolonged in patients receiving long-term lithium therapy.

CLINICAL FEATURES

- The most common adverse effects are hand tremor, polyuria, and rash.
- Nephrogenic diabetes insipidus develops in up to 40% of patients on long-term lithium treatment. Incomplete distal renal tubular acidosis may also be noted.
- Neurologic effects include memory loss, decreased mental status, fatigue, ataxia, and dysarthria.
- Nausea, vomiting, and diarrhea are common at initiation of treatment.

- In acute toxicity, patients present with muscle fasciculations or weakness, ataxia, agitation, lethargy, or coma.
- Acute renal failure may develop, especially in the elderly and those with preexisting renal impairment, diabetes, hypertension, or dehydration.
- GI symptoms include nausea, vomiting, diarrhea, or generalized abdominal pain.
- Cardiac abnormalities include hypotension, conduction delays, and ventricular dysrhythmias. ECG changes include QT prolongation, ST-segment depression, or T-wave inversion.

DIAGNOSIS AND DIFFERENTIAL

- Acute lithium overdoses classically cause more GI toxicity and less neurologic toxicity. Serum lithium levels often do not correlate well with either symptom severity or prognosis.
- Chronic toxicity often displays earlier and greater neurologic effects associated with lower serum levels. Serum lithium levels correlate better with degree of toxicity and prognosis in chronic toxicity.
- The best guideline for therapy is generally the patient's clinical condition.
- Monitoring of lithium serum levels is important, and serial measurements are useful to determine treatment and disposition options.

EMERGENCY DEPARTMENT CARE AND DISPOSITION

- Initial management is supportive.
- Establish vascular access and initiate cardiac monitoring and obtain an ECG.
- Administer normal saline, as most patients with significant toxicity have some sodium and total volume deficits. Typical adult dosing is a 2 L IV bolus over 30 to 60 minutes followed by a 200 mL/h continuous IV infusion.
- Treat seizures with benzodiazepines, followed by phenobarbital or general anesthesia.
- Activated charcoal does not absorb lithium but may be indicated in multidrug ingestions.
- Gastric lavage may be considered with massive ingestions (>4 grams in an adult), if it can be performed within 1 hour of exposure.
- Whole-bowel irrigation may be helpful in ingestions of sustained-release lithium products.
- Laboratory studies should include renal function tests, electrolyte levels, CBC, serum lithium levels, and serum acetaminophen and aspirin levels.
- Indications for hemodialysis include serum lithium levels of >4 mEq/L in acute overdose (3.5 mEq/L in chronic toxicity), or little change in serum level after 6 hours of IV saline. In addition, patients with renal failure, rapidly increasing serum levels, and those who have ingested sustained-release preparations should be considered for hemodialysis. The goal of treatment is to reduce the lithium level to <1 mEq/L. Serum level should be monitored for up to 8 hours following a dialysis session. If the level rises to >1 mEq/L, dialysis should be reinstituted.
- Monitor patients with acute ingestions for 4 to 6 hours, even if asymptomatic.
- Admit patients with serum lithium levels of >1.5 mEq/L following acute ingestion and all patients with ingestion of a sustained-release preparation.
- Patients with minor chronic toxicity and no additional risk factors can be managed with IV saline for 6 to 12 hours, often in an observation unit; once serum lithium levels decrease to <1.5 mEq, they can safely be discharged.

For further reading in Tintinalli's *Emergency Medicine: A Comprehensive Study Guide*, 7th ed., see Chapter 171, "Cyclic Antidepressants," by Kirk C. Mills; Chapter 172, "Atypical Antidepressants, Serotonin Reuptake Inhibitors, and Serotonin Syndrome," by Kirk C. Mills and Keenan M. Bora; Chapter 173, "Monoamine Oxidase Inhibitors," by Kirk C. Mills; Chapter 174, "Antipsychotics," by Michael Levine and Frank LoVecchio; and Chapter 175, "Lithium," by Sandra M. Schneider and Daniel J. Cobaugh.

105 SEDATIVE AND HYPNOTICS

L. Keith French

BARBITURATES

EPIDEMIOLOGY

- Barbiturate use has declined with the adoption of safer sedative-hypnotic agents and second-generation anticonvulsants.
- In 2008, the American Association of Poison Control Centers (AAPCC) received 1523 reports of isolated barbiturate exposures with only four indentified deaths.

PATHOPHYSIOLOGY

- Barbiturates depress activity in the nervous and musculoskeletal systems.

- Within the central nervous system, barbiturates enhance the action of the neurotransmitter γ-aminobutryic acid (GABA). This leads to prolonged opening of chloride channels on postsynaptic neurons, decreasing the resting membrane potential and making it more difficult to bring the neuron to an excitatory threshold.
- Barbiturates decrease vascular tone, which can lead to hypotension.
- Barbiturates are classified according to their duration of action: long-acting (barbital, phenobarbital, duration of action >6 hours), intermediate-acting (amobarbital, butalbital, duration of action 3-6 hours), short-acting (pentobarbital, secobarbital, duration of action <3 hours), and ultrashort-acting (thiopental, methohexital, duration of action <10 minutes).
- Elimination half-life can be shortened in the very young and extended in the very old.
- Chronic barbiturate use induces hepatic P-450 enzymes and may be responsible for several adverse drug–drug interactions (including oral contraceptives, anticoagulants, and corticosteroids).

CLINICAL FEATURES

- Mild to moderate barbiturate toxicity resembles acute intoxication with ethanol or other sedative-hypnotics: drowsiness, disinhibition, ataxia, slurred speech, and confusion.
- Severe intoxication manifests as a range of cognitive decline from stupor to coma, and may include absent corneal and deep tendon reflexes.
- The most common vital sign abnormalities are respiratory depression (usually the first altered vital sign), hypothermia, and hypotension.
- Gastrointestinal (GI) motility is slowed and gastric emptying is delayed.
- Hypoglycemia can occur.
- Heart rate, nystagmus, pupil size, and reactivity are variable.
- Common complications include aspiration pneumonia, pulmonary edema, and acute lung injury.
- Skin bullae, also known as "barbiturate blisters," can be present, but are neither sensitive nor specific for barbiturate overdoses.
- Severe poisoning is likely to occur following ingestion of ten or more times the therapeutic dose.

DIAGNOSIS AND DIFFERENTIAL

- Serum barbiturate concentrations can help establish a diagnosis, but do not exclude alternative etiologies for altered mental status or hypotension; serum levels of potential coingestants (eg, acetaminophen and aspirin) should be obtained.
- Additional tests to consider included ECG, chest radiography, a complete blood count, serum chemistries, creatinine phosphokinase concentration, blood ethanol concentrations, and arterial blood gas analysis.
- The differential diagnosis includes acute ethanol intoxication or toxicity from other sedative-hypnotic agents.

EMERGENCY DEPARTMENT CARE AND DISPOSITION

- Assessment and stabilization of the airway, breathing, and circulation remain the priority for all patients with barbiturate poisoning.
- Activated charcoal (1 gram/kg) may decrease the absorption of barbiturates and should be given to cooperative, stable patients if presenting <1 hour after overdose.
- In life-threatening phenobarbital overdoses, consider multidose activated charcoal (12.5-25 grams via nasogastric tube every 4 hours × 3 doses) once the airway has been secured (generally via endotracheal intubation).
- Treat hypotension with isotonic crystalloids; administer norepinephrine or dopamine for refractory hypotension.
- Treat hypothermia <36°C with aggressive rewarming measures.
- Urinary alkalinization is not considered a first-line therapy, but may be considered in serious phenobarbital or primidone overdoses.
- There is no role for forced dieresis.
- Consider extracorporeal elimination (hemodialysis, hemoperfusion, and hemodiafiltration) in patients with life-threatening phenobarbital overdoses who deteriorate despite aggressive supportive care.
- Observe patients for at least 6 to 8 hours following barbiturate overdose; patients can be safely discharged if they are improving, are minimally symptomatic, and have stable vital signs without supportive measures.
- Evidence of toxicity beyond 6 hours following overdose requires hospital admission, potentially to intensive care.

BENZODIAZEPINES

EPIDEMIOLOGY

- In 2008, the AAPCC received 30,856 reports of isolated benzodiazepine exposures.
- Mortality from isolated benzodiazepine overdoses is rare. However, when benzodiazepines are combined with other sedative-hypnotics, morbidity increases.

PATHOPHYSIOLOGY

- Benzodiazepines stimulate the α-subunit of the postsynaptic GABA receptor in the central nervous system rendering neurons less excitable.
- Benzodiazepines are relatively lipid soluble, but differ individually in time to peak effect, elimination half-life, and duration of action. Many benzodiazepines have active metabolites.
- Most benzodiazepines are classified as category D for teratogenicity, except for flurazepam, quazepam, temazepam, and triazolam, which are characterized as category X.

CLINICAL FEATURES

- Stimulation of the GABA receptor leads to inhibitory effects, typically producing sedation, anxiolysis, anticonvulsant activity, and striated muscle relaxation.
- The predominant clinical features include somnolence, dizziness, slurred speech, confusion, ataxia, incoordination, and general impairment of intellectual function.
- Paradoxical reactions consisting of anxiety, aggression, hostile behavior, rage, and delirium are uncommon but can occur.
- Deaths from isolated benzodiazepine overdoses are more common with short-acting agents such as alprazolam, temazepam, and triazolam.
- The effects of benzodiazepines may be prolonged in patients with liver disease, with protein deficiencies, or at the extremes of age.
- Short-term anterograde amnesia, a potentially desirable effect, is common with lorazepam, midazolam, and triazolam, but may occur with any benzodiazepine.
- Respiratory depression and hypotension may occur after IV administration or in the presence of co-ingestants.
- Metabolic acidosis following high-dose infusions of lorazepam or diazepam may result as a complication of the diluent propylene glycol.

DIAGNOSIS AND DIFFERENTIAL

- The clinical presentation of benzodiazepine intoxication is nonspecific and shares many features of intoxication from other sedative-hypnotics.
- Urine drug screens may detect the presence of benzodiazepines; however, remote exposure may not be the etiology of an acute sedative-hypnotic toxidrome.
- Serum drug screens have no role in active management of a patient with an unknown sedative-hypnotic overdose, but may play a role in forensic investigations or potential child endangerment cases.

EMERGENCY DEPARTMENT CARE AND DISPOSITION

- Assessment and stabilization of the airway, breathing, and circulation remain the priority in management of all patients with benzodiazepine poisoning.
- Endotracheal intubation and mechanical ventilation may be necessary in the obtunded patient.
- Activated charcoal (1 gram/kg) may decrease the absorption of benzodiazepines and should be given to cooperative, stable patients if presenting <1 hour after overdose. There is no role for multidose activated charcoal.
- Gastric lavage, forced dieresis, and hemodialysis are ineffective and generally unwarranted.
- Flumazenil (0.2 milligram IV titrated to effect or a total dose of 3 milligrams), a selective antagonist of the central effects of benzodiazepines, has a limited role in the management of benzodiazepine poisoning.
- Contraindications to the use of flumazenil include overdoses of unknown agents, suspected or known dependence on benzodiazepines, suspected co-ingestions with another seizure-inducing agent (such as tricyclic antidepressants), a known seizure disorder, or suspected increased intracranial pressure.
- If used and effective, benzodiazepine toxicity may recur once the effects of flumazenil have worn off.
- Admit all patients with significant alterations in mental status, respiratory depression, and hypotension to the hospital.
- Although many clinicians use the 6-hour principle for observation and discharge of asymptomatic patients, there is limited data regarding the specific duration of ED observation following benzodiazepine exposure.

NONBENZODIAZEPINE SEDATIVES

EPIDEMIOLOGY

- In 2008, the AAPCC received 13,054 reports of isolated exposures to nonbenzodiazepine sedatives.
- Three sedative-hypnotics, ethchlorvynol, glutethimide, and methaqualone, have been removed from US and Canadian markets.

PATHOPHYSIOLOGY

- The sedative-hypnotic effects of the many nonbenzodiazepines do not share a common mechanism of action, and with some agents, the underlying mechanism of action is unknown.

CLINICAL FEATURES

Buspirone

- Common adverse effects include sedation, GI discomfort, vomiting, and dizziness.
- The effects in overdose exaggerate the clinical effects observed with therapeutic dosing.
- Seizures are rare.
- Buspirone has been associated with serotonin syndrome.

Carisoprodol and Meprobamate

- Meprobamate is the active metabolite of carisoprodol.
- Following carisoprodol and meprobamate overdose, sedation, coma, cardiovascular collapse, and pulmonary edema have been reported.
- Myoclonic jerks are commonly observed following carisoprodol overdose, but are not seen with meprobamate.
- Meprobamate overdose has resulted in gastric bezoar formation and prolonged coma.

Chloral Hydrate

- At therapeutic doses, chloral hydrate produces mental status depression, but airway and respiratory reflexes are maintained. In overdose, however, chloral hydrate can produce coma.
- Vomiting and paradoxical hyperactivity occur in approximately 5% of children.
- Cardiovascular toxicity, specifically decreased cardiac contractility, myocardial electrical instability, and increased sensitivity to catecholamines are important features of chloral hydrate toxicity. Cardiac arrhythmias include premature ventricular contractions, ventricular fibrillation, torsades de pointes, and asystole.
- The sedative effects of chloral hydrate are exaggerated when co-ingested with ethanol.
- A pear-like odor is often present and may be a diagnostic clue in a patient presenting with a sedative-hypnotic toxidrome.

γ-Hydroxybutyrate

- γ-Hydroxybutyrate (GHB) effects are dose dependent and range from short-term amnesia and sedation at low doses to seizures, coma, respiratory depression, and cardiac depression with higher doses.
- Bradycardia, hypothermia, and either miosis or mydriasis can occur.
- Agitation with stimulation or sternal rub is common.
- During recovery, which is generally within 6 hours, a patient may suddenly awaken and become aggressive.
- GHB has a very short half-life and is difficult to detect in urine >6 hours after ingestion; thus urine or serum drug screening has a limited role in management.
- Two other compounds, 1,4-butanediol and γ-butyrolactone, are metabolized to GHB and may produce similar effects.

Zolpidem, Zaleplon, and Zopiclone

- All three agents are used for the treatment of insomnia and are generally considered safer than benzodiazepines.
- Adverse effects include somnolence, nausea, and psychomotor impairment. Sleep walking/driving and vivid dreams are commonly reported.

DIAGNOSIS AND DIFFERENTIAL

- Poisoning from nonbenzodiazepines share many overlapping features and can be difficult to distinguish from one another.
- Diagnostic adjuncts to consider included electrocardiography; chest radiography; a complete blood count; serum chemistries; creatinine phosphokinase concentration; salicylate, acetaminophen, and blood ethanol concentrations; and arterial blood gas analysis.
- There is almost no role for serum or urine drug screening in the management of poisonings from nonbenzodiazepines.

EMERGENCY DEPARTMENT CARE AND DISPOSITION

- Assessment and stabilization of the airway, breathing, and circulation remain the priority in management of all patients with nonbenzodiazepine poisoning.
- Routine use of flumazenil or fomepizole for managing overdoses of any of the nonbenzodiazepine sedatives is not recommended.
- IV β-adrenergic blockers should be used to treat ventricular arrhythmias seen with chloral hydrate overdose.

SEDATIVE-HYPNOTIC WITHDRAWAL

- Withdrawal states have been described with chronic use of barbiturates, benzodiazepines, carisoprodol and meprobamate, chloral hydrate, GHB, and zaleplon/zopiclone/zolpidem.
- Within a given class, shorter acting agents are more likely to produce withdrawal states.
- The onset or duration of withdrawal symptoms vary among agents and may occur hours to days after last use, and last days to weeks.

- Common features of sedative-hypnotic withdrawal include agitation, tremor, insomnia, anxiety, GI distress, and anorexia, and in severe states, may be associated with delirium and seizures.
- Barbiturate withdrawal can occur in neonates born to dependent mothers.
- Treatment requires reintroduction of the dependent drug with a slow, controlled taper. Barbiturate, benzodiazepine, and GHB withdrawal may require hospitalization for management.

For further reading in Tintinalli's *Emergency Medicine: A Comprehensive Guide*, 7th ed., see Chapter 176, "Barbiturates," by Chip Gresham and Frank LoVecchio; Chapter 177, "Benzodiazepines," by Dan Quan; and Chapter 178, "Nonbenzodiazepine Sedatives" by Michael Levine and Dan Quan.

106 ALCOHOLS

Michael P. Kefer

- All alcohols have toxic potential, either from the parent compound or toxic metabolites.
- The presence of an osmolal gap suggests a low-molecular-weight substance such as ethanol, isopropanol, methanol, or ethylene glycol. An understanding of the osmolal gap is important in discussing the toxicity of these common alcohols.
- The osmolal gap = osm measured − osm calculated (normal <10 mOsm/L).

Osm measured = Laboratory determination by freezing point depression

Osm calculated = 2 (Na) + BUN/2.8 + glucose/18

ETHANOL

EPIDEMIOLOGY

- Ethanol is the most frequently ingested intoxicant in the United States and contributes to about 100,000 deaths per year. Roughly 3% of all ED visits are related to ethanol use.

PATHOPHYSIOLOGY

- Ethanol is a central nervous system (CNS) and respiratory depressant through complex mechanisms. Although acute ethanol intoxication may cause death from respiratory depression, morbidity and mortality are usually related to accidental injury resulting from impaired cognitive function.
- The major site of absorption is in the proximal small bowel, and is metabolized in the liver by alcohol dehydrogenase. Approximately 10% is excreted unchanged through the lungs and urine.
- On average, nondrinkers eliminate ethanol from the bloodstream at a rate of 15 to 20 milligrams/dL/h and chronic drinkers at a rate of up to 30 milligrams/dL/h.

CLINICAL FEATURES

- Signs and symptoms of ethanol intoxication include slurred speech, disinhibited behavior, CNS depression, and altered coordination. Lowering of blood pressure with reflex tachycardia may be seen.

DIAGNOSIS AND DIFFERENTIAL

- Diagnosis is based on clinical presentation with confirmation of ethanol intake by history or serum ethanol level.
- The differential diagnosis is broad and includes other CNS depressants such as benzodiazepines, barbiturates, narcotics, as well as other toxic alcohols. Head injury or hypoglycemia can present with altered mental status, and their identification can be complicated by ethanol intoxication.

EMERGENCY DEPARTMENT CARE AND DISPOSITION

- The mainstay of treatment is observation and supportive care.
- Exclude hypoglycemia by measuring fingerstick glucose. IV glucose should be administered as needed, and is unlikely to precipitate acute Wernicke encephalopathy, although prior administration of thiamine (100 milligrams IV/IM) is commonly used in chronic alcoholics.
- Complicating injury or illness must be excluded, and deterioration or lack of improvement during observation should be considered secondary to causes other than ethanol and managed accordingly.
- IV fluids do not alter alcohol elimination and are not required for ethanol intoxication alone; there is little evidence to support the use of IV fluids containing magnesium, folate, thiamine, and multivitamins ("banana bag") for acute intoxication.
- Discharge criteria include sobriety to the extent that there is no threat of harm to self or others.

ISOPROPANOL

EPIDEMIOLOGY

- Isopropanol is commonly found in rubbing alcohol, solvents, skin and hair products, paint thinners, and antifreeze.

PATHOPHYSIOLOGY

- Most isopropanol is rapidly absorbed with peak blood levels 30 to 120 minutes after ingestion.
- The CNS depressant effects are twice as potent and twice as long lasting as ethanol.
- Isopropanol is metabolized in the liver to acetone. Acetone is further metabolized to acetate and formate, but not in amounts that cause a significant metabolic acidosis.

CLINICAL FEATURES

- Isopropanol intoxication manifests similarly to that of ethanol except the duration is longer and the CNS depressant effects are more profound.
- The smell of rubbing alcohol or the fruity odor of ketones may be noted on the patient's breath.
- Severe poisoning is marked by coma, respiratory depression, and hypotension.
- Hemorrhagic gastritis is a characteristic finding that causes nausea, vomiting, abdominal pain, and upper gastrointestinal (GI) bleeding, which can be severe.

DIAGNOSIS AND DIFFERENTIAL

- Diagnosis is based on clinical features and an elevated isopropanol level. Accumulation of acetone may cause mild ketonemia and ketonuria without hyperglycemia or glycosuria.
- Mild acidosis may be present as well as an elevated osmolar gap.
- Isopropanol intoxication is typically distinguished from that of other alcohols by the significant osmolal gap without a significant anion gap metabolic acidosis and a negative ethanol level.

EMERGENCY DEPARTMENT CARE AND DISPOSITION

- General supportive measures are indicated, including consideration of administration of glucose, thiamine, and naloxone as with any patient who presents with altered mental status.
- Hypotension usually responds to IV fluids, but vasopressors may be necessary.
- Severe hemorrhagic gastritis may require transfusion.
- Hemodialysis removes both isopropanol and acetone and is indicated for refractory hypotension or a serum isopropanol level greater than 400 milligrams/dL.
- Patients with prolonged CNS depression require admission. Those who are asymptomatic after 4 to 6 hours of observation can be discharged or referred for psychiatric evaluation if indicated.

METHANOL AND ETHYLENE GLYCOL

EPIDEMIOLOGY

- Methanol is commonly found as a solvent in paint products, windshield wiper fluid, and antifreeze.
- Ethylene glycol is commonly used as antifreeze, and is found in polishes and detergents.

PATHOPHYSIOLOGY OF METHANOL

- Methanol is metabolized in the liver by alcohol dehydrogenase to the toxic compounds formaldehyde and then formic acid. In the presence of folate, formic acid is converted to carbon dioxide and water.
- Methanol accumulation results in an elevated osmolal gap.
- Formaldehyde accumulation in the retina causes edema and optic papillitis.
- Formic acid accumulation results in a high anion gap metabolic acidosis.
- Methanol is a potent GI mucosal irritant and causes pancreatitis and gastritis.

PATHOPHYSIOLOGY OF ETHYLENE GLYCOL

- Ethylene glycol is metabolized in the liver by alcohol dehydrogenase to the toxic compound glycoaldehyde. This is further metabolized to glycolic acid, and then glyoxylic acid. The major pathway after this converts it to oxalic acid. In the presence of thiamine or pyridoxine, glyoxylic acid is converted to nontoxic metabolites.
- Ethylene glycol accumulation results in a high osmolal gap, *although toxicity can occur with a normal osmolal gap*.
- Acid metabolite accumulation eventually causes an anion gap metabolic acidosis.
- Oxalic acid precipitates with calcium to form calcium oxalate crystals found in the urine and tissues.

CLINICAL FEATURES OF METHANOL POISONING

- Symptoms may not appear for 12 to 24 hours after ingestion and may be delayed further if ethanol is consumed, as ethanol inhibits methanol metabolism.
- Symptoms include altered mental status, visual disturbances (classically, feeling as if one is looking at a snowstorm), abdominal pain, nausea, and vomiting.
- GI symptoms may be caused by direct mucosal irritation or pancreatitis.
- Physical examination reveals varying degrees of CNS depression.
- Funduscopic examination may reveal papilledema.

CLINICAL FEATURES OF ETHYLENE GLYCOL POISONING

- Ethylene glycol poisoning often exhibits three distinct clinical phases:
  - In the first 12 hours, CNS effects predominate: patients appear intoxicated without the odor of ethanol on the breath.
  - Twelve to 24 hours after ingestion, cardiopulmonary effects predominate: tachycardia, tachypnea, and hypertension are common; congestive heart failure, acute respiratory distress syndrome, and circulatory collapse may develop.
  - Twenty-four to 72 hours after ingestion, renal effects predominate characterized by flank pain, costovertebral angle tenderness, and acute tubular necrosis with acute renal failure.
- Hypocalcemia may result from precipitation of calcium oxalate into tissues and can cause tetany and ECG changes (prolonged QT interval).

DIAGNOSIS AND DIFFERENTIAL

- Diagnosis is based on clinical presentation and laboratory findings. Serum methanol or ethylene glycol levels provide definitive diagnosis, although may not be readily available. Metabolic acidosis with elevated anion gap and an elevated osmolal gap are often present (although dependent on the time of ingestion, and potentially absent even with toxic levels) and can be useful diagnostic clues.
- Other laboratory abnormalities include hypocalcemia, leukocytosis, and calcium oxalate crystals in the urine (ethylene glycol).
- Ethylene glycol poisoning differs from methanol poisoning in that visual disturbances and funduscopic abnormalities are absent and calcium oxalate crystals are present in the urine.
- Differential diagnosis includes other causes of an anion gap metabolic acidosis such as iron, salicylate, or isoniazid toxicity; diabetic or alcoholic ketoacidosis; uremia; and lactic acidosis.

EMERGENCY DEPARTMENT CARE AND DISPOSITION

- General supportive measures are indicated, including support of the airway, breathing, and circulation, and the administration of glucose, thiamine, and naloxone in the undifferentiated patient with altered mental status.
- Charcoal does not bind toxic alcohols and has no role in isolated methanol or ethylene glycol poisoning.
- Specific treatment is directed toward preventing formation and removing toxic metabolites.
- Both fomepizole and ethanol have a greater affinity for alcohol dehydrogenase than methanol or ethylene glycol and therefore block metabolism to toxic compounds. Indications for initiating metabolic blockade are listed in Table 106-1.
  - Administer fomepizole 15 milligrams/kg IV load over 30 minutes followed by 10 milligrams/kg every 12 hours. Fomepizole is a potent inhibitor of alcohol dehydrogenase with greater affinity and fewer side effects than ethanol.
  - If fomepizole is not available, or the patient allergic, use ethanol 800 milligrams/kg IV load, followed by a continuous infusion of 100 milligrams/kg/h in the average drinker and 150 milligrams/kg/h in the heavy drinker. The continuous infusion is adjusted to maintain blood ethanol levels of 100 to 150 milligrams/dL.

TABLE 106-1 Indications for Metabolic Blockade with Fomepizole or Ethanol

1. Documented plasma methanol or ethylene glycol concentration of >20 milligrams/dL
2. If methanol or ethylene glycol level not immediately available:

   A. Documented or suspected significant methanol or ethylene glycol ingestion with ethanol level lower than approximately 100 milligrams/dL*

   B. Coma or altered mental status in patient with unclear history and:

   (1) Unexplained serum osmolar gap of >10 mOsm/L

   or

   (2) Unexplained metabolic acidosis *and* ethanol level of <100 milligrams/dL*

*If serum ethanol level is >100 milligrams/dL, patient will be protected from the formation of toxic metabolites by coingestion of ethanol and specific metabolic blockade treatment can be delayed until toxic alcohol level is available. However, if ethanol level is likely to fall to <100 milligrams/dL, metabolic blockade treatment should be initiated.

TABLE 106-2	Indications for Urgent Hemodialysis after Methanol or Ethylene Glycol Ingestion
Refractory metabolic acidosis: pH <7.25 with anion gap >30 mEq/L and/or base deficit less than −15	
Visual abnormalities*	
Renal insufficiency	
Deteriorating vital signs despite aggressive supportive care	
Electrolyte abnormalities refractory to conventional therapy	
Serum methanol or ethylene glycol level of >50 milligrams/dL†	

*Applies only to methanol; visual abnormalities may not resolve immediately, so their persistence in the absence of other indications once hemodialysis is started is *not* an indication for continued hemodialysis.
†Although previously considered an indication for hemodialysis, there are reports of patients with levels of ≥50 milligrams/dL successfully treated with fomepizole with or without bicarbonate and no hemodialysis.

- If necessary, oral therapy with commercial 80 proof liquor can be initiated with a loading dose of 1.5 to 2.0 mL/kg followed by a maintenance dose of 0.2 to 0.5 mL/kg/h. Alternatively, a load of 3 to 4 "shots" with maintenance of 1 to 2 "shots" per hour is a typical dose for a 70-kg patient.
- Glucose levels are monitored during treatment with ethanol as hypoglycemia may occur, especially in children.

- Dialysis eliminates both methanol and ethylene glycol and their toxic metabolites. Indications for dialysis are listed in Table 106-2.
- Use of fomepizole or ethanol does not affect indications for dialysis. Both fomepizole and ethanol are removed by dialysis; therefore, dosing of fomepizole is increased to every 4 hours and the continuous infusion rate of ethanol is doubled initially and readjusted to maintain therapeutic serum levels. Serum ethanol levels should be checked every 1 to 2 hours.
- Continue dialysis, fomepizole, or ethanol until the methanol or ethylene glycol level is less than 20 milligrams/dL and acidosis has resolved.
- In methanol poisoning, folate 1 milligram/kg (up to 50 milligrams) IV should be given every 4 hours.
- In ethylene glycol poisoning, pyridoxine 50 to 100 milligrams and thiamine 100 milligrams IV are administered every 6 hours for 2 days to drive the conversion of toxic to nontoxic metabolites.
- Even asymptomatic individuals should be admitted for observation because of possible delayed onset of toxic symptoms.

For further reading in Tintinalli's *Emergency Medicine: A Comprehensive Study Guide*, 7th ed., see Chapter 179, "Alcohols," by Jennifer C. Smith and Dan Quan.

107 DRUGS OF ABUSE

Shana Kusin

OPIOIDS

EPIDEMIOLOGY

- The term *opioid* refers broadly to all opium-related compounds that possess analgesic and sedative properties. The term *narcotic* is used by law enforcement to designate a broad variety of controlled substances and is not clinically relevant.
- Opioids can be categorized as *opiates* (naturally occurring compounds), semisynthetic (chemical modifications of natural compounds), or synthetic (completely artificial).
- ED visits associated with opioid abuse increased by 43% between 2004 and 2006. The opioids most commonly involved are, in order, heroin, oxycodone, hydrocodone, and methadone.

PATHOPHYSIOLOGY

- Opioids modulate nociception in the terminals of afferent nerves in the central nervous system, peripheral nervous system, and the gastrointestinal (GI) tract. They function as agonists at three primary receptors: μ (mu), κ (kappa), and δ (delta).
- Stimulation of μ-receptors results in analgesia, sedation, miosis, respiratory depression, cough suppression, euphoria, and decreased GI motility. Stimulation of κ- and δ-receptors results in some, but generally weaker, analgesia, and κ-receptor stimulation may cause dysphoria or hallucinations. All currently available opioids have some activity at the μ-receptor and cause some degree of respiratory depression.
- Standard formulations of opioids are readily absorbed and achieve peak blood levels 30 to 60 minutes after ingestion. Most opioids undergo first-pass hepatic metabolism and have widely varied bioavailability, ranging from 10% to 80%.
- The metabolism of codeine, morphine, propoxyphene, oxycodone, meperidine, and methadone is mostly hepatic and is subject to drug interactions and genetic variations.

CLINICAL FEATURES

- Opioids cause varying degrees of respiratory and mental status depression, miosis, orthostatic hypotension, nausea, vomiting, histamine release, decreased GI motility, and urinary retention.

- Although clasically considered a part of the opioid toxidrome, miosis is not always present. Meperidine, morphine, propoxyphene, pentazocine, and diphenoxylate have been associated with normal or enlarged pupils, and mydriasis may signal severe cerebral hypoxia or coingestants.
- Opioid withdrawal usually manifests in anxiety, insomnia, yawning, lacrimation, diaphoresis, rhinorrhea, myalgia, piloerection, mydriasis, vomiting, diarrhea, and abdominal cramping.

DIAGNOSIS AND DIFFERENTIAL

- Opioid intoxication or withdrawal is a clinical diagnosis.
- The triad of coma, miosis, and respiratory depression strongly suggests opioid intoxication.
- Detection of opioids in the urine may aid in diagnosis; however, many synthetic and semisynthetic opioids are not routinely detected by this modality, and false positives have been associated with poppy seeds and some antibiotics.
- An acetaminophen level should be obtained in all cases of opioid-acetaminophen overdoses as well as in any intentional suicidal ingestion.
- The differential diagnosis of opioid overdose includes toxicologic exposure to agents producing similar symptoms, such as clonidine, organophosphates and carbamates, phenothiazines, sedative-hypnotic agents, gamma-hydroxybutyrate (GHB), or carbon monoxide; hypoglycemia; central nervous system infection; postictal states; and pontine and intracranial hemorrhage.
- The differential diagnosis of opioid withdrawal includes drugs and toxins that promote an adrenergic state, other drug withdrawal, and hyperthyroidism.

EMERGENCY DEPARTMENT CARE AND DISPOSITION

- Airway protection and ventilatory management are the most important treatment for opioid-intoxicated patients. Bag-valve-mask support may be used to maintain oxygenation while naloxone and/or endotracheal intubation are being prepared.
- Activated charcoal should be considered at a dose of 1 gram/kg PO if the ingestion occurred within 1 hour.
- Naloxone is a pure competitive antagonist at all opioid receptors with particular affinity for the μ-receptor. It can be given by injection (IV, SC, or IM). Onset after IV administration is 1 to 2 minutes and its duration of action is 20 to 90 minutes.
- Patients presenting with decreased mental status but minimal respiratory depression should receive a lower naloxone dose of 0.4 milligram IV, repeated until desired effect is reached. Opioid-dependent patients in this scenario should receive an even smaller starting dose of 0.05 milligram IV in order to avoid precipitation of opioid withdrawal.
- Patients presenting with significant respiratory depression should receive an initial naloxone dose of 2 milligrams IV, with repeated doses of 2 milligrams IV given every 3 minutes as needed until respiratory depression is reversed or a maximum of 10 milligrams IV has been reached.
- Sustained preparations and synthetic opioids such as propoxyphene, fentanyl, pentazocine, and dextromethorphan may require larger doses of naloxone.
- A continuous naloxone infusion should be considered if the patient has required multiple boluses of naloxone. The IV infusion should be started at an hourly rate that is two-thirds of the total reversal dose required. Patients on naloxone infusions may require additional bolus doses and upward or downward adjustments in the infusion rate.
- An ED observation period of 4 to 6 hours is recommended for most cases of opioid exposure.
- Patients receiving naloxone in the setting of IV heroin use may be safely discharged 1 to 2 hours following naloxone administration if they meet the following criteria: independently mobile, oxygen saturation >92% on room air, respiratory rate >10 breaths/min, pulse rate >50 beats/min, normal temperature, Glasgow Coma Scale score of 15.
- Admit moderate to severely symptomatic patients requiring continued naloxone administration to a monitored setting.
- Opioid withdrawal is rarely life threatening. Supportive care with clonidine 2 to 5 micrograms/kg PO, antiemetics, and antidiarrheals may alleviate discomfort.

SPECIAL CONSIDERATIONS

- Buprenorphine is a long-acting partial agonist at μ-receptors. It can precipitate an opioid toxidrome in opioid-naive patients or a withdrawal syndrome in opioid-dependent patients. Naloxone may be partially successful in treating intoxication, but prolonged or repeated dosing may be necessary.
- Methadone can prolong the QT interval and predispose to cardiac dysrhythmia such as torsades de pointes.
- Propoxyphene overdose has been associated with QRS prolongation, heart block, prolonged QT interval, ventricular bigeminy, and seizures. QRS prolongation should be treated with sodium bicarbonate (1 milligram/kg IV). Naloxone may terminate propoxphene-induced seizures but will not reverse ECG changes.

- Tramadol overdose is associated with agitation, hypertension, seizures, and death, particularly at doses >500 milligrams in adults. Naloxone is not effective in reversing tramadol-induced seizures.
- Serotonin syndrome can result from combining meperidine, dextromethorphan, or tramadol with monoamine oxidase inhibitors, selective serotonin reuptake inhibitors, or linezolid.
- Acute lung injury is a rare but serious complication of heroin overdose. It can be delayed up to 24 hours. Treatment includes oxygenation, ventilatory support, and use of positive end-expiratory pressure ventilation. Naloxone, diuretics, and digoxin are not indicated.

COCAINE, AMPHETAMINES, AND OTHER STIMULANTS

EPIDEMIOLOGY

- One-third of drug-related ED visits in the United States are related to cocaine use.
- Methamphetamine is the second most commonly abused drug worldwide, following cannabis, and is used by 0.6% of the global population.

PATHOPHYSIOLOGY

Cocaine

- Cocaine is a water-soluble hydrochloride salt that is rapidly absorbed across all mucous membranes. It can be topically applied, insufflated (snorted), swallowed, or injected IV. Crack cocaine is a free-base form that is stable to pyrolysis and can be smoked.
- Insufflation causes a peak effect within 30 minutes and a duration of effect of 1 to 2 hours. Both the IV and inhalational routes produce a rapid onset of action (less than 1 minute) with a duration of 30 to 60 minutes.
- Cocaine causes sympathetic nervous system activation via enhanced effects of excitatory amino acids and blockade of presynaptic uptake of norepinephrine, dopamine, and serotonin. This produces its characteristic effects of mydriasis, tachycardia, hypertension, and diaphoresis.
- Cocaine is also a local anesthetic and inhibits nerve conduction by blockade of fast sodium channels. It has quinidine-like effects on cardiac conduction, which may widen the QRS complex and prolong the QT interval. In large doses, myocardial toxicity may result in negative inotropy, wide complex dysrhythmia, bradycardia, and hypotension.

Amphetamines

- Amphetamines comprise a broad class of structurally similar derivatives of phenylethylamine. Modification of the basic amphetamine structure may produce substances with additional psychoactive properties; these drugs comprise the "designer" amphetamines.
- Amphetamines enhance release and block reuptake of catecholamines and may directly stimulate catecholamine receptors. Some amphetamine metabolites inhibit monoamine oxidase. Some derivatives may also induce serotonin release, causing hallucinogenic effects.
- Methamphetamine may be ingested, injected IV, inhaled, or insufflated. As with cocaine, absorption and peak effects occur rapidly via these routes.
- Stimulants such as methylphenidate, ephedrine, and phenylpropanolamine produce toxic effects similar to cocaine and amphetamines.

CLINICAL FEATURES

- The cocaine- or amphetamine-intoxicated patient may demonstrate tachycardia, tachypnea, hypertension, hyperthermia, and any degree of altered mental status. Common symptoms include chest pain, palpitations, dyspnea, headache, and focal neurologic complaints.
- Even at low doses, cocaine can produce coronary artery vasoconstriction resulting in chest pain. This effect is potentiated by cigarette smoking.
- Cocaine induces a variety of cardiotoxic effects, including dysrhythmias, myocarditis, cardiomyopathy, myocardial ischemia and infarction, aortic rupture, aortic and coronary artery dissection, and acelerated or increased atherogenesis.
- The increased adrenergic tone associated with cocaine and amphetamine can lead to seizures, intracranial hemorrhage, and cerebral infarction as well as other neurologic sequelae.
- Crack cocaine use has been associated with pulmonary hemorrhage, pneumonitis, asthma, pulmonary edema, pneumomediastinum, pneumothorax, and pneumopericardium.
- Cocaine-induced mesenteric vasospasm can cause intestinal ischemia, bowel necrosis, ischemic colitis, GI bleeding, bowel perforation, and splenic infarction.
- Rhabdomyolysis may occur with cocaine or amphetamine use and can lead to renal failure.
- Cocaine abuse during pregnancy increases the risk of spontaneous abortion, abruptio placentae, fetal prematurity, and intrauterine growth retardation. Methamphetamine abuse also has detrimental effects on fetal growth.

- Mortality is most commonly the result of severe hyperthermia, dysrhythmias, intractable seizures, or hypertension leading to intracranial infarction, hemorrhage, or encephalopathy.

DIAGNOSIS AND DIFFERENTIAL

- Diagnosis of cocaine, amphetamine, and stimulant intoxication is usually made clinically by recognition of the sympathomimetic toxidrome in the correct clinical context.
- Concomitant use of substances such as alcohol or opioids may significantly alter the presentation.
- The differential diagnosis includes intoxication with other sympathomimetic substances, withdrawal syndromes, and infection. Occult trauma and hypoglycemia should be considered.
- Patients with hyperthermia or significant agitation should be evaluated for acidosis, renal failure, and rhabdomyolysis with a basic chemistry panel and creatine kinase (CK).
- An ECG, chest radiograph, and cardiac enzymes should be considered in cocaine- or amphetamine-intoxicated patients presenting with chest pain or dyspnea.
- Urine drug screening for cocaine is fairly specific and exhibits little cross reactivity. It is usually positive for up to 72 hours following exposure.
- Urine drug screens for amphetamines are not specific and have high false-negative and false-positive results.

EMERGENCY DEPARTMENT CARE AND DISPOSITION

- The mainstay of treatment of cocaine and amphetamine toxicity involves adequate sedation and monitoring of vital signs. Benzodiazepines, such as lorazepam 2 milligrams IV or diazepam 5 milligrams IV, will often improve tachycardia, hypertension, and agitation.
- Antipsychotics should be avoided due to the risk of lowering the seizure threshold and contributing to hyperthermia or dysrhythmias.
- Active cooling with mist spray and fanning is used to treat moderate or severe hyperthermia.
- Seizures should be treated with benzodiazepines; for refractory seizures, phenobarbital or neuromuscular blockade should be considered. CT of the brain should be performed to assess for a structural central nervous system (CNS) lesion such as hemorrhage or infarction.
- Cardiac ischemia or infarction should be treated with aspirin, nitrates, morphine, and benzodiazepines. β-Blockers are contraindicated. Fibrinolytic therapy should be used with caution since cocaine-associated intracranial hemorrhage and aortic or coronary artery dissection is a contraindication to thrombolysis.
- Treat cocaine-induced wide complex tachydysrhythmias and QRS interval prolongation by alkalinizing the serum to a pH of 7.45 to 7.5 with sodium bicarbonate.
- Treat hypertensive emergencies with nitroprusside or phentolamine.
- Asymptomatic "body packers" (individuals who ingest prepared packets of cocaine with the intent to transport it) may be treated with whole-bowel irrigation using polyethylene glycol electrolyte solution. If these patients exhibit any signs of intoxication, then administer benzodiazepines and have immediate surgical consultation for laparotomy and packet removal.
- Acidification of the urine for amphetamine intoxication is not recommended.
- Many amphetamines have a longer duration of effect than cocaine, and intoxicated patients may require longer periods of observation or hospital admission.
- Patients with significant laboratory or vital sign abnormalities, ECG changes consistent with myocardial ischemia, or concern for CNS injury should be hospitalized in an intensive care unit setting.

HALLUCINOGENS

EPIDEMIOLOGY

- After ethanol, marijuana (cannabis) is currently the most prevalent psychoactive substance abused by young people.

PATHOPHYSIOLOGY

- The term "hallucinogen" has clasically referred to indole alkylamines such as lysergic acid diethylamide (LSD) and psilocybin and phenylethylamines such as methylenedioxymethamphetamine (MDMA, "ecstasy") and mescaline. Other drugs such as phencyclidine (PCP) and marijuana are also frequently abused for the purpose of alteration of sensory perception.
- Table 107-1 summarizes the classification, mechanism, typical dose, duration of action, features,

TABLE 107-1 Commonly Abused Hallucinogens

DRUG	TYPICAL DOSE	DURATION OF ACTION	CLINICAL FEATURES	COMPLICATIONS	SPECIFIC TREATMENT
Lysergic acid diethylamide (LSD)	20-80 micrograms	8-12 h	Mydriasis Tachycardia Anxiety Muscle tension	Coma Hyperthermia Coagulopathy Persistent psychosis Hallucinogen persisting perception disorder	Supportive Benzodiazepines Haloperidol
Psilocybin	5-100 mushrooms 4-6 milligrams of psilocybin	4-6 h	Mydriasis Tachycardia Muscle tension Nausea and vomiting	Seizures (rare) Hyperthermia (rare)	Supportive Benzodiazepines
Mescaline	3-12 "buttons" 200-500 milligrams of mescaline	6-12 h	Mydriasis Abdominal pain Nausea and vomiting Dizziness Nystagmus Ataxia	Rare	Supportive Benzodiazepines
Methylenedioxymethamphetamine (MDMA, "ecstasy")	50-200 milligrams	4-6 h	Mydriasis Bruxism Jaw tension Ataxia Dry mouth Nausea	Hyponatremia Hypertension Seizures Hyperthermia Arrhythmias Rhabdomyolysis	Benzodiazepines Hydration Active cooling Serotonin antagonists
Phencyclidine (PCP, "angel dust")	1-9 milligrams	4-6 h	Small or midsized pupils Nystagmus Muscle rigidity Hypersalivation Agitation Catatonia	Coma Seizures Hyperthermia Rhabdomyolysis Hypertension Hypoglycemia	Benzodiazepines Hydration Active cooling
Marijuana (cannabis)	5-15 milligrams of tetrahydrocannabinol	2-4 h	Tachycardia Conjunctival injection	Acute psychosis (rare) Panic reactions (rare)	Supportive Benzodiazepines

complications, and specific treatments of commonly abused hallucinogens.

- There are a number of "natural" hallucinogens being encountered with increased frequency, partly due to dissemination of information on and ease of procurement via the Internet.

CLINICAL FEATURES

- LSD is rapidly absorbed with onset of symptoms within 30 minutes. Sympathomimetic symptoms usually precede psychedelic effects. Acute adverse psychological effects can lead to dangerous behavior or potential trauma. Massive overdoses may produce coma, respiratory arrest, hyperthermia, and coagulopathy.
- Psilocybin causes symptoms similar to, but less severe than, LSD. Serious medical side effects are rare, but seizures and hyperthermia have been reported.
- Mescaline causes hallucinogenic effects similar to, but weaker than, LSD. These effects are usually preceded by GI symptoms, dizziness, and headache, are delayed in onset, and persist for 6 to 12 hours. Significant morbidity and mortality is rare.
- MDMA or "ecstasy" is structurally related to both amphetamines and mescaline. Effects include intensification of sensory stimuli and mood as well as hallucinations. Physical manifestations include sympathomimetic effects such as mydriasis and elevations of pulse and blood pressure. Nausea, bruxism, myalgias, and ataxia also occur.

- Death associated with MDMA use has been attributed to severe hypertension, intracranial hemorrhage, hyponatremia, hyperthermia, and arrhythmias.
- PCP is a piperidine derivative that is structurally related to ketamine. It has dissociative properties and causes clouding, rather than heightening, of the sensorium. It has been used as an adulterant in other drugs, and patients may be unwittingly exposed.
- The clinical presentation of PCP is variable and can include CNS stimulation or depression, violent behavior, catatonia, and a combination of cholinergic, anticholinergic, and sympathomimetic effects. Nystagmus and hypertension are frequent findings.
- Rhabdomyolysis, renal failure, seizure, ataxia, muscle rigidity, hypoglycemia, and elevated CPK levels are common complications of PCP abuse.
- Marijuana use most commonly causes drowsiness, euphoria, heightened sensory awareness, paranoia, and distortions of time and space. Significant medical complications are rare.

DIAGNOSIS AND DIFFERENTIAL

- The differential diagnosis of hallucinogen intoxication includes alcohol and benzodiazepine withdrawal, hypoglycemia, anticholinergic poisoning, thyrotoxicosis, CNS infections, structural CNS lesions, and acute psychosis.
- Routine drug screens will not detect psilocybin or mescaline.
- Urine drug screens for MDMA, like other amphetamine drug screens, have low specificity and frequent false positives for a number of pharmaceutical agents.
- Urine tests for PCP and marijuana may be positive for days to weeks after use and are not useful for diagnosing acute intoxication. The PCP screen also has a high rate of false positives.

EMERGENCY DEPARTMENT CARE AND DISPOSITION

- Initial management of patients with hallucinogen intoxication is support of airway, breathing, and circulation. Hypoxia and hypoglycemia must be diagnosed and treated immediately.
- Most hallucinogens are rapidly absorbed, but activated charcoal may be considered for ingestions within the previous hour.
- Calm reassurance is often sufficient to soothe the agitated patient. Benzodiazepines are the mainstay of pharmacologic treatment. Haloperidol may be considered as a second-line agent but should be used with caution because it has anticholinergic properties and can lower the seizure threshold. Physical restraints should be avoided if possible as they can exacerbate agitation and contribute to rhabdomyolysis and hyperthermia.
- Tachycardia and hypertension often respond to sedation with benzodiazepines. Severe hypertension can be treated with nitroprusside.
- MDMA-associated hyponatremia can be significant. Administration of 3% saline to prevent brain stem herniation and death may be necessary in severe cases (serum sodium concentration <115 mEq/L, seizure, or coma).
- Hyperthermia should be treated with rapid cooling. Severe cases may require neuromuscular paralysis and intubation.
- Seizures are treated with benzodiazepines. Refractory seizures may require propofol or barbiturates.
- Most patients with hallucinogen intoxication can be safely discharged from the ED after a period of observation. Patients with medical complications should be admitted to the hospital.

For further reading in Tintinalli's *Emergency Medicine: A Comprehensive Study Guide,* 7th ed., see Chapter 180, "Opioids," by Suzanne Doyon; Chapter 181, "Cocaine, Methamphetamine, and Other Amphetamines," by Jane M. Prosser and Jeanmarie Perrone; and Chapter 182, "Hallucinogens," by Katherine M. Prybys and Karen N. Hansen.

108 ANALGESICS

Joshua Nogar

ASPIRIN AND SALICYLATES

EPIDEMIOLOGY

- In 2008, aspirin and salycilates (ASA) were involved in 20,000 toxic exposures and 48 deaths.
- Many over-the-counter medications (eg, Pepto-Bismol, oil of wintergreen [methyl salicylate], liniments used in vaporizers) contain large amounts of salicylates, and ingestion or application of even small amounts can lead to inadvertent salicylate toxicity.

PATHOPHYSIOLOGY

- Absorption of ASA may be delayed or erratic. Peak serum levels may be significantly delayed, but toxic levels are usually apparent within 6 hours. Peak levels from ingestion of enteric-coated or sustained-release aspirin have been reported up to 60 hours after ingestion.

- ASA may form a gelatinous gastric mass, and large amounts of aspirin may remain in the stomach long after an overdose. In addition, aspirin has an inhibitory effect on gastric emptying. The result is a salicylate level that may vascilate before ultimately trending down.
- At physiologic pH (7.40), essentially all salicylate molecules are ionized. A decrease in pH (acidosis) increases the proportion of nonionized salicylate. Nonionized salicylate molecules cross cell membranes, including the blood-brain barrier. Therefore, acidemia increases intracellular salicylate concentration.
- Mortality from ASA toxicity correlates directly with brain salicylate concentration.
- A urinary pH above 8.0 ionizes salicylate in the urine and impairs reabsorption across the urinary tubules, resulting in enhanced urinary elimination.
- ASA toxicity causes respiratory alkalosis due to an elevated respiratory rate through a direct effect on the medullary respiratory center.
- ASA toxicity causes uncoupling of oxidative phosphorylation and inhibition of various Krebs' cycle enzymes. This results in increased catabolism and elevated carbon dioxide and heat production, increased glycolysis and demand for glucose, and production of organic acids including lactate, pyruvate, and ketoacids, which contribute to the metabolic acidosis of salicylate poisoning.
- Normoglycemia, hyperglycemia, or hypoglycemia may be seen. Hypoglycemia in brain cells may occur despite normal serum glucose levels.
- Chronic administration of large doses of salicylates when the serum salicylate level is greater than 60 milligrams/dL results in hypoprothrombinemia and an elevated prothrombin time (PT).

CLINICAL FEATURES

- ASA toxicity is a clinical diagnosis made in conjunction with the patient's acid–base status. The manifestations of salicylate toxicity depend on the dose, whether exposure is acute or chronic, and the patient's age (Table 108-1).
- ASA blood concentrations may correlate poorly with toxicity, and relying on drug levels as a measure of toxicity is the most common pitfall to avoid when managing ASA overdoses.
- Acute ingestion of less than 150 milligrams/kg usually produces mild toxicity with nausea, vomiting, and gastrointestinal (GI) irritation.
- Acute ingestion of 150 to 300 milligrams/kg usually results in moderate toxicity with vomiting, hyperventilation, sweating, and tinnitus. In adults, these findings often coincide with salicylate levels >30 milligrams/dL.
- Toxicity from ingestion of more than 300 milligrams/kg is usually severe.
- The pathognomonic acid–base disturbance of salicylate toxicity is increased anion gap metabolic acidosis, metabolic alkalosis (due to volume contraction), and respiratory alkalosis.
- The most common clinical picture is combined respiratory alkalosis and increased anion gap metabolic acidosis, although a normal anion gap does not exclude salicylate toxicity in patients with an unknown ingestion. In addition, co-ingestion of sedative drugs may impair the respiratory drive and result in respiratory acidosis.
- ASA toxicity can be misdiagnosed as sepsis, particularly in the elderly population (lactic acidosis, contraction metabolic acidosis, and respiratory alkalosis).
- Uncommon manifestations of severe acute ASA toxicity include hyperthermia, neurologic dysfunction, renal failure, pulmonary edema, and acute respiratory distress syndrome (ARDS). Rarely, rhabdomyolysis, gastric perforation, and GI hemorrhage occur.
- Fatality is more likely with advanced age. Unconsciousness, hyperthermia, severe acidosis, seizures, and dysrhythmias are also associated with increased mortality risk. Toxicity may present with hyperventilation, tremor, papilledema, agitation, paranoia, bizarre behavior, memory loss, confusion, and stupor.
- Chronic ASA toxicity tends to develop at lower drug concentrations as compared to acute overdoses.
- Patients taking carbonic anhydrase inhibitors (CAIs) to treat glaucoma are at increased risk for chronic salicylism. CAIs cause a metabolic acidosis, which

TABLE 108-1 Severity Grading of Salicylate Toxicity in Adults

	MILD	MODERATE	SEVERE
Acute ingestion (dose)	<150 milligrams/kg	150-300 milligrams/kg	>300 milligrams/kg
End-organ toxicity	Tinnitus Hearing loss Dizziness Nausea/vomiting	Tachypnea Hyperpyrexia Diaphoresis Ataxia Anxiety	Abnormal mental status Seizures Acute lung injury Renal failure Cardiac arrhythmias Shock

increases the volume of distribution of salicylates, leading to increased central nervous system (CNS) salicylate levels and possible toxicity despite a "therapeutic" serum salicylate level.

- In children, acute ASA overdoses generally present within a few hours of ingestion.
- Children under 4 years of age tend to develop metabolic acidosis (pH <7.38), whereas children over 4 years usually have mixed acid–base disturbance as in adults.
- In children, chronic salicylate toxicity is usually more serious than acute toxicity, and more likely to be lethal. Symptoms may take days to appear, and there may be an underlying illness that promts salicylate administration.
- Hyperthermia indicates a worse prognosis. Renal failure is a severe complication. Pulmonary edema is rare in pediatric patients.

DIAGNOSIS AND DIFFERENTIAL

- Salicylate levels should be interpreted cautiously since severe toxicity may be present despite a "therapeutic" or declining level.
- The use of the Done nomogram, which was developed to predict toxicity after acute ingestion within a known time frame, may be misleading and is no longer recommended.
- Enteric-coated aspirin may be visible on plain radiographs; however, a negative radiograph does not exclude the ingestion.
- The differential diagnosis of salicylate toxicity includes theophylline toxicity, caffeine overdose, acute iron poisoning, Reye's syndrome, diabetic ketoacidosis, sepsis, and meningitis.
- Chronic salicylism may be mistaken for an infectious process in an adult or child; it may present with hyperventilation, volume depletion, acidosis, marked hypokalemia, and CNS disturbances.
- Chronic salicylism should be considered in any patient with unexplained nonfocal neurologic and behavioral abnormalities, especially with coexisting acid–base disturbance, tachypnea, dyspnea, or noncardiogenic pulmonary edema.

EMERGENCY DEPARTMENT CARE AND DISPOSITION

- Emergent priorities remain airway, breathing, and circulation. Cardiac monitoring and an intravenous (IV) access should be instituted.
- Administer activated charcoal 1 gram/kg to minimize absorption and hasten elimination. Multiple doses are probably not beneficial.
- Whole-bowel irrigation may be effective when toxicity is due to sustained-release or enteric-coated aspirin.
- Intravenous normal saline should be administered to patients with evidence of volume depletion. Except for the initial saline resuscitation, all subsequent fluids should contain at least 5% dextrose; if hypoglycemia or neurologic symptoms are present, then administration of IV fluids with 10% dextrose should be considered.
- After adequate urine output (1-2 mL/kg/h) is established, and if not contraindicated by initial electrolyte and renal function test results, potassium chloride 40 mEq/L should be added to the patient's IV fluids.
- Alkalinization of the serum and urine enhances ASA protein binding and urinary elimination.
- Administer a bolus of 1 to 2 mEq/kg of sodium bicarbonate followed by 150 mEq (three ampules) of sodium bicarbonate added to a liter of D5W and infused at 1.5 to 2.0 times the patient's maintenance rate; adjust the infusion to maintain urine pH above 7.5.
- Severe ASA toxicity may result in significant volume depletion and metabolic abnormalities; during resuscitation frequent clinical evaluations as well as at hourly monitoring of urine pH, salicylate levels, electrolytes, glucose, and acid–base status is indicated.
- Bicarbonate administration can exacerbate hypokalemia. Failure to maintain normokalemia can limit effective alkalinization.
- Cardiac monitoring and an intravenous (IV) line should be instituted early, but airway management deserves special consideration in ASA-poisoned patients. A sudden drop in serum pH due to respiratory failure can precipitously worsen ASA toxicity. If intubation is required, ventilator settings should attempt to maximize minute ventilation. Respiratory acidosis occuring after a mechanical ventilator is set to "normal" rate/volume parameters can be a premorbid event.
- Consider hemodialysis for all cases with ASA levels in excess of 100 milligrams/dL, although no absolute threshold exists. Significant chronic toxicity requiring hemodialysis can occur at levels as low as 60 to 80 milligrams/dL. Also consider hemodialysis for clinical deterioration despite supportive care and alkalinization, renal insufficiency, severe acid–base disturbance, altered mental status, or ARDS.
- Check ASA levels every 2 hours until a peak is identified and then every 4 to 6 hours until the level is nontoxic. In severe ingestions, hourly levels correlated with clinical status are indicated.
- Hemorrhage due to prolonged PT in chronic salicylism is rarely seen, but may be treated with fresh frozen plasma.

- Treat dysrhythmias by correcting metabolic abnormalities and with standard ALS protocols.
- With the exception of enteric-coated or sustained-release formulations, a patient may be discharged from the ED if there is progressive clinical improvement, no significant acid–base abnormality, and declinig serial ASA levels toward a therapeutic range.
- With enteric-coated and sustained-release ASA, peak serum levels may not occur until 10 to 60 hours after ingestion, and observation is warrented.
- In potentially large ingestions, admit the patient for at least 24 hours to assure declining serial salicylate levels and improving clinical status.

ACETAMINOPHEN

EPIDEMIOLOGY

- Acetaminophen (APAP) is the most popular over-the-counter analgesic in the United States.
- In 2008, the American Association of Poison Control Centers received reports of approxamately 150,000 single-agent and combination-agent exposures to APAP.

PATHOPHYSIOLOGY

- APAP is rapidly absorbed from the GI tract. In overdose, peak serum levels usually occur within 2 hours. However, delayed absorption may occur with APAP preparations containing propoxyphene or diphenhydramine and with "extended relief" preparations.
- APAP is primarily metabolized by the liver, while a small percentage (<5%) undergoes direct renal elimination.
- The majority of APAP is metabolized through sulfation and glucuronidation, but a small percentage of APAP is oxidized by cytochrome P450 to a toxic metabolite, N-acetyl-p-benzoquinoneimine (NAPQI). NAPQI is detoxified by hepatic glutathione to a nontoxic compound that undergoes renal elimination.
- In APAP overdose, hepatic glucuronidation and sulfation are quickly saturated, and a higher percentage of APAP is metabolized by cytochrome P450 to NAPQI. When hepatic glutathione stores are depleted to less than 30% of normal, NAPQI accumulates, and hepatic toxicity ensues.
- NAPQI causes hepatocellular injury, and typically produces centrilobular necrosis.
- Patients with low glutathione stores (alcoholics and AIDS patients) and those with induced cytochrome P450 activity (alcoholics and individuals on anticonvulsant or antituberculosis drugs) are at greater risk of developing APAP toxicity.
- N-acetylcysteine (NAC) is a specific antidote for APAP. Among other actions, NAC inhibits binding of NAPQI to hepatic proteins, may act as a glutathione precursor or substitute, and may directly reduce NAPQI back to APAP.

CLINICAL FEATURES

- Acute APAP toxicity presents in four stages. During the first 24 hours, the patient may be asymptomatic or have nonspecific symptoms such as anorexia, nausea, vomiting, and malaise.
- On days 2 and 3, nausea and vomiting may improve, but evidence of hepatotoxicity, such as right upper quadrant abdominal pain and tenderness with elevated transaminases and bilirubin, may be present.
- On days 3 and 4, there may be progression to fulminant hepatic failure with lactic acidosis, coagulopathy, renal failure, and encephalopathy, as well as recurrent nausea and vomiting.
- Those who survive hepatic failure will begin to recover over the next weeks with total resolution of hepatic dysfunction.
- Massive APAP ingestion (4-hour APAP level >800 micrograms/mL) may be associated with acute onset of either coma or agitation and lactic acidosis.

DIAGNOSIS AND DIFFERENTIAL

- APAP toxicity may occur with acute ingestion of more than 140 milligrams/kg or when more than 7.5 grams are ingested by an adult in a 24-hour period. The diagnosis of a significant ingestion depends on laboratory testing, since symptoms may initially be absent or nonspecific.
- An APAP level should be measured in all patients presenting with any drug overdose since APAP is a common co-ingestant.
- An APAP level, drawn as soon as possible within 4 to 24 hours of ingestion, will guide subsequent ED management. Serum levels above 150 micrograms/dL at 4 hours post ingestion are potentially toxic (see Table 108-2). After 24 hours, a detectable APAP level or the presence of elevated transaminases may predict toxicity.
- When multiple ingestions have occurred over a period of time, assessment is problematic. Consultation with a toxicologist is warrented in these cases.
- Clinical experience with extended relief ingestions is limited. If a 4- to 8-hour level is in the toxic range (Table 108-2), then therapy should be initiated. If the 4- to 8-hour level is elevated but below the toxicity cutoff, then a second level 4 to 6 hours later should

TABLE 108-2 Potentially Toxic Serum APAP Levels in Acute Ingestion

TIME AFTER INGESTION (HOURS)	SERUM APAP LEVEL (MICROGRAMS/ML)
4	200
8	100
12	50
16	25
20	15
24	6

be obtained and therapy initiated if the second level is in the toxic range.

- Obtain additional laboratory studies, including a CBC, coagulation studies, renal function tests, liver function tests, electrolytes, and additional toxicologic studies for possible coingestion.
- The differential diagnosis of APAP toxicity includes viral and alcoholic hepatitis, other drug- or toxin-induced hepatitides, and hepatobiliary disease.
- Acute APAP poisoning can often be distinguished from other forms of hepatitis by its acute onset, rapid progression, and markedly elevated transaminase levels.

EMERGENCY DEPARTMENT CARE AND DISPOSITION

- Emergent priorities remain airway, breathing, and circulation. Cardiac monitoring and an IV line should be instituted.
- NAC is a specific antidote for APAP toxicity and can prevent toxicity if administered within 8 hours of ingestion, and significantly reduce hepatotoxicity if administered within 24 hours of ingestion. There may be benefit from NAC, even when administered after 24 hours.
- Begin NAC therapy empirically if there is any delay in obtaining a serum APAP or in patients with toxic serum levels.
- NAC is administered orally or by nasogastric tube as a 140 milligram/kg loading dose, followed by 70 milligrams/kg every 4 hours for 17 additional doses. It can be given IV as a 150 milligram/kg loading dose, followed by 50 milligrams/kg over the next 4 hours, and then 100 milligrams/kg over the next 16 hours.
- NAC can be administered immediately after activated charcoal; there is no evidence that activated charcoal decreases its effectiveness.
- NAC is safe in pregnancy.
- Nausea and vomiting during NAC therapy may be reduced by diluting it in a beverage or with administration of antiemetics such as metoclopramide or ondansetron.
- Treatment of fulminant hepatic failure includes NAC therapy, correction of coagulopathy and acidosis, treatment of cerebral edema, supportive measures for multiorgan system failure, and early referral to a liver transplant center.
- Patients with nontoxic APAP levels below the toxic range (Table 108-2) can be discharged from the ED if there is no evidence of other drug ingestion or intent of self-harm.

NONSTEROIDAL ANTI-INFLAMMATORY DRUGS

EPIDEMIOLOGY

- Morbidity due to nonsteroidal anti-inflammatory drug (NSAID) exposure is far more significant from therapeutic dosing than after overdoses. NSAID-related GI bleeding is estimated to cause 103,000 hospitalizations and 16,500 deaths annually in the United States. NSAIDs have also been implicated in a significant proportion of cases of drug-induced renal failure.

PATHOPHYSIOLOGY

- NSAIDs inhibit the enzyme cyclooxygenase (COX), which produces prostaglandins from arachidonic acid. There are at least two forms of cyclooxygenase, COX-1 and COX-2. COX-1 is responsible for most of the adverse effects of NSAIDs.
- There are three types of cyclooxygenase inhibitors: nonselective (which inhibit both COX-1 and COX-2), which comprise the majority of NSAIDs; partially selective (which preferentially inhibit COX-2 only at low doses), such as etodolac and meloxicam; and selective (which preferentially inhibit COX-2), including valdecoxib, rofecoxib, and celecoxib.
- NSAIDs are rapidly absorbed from the GI tract. Most NSAIDs undergo at least partial hepatic metabolism before elimination in the urine or feces.
- Plasma half-lives of NSAIDs range from 2 to 4 hours for ibuprofen, to approximately 15 hours for the new COX-2 inhibitors, and more than 50 hours for piroxicam and phenylbutazone.
- Phenylbutazone and naproxen may displace warfarin from plasma proteins, resulting in elevated PT times. Phenylbutazone also decreases the elimination of warfarin. The selective COX-2 inhibitors have been reported to slightly elevate the PT at therapeutic doses.
- Other NSAIDs do not interact in these ways with warfarin, but nonselective NSAID use is contraindicated with warfarin because NSAID platelet aggregation inhibition may significantly increase the risk of bleeding.

- NSAIDs may decrease the effectiveness of antihypertensives, including diuretics, α-adrenergic blockers, angiotensin-converting enzyme inhibitors, and β-adrenergic blockers.
- NSAIDs inhibit the renal clearance of lithium and methotrexate and may cause toxicity from these drugs.

CLINICAL FEATURES

- Toxicity associated with therapeutic use of NSAIDs is more common than acute overdose. The most frequent problems are GI bleeding and renal insufficiency.
- CNS effects such as headache, mental status changes, and aseptic meningitis may be seen. Seizures have been reported with large ingestions, especially of mefenamic acid.
- Pulmonary manifestations such as bronchospasm and hypersensitivity pneumonitis can occur.
- Hepatic dysfunction, especially in the elderly and in patients with autoimmune disease, is possible.
- Inhibition of platelet aggregation may lead to bleeding. The COX-2 inhibitors (eg, rofecoxib, celecoxib) have less antiplatelet effect than conventional NSAIDs; the lack of platelet inhibition with COX-2 inhibitors may increase the risk of acute coronary syndrome or thromboembolic stroke in at-risk patients who were previously on conventional NSAIDs.
- Bone marrow suppression, including aplastic anemia, has been reported.
- NSAIDs account for approximately 10% of cutaneous drug reactions, ranging from benign rashes and phototoxic reactions to severe Stevens–Johnson syndrome and toxic epidermal necrolysis.
- Fetal NSAID exposure may lead to premature closure of the ductus arteriosus, oligohydramnios, renal dysfunction, necrotizing enterocolitis, and CNS hemorrhage.
- Acute NSAID overdose generally has low morbidity, and usually becomes clinically apparent within 4 hours of ingestion.
- Abdominal pain, nausea, and vomiting may occur.
- CNS manifestations include altered mental status, diplopia, nystagmus, headache, and rarely seizures. Hypotension and bradydysrhythmias have been reported.
- Renal failure may occur and are often associated with serum electrolyte abnormalities and volume overload.

DIAGNOSIS AND DIFFERENTIAL

- The manifestations of NSAID toxicity are nonspecific.
- NSAID levels are not readily available and are not clinically useful in assessing toxicity.
- Laboratory evaluation should include electrolytes, glucose, BUN/creatinine, liver function tests, and an APAP level.

EMERGENCY DEPARTMENT CARE AND DISPOSITION

- Emergent priorities remain airway, breathing, and circulation. Cardiac monitoring and an IV line should be instituted.
- Activated charcoal 1 gram/kg is indicated for GI decontamination when early overdoses are identified.
- Volume resuscitation, correction of acid–base and electrolyte disorders, and standard treatment of other complications such as seizures, dysrhythmias, and renal failure should be performed as indicated.
- Patients with asymptomatic NSAID ingestions may be safely discharged from the ED after screening for co-ingestants and a 4- to 6-hour observation period. In deliberate overdoses, a psychiatric consultation should be obtained prior to discharge.

For further reading in Tintinalli's *Emergency Medicine: A Comprehensive Study Guide*, 7th ed., see Chapter 183, "Aspirin and Salicylates," by Luke Yip; Chapter 184, "Acetaminophen," by Oliver L. Hung and Lewis S. Nelson; and Chapter 185 "Nonsteroidal Anti-Inflammatory Drugs," by Joseph G. Rella and Wallace A. Carter.

109 METHYLXANTHINES AND NICOTINE

L. Keith French

EPIDEMIOLOGY

- Theophylline poisoning is waning as its use has become less common.
- Life-threatening theophylline overdoses are more likely in elderly patients on chronic therapy than in younger patients following acute overdose.
- Caffeine is the most commonly used psychoactive drug in the world.
- In 2008, the American Association of Poison Control Centers (AAPC) received 4852 reports of caffeine exposures, including one death.
- Approximately one-third of the US population uses nicotine in some form.
- In 2008, the AAPC received 8356 reports of exposure.

PATHOPHYSIOLOGY

- Methylxanthines (theophylline, aminophylline, caffeine, theobromine) have three distinct pathophysiologic features: adenosine antagonism, increased adrenergic stimulation, and phosphodiesterase inhibition.
- Nicotine binds and, in low doses, agonizes nicotinic acetylcholine receptors within the central nervous, autonomic, and neuromuscular systems, thereby augmenting neurotransmitter release. At high doses, neurotransmitter release from the same neurons may become inhibited.

CLINICAL FEATURES

- The main systems affected by methylxanthines are GI, neurologic, cardiovascular, and metabolic.
- Nausea and vomiting are common with methylxanthines overdose and occur in >70% of patients following acute exposure.
- Headache, agitation, tremor, and seizure are characteristic neurologic features.
- The incidence of seizures is approximately 50% in patients with serum levels >40 micrograms/mL in chronic theophylline exposure or >120 micrograms/mL following acute exposure.
- Cardiovascular effects include tachycardia, atrial arrhythmias (multifocal atrial tachycardia, atrial fibrillation or flutter), ventricular arrhythmias, and hypotension.
- Hypokalemia, hyperglycemia, and metabolic acidosis are common metabolic derangements with methylxanthine exposures.
- In overdoses, nicotine mainly affects the GI, neurologic, cardiovascular, and respiratory systems.
- Nausea and vomiting are the most common effects following significant nicotine exposure.
- Tremor, dizziness, tachycardia, salivation, and bronchorrhea are early features following nicotine poisoning.
- Delayed effects of nicotine, particularly in large overdoses, include bradycardia, arrhythmias, hypoventilation, seizures, weakness, and coma.

DIAGNOSIS AND DIFFERENTIAL

- Therapeutic theophylline concentrations are 5 to 15 micrograms/mL, although serum concentrations do not always correlate with clinical findings.
- The best predictor of major theophylline toxicity following acute overdose is peak serum concentration, while the best predictor of toxicity in chronic exposures is patient age.
- Caffeine serum concentrations greater than 120 micrograms/mL are likely to cause life-threatening signs and symptoms; however, levels are not readily available in most institutions.
- Nicotine and its major metabolite, cotinine, can be detected in the urine, but do not provide quantitative information and do not correlate with acute exposure.
- Coingestants, such as acetaminophen or aspirin, should be considered in any patient who presents after an acute, intentional overdose.

EMERGENCY DEPARTMENT CARE AND DISPOSITION

- Treatment for both methylxanthine and nicotine poisoning begins with IV access, cardiac monitoring, noninvasive blood pressure measurement, and fluid administration.
- Activated charcoal is indicated for methylxanthine overdoses if conditions are appropriate (protected airway, no plan for endoscopy, no concomitant hydrocarbon ingestion, present bowel sounds). Consider whole-bowel irrigation following ingestions of sustained-release products.
- Nausea and vomiting generally limit the utility of activated charcoal in nicotine ingestions, although it may theoretically reduce nicotine absorption.
- Ondansetron is the antiemetic of choice. Avoid phenothiazines (which lower the seizure threshold) and cimetidine (which prolongs the half-life of methylxanthines).
- Benzodiazepines are the first-line agents for seizures. Methylxanthines may generate refractory seizures, and in this instance, barbiturates or sedation/paralysis/intubation may be necessary.
- Use cardioselective β-blockers, such as metoprolol or esmolol, for tachyarrhythmias associated with methylxanthine overdose.
- Consider hemodialysis in theophylline poisonings associated with serum concentrations >90 micrograms/mL in acute exposures or >40 micrograms/mL in chronic exposures, or in any patient with life-threatening events such as seizures or tachyarrhythmias.
- Intubation and mechanical ventilation may be necessary in the severely nicotine-poisoned patient who exhibits profound weakness or respiratory failure.
- Asymptomatic patients may be safely discharged after 6 hours of observation following exposure to immediate release methylxanthines, 12 hours of observation following exposure to sustained release methylxanthines, and 3 hours of observation following nicotine exposures.

For further reading in Tintinalli's *Emergency Medicine: A Comprehensive Guide*, 7th ed., see Chapter 186, "Methylxanthines and Nicotine," by Chip Gresham and Daniel E. Brooks.

110 CARDIAC MEDICATIONS

D. Adam Algren

DIGITALIS GLYCOSIDES

EPIDEMIOLOGY

- Digitalis preparations are used in the treatment of supraventricular tachydysrhythmias and congestive heart failure.
- The annual incidence of digoxin toxicity is slowly decreasing due to declining use of digoxin.

PATHOPHYSIOLOGY

- Digitalis inhibits the sodium–potassium–adenosine triphosphate (Na^+-K^+-ATPase) pump. Ultimately, intracellular calcium concentrations increase, which is responsible for the inotropic effect of digitalis. Elevated intracellular calcium also increases automaticity and can result in spontaneous depolarization and tachyarrhythmias.
- Digitalis increases vagal tone and decreases conduction through the atrioventricular node, resulting in bradycardia.

CLINICAL FEATURES

- Toxicity can occur following an acute ingestion or develop during chronic therapy (Table 110-1).
- Chronic toxicity is more common in the elderly and occurs in those with predisposing illnesses (heart disease, renal/liver failure, hypothyroidism, chronic obstructive pulmonary disease), electrolyte disturbances (hypokalemia, hypomagnesemia), or drug interactions (quinidine, amiodarone, spironolactone, calcium channel blockers, macrolide antibiotics).

DIAGNOSIS AND DIFFERENTIAL

- Hyperkalemia is often seen in acute poisoning but may be absent in chronic toxicity.
- Serum digoxin levels are neither sensitive nor specific for toxicity. However, patients with higher digoxin levels (>2 nanograms/mL) are more likely to experience toxicity.
- The differential diagnosis includes sinus node disease or toxicity from calcium channel blockers, β-blockers, class IA antidysrhythmics (quinidine, procainamide), clonidine, organophosphates, or cardiotoxic plants, such as rhododendron or yew berry.

TABLE 110-1 Clinical Presentation of Digitalis Glycoside Toxicity

Acute toxicity	
Clinical history	Intentional or accidental ingestion
GI effects	Nausea and vomiting
Central nervous system effects	Headache, dizziness, confusion, coma
Cardiac effects	Bradyarrhythmias or supraventricular tachyarrhythmias with atrioventricular block
Electrolyte abnormalities	Hyperkalemia
Digoxin level	Marked elevation (if obtained within 6 h)
Chronic toxicity	
Clinical history	Typically in elderly cardiac patients taking diuretics; may have renal insufficiency
GI effects	Nausea, vomiting, diarrhea, abdominal pain
Central nervous system effects	Fatigue, weakness, confusion, delirium, coma
Cardiac effects	Almost any ventricular or supraventricular dysrhythmia can occur; ventricular dysrhythmias are common
Electrolyte abnormalities	Normal or decreased serum potassium, hypomagnesemia
Digoxin level	Minimally elevated or within "therapeutic" range

EMERGENCY DEPARTMENT CARE AND DISPOSITION

- Management priorities include supportive care, prevention of further absorption in cases of an acute ingestion, and antidote administration, if indicated. All patients require continuous cardiac monitoring, vascular access, and frequent reevaluation.
- Consider activated charcoal, 1 gram/kg following acute ingestions.
- Use atropine, 0.5 to 2.0 milligrams (0.02 milligram/kg) IV, and cardiac pacing to treat bradydysrhythmias.
- Digoxin-specific Fab is indicated for ventricular dysrhythmias, hemodynamically significant bradydysrhythmias, and hyperkalemia greater than 5.5 mEq/L. Dosing of digoxin-specific Fab is calculated according to Table 110-2.
- Treat ventricular dysrhythmias with phenytoin, 15 milligrams/kg, infused no faster than 25 milligrams/min; lidocaine, 1 milligram/kg, or magnesium sulfate, 2 to 4 grams IV, are alternatives.
- Electrocardioversion may induce refractory ventricular dysrhythmias and should be considered only as a last resort. The initial setting should be 10 to 25 J.

TABLE 110-2 Calculation of Digoxin-Specific Fab Antibody Fragment Dose

Calculate total-body load
Based on history of amount ingested: total-body load = amount ingested (milligrams) × 0.80 (bioavailability)
Based on serum digoxin concentration: total-body load = [serum digoxin level (nanograms/mL) × 5.6 L/kg × patient's weight (kg)]/1000
Calculate number of vials of digoxin-specific Fab antibody fragments needed to neutralize the calculated total-body load
An equimolar dose is required for neutralization—one vial contains 38 or 40 milligrams of digoxin-specific Fab antibody fragments that will bind approximately 0.5 milligram of digoxin*
Number of vials = total-body load/0.5
A simple and accurate variation using serum digoxin level
Number of vials = [serum digoxin level (nanograms/mL) × patient's weight (kg)]/100

Abbreviation: Fab = antigen-binding fragment.
*The digoxin-specific Fab antibody fragments commercially available in the United States contain 38 or 40 milligrams per vial, depending in the manufacturer, but both bind approximately 0.5 milligram of digoxin.

- Treat hyperkalemia with glucose followed by insulin; other options are sodium bicarbonate, potassium-binding resin, or hemodialysis. Historically, calcium administration in the setting of digoxin toxicity was thought to be associated with an increased incidence of ventricular dysrhythmias and death. However, recent literature suggests that use of calcium is likely safe.
- Admit patients with signs of mild toxicity to a monitored setting, and those with significant toxicity should be managed in an intensive care unit. Repeat digoxin levels following digoxin Fab are not accurate and should not be obtained.
- Discharge patients not requiring digoxin Fab if they remain asymptomatic with normal serum potassium and digoxin levels after 6 to 12 hours of observation.

β-BLOCKERS

EPIDEMIOLOGY

- β-Blockers are used in the treatment of various cardiovascular, neurologic, ophthalmologic, and psychiatric disorders.
- In 2008, the American Association of Poison Centers received 21,282 reports of β-blocker exposures resulting in six deaths.

PATHOPHYSIOLOGY

- β-Blockers alter activity of myocardial, vascular, and smooth muscle cells by attenuating calcium entry into the cell. In cases of toxicity, their negative inotropic and chronotropic effects result in progressive bradycardia and hypotension.
- Different agents possess varying pharmacologic properties including β-receptor selectivity, membrane-stabilizing activity (sodium channel blockade), lipid solubility, and partial agonist activity. These different properties influence the clinical spectrum and severity of toxicity.
- Sotalol is unique in that it is also a class III antiarrhythmic because of its ability to block potassium channels.

CLINICAL FEATURES

- Toxicity usually develops within 6 hours of ingestion of an immediate-release product. In the case of sustained-release preparations, toxicity may be delayed up to 12 hours.
- The primary effects of toxicity involve the cardiovascular system and include hypotension, bradycardia, conduction abnormalities, cardiogenic shock, and asystole.
- Sotalol is unique in that it can produce QT interval prolongation and is associated with ventricular dysrhythmias such as torsades de pointes.
- Noncardiac manifestations of toxicity include altered mental status, psychosis, seizures, hypoglycemia, and bronchospasm.

DIAGNOSIS AND DIFFERENTIAL

- The diagnosis is clinical. Drug levels are not commonly available and do not help in acute management.
- An ECG should be obtained in all cases. Laboratory studies are directed at identifying underlying medical conditions or complications.
- The differential diagnosis includes overdose of calcium channel blockers, α_2-agonists, digoxin, organophosphates, and cardiotoxic plants (such as oleander, foxglove, and rhododendron).

EMERGENCY DEPARTMENT CARE AND DISPOSITION

- The goal of treatment is restoration of perfusion to critical organs by increasing heart rate and myocardial contractility.
- All patients should have continuous cardiac monitoring and vascular access established. Administer crystalloid boluses to treat hypotension.
- Obtain bedside serum glucose in the setting of altered mental status.

- Administer activated charcoal, 1 gram/kg, within 1 to 2 hours of ingestion if no contraindications are present. Gastric lavage prior to administration of charcoal may be beneficial if performed within 1 to 2 hours of ingestion. Whole-bowel irrigation can be considered in cases of sustained-release preparations.
- Atropine, 0.5 to 1 milligram (0.02 milligram/kg, minimum dose 0.1 milligram) IV, can be given for bradycardia, but it is unlikely to be of benefit in cases of severe β-blocker–induced bradycardia or hypotension.
- Glucagon has inotropic and chronotropic effects and is the agent of choice for the treatment of toxicity. It is administered as an IV bolus of 3 to 5 milligrams (0.05 milligram/kg). This is followed by a continuous infusion of 1 to 10 milligrams/h. Nausea and vomiting are common side effects of glucagon.
- Vasopressors, such as norepinephrine (2-30 micrograms/kg/min), epinephrine (1-20 micrograms/kg/min), and/or dopamine (2.5-20 micrograms/kg/min), can be used for refractory bradycardia and hypotension.
- Hyperinsulinemia-euglycemia (HIE) therapy can improve myocardial contractility (Table 110-3).
- Calcium may be of limited benefit in cases of refractory hypotension. Either calcium gluconate or calcium chloride may be administered (10 mL of 10% [0.15 mL/kg] repeated three to six times as necessary). Although calcium chloride contains more elemental calcium than calcium gluconate, it is very irritating to soft tissues and should ideally be administered via a central line.
- Cardiac pacing may be attempted for refractory bradycardia, but is not always successful and may not reverse hypotension.
- Use lidocaine, magnesium sulfate, isoproterenol, and overdrive pacing to treat sotalol-induced ventricular dysrhythmias.

TABLE 110-3 Protocol for Hyperinsulin/Euglycemia Therapy in Severe Calcium Channel Blocker Overdose

Administer 50 mL of 50% glucose (0.5 gram/mL) in water IV.
Administer regular insulin 1 unit/kg IV bolus.
Begin regular insulin infusion at 0.5-1.0 unit/kg/h along with glucose 10% (0.1 gram/mL) in water at 200 mL/h (adult) or 5 mL/kg/h (pediatric).
Monitor serum glucose every 20 min. Titrate glucose infusion rate to maintain serum glucose level between 150 and 300 milligrams/dL.
Once infusion rates have been stable for 60 min, glucose monitoring may be decreased to hourly.
Monitor serum potassium level and start IV potassium infusion if serum potassium level is <3.5 mEq/L.

- Hemodialysis may be of benefit in cases involving acebutolol, atenolol, nadolol, or sotalol.
- Admit patients who develop bradycardia, hypotension, conduction disturbances, or altered mental status to an ICU.
- Admit patients who have ingested a sustained-release preparation or sotalol to a monitored setting due to concern for delayed toxicity.
- Those patients who remain asymptomatic 6 hours following ingestion of an immediate-release preparation can be medically cleared.

CALCIUM CHANNEL BLOCKERS

EPIDEMIOLOGY

- Calcium channel blockers are used in the treatment of hypertension, angina, vasospasm, and supraventricular dysrhythmias.
- Calcium channel blockers are associated with more deaths than any other class of cardiovascular drugs.
- In 2008, the American Association of Poison Control Centers received 10,398 calcium channel blocker exposure reports that were associated with 12 deaths.

PATHOPHYSIOLOGY

- Intracellular calcium is the primary stimulus and determinant for cardiac and vascular smooth muscle contraction. It is also responsible for stimulating impulse formation in the sinoatrial pacemaker cells.
- Calcium channel blockers block L-type calcium channels and prevent entry of calcium into cells, resulting in smooth muscle relaxation, decreased cardiac contractility, blunted cardiac automaticity, and intracardiac conduction delay.
- The three classes of calcium channel blockers are the phenylalkylamines (eg, verapamil), benzothiazepines (eg, diltiazem), and dihydropyridines (eg, nifedipine, amlodipine, etc.).

CLINICAL FEATURES

- Toxicity primarily involves the cardiovascular system and can result in bradydysrhythmias, atrioventricular blocks, and hypotension.
- In cases of dihydropyridine overdose, reflex tachycardia may develop initially.
- In severe cases, all classes of calcium channel blockers can cause complete heart block, depressed myocardial contractility, and vasodilatation ultimately resulting in cardiovascular collapse. Verapamil is the most cardiotoxic.

- Noncardiac consequences include hyperglycemia, lactic acidosis, and noncardiogenic pulmonary edema.
- Altered mental status is usually due to hypoperfusion. If noted in the setting of a normal blood pressure, other etiologies should be considered.

DIAGNOSIS AND DIFFERENTIAL

- The diagnosis is clinical. Identification of the formulation type (ie, immediate vs. sustained-release preparation) is helpful in anticipating the clinical course and disposition.
- In the setting of dihydropyridine overdose, vasodilatation may result in flushed skin, hypotension, and tachycardia.
- Hypoperfusion may result in lactic acidosis.
- Hyperglycemia is common and helps to distinguish calcium channel blocker from β-blocker toxicity, which is often associated with hypoglycemia.
- The differential diagnosis for bradycardia and hypotension includes hypothermia, acute coronary syndrome, hyperkalemia, and toxicity due to cardiac glycosides, β-blockers, class IA and IC antidysrhythmics, and central α_2-adrenergic agonists (clonidine).

EMERGENCY DEPARTMENT CARE AND DISPOSITION

- All patients require supplemental oxygen, cardiac monitoring, and vascular access. Bedside glucose testing should be performed in patients with alerted mental status.
- The goal of treatment is to improve cardiac output and systemic vascular resistance.
- Administer activated charcoal, 1 gram/kg within 1 to 2 hours of ingestion if no contraindications exist. Gastric lavage may be beneficial if performed within 1 hour of ingestion. Whole-bowel irrigation can be considered for cases involving sustained-release preparations.
- Administer crystalloids for hypotension, with care taken to avoid fluid overload.
- Atropine 0.5 to 1 milligram (0.02 milligram/kg, minimum dose 0.1 milligram) and calcium may be of limited benefit in cases of severe toxicity. Either calcium gluconate or calcium chloride can be administered (10 mL of 10% [0.15 mL/kg] repeated 3-6 times as necessary). Although calcium chloride contains more elemental calcium than calcium gluconate, it is very irritating to soft tissues and should ideally be administered via a central line.
- Norepinephrine (2-30 micrograms/kg/min), epinephrine (1-20 micrograms/kg/min), or dopamine (2.5-20 micrograms/kg/min) can be used for refractory bradycardia and hypotension.
- Hyperinsulinemia-euglycemia (HIE) therapy can improve myocardial contractility and blood pressure (Table 110-3).
- Glucagon is variably successful in the treatment of calcium channel blocker toxicity. It is administered as an IV bolus of 3 to 5 milligrams (0.05 milligram/kg) followed by a continuous infusion of 1 to 10 milligrams/h. Nausea and vomiting are common side effects.
- IV fat emulsion (20% solution) has shown promising results in the treatment of severe toxicity. A bolus of 1.5 mL/kg IV is followed by a continuous infusion of 0.25 mL/kg/min.
- Admit patients with bradycardia, hypotension, or conduction disturbances to an ICU. Admit patients who have ingested a sustained-release preparation to a monitored setting due to concern for delayed toxicity.
- Patients who remain asymptomatic 6 hours after ingestion of an immediate release agent can be medically cleared.

ANTIHYPERTENSIVE AGENTS

EPIDEMIOLOGY

- Multiple classes of medications are used in the treatment of hypertension. Given the high prevalence of hypertension, these agents are commonly prescribed.
- Toxicity can occur following an acute ingestion, or complications may develop during chronic therapy.
- For a majority of agents, life-threatening toxicity is not expected with acute overdose.

DIURETICS

- Diuretics include thiazides (hydrochlorothiazide), loop diuretics (furosemide, bumetanide, ethacrynic acid, torsemide), potassium-sparing diuretics (spironolactone, triamterene, amiloride), and carbonic anhydrase inhibitors (acetazolamide).

CLINICAL FEATURES

Thiazides and Loop Diuretics

- Patients may present with hypotension, tachycardia, hyponatremia, hypokalemia, hypocalcemia (loop diuretics), hypomagnesemia, hyperuricemia (thiazides), and hypochloremic metabolic alkalosis.

Potassium-Sparing Diuretics

- Toxicity manifests as volume depletion, hyperkalemia, hyponatremia, and hypochloremia.

Carbonic Anhydrase Inhibitors

- Overdose may result in volume depletion, electrolyte disturbances, and non–anion gap metabolic acidosis.

EMERGENCY DEPARTMENT CARE AND DISPOSITION

- Management is supportive and includes fluid resuscitation and correction of electrolyte and pH abnormalities.
- Use IV normal saline to correct hypovolemia, hyponatremia, and alkalosis.
- Asymptomatic patients can be medically cleared after several hours of observation.
- Admit patients with hypotension or significant electrolyte abnormalities.

SYMPATHOLYTIC AGENTS

EPIDEMIOLOGY

- These agents work to decrease central sympathetic outflow and act as peripheral α_1-receptor antagonists.

CLINICAL FEATURES

- Peripheral α_1-adrenergic receptor antagonists (ie, doxazosin, prazosin, terazosin) may produce hypotension with reflex tachycardia.
- Clonidine and other α_2-agonists produce hypotension and bradycardia. Other findings include respiratory depression, hypothermia, CNS depression, and miosis.
- Guanabenz, guanfacine, methyldopa, and reserpine can cause hypotension, symptomatic bradycardia, dry mouth, and mental status changes.

EMERGENCY DEPARTMENT CARE AND DISPOSITION

- Treatment involves aggressive supportive care. All patients require continuous cardiac monitoring and vascular access.
- Recurrent apnea from clonidine, most commonly seen in children, may necessitate endotracheal intubation.
- Administer crystalloid for hypotension.
- Dopamine or norepinephrine may be necessary in cases of refractory hypotension.
- Atropine is indicated for management of symptomatic bradycardia associated with clonidine.
- Naloxone may be effective for refractory cases of clonidine-induced hypotension or CNS/respiratory depression. If utilized, large doses (up to 10 milligrams) are often required.

ANGIOTENSIN-CONVERTING ENZYME INHIBITORS AND ANGIOTENSIN II RECEPTOR ANTAGONISTS

- Hyperkalemia may develop during chronic therapy. Angioedema is the most severe adverse effect associated with angiotensin-converting enzyme inhibitors (ACEIs) and angiotensin II receptor antagonists (ARBs).
- Although uncommon, hypotension is the most common concern in overdose.
- Care is supportive. Hypotension may be treated with IV normal saline, followed by vasopressors such as dopamine.
- Naloxone has been reported to reverse ace inhibitor-induced hypotension, although it is not always effective.

DIRECT VASODILATORS

CLINICAL FEATURES

- Toxicity from hydralazine is uncommon. Hypotension is the most common presentation. Symptomatic tachycardia and/or myocardial ischemia may also be noted.
- Minoxidil causes hypotension and tachycardia.
- Toxicity from sodium nitroprusside includes hypotension. With high doses, cyanide toxicity may develop. Shock and lactic acidosis are the hallmarks of cyanide toxicity.
- Thiocyanate, a detoxification byproduct of nitroprusside, can also accumulate in patients with renal failure resulting in altered mental status, nausea, and abdominal pain.

EMERGENCY DEPARTMENT CARE AND DISPOSITION

- Use IV fluids to treat nitroprusside-related hypotension. Given the short half-life of the drug, immediate discontinuation is typically all that is required.
- Use IV fluids and vasopressors to treat hypotension related to hydralazine and minoxidil. Norepinephrine and phenylephrine are vasopressors of choice.
- Avoid thiocyanate toxicity by limiting the duration of infusion and restricting the use of nitroprusside

in patients with renal insufficiency. In severe cases, thiocyanate may be removed by dialysis.
- Avoid cyanide toxicity by coadministration of sodium thiosulfate or by limiting the duration of infusion.

For further reading in Tintinalli's *Emergency Medicine: A Comprehensive Study Guide*, 7th ed., see Chapter 187, "Digitalis Glycosides," by Jennifer S. Boyle and Mark A. Kirk; Chapter 188, "β-Blockers," by Jennifer L. Englund and William P. Kerns II; Chapter 189, "Calcium Channel Blockers," by Alicia B. Minns and Christian Tomaszewski; and Chapter 190, "Antihypertensive Agents," by Andrew Stolbach and Arjun Chanmugam.

111 ANTICONVULSANTS

Alicia B. Minns

- First-generation anticonvulsants such as phenytoin and phenobarbital have potential for serious toxicity, especially in overdose. The newer, second-generation anticonvulsants generally have fewer adverse effects in overdose.

PHENYTOIN AND FOSPHENYTOIN

EPIDEMIOLOGY

- Most phenytoin-related deaths have been caused by rapid IV administration or hypersensitivity reactions.

CLINICAL FEATURES

- Toxicity depends upon the duration of exposure, dosage taken, and most importantly, route of administration.
- Life-threatening effects such as hypotension, bradycardia, conduction delays, ventricular dysrhythmias, and asystole can be seen with IV administration, and are secondary to the diluent propylene glycol. This morbidity can be avoided by slowing the rate of administration.
- Clinical manifestations in oral overdose are dose related and present with central nervous system (CNS) toxicity. Symptoms include nystagmus, depressed level of consciousness, nausea, vomiting, ataxic gait, dysarthria, and confusion. Seizures, coma, and apnea may occur in large overdoses. Death from oral overdose alone is extremely rare.
- Cardiovascular toxicity is usually associated with IV administration. In an otherwise healthy patient, cardiac toxicity has never been reported after an oral overdose of phenytoin; when observed, this requires assessment for other causes.
- Phenytoin causes significant soft tissue toxicity. Intramuscular injection can result in localized crystallization of the drug, hematoma, sterile abscess, and myonecrosis.
- Reported complications of extravasation after IV infusion have included skin and soft tissue necrosis, compartment syndrome, gangrene, and death.
- Fosphenytoin, a prodrug of phenytoin, is more soluble and less irritating to tissues. Fosphenytoin is well tolerated intramuscularly or intravenously, although intravenous fosphenytoin can cause pruritus and hypotension. The toxic effects of propylene glycol are not present.
- Hypersensitivity reactions usually occur within 1 to 6 weeks of initiating phenytoin therapy. Reactions can include systemic lupus erythematosus, erythema multiforme, toxic epidermal necrolysis, Stevens–Johnson syndrome, hepatitis, rhabdomyolysis, acute interstitial pneumonitis, lymphadenopathy, leukopenia, disseminated intravascular coagulation, and renal failure.
- Gingival hyperplasia is a common side effect of phenytoin and its absence may suggest poor compliance.
- Phenytoin is teratogenic and should never be initiated in a pregnant patient without consulting a neurologist and obstetrician.

DIAGNOSIS AND DIFFERENTIAL

- Therapeutic levels are between 10 and 20 micrograms/mL (40-80 micromoles/L). Some patients require levels above 20 micrograms/mL for adequate seizure control. Patients with underlying brain disease are predisposed to toxicity and may become toxic at low levels.
- Toxicity generally correlates with increasing plasma levels (Table 111-1). Due to erratic absorption, serial phenytoin levels should be obtained to identify peak levels.
- Almost any CNS-active drug, such as ethanol, carbamazepine, benzodiazepines, barbiturates, and lithium, can mimic phenytoin toxicity.
- Disease states that resemble phenytoin toxicity include hypoglycemia, Wernicke's encephalopathy, and posterior fossa hemorrhage or tumor.

TABLE 111-1 Correlation of Plasma Phenytoin Level and Side Effects

PLASMA LEVEL (MICROGRAMS/ML)	SIDE EFFECTS
<10	Usually none
10-20	Occasional mild nystagmus
20-30	Nystagmus
30-40	Ataxia, slurred speech, nausea and vomiting
40-50	Lethargy, confusion
>50	Coma, seizures

- Seizures from phenytoin toxicity are uncommon, and other causes should be investigated, such as trauma or alcohol withdrawal.

EMERGENCY DEPARTMENT CARE AND DISPOSITION

- Place patients on a cardiac monitor, noninvasive blood pressure device, and pulse oximeter. Establish vascular access.
- Correct acidosis (respiratory or metabolic) to decrease the active free phenytoin fraction.
- Treat hypotension from IV administration of phenytoin with isotonic crystalloids and discontinuation of the infusion.
- For an acute oral overdose, give multiple doses of oral activated charcoal (1 gram/kg) initially and then every 4 hours for the first 24 hours.
- Consider atropine or cardiac pacing for bradydysrhythmias.
- Treat seizures with a benzodiazepine or phenobarbital.
- Hemodialysis and hemoperfusion are of no benefit.
- Admit patients following oral ingestion, if serious complications (eg, seizures, coma, altered mental status, and ataxia) are present.
- Observe patients with mild symptoms in the ED and discharge home if serum levels are declining. Cardiac monitoring after isolated oral ingestion is unnecessary.
- After IV administration of phenytoin, admit patients with significant or persistent complications for observation on a telemetry unit. Discharge those with transient effects.
- Admit patients with symptomatic chronic intoxication for observation unless the toxic effects are minimal, adequate care can be obtained at home, drug levels are decreasing, and patients are 6 to 8 hours from their last dose. Phenytoin should be stopped and levels rechecked in 2 to 3 days.

CARBAMAZEPINE

CLINICAL FEATURES

- In acute toxicity, delayed and erratic absorption due to carbamazepine's anticholinergic properties and lower water solubility can cause delayed clinical deterioration.
- Manifestations of acute toxicity include coma, respiratory failure, ataxia, nystagmus, miosis or mydriasis, ileus, bowel obstruction, hypertonicity, increased deep tendon reflexes, dystonic reactions, and anticholinergic toxidrome.
- Seizures may occur at high concentrations.
- Although cardiac arrhythmias are rare, carbamazepine is one of the few anticonvulsants that can cause a wide QRS and seizures.

DIAGNOSIS AND DIFFERENTIAL

- Serum carbamazepine concentrations do not accurately correlate with the severity of the poisoning; however, concentrations of >40 micrograms/mL may be associated with an increased risk of serious complications and concentrations higher than 60 to 80 micrograms/mL may be fatal.
- Obtain an ECG to evaluate the QRS interval in suspected carbamazepine toxicity.
- A false-positive tricyclic antidepressant result on urine drug screen can occur due to structural similarity.

EMERGENCY DEPARTMENT CARE AND DISPOSITION

- Consider activated charcoal if the patient is not obtunded and presents within 1 hour of ingestion.
- Hemodialysis or hemodiafiltration are effective in life-threatening overdose.
- Give sodium bicarbonate for widening of the QRS.
- Asymptomatic patients may be medically cleared if at least two carbamazepine levels obtained a few hours apart are decreasing.

VALPROATE

CLINICAL FEATURES

- In acute overdose, the most frequent sign is central nervous system depression. Other findings include respiratory depression, hypotension, hypoglycemia, hypernatremia, hypophosphatemia, and an anion gap metabolic acidosis that may persist for days.
- Liver toxicity leads to elevated serum aminotransferases, ammonia, and lactate. Hepatic failure (microvesicular steatosis) occurs in about 1 in 20,000 patients on

long-term therapy. Children <3 years of age on multiple antiepileptics with multiple medical problems are at increased risk of hepatotoxicity.
- Hyperammonemia in the absence of liver failure has been reported following both overdose and long-term therapeutic use.
- Pancreatitis and thrombocytopenia may occur.
- Cerebral edema has been observed after acute overdose.

DIAGNOSIS AND DIFFERENTIAL

- Therapeutic valproate concentrations are between 50 and 100 micrograms/mL. Adverse effects increase as concentrations rise above 150 micrograms/mL, and frank coma may occur with levels above 800 micrograms/mL.
- Obtain serum ammonia and bedside glucose concentrations in patients with altered level of consciousness. Consider a CBC, electrolytes, liver function tests, and serum lactate.

EMERGENCY DEPARTMENT CARE AND DISPOSITION

- Consider multidose activated charcoal after ingestion of enteric-coated delayed-release preparations. Consider whole-bowel irrigation in extended-release preparations.
- Measure serial concentrations due to delayed peak serum concentration.
- Administer L-carnitine, 50 milligrams/kg/d, to patients with lethargy, coma, hyperammonemia, and hepatic dysfunction.
- Initiate hemoperfusion or hemodiafiltration for severe overdose.
- A patient should be asymptomatic with a decline in levels before considered stable for discharge.

SECOND-GENERATION ANTICONVULSANTS

As a group, the second-generation anticonvulsants possess little toxicity in acute overdose.

- **Felbamate** may cause aplastic anemia and hepatic failure with therapeutic use. In large overdose, it can crystallize in the kidney, causing acute renal failure.
- **Gabapentin** produces little toxicity in overdose—usually drowsiness, ataxia, nausea, and vomiting that resolve in about 10 hours.
- **Lacosamide** can cause dizziness, headache, nausea, and diplopia in therapeutic use. Clinical experience in overdose is limited.
- **Lamotrigine** has been associated with autoimmune reactions, such as Stevens–Johnson syndrome during therapeutic use. The most common effects in overdose are drowsiness, vomiting, ataxia, and dizziness. Seizures, coma, cardiac toxicity (QRS and QT-interval prolongation), and acute pancreatitis have been reported with lamotrigine overdose. Treatments include sodium bicarbonate and IV lipid emulsion.
- **Levetiracetam** can cause lethargy, coma, and respiratory depression.
- **Oxcarbazepine** may cause hyponatremia and a drug rash with therapeutic use. There is little toxicity from isolated overdose.
- **Pregabalin** can cause somnolence and dizziness in long-term therapeutic use. There is little experience with overdose.
- **Rufinamide** may cause headache, dizziness, fatigue, and somnolence in long-term therapy. Clinical experience in overdose is limited.
- **Tiagabine** overdose can cause rapid onset of neurologic toxicity, including lethargy, coma, and seizures (status epilepticus, even in patients without an underlying seizure disorder, may be seen). Other findings in overdose include myoclonus, muscular rigidity, and delirium.
- **Topiramate** can promote renal stone formation and glaucoma in therapeutic use. In overdose, topiramate can cause somnolence, vertigo, agitation, and mydriasis. Seizures and status epilepticus have been reported. It can produce a metabolic acidosis, which can last up to 7 days due to the long half-life of the drug.
- **Zonisamide** can promote renal stone formation and cause a drug rash in therapeutic use. Clinical experience in overdose is limited.

For further reading in Tintinalli's *Emergency Medicine: A Comprehensive Study Guide*, 7th ed., see Chapter 191, "Anticonvulsants," by Frank LoVecchio and Jennifer C. Smith.

112 IRON

O. John Ma

EPIDEMIOLOGY

- Iron toxicity from intentional or accidental ingestion is a common poisoning.
- Significantly fewer poison center calls and deaths caused by ingestion of iron supplements were reported after the US Food and Drug Administration issued a regulation for unit-dose packaging.

PATHOPHYSIOLOGY

- Iron is a direct gastrointestinal (GI) irritant and causes vomiting, diarrhea, abdominal pain, mucosal ulceration, and GI bleeding after a significant ingestion.
- Vomiting and diarrhea from iron toxicity can lead to hypovolemia, which in turn may produce hypotension, tissue hypoperfusion, and metabolic acidosis.
- Toxic effects have been reported following oral doses as low as 10 to 20 milligrams/kg of elemental iron. Moderate toxicity occurs at doses of 20 to 60 milligrams/kg of elemental iron, and severe toxicity can be expected following doses greater than 60 milligrams/kg.

CLINICAL FEATURES

- Based on clinical findings, iron poisoning can be divided into five stages. Patients can die in any stage of iron poisoning.
- The first stage develops within the first few hours after the ingestion. The direct irritative effects of iron on the GI tract produce abdominal pain, vomiting, and diarrhea. Hematemesis is not unusual. Vomiting is the clinical sign most consistently associated with acute iron toxicity. The absence of these symptoms within 6 hours of ingestion essentially excludes a diagnosis of significant iron toxicity.
- During the second stage, which can continue up to 24 hours following ingestion, the patient's GI symptoms may temporarily resolve, thereby giving a false sense of security despite toxic amounts of absorbed iron. Although potentially asymptomatic, patients appear ill, and may have abnormal vital signs and evidence of poor tissue perfusion because of ongoing volume loss and worsening metabolic acidosis.
- The third stage can either appear very early or develop hours after the second stage: shock and lactic acidosis develop. Iron-induced coagulopathy may worsen bleeding and hypovolemia. Hepatic dysfunction, cardiomyopathy, and renal failure also may occur.
- The fourth stage develops 2 to 5 days after ingestion and manifests as elevation of aminotransferase levels that may progress to hepatic failure.
- The fifth stage, which occurs 4 to 6 weeks after ingestion, involves gastric outlet obstruction secondary to corrosive effects of iron on the pyloric mucosa.

DIAGNOSIS AND DIFFERENTIAL

- The diagnosis of iron poisoning is based on the clinical picture and history provided by the patient, significant others, or EMS providers.
- Order a basic metabolic panel, coagulation studies, complete blood count, hepatic enzymes, and a serum iron level.
- It is crucial to note that a single serum iron level does not reflect what iron levels have been previously, what direction they are going, or the degree of iron toxicity in tissues. A single low serum level does not exclude the diagnosis of serious iron toxicity since peak levels following ingestion of different iron preparations are variable in timing.
- Serum iron levels have limited use in directing management since toxicity is intracellular.
- In general, serum iron levels between 300 and 500 micrograms/dL correlate with mild systemic toxicity and iron levels between 500 and 1000 micrograms/dL correlate with moderate systemic toxicity. Levels greater than 1000 micrograms/dL are associated with severe toxicity and increased morbidity.
- The total iron-binding capacity (TIBC) does not aid in the assessment of iron-poisoned patients because it becomes falsely elevated in the presence of elevated serum iron levels or deferoxamine.
- A plain radiograph may reveal iron in the GI tract; however, many iron preparations are not routinely detected, so negative radiographs do not exclude iron ingestion.

EMERGENCY DEPARTMENT CARE AND DISPOSITION

- Patients who have remained asymptomatic for 6 hours after ingestion of iron and who have a normal physical examination do not require medical treatment for iron toxicity.
- Patients whose symptoms resolve after a short period of time and have normal vital signs usually have mild toxicity and require only supportive care. This subset of patients still requires an observation period.
- Patients who are symptomatic or demonstrate signs of hemodynamic instability after iron ingestion should be managed aggressively in the ED.
- Place the patient on supplemental oxygen and a cardiac monitor, and secure intravenous (IV) access.
- Administer aggressive IV crystalloids to help correct hypovolemia and hypoperfusion.
- Perform gastric lavage in patients who present within 60 minutes of ingestion. Activated charcoal is not recommended.
- Whole-bowel irrigation with a polyethylene glycol solution is efficacious. Administer 250 to 500 mL/h in children or 2 L/h in adults via nasogastric tube, which may clear the GI tract of iron pills before absorption occurs.

- Administer antiemetics such as ondansetron (4 milligrams IV in adults; 0.1 milligram/kg IV to a maximum dose of 4 milligrams in children) or promethazine (25 milligrams IV in adults; 0.25 milligram/kg IV in pediatric patients).
- Correct coagulopathy with vitamin K_1 (5-10 milligrams SC) and fresh frozen plasma (10-25 mL/kg in adults; 10 mL/kg in pediatric patients). Order blood for type and screen or crossmatch, as necessary.
- Deferoxamine is a chelating agent that removes iron from tissues and plasma. Deferoxamine is safe to administer to children and pregnant women. Deferoxamine therapy is indicated in patients with systemic toxicity, metabolic acidosis, worsening symptoms, or a serum iron level predictive of moderate or severe toxicity.
- Intravenous infusion is the preferred route of deferoxamine administration because IM absorption is unpredictable in the hypovolemic patient. The recommended initial dose is 1000 milligrams IV. Since hypotension is the rate-limiting factor for IV infusion, it is recommended to begin with a slow IV infusion at 5 milligrams/kg/h. The rate can be increased to 15 milligrams/kg/h, as tolerated, within the first hour of treatment.
- The recommended total amount of deferoxamine is 360 milligrams/kg or 6 grams during the first 24 hours.
- Initiate deferoxamine therapy without waiting for the serum iron level in any clinically ill patient with a known iron ingestion.
- Evaluate the efficacy of deferoxamine treatment through serial urine samples. As ferrioxamine is excreted, urine changes to a classic *vin rose* appearance. Clinical recovery is the most important factor guiding termination of deferoxamine therapy.
- Patients who remain asymptomatic after 6 hours of observation have a normal physical examination, and a reliable history of an insignificant ingestion can be considered for discharge.
- Patients initially symptomatic who become asymptomatic should be admitted for further evaluation since this may represent the second stage of iron toxicity.
- Admit all patients who receive deferoxamine therapy to an intensive care setting.
- Assess all patients for suicide risk. Consider child abuse or neglect in pediatric cases.

For further reading in Tintinalli's *Emergency Medicine: A Comprehensive Study Guide*, 7th ed., see Chapter 192, "Iron," by Stephanie H. Hernandez and Lewis S. Nelson.

113 HYDROCARBONS AND VOLATILE SUBSTANCES

Allyson A. Kreshak

EPIDEMIOLOGY

- Hydrocarbons are among the 25 most frequent exposures reported to the American Association of Poison Control Centers.
- Approximately 3.5% to 10% of young people have tried volatile substance inhalation.

PATHOPHYSIOLOGY

- Products containing hydrocarbons are found in many household and workplace settings; these include fuels, lighter fluids, paint removers, pesticides, polishers, degreasers, and lubricants.
- Volatile substances containing hydrocarbons such as glue, propellants, and gasoline are occasionally used for recreational abuse.
- Pulmonary toxicity manifests as chemical pneumonitis which results from direct parenchymal injury and altered surfactant function. This results either from aspiration of a low-viscosity compound or from inhalation of a high-volatility compound.
- Cardiac toxicity manifests as dysrhythmias that are mediated by endogenous catecholamines.
- Central nervous system (CNS) toxicity can be caused directly by systemically absorbed hydrocarbon, or indirectly from hypoxia due to pulmonary toxicity.
- Peripheral neuropathy secondary to demyelination and retrograde axonal degeneration results from P450 metabolism of six-carbon hydrocarbons to the toxic metabolite 2,5-hexanedione.
- Chlorinated hydrocarbons can cause lipid peroxidation and hepatic injury.
- With methylene chloride exposure, carbon monoxide formation may continue after cessation of exposure; this is caused by gradual release of methylene chloride from the tissues prior to its metabolism to carbon monoxide.

CLINICAL FEATURES

- Toxicity depends on the route of exposure (ingestion, inhalation, or dermal), physical characteristics of the agent (volatility, viscosity, and surface tension), chemical characteristics (aliphatic, aromatic, or hydrogenated), and the presence of toxic additives (eg, lead or pesticides).

TABLE 113-1 Clinical Manifestations of Hydrocarbon Exposure

SYSTEM	CLINICAL MANIFESTATIONS
Pulmonary	Tachypnea, grunting respirations, wheezing, retractions
Cardiac	Ventricular dysrhythmias (may occur after exposure to halogenated hydrocarbons and aromatic hydrocarbons)
Central nervous	Slurred speech, ataxia, lethargy, coma
Peripheral nervous	Chronic numbness and paresthesias in the extremities
GI and hepatic	Nausea, vomiting, abdominal pain, loss of appetite (mostly with halogenated hydrocarbons)
Renal and metabolic	Muscle weakness or paralysis secondary to hypokalemia in patients who abuse toluene
Hematologic	Lethargy (anemia), shortness of breath (anemia), neurologic depression/syncope (carbon monoxide from methylene chloride), cyanosis (methemoglobinemia from amine-containing hydrocarbons)
Dermal	Local erythema, papules, vesicles, generalized scarlatiniform eruption, exfoliative dermatitis, "huffer's rash," cellulitis

- Table 113-1 lists the most common clinical manifestations of hydrocarbon toxicity; pulmonary and cardiac effects are most common.
- Aspiration of highly volatile aliphatic substances such as gasoline, kerosene, methane, or butane may result in chemical pneumonitis, pneumodeiastinum, pneumothorax, and pneumatocele.
- Patients may present with coughing, dyspnea, choking, and gasping. Physical examination may reveal tachypnea, wheezing, grunting, and decreased breath sounds. Chest radiographic findings lag behind the clinical picture by 4 to 6 hours.
- Cardiac toxicity from aromatic and halogenated hydrocarbons is due to sensitization of the myocardium to catecholamines that may cause serious or fatal dysrhythmias.
- CNS toxicity occurs most commonly with the volatile petroleum distillates such as toluene and trichloroethane. Symptoms range from giddiness, slurred speech, ataxia, and hallucinations to seizures, lethargy, obtundation, and coma. Chronic exposure can cause cerebellar ataxia and mood lability.
- Halogenated hydrocarbons such as carbon tetrachloride and chloroform cause direct hepatocellular injury. Liver enzymes may be elevated within 24 hours, and right upper quadrant abdominal pain and jaundice develop within 48 to 96 hours. Chronic exposure causes cirrhosis and hepatoma.
- Hematologic toxicity from gasoline, kerosene, and trichloroethane can lead to hemolysis. Chronic benzene abuse can cause aplastic anemia and hematologic malignancies.
- Dermal toxicity includes rashes (erythema, papules, vesicles, or scarlatiniform rash), eczematous dermatitis, and burns.
- Carbon monoxide poisoning from methylene chloride metabolism may result in a metabolic acidosis.

DIAGNOSIS AND DIFFERENTIAL

- Diagnosis is made by history and the accompanying physical examination findings.
- Helpful laboratory tests include arterial blood gas, liver function panel, BUN, creatinine, hematocrit, and carboxyhemoglobin level (in methylene chloride exposure).
- A chest radiograph should be ordered to evaluate for aspiration pneumonitis immediately in symptomatic patients and after a 6-hour observation in asymptomatic patient.
- A kidney, ureter, and bladder radiograph (KUB) may show the presence of chlorinated hydrocarbons (eg, carbon tetrachloride) in the gastrointestinal (GI) tract as polyhalogenated substances are radiopaque.

EMERGENCY DEPARTMENT CARE AND DISPOSITION

- Decontamination of the patient should follow standard HAZMAT measures, and should preferably occur in the out-of-hospital setting.
- Administer supplemental oxygen and place all symptomatic patients on a cardiac monitor.
- Consider endotracheal intubation for patients with significant respiratory distress. Positive end-expiratory pressure may be added to improve oxygenation, but pneumothorax or pneumatocele are potential complications.
- In severe pulmonary aspiration with refractory hypoxemia, successful treatment with extracorporeal membrane oxygenation or high-frequency jet ventilation has been reported.
- Treat hypotension with IV crystalloid infusion. Catecholamines may precipitate life-threatening dysrhythmias and should be avoided, except in cases of cardiac arrest.
- Treat tachydysrhythmias with a beta-adrenergic antagonist (eg, propranolol 1 milligram, which can be repeated if well tolerated).
- Seizures are managed using standard regimens.
- Hydrocarbons referred to with the CHAMP acronym (camphor, halogenated hydrocarbons, aromatic hydrocarbons, metals, pesticides) have potential

inherent systemic toxicity or solubilize into toxic agents. GI decontamination using gastric emptying should be considered when exposure to these hydrocarbons has occurred, but is generally contraindicated in other hydrocarbon ingestions.

- The majority of hydrocarbon ingestions, which consist of aliphatic mixtures, are poorly absorbed from the GI tract and carry a risk of aspiration during GI decontamination measures.
- Activated charcoal and cathartics are of no benefit for any hydrocarbon ingestion.
- Hyperbaric oxygen therapy may be indicated for patients who develop significant carbon monoxide toxicity after exposure to methylene chloride.
- Because most fatalities occur in the first 24 to 48 hours, admit all patients who are symptomatic at the time of evaluation.
- Asymptomatic patients with a normal chest radiograph who remain symptom-free after 6 hours of observation can be discharged. All discharged patients should receive close follow-up for delayed toxicity.

For further reading in Tintinalli's *Emergency Medicine: A Comprehensive Study Guide*, 7th ed., see Chapter 193, "Hydrocarbons and Volatile Substances," by Paul M. Wax and Stella C. Wong.

114 CAUSTICS

Christian A. Tomaszewski

EPIDEMIOLOGY

- Caustic exposures in the United States totaled more than 130,000 in 2008. They consist of three groups: (1) intentional ingestions in adolescents and adults; (2) unintentional exposures in children; and (3) accidental exposures, often occupational. Although a minority, intentional exposures caused the most morbidity.
- Alkali exposures mainly result from cleaners, such as sodium hydroxide in drain openers and ammonium hydroxide in fertilizers. Acid exposures involve household and toilet cleaners, such as sulfuric and hydrochloric acid, and the more insidious rust remover, hydrofluoric acid, which is potentially lethal through dermal exposure.
- The most common caustic exposure is household bleach, with approximately 37,000 annual exposures. Although potentially lethal in large intentional ingestions, it rarely results in any morbidity among the countless incidental pediatric exposures each year.

PATHOPHYSIOLOGY

- The strength of a caustic and duration of the exposure determine the extent of injury. As a rule of thumb, injuries can be expected at pH <3 or >11.
- Alkalis penetrate deeply into tissue through liquefaction necrosis. Liquid alkali ingestions cause proximal damage to the esophagus, which may lead to stricture formation or perforation.
- Strong acids produce coagulation necrosis, with early eschar formation, which usually protects against deeper esophageal injury. Regardless, both esophageal and gastric injury can occur with acid ingestion.
- Hydrofluoric acid is a weak acid (pKa = 3.2) that can cause delayed morbidity from the fluoride component, which penetrates deeply into tissues, complexes with calcium and magnesium, and leads to cell death.

CLINICAL FEATURES

- Caustics can cause injury at various levels. Laryngotracheal injury is suggested by dysphonia or stridor. Injury to the GI tract usually manifests as dysphagia, odynophagia, epigastric pain, or vomiting. Direct injury to the lungs can occur from aspiration or inhalation of acid fumes.
- Esophageal injuries from caustic ingestion are classified by endoscopy as grades 1 to 3: (1) edema and hyperemia; (2) ulceration, blisters, and exudates (2A are non-circumferential and 2B circumferential or deeper); and (3) deep ulcerations and necrosis. Higher grades of injury are more likely to result in stricture or perforation in the first 1 to 2 weeks.
- Intentional injuries can cause severe GI tract injury without clinically obvious signs.
- Unintentional injuries, usually in children, may have esophageal injury even when asymptomatic, although stridor, drooling, or vomiting usually accompany serious esophageal injury (grade 2 or 3).
- Complications of severe caustic injury include shock from GI bleeding or perforation. Chest discomfort may signify mediastinitis.
- Dermal exposures usually produce local pain and irritation. However, hydrofluoric acid differs in its ability to cause deep and delayed tissue necrosis. At concentrations <20%, pain and erythema may not develop for 24 hours; at 20% to 50%, burns typically evolve within 8 hours. Burns from concentrations >50% can cause systemic toxicity with hypocalcemia, hypomagnesemia, and hyperkalemia, which can cause fatal ventricular dysrhythmias. Oral ingestions of

hydrofluoric acid result in earlier mortality through similar mechanisms.

DIAGNOSIS AND DIFFERENTIAL

- Accidental ingestions of household caustics in children usually require no workup if asymptomatic.
- Intentional ingestions, or ingestions of strong caustics may require the following labs: blood gas, electrolyte panel, hepatic profile, CBC, coagulation profile, lactate, and serum type and screen.
- Obtain serum calcium and magnesium levels and perform an ECG to evaluate for prolonged QT intervals or changes suggestive of hyperkalemia in cases of hydrofluoric acid exposure.
- Upright chest radiograph can be used to detect peritoneal or mediastinal free air. CT is useful when GI perforation is suspected.

EMERGENCY DEPARTMENT CARE AND DISPOSITION

- Administer 100% oxygen to any patient with respiratory symptoms. Strongly consider early intubation in patients with respiratory distress since rapid deterioration can develop and control of the airway can become difficult.
- Gastric decontamination is contraindicated in caustic ingestions. In cases of large ingestions of strong acids, a nasogastric tube can be inserted for removal of stomach contents.
- Dilution is only indicated if it can be performed within 30 minutes of ingestion in patients who can swallow without pain. Neutralization is not routinely recommended.
- Early diagnostic endoscopy is indicated after intentional caustic ingestions. In unintentional ingestions, endoscopy is recommended only if the patient is symptomatic with stridor, significant oropharyngeal burns, vomiting, drooling, or food refusal. Endoscopy should be performed within 12 hours of ingestion to avoid iatrogenic perforation.
- Steroids to decrease strictures are controversial and not routinely recommended.
- Prophylactic antibiotics are not indicated.
- Emergency laparotomy may be indicated for peritoneal signs or free air. Esophageal injuries with perforation may require surgery for mediastinitis. Delayed esophageal dilation or stenting may be necessary for strictures.
- Systemic toxicity from acid ingestions such as acidosis, hemolysis, coagulopathy, and renal failure should be appropriately managed.
- Treat ocular exposures, especially alkali, with copious irrigation and reassessment every 15 minutes. Conjunctival pH should be below 7.5 to 8.0 before irrigation is discontinued. Presence of corneal haziness or opacity, or limbal ischemia, requires ophthalmologic evaluation for possible anterior chamber irrigation.
- Dermal exposures to caustics require copious irrigation with water. Exceptions include exposures to lime or caustic powders such as cement, which must be brushed off before irrigation.
- Admit patients with symptomatic caustic ingestion. Grade 1 injuries of the esophagus can be discharged if tolerating oral intake. Grade 2A injuries require observation. Grade 2B and 3 injuries are at risk for perforation or bleeding and require admission to intensive care. Severe dermal burns may also require admission.
- Hydrofluoric acid dermal exposures require additional treatment after irrigation. Treat small areas of exposed skin with topical calcium gluconate gel (commercially available or use 3.5 grams of powder mixed with five ounces of water-soluble surgical lubricant), applied to the area for 10 to 15 minutes until pain control is achieved and repeated every 4 to 8 hours as needed.
- In non-digital areas, if relief is not obtained through topical application, or in cases of extensive exposure, consider intradermal calcium gluconate 5% (1:1 mix with NS) injected into the burn area with a maximum dose of 0.5 mL/cm^2. In digits and hands, calcium gluconate (10 mL of 10% in 40 mL of NS or D5W) can be infused into the radial artery of the affected extremity over 4 hours.
- Oral ingestions of hydrofluoric acid and severe dermal exposures (>20% concentration) require aggressive treatment: nasogastric aspiration of stomach contents within 60 minutes of ingestion followed by instillation of 300 mL of 10% calcium gluconate may be helpful; monitor serum calcium and magnesium levels closely and replace as needed; monitor and treat for hyperkalemia.
- Suspected disc battery ingestions require a chest radiograph to exclude esophageal entrapment, which requires prompt endoscopic removal to prevent esophageal perforation from local pressure necrosis and alkaline release. Batteries in the stomach can be managed expectantly with a repeat radiograph in 24 to 48 hours to insure distal passage.

For further reading in Tintinalli's *Emergency Medicine: A Comprehensive Study Guide*, 7th ed., see Chapter 194, "Caustics," by Nicole C. Bouchard and Wallace A. Carter.

115 PESTICIDES

Christian A. Tomaszewski

INSECTICIDES

- Pesticides include insecticides, herbicides, and rodenticides. Insecticides are responsible for over half of the poisonings and deaths.

ORGANOPHOSPHATES

EPIDEMIOLOGY

- The most common organophosphates are diazinon, acephate, malathion, parathion, and chlorpyrifos. Nerve gas agents, such as sarin and VX, are organophosphates used in terrorist attacks.

PATHOPHYSIOLOGY

- Organophosphates bind irreversibly to and inhibit cholinesterases in the nervous system and skeletal muscle, which leads to the accumulation of acetylcholine at synapses and neuromuscular junctions.
- Aging refers to the irreversible binding of the compound to the cholinesterase; once this occurs, antidotes are ineffective.

CLINICAL FEATURES

- Patients usually become symptomatic within 8 hours of dermal exposure to organophosphates; nerve gas agents (eg, VX gas) can cause immediate effects via dermal or inhalational routes. Fat-soluble agents (eg, fenthion) can cause delayed or persistent symptoms.
- Muscarinic overstimulation from cholinesterase inhibition results in a classic cholinergic crisis (Table 115-1). Exposure to nerve gas agents may lead initially to blurred vision with miosis.
- Nicotinic stimulation leads to muscle fasciculations and weakness, which is most pronounced in the respiratory system already compromised by excessive secretions from muscarinic effects. Nicotinic effects can also lead to paradoxical tachycardia and mydriasis.
- Central nervous system (CNS) effects, which often predominate in children, include tremor, restlessness, confusion, seizures, and coma.
- An intermediate syndrome, which occurs 1 to 4 days after acute poisoning, may present with paralysis or weakness of neck, facial, and respiratory muscles. Since cholinergic excess may not be evident, it can be missed and result in respiratory arrest if not treated.

TABLE 115-1	SLUDGE, DUMBELS, and "Killer Bees" Mnemonics for the Muscarinic Effects of Cholinesterase Inhibition
S	Salivation
L	Lacrimation
U	Urinary incontinence
D	Defecation
G	GI pain
E	Emesis
D	Defecation
U	Urination
M	Muscle weakness, miosis
B	Bradycardia, bronchorrhea, bronchospasm
E	Emesis
L	Lacrimation
S	Salivation
Killer Bees	Bradycardia, bronchorrhea, bronchospasm

- Delayed organophosphate-induced neuropathy occurs 1 to 3 weeks after acute poisoning from inhibition of neuronal esterase, causing a distal motor-sensory polyneuropathy.

DIAGNOSIS AND DIFFERENTIAL

- The diagnosis of organophosphate poisoning is clinical and based on recognition of the classic toxidrome. An odor of garlic or hydrocarbons may suggest exposure.
- Other clues to organophosphate poisoning include pulmonary edema on chest radiograph and prolonged QT, which is an independent predictor of toxicity.
- Although plasma and erythrocyte cholinesterase levels can confirm exposure, they are not clinically useful in the acute setting.

EMERGENCY DEPARTMENT CARE AND DISPOSITION

- Table 115-2 outlines the treatment for organophosphate poisoning.
- Primary decontamination and personal protective equipment (neoprene or nitrile) for health care workers is essential to prevent secondary contamination.
- Support airway and breathing with 100% oxygen, suctioning, and endotracheal intubation and mechanical ventilation when necessary; avoid succinylcholine

TABLE 115-2 Treatment for Organophosphate Poisoning

Decontamination	Protective clothing must be worn to prevent secondary poisoning of health care workers. Handle and dispose of all clothes as hazardous waste. Wash patient with soap and water. Handle and dispose of water runoff as hazardous waste.
Monitoring	Cardiac monitor, pulse oximeter, 100% oxygen.
Gastric lavage	No proven benefit (see text).
Activated charcoal	No proven benefit (see text).
Urinary alkalinization	No proven benefit (see text).
Atropine	1 milligram or more IV in an adult or 0.01-0.04 milligram/kg (but never <0.1 milligram) IV in children. Repeat every 5 min until tracheobronchial secretions attenuate.
Pralidoxime	1-2 grams for adults or 20-40 milligrams/kg (up to 1 gram) in children, mixed with normal saline and infused IV over 5-10 min. Continuous infusion often necessary.
Seizures	Benzodiazepines.

during RSI because of prolonged paralysis in organophosphate poisoning.

- Use atropine to reverse the muscarinic and central effects from parasympathetic stimulation. It is used in large amounts, titrating to drying of tracheobronchial secretions. Tachycardia is not a contraindication to its use.
- Response to pralidoxime is measured by clinical improvement in muscle weakness and fasciculations. It can be used for up to 48 hours post-poisoning, but its efficacy wanes with time. Pralidoxime is not recommended in asymptomatic patients.
- Watch mild asymptomatic exposures 6 to 8 hours in the ED. Contaminated clothing, especially leather, are potential sources of exposure and should be discarded.
- Significant poisonings will need admission to the ICU. The first 24 to 48 hours are critical and patients usually survive if they respond to treatment during that time period.

CARBAMATES

EPIDEMIOLOGY

- Carbamates are cholinesterase inhibitors and include the pesticides carbaryl, pirimicarb, propoxur, and trimethacarb as well as the pharmacological agents physostigmine, pyridostigmine, and neostigmine.

PATHOPHYSIOLOGY

- Like organophosphates, carbamates are absorbed through ingestion, inhalation, and dermal contact.
- Unlike organophosphates, carbamates bind only transiently to cholinesterase.

CLINICAL FEATURES

- Acute carbamate poisoning produces a cholinergic syndrome similar to organophosphates, but of shorter duration and less neurotoxicity.

DIAGNOSIS AND DIFFERENTIAL

- The diagnosis is clinical. Cholinesterase activity is of no clinical value.

EMERGENCY DEPARTMENT CARE AND DISPOSITION

- Initial treatment is the same as for organophosphates (Table 115-2).
- Use atropine for muscarinic symptoms.
- Pralidoxime is usually not indicated because symptoms typically resolve within 24 hours, and pralidoxime may exacerbate carbaryl poisoning.
- Mild poisonings can be discharged.
- Observe moderately symptomatic poisonings for up to 24 hours.

ORGANOCHLORINES

EPIDEMIOLOGY

- Organochlorines include DDT (dichlorodiphenyltrichloroethane), methoxychlor, endosulfan, toxaphene, and the therapeutic agent lindane.

PATHOPHYSIOLOGY

- Organochlorines are toxic via inhalation, ingestion, and dermal exposure. Through antagonism of γ-aminobutyric acid (GABA) at membranes, sodium channel permeability is decreased resulting in neuronal hyperexicitability. These agents can accumulate because of high lipid solubility.

CLINICAL FEATURES

- Acute poisoning primarily produces CNS stimulation and fever.
- Mild exposures can cause dizziness, ataxia, headache, tremor, and myoclonus.

- Severe exposures can cause seizures, coma, respiratory distress, and death.
- Exposure to concomitant hydrocarbon solvent causes cardiac sensitization to catecholamines and dysrhythmias.

DIAGNOSIS AND DIFFERENTIAL

- The diagnosis is clinical.

EMERGENCY DEPARTMENT CARE AND DISPOSITION

- Support airway and breathing as needed.
- Remove clothing and wash skin with soap and water.
- Consider activated charcoal or gastric lavage in recent, large ingestions. Cholestyramine may be useful in cases of chlordecone ingestion.
- Use benzodiazepines to treat seizures.
- Treat arrhythmias per Advanced Cardiac Life Support (ACLS) protocols, but avoid epinephrine due to toxic cardiac sensitization to catecholamines.

PYRETHRINS AND PYRETHROIDS

EPIDEMIOLOGY

- Natural pyrethrins and synthetic pyrethroids have replaced organophosphates as home insecticides because of their relative safety.

PATHOPHYSIOLOGY

- Toxicity occurs primarily through inhalation, although dermal or oral exposure can also occur.
- These agents block sodium channels in neurons, leading to neuronal excitability and repetitive discharge.

CLINICAL FEATURES

- The most common effect from these agents is allergic hypersensitivity, including dermatitis, bronchospasm, and anaphylaxis.
- In massive ingestions, gastrointestinal (GI) distress, and rarely tremors, paresthesias, and seizures can occur.

EMERGENCY DEPARTMENT CARE AND DISPOSITION

- Decontaminate eyes, skin, and GI tract.
- Treat symptomatic allergic reactions.

N,N-DIETHYL-3-METHYLBENZAMIDE

- *N,N*-diethyl-3-methylbenzamide (DEET) is an over-the-counter insect repellant toxic through dermal absorption.
- Systemic toxicity includes confusion, ataxia, tremors, and seizures. Large ingestions can cause hypotension and bradycardia.
- Decontaminate the skin with mild soap and water; administer activated charcoal for recent ingestions.
- Treat seizures with benzodiazepines.

HERBICIDES

- Herbicides are used as weed killers, and may be mixed in solvents, surfactants, and preservatives, all of which have potential toxicity.

CHLOROPHENOXY HERBICIDES

EPIDEMIOLOGY

- Chlorophenoxy compounds are synthetic plant hormones that kill broadleaf weeds.

CLINICAL FEATURES

- Local exposure can cause eye and mucous membrane irritation.
- Inhalation can cause dyspnea and pulmonary edema.
- Ingestion can lead to nausea, vomiting, and diarrhea.
- With severe systemic toxicity hypotension, dysrhythmias, altered mental status, seizures, and rhabdomyolysis can occur.

DIAGNOSIS AND DIFFERENTIAL

- The diagnosis is clinical.
- Laboratory findings may include metabolic acidosis, rhabdomyolysis, and hepatorenal dysfunction.

EMERGENCY DEPARTMENT CARE AND DISPOSITION

- Care is primarily supportive and includes decontamination and respiratory assistance.
- Consider alkalinization of the urine with intravenous sodium bicarbonate to increase elimination.
- Consider hemodialysis for massive ingestions.
- Observe mild exposures for 4 to 6 hours prior to discharge.

BIPYRIDYL HERBICIDES

PATHOPHYSIOLOGY

- Paraquat and diquat are caustic, causing local irritation and burns, as well as systemic toxicity leading to multiorgan failure.

CLINICAL FEATURES

- Paraquat is extremely caustic to skin, mucous membranes, and cornea causing ulceration. Inhalation can cause cough, dyspnea, chest pain, pulmonary edema, epistaxis, and hemoptysis that can last for weeks.
- Ingestion causes mucosal and esophageal ulceration, abdominal pain, vomiting, and potential hypovolemia.
- Systemic effects include acute renal, cardiac, and hepatic failure followed by multiorgan dysfunction.
- Delayed effects include progressive pulmonary fibrosis with refractory hypoxemia.

DIAGNOSIS AND DIFFERENTIAL

- Differential includes other corrosives and herbicides.
- Qualitative and quantitative urine and blood paraquat levels are available; plasma levels >0.4 milligram/L 10 hours postingestion predict death.
- Chest radiography early on may show pneumomediastinum from esophageal perforation followed by lung parenchyma consolidation.
- Additional laboratory findings include evidence of multiorgan failure.
- Esophagoscopy may be indicated to define the extent of upper GI corrosive injury.

EMERGENCY DEPARTMENT CARE AND DISPOSITION

- Early aggressive decontamination with activated charcoal (1-2 grams/kg) should be repeated every 4 hours.
- Institute charcoal hemoperfusion early for paraquat poisoning.
- Use low inspired oxygen fraction (<21%) to reduce pulmonary injury.

RODENTICIDES

EPIDEMIOLOGY

- Rodenticides are classified as non-anticoagulants (Table 115-3) or anticoagulants.
- Warfarin rodenticides can contain simple warfarin or, due to rodent resistance, superwarfarin, which includes bordifacoum, diphenacoum, coumafuryl, and bromadoline.

CLINICAL FEATURES

- Most one-time ingestions of warfarin anticoagulants do not cause bleeding problems.
- Anticoagulant effects develop within 12 to 24 hours for warfarin anticoagulants and 24 to 48 hours for superwarfarins.
- The duration of action is short for regular warfarin, with a half-life of 42 hours, while superwarfarins that have a half-life or 120 days.
- Toxicity from anticoagulants can be manifested as ecchymosis, mucosal bleeding, hemoptysis, hematuria, and pelvic or GI bleeding.

TABLE 115-3 Non-Anticoagulant Rodenticides

AGENT	TOXICITY	CLINICAL EFFECTS	TREATMENT
Arsenic	Severe	Vomiting and diarrhea, cardiovascular collapse	Succimer
Barium carbonate	Severe	Vomiting and diarrhea, dysrhythmia, respiratory failure, paralysis	Gastric lavage with sodium or magnesium sulfate; potassium replacement
Phosphorus	Severe	Burns, cardiovascular collapse	Lavage with potassium permanganate
N-3-Pyridylmethyl-*N*′-p-nitrophenyl urea (Vacor)	Severe	GI symptoms, insulin deficient hyperglycemia, and Diabetic Ketoacidosis (DKA)	Nicotinamide IV
Sodium fluoroacetate	Severe	Vomiting, respiratory depression, pulmonary	Supportive care
Strychnine	Severe	Awake seizure-like activity	Benzodiazepines
Thallium	Severe	Early GI, respiratory failure, and dysrhythmias	Oral Prussian blue
Zinc phosphide	Severe	Vomiting, shock, hypocalcemia	Intragastric alkalinization
α-Naphthyl-thiourea	Moderate	Pulmonary edema	Supportive care
Cholecalciferol	Moderate	Hypercalcemia	Saline, furosemide, steroids
Bromethalin	Low	Tremors, focal seizures	Benzodiazepines
Norbormide	Low	Vasoconstrictive tissue hypoxia	Supportive care
Red squill	Low	Vomiting, diarrhea, hyperkalemia, heart block with ventricular dysrhythmias	Treat as digoxin

DIAGNOSIS AND DIFFERENTIAL

- The presence of an unexplained coagulopathy suggests possible anticoagulant poisoning.
- Prolongation of the INR can be seen with moderate ingestions and large doses can prolong the PTT as well.
- In suspected ingestions, INR should be checked postingestion at 12 to 24 hours for warfarin, and 24 to 48 hours for superwarfarin.

EMERGENCY DEPARTMENT TREATMENT AND DISPOSITION

- Treat elevated INR with vitamin K_1. For regular warfarin ingestions, the oral daily dose is 20 milligrams (1-5 milligrams in children) divided in two to four doses. The same starting dose can be used for superwarfarins; however, daily divided doses of up to 100 milligrams for many months may be required.
- After initiating treatment with vitamin K_1, follow INR regularly—at least every 24 hours. When discontinuing the therapy, a follow up INR should be obtained in 24 to 48 hours.
- Active hemorrhage requires aggressive therapy with intravenous vitamin K_1 and fresh frozen plasma. Consider prothrombin complex concentrate or recombinant activated factor VII for refractory bleeding.
- Asymptomatic accidental ingestions of large amounts of superwarfarin can be managed as an outpatient with an INR checked 24 to 48 hours postingestion.

For further reading in Tintinalli's *Emergency Medicine: A Comprehensive Study Guide*, 7th ed., see Chapter 195, "Pesticides," by Walter C. Robey III and William J. Meggs.

116 METALS AND METALLOIDS

D. Adam Algren

LEAD

EPIDEMIOLOGY

- Lead is the most common chronic metal poisoning. Both ingestion and inhalation can result in clinical lead toxicity.

PATHOPHYSIOLOGY

- Lead toxicity results in injury to multiple organ systems but primarily involves the nervous, cardiovascular, hematologic, and renal systems.
- Central nervous system (CNS) neuronal injury results in cerebral edema and increased intracranial pressure. Lead toxicity may also produce peripheral neuropathies.
- Lead interferes with porphyrin metabolism and heme synthesis causing anemia.

CLINICAL FEATURES

- Table 116-1 lists the common signs and symptoms of lead poisoning by organ system.

DIAGNOSIS AND DIFFERENTIAL

- Though an elevated serum lead level (>10 micrograms/dL) confirms the diagnosis, results are often not immediately available.
- Radiopaque material may be present in the gastrointestinal (GI) tract following acute ingestion. With chronic exposure, children may develop horizontal metaphyseal bands in long bones, especially involving the knee ("lead lines").
- Other laboratory findings suggestive of lead poisoning include anemia with basophilic stippling of erythrocytes, hemolytic anemia, nephritis, and/or hepatitis.

TABLE 116-1 Common Manifestations of Lead Poisoning

SYSTEM	CLINICAL MANIFESTATIONS
Central nervous system	Acute toxicity: encephalopathy, seizures, altered mental status, papilledema, optic neuritis, ataxia Chronic toxicity: headache, irritability, depression, fatigue, mood and behavioral changes, memory deficit, sleep disturbance
Peripheral nervous system	Paresthesias, motor weakness (classic is wrist drop), depressed or absent deep tendon reflexes, sensory function intact
GI	Abdominal pain (mostly with acute poisoning), constipation, diarrhea, toxic hepatitis
Renal	Acute toxicity: Fanconi syndrome (renal tubular acidosis with aminoaciduria, glucosuria, and phosphaturia) Chronic toxicity: interstitial nephritis, renal insufficiency, hypertension, gout
Hematologic	Hypoproliferative and/or hemolytic anemia; basophilic stippling (rare and nonspecific)
Reproductive	Decreased libido, impotence, sterility, abortions, premature births, decreased or abnormal sperm production

EMERGENCY DEPARTMENT CARE AND DISPOSITION

- Consider whole-bowel irrigation with polyethylene glycol solution for lead ingestion, especially when radiopaque material is visible on a radiograph. The adult rate of instillation is 1500 to 2000 mL/h, and the pediatric rate of instillation is 500 to 1000 mL/h.
- Guidelines for chelation therapy are presented in Table 116-2.
- Patients requiring parenteral chelation therapy or whose only option is to return to the environment producing the lead exposure should be admitted to the hospital.

ARSENIC

EPIDEMIOLOGY

- Arsenic is found in agricultural chemicals, insecticides, contaminated well water, and mining/smelting operations.
- Exposure to inorganic arsenic can result in significant toxicity whereas organic arsenic is minimally toxic.

PATHOPHYSIOLOGY

- Arsenic inhibits multiple enzymes and uncouples oxidative phosphorylation with effects on multiple organ systems.

CLINICAL FEATURES

- Clinical features of arsenic toxicity are summarized in Table 116-3.
- Chronic poisoning causes stocking glove peripheral neuropathies, hyperkeratosis, peripheral vascular disease, malaise, myalgia, abdominal pain, memory loss, and personality changes.

DIAGNOSIS AND DIFFERENTIAL

- Consider arsenic poisoning in patients with severe vomiting and diarrhea causing hypotension.
- Other diagnoses to consider include septic shock, encephalopathy, Guillain–Barre syndrome, Addison's disease, hypo- and hyperthyroidism, porphyria, and other metal poisonings.
- Acutely, the electrocardiogram (ECG) may demonstrate a prolonged QT interval; abdominal radiographs may reveal radiopaque arsenic.
- Transverse white lines of the nails (Mees' lines) may occur 4 to 6 weeks following ingestion.

TABLE 116-2 Guidelines for Chelation Therapy in Lead-Poisoned Patients*

SEVERITY [BLOOD LEAD LEVEL (MICROGRAMS/DL)]	DOSE
Encephalopathy	Dimercaprol, 75 milligrams/m^2 (or 4 milligrams/kg) IM every 4 h for 5 d *and* Edetate calcium disodium, 1500 milligrams/m^2/d, for 5 d as a continuous IV infusion started 4 h after dimercaprol
Symptomatic Adults: blood lead >100 Children: blood lead >69	Dimercaprol *and* Edetate calcium disodium (as described above) *or* Edetate calcium disodium (alone) *or* Succimer (as described below)
Asymptomatic Adults: blood lead 70-100 Children: blood lead 45-69	Succimer, 350 milligrams/m^2 (or 10 milligrams/kg) PO every 8 h for 5 d, then every 12 h for 14 d
Asymptomatic Adults: blood lead <70 Children: blood lead <45	Routine chelation not indicated Remove patient from source of exposure

*General guidelines. Consult with medical toxicologist or regional poison center for specifics and dosing.

TABLE 116-3 Clinical Features of Arsenic Toxicity

ONSET OF SYMPTOMS	CLINICAL FEATURES BY ORGAN SYSTEM
Acute toxicity (10 min to several hours)	GI: nausea, vomiting, cholera-like diarrhea Cardiovascular: hypotension; tachycardia; dysrhythmias, including torsades de pointes; secondary myocardial ischemia Pulmonary: acute lung injury (noncardiogenic pulmonary edema) Renal: acute renal failure Central neurologic: encephalopathy
Subacute toxicity (1-3 wk after acute exposure or with chronic exposure)	Central neurologic: headache, confusion, delirium, personality changes Peripheral neurologic: sensory and motor neuropathy Cardiovascular: QT-interval prolongation Pulmonary: cough, alveolar infiltrates Dermatologic: rash, alopecia, Mees' lines
Chronic toxicity (ongoing low-level occupational or environmental exposure)	Dermatologic: hyperpigmentation, keratoses, Bowen disease, squamous and basal cell carcinoma Cardiovascular: hypertension, peripheral arterial disease Endocrine: diabetes mellitus Oncologic: lung and skin cancer

TABLE 116-4	Guidelines for Chelation Therapy in Arsenic-Poisoned Patients
CHELATOR	DOSE
Dimercaprol	3-5 milligrams/kg IM every 4 h for 2 d, followed by 3-5 milligrams/kg IM every 6-12 h until able to switch to succimer
Succimer	10 milligrams/kg PO every 8 h for 5 d, followed by 10 milligrams/kg PO every 12 h

- Definitive diagnosis depends on 24-hour urine arsenic levels.

EMERGENCY DEPARTMENT CARE AND DISPOSITION

- Treat hypotension with aggressive volume resuscitation with isotonic crystalloid, and vasopressors for fluid-refractory shock.
- Manage dysrhythmias according to Advanced Cardiac Life Support (ACLS) protocols, but avoid drugs that prolong the QT interval (class IA, IC, and III agents).
- Consider gastric lavage if the patient presents early following acute ingestion. Whole-bowel irrigation with polyethylene glycol solution is indicated for patients in whom abdominal radiographs demonstrate radiopaque material.
- Guidelines for inpatient chelation therapy with dimercaprol and outpatient treatment of stable patients with succimer are presented in Table 116-4.
- Hospitalization is recommended for patients with severe symptoms, those requiring parenteral chelation, and those with suicidal or homicidal intent.

MERCURY

EPIDEMIOLOGY

- Elemental mercury is present in older thermometers and exposures occur via inhalation, especially when vacuumed or heated. Ingestion of elemental mercury typically does not result in toxicity.
- Organic mercury is used in wood preservatives, fungicides, pesticides, and is also found in contaminated seafood. Absorption primarily occurs via the GI tract.

PATHOPHYSIOLOGY

- Similar to other heavy metals, mercury binds to sulfhydryl groups and affects multiple enzymes and organ systems.

CLINICAL FEATURES

- Inhalation of elemental mercury can result in fever, cough, dyspnea, vomiting, and headache that can progress to acute respiratory failure.
- Ingestion of inorganic mercury salts results in corrosive injury to the GI tract: vomiting, diarrhea, abdominal pain, and GI bleeding may occur. Acute renal failure often accompanies significant toxicity.
- Chronic inorganic mercury toxicity is associated with multiple neurologic effects including tremor, fatigue, depression, and headaches. Erethism refers the constellation of emotional lability, shyness, irritability, insomnia, and blushing. Acrodynia ("pink disease") is characterized by a generalized rash, edema/erythema of the palms/soles, excessive sweating, fever, irritability, and muscle weakness.
- Organic mercury poisoning is usually seen with chronic ingestion and is associated with headache, tremor, fatigue, ataxia, blindness, muscle spasticity, and dementia.

DIAGNOSIS AND DIFFERENTIAL

- A history of exposure or physical findings of erethism or acrodynia may suggest the diagnosis.
- An elevated 24-hour urine mercury level confirms the diagnosis in cases of elemental and inorganic mercury exposures. An elevated whole blood mercury level is necessary to confirm poisoning from organic mercury compounds.
- The differential diagnosis of symptoms caused by mercury poisoning is extensive and includes other causes of encephalopathy, tremor, gastroenteritis, and acute renal failure.

EMERGENCY DEPARTMENT CARE AND DISPOSITION

- Supportive care and removal from exposure are the most important aspects in managing mercury poisoning. Intubation may be necessary in cases of respiratory failure associated with elemental mercury vapor exposure.
- Chelation is most effective in cases of elemental and inorganic mercury poisoning and should be considered in cases with significant symptoms (Table 116-5). Parenteral chelation is contraindicated in cases of organic mercury poisoning due to the potential to exacerbate CNS symptoms.

TABLE 116-5 Guidelines for Chelation Therapy in Mercury-Poisoned Patients

	INORGANIC MERCURY, ELEMENTAL MERCURY	ORGANIC MERCURY
Severe poisoning	Dimercaprol, 5 milligrams/kg IM every 4 h for 2 d, followed by 2.5 milligrams/kg IM every 6 h for 2 d, followed by 2.5 milligrams/kg IM every 12-24 h until clinical improvement occurs or until able to switch to succimer therapy	Succimer, 10 milligrams/kg PO every 8 h for 5 d, then every 12 h for 14 d
Mild poisoning and chronic poisoning	Succimer, 10 milligrams/kg PO every 8 h for 5 d, then every 12 h for 14 d	No proven benefit for chelation therapy

For further reading in Tintinalli's *Emergency Medicine: A Comprehensive Study Guide*, 7th ed., see Chapter 197, "Metals and Metalloids," by Heather Long and Lewis S. Nelson.

117 INDUSTRIAL TOXINS AND CYANIDE

Christian A. Tomaszewski

EPIDEMIOLOGY

- Chemicals are considered hazardous if they present a risk to health or physical safety.
- Children have increased sensitivity to hazardous materials due to higher minute volumes and smaller airways that increase susceptibility to respiratory toxicity, and thinner skin and larger surface area, that increase dermal absorption.
- Common industrial toxins that cause respiratory and metabolic toxicity are listed in Table 117-1.

RESPIRATORY TOXINS

- Toxicity from airborne agents is affected by concentration, duration, and exposure in an enclosed space. Host factors such as metabolic rate, preexisting lung disease, and allergies are also important.
- Treatment starts with removal of the victim from the source, delivery of 100% oxygen, and bronchodilators for bronchospasm.
- Physical examination should focus on the presence of burns, singed nasal hairs, soot, hoarseness, cough, carbonaceous sputum, and respiratory difficulty.

TABLE 117-1 Common Signs and Symptoms of Exposure to Hazardous Chemicals

TOXIN	SUBSTANCES	SYMPTOMS	ANTIDOTES
Respiratory	Phosgene Chlorine Vinyl chloride Nitrogen oxides Ammonia	Respiratory distress Pulmonary edema	Supportive care
Metabolic	Cyanide Hydrogen sulfide Carbon monoxide	Coma Seizures Cardiac arrest	Hydroxocobalamin or cyanide kit for cyanide Sodium nitrite for hydrogen sulfide Oxygen (hyperbaric) for carbon monoxide

- Antibiotics and steroids are usually not indicated in toxic inhalations, except possibly in nitrogen dioxide exposure or in patients with preexisting asthma and bronchospasm.
- Appropriate laboratory tests include carboxyhemoglobin, methemoglobin, lactate, ECG, and chest radiography.

PHOSGENE

- Phosgene is widely used in the production of plastics, dyes, polyurethane, and pesticides.
- Phosgene forms hydrochloric acid, causing lower airway burns with noncardiogenic pulmonary edema that can be delayed as much as 24 hours.
- The main symptoms after inhalation are dyspnea and chest tightness.
- Large exposures can cause mucous membrane irritation with pulmonary edema within 4 hours.
- Care is supportive. A 24-hour observation period is recommended for asymptomatic patients with definite exposure. Recovery can be expected in 3 to 4 days.

CHLORINE

- Chlorine is widely available and used in water treatment, paper manufacturing, and industrial lab work.
- Chlorine is a green-yellow gas with good warning properties because of its acrid, pungent odor. Because of its intermediate water solubility, it can cause both airway damage and pulmonary edema.
- Chlorine gas forms hydrochloric and hypochlorous acids and oxidants on contact with moist membranes.
- Early eye and upper airway irritation accompany mild exposures.

- Severe exposures cause coughing, hoarseness, and pulmonary edema, usually within 6 hours.
- Provide supportive care with humidified oxygen and bronchodilators as needed.
- The use of nebulized sodium bicarbonate and steroids is controversial.

NITROGEN OXIDES

- Nitrogen dioxide and other nitrogen oxides are found in silo gas ("silo filler disease"), combustion, blast weapons, obscurants, and certain industrial processes.
- Oxides of nitrogen have low water solubility leading primarily to lower airway toxicity.
- Nitrogen dioxide is slowly converted to nitric acid in the alveoli.
- A triphasic response to toxicity starts with mild discomfort even with high concentrations, accompanied by dyspnea and flu-like symptoms.
- Patients then have mild improvement or persistent symptoms.
- Finally, 24 to 72 hours later, there may be worsening dyspnea due to ensuing pulmonary edema.
- Methemoglobinemia may occur after nitrogen oxide exposure.
- Although unproven, early corticosteroids have been used for acute lung injury.

AMMONIA

- Ammonia is a common component of various chemicals and fertilizers, as used in the production of plastics.
- It is highly water-soluble, forming ammonium hydroxide on contact with wet surfaces.
- Immediate symptoms include mucous membrane, eye, and throat irritation.
- Massive exposures, especially in enclosed spaces, can lead to lower airway irritation with bronchospasm and pulmonary edema.
- Supportive care with humidified oxygen and bronchodilators is the main treatment.
- Eye exposures to concentrated ammonia require aggressive ocular irrigation and evaluation for corneal burns.

METABOLIC TOXINS

HYDROGEN SULFIDE

- Hydrogen sulfide is a colorless gas found in petroleum industry and sites of organic decomposition, such as sewers and manure pits.
- It is the most common cause of fatal gas inhalational exposure.
- Hydrogen sulfide inhibits cytochrome oxidase a_3, uncoupling oxidative phosphorylation, which causes lactic acidosis from cellular asphyxia.
- High concentrations or prolonged exposure blunts the ability to detect the characteristic rotten egg odor.
- Respiratory and ocular irritation is common after exposure.
- High concentrations can lead to syncope, seizures, and death within a few breaths.
- Delayed pulmonary edema and corneal ulceration can occur after massive exposure.
- Treatment is primarily supportive and includes prompt removal from the scene, dermal and ocular decontamination, and administration of 100% oxygen.
- Consider administration of the nitrite component of the cyanide antidote kit (see below) withholding the thiosulfate portion.

CYANIDE

- Cyanide is found in chemical laboratories and in industry, particularly plastics, electroplating, mining, precious metal reclamation, and hide preparation. It is also used as a rodenticide, fumigant, and fertilizer.
- The burning of wool, synthetic fabrics, and certain plastics can result in liberation of hydrogen cyanide.
- Cyanide avidly binds to cytochrome a_3, shutting down oxidative phosphorylation for cellular respiration; therefore, tissues like the brain and heart with high oxygen consumption are the most affected.
- Chronic low dose exposure to cyanogens can occur from foods and inhalation of cigarette smoke. Detoxification in these cases occurs naturally through enzymatic transformation of thiocyanate by rhodanese.
- Inhalational exposure to hydrogen cyanide gas causes immediate symptoms. At concentrations less than 50 ppm, patients may experience anxiety, dyspnea, palpitations, and headache. Higher concentrations can cause severe dyspnea, syncope, seizures, and dysrhythmias. Continued exposure or higher concentrations can cause coma, cardiovascular collapse, and death.
- Ingestion of cyanide usually leads to symptoms within minutes.
- Signs and symptoms of acute cyanide toxicity are listed in Table 117-2.
- Delayed cyanide toxicity may be seen after ingestion of acetonitrile, a cosmetic nail polish remover, and amygdalin from apricot pits. Prolonged infusions of sodium nitroprusside can also lead to mild cyanide toxicity.

TABLE 117-2 Signs and Symptoms of Acute Cyanide Toxicity

Cardiovascular	
Tachycardia	Mild
Hypertension	↓
Bradycardia	↓
Hypotension	↓
Cardiovascular collapse	↓
Asystole	Severe
Central nervous system	
Headache	Mild
Drowsiness	↓
Seizures	↓
Coma	Severe
Pulmonary	
Dyspnea	Mild
Tachypnea	↓
Apnea	Severe

- The diagnosis of cyanide poisoning is primarily clinical.
- The odor of bitter almonds supports the diagnosis of cyanide toxicity, but only 60% to 80% of the populations can smell this.
- Table 117-3 lists the laboratory findings in cyanide poisoning. The hallmark is an unexplained metabolic acidosis and plasma lactate levels >10 mmol/L are predictive of toxic cyanide levels.
- Treatment of cyanide toxicity should not wait for whole blood cyanide levels, but should be administered promptly and empirically when exposure is suspected and signs and symptoms present.
- Initially, treatment should focus on aggressive supportive care: provide 100% oxygen to all patients and support the airway and breathing.
- Treat hypotension with crystalloids and pressors.
- Consider sodium bicarbonate in severe acidosis, which may enhance efficacy of cyanide antidotes.
- Table 117-4 lists the specific antidotal treatment for cyanide poisoning in the adult, and Table 117-5 lists the hemoglobin-based dosing of sodium nitrite recommended for children.
- Amyl nitrite can be administered via inhalation when vascular access is not immediately obtained.
- The FDA has approved a new antidote for cyanide, hydroxocobalamin (vitamin B_{12A}). Due to its low toxicity, it is ideal for questionable cases and smoke inhalation victims where methemoglobin formation from nitrite therapy may be detrimental. Administer 2 vials, each 2.5 grams reconstituted in 100 mL NS, over 7.5 minutes, for a total dose of 5 grams in 200 mL NS over 15 minutes. Although not approved for pediatric use, a dose of 70 milligrams/kg has been suggested. Side effects include red discoloration of the skin and urine, transient hypertension, and rarely, anaphylactoid reactions.
- Hyperbaric oxygen is recommended only for cyanide-poisoned patients with concomitant carbon monoxide poisoning.
- Observe patients with mild to moderate symptoms from cyanide exposure prior to initiating treatment.

TABLE 117-3 Anticipated Laboratory Findings in Cyanide Poisoning

TEST	RESULT	CAUSE
Serum electrolytes	Elevated anion gap	Lactic acidosis from anaerobic metabolism
Arterial blood gases	Metabolic acidosis Normal Pao_2	Oxygenation initially normal
Lactate	>10 mmol/L	Correlates with toxic cyanide level
Measured oxygen saturation by co-oximetry	Normal	Hemoglobin retains normal oxygen-carrying capacity
Measured arterial-mixed venous oxygen difference	Decreased	Decreased tissue oxygen consumption
Whole-blood cyanide level	Toxic >0.5 microgram/mL Fatal >2.5 micrograms/mL	Note: plasma cyanide levels are roughly one tenth of the whole-blood cyanide levels
Fire victims	Elevated carboxyhemoglobin level	Carbon monoxide generated by incomplete combustion Synergistic toxicity with cyanide

TABLE 117-4 Treatment of Cyanide Poisoning in Adults

	ROUTE	TREATMENT
Prehospital	Inhaled	Amyl nitrite: crack vial and inhale over 30 s*
Traditional	IV	(1) Sodium nitrite 3% solution: 10 mL (300 milligrams) IV given over no less than 5 min† (2) Sodium thiosulfate 25% solution: 50 mL (12.5 grams) IV (may repeat sodium thiosulfate once at half dose 25 mL if symptoms persist)
Alternate	IV	Hydroxocobalamin 5 grams over 15 min (may combine with sodium thiosulfate)

*Not necessary if IV is in place.
†Avoid nitrites in the presence of severe hypotension if diagnosis is unclear.

TABLE 117-5 Treatment of Cyanide Poisoning in Children

100% oxygen	
Sodium nitrite 3% solution: adjusted according to hemoglobin level, given IV over no less than 5 min*	
HEMOGLOBIN (GRAMS/100 ML)	SODIUM THIOSULFATE 3% SOLUTION (ML/KG)
7	0.19
8	0.22
9	0.25
10	0.27
11	0.30
12	0.33
13	0.36
14	0.39
Sodium thiosulfate 25% solution: 1.65 mL/kg IV	
Repeat sodium thiosulfate once at half dose (0.825 mL/kg) if symptoms persist	
Monitor methemoglobin and keep level <30%	

*Avoid nitrites in the presence of severe hypotension if diagnosis is unclear.

- Treat severely ill patients with altered mental status and bradycardia or hypotension immediately if cyanide is suspected. Hypotension is not a contraindication for nitrite therapy, but one may want to substitute hydroxocobalamin, especially for smoke inhalation cases with high carboxyhemoglobin levels.

For further reading in Tintinalli's *Emergency Medicine: A Comprehensive Study Guide*, 7th ed., see Chapter 198, "Industrial Toxins," by Chip Gresham and Frank LoVecchio.

118 VITAMINS AND HERBALS

Christian A. Tomaszewski

VITAMINS

- The fat-soluble vitamins A, D, and E are the most toxic vitamins (Table 118-1).
- The water-soluble vitamins niacin (B_3), pyridoxine (B_6), and ascorbate (C) have toxic potential.

TABLE 118-1 Symptoms of Hypervitaminosis

VITAMIN	SYMPTOMS
Vitamin A	Chronic toxicity: blurred vision, appetite loss, abnormal skin pigmentation, hair loss, dry skin, pruritus, long-bone pain, bone fractures, rare cases of pseudotumor cerebri and hepatic failure
Vitamin D	Subacute toxicity: hypercalcemia, anorexia, nausea, abdominal pain, lethargy, weight loss, polyuria, constipation, confusion, and coma
Vitamin E	Chronic toxicity: nausea, fatigue, headache, weakness, and blurred vision
Vitamin B_1 (thiamine)	No toxicity observed, even with ingestion of large doses over prolonged periods
Vitamin B_2 (riboflavin)	No toxicity observed, regardless of amount ingested
Vitamin B_3 (niacin)	Acute toxicity: niacin flush, dose >100 milligrams, redness, burning, and itching of the face, neck, and chest, rarely hypotension Chronic toxicity: doses >2000 milligrams/d, abnormalities of liver function, impaired glucose tolerance, hyperuricemia, skin dryness, and discoloration
Vitamin B_6 (pyridoxine)	Subacute and chronic toxicity: doses >5 grams/d or more over several weeks, peripheral neuropathy with unstable gait, numbness of the feet, similar symptoms in the hands and arms, marked loss of position and vibration senses
Vitamin B_{12}	No toxicity observed, even with ingestion of large doses
Folate	No toxicity observed, even with ingestion of large doses
Vitamin C (ascorbate)	Chronic toxicity: attacks of gout, nephrolithiasis, intrarenal deposition of oxalate crystals with renal failure, large doses can produce diarrhea and abdominal cramps

FAT-SOLUBLE VITAMINS (A, D, E, K)

EPIDEMIOLOGY

- Hypervitaminosis A usually occurs in children given excessive high-potency supplements; in adults, high doses of vitamin A must be ingested chronically to cause toxicity.
- Wheat germ, corn, soybean, sunflower seed, and cod liver are foods naturally high in vitamin E content.
- Vitamin D activity comes from calciferol (D_3), which is converted in the body to 1,25-dihydroxycholecalciferol, the physiologically active form of vitamin D, and ergocalciferol (D_2).
- Vitamin K is absorbed from the diet and produced by enteric bacteria.

PATHOPHYSIOLOGY

- Dietary vitamin A is converted to retinyl esters, absorbed, and stored in the liver. When liver storage capacity is exceeded, blood levels of retinyl ester circulate in the blood and can cause cell membrane injury.
- The final metabolite of vitamin D, 1,25-dihydroxyhydrocalciferol, causes increased serum calcium and phosphorus levels, which are responsible for the toxic effects of hypervitaminosis D.
- Vitamin E is metabolized to a toxic compound in high doses that acts as a competitive inhibitor of vitamin K–dependent gamma-carboxylation, thereby increasing daily vitamin K requirement. High levels of vitamin E inhibit platelet aggregation through the production of thromboxane.
- Unlike other fat-soluble vitamins, vitamin K is not stored by the body, but excreted in the bile and urine. Megadoses of menadione (vitamin K_3) can cause cellular toxicity.

CLINICAL FEATURES

- Symptoms of hypervitaminosis are listed in Table 118-1.

EMERGENCY DEPARTMENT CARE

- Discontinuation of exogenous fat-soluble vitamins usually leads to resolution of symptoms without specific treatment.
- Treat hypercalcemia from hypervitaminosis D by decreasing oral calcium intake and administering IV saline and the bisphosphonate, pamidronate disodium.
- Consider monitoring coagulation and liver function in overdoses of vitamin K.

B VITAMINS

- Vitamins B_1 (thiamine) and B_2 (riboflavin) are not stored in the body and therefore are nontoxic in overdose. Due to rate-limited GI absorption, excessive ingestion of vitamin B_{12} (cyanocobalamin) is nontoxic, though parenteral (IM) overdoses can lead to temporary skin changes.
- Vitamin B_3 (niacin) consists of water-soluble nicotinic acid and its active metabolite nicotinamide.
- Vitamin B_6 inactivates levodopa, which may be problematic in patients with Parkinson's disease.
- Discontinue exogenous intake of vitamins B_3 and B_6, which will improve symptoms without further specific treatment.

HERBALS

- Up to one-third of US patients use complementary and alternative medicines, many of which contain herbal preparations. Less than a third of patients divulge their use of herbal medications to their physicians.
- Herbal products may cause harm through toxic compounds (eg, digitoxin in foxglove) or contaminants (eg, lead).
- Many herbal products can interact with prescription medications. For example, gingko increases the risk of bleeding with aspirin and warfarin; grapefruit juice inhibits metabolism of multiple drugs through intestinal CYP3A4; St. John's wort decreases serum levels of cyclosporine and digoxin.
- Table 118-2 lists potential toxic effects of a number of herbal compounds.

TABLE 118-2 Some Potentially Toxic Herbal Agents

AGENT	GENERAL USE	ADVERSE EFFECT
Black cohosh	To delay or treat menopause	Nausea, vomiting, dizziness, weakness
Chaparral (creosote bush)	Antioxidant effects, analgesia	Potentially hepatotoxic and nephrotoxic
Comfrey	Bone and teeth building, variety of other uses	Potentially hepatotoxic
Ephedra	Weight loss	Hypertension, contraindicated for patients with hypertension, diabetes, or glaucoma
Hawthorn	Congestive heart failure	Additive toxicity with prescribed cardioactive steroids
Juniper	Diuretic	Hallucinogenic, may also cause renal toxicity, nausea, and vomiting
Lobelia	As an expectorant or for treatment of asthma	Anticholinergic syndrome
Nutmeg	Dyspepsia, muscle aches, and arthritis	Hallucinations, GI upset, agitation, coma, miosis, and hypertension
Pennyroyal	Rubefacient, delaying menses, abortifacient	Hepatotoxicity
Pyrrolizidine alkaloids	Pulmonary ailments	Hepatic veno-occlusive disease
Sabah	Weight loss	Pulmonary toxicity
Wormwood	Dyspepsia	Absinthism: restlessness, vertigo, tremor, paresthesias, delirium
Yohimbe	Aphrodisiac	Hallucinations, weakness, hypertension, and paralysis

For further reading in Tintinalli's *Emergency Medicine: A Comprehensive Study Guide*, 7th ed., see Chapter 199, "Vitamins and Herbals," by G. Richard Braen and Prashant Joshi.

119 DYSHEMOGLOBINEMIAS

Kristine L. Bott

- Dyshemoglobinemias are a group of disorders caused by functionally altered hemoglobin that is unable to bind to oxygen. The most clinically significant dyshemoglobinemias are methemoglobin, sulfhemoglobin, and carboxyhemoglobin.

METHEMOGLOBINEMIA

PATHOPHYSIOLOGY

- Methemoglobinemia can develop in the presence of oxidant stress caused by drugs or chemicals. There is also a hereditary form.
- Methemoglobinemia causes a shift of the oxyhemoglobin dissociation curve, causing more avid oxygen binding that leads to tissue hypoxia.
- Medications that can precipitate methemoglobinemia include phenazopyridine (Pyridium), benzocaine (a topical anesthetic) along with other local anesthetics, and dapsone (an antibiotic often used in HIV-related therapy). There may be a significant time delay from exposure to symptoms with some agents.
- Nitrates (in well water and vegetables) and nitrite salts can cause epidemic methemoglobinemia.
- All age groups are affected, but neonates and infants are more susceptible due to an underdeveloped methemoglobin reduction mechanism. Gastroenteritis can precipitate methemoglobinemia in infants.

CLINICAL FEATURES

- Clinical suspicion for methemoglobinemia should be raised when pulse oximetry approaches 80% to 85% without a response to supplemental oxygen. Patients may display gray discoloration of the skin.
- "Chocolate brown" discoloration of the blood is seen with methemoglobin levels above 20%.
- Patients with normal hemoglobin concentrations do not develop clinically significant effects until methemoglobin levels exceed 20%.
- Patients may seek evaluation for cyanosis that occurs when the methemoglobin level approaches 1.5 grams/dL; this is approximately 10% of the total hemoglobin in normal individuals.
- Patients with anemia require a higher percentage of methemoglobin to develop symptoms as the absolute concentration (1.5 grams/dL) determines cyanosis.
- Symptoms of anxiety, headache, weakness, and lightheadedness develop when levels reach 20% to 30%. Tachypnea and sinus tachycardia may occur.
- Methemoglobin concentrations of 50% to 60% impair oxygen delivery to tissues, causing myocardial ischemia, dysrhythmias, depressed mental status (including coma), seizures, and lactic acidosis.
- Levels above 70% are typically fatal.
- Patients with anemia and those with preexisting diseases that impair oxygen delivery (eg, emphysema, congestive heart failure) may be symptomatic at lower concentrations of methemoglobin.

DIAGNOSIS AND DIFFERENTIAL

- Methemoglobinemia must be considered in any patient who presents with cyanosis, especially when unresponsive to supplemental oxygen.
- Pulse oximetry must be interpreted with caution, as it cannot properly differentiate oxyhemoglobin from methemoglobin and may therefore appear falsely elevated. Pulse oximetry trends toward 80% to 85% in those with methemoglobin levels above 30%.
- The oxygen saturation obtained from an arterial blood gas analysis is falsely reassuring, as it is calculated from dissolved oxygen tension rather than bound oxygen, and is typically normal.
- Definitive diagnosis of methemoglobinemia is made using co-oximetry, which is widely available and requires only venous blood (although arterial blood can be used). It can differentiate oxyhemoglobin, deoxyhemoglobin, carboxyhemoglobin, and methemoglobin.

EMERGENCY DEPARTMENT CARE AND DISPOSITION

- Treatment of patients with methemoglobinemia begins with supportive measures to ensure oxygen delivery.

- The effectiveness of gastric decontamination is limited since there is often a substantial delay between exposure and development of methemoglobin. If an ongoing source of exposure exists, a single dose of oral activated charcoal 1 gram/kg PO is indicated. Decontamination of the skin may also be necessary.
- Methylene blue therapy is reserved for patients with documented methemoglobinemia or a high clinical suspicion of disease. Unstable patients should receive methylene blue, but may require blood transfusion or exchange transfusion for immediate improvement of oxygen delivery.
- The initial dose of methylene blue is 1 to 2 milligrams/kg IV. It should be administered slowly over 15 minutes, as rapidly administered high doses (>7 milligrams/kg) may actually induce methemoglobin formation. Improvement should be seen within 20 minutes. Repeat dosing may be necessary.
- Treatment failures occur in some patients, including those with glucose-6-phosphate dehydrogenase (G6PD) deficiency and other enzyme deficiencies, and may occur in the presence of hemolysis.
- Agents with long half-lives, such as dapsone, may require repetitive dosing of methylene blue.
- In patients with methemoglobinemia due to dapsone, inhibition of formation of the hydroxylamine metabolite with cimetidine will reduce toxicity.
- Patients with methemoglobinemia unresponsive to methylene blue are treated supportively. In unstable patients, perform simple or exchange transfusions. If newly transfused red blood cell hemoglobin undergoes oxidation, it will likely respond to methylene blue therapy.

SULFHEMOGLOBINEMIA

- Sulfhemoglobinemia is caused by many of the same agents that cause methemoglobinemia, as well as metoclopromide and sumatriptan.
- Sulfhemoglobinemia is clinically less concerning than methemoglobinemia, as the oxygen dissociation curve is shifted rightward. This favors the release of oxygen in tissues and lessens the degree of tissue hypoxia.
- The pigmentation of blood by sulfhemoglobin is substantially more intense than in methemoglobinemia. The color of the blood on venipuncture has been described as dark greenish-black.
- Cyanosis may occur at levels of 0.5 gram/dL due to increased pigmentation.
- Standard pulse oximetry tends to report a falsely low value for arterial oxygen saturation.
- Standard co-oximetry may not differentiate sulfhemoglobin from methemoglobin because of similar spectral absorbance. Specialized testing is needed to confirm the diagnosis reliably.
- Sulfhemoglobinemia persists for the life of the red blood cell and patients do not respond to methylene blue. Supportive treatment is indicated, and blood transfusions may be required in cases of severe toxicity.

For further reading in Tintinalli's *Emergency Medicine: A Comprehensive Guide*, 7th ed., see Chapter 201, "Dyshemoglobinemias" by Brenna M. Farmer and Lewis S. Nelson.

Section 13
ENVIRONMENTAL INJURIES

120 FROSTBITE AND HYPOTHERMIA

Michael C. Wadman

EPIDEMIOLOGY

- Extremes of age increase the risk of hypothermia.
- Alcohol and drug intoxication and psychiatric illness impair behavioral responses to a cold environment, increasing the risk of hypothermia.
- Military personnel, outdoor workers, the elderly, the homeless, drug and alcohol abusers, and psychiatric patients are at increased risk for frostbite.
- Wind increases frostbite injury rates, most notably when temperatures fall below −12°C (10.4°F) and wind speeds exceed 4.5 m/s (10 mph).

PATHOPHYSIOLOGY

- Heat loss results from conduction, convection, radiation, or evaporation.
- Heat gain and conservation are generally controlled in the hypothalamus. Heat is generated by shivering and thyroid-mediated increase in metabolic rate. Heat is conserved by peripheral vasoconstriction and behavioral responses (ie, dressing appropriately and seeking shelter).
- Acid-base disturbances are usually present but do not follow a uniform pattern.
- Renal concentrating abilities are impaired, resulting in a 'cold diuresis' and possible volume depletion.
- Hemoconcentration and volume depletion may lead to intravascular thrombosis and disseminated intravascular coagulation. Platelet function is impaired and the enzymatic reactions of the coagulation cascade.
- Prolonged immobility increases the risk of rhabdomyolysis and acute renal failure.
- The oxyhemoglobin dissociation curve is shifted to the left, resulting in impaired oxygen release to the tissues.
- Non-freezing cold injuries, such as trench foot and chilblains (pernio), result from prolonged cooling accelerated by wet conditions and are characterized by mild inflammatory skin lesions.
- Frostbite occurs in freezing temperatures, most often below −20°C (−4°F). Thawing of frozen tissue initiates an arachidonic acid cascade promoting vasoconstriction, platelet aggregation, leukocyte sludging, and erythrostasis, resulting in thrombosis and subsequent ischemia.

CLINICAL FEATURES

- Mild hypothermia, 32°C (89.6°F) to 35°C (95.0°F), results in an excitatory phase characterized by shivering and increases in heart rate and blood pressure.
- Shivering ceases when core temperatures drop below 30°C to 32°C (86.0°F to 89.6°F). A slowing (adynamic) phase then occurs, with decreased heart rate, respiratory rate, and blood pressure. Mild incoordination is followed by confusion, lethargy, and coma. Bronchorrhea and depression of cough and gag reflexes make aspiration pneumonia a common complication. Below 30°C, dysrhythmias begin to occur.
- The ECG may show PR-, QRS-, and QT-interval prolongations and Osborn J waves. Cardiac rhythm progresses from sinus bradycardia to atrial fibrillation with a slow ventricular response, to ventricular fibrillation, and ultimately to asystole.
- First-degree frostbite (frostnip), partial skin freezing, is characterized by erythema, mild edema, lack of blisters, and occasional late skin desquamation. Patients complain of stinging and burning, followed by throbbing.
- Second-degree frostbite, full-thickness skin freezing, is characterized by substantial edema, and clear blisters that usually desquamate and form black eschars over several days. Patients complain of numbness followed by aching and throbbing.
- Third-degree frostbite, injury involving the deeper subdermal plexus, is characterized by hemorrhagic blisters, necrosis, and blue-gray discoloration of the skin. Patients complain of the affected part felling like 'a block of wood', followed by burning, throbbing, and shooting pains.
- Fourth-degree frostbite, injury involving the subcutaneous tissue, muscle, tendon, and bone, is characterized by little edema, mottled skin with non-blanching cyanosis, and eventual formation of black, mummified eschar. Patients may complain of a deep, aching joint pain.
- Trench foot results in a pale, mottled, anesthetic, pulseless foot. Long-term hyperhidrosis and cold insensitivity are common, and anesthesia may be prolonged or permanent.

- Chilblains, presents with painful and inflamed skin lesions caused by chronic, intermittent exposure to damp, nonfreezing ambient temperatures. Once affected by chilblains or frostbite, the involved body part becomes more susceptible to re-injury.

DIAGNOSIS AND DIFFERENTIAL

- Hypothermia is diagnosed when the core body temperature is below 35.0°C (95.0°F).
- Other underlying disease states that may result in hypothermia include thyroid deficiency, adrenal insufficiency, CNS dysfunction, infection, sepsis, dermal disease, drug intoxication, and metabolic derangements.

EMERGENCY DEPARTMENT CARE AND DISPOSITION

- Chilblains is managed with rewarming, elevation, and bandaging of the affected tissues. **Nifedipine** 20 milligrams PO three times daily, **pentoxifyline** 400 milligrams PO three times daily, topical corticosteroids, prednisone, and prostaglandin E1 (**limaprost** 20 micrograms PO three times daily) may be helpful.
- Trench foot is managed with rewarming, drying, and elevation.
- Frostbite is treated by rapid rewarming with circulating water at 40.0°C-42.0°C (104.0°F-107.6°F) for 20 to 30 minutes (until the area is pliable and erythematous) for extremities. Use compresses soaked in warm water for faces.
- Dry air rewarming may cause further tissue injury and should be avoided.
- Patients should receive narcotics, ibuprofen, and tetanus immunization if not current. **Penicillin G** 500,000 units IV every 6 hours for 48 to 72 hours has been shown to be beneficial.
- Debridement of blisters is controversial. Some recommend debridement or aspiration of clear blisters to limit the potential damage caused by blister fluid prostaglandins and thromboxane. Hemorrhagic blisters should be left intact. Both types should be treated with topical aloe vera to combat the arachidonic acid cascade.
- Other treatment options for frostbite include sympathetic blockade using a long-acting anesthetic (bupivacaine) to improve blood flow to the hand, reduce pain, and speed recovery. **Tissue plasminogen activator** administered IV after rapid rewarming reduces predicted digit amputations. Heparin and hyperbaric oxygen therapy appear to be of little value.
- Hypothermia is treated by rewarming using passive, active external, and active core techniques.
- All patients should be removed from the cold environment, have wet clothing removed, and skin dried. Patients should be handled in a gentle manner to minimize the likelihood of ventricular fibrillation.
- Mild hypothermia is treated with passive warming using insulating blankets.
- All patients with severe hypothermia, hypothermia secondary to an underlying illness, or hypothermia causing cardiovascular compromise require active rewarming.
- Active external rewarming is the application of exogenous heat to the body surface, through the use of heating blankets set at 40.0°C (104.0°F), radiant heat, or heated air forced through slits in commercially available plastic blankets.
- Active core rewarming techniques include inhalation (with temperature of gas at 40.0°C (104.0°F), administration of IV fluids warmed to 40.0°C (104.0°F), GI tract lavage, bladder lavage, peritoneal lavage, pleural lavage, mediastinal lavage via thoracotomy, and extracorporeal warming.
- At temperatures >30.0°C (>86.0°F) the incidence of dysrhythmias is low and rapid rewarming is rarely necessary. For patients with core temperature below 30.0°C, cardiovascular status is the most important consideration. Some recommend passive rewarming and non-invasive active rewarming for all patients with stable cardiac rhythm (including sinus bradycardia and atrial fibrillation) and stable vital signs. Others recommend rapid rewarming of all profoundly hypothermic patients utilizing extracorporeal rewarming or a combination of other active rewarming techniques. For hypothermic patients with cardiovascular instability, rapid rewarming via active core techniques is required.
- Patients with suspected thiamine depletion and alcoholism should receive **thiamine** 100 milligrams IV or IM and **50% glucose in water** 50 to 100 mL IV if rapid glucose testing is not available or if glucose is low.
- Patients with suspected hypothyroidism or adrenal insufficiency may require IV thyroxine and **hydrocortisone** 100 milligrams.
- Ventricular fibrillation is usually refractory to defibrillation until a temperature of 30.0°C (86.0°F) is obtained, although a single defibrillation attempt is recommended.
- All patients with more than isolated superficial frostbite or mild hypothermia should be admitted to the hospital. A patient should not be discharged unless they can return to a warm environment.

For further reading in Tintinalli's *Emergency Medicine: A Comprehensive Study Guide*, 7th ed., see Chapter 202, "Frostbite and Other Localized Cold Injuries," by Tiina M. Ikaheimo, Juhani Junila, Jorma Hirvonen, and Juhani Hassi, and Chapter 203, "Hypothermia," by Howard Bessen and Bryan Ngo.

121 HEAT EMERGENCIES

T. Paul Tran

EPIDEMIOLOGY

- Heat-related illnesses cause approximately 400 deaths annually in the United States.
- Risks for heat-related deaths are highest among children and the elderly, those with predisposing medical conditions, and those on medications that interfere with the thermoregulatory response.
- Heat-related illnesses and deaths are preventable and are closely correlated with high environmental temperature and urban heat waves, which are defined as three or more consecutive days with ambient temperatures >32.2°C.

PATHOPHYSIOLOGY

- Body heat generated by metabolism and heat gained from the hot environment must be dissipated to maintain body temperature at or near 37°C.
- Externally, body heat is thermodynamically dissipated through radiation, convection, evaporation, and conduction.
- While radiation is the primary mechanism for heat loss in a cold environment (accounting for 65% of total heat loss), evaporation becomes the primary mechanism for heat dissipation in a hot environment.
- Internally, thermoregulatory homeostasis is accomplished via the body's thermoregulatory response, acute phase response, and heat shock protein response.
- Upon exposure to heat stress, cardiac output is augmented, core blood circulation is shifted to the peripheral circulation, vasodilatation occurs, and thermal sweating is augmented.
- Several inflammatory cytokines and heat shock proteins are released to improve tissue repair and protect against tissue injury and protein denaturation.
- Heat stroke is a life-threatening injury pathogenetically characterized by thermoregulatory breakdown, endothelial injury, coagulation disorder, microcirculatory derangement, and multiorgan failure. It is the final result of interplay among thermoregulatory response failure, exaggerated acute phase response, and altered heat shock protein response.
- Clinically heat stroke is characterized by hyperthermia and central nervous system (CNS) dysfunction.

CLINICAL FEATURES

- Patients with heat stroke usually present with a history of environmental or occupational heat exposure.
- On physical examination, patients usually have altered mental status and an elevated body temperature. Core temperature ranges from 40°C to 47°C.
- Neurologic abnormalities include ataxia, confusion, bizarre behavior, agitation, seizures, obtundation, and coma. Anhidrosis is not invariably present.
- Risk factors for heat-related injuries include extremes of age (<4 years and >75 years), predisposing conditions (heart failure, psychiatric illnesses, alcohol abuse, dehydration, poverty, social isolation), medications (anticholinergics, β-blockers, calcium channel blockers), and host-environment factors (lacking access to air conditioning, poor physical fitness, inadequate acclimatization to hot weather).

DIAGNOSIS AND DIFFERENTIAL

- Heat stroke is a true time-dependent medical emergency. It should be considered in the clinical context of environmental heat stress, hyperthermia, and altered mental status.
- Patients are tachycardic, are hyperventilating, and have respiratory alkalosis.
- About 20% of heat stroke patients are hypotensive.
- In contrast to classic heat stroke, patients with exertional heat stroke may have both respiratory alkalosis and lactic acidosis.
- Exertional heat stroke patients may present with rhabdomyolysis, hyperkalemia, hyperphosphatemia, and hypocalcemia.
- Neuroimaging studies and other evaluation (eg, septic workup) can be individualized as clinically indicated.
- Differential diagnosis includes infection (sepsis, meningitis, encephalitis, malaria, typhoid fever), toxins (serotonin syndrome, anticholinergics, phenothiazine, salicylate, phencyclidine (PCP), sympathomimetic abuse, alcohol withdrawal), metabolic and endocrinologic emergencies (thyrotoxicosis, diabetic ketoacidosis), CNS disorders (status epilepticus, stroke syndrome), neuroleptic malignant syndrome, and malignant hyperthermia.

EMERGENCY DEPARTMENT CARE AND DISPOSITION

- Emergent priorities remain airway, breathing, and circulation. Cardiac monitoring and an IV line should be established.
- Along with the ABC, immediate cooling measures must be immediately instituted. The goal in the treatment of heat stroke is to bring the core temperature down by 0.2°C/min, to a core temperature <39°C.
- Cooling measures should be stopped when core temperature reaches 39°C to avoid overcooling and hypothermia.

- Patients should have clothes removed. Ice packs are placed on neck, axillae, and groins of patient. Tepid or ice water can be sprayed on patients. Fans are positioned near the completely disrobed patient.
- High-flow supplemental oxygen should be administered. Patients with significantly altered mental status, diminished gag reflex, and hypoxia are candidates for definitive airway management (eg, endotracheal intubation).
- Core temperature should immediately be obtained with a rectal (or bladder) probe and continuously monitored.
- Volume-depleted patients should be rehydrated with IV normal saline or lactated Ringer's solution to maintain mean arterial pressure >60 mm Hg or a urine output of ≥0.5mL/kg/h. Inotropic support and pressors may be required. Care should be exercised not to volume overload the patient.
- Spraying with ice water may cause shivering, which induces thermogenesis. Excessive shivering can be treated with short-acting benzodiazepines (**midazolam** 2 milligrams IV).
- Other methods of cooling such as immersion cooling, cold water gastric and urinary bladder lavage, peritoneal or thoracostomy lavage, cold IV fluid infusion, cooling blanket, and cardiopulmonary bypass may be considered as clinically indicated and logistically feasible.
- Seizures can be treated with benzodiazepines.
- Treat rhabdomyolysis with IV hydration. To date, no prospective control studies have shown improved outcomes from alkalinization of the urine or forced diuresis with mannitol or loop diuretics.
- Hyperkalemia should be treated with standard regimens. The patient's electrolytes should be monitored every hour initially.
- Heat stroke patients need to be admitted to an intensive care unit for further observation and monitoring.

OTHER HEAT ILLNESSES

HEAT EXHAUSTION

- Heat exhaustion is a clinical syndrome that results from heat exposure in an individual who is volume depleted, sodium depleted, or both.
- It is characterized by nonspecific signs and symptoms, including malaise, fatigue, weakness, dizziness, syncope, headache, nausea, vomiting, myalgias, diaphoresis, tachypnea, tachycardia, and orthostatic hypotension.
- Core body temperature is frequently elevated, but usually doesn't exceed 40°C (104°F).
- Although patients may complain of neurologic symptoms, patients' sensorium and neurologic examination should be normal.
- Laboratory examination usually demonstrates hemoconcentration. A creatinine kinase level should be checked to exclude rhabdomyolysis.
- Treatment consists of rest, evaporative cooling, and administration of IV normal saline or oral electrolyte solution, depending upon the clinical situation.
- Since heat exhaustion has the potential to evolve into heat stroke, patients should be aggressively treated and observed until symptoms resolve.
- The majority of patients can be discharged home. Those patients with significant comorbid conditions (heart failure, poor social support) or severe electrolyte abnormality may require hospitalization.

HEAT SYNCOPE

- Heat syncope results from volume depletion, peripheral vasodilation, and decreased vasomotor tone.
- It occurs most commonly in the elderly and poorly acclimatized individuals.
- Postural vital signs may or may not be demonstrable on presentation to the ED.
- Patients should be evaluated for any trauma resulting from a fall.
- Potentially serious causes of syncope (eg, cardiovascular, neurologic, infectious, endocrine, and electrolyte abnormalities) should be investigated, especially in the elderly.
- Treatment for heat syncope consists of rest and oral or IV rehydration.

HEAT CRAMPS

- Heat cramps are characterized by painful muscle spasms, especially in the calves, thighs, and shoulders.
- Common during athletic events, they are thought to result from dilutional hyponatremia as individuals replace evaporative losses with free water but not salt.
- Core body temperature may be normal or elevated.
- Treatment consists of rest and administration of oral electrolyte solution or IV normal saline. Patients should be instructed to replace future fluid losses with a balanced electrolyte solution.

HEAT TETANY

- Heat tetany is due to the effects of respiratory alkalosis that result when an individual hyperventilates in response to an intense heat stress.

- Patients may complain of paresthesia of the extremities, circumoral paresthesia, and carpopedal spasm. Muscle cramps are minimal or nonexistent.
- Treatment consists of removal from the heat stress and self-rebreathing through a paper bag.

HEAT EDEMA

- Heat edema is a self-limited, mild swelling of dependent extremities (hands and feet) that occurs in the first few days of exposure to a new hot environment.
- It is due to cutaneous vasodilation and pooling of interstitial fluid in dependent extremities.
- Treatment consists of elevation of the extremities, and in severe cases, application of compressive stockings. Administration of diuretics may exacerbate volume depletion and should be avoided.

HEAT RASH

- Heat rash (prickly heat) is a maculopapular eruption that is most commonly found over clothed areas of the body.
- It results from inflammation and obstruction of sweat ducts.
- Early stages present with a pruritic, erythematous rash best treated with antihistamines and **chlorhexidine cream or lotion**.
- Continued blockage of pores results in a nonpruritic, nonerythematous, whitish papular rash known as the profunda stage of prickly heat.
- This is best treated with antistaphylococcal antibiotics and application of **1% salicylic acid** to affected areas three times daily.

For further reading in Tintinalli's *Emergency Medicine: A Comprehensive Study Guide*, 7th ed., see Chapter 204, "Heat Emergencies," by Thomas A. Waters and Majid A. Al-Salamah.

122 BITES AND STINGS

Burton Bentley II

WASPS, BEES, AND STINGING ANTS (*HYMENOPTERA*)

EPIDEMIOLOGY

- More fatalities result from stings by Hymenoptera than by stings or bites by any other arthropod.

CLINICAL FEATURES

- Wasps, bees, and stinging ants are members of the order Hymenoptera. Both local and generalized reactions may occur in response to an encounter.
- Most allergic reactions from Hymenoptera occur from Vespidae (wasp, hornet, and yellow jacket) stings.
- Local reactions consist of pain, erythema, edema, and pruritus at the sting site. Local reactions cause no systemic symptoms.
- Severe local reactions increase the likelihood of serious systemic reactions in the event of recurrent envenomation.
- Toxic reactions are a nonantigenic response to multiple stings. They have many of the same features of true systemic (allergic) reactions, but there is a greater frequency of gastrointestinal disturbances. Bronchospasm and urticaria do not occur.
- Systemic or anaphylactic reactions are true allergic reactions that range from mild to fatal. In general, the shorter the interval between the sting and the onset of symptoms, the more severe the reaction.
- Initial symptoms of anaphylaxis consist of itchy eyes, urticaria, and cough. As the reaction progresses, patients may experience respiratory failure and cardiovascular collapse.
- The majority of anaphylactic reactions occur within the first 15 minutes and nearly all occur within 6 hours. There is no correlation between a systemic reaction and the number of stings.
- Delayed reactions may appear 10 to 14 days after a sting. Symptoms of delayed reactions resemble serum sickness and include fever, malaise, headache, urticaria, lymphadenopathy, and polyarthritis.

EMERGENCY DEPARTMENT CARE AND DISPOSITION

- The treatment of all Hymenoptera encounters is the same. Remove retained stingers and cleanse all wounds.
- Erythema and swelling seen in local reactions may be difficult to distinguish from cellulitis. As a general rule, infection is present in a minority of cases.
- For minor local reactions, oral antihistamines and analgesics typically suffice.
- Treat severe reactions with **1:1000 epinephrine** intramuscularly (IM); 0.3 to 0.5 mL for an adult and 0.01 mL/kg for a child (0.3 mL maximum). Some patients may require a second dose in 10 to 15 minutes.
- Parenteral H1- and H2-receptor antagonists (eg, diphenhydramine and ranitidine) and steroids (eg, methylprednisolone) should be rapidly administered.
- Bronchospasm responds to courses of inhaled β-agonists (eg, albuterol).

- Hypotension should be treated aggressively with crystalloid, although dopamine and epinephrine infusions may be required.
- Patients with minor symptoms who respond to conservative measures may be discharged after monitoring for several hours. Patients with severe reactions require hospitalization.
- All patients with Hymenoptera reactions should be prescribed a premeasured epinephrine injector (EpiPen) and referred to an allergist for further evaluation.

SPIDERS, SCABIES, CHIGGERS, AND SCORPIONS (*ARACHNIDA*)

BROWN RECLUSE SPIDER (*LOXOSCELES RECLUSA*)

Clinical Features

- The bite of the brown recluse causes an erythematous lesion that may become firm and heal over several days to weeks.
- Occasionally, a severe reaction with immediate pain, blister formation, and bluish discoloration may occur. These lesions often become necrotic over 3 to 4 days.
- Loxoscelism is a systemic reaction that may occur 1 to 2 days after envenomation. Signs and symptoms include fever, chills, vomiting, arthralgias, myalgias, petechiae, and hemolysis; severe cases progress to seizure, renal failure, disseminated intravascular coagulation (DIC), and death.
- The diagnosis of envenomation is made on clinical grounds since the bite is often unwitnessed.

Emergency Department Care and Disposition

- Treatment of a brown recluse spider bite includes routine wound care, tetanus prophylaxis, and analgesics. Antibiotics may be offered when appropriate. Currently, there is no commercially available antivenin.
- Most wounds heal without intervention. Surgery is reserved for lesions greater than 2 cm in size and is deferred for 2 to 3 weeks following the bite.
- The role of **dapsone** (50-200 milligrams per day) and hyperbaric oxygen has recently been challenged, but these may prevent some ongoing local necrosis.
- Patients with systemic reactions and hemolysis must be hospitalized for consideration of blood transfusion and hemodialysis.

HOBO SPIDERS (*TEGENARIA AGRESTIS*)

- The hobo spider bite causes clinical signs and symptoms that are quite similar to those of the brown recluse spider bite.
- The skin site is initially painless before developing induration, erythema, blistering, and necrosis. Victims also may experience headache, vomiting, and fatigue.
- There is no specific diagnostic test or therapeutic intervention for hobo spider bites. Surgical repair may be required, although it must be delayed until the necrotizing process is complete.

BLACK WIDOW SPIDER (*LATRODECTUS MACTANS*)

Clinical Features

- Black widow spider bites induce an immediate pinprick sensation that often allows the victim to identify the offending spider.
- Within 1 hour, the patient may experience erythematous skin lesions (often target-shaped), swelling, and diffuse muscle cramps.
- Large muscle groups are involved, resulting in painful cramping of the abdominal wall musculature that may mimic peritonitis. Severe pain may wax and wane for up to 3 days, but muscle weakness and spasm can persist for weeks to months.
- Serious acute complications include hypertension, respiratory failure, shock, and coma.

Emergency Department Care and Disposition

- Initial therapy includes local wound treatment and supportive care. Analgesics and benzodiazepines relieve cramping and pain.
- Severe envenomation may necessitate hospitalization for parenteral pain medication and antivenin therapy.
- A commercially available horse-derived antivenin is rapidly effective for severe envenomation. The package insert provides dosing instructions. Following antivenin treatment, patients may be observed and discharged if they are asymptomatic.

TARANTULAS

- When threatened, tarantulas may flick barbed hairs into their victim. These hairs can embed deeply into the conjunctiva and cornea resulting in an inflammatory response.
- Tarantulas also render a painful bite causing erythema, swelling, and local joint stiffness. The treatment is local wound care and appropriate analgesia.
- Any patient complaining of ocular symptoms after exposure to a tarantula should undergo a thorough slit lamp examination.
- Treatment includes topical steroids and consultation with an ophthalmologist for surgical removal of the hairs.

SCORPIONS (*SCORPIONIDA*)

Clinical Features

- Of all North American scorpions, only the bark scorpion (*Centruroides exilicauda*) of the western United States is capable of producing systemic toxicity.
- *Centruroides exilicauda* venom causes immediate burning and stinging without any visible local injury. Systemic effects are infrequent and mainly occur at the extremes of patient age.
- Findings may include tachycardia, excessive secretions, roving eye movements, opisthotonos, and fasciculations.
- The diagnosis may be elusive if the scorpion is not seen. Roving eye movements are nearly pathognomonic. A positive "tap test" (ie, exquisite local tenderness when the area is lightly tapped) is also suggestive.

Emergency Department Care and Disposition

- Treatment includes local wound care and reassurance to allay misconceptions about the lethality of scorpion stings.
- The application of ice may provide relief of local pain. Muscle spasm and fasciculations respond promptly to benzodiazepines.
- Severe toxicity warrants an immediate three-vial dose of ***Centruroides*-specific antivenin** (**Centruroides Immune Fab**). Patients who respond to antivenin therapy may be released.

SCABIES (*SARCOPTES SCABIEI*)

Clinical Features

- Scabies often localize to the interdigital web spaces, penis, and female nipple. In children, the face and the scalp are commonly affected.
- Transmission is typically by direct contact.
- The distinctive feature of scabies is intense pruritus with burrows. The mites form white, threadlike channels with zigzag patterns and a small gray spot at the closed end.
- Associated vesicles, papules, crusts, and eczematization may obscure the diagnosis. However, in undisturbed burrows the female mite may be scraped out with a blade edge.

Emergency Department Care and Disposition

- Treatment of adults with scabies infestation consists of a thorough application of **permethrin** (Elimite) from the neck down; infants may require additional application to the scalp, temple, and forehead.
- Reapplication is only necessary if mites are found 2 weeks following treatment, although the pruritus may last for several weeks after successful therapy.
- Oral **ivermectin** is an alternative treatment.

CHIGGERS (*TROMBICULIDAE*)

Clinical Features

- Chiggers are tiny mite larvae that cause intense pruritus.
- Itchiness begins within hours, followed by a papule that enlarges to a nodule over the next 1 to 2 days. Infestation has been associated with fever and erythema multiforme.
- Children who have been sitting on lawns are prone to chigger lesions in the genital area.
- The diagnosis of chigger bites is based on typical skin lesions in the context of a known outdoor exposure.

Emergency Department Care and Disposition

- Treatment consists of symptomatic relief with oral or topical antihistamines; oral steroids may be required in more severe cases.
- Annihilation of the mites requires topical application of lindane, permethrin, or crotamiton.

FLEAS (*SIPHONAPTERA*)

- Flea bites cause intensely pruritic zigzag lines, especially on the legs and waist. The lesions have hemorrhagic puncta surrounded by erythematous and urticarial patches.
- Oral antihistamines, starch baths, calamine lotion, and topical steroids relieve discomfort. If secondary infection develops, topical or oral antibiotics may be needed.

LICE (*ANOPLURA*)

- Body lice are transmitted by direct contact with infected people or fomites (eg, clothing) and typically concentrate around the waist, shoulders, axillae, and neck. Pubic lice are spread by sexual contact. Infestation induces intensely pruritic papules and wheals.
- **Permethrin** is the primary treatment of body lice infestation. Treatment of hair infestation requires a thorough shampoo with **pyrethrin with piperonyl butoxide**; reapplication is mandatory in 10 days.
- Clothing, bedding, and personal articles must be sterilized in hot (>52°C) water to prevent reinfestation.

KISSING BUGS AND BEDBUGS (*HEMIPTERA*)

- Kissing bugs (conenose beetles) and bedbugs feed on blood as they attack the exposed surface of a sleeping victim.
- The initial bite is painless. Wheals, hemorrhagic papules, and bullae may follow. Anaphylaxis is common in the sensitized individual.
- Treatment consists of local wound care and analgesics. Allergic reactions must be treated as previously outlined for Hymenoptera envenomation.

PIT VIPER (*CROTALIDAE*) BITES

EPIDEMIOLOGY

- There are approximately 8000 venomous snakebites each year in the United States, but only about 10 deaths result. Twenty-five percent of bites are "dry strikes" with no effect from venom.
- Except for imported species and coral snakes, the only venomous North American snakes are members of the Crotalidae family (eg, rattlesnakes, copperheads, water moccasins, and massasaugas).
- Crotalid snakes, commonly known as pit vipers, are identified by their retractable fangs and by heat-sensitive depressions (pits) located between each eye and nostril.

CLINICAL FEATURES

- The effects of crotalid envenomation depend on the size and species of the snake, the age and size of the victim, the time elapsed since the bite, and the characteristics of the bite itself.
- The hallmark of pit viper envenomation is fang marks with local pain and swelling.
- There are three classes of criteria that determine the severity of a rattlesnake bite: (1) degree of local injury (swelling, pain, ecchymosis), (2) degree of systemic involvement (hypotension, tachycardia, paresthesia), and (3) evolving coagulopathy (thrombocytopenia, elevated prothrombin time, hypofibrinogenemia). Abnormalities in any of these three areas indicate that envenomation has occurred.
- Conversely, the absence of any clinical findings after 8 to 12 hours effectively rules out venom injection.
- It is crucial to remember that initially benign-appearing bites may still evolve with devastating complications.

DIAGNOSIS AND DIFFERENTIAL

- The diagnosis of crotalid envenomation is based on clinical findings and corroborating laboratory data.
- In general, envenomated patients will have swelling within 30 minutes, although some may take up to 12 hours.
- Minimal envenomation describes cases with local swelling, no systemic signs, and no laboratory abnormalities.
- Moderate envenomation causes increased swelling that spreads from the site. These patients also may have systemic signs such as nausea, paresthesia, hypotension, and tachycardia. Coagulation parameters may be abnormal, but there is no significant bleeding.
- Severe envenomation causes extensive swelling, potentially life-threatening systemic signs (eg, hypotension, altered mental status, respiratory distress), and markedly abnormal coagulation parameters that may result in hemorrhage.

EMERGENCY DEPARTMENT CARE AND DISPOSITION

- All pit viper bites require medical attention; first aid measures must not delay definitive care. The patient should minimize physical activity and immobilize the bitten extremity in a neutral position below the level of the heart.
- Local wound care and tetanus immunization should be given, but prophylactic antibiotics and steroids have no proven benefit.
- Limb circumference at several sites above and below the wound should be checked and documented every 30 minutes. The border of advancing edema should be marked.
- Any patient with progressive local swelling, systemic effects, or coagulopathy should receive antivenin therapy immediately.
- **Polyvalent Crotalidae Immune Fab (FabAV),** a sheep-derived antivenin, is administered as an initial dose of four to six vials IV; there is no need for a prior skin testing.
- The initial dose of **FabAV** is infused IV over 1 hour. Since allergic reactions may occur, the infusion should proceed at a slow rate of 25 to 50 mL/h for the first 10 minutes. If the patient remains stable, the infusion rate may be increased to the full 250-mL/h rate.
- Since the goal of therapy is to neutralize existing venom, dosing regimens are exactly the same for both children and adults (although the amount of diluent will need proper adjustment).
- One hour after the initial dose has been administered, the patient must be reexamined to determine if local swelling has been arrested, coagulation tests have normalized, and systemic symptoms have abated. If

the initial dose was ineffective in any of these three areas, then a repeat dose of four to six vials should be administered.

- Laboratory determinations are repeated every 4 hours or after each course of antivenin, whichever is more frequent.
- Since the end point of antivenin therapy is the arrest of progressive symptoms and coagulopathy, the administration of antivenin must continue until complete control of the envenomation is achieved.
- Once initial control has been achieved, the protocol is completed by administering additional two-vial doses every 6 hours for a total of three more doses.
- Compartment syndrome (pressure >30 mm Hg) may occur secondary to envenomation. Repeated dosing of antivenin is the most effective therapy for elevated compartment pressures. Limb elevation, IV mannitol, and surgical fasciotomy may be required.
- The mainstay of coagulopathy remains antivenin therapy. Severe active bleeding due to coagulopathy may require additional transfusion of blood products.
- Any patient with a pit viper bite must be observed for at least 8 hours. Patients with no evidence of envenomation after 8 to 12 hours may be discharged.
- Serum sickness occurs in 5% of patients within 1 to 2 weeks of FabAV therapy. Oral prednisone is the standard treatment.

CORAL SNAKE BITE

CLINICAL FEATURES

- True coral snakes have a yellow band directly touching a red band; nonpoisonous impostors have an intervening black band. This distinctive pattern establishes the mnemonic for North American snakes: "Red on yellow, kill a fellow; red on black, venom lack."
- Only the bite of the eastern coral snake (*Micrurus fulvius fulvius*) requires significant treatment; the bite of the Sonoran (Arizona) coral snake is mild and only needs local care.
- Eastern coral snake venom is a potent neurotoxin capable of causing tremor, salivation, respiratory paralysis, seizures, and bulbar palsies (eg, dysarthria, diplopia, and dysphagia).

EMERGENCY DEPARTMENT CARE AND DISPOSITION

- Patients with possible envenomation must be admitted to the hospital for 24 to 48 hours of observation. In the absence of antivenin therapy, the toxic effects of coral snake venom are not easily reversed.
- The manufacture of coral snake antivenin has ceased and current lots are expiring. If treatment is required, immediately contact a poison control center for current information on availability.

GILA MONSTERS

- Gila monsters are slow-moving poisonous lizards that are indigenous to the desert of the southwestern United States.
- Gila monsters have a tenacious bite and may be difficult to remove from the bitten extremity.
- Most bites result in local pain and swelling that worsens over several hours before subsiding.
- Patients rarely experience systemic toxicity, including weakness, lightheadedness, paresthesia, diaphoresis, or severe hypertension.
- Treatment involves removal of the reptile from the bite site. The Gila monster often will loosen its grip when no longer suspended in midair. Other reported methods include submersion, cast spreaders, or application of an irritating flame.
- The only requisite treatment is local wound care and a careful search for implanted teeth.

For further reading see Tintinalli's *Emergency Medicine: A Comprehensive Study Guide,* 7th ed., see Chapter 205, "Bites and Stings," by Aaron B. Schneir and Richard F. Clark, and Chapter 206, "Reptile Bites," by Richard C. Dart and Frank F. S. Daly.

123 TRAUMA AND ENVENOMATION FROM MARINE FAUNA

Christian A. Tomaszewski

EPIDEMIOLOGY

- The population growth along coastal areas has made exposure to hazardous marine fauna increasingly common.
- The popularity of home aquariums generates additional exposures inland.
- Marine fauna can inflict injury through direct traumatic bite or envenomation, usually via a stinging apparatus.

CLINICAL FEATURES

- Marine trauma includes bites from sharks, barracudas, moray eels, seals, crocodiles, needlefish, wahoos, piranhas, and trigger fish.
- Shark bites may also cause substantial tissue loss with hemorrhagic shock and delayed infection.
- Minor trauma is usually due to cuts and scrapes from coral that can cause local stinging pain, erythema, urticaria, and pruritus.
- Marine wounds can be infected with routine skin flora, such as *Staphylococcus* and *Streptococcus*, along with bacteria unique to the marine environment.
  - The most serious halophilic organism is the gram-negative bacillus *Vibrio*, which can cause rapid infections marked by pain, swelling, hemorrhagic bullae, vasculitis, and even necrotizing fascitis and sepsis.
  - Immunosuppressed patients, particularly those with liver disease, are susceptible to sepsis and death (up to 60%) from *Vibrio vulnificus*.
  - Another bacterium, *Erysipelothrix rhusiopathiae*, implicated in fish handler's disease, can cause painful, marginating plaques after cutaneous puncture wounds.
  - The unique marine bacterium *Mycobacterium marinum*, an acid-fast bacillus, can cause a chronic cutaneous granuloma 3 to 4 weeks after exposure.
- Numerous invertebrate and vertebrate marine species are venomous.
- The invertebrates belong to five phyla: Cnidaria, Porifera, Echinodermata, Annelida, and Mollusca.
  - The four classes of Cnidaria all share stinging cells, known as nematocysts, which deliver venom subcutaneously when stimulated.
  - The most common effects are pain, swelling, pruritus, urticaria, and even blistering and necrosis in severe cases.
  - The Hydrozoans include hydroids, *Millepora* (fire corals), and *Physalia* (Portuguese man-of-war).
    - The latter causes a linear erythematous eruption and rarely can cause respiratory arrest, possibly from anaphylaxis.
    - In addition to local tissue injury, the Scyhozoans (true jellyfish) include Atlantic Ocean larval forms that can cause a persistent dermatitis under bathing suits lasting days after exposure (Seabather's eruption).
  - The Cubozoans (box jellyfish), in particular *Chironex fleckeri* in Australia and *Chiropsalmus* in the Gulf of Mexico, can cause death after severe stings.
  - A Hawaiian species, *Carybdea,* has been implicated in painful stings but no deaths.
  - Another Australian box jellyfish, *Carukia barnesi,* can cause Irukandji syndrome, characterized by diffuse pain, hypertension, tachycardia, diaphoresis, and even pulmonary edema.
  - The most innocuous cnidaria are the Anthozoans (anemones) that occasionally cause a mild local reaction.
- Porifera (the sponges) can produce a stinging, pruritic dermatitis.
  - Spicules of silica or calcium carbonate can become embedded in the skin along with toxic secretions from the sponge.
- Echinodermata include sea urchins and sea stars.
  - Sea urchin spines produce immediate pain with trauma; some contain venom that leads to erythema and swelling.
  - Retained spines can lead to infection and granuloma formation.
  - The crown-of-thorns sea star, *Acanthaster planci,* has sharp rigid spines that cause burning pain and local inflammation.
- Annelida include bristle and fire worms, which embed bristles in the skin, causing pain and erythema.
- Mollusca include gastropods and octopuses.
  - Both the Indo-Pacific cone shell, *Conus,* and the blue-ringed octopus, *Hapalochalena,* can deliver paralytic venom that can quickly lead to respiratory paralysis.
- Vertebrate envenomations are primarily due to stingrays (order Rajiformes) and spined venomous fish (scorpion fish, lion fish, catfish, and weeverfish).
  - The stingray whip tail has venomous spines, which puncture or lacerate causing an intense painful local reaction.
  - The spines of venomous fish have glands that force venom into the wound after puncture and cause local pain, erythema, and edema.
  - Retention of a spine can lead to infection.

EMERGENCY DEPARTMENT CARE AND DISPOSITION

- Copiously irrigate lacerations, punctures, and bite wounds; explore for foreign matter and debride devitalized tissue. Soft tissue radiographs or ultrasound may help locate foreign bodies, which usually require removal, especially if intra-articular. Leave lacerations open for delayed primary closure. Update tetanus, if needed.
- Prophylactic antibiotic therapy is not indicated for routine minor wounds in healthy patients but may be considered in selected patients (Table 123-1).
- Antibiotic therapy for infected wounds is first directed toward likely pathogens and later by culture and sensitivity results.

TABLE 123-1 Recommendations for Antibiotic Treatment of Marine-Associated Wounds

NO ANTIBIOTICS INDICATED	PROPHYLACTIC/ OUTPATIENT ANTIBIOTICS	HOSPITAL ADMISSION FOR IV ANTIBIOTICS
Healthy patient	Late wound care	Predisposing medical conditions
Prompt wound care	Large lacerations or injuries	Long delays before definitive wound care
No foreign body	Early or local inflammation	Deep wounds, significant trauma
No bone or joint involvement		Wounds with retained foreign bodies
Small or superficial injuries		Progressive inflammatory change
		Penetration of periosteum, joint space, or body cavity
		Major injuries associated with envenomation
		Systemic illness

- Cover *Staphylococcus* and *Streptococcus* species with a first-generation cephalosporin, such as **cephalexin** 500 milligrams 4 times daily or **cefazolin** 1 to 2 grams every 8 hours, or **clindamycin** 300 milligrams PO/600 milligrams IV 4 times daily or **doxycycline** 100 milligrams PO/IV twice daily. Addition of a third-generation cephalosporin, such as **ceftriaxone** 1 gram IV daily or **cefotaxime** 2 grams IV every 8 hours, or a fluoroquinolone, such as **levofloxacin** 500 milligrams PO/IV daily, will cover ocean-related infections from *Vibrio*.
- A **fluoroquinolone** or **third-generation cephalosporin**, or **trimethoprim-sulfamethoxazole double strength**, 1 tablet PO twice daily, or **imipenem**, 500 milligrams IV every 6 hours, will cover fresh water infections from *Aeromonas*. Granulomas from *M. marinum* require several months of treatment with **clarithromycin** or **rifampin plus ethambutol.**
- See Table 123-2 for early treatment of envenomations.

For further reading in Tintinalli's *Emergency Medicine: A Comprehensive Study Guide*, 7th ed., see Chapter 207, "Trauma and Envenomation from Marine Fauna," by Geoffrey K. Isbister.

TABLE 123-2 Early Treatment of Marine Envenomations

MARINE ORGANISM	DETOXIFICATION	FURTHER TREATMENT
Catfish, lionfish, scorpionfish, stingray	Submerge injury in hot water [45°C (113°F)] for up to 90 min.	Irrigate with normal saline (0.9%). Explore and debride wound. Administer antibiotics and analgesics. Update tetanus immunization if needed. Elevate extremity. Observe for development of systemic symptoms.
Stonefish	Submerge injury in hot water [45°C (113°F)] for up to 90 min.	Irrigate with normal saline (0.9%). Explore and debride wound. Administer antibiotics and analgesics. Update tetanus immunization if needed. Elevate extremity. Administer stonefish antivenin if severe systemic reaction occurs.
Sea snake	—	Use pressure immobilization. Administer antivenom if severe systemic reaction occurs. Provide supportive care.
Fire coral, hydroids, anemones	Blot area. Irrigate with saline. Apply 5% acetic acid (vinegar) topically.	Apply topical antihistamines or corticosteroid cream for itching.
Portuguese man-of-war, blue bottles	Blot area. Submerge injury in hot water [45°C (113°F)] for 20–30 min. Remove tentacles.	Apply topical antihistamines or corticosteroid cream for itching. Observe for development of systemic symptoms. Provide supportive care.
Box jellyfish	Blot area. Irrigate with saline. Apply 5% acetic acid (vinegar) topically. Remove tentacles.	Apply topical antihistamines or corticosteroid cream for itching. Observe for development of systemic symptoms. Provide supportive care. Administer *Chironex* antivenin.
Australian blue-ringed octopus	—	Use pressure immobilization. Provide supportive care.
Cone snail	—	Use pressure immobilization. Provide supportive care.

(Continued)

TABLE 123-2 Early Treatment of Marine Envenomations (Continued)

MARINE ORGANISM	DETOXIFICATION	FURTHER TREATMENT
Cone snail	—	Use pressure immobilization. Provide supportive care.
Sea urchin	Submerge injury in hot water [45°C (113°F)] for up to 90 min. Remove visible spines or pedicellariae.	Explore wound and remove any spines.
Sponge	Irrigate with water. Apply cold compresses.	Administer oral analgesics. Consider topical or oral antihistamines.
Fireworms	Apply 5% acetic acid (vinegar) topically. Remove bristles.	Consider topical corticosteroids.

124 HIGH-ALTITUDE MEDICAL PROBLEMS

Shaun D. Carstairs

EPIDEMIOLOGY

- The incidence of acute mountain sickness (AMS), as well as high-altitude cerebral edema (HACE) and high-altitude pulmonary edema (HAPE), is influenced primarily by the rapidity of ascent and sleeping altitude.
- The incidence of AMS is 17% and 40% at resorts with altitudes between 2200 and 2700 m (7200 and 9000 ft).
- The incidence of HAPE is much lower than that of AMS. HAPE has been reported in less than 1 in 10,000 skiers in Colorado, and 2% to 3% of climbers on Mt. McKinley. The incidence of HACE is lower than that of HAPE.

PATHOPHYSIOLOGY

- AMS is caused by hypobaric hypoxia, and HAPE and HACE can be viewed as extreme progressions of the same pathophysiology.
- Hypobaric hypoxemia increases cerebral blood flow and cerebral capillary hydrostatic pressure, contributing to fluid shifts, and cerebral edema (mild in AMS, severe in HACE). In addition, increased permeability of capillaries as a result of inflammatory endothelial activation may also play a role, especially in the brain.
- Hypoxemia elevates sympathetic nervous system activity, which promotes uneven pulmonary vasoconstriction and increases pulmonary capillary pressure.
- Increased sympathetic nervous system activity is associated with decreased urine output, mediated by increased renin-angiotensin, aldosterone, and antidiuretic hormone (ADH). This leads to fluid retention and results in elevated capillary hydrostatic pressure in lungs, brain, and peripheral tissues.
- Susceptibility to AMS is linked to a low hypoxic ventilatory response and low vital capacity; susceptible individuals are prone to recurrence on return to high altitude.
- Partially acclimatized individuals who live at intermediate altitudes of 1000 to 2000 m are less likely to develop AMS on ascent to higher altitude.

CLINICAL FEATURES

- AMS is usually seen in unacclimated people making a rapid ascent to over 2000 m (6600 ft) above sea level. The earliest symptoms are light-headedness and mild breathlessness.
- Symptoms similar to a hangover may develop within 6 hours after arrival at altitude, but may be delayed as long as 24 hours. Symptoms may include bifrontal headache, anorexia, nausea, weakness, and fatigue.
- Worsening headache, vomiting, oliguria, dyspnea, and weakness can indicate progression of AMS.
- There are few specific physical examination findings in AMS. Postural hypotension and peripheral and facial edema may occur. Localized rales are noted in 20% of cases. Funduscopy can reveal tortuous and dilated veins; retinal hemorrhages are common at altitudes over 5000 m.
- HACE is an extreme progression of AMS and is usually associated with pulmonary edema. It presents with altered mental status, ataxia, stupor, and progression to coma. Focal neurologic signs such as third and sixth cranial nerve palsies may be present.
- HAPE is the most lethal of the high-altitude syndromes. Risk factors include heavy exertion, rapid ascent, cold exposure, excessive salt intake, use of sleeping medications, and previous history of HAPE.
- Individuals with pulmonary hypertension as well as children with acute respiratory infections may be more susceptible to HAPE.
- Early findings of HAPE include a dry cough, impaired exercise capacity, and localized rales, usually in the right mid-lung field.
- Progression of HAPE leads to tachycardia, tachypnea, resting dyspnea, severe weakness, productive cough, cyanosis, and generalized rales. Low-grade fever is common.

- As hypoxemia worsens, consciousness is impaired, and without treatment, coma and death usually follow.
- Other findings of HAPE may include signs of pulmonary hypertension such as a prominent P2 and right ventricular heave on cardiac examination, as well as right axis deviation and a right ventricular strain pattern on electrocardiogram (ECG).
- Early recognition of HAPE, and descent and treatment are essential to prevent progression.
- High altitude may adversely affect patients with chronic obstructive pulmonary disease (COPD), heart disease, sickle-cell disease, and pregnancy.
- COPD patients may require supplemental O_2 or an increase in their usual O_2 flow rate.
- Patients with atherosclerotic heart disease do surprisingly well at high altitude, but there may be a risk of earlier onset of angina and worsening of heart failure.
- Ascent to 1500 to 2000 m may cause a vaso-occlusive crisis in individuals with sickle-cell disease or sickle thalassemia.
- Individuals with sickle-cell trait usually do well at altitude, but splenic infarction has been reported during heavy exercise.
- Pregnant long-term high-altitude residents have an increased risk of hypertension, low-birth-weight infants, and neonatal jaundice, but no increase in pregnancy complications has been reported in pregnant visitors to high altitude who engage in reasonable activities.
- It is reasonable to advise pregnant women to avoid altitudes above which oxygen saturation falls below 85%; this corresponds to a sleeping altitude of approximately 10,000 ft.

DIAGNOSIS AND DIFFERENTIAL

- The differential diagnosis of the high-altitude syndromes includes hypothermia, carbon monoxide poisoning, pulmonary or central nervous system infections, dehydration, and exhaustion.
- HACE may be difficult to distinguish in the field from other high-altitude neurologic syndromes.
- Strokes due to arterial or venous thrombosis or arterial hemorrhage have been reported at high altitude in individuals without classic risk factors.
- Reversible focal neurologic signs or symptoms may occur and may be due to vasospasm, migraine headache, or transient ischemic attack. These syndromes typically have more focal findings than HACE.
- Previously asymptomatic brain tumors may be unmasked by ascent to high altitude.
- Underlying epilepsy may be worsened by hyperventilation, which is part of the normal acclimatization response.
- HAPE must be distinguished from pulmonary embolus, cardiogenic pulmonary edema, and pneumonia. Low-grade fever is common in HAPE and may make it difficult to distinguish from pneumonia.
- A key to diagnosis is the clinical response to treatment.

CARE AND DISPOSITION IN THE FIELD AND EMERGENCY DEPARTMENT

- AMS can usually be avoided by gradual ascent. A reasonable recommendation for sea-level dwellers is to spend a night at 1500 to 2000 m before sleeping at altitudes above 2500 m.
- High-altitude trekkers should allow two nights for each 1000-m gain in sleeping altitude starting at 3000 m.
- Eating a high-carbohydrate diet and avoiding overexertion, alcohol, and respiratory depressants may also help prevent AMS.
- Mild AMS usually improves or resolves in 12 to 36 hours if further ascent is delayed and acclimatization is allowed. A decrease in altitude of 500 to 1000 m may provide prompt relief of symptoms.
- Oxygen relieves symptoms of mild AMS, and nocturnal low-flow O_2 (0.5-1 L/min) is helpful.
- Patients with mild AMS should not ascend to a higher sleeping elevation. Descent is indicated if symptoms persist or worsen.
- Immediate descent and treatment is indicated if there is a change in the level of consciousness, or if there is ataxia or pulmonary edema.
- **Acetazolamide** causes a bicarbonate diuresis, leading to a mild metabolic acidosis. This stimulates ventilation and pharmacologically produces an acclimatization response. It is effective for prophylaxis and treatment.
- Specific indications for acetazolamide are (1) prior history of altitude illness; (2) abrupt ascent to over 3000 m (10,000 ft); (3) treatment of AMS; and (4) symptomatic periodic breathing during sleep at altitude.
- The adult dose of **acetazolamide** is 125 to 250 milligrams PO twice daily; it is continued until symptoms resolve or is started 24 hours before ascent and continued for 2 days at altitude as prophylaxis.
- Acetazolamide should be restarted if symptoms recur. Acetazolamide is contraindicated in sulfa-allergic patients.
- **Dexamethasone** 4 milligrams PO, IM, or IV every 6 hours, is effective in moderate to severe AMS. Tapering of the dose over several days may be necessary to prevent rebound.
- Aspirin or acetaminophen may improve headache in AMS. **Ondansetron** 4 milligrams PO (disintegrating tablet) every 6 hours may help with nausea and vomiting.

- Diuretics may be useful for treating fluid retention, but should be used with caution to avoid intravascular volume depletion.
- HACE mandates immediate descent or evacuation. Oxygen and **dexamethasone**, 8 milligrams PO, IM, or IV initially, then 4 milligrams every 6 hours, should be administered.
- Intubation and hyperventilation may be necessary in severe cases of HACE. Careful monitoring of arterial blood gases is needed to prevent excessive lowering of P_{CO_2} (below 30 mm Hg), which may cause cerebral ischemia. Mannitol should also be considered.
- HAPE should also be treated with immediate descent. Oxygen may be life-saving if descent is delayed. The patient should be kept warm and exertion minimized.
- For HAPE, drugs are second-line treatment after descent and oxygen. **Nifedipine**, 20 to 30 milligrams extended release PO every 12 hours, may be effective. **Sildenafil**, 50 milligrams PO three times daily, and **tadalafil**, 10 milligrams PO twice daily, both blunt hypoxic pulmonary vasoconstriction and may be considered. Inhaled **albuterol** 2 to 4 puffs every 6 hours may also be considered but is not well studied.
- HAPE patients are usually volume depleted, and care should be taken to avoid precipitating drug-induced hypotension.
- An expiratory positive airway pressure (EPAP) mask may be useful in the field, and without supplemental O_2 can increase oxygen saturation by 10% to 20%.
- Portable fabric inflatable hyperbaric chambers may be effective in the field when immediate descent is not possible.
- In individuals with prior episodes of HAPE, **nifedipine**, 20 milligrams extended release PO every 12 hours, every 8 hours during ascent may be effective as prophylaxis.

MISCELLANEOUS HIGH-ALTITUDE SYNDROMES

- Acute hypoxia may occur with decompression of an aircraft or failure of a mountaineer's oxygen delivery system. Symptoms include dizziness, lightheadedness, and dimming of vision progressing to loss of consciousness.
- A sudden drop in oxygen saturation to 50% or 60% will usually result in unconsciousness. Deliberate hyperventilation may increase the period of useful consciousness in the setting of acute hypoxia.
- High-altitude retinopathy includes retinal edema, tortuous and dilated retinal veins, disc hyperemia, retinal hemorrhages, and less frequently, cotton wool exudates.
- Except for macular hemorrhages, retinal hemorrhages are usually asymptomatic and descent is not indicated unless visual changes occur; hemorrhages usually resolve in 10 to 14 days.
- High-altitude pharyngitis and bronchitis are due to local irritation and drying of mucus membranes from breathing high volumes of cold, dry air. Severe coughing spasms and bronchospasm may be present. Symptomatic treatment as well as hydration, lozenges to encourage salivation, and breathing of steam or through a scarf to trap moisture and heat may provide some relief.
- Chronic mountain polycythemia in long-term high-altitude residents may be attributed to underlying diseases (such as COPD or sleep apnea) that worsen hypoxia at altitude in half of patients, or may be linked to idiopathic hypoventilation due to a diminished respiratory drive.
- Symptoms of chronic mountain polycythemia include impaired cognition, sleep, and peripheral circulation, as well as headache, drowsiness, and chest congestion, along with abnormally elevated hemoglobin levels, usually over 20 to 22 grams/dL.
- Treatment options for chronic mountain polycythemia include moving to a lower altitude, phlebotomy, home oxygen, and respiratory stimulants such as acetazolamide and medroxyprogesterone.
- Ultraviolet keratitis (snow blindness) may affect unprotected eyes in as little as 1 hour at high altitude. Findings include severe pain, photophobia, tearing, conjunctival erythema, chemosis, and eyelid swelling.
- Cold compresses, analgesics, and occasionally eye patching are generally adequate symptomatic treatment for ultraviolet keratitis; the keratitis usually heals in 24 hours. Prevention with adequate sunglasses that transmit less than 10% of UVB light is essential.

For further reading in Tintinalli's *Emergency Medicine: A Comprehensive Study Guide*, 7th ed., see Chapter 216, "High Altitude Medical Problems," by Peter H. Hackett and Jenny Hargrove.

125 DYSBARISM AND COMPLICATIONS OF DIVING

Christian A. Tomaszewski

EPIDEMIOLOGY

- Dysbarism is commonly encountered in scuba divers and refers to complications associated with changes in environmental ambient pressure while breathing compressed gases.

- To understand diving injuries, one must be familiar with the three gas laws: Boyle's, Dalton's, and Henry's.
- Boyle's law states that pressure and volume are inversely related. Therefore, if air-filled spaces that are fixed in size are not equilibrated during descent or ascent, barotrauma can ensue.
- Dalton's law states that the total pressure exerted by a mixture of gases is the sum of the partial pressures of each gas. This helps explains the uptake of inert gas into tissue with depth.
- Henry's law states that, at equilibrium, the quantity of gas in solution is proportional to the partial pressure of that gas. This, along with Dalton's law, explains the release of inert gas, that is, nitrogen, from tissue with ascent.
- Divers using compressed air, caisson (tunnel) workers, and high-altitude pilots can all present with decompression sickness (DCS). In divers, this usually results from exceeding the dive table limits for depth and time.
- Sport divers are more prone to DCS of the spinal cord, while professional divers, caisson workers, and aviators tend more often to DCS of the joints.
- DCS can occur within minutes to hours of surfacing, rarely days later. It may be precipitated by flying within 24 hours of diving.

PATHOPHYSIOLOGY

- Barotrauma of descent includes squeezes of the ears, face, and teeth along with inner ear and sinus barotraumas (Table 125-1).
- Gas-filled areas are subjected to decreases in volume with descent. If such areas are not equilibrated, for example, by Valsalva maneuver for the middle ear, a "squeeze" can result with pain and injury to surrounding structures, that is, tympanic membrane.
- Barotrauma during ascent is due to expansion of gas in body cavities.
- Clinical conditions associated with ascent include alternobaric vertigo, pulmonary barotrauma, cerebral arterial gas embolism, and DCS (Table 125-1).
- DCS is due to release of inert gas (nitrogen) within tissues or the circulation. This usually occurs from saturated tissue during or immediately after ascent. In extreme amounts, these bubbles can cause both acute occlusive and delayed inflammatory effects.
- Spinal cord DCS, a form of type II DCS, occurs when autochthonous bubbles form *in situ* in various sites throughout the cord. Therefore, there may not be a distinct spinal cord syndrome and patients can present with ascending paralysis or spotty deficits with autonomic dysfunction, including incontinence or retention.

TABLE 125-1 Summary of Barotrauma of Descent and Ascent

BAROTRAUMA OF DESCENT	CLINICAL FEATURES	TREATMENT
Otic barotrauma ("ear squeeze")	Pain, fullness, vertigo, conductive hearing loss from inability to equalize middle ear pressure	Decongestants, consider antibiotics.
Sinus barotrauma ("sinus squeeze")	Pain over affected sinus, possible bleeding from nare	Decongestants, consider antibiotics.
Inner ear barotrauma	Sudden onset of sensorineural hearing loss, tinnitus, severe vertigo after forced Valsalva	Head of bed up, no nose blowing, antivertigo medications, urgent otolaryngology consultation as some surgeons advocate early exploration.
BAROTRAUMA OF ASCENT	**CLINICAL FEATURES**	**TREATMENT**
Pulmonary barotrauma	Dyspnea, chest pain, subcutaneous air, extra-alveolar air on radiograph; usually occurring secondary to rapid or uncontrolled ascent	Pneumomediastinum requires only symptomatic care and does not require recompression. Pneumothorax requires drainage and does not require recompression (if recompression is instituted for treatment of arterial gas embolism, then the pneumothorax must be drained before recompression).
Arterial gas embolism	Neurologic symptoms occurring immediately after uncontrolled or rapid ascent or neurologic symptoms in the setting of pulmonary barotrauma	Airway, breathing, circulation, high-flow oxygen, IV hydration, immediate recompression (hyperbaric oxygen), consider adjunctive lidocaine. Any neurologic symptom in the setting of documented pulmonary barotrauma must be treated as an arterial gas embolism.

CLINICAL FEATURES

BAROTRAUMA OF DESCENT (SEE TABLE 125-1)

- The most common form of barotrauma occurs during descent and is middle ear squeeze, or barotitis media. It is caused by inability to equalize pressure causing tympanic membrane bleeding or rupture and may result in conductive hearing loss.

- A forceful Valsalva during equalization can cause inner ear barotrauma with rupture of the round or oval window. Symptoms include tinnitus, sensorineural hearing loss, and vertigo.
- If the sinus ostia are occluded on descent, an impending squeeze can cause bleeding from the maxillary or frontal sinuses, resulting in pain and epistaxis.
- Other gas-filled areas can be subjected to squeeze with descent. Facial bruising and subconjunctival hemorrhages may result when air is not added to a face mask. A dry-suit squeeze can result when folds compress down on underlying skin producing painful red skin lines.

BAROTRAUMA OF ASCENT (SEE TABLE 125-1)

- In the middle ear, the pressure differential from asymmetrical expansion can cause alternobaric vertigo. This is a temporary condition due to unequal pressure between both vestibular complexes.
- Although rare, "reverse squeeze" may affect the ear or sinuses during ascent with rupture.
- Pulmonary overinflation or burst lung can occur during rapid, panicked ascents if divers fail to exhale or if intrinsic pulmonary air trapping exists (eg, COPD). This may be manifested by pneumomediastinum, subcutaneous emphysema, or pneumothorax.
- The most serious consequence of pulmonary overinflation is cerebral arterial gas embolism (CAGE). Air transgresses into the pulmonary venous circulation, thereby embolizing to the brain. Any neurologic symptoms that occur on ascent or immediately upon surfacing should be considered secondary to CAGE. Such symptoms may include loss of consciousness, seizure, blindness, disorientation, hemiplegia, or other signs of stroke.

DECOMPRESSION SICKNESS (SEE TABLE 125-2)

- DCS presents as one of two types. Type I is "pain only," and type II is more "serious."
- Type I DCS includes mottled skin ("cutis marmorata") or deep pain of the joints, usually the shoulder or knee, that is unaffected by movement.
- Type II DCS is primarily associated with the central nervous system, typically the spine. Patients may initially complain of truncal constriction with ascending paralysis. Prolonged exposure at depth can also lead to cardiopulmonary "chokes" or vestibular "staggers." In chokes, massive numbers of pulmonary artery bubbles can cause cough, hemoptysis, dyspnea, and substernal chest pain. Staggers, from vestibular DCS, is manifested by vertigo, hearing loss, tinnitus, and disequilibrium.
- A third type of DCS has been described (Table 125-2). It occurs when arterial gas embolism promotes release of tissue gas and can have features of cerebral arterial gas embolism.
- Because DCS and CAGE can be difficult to distinguish, or present simultaneously, the inclusive term "decompression illness (DCI)" is often typically used.

TABLE 125-2 Classification of Decompression Sickness

CLASSIFICATION	CLINICAL FEATURES	COMMENTS
Type I: "pain-only" DCS	Deep pain in joints and extremities, unrelieved but not worsened with movement.	Usually single joint, most commonly knees and shoulders.
	Skin changes—mottling, pruritus, color changes.	Lymphatic obstruction can occur and takes days to resolve despite recompression therapy.
Type II: "serious" DCS	Pulmonary ("chokes")—cough, hemoptysis, dyspnea, and substernal chest pain.	—
	Cardiovascular collapse can occur.	—
	Neurologic—sensation of truncal constriction → ascending paralysis, usually rapid in onset.	Has a tendency to affect the lower cervical and thoracic regions → may see scattered lesions. Autonomic dysfunction seen
	Vestibular ("staggers")—vertigo, hearing loss, tinnitus, and dysequilibrium.	Usually occurs after deep, long dives.
Type III: combination of DCS and arterial gas embolism	Symptoms of DCS II noted above +	—
	Variety of stroke syndromes, symptoms, and signs	Symptoms occur on ascent or immediately upon surfacing. Symptoms may spontaneously resolve.

Abbreviation: DCS = decompression sickness.

DIAGNOSIS AND DIFFERENTIAL

- Dive profile (depth, duration, and repetitiveness) and time of symptom onset are the most useful historical factors in distinguishing dysbarism from other disorders.
- During descent, the most common maladies are the squeezes. A fistula test, insufflation of the tympanic membrane on the affected side causing the eyes to deviate to the contralateral side, may help diagnose inner ear barotrauma.
- During ascent, barotrauma or alternobaric vertigo is most likely to occur. A chest radiograph may reveal pneumomediastinum, pneumothorax, or subcutaneous air after pulmonary overinflation. If accompanied by early neurological symptoms, CAGE should be considered.
- The differential diagnosis for DCS is broad. Musculoskeletal complaints could be joint strain or symptomatic herniated cervical disk. Chest pain may represent cardiac ischemia from overexertion. Immersion pulmonary edema from non-cardiogenic causes can occur during strenuous dives, particularly in cold water. Seizures at depth can result from breathing-enriched mixtures of oxygen exceeding 1.4 atmospheres absolute.
- If DCS is suspected, a trial of pressure with hyperbaric oxygen usually results in some improvement.

EMERGENCY DEPARTMENT CARE AND DISPOSITION

- Both middle ear and sinus barotrauma can be treated with decongestants and analgesics (Table 125-1). One can consider antibiotics. Advise patients against diving until healing is completed, especially for tympanic trauma. The patient should be able to equalize pressures within the ears effectively in order to return to diving.
- Inner ear barotrauma requires bed rest with the head upright until otolaryngologic evaluation for possible surgical exploration.
- Alternobaric vertigo requires no specific treatment because of its transient nature.
- All cases of DCI, both DCS and CAGE, deserve immediate 100% oxygen and IV fluids.
- If CAGE is suspected, place the patient in the supine position, not Trendelenburg. If vomiting occurs, readjust to the left lateral decubitus position to prevent aspiration.
- In all cases of DCI, particularly if serious, rapidly arrange for recompression therapy (hyperbaric oxygen). Hyperbaric oxygen therapy can decrease bubble size, increase nitrogen washout, decrease tissue edema and ischemia, and prevent neutrophil adherence with inflammation. Divers Alert Network (1-919-684-8111) may help provide chamber locations.
- **Lidocaine** 1 milligram/kg IV bolus followed by a continuous infusion at 1 milligram/min may provide neuroprotection, especially in cases of CAGE.
- Pulmonary overinflation with ascent may require **needle decompression** or **tube thoracostomy** if a pneumothorax develops.

SPECIAL CONSIDERATIONS

- Immersion pulmonary edema can occur during strenuous diving, particularly in cold water. Clinical features include dyspnea, chest pain, and frothy pink sputum, with pulmonary edema on radiography. Although a cardiac evaluation may be warranted, this condition is usually not associated with any abnormality and does not require treatment beyond symptomatic care.
- Nitrogen narcosis occurs when breathing air at depths greater than 100 ft of seawater. High-order mental function and motor skills are temporarily disabled. This effect resolves with ascent or breathing of alternate gas mixtures.
- Oxygen toxicity can affect the pulmonary and/or cerebral systems. Pulmonary oxygen toxicity is unusual in diving because prolonged exposures are required. But cerebral oxygen toxicity can occur with partial pressures of oxygen just exceeding 1.4 ATA. Manifestations of this include twitching, nausea, paresthesias, dizziness, and even seizures. Although rare, cerebral oxygen toxicity can occur in divers breathing enhanced oxygen concentrations or patients during hyperbaric oxygen therapy sessions.

For further reading in Tintinalli's *Emergency Medicine: A Comprehensive Study Guide,* 7th ed., see Chapter 208, "Dysbarism and Complications of Diving," by Brain Snyder and Tom Neuman.

126 DROWNING

Richard A. Walker

EPIDEMIOLOGY

- The three age-related peaks for drowning are (1) toddlers and young children, (2) adolescents and young adults, and (3) the elderly.

- The elderly are at increased risk of bathtub drowning.
- Warm, freshwater drowning (especially swimming pools) is more common than salt water drowning, even in coastal areas.

PATHOPHYSIOLOGY

- Prognosis after submersion injuries depends on the degree of pulmonary and central nervous system injury.
- The diving reflex is strongest in infants <6 months old, but decreases with age and may not provide as much cerebral protection as once thought.
- Cerebral protection in cold water submersion may result from rapid central nervous system (CNS) cooling.
- "Dry drowning" results from laryngospasm that causes hypoxemia and varying degrees of neurologic insult, and represents up to 20% of submersion injuries.
- "Wet drowning" consists of aspiration of water into the lungs, causing washout of surfactant, which results in diminished alveolar gas transfer, atelectasis, and ventilation-perfusion mismatch.
- The majority of patients who arrive at the hospital with stable cardiovascular signs and awake, alert neurologic function survive with minimal disability.
- Those who arrive with unstable cardiovascular function and coma do poorly because of the hypoxic, ischemic CNS insult.

CLINICAL FEATURES

- Transient hemodilution may occur in freshwater drownings with large-volume aspiration resulting in hemolysis and hyponatremia.
- Hemoconcentration, hypernatremia, and hyperkalemia may occur in salt water drowning.
- Noncardiogenic pulmonary edema results from moderate to severe aspiration of water in "wet drowning" cases.
- Physical examination may reveal clear lungs, rales, rhonchi, or wheezes.
- Mental status may range from normal to comatose.

DIAGNOSIS AND DIFFERENTIAL

- Injuries or disorders that precipitate or are associated with submersion events are shown in Table 126-1.
- Laboratory findings may include metabolic acidosis and electrolyte abnormalities if there is associated renal injury from hypoxemia, hemoglobinuria, or myoglobinuria.
- Disseminated intravascular coagulation is rare.

TABLE 126-1 Injuries and Disorders Associated with Submersion Events
Spinal cord injuries that occur after diving into shallow water or in boating mishaps
Hypothermia
Panicking
Syncope (eg, due to hyperventilation prior to underwater diving)
Seizures
Other premorbid conditions (eg, dysrhythmias, heart disease)

- The chest radiograph may be normal or show generalized pulmonary edema or perihilar infiltrates.
- Since the chest radiograph findings may not correlate with the arterial Po_2, an arterial blood gas (ABG) analysis to assess oxygen saturation and metabolic acidosis is important.

EMERGENCY DEPARTMENT CARE AND DISPOSITION

- Treatment for submersion events is summarized in Fig. 126-1.
- All patients should have their airway, ventilation, and oxygenation status assessed. The cervical spine should be stabilized and evaluated in cases of diving accidents, multiple trauma, or if the circumstances are unknown.
- Warmed IV normal saline and warming adjuncts (overhead warmer, bear hugger, etc.) should be used if the patient is hypothermic. The patient's core temperature should be monitored.
- Patients with a Glasgow Coma Scale (GCS) score ≥14 and oxygen saturation (Sao_2) ≥95% may be discharged home after a 4- to 6-hour observation period as long as their pulmonary and neurologic examinations and Sao_2 remain normal.
- The patient with an oxygen requirement or abnormal pulmonary examination after 4 to 6 hours should be admitted.
- Patients with a GCS <14 should be administered supplemental oxygen. Intubation and mechanical ventilation are indicated if the Pao_2 cannot be maintained >60 mm Hg in adults or >80 mm Hg in children, despite high-flow oxygen (40-60%).
- Antibiotics are usually administered to treat pulmonary aspiration and possible contamination with Aeromonas species, but there is no data to support or refute this practice.
- Childhood victims of freshwater near drowning rarely develop dilutional hyponatremia and seizures, which are usually easily controlled by correction of the electrolyte abnormality.

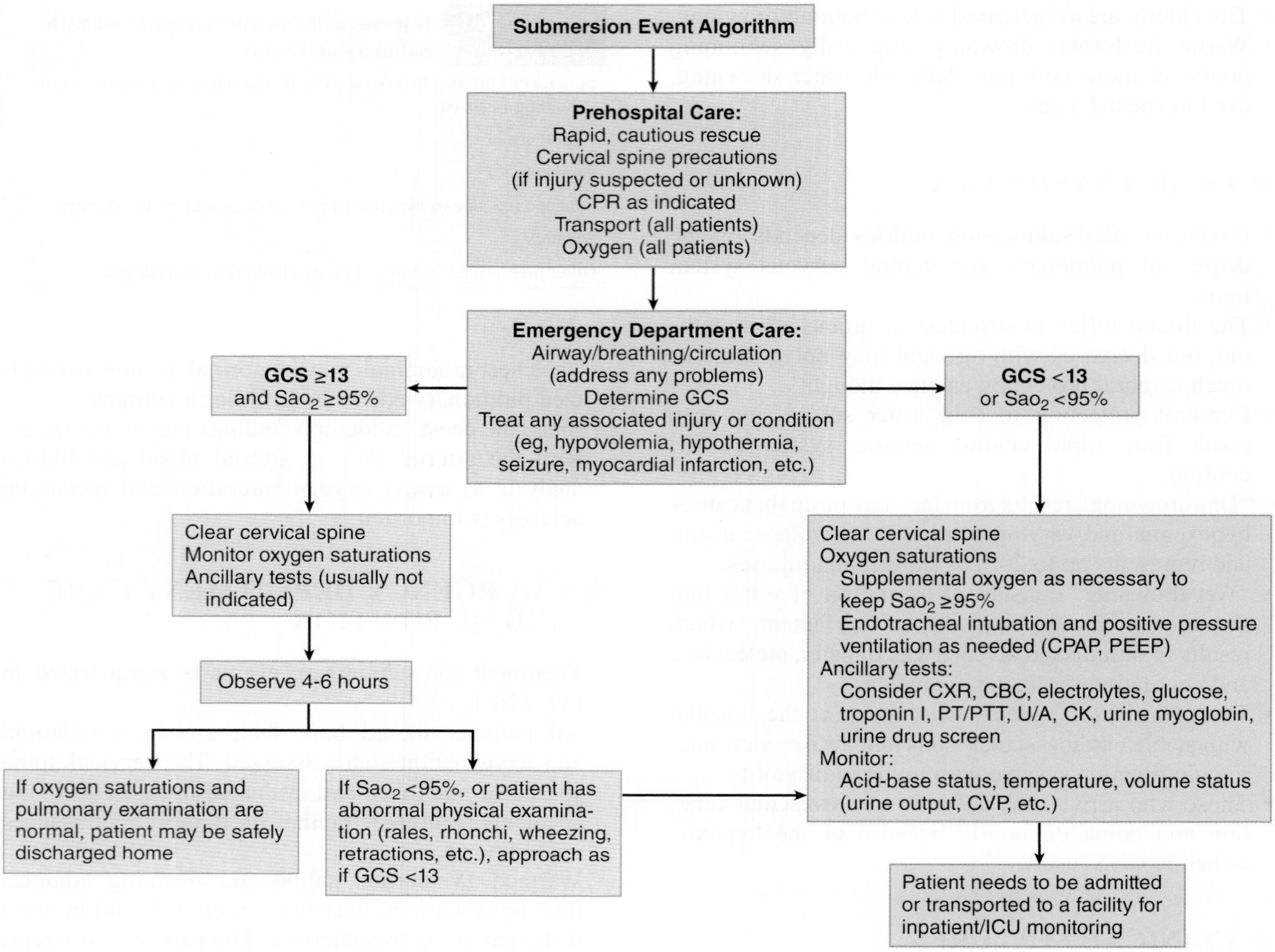

FIG. 126-1. Submersion event algorithm. CBC = complete blood count; CK = creatine kinase; CPAP = continuous positive airway pressure; CVP = central venous pressure; CXR = chest radiograph; GCS = Glasgow Coma Scale score; ICU = intensive care unit; PEEP = positive end-expiratory pressure; PT = prothrombin time; PTT = partial thromboplastin time; Sao_2 = oxygen saturation (via pulse oximetry); U/A = urinalysis.

- Efforts at "brain resuscitation," including the use of mannitol, loop diuretics, hypertonic saline, fluid restriction, mechanical hyperventilation, controlled hypothermia, barbiturate coma, and intracranial pressure monitoring have not shown benefit.
- Continuous infusion of vasopressors may be required in the postresuscitation phase.
- Factors associated with after a poor prognosis in warm-water drowning include bystander CPR at the scene, cardiopulmonary resuscitation (CPR) in the ED, and asystole at the scene or in the ED.
- Consideration should be given to withholding resuscitation in patients with prolonged submersion and transport.
- Reports of complete and near-complete neurologic recovery after asystole in adults and children have been reported in prolonged icy-water submersion.
- Hypothermic victims of cold-water submersion in cardiac arrest should undergo prolonged and aggressive resuscitation maneuvers until they are normothermic or considered not viable.

For further reading in Tintinalli's *Emergency Medicine: A Comprehensive Study Guide,* 7th ed., see Chapter 209, "Near Drowning," by Alan L. Causey and Mark A. Nichter.

127 THERMAL AND CHEMICAL BURNS

Sandra L. Werner

THERMAL BURNS

EPIDEMIOLOGY

- Approximately 500,000 Americans are treated for burns annually, and 40,000 are hospitalized. Most ED burn patients are treated and discharged. Of those patients requiring hospitalization, over 60% are admitted to one of the country's 125 burn centers.
- The risk of burns is highest in the 18- to 35-year-old age group. There is a male–female ratio of 2:1 for both injury and death. Scald injuries are more common in the pediatric and elderly populations.
- The death rate in patients over 65 years of age is much higher than in the overall burn population.
- The risk of death from a major burn is associated with increased burn size, increased age, concomitant inhalation injury, and female sex.
- Significant advances in burn management have decreased the mortality rate for major thermal burns to 4%.

PATHOPHYSIOLOGY

- Thermal injury results in local and systemic homeostatic derangements including disruption of cell membrane function, hormonal alterations, changes in tissue acid–base balance, as well as hemodynamic and hematologic affects, all of which contribute to burn shock.
- Fluid and electrolyte abnormalities in burn shock are caused by dysfunction of the sodium pump and include a cellular influx of sodium and fluid, and extracellular migration of potassium.
- Significant metabolic acidosis may be present in large burns. Patients with burns covering >60% total body surface area (TBSA) may have depression myocardial activity.
- Hematologic derangements include an early increase in hematocrit and viscosity, followed by anemia in the later phases.
- Thermal injury is progressive. Initial local effects include release of vasoactive substances, cellular dysfunction, and edema. The systemic response results in changes in the neurohormonal axis and alterations in all organ systems. The released neurohormonal and vasoactive substances act at the local level, causing progression of the burn wound.
- A full-thickness burn has three zones:

  Coagulation—tissue is irreversibly destroyed by thrombosis of blood vessels
  Stasis—tissue is viable but there is stagnation of circulation
  Hyperemia—tissue is viable and there is increased blood flow
- Inadequate resuscitation results in increased tissue damage within the zone of stasis.
- Prognosis of burn patients is most affected by the severity of the burn, presence of inhalation injury, associated injuries, patient's age, preexisting conditions, and acute organ failure.

CLINICAL FEATURES

- Burns are categorized by their size and depth. Burn size is calculated as the percentage of total body surface area (BSA) involved.
- The most common method to estimate the percentage of BSA burned is the "rule of nines" (Fig. 127-1).
- A more accurate tool to determine the percentage of BSA burned, especially in infants and children, is the Lund and Browder burn diagram (Fig. 127-2).
- For smaller burns, the patient's hand can be used as a "ruler" to estimate percent BSA. This area represents approximately 1% of the patient's BSA.
- Burn depth has historically been described in degrees: first, second, third, and fourth.

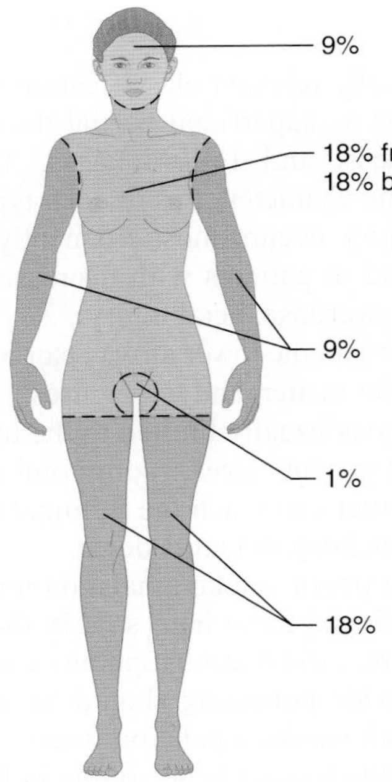

FIG. 127-1. Rule of nines to estimate the percentage of burn.

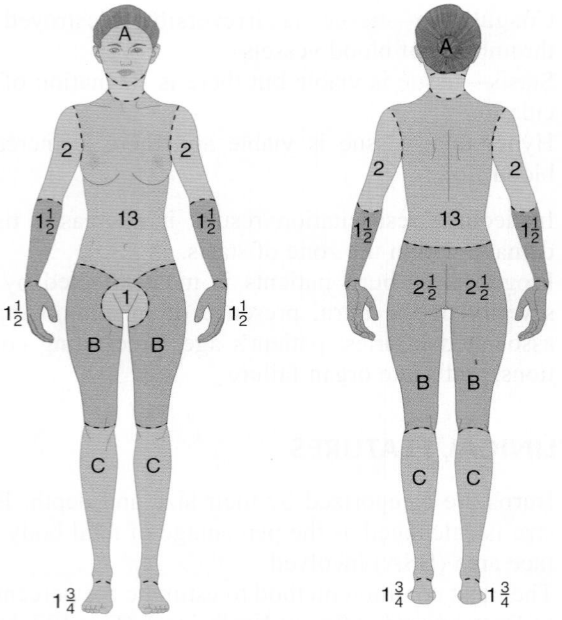

Relative percentages of areas affected by growth (age in years)

	0	1	5	10	15	Adult
A: half of head	9½	8½	6½	5½	4½	3½
B: half of thigh	2¾	3¼	4	4¼	4½	4¾
C: half of leg	2½	2½	2¾	3	3¼	3½

Second-degree ________________ and

Third-degree ________________ =

Total percent burned ______

FIG. 127-2. Lund and Browder diagram to estimate the percentage of a burn.

- A more clinically relevant classification scheme categorizes burns as superficial partial-thickness, deep partial-thickness, and full-thickness. Table 127-1 summarizes the characteristics of each type of burn.
- Inhalation injury occurs most frequently in closed-space fires and in patients with decreased cognition (intoxication, overdose, head injury).
- Both the upper and the lower airway can be injured by heat, particulate matter, and toxic gases.
- Thermal injury is usually limited to the upper airway and can result in acute airway compromise.
- Particulate matter can reach the terminal bronchioles and cause bronchospasm and edema.
- Clinical indicators of smoke inhalation injury include facial burns, singed nasal hair, soot in the upper airway, hoarseness, carbonaceous sputum, and wheezing.
- Carbon monoxide poisoning should be suspected in all patients with smoke inhalation injury.
- Consider hydrogen cyanide poisoning in fires involving nitrogen-containing polymer products such as wool, silk, polyurethane, and vinyl.

TABLE 127-1 Burn Depth Features Classified by Degree of Burn

BURN DEPTH	HISTOLOGY/ ANATOMY	EXAMPLE	HEALING
First degree	Epidermis No blisters, painful	Sunburn	7 d
Superficial second degree or superficial partial thickness	Epidermis and superficial dermis Blisters, very painful	Hot water scald	14-21 d, no scar
Deep second degree or deep partial thickness	Epidermis and deep dermis, sweat glands, and hair follicles Blisters, very painful	Hot liquid, steam, grease, flame	3-8 wk, permanent scar
Third degree	Entire epidermis and dermis charred, pale, leathery; no pain	Flame	Months, severe scarring, skin grafts necessary
Fourth degree	Entire epidermis and dermis, as well as bone, fat, and/or muscle	Flame	Months, multiple surgeries usually required

DIAGNOSIS AND DIFFERENTIAL

- Burns are classified as major, moderate, or minor. Table 127-2 summarizes the American Burn Association (ABA) burn classifications and recommended patient dispositions.
- Inhalation injury is diagnosed based on clinical history of an enclosed-space fire and presence of facial burns, singed nasal hairs, carbonaceous sputum, soot in the upper airway, and/or wheezing on examination.
- The chest radiograph in smoke inhalation injury may be normal initially. Flexible fiberoptic bronchoscopy can confirm the diagnosis.
- Obtain carboxyhemoglobin levels if carbon monoxide poisoning is suspected.

EMERGENCY DEPARTMENT CARE AND DISPOSITION

- Management of patients with moderate to major burns is divided into three phases: prehospital care, ED resuscitation, and transfer to a burn center.
- Prehospital care consists of stopping the burning process, establishing an airway, initiating fluid resuscitation, relieving pain, and protecting the burn wound.
- In the ED, reevaluate the airway and administer 100% oxygen.

TABLE 127-2 Burn Depth Features: American Burn Association Burn Classification

BURN CLASSIFICATION	BURN CHARACTERISTICS	DISPOSITION
Major burn	Partial thickness >25% BSA, age 10-50 y Partial thickness >20% BSA, age <10 y or >50 y Full thickness >10% BSA in anyone Burns involving hands, face, feet, or perineum Burns crossing major joints Circumferential burns of an extremity Burns complicated by inhalation injury Electrical burns Burns complicated by fracture or other trauma Burns in high-risk patients	Burn center treatment
Moderate burn	Partial thickness 15-25% BSA, age 10-50 y Partial thickness 10-20% BSA, age <10 y or >50 y Full thickness burns ≤10% BSA in anyone No major burn characteristics present	Hospitalization
Minor burn	Partial thickness <15% BSA, age 10-50 y Partial thickness <10% BSA, age <10 y or >50 y Full thickness <2% in anyone No major burn characteristics present	Outpatient treatment

Abbreviation: BSA = body surface area.

- Intubate and ventilate the patient if indicated by the presence of oral/perioral burns, circumferential neck burns, stridor, depressed mental status, or respiratory distress. Obtain an ABG with co-oximetry and a CXR.
- Establish at least two IV lines in unburned areas and initiate fluid resuscitation using the Parkland or similar burn formula.
- The Parkland formula calls for Lactated Ringers, 4 mL/kg times the percentage of BSA burned, given over 24 hours. Give half the calculated amount in the first 8 hours post injury and the remainder over the next 16 hours.
- The 24-hour time interval begins at the time the patient sustained the burn, not the time of resuscitation onset. The percentage BSA used in this calculation includes only second- and third-degree burns.
- Further fluid resuscitation is guided by vital signs, cerebral and peripheral perfusion, and adequate urine output.
- Evaluate and treat traumatic injures using standard trauma resuscitation guidelines (see Chapter 158, Trauma in Adults; Chapter 159, Trauma in Children; and Chapter 160, Geriatric Trauma).

TABLE 127-3 American Burn Association Burn Unit Referral Criteria

Third-degree burns in any age group
Electrical burns, including lightning injury
Chemical burns
Inhalation injury
Burn injury in patients with preexisting medical disorders that could complicate management, prolong recovery, or affect mortality
Burn injury in any patients with concomitant trauma (such as fractures) in whom the burn injury poses the greatest risk of morbidity or mortality
Burn injury in children in hospitals without qualified personnel or equipment to care for children
Burn injury in patients who will require special social, emotional, or long-term rehabilitative intervention
Burn injury in children <10 y and adults >50 y of age

- After initiating resuscitation, address burn wounds. Apply cool compresses to small burns. Cover large burns with sterile, dry sheets, as saline-soaked sheets may cause hypothermia.
- Administration of empiric intravenous antibiotics and application of topical antibiotics is not recommended.
- Administer intravenous opiod analgesia early and titrate to relief of pain.
- Treat inhalation injury with humidified oxygen, intubation and ventilation, bronchodilators, and pulmonary toilet. Treat severe carbon monoxide poisoning with hyperbaric oxygen therapy.
- Perform escharotomy as indicated for circumferential burns of the neck, chest, or extremities.
- Update tetanus prophylaxis, if needed. Give tetanus immune globulin to patients without primary immunization.
- Hospitalize patients with moderate and major burns. The ABA's criteria for burn center referral are listed in Table 127-3.
- Minor burns can be treated on an outpatient basis. Table 127-4 summarizes the care of minor burns.

TABLE 127-4 ED Care of Minor Burns

Provide appropriate analgesics before burn care and for outpatient use
Cleanse burn with mild soap and water or dilute antiseptic solution
Debride wound as needed
Apply topical antimicrobial:
1% silver sulfadiazine cream (not on the face or in patients with a sulfa allergy)
Bacitracin ointment
Triple-antibiotic ointment (neomycin, polymyxin B, bacitracin zinc)
Consider use of synthetic occlusive dressings
Provide detailed burn care instructions with follow-up in 24-48 h

Patients with minor burns may be discharged from the ED, provided close follow-up is available.

CHEMICAL BURNS

EPIDEMIOLOGY

- Chemical burn injuries account for 5% to 10% of burn center admissions.
- Common household chemical burns are usually minor and are caused by lye (drain cleaner), halogenated hydrocarbons (paint removers), phenols (deodorizers, disinfectants), sodium hypochlorite (bleach), and sulfuric acid (toilet bowl cleaner).
- Alkalis and acids are commonly used in numerous industrial processes including tanning, curing, extracting, and preserving.
- White phosphorus has been used in military munitions and may be found in rodenticides, pesticides, and fireworks.
- Body sites most often burned by chemicals are the face, eyes, and extremities.
- Although chemical burns are smaller and have a lower mortality rate than thermal burns, wound healing and hospital length of stay are longer.

PATHOPHYSIOLOGY

- Contact with chemical agents can result in burns, irritant contact dermatitis, allergic reaction, thermal injury, or systemic toxicity.
- Skin damage by chemicals can be similar to thermal injury, ranging from superficial erythema to full-thickness loss. Chemical burns may initially appear deceptively mild, but progress to more extensive skin damage and systemic toxicity.
- Factors that influence tissue damage include the quantity and strength/concentration of the agent, manner and duration of contact, phase of the agent, mechanism of action, and extent of penetration.
- Factors that influence percutaneous absorption of chemicals include the body site exposed, integrity and condition of the skin, nature of the chemical, and occlusion of the exposed area.
- The majority of chemical burns are caused by acids or alkalis. Alkalis usually produce far more tissue damage than acids.
- Acids typically cause coagulation necrosis, which produces a leathery eschar that limits further damage.
- Alkalis cause liquefaction necrosis, allowing deeper tissue damage to occur.

CLINICAL FEATURES

- Skin damage from chemical burns depends on the type of agent, concentration, volume, and duration of exposure.
- Hydrofluoric (HF) acid is a special case as it rapidly penetrates intact skin and causes progressive pain and deep tissue destruction without obvious superficial damage.
- Chemical burns of the eye are true ocular emergencies.
- Acid ocular burns quickly precipitate proteins in the superficial eye structures, resulting in a "ground glass" appearance.
- Alkali ocular burns are more severe due to deeper, ongoing penetration. Severe chemosis, blanched conjunctiva, and an opacified cornea can occur. Blindness can result from retinal penetration with destruction of sensory elements.
- Lacrimators (tear gas and pepper mace) cause ocular, mucous membrane, and pulmonary irritation.

DIAGNOSIS AND DIFFERENTIAL

- Diagnosis is usually made by history of exposure to a chemical agent.
- Chemical topical exposure should be considered in all cases of skin irritation/pain.
- For ocular exposures, pH paper can help distinguish alkali from acid exposure.

EMERGENCY DEPARTMENT CARE AND DISPOSITION

- The first priority in treatment of chemical burns is to terminate the burning process.
- Remove garments. Brush off dry chemical particles. Immediately irrigate the skin copiously with water.
- Cover elemental metals (sodium, lithium, calcium, magnesium) with mineral oil because exposure to water may cause a severe exothermic reaction.
- For ocular burns, begin irrigation with 1 to 2 L of normal saline. In patients with acid or alkali burns, continue irrigation until pH is normal.
- Patients with alkali burns will require prolonged irrigation.
- Visual acuity check and pH testing should follow, not precede, ocular irrigation.
- Consult with an ophthalmologist.
- Treatment for specific chemical burns is provided in Table 127-5.
- Options for treating cutaneous HF acid burns are provided in Table 127-6. Consult with a plastic surgeon for patients with HF acid burns of the hands, feet, digits, or nails.
- After initial decontamination, initiate IV fluid resuscitation, analgesia, and tetanus immunoprophylaxis, and address systemic toxicity, as needed.

TABLE 127-5 Treatment of Select Chemical Burns

CHEMICAL	TREATMENT	COMMENTS
Acids		
All acid burns require prompt decontamination and copious irrigation with water.		
Acetic acid	Copious irrigation.	Consider systemic antibiotics for extensive scalp burns.
Phenol (carbolic acid)	Copious irrigation. Swab with polyethylene glycol 300 and industrial methylated spirits in a 2:1 mixture.	Isopropyl alcohol may also be used.
Chromic acid	Copious irrigation. 5% thiosulfate soaks or ascorbic acid creams.	Observe for systemic toxicity.
Formic acid	Copious irrigation.	Dialysis may be needed for severe toxicity.
Hydrofluoric acid	Copious irrigation. Calcium gluconate gel.	Consider SC or intradermal injection of 5% calcium gluconate or intra-arterial calcium gluconate for severe cases.
Nitric acid	Copious irrigation.	Consult with burn specialist.
Oxalic acid	Copious irrigation.	Evaluate serum electrolytes and renal function.
	IV calcium may be required.	Cardiac monitoring for serious dermal exposure.
Alkalis		
All alkali burns require prompt decontamination and copious, prolonged irrigation with water.		—
Portland cement	Prolonged copious irrigation.	May need to remove cement particles with a brush, such as a pre-operative scrubbing brush.
Elemental Metals		
Water is generally contraindicated in extinguishing burning metal fragments embedded in the skin.		
Elemental metals (sodium, lithium, potassium, magnesium, aluminum, and calcium)	Cover metal fragments with sand, foam from a Class D fire extinguisher, or with mineral oil. Excise metal fragments that cannot be wiped away.	—
Hydrocarbons		
Gasoline	Decontamination.	—
Tar	Cool before removal.	Mayonnaise can be used.
	Remove using ointment containing polyoxylene sorbitan (polysorbate) or De-solv-it.	
Vesicants		
Mustards	Decontaminate. Copious irrigation.	If limited water supply, adsorbent powders (flour, talcum powder, fuller's earth) can be applied to the mustard and then wiped away with a moist towel.
Reducing Agents		
Alkyl mercury compounds	Copious irrigation. Debride, drain, and copiously irrigate blisters.	Blister fluid is high in metallic mercury content.
Lacrimators		
Tear gas	Copious irrigation.	May cause respiratory symptoms if inhaled.
Pepper spray	Copious irrigation.	May cause respiratory symptoms if inhaled.
Miscellaneous		
White phosphorus	Remove clothing. Copious irrigation. Debride visible particles.	Systemic toxicity is a significant concern.
Airbag	Prolonged copious irrigation.	—

TABLE 127-6 Options for Treatment of Hydrofluoric Acid Skin Burns

1. Copious irrigation for 15-30 min immediately.
2. Application of calcium gluconate gel, 25 mL of 10% calcium gluconate in 75 mL of sterile water-soluble lubricant.
3. Further treatment options as dictated by patient response:
   a. Dermal injection of 5% calcium gluconate up to a maximum of 1 mL per cm^2 of skin surface using a small gauge needle.
   b. Regional block using Bier's method with 40 mL 10% calcium gluconate.
   c. Arterial infusion over 2-4 h (40 mL of 5% dextrose in water with 10 mL of 10% calcium gluconate).
   d. Consider supplemental magnesium IV.

For further reading in Tintinalli's *Emergency Medicine: A Comprehensive Study Guide,* 7th ed., see Chapter 210, "Thermal Burns," by Lawrence R. Schwartz and Chenicheri Balakrishnan, and Chapter 211, "Chemical Burns," by Fred P. Harchelroad Jr. and David M. Rottinghaus.

128 ELECTRICAL AND LIGHTNING INJURIES

Sachita P. Shah

ELECTRICAL INJURIES

EPIDEMIOLOGY

- At-risk groups for electrical injuries include young children (low-voltage injuries) from contact with electrical cords and appliances, and adult professionals working with high-voltage electricity.

PATHOPHYSIOLOGY

- Electrical injuries are arbitrarily classified as low voltage (≤1000 V) and high voltage (>1000 V).
- Current can either be continuous in one direction (direct current, DC) or be in alternating directions (alternating current, AC).
- Factors associated with severity of electrical injuries include the amount, duration, type (AC or DC), the current path through the body, and environmental factors (eg, water immersion).
- Electrical energy in tissues can cause burns (entry and exit), thermal heating, flash and arc burns, blunt trauma, and muscular tetany.
- Low-voltage AC current will cause muscular tetany, causing the injured person to continually grasp the source, increasing contact time.
- High-voltage AC and DC currents cause a single violent muscular contraction, which tends to throw the victim from the source, thus increasing the risk of blunt trauma and blast injuries.
- Electricity causes damage by direct tissue damage from electrical energy, thermal damage from the heat generated by the resistance of tissue, and mechanical injury due to fall or muscular tetany.
- Energy is greatest at the contact point; thus the skin often has the greatest visible damage, although evaluation for deeper injury must be performed.

CLINICAL FEATURES

- As current flows through the body, the greatest damage is sustained by nerves, blood vessels, and muscles causing coagulation necrosis, neuronal death, and damage to blood vessels. As a result, the overall picture often resembles a crush injury more than a thermal burn.
- Traumatic injuries frequently accompany electrical injuries.
- Specific complications of electrical injuries are summarized in Table 128-1.
- Immediate life-threatening features include cardiac arrhythmias including ventricular fibrillation (low voltage) and asystole (high voltage), respiratory arrest, seizures, and severe burns.
- Oral burns in children may have delayed labial artery bleeding (up to 2 weeks later).

DIAGNOSIS AND DIFFERENTIAL

- Diagnosis of electrical injury is usually based on history.
- In unclear cases, characteristic skin or oral lesions in children may be helpful.
- Laboratory and radiographic evaluation of high-voltage injures should follow standard trauma guidelines.
- The creatine kinase (CK-MB) may be elevated without myocardial damage due to extensive muscle injury with potential for rhabdomyolysis. Urine myoglobin and total CPK should be obtained.
- Electrocardiogram (ECG) may show atrial or ventricular arrhythmias, bradyarrhythmias, prolonged QT intervals, or ST–T wave abnormalities
- Computed tomographic (CT) scanning of the head is indicated for those with severe head injury, coma, or unresolving mental status changes.

TABLE 128-1	Complications of Electrical Injuries
Cardiovascular	Sudden death (ventricular fibrillation, asystole), chest pain, dysrhythmias, ST–T segment abnormalities, bundle-branch block, myocardial damage, ventricular dysfunction, myocardial infarction (rare), hypotension (volume depletion), hypertension (catecholamine release)
Neurologic	Altered mental status, agitation, coma, seizures, cerebral edema, hypoxic encephalopathy, headache, aphasia, weakness, paraplegia, quadriplegia, spinal cord dysfunction (maybe delayed), peripheral neuropathy, cognitive impairment, insomnia, emotional lability
Cutaneous	Electrothermal contact injuries, noncontact arc and "flash" burns, secondary thermal burns (clothing ignition, heating of metal)
Vascular	Thrombosis, coagulation necrosis, disseminated intravascular coagulation, delayed vessel rupture, aneurysm, compartment syndrome
Pulmonary	Respiratory arrest (central or peripheral; eg, muscular tetany), aspiration pneumonia, pulmonary edema, pulmonary contusion, inhalation injury
Renal/metabolic	Acute renal failure (due to heme pigment deposition and hypovolemia), myoglobinuria, metabolic (lactic) acidosis, hypokalemia, hypocalcemia, hyperglycemia
Gastrointestinal	Perforation, stress ulcer (Curling's ulcer), GI bleeding, GI tract dysfunction, various reports of lethal injuries at autopsy
Musculoskeletal	Myonecrosis, compartment syndrome, vertebral compression fractures, long bone fractures, shoulder dislocations (anterior and posterior), scapular fractures
Obstetric	Spontaneous abortion, fetal death
Ophthalmologic	Corneal burns, delayed cataracts, intraocular hemorrhage or thrombosis, uveitis, retinal detachment, orbital fracture
Auditory	Hearing loss, tinnitus, tympanic membrane perforation (rare), delayed mastoiditis, or meningitis
Oral burns	Delayed labial artery hemorrhage, scarring and facial deformity, delayed speech development, impaired mandibular/dentition development

EMERGENCY DEPARTMENT CARE AND DISPOSITION

- The airway, breathing, and circulation should be stabilized. Spinal immobilization should be instituted for any unwitnessed events or when there is a potential for spine injury.
- High-flow oxygen should be administered by face mask.
- Patients should have continuous cardiac monitoring, pulse oximetry, noninvasive blood pressure monitoring, and preferably two large-bore IV lines.
- Ventricular fibrillation, asystole, or ventricular tachycardia should be treated by standard Advanced Cardiac Life Support (ACLS) protocols. Other dysrhythmias are usually transient and do not need immediate therapy.
- IV crystalloid fluid should be given with an initial bolus of 20 to 40 mL/kg over the first hour. Fluid requirements are generally higher than those of thermal burn patients.
- Monitor for rhabdomyolysis, compartment syndrome, and renal failure. Treat rhabdomyolysis with aggressive fluid rehydration aiming for a urine output of 2 mL/kg/h.
- Tetanus prophylaxis should be given. Prophylactic antibiotics are not necessary initially unless large open wounds are present.
- Seizures are treated with standard therapy.
- It is appropriate to consult a general surgeon if there is evidence of systemic or deep tissue injury. These patients may require formal wound exploration, debridement, fasciotomy, and long-term care.
- Children with oral injuries should be evaluated by an ENT specialist or plastic surgeon.
- All pregnant patients should undergo obstetric consultation for admission and fetal monitoring.
- Table 128-2 summarizes admission criteria. Patients with an unclear history of exposure or degree of injury should be admitted.
- Children with isolated oral injuries or isolated hand wounds can usually be discharged. Parents should be given instructions for controlling delayed labial artery bleeding.
- Asymptomatic patients with household voltage exposure (110-220 V), a normal ECG, and a normal examination may be discharged.

TABLE 128-2 Indications for Admission for Patients with Electrical Injuries
High voltage >600 V
Symptoms suggestive of systemic injury
Cardiovascular: chest pain, palpitations
Neurologic: loss of consciousness, confusion, weakness, headache, paresthesias
Respiratory: dyspnea
Gastrointestinal: abdominal pain, vomiting
Evidence of neurologic or vascular injury to a digit or extremity
Burns with evidence of subcutaneous tissue damage
Dysrhythmia or abnormal electrocardiogram
Suspected foul play, abuse, suicidal intent, or unreliable social situation
High-risk exposures
Associated injuries requiring admission
Comorbid diseases (cardiac, renal, neurologic)

- Electronic control devices, such as the cattle prod, stun gun, and the TASER®, emit electrical pulses that induce involuntary muscle contraction, neuromuscular incapacitation, and/or pain. Serious injury is rare, and cardiac monitoring is usually not necessary.

LIGHTNING INJURIES

EPIDEMIOLOGY

- There are about 300 lightning injuries reported each year in the United States, with approximately 100 deaths.
- Unlike electrical injuries, extensive tissue damage and renal failure are rare, although as many as 75% of survivors sustain significant morbidity and permanent sequelae.
- Sports, particularly water sports, and transportation are associated with increased risk of lightning injury.

PATHOPHYSIOLOGY

- Lightning is DC imparting a single extremely high-voltage discharge of energy.
- Lightning injures can result via direct strike, side flash (current flows over from another struck object), contact strike (a person touching a struck object), ground current (passing through the ground and transferred to a standing person), or step potential (ground strike passes up a person's leg and down through the other leg).

CLINICAL FEATURES

- Lightning injuries can vary in severity depending on the circumstances of the strike, and range from minor injuries to cardiac or respiratory arrest.
- Minor injuries include confusion, amnesia, short-term memory problems, headache, muscle pain, paresthesias, tympanic membrane damage, and temporary visual or auditory problems.
- Most patients with minor lightning injuries have a gradual improvement and few long-term sequelae.
- Feathering or fern-shaped burns on the skin are pathognomonic of lightning.
- Complications associated with lightning injuries are summarized in Table 128-3.

DIAGNOSIS AND DIFFERENTIAL

- The diagnosis of lightning injury is based on history and should be considered in a patient found unconscious or in arrest who was outside during appropriate weather conditions.

TABLE 128-3 Complications Associated with Lightning Injuries

SYSTEM	INJURY
Cardiovascular	Dysrhythmias (asystole, ventricular fibrillation/tachycardia, premature ventricular contractions), electrocardiographic changes, myocardial infarction (unusual)
Neurologic	(Immediate or delayed, permanent or transient) Loss of consciousness, confusion, amnesia, intracranial hemorrhage, hemiplegia, amnesia, respiratory center paralysis, cerebral edema, neuritis, seizures, parkinsonian syndromes, cerebral infarction, myelopathy, progressive muscular atrophy, progressive cerebellar syndrome, transient paralysis, paresthesias, myelopathy, autonomic dysfunction
Cutaneous	Burns (first- to third-degree), scars, contractures
Ophthalmologic	Cataracts (often delayed), corneal lesions, uveitis, iridocyclitis, vitreous hemorrhage, macular degeneration, optic atrophy, diplopia, chorioretinitis, retinal detachment, hyphema
Otologic	Tympanic membrane rupture, temporary or permanent deafness, tinnitus, ataxia, vertigo, nystagmus
Renal	Myoglobinuria, hemoglobinuria, renal failure (rare)
Obstetric	Fetal death, placental abruption
Miscellaneous	Secondary blunt trauma, compartment syndrome, disseminated intravascular coagulation

- Pupillary dilatation or anisocoria may occur and has no prognostic value.
- Ruptured tympanic membranes or fernlike erythematous skin markings should alert the physician to potential lightning injury.
- Misdiagnoses include stroke or intracranial hemorrhage, seizure disorder, and cerebral, spinal cord, or other neurologic trauma.

EMERGENCY DEPARTMENT CARE AND DISPOSITION

- Aggressive resuscitation measures are indicated, as survival has been reported after prolonged respiratory arrest.
- Respiratory arrest may outlast initial cardiac arrest, and adequate ventilation can prevent hypoxic injury until return of spontaneous circulation.
- Spinal immobilization should be used in unwitnessed events or when there is potential spine injury.
- Continuous cardiac monitoring, pulse oximetry, non-invasive blood pressure monitoring, and at least one large-bore IV should be utilized.
- Hypotension is unexpected and should prompt investigation for hemorrhage.

- High-flow oxygen should be administered by face mask.
- Ventricular tachycardia or fibrillation and asystole should be treated with standard ACLS protocols.
- Fluid resuscitation is usually unnecessary.
- Tetanus prophylaxis should be given.
- Seizures may be treated with standard therapy.
- Those with moderate or severe injuries should be admitted to a critical care unit with appropriate consultation.
- Most patients with minor injuries should be admitted for close monitoring of cardiac and neurologic status.
- All pregnant patients should be admitted and undergo fetal monitoring.

For further reading in Tintinalli's *Emergency Medicine: A Comprehensive Study Guide*, 7th ed., see Chapter 126, "Electrical and Lightning Injuries," by Sachita P. Shah.

129 CARBON MONOXIDE

Christian A. Tomaszewski

EPIDEMIOLOGY

- Carbon monoxide (CO) is probably the most common cause of fatal poisoning, both intentionally and accidentally, with peak incidence in the fall and winter.
- Potential sources of CO include incomplete combustion from such things as kerosene heaters, gas furnaces, wood burning stoves, charcoal grills, forklifts, generators, and automobiles. With inadequate ventilation any gasoline or natural gas-powered machinery can contribute to a high ambient CO.
- Carbon monoxide contributes to fire deaths through smoke inhalation.
- Methylene chloride can cause delayed, up to 8 hours post exposure, elevations of carboxyhemogoblin (COHb) because it is metabolized in the liver to CO.

PATHOPHYSIOLOGY

- CO is an odorless, colorless gas. Ambient levels are usually around 10 ppm.
- The permissible level of CO is 50 ppm averaged over an 8 hour shift (OSHA). Toxicity is usually seen at 100 ppm.
- CO has an affinity for hemoglobin approximately 200 times that of oxygen. The half-life of COHb on room air is 250 to 320 minutes, reducing to about 85 minutes on 100% oxygen. The half-life of COHb from methylene chloride is longer and approaches 13 hours.
- COHb cannot carry oxygen and it shifts the oxygen dissociation curve to the left for the remaining oxyhemoglobin, thereby providing less oxygen release to cells.
- COHb does not account for all of the toxicity associated with CO poisoning. Ten percent to 15% of CO is dissolved in plasma. It binds to both myoglobin and cytochrome oxidase, interfering with cellular respiration in the heart and brain. CO also causes endothelial dysfunction and indirect vasodilation from nitric oxide release.
- Delayed effects of CO include ischemic-reperfusion injury with attraction of neutrophils that trigger an inflammatory cascade with neuronal cell loss, particularly in the basal ganglia.

CLINICAL FEATURES

- Clinical features of CO are varied, but commonly relate to hypoxic effects on the neurological and cardiovascular systems (Table 129-1). Symptoms range from "flu-like" symptoms, such as headache, dizziness, nausea, and vomiting, to coma. Older patients may present with syncope or cardiac ischemia.
- A history of exposure to gas heat or smoke inhalation, or multiple victims with altered mental status, acidosis, or coma, should alert one to the possibility of CO poisoning.
- Physical examination may reveal tachycardia, tachypnea, or hypotension. The hallmark neurological manifestations of CO poisoning beyond headache include confusion, irritability, seizures, focal neurological deficits, or coma. The "classic finding" of cherry red lips is rarely seen in living patients.

TABLE 129-1 Signs and Symptoms of Acute Carbon Monoxide Poisoning
Headache
Visual disturbances
Vomiting
Confusion
Ataxia
Dyspnea/tachypnea
Seizure
ECG changes/dysrhythmias
Syncope
Retinal hemorrhage
Chest pain
Bullous skin lesions
Focal neurologic deficit

- Patients with significant poisoning from acute or even chronic exposure may go on to experience long-term neuropsychiatric problems including memory loss and inability to concentrate.

DIAGNOSIS AND DIFFERENTIAL

- A venous, or arterial, blood sample for measurement of COHb on co-oximetry is the most reliable test to diagnose carbon monoxide poisoning. The use of bedside pulse co-oximetry in the ED to screen for CO exposure is still under investigation.
- Although COHb levels confirm exposure, they do not necessarily correlate with symptoms or prognosis. CO poisoning is usually detected by measuring COHb levels. Normal COHb levels are around 1% but may be as high as 3% in nonsmokers and 10% in smokers. Higher levels are suggestive of CO exposure.
- Standard pulse oximetry is unreliable in the presence of increasing COHb as oxygen saturation readings will be artificially high.
- Additional lab abnormalities seen in symptomatic patients may include elevated anion gap metabolic acidosis, creatinine phosphokinase, or lactate. The latter may be indicative of concomitant cyanide poisoning in smoke inhalation victims.
- Cardiac toxicity may be manifested by elevated troponin or signs of ischemia on ECG.
- Radiographic imaging is more useful for exploring alternate diagnoses. Early CT scanning of the brain is not very sensitive, but may show globus pallidus lesions in severely poisoned patients.
- The differential diagnosis for CO poisoning is wide due to the nonspecific nature of the symptoms and includes flu-like illness, gastroenteritis, exposure to other toxins, and infectious causes of mental status changes. Cardiovascular compromise after poisoning may represent a concomitant myocardial infarction.

EMERGENCY DEPARTMENT CARE AND DISPOSITION

- Remove patients from the source of exposure and address airway, breathing, and circulation.
- Begin treatment in all patients suspected of CO poisoning with the highest concentration of supplemental oxygen available (eg, 100% oxygen via facemask with reservoir) and continue until the patient is asymptomatic. Provide continuous monitoring of vital signs, heart rate, and rhythm. Establish IV access for seriously poisoned patients.
- Guidelines for hyperbaric oxygen therapy (HBO) in patients with severe poisoning are the same in adults and children (Table 129-2). The threshold COHb for initiating HBO in pregnant patients is lower because of concerns for the fetus. Consult with a hyperbaric specialist.

TABLE 129-2 Commonly Utilized Indications for Referral for Hyperbaric Oxygen Treatment
Syncope
Confusion/altered mental status
Seizure
Coma
Focal neurologic deficit
Pregnancy with carboxyhemoglobin level >15%
Blood level >25%
Evidence of acute myocardial ischemia

- Patients should have a secure airway and stable hemodynamics before transport and treatment with HBO as access may be limited en route and in the chamber.
- Guidelines for disposition of CO victims are based on severity of presentation (Table 129-3).
- Symptomatic patients that do not require HBO treatment can be observed for approximately 4 hours while being treated with oxygen. If symptoms resolve and their neurological examination is normal, they can be discharged provided the home or work environment is no longer a source of carbon monoxide exposure.

TABLE 129-3 Disposition Considerations

SYMPTOM SEVERITY	DISPOSITION	COMMENTS
Minimal or no symptoms	Home.	Assess safety issues.
Headache Vomiting	Home after symptom resolution.	Administer 100% oxygen in ED. Observe 4 h.
Elevated carbon monoxide level		Assess safety issues.
Ataxia, seizure, syncope, chest pain, focal neurologic deficit, dyspnea, ECG changes	Hospitalize. Consult with hyperbaric specialist.	Administer 100% oxygen in ED. Carbon monoxide level, comorbid conditions—including pregnancy—and age; stability of the patient must be considered if considering transfer for hyperbaric oxygen.

For further reading in Tintinalli's *Emergency Medicine: A Comprehensive Study Guide*, 7th ed., see Chapter 217, "Carbon Monoxide Poisoning," by Gerald Maloney.

130 POISONOUS PLANTS AND MUSHROOMS

B. Zane Horowitz

EPIDEMIOLOGY

- Plants are very common ingestions; young children account for 70% to 80% of all plant-related exposures. Fatalities are extremely rare.
- Mushroom ingestions account for 8000 exposures annually, and less than 5 deaths per year.
- *Amanita* species are responsible for 95% of fatalities associated with mushrooms in the United States.

PATHOPHYSIOLOGY

- Toxins found in plants and mushrooms produce effects that range from mild gastrointestinal (GI) symptoms to organ failure and death.
- Mushrooms with psilocybin- and psilocin-containing toxins have neuroactive chemicals with effects similar to lysergic acid diethylamide (LSD), producing hallucinogenic effects; they are often intentionally ingested for their mind-altering effects.
- Mushrooms that contain gyromitrin, a compound that is broken down to monomethyl hydrazine, can cause seizures. It inhibits the enzyme pyridoxal phosphate, which is responsible for formation of vitamin B_6. Without vitamin B_6, the CNS neurotransmitter GABA cannot be formed, and refractory seizures occur.
- *Amanita phalloides* contain amanitin, which is well absorbed in the intestines, is actively transported into the liver, and undergoes enterohepatic circulation. Amanitin binds to hepatocytes and inhibit formation of messenger RNA, leading to delayed onset of liver failure.
- *Coprinus atramentarius* (inky cap) mushrooms contain the amino acid coprine, which is converted to L-aminocyclopropanol by the liver. This compound inhibits aldehyde dehydrogenase, preventing breakdown of alcohol, identical in its mechanism of action to an Antabuse (disulfiram) reaction.
- Ricin, a potent toxalbumin found in castor beans, produces severe cytotoxic effects in multiple organ systems.
- Amygdalin, found in the pits of peaches, apricots, pears, crab apples, and hydrangea, is metabolized to hydrocyanic acid, and can lead to acute cyanide poisoning if the pits are crushed and ingested in sufficient quantities.
- Cardiogenic glycosides are found in foxglove, oleander, and lily of the valley (Table 130-1).

TABLE 130-1 Symptoms and Treatment of Severely Poisonous Plant Ingestions

PLANT	SYMPTOMS	TREATMENT
Castor bean (*Ricinus communis*)	Delayed gastroenteritis, delirium, seizures, coma, death	Whole-bowel irrigation Supportive care
Coyotillo (*Karwinskia humboldtiana*)	Ascending paralysis	Supportive care
Foxglove (*Digitalis purpurea*)	Nausea, vomiting, diarrhea, abdominal pain, confusion, cardiac dysrhythmias	GI decontamination with activated charcoal Monitoring of potassium level Antidysrhythmics Digoxin-specific Fab antibody for dysrhythmias
Jequirity bean (*Abrus precatorius*)	Delayed gastroenteritis, delirium, seizures, coma, death	Whole-bowel irrigation Supportive care
Oleander (*Nerium oleander*)	Nausea, vomiting, diarrhea, abdominal pain, confusion, cardiac dysrhythmias	GI decontamination with activated charcoal Monitoring of potassium level Antidysrhythmics Digoxin-specific Fab antibody for dysrhythmias
Poison hemlock (*Conium maculatum*)	Tachycardia, tremors, diaphoresis, mydriasis, muscle weakness, seizures, neuromuscular blockade	GI decontamination with activated charcoal Supportive care
Water hemlock (*Cicuta maculata*)	Nausea, vomiting, abdominal pain, delirium, seizures, death	GI decontamination Supportive care
Yew (*Taxus* species)	Common: nausea, vomiting, abdominal pain Rare: seizures, cardiac dysrhythmias, coma	GI decontamination with activated charcoal Consider whole-bowel irrigation Supportive care

CLINICAL FEATURES

- Cicutoxin, found in water hemlock, produces severe GI symptoms, followed by delirium, seizures, and death.
- Direct irritation and chemical burns to the oropharynx have been reported after ingestion of *Abrus* (rosary pea), *Capsicum* (ornamental peppers), *Daphne*, *Dieffenbachia*, and *Rhododendron*.
- Cardiovascular symptoms, including hypotension, dysrhythmias, and conduction defects, have been

reported after ingestion of aconitine, *Convallaria*, *Taxus*, *Rhododendron*, and oleander, and may be life threatening.

- Jimson weed, henbane, and nightshade berries contain atropine-like alkaloids that can cause an acute anticholinergic crisis.
- Urushiol, found in *Toxicodendron* species (poison ivy, oak, and sumac), produces a contact dermatitis in sensitized individuals.
- Seizures may be seen after ingestion of *Conium,* water hemlock, and gyromitrin-containing mushrooms.
- Ingestion of *Amanita* species of mushrooms produces delayed onset of GI symptoms 6 to 48 hours after ingestion. Manifestations of hepatic failure develop 1 to 3 days after exposure.
- *Cortinarius orellanus* and *Amanita smithiana* mushrooms contain nephrotoxic compounds, which result in delayed onset of renal failure.
- Consuming alcohol after ingestion of coprine-containing mushrooms will result in a disulfiram-like reaction. Facial flushing, nausea and vomiting, diaphoresis, palpitations, hypotension, and weakness can be observed 2 to 72 hours after ingestion.
- Mushrooms with ibotenic acid and muscimol cause early-onset stimulatory neurologic symptoms, followed by sedation.
- *Inocybe* and *Clitocybe* species containing muscarine cause early-onset cholinergic effects, characterized by the SLUDGE syndrome (*s*alivation, *l*acrimation, *u*rination, *d*efecation, *g*astrointestinal hypermotility, and *e*mesis).

DIAGNOSIS AND DIFFERENTIAL

- Diagnosis of plant and mushroom poisoning is clinical, based on history of ingestion, with confirmation by a mycologist or botanist.
- Early GI toxicity of mushroom poisoning (within 1-2 hours of ingestion) generally indicates a benign course.
- Delayed GI toxicity of mushroom poisoning (greater than 6 hours) suggests a more toxic ingestion, which can lead to hepatic failure, renal failure, and even death (Table 130-2).

TABLE 130-2 Mushrooms: Symptoms, Toxicity, and Treatment

SYMPTOMS	MUSHROOMS	TOXICITY	TREATMENT
GI symptoms			
Onset <2 h	*Chlorophyllum molybdites* *Omphalotus illudens* *Cantharellus cibarius* *Amanita caesarea*	Nausea, vomiting, diarrhea (occasionally bloody)	IV hydration Antiemetics
Onset 6-24 h	*Gyromitra esculenta* *A. phalloides*, *A. bisporigera*	Initial: nausea, vomiting, diarrhea Day 2: rise in AST, ALT levels Day 3: hepatic failure	IV hydration, glucose; monitor AST, ALT, bilirubin, blood urea nitrogen, and creatinine levels, prothrombin time, partial thromboplastin time For *Amanita:* activated charcoal Consider penicillin G, 300,000-1,000,000 units/kg/d Silymarin, 20-40 milligrams/kg/d Consider cimetidine, 4-10 grams/d
Muscarinic syndrome Onset <30 min	*Inocybe* *Clitocybe*	SLUDGE syndrome (*s*alivation, *l*acrimation, *u*rination, *d*efecation, *G*I hypermotility, and *e*mesis)	Supportive; atropine, 0.01 milligram/kg, repeated as needed for severe secretions
Central nervous system excitement Onset <30 min	*A. muscaria* *A. pantherina*	Intoxication, dizziness, ataxia, visual disturbances, seizures, tachycardia, hypertension, warm dry skin, dry mouth, mydriasis (anticholinergic effects)	Supportive; sedation with diazepam, 0.1 milligram/kg IV for children; diazepam, 2-5 milligrams IV
Hallucinations Onset <30 min	*Psilocybe* *Gymnopilus*	Visual hallucinations, ataxia	Supportive; sedation with diazepam, 0.1 milligram/kg or 5 milligrams IV for adults
Disulfiram reaction 2-72 h after mushroom, and <30 min after alcohol	*Coprinus*	Headache, flushing, tachycardia, hyperventilation, shortness of breath, palpitations	Supportive; IV hydration β-Blockers for supraventricular tachycardia Norepinephrine for refractory hypotension

Abbreviations: ALT = alanine aminotransferase; AST = aspartate aminotransferase.

- Physical examination should include a search for evidence of cholinergic, anticholinergic, or sympathetic nervous system stimulation.
- If delayed-onset GI symptoms suggest cytotoxic mushroom poisoning, electrolytes, blood urea nitrogen, creatinine, liver enzymes, and coagulation studies should be obtained.
- Ingestion of cardiotoxic plants warrants ECG monitoring and serial potassium levels.

EMERGENCY DEPARTMENT CARE AND DISPOSITION

- Initial treatment for plant-related and mushroom poisoning is supportive, with priority given to airway management, ventilation, fluid resuscitation, and seizure control.
- Activated charcoal should be considered only for suspected plants and mushrooms of high toxicity if presenting within 1 to 2 hours of ingestion.
- Controversy exists as to the best treatment for amanitin-containing mushrooms but generally utilized modalities include **silimarin,** 1 gram PO four times daily, or its purified alkaloid, **silibinin,** 5 milligrams/kg IV over 1 hour, followed by 20 milligrams/kg/d as a constant infusion.
- High-dose **penicillin therapy**, 0.3 to 1.0 million units/kg/d of penicillin G, is recommended for amatoxin poisoning; it blocks the uptake of amatoxin into the liver.
- Intravenous *N*-acetylcysteine is often used for amanitin toxins at the same doses used to treat acetaminophen poisoning.
- Rapid progression to hepatic encephalopathy, hepatorenal syndrome, and coagulopathy are indications for liver transplantation. Consider transfer to a liver transplant setting and ICU care early in the course of mushroom ingestions.
- High-dose **pyridoxine**, 25 milligrams/kg IV, is recommended for patients presenting with neurologic symptoms and seizures associated with gyromitrin.
- Fluid and electrolyte replacement and hemodialysis are the mainstays of treatment for renal failure.
- Patients with potential amanitin, gyromitrin, or orellanine poisoning, or those with refractory symptoms, require admission and monitoring for at least 48 hours. All other patients who are asymptomatic after 6 to 8 hours of treatment and observation can be discharged.
- Atropine may be administered to patients with severe muscarinic symptoms.
- Digoxin-specific Fab antibodies can be used for heart block and dysrhythmias from cardiogenic glycoside containing plants.
- Jimson weed ingestions with anticholinergic delirium may be treated with physostigmine.

For further reading in Tintinalli's *Emergency Medicine: A Comprehensive Study Guide,* 7th ed., see Chapter 214, "Mushroom Poisoning," by Anne F. Brayer, Sandra M. Schneider, and Arif Alper Cevik, and Chapter 215, "Poisonous Plants," by Mark A. Hostetler and Sandra M. Schneider.

Section 14
ENDOCRINE EMERGENCIES

131 DIABETIC EMERGENCIES

Michael P. Kefer

HYPOGLYCEMIA

EPIDEMIOLOGY

- Patients with diabetes mellitus, alcoholism, sepsis, adrenal insufficiency, or malnutrition are at risk for hypoglycemia.
- Hypoglycemia occurs most commonly in diabetics treated with insulin or sulfonylureas (chlorpropamide, glyburide, glipizide). It is less common with the glinides (repaglinide, nateglinide) and unlikely from monotherapy with the α-glucosidase inhibitors (acarbose, miglitol), the glitazones (rosiglitazone, pioglitazone), and the biguanide, metformin.

PATHOPHYSIOLOGY

- Glucose is the main energy source of the brain. Severe hypoglycemia can cause brain damage or death.
- Serum glucose is dependent on the balance between insulin and the counter-regulatory hormones: epinephrine, glucagon, cortisol, and growth hormone. Excess insulin, either relative or absolute, will result in decreased glucose production and utilization.

CLINICAL FEATURES

- Typical symptoms of hypoglycemia include sweating, shakiness, anxiety, nausea, dizziness, confusion, blurred vision, headache, and lethargy.
- Typical signs include diaphoresis, tachycardia, and almost any neurologic finding, ranging from altered mental status or tremor to focal neurologic deficit or seizure.

DIAGNOSIS AND DIFFERENTIAL

- Diagnosis is based on a low serum glucose level in conjunction with the clinical features that resolve with treatment.
- Differential diagnosis is wide due to the nonspecific features. It can be misdiagnosed as a primary neurologic, psychiatric, or cardiovascular condition (Table 131-1).

EMERGENCY DEPARTMENT CARE AND DISPOSITION

- Glucose is administered orally in mild cases.
- Advanced cases are treated with 50% dextrose 50 mL intravenously (IV).
- Continuous infusion of 10% dextrose solution may be required to maintain the serum glucose level above 100 milligrams/dL.
- If no IV access is obtained, give glucagon 1 milligram intramuscularly (IM) or subcutaneously (SC).
- Sulfonylureas can cause refractory hypoglycemia that may respond to octreotide 50 to 100 micrograms SC. Subsequent dosing every 6 hours or continuous infusion of 125 micrograms/h may be required.
- Check blood glucose every 30 minutes initially to monitor for rebound hypoglycemia.
- Factors considered in determining disposition include the patient's response to treatment, etiology of hypoglycemia, existing comorbid conditions, and social situation.

TABLE 131-1 Differential Diagnosis of Hypoglycemia
Stroke
Transient ischemic attack
Seizure disorder
Traumatic head injury
Brain tumor
Narcolepsy
Multiple sclerosis
Psychosis
Sympathomimetic drug ingestion
Hysteria
Altered sleep patterns and nightmares
Depression

TABLE 131-2	Disposition/Guidelines for Hospital Admission
Inpatient care for type 2 diabetes mellitus is generally appropriate for the following clinical situations:	
Life-threatening metabolic decompensation such as diabetic ketoacidosis or hyperglycemic hyperosmolar nonketotic state	
Severe chronic complications of diabetes, acute comorbidities, or inadequate social situation	
Hyperglycemia (>400 milligrams/dL) associated with severe volume depletion or refractory to appropriate interventions	
Hypoglycemia with neuroglycopenia (altered level of consciousness, altered behavior, coma, seizure) that does not rapidly resolve with correction of hypoglycemia	
Hypoglycemia resulting from long-acting oral hypoglycemic agents	
Fever without an obvious source in patients with poorly controlled diabetes	

- Most diabetics with insulin reactions respond rapidly to treatment. They can be discharged with instructions to continue oral intake of carbohydrates and to closely monitor their fingerstick glucose level.
- Admission guidelines are listed in Table 131-2.

DIABETIC KETOACIDOSIS

EPIDEMIOLOGY

- Diabetic ketoacidosis (DKA) occurs predominantly in type 1 insulin-dependent diabetics, but may occur in type 2 non–insulin-dependent diabetics.
- Table 131-3 lists important causes of DKA.

TABLE 131-3	Important Causes of Diabetic Ketoacidosis
Omission or reduced daily insulin injections	
Dislodgement/occlusion of insulin pump catheter	
Infection	
Pregnancy	
Hyperthyroidism	
Substance abuse (cocaine)	
Medications: steroids, thiazides, antipsychotics, sympathomimetics	
Heat-related illness	
Cerebrovascular accident	
GI hemorrhage	
Myocardial infarction	
Pulmonary embolism	
Pancreatitis	
Major trauma	
Surgery	

PATHOPHYSIOLOGY

- DKA results from a relative insulin deficiency and counter-regulatory hormone excess, resulting in cellular starvation.
- Insulin acts on the liver to promote glucose storage as glycogen, on adipose tissue to promote storage of triglycerides, and on skeletal muscle to promote protein synthesis.
- Although serum glucose levels are high, in the absence of insulin, cells cannot use glucose as fuel.
- The counter-regulatory hormones epinephrine, glucagon, cortisol, and growth hormone have the opposite effect of insulin. Glycogenolysis releases glucose stores. Proteolysis and lipolysis result in release of amino acids and glycerol, respectively, for gluconeogenesis to synthesize more glucose.
- Free fatty acids are metabolized in the liver to the ketone bodies β-hydroxybutyrate, acetoacetate, and acetone. However, these also are unavailable for use as fuel by cells in the absence of insulin.
- Hyperglycemia causes an osmotic diuresis with volume depletion and electrolyte loss.
- Ketonemia results in a high anion gap metabolic acidosis with myocardial depression, vasodilation, and compensatory hyperpnea (Kussmaul respiration).

CLINICAL FEATURES

- Clinical manifestations are directly related to metabolic derangements.
- Dehydration, hypotension, and tachycardia result from osmotic diuresis.
- Ketonemia causes a metabolic acidosis with myocardial depression, vasodilation, and compensatory Kussmaul respiration. Nausea, vomiting, and abdominal pain are common.
- Acetone excretion via the lungs causes the characteristic fruity odor of the breath.
- Inappropriate normothermia may occur, so infection must be considered even in the absence of fever.

DIAGNOSIS AND DIFFERENTIAL

- Diagnosis of DKA is based on the clinical presentation and laboratory values of a serum glucose >250 milligrams/dL, serum bicarbonate <15 mEq/L, pH <7.3, and moderate ketonemia.
- β-Hydroxybutyrate is the reduced form of acetoacetate. In DKA, reduction of acetoacetate to β-hydroxybutyrate is favored. As a result, in advanced cases, acetoacetate levels are low and β-hydroxybutyrate levels are high.

- If the nitroprusside test is used to detect serum or urine ketones, results may be falsely low or negative because this test detects acetoacetate and not β-hydroxybutyrate.
- Sodium, chloride, calcium, phosphorus, and magnesium levels may be low from osmotic diuresis.
- Pseudohyponatremia is common: for each 100 milligrams/dL increase in the glucose level, there is a 1.6 mEq/L decrease in sodium.
- Serum potassium may be low (from osmotic diuresis and vomiting), normal, or high (from acidosis since acidosis drives potassium out of cells). The patient who is acidotic with a normal or low potassium level has a marked depletion of total body potassium.
- Laboratory investigation includes serum pH, glucose, electrolytes, blood urea nitrogen, creatinine, phosphorus, magnesium, complete blood count, urinalysis, pregnancy if indicated, electrocardiogram, and chest radiograph to assess the severity of DKA and search for the underlying cause. When ordering serum pH, consider that venous pH correlates closely with arterial pH and avoids the pain and risk of arterial puncture.
- Differential diagnosis includes other causes of an anion gap metabolic acidosis (Table 131-4). Hypoglycemia and hyperosmolar hyperglycemic state should also be considered.

EMERGENCY DEPARTMENT CARE AND DISPOSITION

- The goal of treatment is to correct hypovolemia, ketonemia, acidosis, and electrolyte abnormalities, and treat the underlying cause (Fig. 131-1).
- Bicarbonate therapy remains controversial as to when the benefits of correcting the effects of acidosis (vasodilation, central nervous system and myocardial depression, hyperkalemia) outweigh the risks of bicarbonate treatment (paradoxical cerebrospinal fluid acidosis, hypokalemia, impaired oxyhemoglobin dissociation, rebound alkalosis, sodium overload). It may be of benefit to treat severe acidosis (pH <6.9). It is indicated to treat severe hyperkalemia.
- Monitor serum glucose, anion gap, potassium, and bicarbonate hourly until recovery is well established.
- Note that if monitoring ketones with the nitroprusside test, there will be a paradoxical increase in levels as the undetectable β-hydroxybutyrate is converted back to acetoacetate during recovery.
- Cerebral edema is a complication of treatment and occurs predominantly in children. It tends to develop 4 to 12 hours into treatment and manifests as a deterioration in neurologic status. Treat with mannitol 1 gram/kg before the diagnosis is confirmed by computed tomography.
- Cerebral edema has been associated with rapid correction of sodium, glucose, and hypovolemia.

TABLE 131-4	Differential Diagnosis for Diabetic Ketoacidosis
Alcoholic ketoacidosis	
Starvation ketoacidosis	
Renal failure	
Lactic acidosis	
Ingestions	
Salicylates	
Ethylene glycol	
Methanol	

HYPEROSMOLAR HYPERGLYCEMIC STATE

EPIDEMIOLOGY

- Hyperosmolar hyperglycemic state (HHS) is distinguished from DKA by the absence of significant ketosis.
- HHS occurs in poorly controlled type 2 diabetics. It is a relatively common presentation of new-onset type 2 diabetes. Precipitating factors are the same as for DKA (Table 131-3).

PATHOPHYSIOLOGY

- HHS develops as a result of (1) insulin resistance, deficiency, or both; (2) increased hepatic gluconeogenesis and glycogenolysis; and (3) osmotic diuresis and dehydration.
- As serum glucose increases, the osmotic gradient pulls intracellular fluid into the intravascular space. Glucosuria also ensues resulting in an osmotic diuresis causing volume depletion.

CLINICAL FEATURES

- The typical patient is elderly with type 2 diabetes, presents with complaints of weakness or mental status changes, and has preexisting renal or heart disease. Because metabolic changes progress slowly, symptoms often signal advanced HHS.
- Physical examination reveals signs of dehydration with orthostasis, dry skin and mucous membranes, and altered mental status. Focal deficits and seizures may occur.

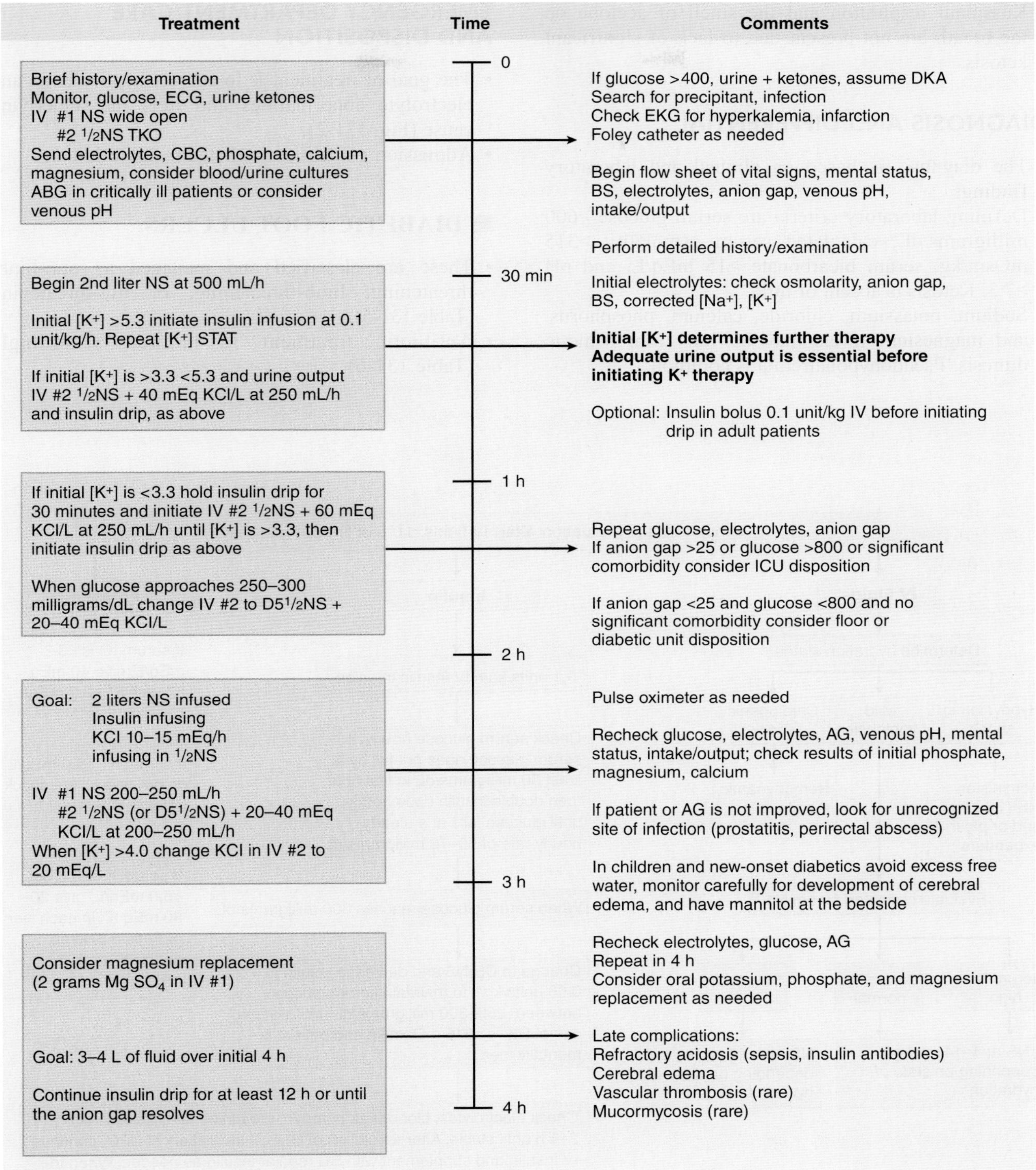
Treatment
Time
Comments
0
Brief history/examination
Monitor, glucose, ECG, urine ketones
IV #1 NS wide open
#2 1/2NS TKO
Send electrolytes, CBC, phosphate, calcium, magnesium, consider blood/urine cultures
ABG in critically ill patients or consider venous pH
If glucose >400, urine + ketones, assume DKA
Search for precipitant, infection
Check EKG for hyperkalemia, infarction
Foley catheter as needed
Begin flow sheet of vital signs, mental status, BS, electrolytes, anion gap, venous pH, intake/output
Perform detailed history/examination
30 min
Begin 2nd liter NS at 500 mL/h
Initial [K+] >5.3 initiate insulin infusion at 0.1 unit/kg/h. Repeat [K+] STAT
If initial [K+] is >3.3 <5.3 and urine output IV #2 1/2NS + 40 mEq KCl/L at 250 mL/h and insulin drip, as above
Initial electrolytes: check osmolarity, anion gap, BS, corrected [Na+], [K+]
Initial [K+] determines further therapy
Adequate urine output is essential before initiating K+ therapy
Optional: Insulin bolus 0.1 unit/kg IV before initiating drip in adult patients
1 h
If initial [K+] is <3.3 hold insulin drip for 30 minutes and initiate IV #2 1/2NS + 60 mEq KCl/L at 250 mL/h until [K+] is >3.3, then initiate insulin drip as above
When glucose approaches 250–300 milligrams/dL change IV #2 to D51/2NS + 20–40 mEq KCl/L
Repeat glucose, electrolytes, anion gap
If anion gap >25 or glucose >800 or significant comorbidity consider ICU disposition
If anion gap <25 and glucose <800 and no significant comorbidity consider floor or diabetic unit disposition
2 h
Goal: 2 liters NS infused
Insulin infusing
KCl 10–15 mEq/h
infusing in 1/2NS
IV #1 NS 200–250 mL/h
#2 1/2NS (or D51/2NS) + 20–40 mEq KCl/L at 200–250 mL/h
When [K+] >4.0 change KCl in IV #2 to 20 mEq/L
Pulse oximeter as needed
Recheck glucose, electrolytes, AG, venous pH, mental status, intake/output; check results of initial phosphate, magnesium, calcium
If patient or AG is not improved, look for unrecognized site of infection (prostatitis, perirectal abscess)
In children and new-onset diabetics avoid excess free water, monitor carefully for development of cerebral edema, and have mannitol at the bedside
3 h
Consider magnesium replacement (2 grams Mg SO4 in IV #1)
Goal: 3–4 L of fluid over initial 4 h
Continue insulin drip for at least 12 h or until the anion gap resolves
Recheck electrolytes, glucose, AG
Repeat in 4 h
Consider oral potassium, phosphate, and magnesium replacement as needed
Late complications:
Refractory acidosis (sepsis, insulin antibodies)
Cerebral edema
Vascular thrombosis (rare)
Mucormycosis (rare)
4 h

FIG. 131-1. Timeline for the typical adult patient with suspected diabetic ketoacidosis. ABG = arterial blood gas; AG = anion gap, BS = blood sugar; CBC = complete blood count; chemistries = sodium, potassium, chloride, CO_2 content, blood urea nitrogen, creatinine; DKA = diabetic ketoacidosis; NS = normal saline; STAT = immediately; TKO = IV infusion just to keep the venous access patent.

- Kussmaul respiration and the smell of acetone on the breath are not present due to lack of significant ketosis.

DIAGNOSIS AND DIFFERENTIAL

- The diagnosis is based on clinical and laboratory findings.
- Defining laboratory criteria are serum glucose >600 milligrams/dL, calculated serum osmolality >315 mOsm/kg, serum bicarbonate >15 mEq/L, and pH >7.3. Ketosis is absent or mild.
- Sodium, potassium, chloride, calcium, phosphorus, and magnesium levels may be low from osmotic diuresis. Pseudohyponatremia is common.

EMERGENCY DEPARTMENT CARE AND DISPOSITION

- The goal of treatment is to correct hypovolemia and electrolyte abnormalities and treat the underlying cause (Fig. 131-2).
- Admission guidelines are listed in Table 131-2.

■ DIABETIC FOOT ULCERS

- These are classified and managed as non-limb-threatening, limb-threatening, or life-threatening (Table 131-5).
- Antibiotic treatment is tailored accordingly (Table 131-6).

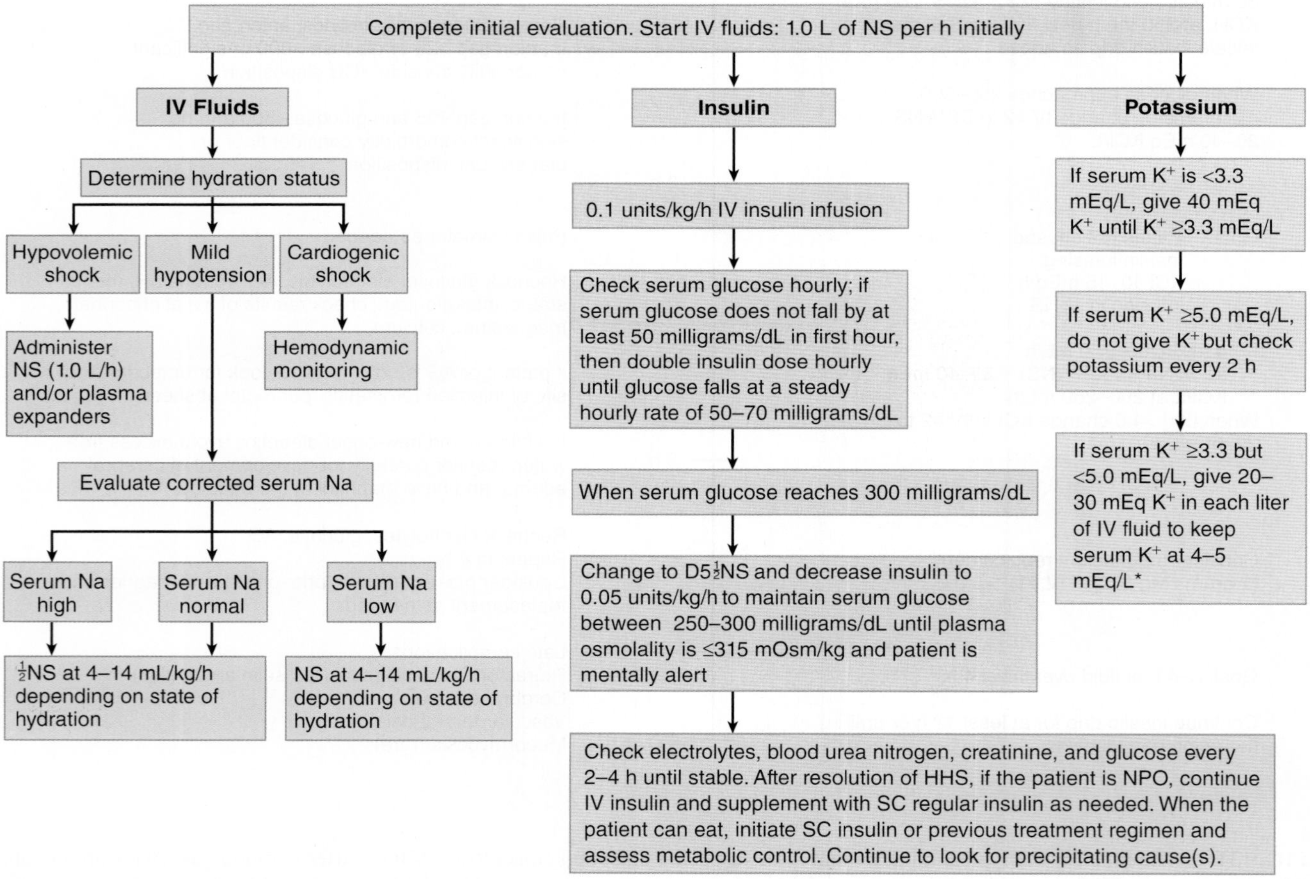

FIG. 131-2. Protocol for the management of severely ill adult patients with hyperosmolar hyperglycemic state (HHS). Diagnostic criteria for HHS: blood glucose >600 milligrams/dL, arterial pH >7.3, bicarbonate >15 mEq/L, mild ketonuria or ketonemia, and effective serum osmolality >320 mOsm/kg of water. *Concentrations of K^+ ≥20 mEq/L should be administered via central line. History and physical examination, appropriate ancillary studies. D5½NS = 5% dextrose in half normal saline; HHS = hyperosmolar hyperglycemic state; NS = normal saline.

TABLE 131-5 Clinical Practice Pathways for Diabetic Foot Ulcer and Infection

EXTENT OF INFECTION	CHARACTERISTICS	DIAGNOSTIC PROCEDURES	TREATMENT
Non–limb-threatening infection	<2 cm cellulitis Superficial ulcer Mild infection No systemic toxicity No ischemic changes No bone or joint involvement Does not probe to bone	Cultures from base of ulcer (with tissue specimen if possible) Diagnostic imaging (radiography, MRI, nuclear scans as indicated) Serologic testing CBC with differential ESR Comprehensive metabolic panel	Outpatient management with follow-up in 24–72 h Debridement of all necrotic tissue and callus Wound care/dressing Empiric antibiotic coverage, modified by culture findings Appropriate off-loading of weightbearing Wound care continued with packs, dressings, and debridement as needed Hospital admission if infection progresses or systemic signs or symptoms develop Refer to podiatrist for follow-up care, special shoes, and prostheses as needed
Life- or limb-threatening infection	>2 cm cellulitis Deep ulcer Odor or purulent drainage from wound Fever Ischemic changes Lymphangitis, edema Sepsis or septic shock	Deep culture from base of ulcer/wound with tissue specimen if possible Diagnostic imaging (radiography, MRI, nuclear scan, bone scan, leukocyte scan, arteriography) Serologic testing CBC with differential ESR Comprehensive metabolic panel Blood cultures	Hospital admission Surgical debridement with resection of all necrotic bone and soft tissue Exploration and drainage of deep abscess Empiric antibiotic coverage, modified by culture findings Surgical resection of osteomyelitis Wound care continued with packs, dressings, debridement as needed Foot-sparing reconstructive procedures Refer to podiatrist for follow-up care, special shoes, and prostheses as needed

Abbreviations: CBC = complete blood cell count; ESR = erythrocyte sedimentation rate.

TABLE 131-6 Antimicrobial Therapy in Infected Diabetes-Related Lower Extremity Ulcers

Non–limb-threatening*

(*May give initial dose as IV equivalent*)

Cephalexin, 500 milligrams PO every 12 h, 10-d course (cefazolin, 1 gram IV)

or

Clindamycin, 300 milligrams PO every 6-8 h, 10-d course (clindamycin, 900 milligrams IV)

or

Dicloxacillin, 500 milligrams PO every 6 h, 10-d course

or

Amoxicillin-clavulanate, 875 milligrams PO twice a day, 10-d course

Limb-threatening*

Oral regimen[†]:

Fluoroquinolone and clindamycin

IV regimens:

Ampicillin-sulbactam, 3 grams IV every 6 h

or

Ticarcillin-clavulanate, 3.1 grams IV every 8 h

or

Second-generation cephalosporin (cefoxitin, cefotetan), 1-2 grams IV every 12 h

or

Clindamycin, 900 milligrams IV every 6 h, plus either ciprofloxacin, 400 milligrams IV every 12 hours, or ceftriaxone, 1 gram IV every 12 h

(*Continued*)

TABLE 131-6 Antimicrobial Therapy in Infected Diabetes-Related Lower Extremity Ulcers (Continued)

Life-threatening*

IV regimens:

Imipenem-cilastatin, 1 gram every 6 h

or

Ampicillin-sulbactam, 3 grams every 6 h, plus antipseudomonal aminoglycoside tobramycin, 5-7 milligrams/kg every day

or

Vancomycin, 1 gram every 12 h, plus metronidazole, 500 milligrams every 6 h, plus aztreonam, 2 grams every 8 h

Note: Adjust all dosages for renal/hepatic function and monitor blood levels where appropriate.

**See the section Lower Extremities and Foot Complications for definitions.*

[†]This approach is acceptable under special circumstances with close follow-up.

For further reading in Tintinalli's *Emergency Medicine: A Comprehensive Study Guide*, 7th ed., see Chapter 218, "Type 1 Diabetes Mellitus," by Nikhil Goyal and Adam B. Schlichting; Chapter 219, "Type 2 Diabetes Mellitus," by Mohammad Jalili; Chapter 220, "Diabetic Ketoacidosis," by Michael E. Chansky and Cary Lubkin; and Chapter 222, "Hyperosmolar Hyperglycemic State," by Charles S. Graffeo

132 ALCOHOLIC KETOACIDOSIS

Michael P. Kefer

EPIDEMIOLOGY

- Alcoholic ketoacidosis (AKA) is a high anion gap metabolic acidosis that can occur after acute cessation of alcohol. It usually occurs in chronic alcoholics, but can occur in first-time drinkers.

PATHOPHYSIOLOGY

- AKA results from heavy ethanol intake, either acute or chronic, and minimal to no food intake. Glycogen stores become depleted and insulin secretion is suppressed.
- To maintain a supply of glucose, the counter-regulatory hormones glucagon, growth hormone, cortisol, and epinephrine are released.
- Fat and ethanol oxidation become the body's primary substrate for energy production, resulting in the formation of the ketone bodies β-hydroxybutyrate, acetoacetate, and acetone.
- Acetone is rapidly excreted by the lungs. Acetoacetate and β-hydroxybutyrate accumulate, resulting in a metabolic acidosis.
- β-Hydroxybutyrate is the reduced form of acetoacetate. In AKA, the reduction of acetoacetate to β-hydroxybutyrate is favored. As a result, in advanced cases, acetoacetate levels are low and β-hydroxybutyrate levels are high.

CLINICAL FEATURES

- AKA presents with nausea, vomiting, orthostasis, and abdominal pain 24 to 72 hours after the last alcohol intake.
- On examination, the patient is acutely ill and dehydrated with a tender abdomen. Abdominal tenderness is diffuse and nonspecific, or is a result of other causes associated with the use of alcohol, such as gastritis, hepatitis, or pancreatitis.
- Presentation may be confounded by other complications of alcoholism, such as infection or alcohol withdrawal.

DIAGNOSIS AND DIFFERENTIAL

- Laboratory investigation reveals an anion gap ($Na^+ - [Cl^- + HCO_3^-] > 12 \pm 4$ mEq/L) metabolic acidosis.
- Serum pH may be low, normal, or high, as these patients often have mixed acid–base disorders, such as a metabolic acidosis from AKA and a metabolic alkalosis from vomiting and volume depletion.
- Blood glucose is low to mildly elevated.
- Blood alcohol level is usually low or zero, as vomiting and abdominal pain limit intake.
- Serum ketones (acetoacetate and β-hydroxybutyrate) are elevated. Although ketones are usually detected in significant amounts, the redox state may be such that most or all acetoacetate is reduced to β-hydroxybutyrate.
- If the nitroprusside test is used to detect serum or urine ketones, results may be falsely low or negative because this test only detects acetoacetate and not β-hydroxybutyrate.
- Diagnosis of AKA is established by criteria listed in Table 132-1.
- Differential diagnosis includes other causes of an anion gap metabolic acidosis such as salicylate, methanol, ethylene glycol, iron, or isoniazid toxicity, diabetic ketoacidosis, uremia, and lactic acidosis.

TABLE 132-1 Diagnostic Criteria for Alcoholic Ketoacidosis*

Low, normal, or slightly elevated serum glucose
Binge drinking ending in nausea, vomiting, and decreased intake
Wide anion gap metabolic acidosis
Positive serum ketones*
Wide anion gap metabolic acidosis without alternate explanation

*The absence of ketones in the serum based on the nitroprusside test does not exclude the diagnosis.

EMERGENCY DEPARTMENT CARE AND DISPOSITION

- Treat with IV infusion of D_5NS. The crystalloid solution restores intravascular volume and glucose administration stimulates endogenous insulin release, which inhibits ketosis.
- Unlike treatment for diabetic ketoacidosis, insulin administration is not necessary.
- Thiamine 100 milligrams IV is recommended before glucose administration to, in theory, prevent precipitation of Wernicke's disease.
- Other electrolytes and vitamins should be supplemented as the condition warrants.
- Treatment should be continued until the acidosis clears, which is usually within 12 to 24 hours.

For further reading in Tintinalli's *Emergency Medicine: A Comprehensive Study Guide*, 7th ed., see Chapter 221, "Alcoholic Ketoacidosis," by William A. Woods and Debra G. Perina.

133 THYROID DISEASE EMERGENCIES

Katrina A. Leone

EPIDEMIOLOGY

- Hypothyroidism is a condition of insufficient thyroid hormone production that causes slowed metabolism.
- Hypothyroidism is more common in women than in men.
- Myxedema coma is a life-threatening expression of severe hypothyroidism. Vast majority of cases occur during the winter months in elderly women with undiagnosed or under-treated hypothyroidism.
- Mortality for myxedema coma ranges from 30% to 60%, depending on the extent of comorbid diseases.

PATHOPHYSIOLOGY

- The most common etiologies of hypothyroidism are primary thyroid failure due to autoimmune disease (Hashimoto's thyroiditis), idiopathic causes, ablative surgery, or iodine deficiency.
- Secondary hypothyroidism is due to a deficiency of thyroid stimulating hormone (TSH) from pituitary tumors, infiltrative disease, or hemorrhage, or a deficiency of thyrotropin-releasing hormone from the hypothalamus.
- Medications that cause hypothyroidism include amiodarone and lithium.
- Precipitating events of myxedema coma include infection, congestive heart failure, drugs, trauma, and exposure to a cold environment.

CLINICAL FEATURES

- Typical signs and symptoms of hypothyroidism include fatigue, weakness, cold intolerance, constipation, weight gain, and deepening of the voice.
- Cutaneous signs include dry skin, non-pitting edema of the face and extremities (myxedema), and thinning eyebrows.
- Cardiac findings include bradycardia, cardiomyopathy, and a low-voltage electrocardiogram.
- Paresthesias, ataxia, and prolongation of the deep tendon reflexes are characteristic neurologic findings.
- A thyroidectomy scar may be present, but a goiter is uncommon.
- In addition to the above features of hypothyroidism, patients with myxedema coma present with hypothermia, hypotension, altered mental status, hyponatremia, hypoglycemia, and respiratory failure.

DIAGNOSIS AND DIFFERENTIAL

- Thyroid tests will typically demonstrate low free thyroxine (FT_4) or triiodothyronine (FT_3) levels and elevated TSH in primary hypothyroidism. Low TSH with low FT_4 and FT_3 indicates secondary hypothyroidism.
- Myxedema coma is a clinical diagnosis that must be suspected based upon the clinical presentation. There is no level of TSH or thyroid hormone that differentiates hypothyroidism from myxedema coma, and treatment should not be delayed to obtain confirmatory laboratory tests.
- The differential diagnosis of myxedema coma includes sepsis, adrenal crisis, hypoglycemia, meningitis, hypercarbia, hyponatremia, environmental hypothermia, congestive heart failure, stroke, and drug overdose.

EMERGENCY DEPARTMENT CARE AND DISPOSITION

- Most patients with uncomplicated symptomatic hypothyroidism may be referred to their primary care physician for further evaluation and initiation of treatment.
- Supportive care for myxedema coma includes airway stabilization and establishment of adequate oxygenation and ventilation. A difficult airway should be anticipated due to macroglossia and oropharyngeal edema.
- Initiate cardiac monitoring, gradual rewarming for hypothermia, and correction of hypoglycemia. Hyponatremia typically responds to fluid restriction.
- Vasopressors are often ineffective and should be reserved for severe hypotension. Sedating drugs should be avoided.
- Investigate and treat precipitating causes.
- Pharmacologic therapy for myxedema coma includes hydrocortisone 100 milligrams IV (to treat possible concurrent adrenal insufficiency) and levothyroxine (T_4) 4 micrograms/kg by slow IV infusion. Add L-triiodothyronine (T_3) 20 micrograms IV for severe symptoms. L-triiodothyronine dosage should be halved (or avoided completely) in patients with cardiovascular disease due to a risk of arrhythmias and myocardial infarction.
- Admit all patients with myxedema coma to an ICU setting.

THYROTOXICOSIS AND THYROID STORM

EPIDEMIOLOGY

- Thyrotoxicosis is a general term for excess circulating thyroid hormone from any cause. Hyperthyroidism is defined as excess circulating thyroid hormone due to thyroid gland hyperactivity.

- Graves' disease is the most common cause of hyperthyroidism (85%) and typically presents in the third and fourth decades of life.
- Thyroid storm is an acute, life-threatening manifestation of thyrotoxicosis most often seen in patients with unrecognized or undertreated hyperthyroidism.
- Thyroid storm mortality is high, even with aggressive treatment.

PATHOPHYSIOLOGY

- Primary hyperthyroidism is caused by excess production of thyroid hormones from the thyroid gland. Secondary hyperthyroidism is due to excess production of thyroid-releasing hormone from the hypothalamus or TSH from the pituitary.
- Other causes of hyperthyroidism include iodine or amiodarone use, ingestion of excessive thyroid hormone, and thyroid hormone production at ectopic sites (ovarian teratoma, hydatidiform mole, metastatic thyroid cancer).
- Precipitants of thyroid storm include infection, trauma, diabetic ketoacidosis (DKA), myocardial infarction, stroke, pulmonary embolism, surgery, withdrawal of thyroid medication, iodine administration, palpation of the thyroid gland, ingestion of thyroid hormone, and idiopathic causes (~25%).

CLINICAL FEATURES

- Symptoms of hyperthyroidism include heat intolerance, palpitations, weight loss, sweating, tremor, nervousness, weakness, fatigue, ophthalmoplegia, exophthalmos, widened pulse pressure, and a palpable goiter.
- The signs and symptoms associated with thyroid storm are related to enhanced sympathetic nervous system activity and include central nervous system disturbance (confusion, delirium, seizure, coma), cardiovascular abnormalities (sinus tachycardia, atrial fibrillation, premature ventricular contractions, congestive heart failure), and stimulated gastrointestinal motility and diarrhea.
- Apathetic thyrotoxicosis is a distinct presentation of thyroid storm in the elderly that includes lethargy, slowed mentation, apathetic facies, goiter, weight loss, and proximal muscle weakness.

DIAGNOSIS AND DIFFERENTIAL

- A suppressed TSH and elevated free FT_4 or FT_3 level confirm the diagnosis of primary hyperthyroidism. In cases of secondary hyperthyroidism, TSH, FT_4, and FT_3 are all elevated.
- Thyroid hormone levels do not differentiate between symptomatic, uncomplicated thyrotoxicosis and thyroid storm.
- The differential diagnosis of thyroid storm includes sepsis, other causes of congestive heart failure, stroke, complications of diabetes (eg, DKA or hypoglycemia), heat stroke, delirium tremens, malignant hyperthermia, neuroleptic malignant syndrome, pheochromocytoma, medication withdrawal, and sympathomimetic or organophosphate overdose.

EMERGENCY DEPARTMENT CARE AND DISPOSITION

- Treatment of thyroid storm can be divided into three areas: (1) general supportive care, including airway assessment, supplemental oxygen, intravenous fluids, and cardiac monitoring; (2) pharmacologic therapy

TABLE 133-1 Drug Treatment of Thyroid Storm

1. Inhibit new thyroid hormone production	**Propylthiouracil** (PTU) 600-1000 milligrams PO loading dose followed by 200-250 milligrams PO every 4 h or **Methimazole** 40 milligrams PO loading dose followed by 25 milligrams PO every 4 h
2. Inhibit thyroid hormone release (give at least 1 h after step 1)	**Lugol's solution** 8-10 drops PO every 6-8 h Or **Potassium iodide** (SSKI) 5 drops PO every 6 h Or **Iopanoic acid** 1 gram IV every 8 h Or **Lithium carbonate*** 300 milligrams PO every 6 h
3. Block peripheral thyroid hormone effects	**Propranolol** 1-2 milligrams IV every 10-15 min Or **Reserpine**† 1 milligram IM test dose followed by 2.5-5 milligrams IM every 4-6 h Or **Guanethidine**† 30-40 milligrams PO every 6 h
4. Prevent conversion of T_4 to T_3	**Hydrocortisone** 100 milligrams IV every 8 h Or **Dexamethasone** 2 milligrams IV every 6 h

*Lithium is preferred over iodine in the setting of iodine or thionamide allergies and iodine- or amiodarone-induced thyrotoxicosis.
†Use if β-blocker is contraindicated and congestive heart failure or hypotension are not present.

to inhibit thyroid hormone synthesis, prevent thyroid hormone release, block peripheral thyroid hormone effects, and prevent peripheral conversion of FT_4 to FT_3 (Table 133-1); and (3) identification and treatment of precipitating events.
- All patients with thyroid storm should be admitted to a monitored or intensive care unit setting.

For further reading in Tintinalli's *Emergency Medicine; A Comprehensive Study Guide*, 7th ed., see Chapter 223, "Thyroid Disorders: Hypothyroidism and Myxedema Crisis," by Alzamani Mohammad Idrose, and Chapter 224, "Thyroid Disorders: Hyperthyroidism and Thyroid Storm," by Alzamani Mohammad Idrose.

134 ADRENAL INSUFFICIENCY AND ADRENAL CRISIS

Michael P. Kefer

PATHOPHYSIOLOGY

- Adrenal insufficiency may be acute or chronic, and results when the physiologic demand for glucocorticoids and mineralocorticoids exceeds the supply from the adrenal cortex.
- The pituitary secretes adrenocorticotropic hormone (ACTH) and associated melanocyte-stimulating hormone (MSH).
- ACTH stimulates the adrenal cortex to secrete cortisol (and aldosterone to a minor degree). Cortisol has negative feedback on the pituitary to inhibit secretion of ACTH and MSH.
- Cortisol is the major glucocorticoid. It has a key role in maintaining blood glucose levels by decreasing glucose uptake and stimulating proteolysis and lipolysis for gluconeogenesis. Cortisol is necessary for the proper function of catecholamines on cardiac muscle and arterioles. Cortisol also controls body water balance.
- Aldosterone is the major mineralocorticoid. The renin-angiotensin system and serum potassium regulate its secretion. ACTH has a minor effect.
- The adrenal cortex as a source of androgens is much more important in women than men.
- Adrenal insufficiency is described as primary or secondary based on whether the insufficiency occurs at the level of the adrenal glands or pituitary, respectively.
- Adrenal crisis is the acute, life-threatening form of adrenal insufficiency.
- Congenital adrenal hyperplasia results from an enzyme deficiency in cortisol production. In 95% of cases the deficient enzyme is 21-hydroxylase.

CLINICAL FEATURES

- Manifestations of primary adrenal insufficiency, which are due to cortisol and aldosterone deficiency, include weakness, dehydration, hypotension, anorexia, nausea, vomiting, weight loss, and abdominal pain.
- Hyperpigmentation of both exposed and nonexposed skin and mucous membranes occurs as a result of uninhibited MSH secretion in conjunction with ACTH.
- Androgen deficiency in women manifests as thinning of pubic and axillary hair.
- Secondary adrenal insufficiency results from inadequate secretion of ACTH (which is accompanied by MSH), with resultant cortisol deficiency. Aldosterone levels are not significantly affected because of regulation through the renin-angiotensin system. Therefore, hyperpigmentation and hyperkalemia are not seen.
- Clinical features of adrenal crisis are as described above, but to the extreme and accompanied by shock and altered mental status.
- Congenital adrenal hyperplasia presents in the first month of life with nonspecific symptoms of lethargy, vomiting, poor feeding, and poor weight gain. Examination reveals dehydration, hyperpigmentation, and, in females, clitoromegaly.

DIAGNOSIS AND DIFFERENTIAL

- All patients with adrenal insufficiency have low plasma cortisol levels.
- Diagnosis of primary adrenal insufficiency and congenital adrenal hyperplasia is based on clinical features and laboratory investigation revealing hyponatremia, hyperkalemia, hypoglycemia, anemia, metabolic acidosis, and prerenal azotemia.
- Secondary adrenal insufficiency is similarly diagnosed except hyperkalemia is not seen as there is no aldosterone deficiency, and hyperpigmentation is not seen as MSH levels are low along with ACTH levels.
- The most common cause of adrenal insufficiency and adrenal crisis is adrenal suppression from prolonged steroid use with either abrupt steroid withdrawal or exposure to increased physiologic stress such as injury, illness, or surgery.
- Adrenal suppression can occur with steroids given by any route (oral, topical, intrathecal, or inhaled).

TABLE 134-1 Causes of Primary Adrenal Insufficiency

PRIMARY ADRENAL INSUFFICIENCY (DISORDERS IN THE ADRENAL GLAND)	EXAMPLES
Autoimmune	Isolated adrenal insufficiency or associated with polyglandular insufficiencies (polyglandular autoimmune syndrome types I or II)
Adrenal hemorrhage or thrombosis	Necrosis caused by meningococcal sepsis Coagulation disorders Overwhelming sepsis (Waterhouse-Friderichsen syndrome)
Drugs	Adrenolytic agents Metyrapone Aminoglutethimide Mitotane Ketoconazole
Infections involving adrenal glands	Tuberculosis Fungal, bacterial sepsis Acquired immunodeficiency syndrome involving adrenal glands
Infiltrative disorders involving adrenal glands	Sarcoidosis Hemochromatosis Amyloidosis Lymphoma Metastatic cancer
Surgery	Bilateral adrenalectomy
Hereditary	Adrenal hypoplasia Congenital adrenal hyperplasia Adrenoleukodystrophy Familial glucocorticoid deficiency
Idiopathic	—

- It may take up to 1 year for the hypothalamic-pituitary-adrenal axis to recover following prolonged suppression with steroid treatment.
- Differential diagnosis of primary and secondary adrenal insufficiency is listed in Tables 134-1 and 134-2, respectively.

EMERGENCY DEPARTMENT CARE AND DISPOSITION

- Treatment of acute adrenal insufficiency is outlined in Table 134-3.
- Neonates with congenital adrenal hyperplasia are treated with normal saline 20 milligrams/kg bolus for hypovolemia, hydrocortisone 25 mg IV/IO for steroid deficiency, and 10% dextrose 5 mL/kg for hypoglycemia.

TABLE 134-2 Causes of Secondary Adrenal Insufficiency

SECONDARY ADRENAL INSUFFICIENCY (HYPOTHALAMIC-PITUITARY DYSFUNCTION)	EXAMPLES
Sudden cessation of prolonged glucocorticoid therapy	Chronic use of steroid inhibits ACTH production
Pituitary necrosis or bleeding	Postpartum pituitary necrosis (Sheehan syndrome)
Exogenous glucocorticoid administration	Causes decreased production of ACTH at pituitary
Brain tumors	Pituitary tumor Hypothalamic tumor Local invasion (craniopharyngioma)
Pituitary irradiation Pituitary surgery Head trauma involving the pituitary gland	Disrupts corticotropin-releasing hormone and ACTH production capacity in hypothalamic-pituitary axis
Infiltrative disorders of the pituitary or hypothalamus	Sarcoidosis Hemosiderosis Hemochromatosis Histiocytosis X Metastatic cancer Lymphoma
Infectious diseases involving organs away from adrenal	Tuberculosis Meningitis Fungus Human immunodeficiency virus

Abbreviation: ACTH = adrenocorticotropic hormone.

TABLE 134-3 Treatment Guide for Adrenal Insufficiency

Begin therapy immediately in any suspected case of adrenal crisis (prognosis is related to rapidity of treatment delivery).

↓

Administer IV fluids

5% dextrose in normal saline is the fluid of choice to correct both hypoglycemia and hyponatremia.

↓

Steroids

Hydrocortisone (100 milligram bolus) is the drug of choice for cases of adrenal crisis or insufficiency (provides both glucocorticoid and mineralocorticoid effects).

or

Dexamethasone, 4 milligram bolus (for accuracy of rapid adrenocorticotropic hormone stimulation test results).

↓

Vasopressors

Administered after steroid therapy in patients unresponsive to fluid resuscitation (norepinephrine, dopamine, or phenylephrine [Neo-Synephrine®] preferred).

↓

(*Continued*)

TABLE 134-3 Treatment Guide for Adrenal Insufficiency (Continued)

Supplementation Patients may require lifelong glucocorticoids ± mineralocorticoid supplementation.
↓
Maintenance Increased maintenance doses of chronic steroids are required during periods of stress (eg, illness, surgery, trauma, etc.) to satisfy increased physiologic need for cortisol.

For further reading in Tintinalli's *Emergency Medicine: A Comprehensive Study Guide*, 7th ed., see Chapter 137, "Hypoglycemia and Metabolic Emergencies in Infants and Children," by Nadeemuddin Qureshi, Mohammed Al-Mogbil, and Osama Y. Kentab and Chapter 225, "Adrenal Insufficiency and Adrenal Crisis," by Alzamani Mohammed Idrose.

Section 15

HEMATOLOGIC AND ONCOLOGIC EMERGENCIES

135 EVALUATION OF ANEMIA AND THE BLEEDING PATIENT

Daniel A. Handel

PATHOPHYSIOLOGY

- Anemia is due to loss of red blood cells (RBCs) by hemorrhage, increased destruction of RBCs, or impaired production of RBCs.
- Bleeding disorders from congenital or acquired abnormalities in the hemostatic system can result in excessive hemorrhage, excessive clot formation, or both.

CLINICAL FEATURES

- The rate of the development of the anemia, the extent of the anemia, and the ability of the cardiovascular system to compensate for the decreased oxygen-carrying capacity determine the severity of the patient's symptoms and clinical presentation.
- Patients may complain of palpitations, dizziness, postural faintness, easy fatigability, exertional intolerance, and tinnitus.
- On physical examination, patients may have pale conjunctiva, skin, and nail beds.
- Tachycardia, hyperdynamic precordium, and systolic murmurs may be present. Tachypnea at rest and hypotension are late signs.
- Use of ethanol, prescription drugs, and recreational drugs may alter the patient's ability to compensate for the anemia.
- Risk factors for underlying bleeding disorders include a family history of bleeding disorder, history of liver disease, and use of aspirin, nonsteroidal anti-inflammatory drugs, ethanol, warfarin, or certain antibiotics.
- Signs of platelet disorders include mucocutaneous bleeding (including petechiae, ecchymoses, purpura, and epistaxis), gastrointestinal or genitourinary bleeding, or heavy menstrual bleeding.
- Signs of coagulation factor deficiencies include delayed bleeding, hemarthrosis, or bleeding into potential spaces (eg, retroperitoneum).
- Patients with combined abnormalities of platelets and coagulation factors, such as disseminated intravascular coagulation, present with both mucocutaneous and deep space bleeding.

DIAGNOSIS AND DIFFERENTIAL

- Decreased RBC count, hemoglobin, and hematocrit are diagnostic of anemia. Hemoccult examination, complete blood cell count, reticulocyte count, review of RBC indices, and examination of peripheral blood smear are necessary for the initial evaluation of the patient with anemia (Table 135-1).
- The mean cellular volume and reticulocyte count can assist in classifying the anemia and can aid in differential diagnosis (Fig. 135-1).
- Complete blood cell count, platelet count, prothrombin time, and partial thromboplastin time are necessary for the initial evaluation of the patient with a suspected bleeding disorder (Table 135-2).

EMERGENCY DEPARTMENT CARE AND DISPOSITION

- Emergent priorities remain airway, breathing, and circulation. Hemorrhage should be controlled with direct pressure.

TABLE 135-1 Laboratory Tests in the Evaluation of Anemia

TEST	INTERPRETATION	CLINICAL CORRELATION
MCV	Measure of the average red blood cell size.	Decreased MCV (microcytosis) is seen in chronic iron deficiency, thalassemia, anemia of chronic disease, lead poisoning. Increased MCV (macrocytosis) can be due to vitamin B_{12} or folate deficiency, alcohol abuse, liver disease, reticulocytosis, and some medications (see Diagnosis section).
Mean corpuscular hemoglobin	Measure of the amount of hemoglobin in average red blood cell.	—
Red cell distribution width	Measures the size variability of the RBC population.	In early deficiency anemia (iron, vitamin B_{12}, or folate), may be increased before the mean corpuscular volume becomes abnormal.
MCHC	Measure of hemoglobin concentration in average RBC.	Low MCHC can be seen in iron deficiency anemia, defects in porphyrin synthesis and hemolytic anemia.
Ferritin	Ferritin is a protein in the body that binds to iron. Serum levels serve as an indication of the amount of iron stored in the body.	Low serum ferritin is associated with iron deficiency anemia and helps differentiate this anemia from other causes.
Reticulocyte count	These RBCs of intermediate maturity are a marker of production by the bone marrow.	Decreased reticulocyte count reflects impaired RBC production. Increased counts are a marker of accelerated RBC production.
Peripheral blood smear	Allows visualization of the RBC morphology. Allows evaluation for abnormal cell shapes. Allows examination of the white blood cells and platelets.	May guide to new diagnosis of diseases such as sickle cell disease. Aids in the diagnosis of entities such as hemolytic anemia. May guide the diagnosis of other diseases that cause anemia.
Direct and indirect Coombs test	Direct Coombs test is used to detect antibodies on RBCs. Indirect Coombs test is used to detect antibodies in the sera.	Direct Coombs test is positive in autoimmune hemolytic anemia, transfusion reactions, and some drug-induced hemolytic anemia. Indirect Coombs test is routinely used in compatibility testing before transfusion.

Abbreviations: MCHC = mean corpuscular hemoglobin concentration; MCV = mean corpuscular volume; RBC = red blood cell.

- Type- and cross-matched blood should be ordered if blood transfusion is anticipated. Packed RBCs should be transfused in symptomatic patients and those who are hemodynamically unstable.
- Patients with anemia and ongoing blood loss should be admitted to the hospital for further evaluation and treatment.
- Patients with chronic anemia or newly diagnosed anemia with unclear etiology require admission if they are hemodynamically unstable, hypoxic, or acidotic, or demonstrate cardiac ischemia.
- Hematology consultation is warranted in patients with suspected bleeding disorders and anemia of unclear etiology.

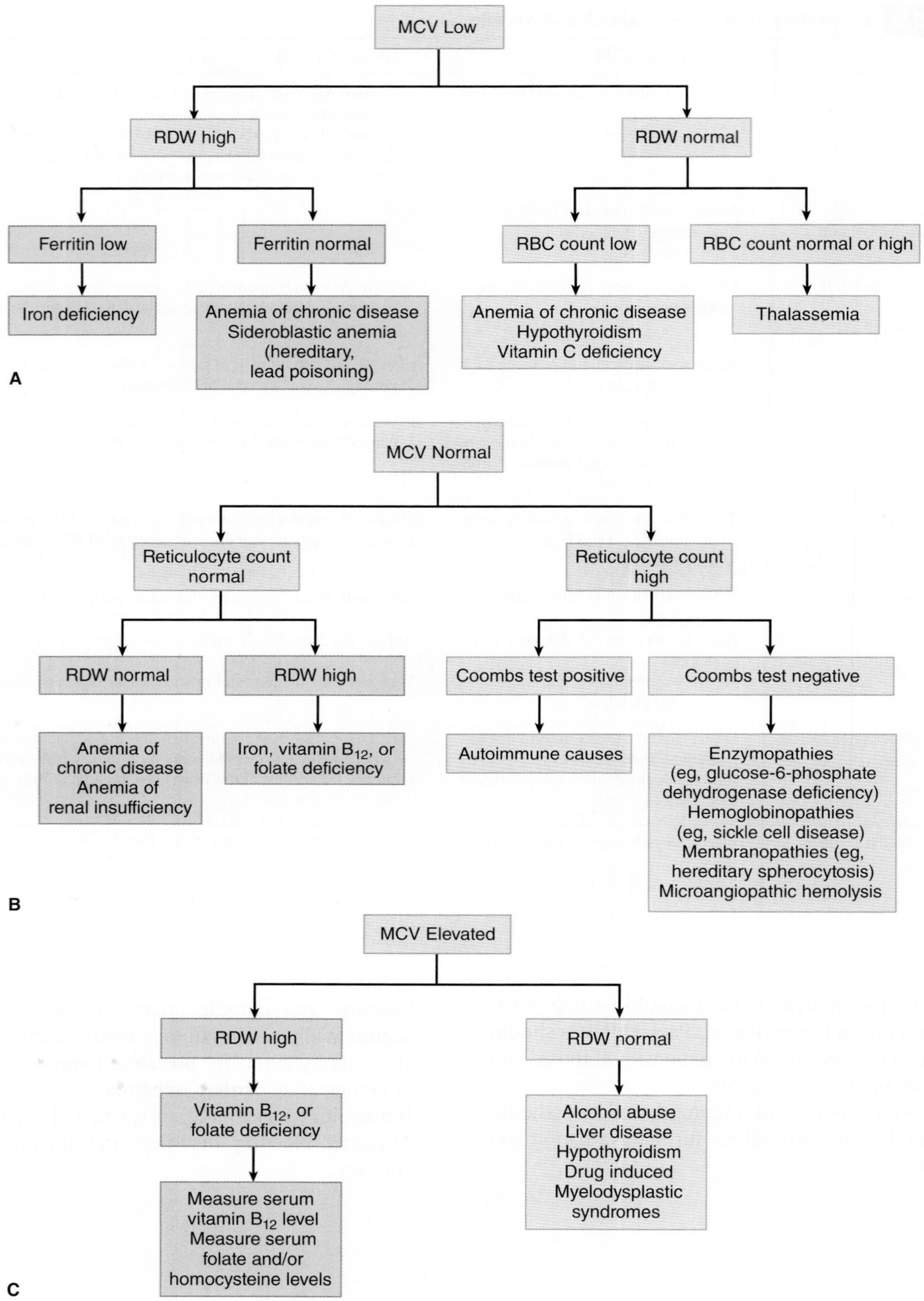

FIG. 135-1. A. Evaluation of microcytic anemia. MCV = mean corpuscular volume; RBC = red blood cell; RDW = red cell distribution width. **B.** Evaluation of normocytic anemia. MCV = mean corpuscular volume; RDW = red cell distribution width. **C.** Evaluation of macrocytic anemia. MCV = mean corpuscular volume; RDW = red cell distribution width.

TABLE 135-2 Initial Tests of Hemostasis

SCREENING TESTS	REFERENCE VALUE	COMPONENT MEASURED	CLINICAL CORRELATIONS/COMMENTS
Primary Hemostasis			
Platelet count	150,000-300,000/mm^3	Number of platelets per mm^3	*Decreased platelet count (thrombocytopenia)*: bleeding usually not a problem until platelet count is <50,000/mm^3; high risk of spontaneous bleeding, including central nervous system bleeding, seen with count of <10,000/mm^3; usually due to decreased production or increased destruction of platelets *Elevated platelet count (thrombocytosis)*: commonly a reaction to inflammation or malignancy, and occurs in polycythemia vera; can be associated with hemorrhage or thrombosis
Bleeding time (BT)	Variable Typically 2.5-10.0 min using a BT template	Interaction between platelets and the subendothelium	*Prolonged BT* caused by: Thrombocytopenia (platelet count <50,000/mm^3) Abnormal platelet function (von Willebrand disease, antiplatelet drugs, uremia, liver disease)
Secondary Hemostasis			
Prothrombin time (PT) and international normalized ratio (INR)	PT: 11-13 s; depends on reagent INR: 1.0	Extrinsic system and common pathway—Factors VII, X, V, prothrombin, and fibrinogen	*Prolonged PT* most commonly caused by: Warfarin (inhibits production of vitamin K–dependent Factors II, VII, IX, and X) Liver disease with decreased factor synthesis Antibiotics that inhibit vitamin K–dependent factors (moxalactam, cefamandole, cefotaxime, cefoperazone)
Activated partial thromboplastin time (aPTT)	22-34 s Depends on type of thromboplastin reagent used "Activated" with kaolin	Intrinsic system and common pathway—Factors XII, XI, IX, VIII, X, V, prothrombin, and fibrinogen	*Prolonged aPTT* most commonly caused by: Heparin therapy Factor deficiencies (factor levels have to be <30% of normal to cause prolongation)
Fibrinogen level	Slightly variable according to specific test Typically 200-400 milligrams/dL	Protein made in liver; converted to fibrin as part of normal coagulation cascade	Low levels seen in disseminated intravascular coagulation Elevated in inflammatory processes (acute-phase reactant)
Thrombin clotting time (TCT)	10-12 s	Conversion of fibrinogen to fibrin monomer	*Prolonged TCT* caused by: Low fibrinogen level Abnormal fibrinogen molecule (liver disease) Presence of heparin, fibrin degradation products, or a paraprotein (multiple myeloma); these interfere with the conversion Occasionally seen in hyperfibrinogenemia
"Mix" testing	Variable	Performed when results on one or more of the above screening tests is prolonged; the patient's plasma ("abnormal") is mixed with "normal" plasma and the screening test is repeated	*If the mixing corrects* the screening test result: one or more factor deficiencies are present *If the mixing does not correct* the screening test result: a circulating inhibitor is present
Fibrin degradation product (FDP) and D-dimer levels	FDP: variable depending on specific test, typically <2.5-10 micrograms/mL D-Dimer: variable depending on specific test, typically <250-500 nanograms/mL	*FDP* test: measures breakdown products from fibrinogen and fibrin monomer D-*Dimer* test: measures breakdown products of cross-linked fibrin	Levels are elevated in diffuse intravascular coagulation, venous thrombosis, pulmonary embolus, and liver disease, and during pregnancy
Factor level assays	60%-130% of reference value (0.60-1.30 units/mL)	Measures the percent activity of a specified factor compared to normal	To identify specific deficiencies and direct therapeutic management
Protein C level	Variable Typically 60%-150% of reference value	Level of protein C in the blood	Vitamin K dependent Increases with age Values higher in males than females Deficiency associated with thromboembolism in people <50 y of age

(*Continued*)

TABLE 135-2 Initial Tests of Hemostasis (Continued)

SCREENING TESTS	REFERENCE VALUE	COMPONENT MEASURED	CLINICAL CORRELATIONS/COMMENTS
Protein S level	Variable Typically 60%-150% of reference value	Level of protein S in the blood	Vitamin K dependent Increases with age Values higher in males than females Deficiency associated with thromboembolism in people <50 y of age
Factor V Leiden (FVL)	Variable	Screening test looks for activated protein C resistance and confirmatory test analyzes DNA sequence of Factor V gene Screening assay uses activated partial thromboplastin time with and without added activated protein C	FVL not inactivated by activated protein C Heterozygotes have 7× and homozygotes have a 20× increased lifetime risk of venous thrombosis Mutation associated with thromboembolism in people <50 yr of age
Antithrombin level	Variable depending on specific test Typically 20-45 milligrams/dL	Measures level of antithrombin in the blood	Not vitamin K dependent; patients with deficiency require higher dosages of heparin for anticoagulation therapy Deficiency associated with thromboembolism in people <50 y of age
Antiphospholipid antibodies	IgG <23 GPL units/mL and IgM <11 MPL units/mL	Tests for antibodies that bind to phospholipids Lupus anticoagulant Anticardiolipin antibody	*Lupus anticoagulant*: elevated in systemic lupus erythematosus (SLE) and other autoimmune diseases *Anticardiolipin antibody*: elevated in SLE, other autoimmune diseases, syphilis, and Behçet syndrome Increased risk of spontaneous abortions, fetal loss, and fetal growth retardation
Anti–Factor Xa activity	Therapeutic: 0.7-1.1 units/mL Prophylactic: 0.2-0.3 units/mL	Inhibition of Factor Xa activity	Used to monitor low-molecular-weight heparin therapy May be elevated in renal dysfunction
Platelet function assay	88-198 s Variable	Tests for platelet adhesion and aggregation	Affected by uremia, anemia, thrombocytopenia, antiplatelet medications, and von Willebrand disease
Peripheral blood smear	Qualitative and quantitative based on visualization	Estimates quantity and appearance of platelets, white blood cells, and red blood cells	Allows identification of clumped platelets, abnormal cells interfering with coagulation (leukemia) Operator dependent
Dilute Russell viper venom time	23-27 s	Venom directly activates Factor X and converts prothrombin to thrombin when phospholipid and Factor V are present	Prolonged in the presence of antiphospholipid antibodies
Inhibitor screens	Variable	Verifies the presence or absence of antibodies directed against one or more of the coagulation factors	*Specific inhibitors*: directed against one coagulation factor, most commonly against Factor VIII *Nonspecific inhibitors*: directed against more than one coagulation factor; example is lupus-type anticoagulant
PIVKA II (proteins induced by vitamin K absence or antagonism) test[16]	Variable	Measures nonfunctional precursors of vitamin K–dependant coagulation factors (II, VII, IX, X)	Increased in vitamin K–deficient states, such as hemorrhagic disease of the newborn, and can differentiate it from nonaccidental trauma Increased in overdoses of warfarin or cholestatic liver diseases that can respond to vitamin K therapy

Abbreviations: GPL = 1 microgram of affinity-purified IgG anticardiolipin antibody from an original index serum; MPL = 1 microgram of affinity-purified IgM anticardiolipin antibody from an original index serum.

For further reading in Tintinalli's *Emergency Medicine: A Comprehensive Study Guide*, 7th ed., see Chapter 226, "Anemia," by Robin R. Hemphill; Chapter 227, "Tests of Hemostasis," by Stephen John Cico and Robin R. Hemphill; and Chapter 232, "Acquired Hemolytic Anemia," by Patricia Chu Klap and Robin R. Hemphill.

136 ACQUIRED BLEEDING DISORDERS

Aaron Barksdale

ACQUIRED PLATELET DEFECTS

PATHOPHYSIOLOGY

- Acquired platelet abnormalities include *qualitative* (dysfunctional) and *quantitative* (thrombocytopenia) defects.
- Thrombocytopenia may be a result of decreased platelet production, increased platelet destruction, increased platelet loss, and splenic sequestration.

CLINICAL FEATURES

- Bleeding due to thrombocytopenia commonly presents as petechiae and mucosal bleeding (gingival, epistaxis).
- Additional findings may include purpura, hemoptysis, menorrhagia, hematuria, or hematochezia.
- Deep tissue bleeding is uncommon.

DIAGNOSIS AND DIFFERENTIAL

- Causes of decreased platelet production include marrow infiltration, aplastic anemia, drugs, viral infections, and chronic alcohol use.
- Causes of increased platelet destruction include idiopathic thrombocytopenic purpura (ITP), thrombotic thrombocytopenic purpura (TTP), hemolytic uremic syndrome (HUS), disseminated intravascular coagulation (DIC), and viral infection, drugs, and HELLP syndrome.
- Thrombocytopenia may also be the result of acute hemorrhage, hemodialysis, and splenic sequestration.
- Qualitative platelet disorders include uremia, liver disease, drugs (aspirin, NSAIDs, clopidogrel), antiplatelet antibodies, DIC, and myeloproliferative disorders.

EMERGENCY DEPARTMENT CARE AND DISPOSITION

- Initial laboratory testing should include a CBC with peripheral smear.
- Consider consultation with hematologist. Some conditions may worsen with platelet transfusion (DIC and TTP).
- Consider platelet transfusion when platelet count <10,000/mm^3 or when active bleeding and platelets <50,000/mm^3.
- Patient's with ITP and platelets >50,000/mm^3 do not require treatment.
- Patients with ITP and platelet count <20,000 to 30,000/mm^3 or active bleeding and platelets <50,000 typically require treatment.
- The initial treatment of ITP is usually corticosteroids, **prednisone** 60 to 100 milligrams PO daily.
- Severe cases of ITP may require **IV immunoglobulin**, 1 gram/kg/d.

BLEEDING IN LIVER DISEASE

PATHOPHYSIOLOGY

- Liver disease increases the risk of bleeding for multiple reasons, including decreased synthesis of vitamin K-dependent coagulation factors (II, VII, IX, and X), thrombocytopenia, and increased fibrinolysis.

EMERGENCY DEPARTMENT CARE AND DISPOSITION

- Patients with liver disease and active bleeding should receive **vitamin K**, 10 milligrams PO or IV.
- Patients with severe bleeding or prior to invasive procedure should receive fresh frozen plasma 15 milliliters/kg IV to temporarily replace coagulation factors.
- Patients with active bleeding and fibrinogen levels <100 milligrams/dL, administer cryoprecipitate, 1 unit/5 kg IV.
- Platelet transfusion may be indicated when severe bleeding and associated thrombocytopenia.
- **Desmopressin** 0.3 microgram/kg SC or IV may shorten bleeding times in some patients.

BLEEDING IN RENAL DISEASE

PATHOPHYSIOLOGY

- Bleeding in renal disease is the result of a variety of hemostatic abnormalities including platelet dysfunction due to uremic toxins, deficiency of coagulation factors, and thrombocytopenia.

EMERGENCY DEPARTMENT CARE AND DISPOSITION

- Treat acute bleeding with the transfusion of packed red blood cells when indicated.
- Hemodialysis improves platelet function transiently for 1 to 2 days.
- **Desmopressin** 0.3 microgram/kg SC or IV shortens bleeding time in most patients.

- **Conjugated estrogen** 0.6 milligram/kg IV improves the bleeding time and active bleeding in the majority of uremic patients.
- Platelet transfusions and cryoprecipitate are indicated for life-threatening bleeding only, and are to be used in conjunction with the previously listed therapies.

DISSEMINATED INTRAVASCULAR COAGULATION

PATHOPHYSIOLOGY

- DIC is an acquired syndrome that results from the activation of both the coagulation and fibrinolytic systems.

CLINICAL FEATURES

- The complications of DIC are related to both bleeding and thrombosis, although one usually predominates.
- The clinical features include bleeding from venipuncture sites and the GI or GU tract, petechiae and ecchymosis, thrombosis, purpura fulminans, and multiple organ failure.
- Patients may also display mental status changes, focal ischemia of the extremities, oliguria, renal cortical necrosis, and adult respiratory distress syndrome (ARDS).

DIAGNOSIS AND DIFFERENTIAL

- The diagnosis is based on the history, clinical presentation, and associated laboratory abnormalities.
- The common conditions associated with DIC are listed in Table 136-1.
- Refer to Table 136-2 for the laboratory abnormalities associated with DIC.

EMERGENCY DEPARTMENT CARE AND DISPOSITION

- Treatment should focus on the underlying illness and hemodynamic support (IV fluid resuscitation, transfusion of red bloods cells, and vasopressors and inotropic agents).
- Administer cryoprecipitate 1 unit/5 kg IV to patients with active bleeding until fibrinogen levels are between 100 and 150 milligrams/dL.
- Transfuse platelets if counts are <20,000/mm^3 or <50,000/mm^3 with active bleeding.
- Transfuse fresh frozen plasma 15 mL/kg IV if active bleeding.
- Patients with active bleeding, administer **vitamin K** 10 milligrams IV/PO and **folate** 1 milligram IV.
- The role of heparin remains unclear.

TABLE 136-1 Common Conditions Associated with Disseminated Intravascular Coagulation (DIC)

CLINICAL SETTING	COMMENTS
Infection Bacterial Viral Fungal	Probably the most common cause of DIC; 10%-20% of patients with gram-negative sepsis have DIC; endotoxins stimulate monocytes and endothelial cells to express tissue factor; Rocky Mountain spotted fever causes direct endothelial damage; DIC more likely to develop in asplenic patients or cirrhosis; septic patients are more likely to have bleeding than thrombosis.
Carcinoma Adenocarcinoma Lymphoma	Malignant cells may cause endothelial damage and allow the expression of tissue factor as well as other procoagulant materials; most adenocarcinomas tend to have thrombosis (Trousseau syndrome), except prostate cancer tends to have more bleeding; DIC is often chronic and compensated.
Acute leukemia	DIC most common with promyelocytic leukemia; blast cells release procoagulant enzymes, there is excessive release at time of cell lysis (chemotherapy); more likely to have bleeding than thrombosis.
Trauma	DIC especially with brain injury, crush injury, burns, hypothermia, hyperthermia, rhabdomyolysis, fat embolism, hypoxia.
Organ injury Liver disease Pancreatitis	May have chronic compensated DIC; acute DIC may occur in the setting of acute hepatic failure, tissue factor is released from the injured hepatocytes. Pancreatitis can activate the coagulation cascade.
Pregnancy	Placental abruption, amniotic fluid embolus, septic abortion, intrauterine fetal death (can be chronic DIC); can have DIC in *h*emolysis-*e*levated *l*iver enzymes-*l*ow *p*latelets (HELLP) syndrome.
Vascular disease	Large aortic aneurysms (chronic DIC can become acute at time of surgery), giant hemangiomas, vasculitis, multiple telangiectasias.
Envenomation	DIC can develop with bites of rattlesnakes and other vipers; the venom damages the endothelial cells; bleeding is not as serious as expected from laboratory values.
Acute lung injury or adult respiratory distress syndrome	Microthrombi are deposited in the small pulmonary vessels, the pulmonary capillary endothelium is damaged; 20% of patients with ARDS develop DIC and 20% of patients with DIC develop ARDS.
Transfusion reactions, such as acute hemolytic reaction	DIC with severe bleeding, shock, and acute renal failure.

Abbreviation: ARDS = acute respiratory distress syndrome.

TABLE 136-2 Laboratory Abnormalities Characteristic of Disseminated Intravascular Coagulation (DIC)

STUDIES	RESULT
Most Useful	
Prothrombin time	Prolonged
Platelet count	Usually low, or dropping
Fibrinogen level	Usually low (fibrinogen is an acute phase reactant, so may actually start out elevated) fibrinogen level <100 milligrams/dL correlates with severe DIC
Helpful	
Activated partial thromboplastin time	Usually prolonged
Thrombin clotting time	Prolonged (not sensitive)
Fragmented red blood cells	Should be present (not specific)
Fibrin degradation products and D-dimer*	Elevated
Specific factor assays	Extrinsic pathway factors are most affected (VII, X, V, and II)
Factor II, V, VII,† X	Low
Factor VIII (acute phase reactant)	Low, normal, high
Factor IX	Low (decreases later than other factors)

*Levels may be chronically elevated in patients with liver or renal disease.
†Factor VII is usually low early because it has the shortest half-life.

CIRCULATING INHIBITORS OF COAGULATION

EPIDEMIOLOGY

- Acquired inhibitors of coagulation are very rare. There are 1.4 cases per 1 million persons per year.
- Most cases of acquired hemophilia occur in the elderly.

PATHOPHYSIOLOGY

- Circulating anticoagulants are antibodies directed against one or more of the coagulation factors.
- The two most common circulating anticoagulants are factor VIII inhibitor (a specific inhibitor directed only against factor VIII) and antiphospholipid antibodies, including lupus anticoagulant and anticardiolipin antibody (nonspecific inhibitors directed against several coagulation factors).

CLINICAL FEATURES

- Patients with factor VIII inhibitor may present with massive spontaneous bruises, ecchymosis, and hematomas.
- Patients with lupus anticoagulant and anticardiolipin antibodies typically develop symptoms associated with thrombosis.

DIAGNOSIS AND DIFFERENTIAL

- Coagulation studies in patients with factor VIII inhibitor will display a normal PT, normal thrombin clot time, and a prolonged PTT that does not correct with mixing studies.
- A factor VIII–specific assay will show low or absent factor VIII activity.

EMERGENCY DEPARTMENT CARE AND DISPOSITION

- Patients with factor VIII inhibitor and acute bleeding should be managed in conjunction with a hematologist.
- Treatment options include factor VIII, factor IX complex, recombinant factor VIIa, desmopressin acetate, prothrombin complex, and plasmapheresis.

CLOTTING DISORDERS

PATHOPHYSIOLOGY

- Hypercoagulable states may be inherited or acquired (see Table 136-3).
- Thrombosis formation may occur in the venous and/or arterial circulation systems.
- "Virchow's triad" increases the risk of venous thrombus formation and includes hypercoagulability, venous stasis, and endothelial injury.

CLINICAL FEATURES

- Features suggestive of a clotting disorder include early thrombosis (<45 years old), recurrent thrombotic events, family history of thrombosis, recurrent fetal loss, and thrombosis in unusual locations (mesenteric, cerebral, axillary, or portal veins).
- Patients may present with signs of a deep venous thrombosis (unilateral swollen and potentially painful extremity).

TABLE 136-3 Hypercoagulable States

INHERITED	ACQUIRED
Activated protein C resistance due to Factor V Leiden mutation	Antiphospholipid syndrome
	Pregnancy
Prothrombin gene mutation 20210A	Oral contraceptives/hormone replacement therapy
Protein C deficiency	Malignancy
Protein S deficiency	Heparin-induced thrombocytopenia
Antithrombin deficiency	
Hyperhomocysteinemia	Warfarin-induced skin necrosis
	Hyperviscosity syndromes

- Patients may present with signs of a pulmonary embolus (dyspnea, tachycardia, hemoptysis, hypoxia, dizziness, and in severe cases hypotension).
- Other potential presenting symptoms include abdominal pain (mesenteric thrombus and/or ischemia), portal hypertension (portal vein thrombosis), or neurologic symptoms (cerebral vein thrombosis or acute CVA).

DIAGNOSIS AND DIFFERENTIAL

- Laboratory tests for hypercoagulable conditions are time consuming, highly specialized, and it is unlikely to acquire results in the acute ED setting.
- A CBC with complete differential and coagulation studies should be ordered.
- Consider heparin-induced thrombocytopenia (HIT) in patients with a drop in platelet count >50% after 5 to 15 days of initiating heparin therapy.
- See Table 136-3 for the differential diagnosis of hypercoagulable states.

EMERGENCY DEPARTMENT CARE AND DISPOSITION

- Patients with new or worsening thrombosis should be started on low molecular weight or unfractionated heparin therapy, and hospital admission.
- In patients with HIT, heparin must be stopped. Another anticoagulant (lepirudin, argatroban, danaparoid) should be initiated in consultation with a hematologist.

For further reading in Tintinalli's *Emergency Medicine: A Comprehensive Study Guide*, 7th ed., see Chapter 228, "Acquired Bleeding Disorders," by Sally A. Santen and Rubin R. Hemphill, and Chapter 229, "Clotting Disorders, " by Jessie G. Nelson and Robin R. Hemphill.

137 HEMOPHILIAS AND VON WILLEBRAND'S DISEASE

Daniel A. Handel

HEMOPHILIA

EPIDEMIOLOGY

- Hemophilia A (factor VIII deficiency) occurs in about 1:10,000 male births.
- Hemophilia B, or Christmas disease, is a factor IX deficiency and occurs in 1:25,000 to 35,000 male births.

PATHOPHYSIOLOGY

- Hemophilia is an inherited disorder of a circulating coagulation protein. Hemophilia A and B are X-linked, recessive disorders, and therefore affect males almost exclusively.
- Deficiency or defect of the factor VIII or IX protein results in abnormal intrinsic coagulation pathway function.

CLINICAL FEATURES

- Patients with hemophilia are categorized as having mild (5-40% of normal factor function), moderate (1-5% of normal function), or severe (<1% of normal function) disease.
- Hemophilia is characterized by easy bruising and bleeding into the muscles and joints.
- The extent, severity, and frequency of bleeding are dependent on the severity of disease (mild, moderate, or severe).
- Trauma, surgical procedures, and spontaneous retroperitoneal or central nervous system bleeding may be life threatening. Traumatic bleeding may be delayed for several hours.
- Unless there is another underlying disease, patients with hemophilia do not have problems with minor cuts and abrasions.
- Compartment syndrome may result from extremity hematoma.

DIAGNOSIS AND DIFFERENTIAL

- Laboratory testing in patients with hemophilia most often shows a normal prothrombin time (PT), prolonged partial thromboplastin time (PTT), and normal bleeding time (BT).
- If more than 30% to 40% of factor activity is present, the PTT may be normal.
- Specific factor assays may be used to differentiate between the types of hemophilia.
- Approximately 10% to 25% of patients with hemophilia A and 1% to 2% of patients with hemophilia B will develop an inhibitor, which is an antibody against the deficient factor.
- An inhibitor is diagnosed by mixing the patient's plasma 50:50 with plasma of a normal control and finding that the mixture still has a prolonged PTT. The quantity of inhibitor is measured by the Bethesda inhibitor assay (BIA) and is reported in BIA units.

EMERGENCY DEPARTMENT CARE AND DISPOSITION

- For major or life-threatening bleeding, the mainstay of therapy is factor replacement (Table 137-1).
- The management of less severe bleeding depends on the severity of hemophilia, presence or absence of inhibitor, and site and severity of bleeding. Replacement guidelines can be found in Table 137-2.
- For severe bleeding the desired factor level is 80% to 100%. For less severe bleeding, the desired factor level is 30% to 50%.
- The amount of factor VIII (FVIII) required is determined by: (Target FVIII − Baseline FVIII)/2 × weight (kg).
- The amount of factor IX (FIX) required is determined by: (Target FIX − Baseline FIX) × weight (kg).
- If factor concentrate is unavailable, or if the type of hemophilia is unknown, fresh frozen plasma (FFP) should be administered. Each milliliter of FFP contains 1 unit of factor VIII. Volume constraints make complete replacement with FFP difficult.
- Desmopressin (DDAVP) may be used to raise factor VIII levels in patients with mild to moderate hemophilia A and no inhibitor.

VON WILLEBRAND'S DISEASE

EPIDEMIOLOGY

- Von Willebrand's disease (vWD) is the most common inherited bleeding disorder, occurring in 1% of the population. However, only 1 in 10,000 people manifests a clinically significant bleeding disorder.

PATHOPHYSIOLOGY

- Von Willebrand's factor (vWF) is a cofactor for platelet adhesion as well as a carrier protein for factor VIII, protecting factor VIII from proteolytic degradation.

TABLE 137-1 Replacement Factor Products for Hemophilia Treatment

HEMOPHILIA TYPE	AVAILABLE PRODUCTS*	COMMENTS
Hemophilia A	*Human plasma-derived Factor VIII products* Koate-HP® (gel chromatography, solvent, and detergent treated) Humate-P® (heat treated) Alphanate® (solvent and detergent treated)	All products have a low risk of HIV and hepatitis transmission.
	Human plasma-derived Factor VIII with immunoaffinity purification Hemofil-M® (monoclonal antibody purification, solvent and detergent treated) Monoclate-P® (monoclonal antibody purification, heat treated)	Both products have reduced amounts of von Willebrand factor. Highly purified source of Factor VIII.
	Recombinant Factor VIII products Recombinate® (recombinant DNA product) Helixate® (recombinant DNA product) Advate® (recombinant DNA product) Kogenate-FS® (recombinant DNA product) Xyntha® (recombinant DNA product)	All products have low to no risk of HIV and hepatitis transmission.
	Porcine Factor VIII product cryoprecipitate fractionation, screened for porcine viruses Hyate:C®	No evidence that human viral infection occurs.
Hemophilia B	*Factor IX complex products* Koyne-80® Factor IX complex (heat treated) Proplex-T® Factor IX complex (heat treated) Profilnine-SD® (solvent and detergent treated)	Thrombotic risk. Low risk of HIV and hepatitis transmission.
	Activated Factor IX complex products Autoplex-T® (heat treated)	Low risk of HIV and hepatitis transmission.
	Purified Factor IX products AlphaNine-SD® (purified, solvent, and detergent treated) Mononine® (monoclonal antibody purification, ultrafiltration)	Low to no transmissions of HIV or hepatitis reported.
	Recombinant Factor IX products BeneFIX® (recombinant DNA product)	No known risk of HIV or hepatitis transmission. Product of choice for patients with significant inhibitor activity.

Abbreviation: HIV = human immunodeficiency virus.
**Commercial trade names provided for ease of specific identification.*

TABLE 137-2 Initial Factor Replacement Guidelines in Severe Hemophilia

SITE	DESIRED INITIAL FACTOR LEVEL (%)	HEMOPHILIA A INITIAL DOSE (UNITS/KG)	HEMOPHILIA B INITIAL DOSE (UNITS/KG)	DETAILS
Skin (deep laceration)	—	—	—	Abrasions and superficial lacerations usually do not require factor replacement. Treat with pressure and topical thrombin.
Deep muscle	40-80	20-40	40-60	Admit, monitor total blood loss, watch for compartment syndrome. Duration of replacement: 1-5 d.
Joint (hemarthrosis)	30-50	15-25	30-40	Orthopedic consult may be required for splinting, physical therapy, and follow-up. Duration of replacement: 1-3 d.
Epistaxis	40-50	20-25	80-100	Local measures should be used. Replacement is given until bleeding resolves.
Oral mucosa	50	25	50	Local measures and antifibrinolytic therapy will decrease need for additional factor replacement.
Hematuria	50	25	50	Common and typically not severe. Rest and hydration are important.
GI bleeding	100	50	100	Consultation with a gastroenterologist for endoscopy to locate potential lesion is appropriate.
Central nervous system	100	50	100	Treat before CT. Early neurosurgical consultation. Lumbar puncture requires factor replacement.

- When exposed to the subendothelial matrix, vWF undergoes a structural change, allowing it to bind to glycoprotein Ib. This leads to platelet activation and adhesion to other platelets and to the damaged endothelium.

CLINICAL FEATURES

- There are three main types of vWD. Type I (70-80% of cases) is a mild form with bleeding episodes usually manifesting as epistaxis, easy bruising, menorrhagia, or dental bleeding. Type II is a qualitative disorder accounting for about 10% to 15% of cases.
- Type III is a severe form accounting for less than 10% of cases. These patients manifest with severe bleeding episodes that may resemble the hemophilias (hemarthrosis and hematomas).
- Unlike patients with hemophilia, patients with vWD often present with skin and mucosal bleeding. Hemarthrosis is not typical unless severe disease (type III) is present.
- In mild cases of vWD, the patient may not be aware of their disease until a traumatic episode or surgical procedure.

DIAGNOSIS AND DIFFERENTIAL

- In patients with vWD, the PT and PTT are usually normal. The BT is prolonged and vWF activity is low.
- Occasionally, the PT and factor VIII level may be abnormal, making it difficult to distinguish vWD from hemophilia A.

EMERGENCY DEPARTMENT CARE AND DISPOSITION

- For most patients with vWD, DDAVP is the mainstay of treatment.
- DDAVP works by stimulating endothelial cells to secrete stored vWF, and possibly by promoting hemostasis via additional endothelial effects.
- The dose of **DDAVP** is 0.3 microgram/kg IV or SC over 30 minutes every 12 to 24 hours for up to four doses. The dose of the concentrated intranasal form of **DDAVP** is one spray in one nostril (150 micrograms) for children over 5 years of age and one spray in each nostril (300 micrograms) for adolescents and adults.
- For type 1 patients who do not respond to DDAVP or for patients with type II or III disease, factor VIII concentrate that has a significant concentration of vWF is required.

- Cryoprecipitate also contains high concentrations of vWF and may be used to treat patients with vWD. There is, however, a greater risk of viral transmission.
- Platelet transfusions may benefit patients with certain types of vWD (type 3) who do not respond to plasma products.
- For women with vWD and menorrhagia, birth control pills may help increase the vWF levels and limit the menstrual bleeding.

For further reading in Tintinalli's *Emergency Medicine: A Comprehensive Study Guide, 7th ed.*, see Chapter 230, "Hemophilias and von Willebrand Disease," by William Manson, Robin R. Hemphill, and Christine L. Kempton.

138 SICKLE CELL DISEASE AND OTHER HEREDITARY HEMOLYTIC ANEMIAS

Jason B. Hack

- Hereditary hemolytic anemias occur when genetic abnormalities cause functional and conformational red blood cell (RBC) abnormalities resulting in increased endogenous removal.
- Most common types are from abnormal Hb structure (eg, sickle cell disease [SCD]) or abnormal Hb production (eg, the thalassemia).
- Anemia occurs when destruction outstrips production.
- Most patients are aware of their dyshemoglobinemia status.

SICKLE CELL DISEASE

CLINICAL FEATURES

- The most common complaints in SCD (homozygous, or trait) are pain, weakness, or infectious complaints.
- Physical examination findings include pale complexion, venous stasis changes, jaundice, hepatosplenomegaly, anemic cardiac flow murmurs, cardiomegaly, and high-output CHF.
- Painful vaso-occlusive crisis in the musculoskeletal system or in the abdomen are the most common presenting complaint in the ED (Table 138-1).
- Crisis results from sickled RBCs mechanically obstructing blood flow, causing ischemia, organ damage, and infarcts.

TABLE 138-1 Guidelines for the Assessment and Management of Acute Vaso-Occlusive Crisis

History	Duration and location of pain History of fever History of focal swelling or redness Precipitation factors for acute episode Medications taken for pain relief
Physical examination	Assess degree of pain Inspect sites of pain, looking for swelling, warmth, redness General: respiratory distress, pallor, hydration, jaundice, rash Vital signs: especially temperature, pulse oximetry Respiratory: chest wall, lung sounds Heart: cardiomegaly and systolic murmur common with chronic anemia Abdomen: tenderness, organomegaly
Ancillary tests	If moderate to severe pain, focal pathology is present, or pain is atypical for acute episode Complete blood count, leukocyte differential, reticulocyte count, urinalysis Chest radiograph, if signs of lower respiratory tract pathology Blood cultures and additional blood tests: as indicated by clinical condition
General management	Bed rest, provide warmth, and a calm, relaxing atmosphere Distractions where appropriate—television, music, etc. Oral fluids: typically about 3 L per day IV fluids to correct dehydration or if reluctant to drink or vomiting is present Oxygen: not routinely required, unless hypoxemia is present Encourage deep breathing, incentive spirometry
Pain management	Use analgesics appropriate to degree of pain Acetaminophen for mild pain NSAID for mild to moderate pain (avoid if renal insufficiency is present) Opioids for moderate to severe pain, typical initial doses include: Morphine, 0.3 milligram/kg PO or 0.1-0.15 milligram/kg IV Hydromorphone, 0.06-0.08 milligram/kg PO or 0.015-0.020 milligram/kg IV Reassess response in 15-30 min, may repeat with one-fourth to one-half initial dose
Disposition and follow-up	Consider admission to the hospital if: Acute chest syndrome is suspected Sepsis, osteomyelitis, or other serious infection is suspected White blood cell count is >30,000/mm^3 Platelet count is <100,000/mm^3 Pain is not under control after two to three rounds of analgesics in the ED Consider discharge if: Pain is under control and patient can take oral fluids and medications Ensure appropriate oral analgesics are available Provide home care instructions Ensure resource for follow-up

- Fever or infection (especially *Haemophilus influenza* or *Pneumococcus*), cold exposure or high altitude, dehydration or overexertion, medication noncompliance or drug use can provoke RBC sickling and crisis.
- Symptomatic anemia results from splenic sequestration or bone marrow failure (aplastic crisis) and presents with weakness, dyspnea, CHF, or shock.
- Life- or limb-threatening crisis include acute chest syndrome (vaso-occlusive pulmonary insult), stroke, renal infarct, mesenteric infarcts, sepsis, osteomyelitis, pneumonia, or priapism (Table 138-2).

DIAGNOSIS AND DIFFERENTIAL

- Workups should be individualized and the degree of illness guides the evaluation of an acute crisis.
- However, protean complaints (pain, weakness, fever) must include a search for a cryptic inciting events.
- Acute worsening anemia may suggest increased splenic sequestration if the reticulocyte count is elevated, or bone marrow failure if the reticulocyte count is depressed.
- Leukocytosis or increased bands suggest infection.
- Pregnancy tests should be obtained in all women of childbearing age.
- Assessment of electrolytes evaluates dehydration and renal function.
- Liver function tests and lipase may help evaluate abdominal pain.
- Febrile SCD patients without localizing symptoms should have blood cultures, urinalysis, and chest radiographs performed.
- Patients presenting with symptoms of acute chest syndrome (chest pain, cough, fever, dyspnea) are critically ill requiring immediate evaluation.
- Chest radiograph, ECG, and arterial blood gas help evaluate degree of hypoxia; type and cross for possible exchange transfusion.
- Radiographs of the skeleton are indicated for atypical focal bone pain.
- Advanced imaging for abdominal pain, or for neurologic manifestations should be considered.
- The differential diagnosis of potentially life-threatening inducers of crisis in SCD patients includes osteomyelitis, bony infarcts, cellulitis, acute arthritides, pancreatitis, hepatitis, cholecystitis, pelvic inflammatory disease, pyelonephritis, pneumonia, pulmonary embolus, and meningitis.

TABLE 138-2 Assessment and Treatment of Acute Chest Syndrome

History	Major presenting symptom: dyspnea, fever, cough Accompanying chest, rib, bone, or joint pain Assess degree or severity of pain Recent or previous sepsis, infection, pneumonia, or hospitalization Prior history of acute chest syndrome, especially if required intubation and ventilatory support Potentially infectious contacts Current medications Immunization history: especially pneumococcal and *Haemophilus influenzae* type b Baseline hemoglobin level and arterial oxygenation saturation
Physical examination	General: respiratory distress, pallor, hydration, jaundice, rash Vital signs: especially temperature, pulse oximetry Respiratory: chest wall, lung sounds Heart: cardiomegaly and systolic murmur common with chronic anemia Abdomen: tenderness, organomegaly
Ancillary tests	Complete blood count, leukocyte differential, reticulocyte count, urinalysis Cross-match sample: if red blood cell transfusion is contemplated Arterial blood gas: if moderate to severe respiratory distress and/or hypoxemia on pulse oximetry Chest radiography Blood cultures Additional blood tests: as indicated by clinical condition
Treatment	Oxygen: adjust according to pulse oximetry Oral hydration: preferable IV hydration: use hypotonic fluids, use a rate and dose at approximately 1.5 of maintenance (over aggressive IV fluids can worsen acute chest syndrome) Analgesics: if needed, generally potent parenteral opioids are used, monitor for signs of respiratory suppression Antibiotics: empiric antibiotics recommended to treat community-acquired pneumonia Bronchodilators: nebulized β_2-adrenergic agonists Chest physiotherapy Transfusion: use if severe acute anemia is present
Exchange transfusion	Consider when Severe acute chest syndrome on admission and past history of requiring ventilatory support: useful to prevent intubation Deterioration despite above management: useful to prevent intensive care unit admission Patient already intubated and on ventilatory support: useful to shorten duration of ventilatory need Suspected or confirmed fat or bone marrow embolism

EMERGENCY DEPARTMENT TREATMENT AND DISPOSITION

- Initial interventions for acute crisis in SCD patients are primarily supportive.
- Judicious pain management and a thorough assessment for the inciting events are required.
- **Opioid pain medications** are often required for severe pain. Individualized **treatment plans** are warranted for patients with frequent crises.

- Oral **rehydration** should be encouraged for suspected dehydration. IV crystalloid may be used at 1.5 times maintenance.
- Supplemental **oxygen** is indicated for hypoxia.
- **ECG** and **cardiac monitoring** is appropriate for patients with cardiopulmonary symptoms.
- **Cultures** should be obtained and **broad-spectrum antibiotics** administered for patient with symptoms of acute infection.
- **Exchange transfusion** should be considered in specific circumstances—aplastic crisis, cardiopulmonary decompensation, pregnancy, stroke, respiratory failure, general surgery, and priapism (requires urologic consultation).
- **Admission** criteria include pulmonary, neurologic, aplastic, or infectious crises; splenic sequestration; intractable pain; persistent nausea and vomiting; or an uncertain diagnosis.
- Arrange close follow-up for patients who are discharged. Give instructions to return immediately for temperature above 38°C or worsening symptoms.

VARIANTS OF SICKLE CELL DISEASE

- Other hemoglobinopathies exist and vary in presentation, asymptomatic to SCD-like depending upon the specific abnormality and whether homozygous, heterozygous, or combined with sickle-cell trait.

THALASSEMIAS

- Thalassemias are hereditary disorders caused by defective synthesis of globin chains, resulting in microcytic, hypochromic, hemolytic anemia.
- The degree of illness depends upon the type and number of genetic abnormalities.
- Patients with β-thalassemia minor have mild microcytic anemia and are generally asymptomatic.
- Patients with β-thalassemia major (Cooley's anemia), develop hepatosplenomegaly, jaundice, and bony changes, are at risk for infection and severe anemia requiring blood transfusions.
- Iron overload from transfusions can occur.

GLUCOSE-6-PHOSPHATE DEHYDROGENASE DEFICIENCY

- Glucose-6-phosphate dehydrogenase (G6PD) deficiency is the most common enzymopathy of RBCs.
- This causes Hb precipitation, RBC removal by the spleen and hemolysis.
- Most patients are asymptomatic.
- Exposure to an oxidative stress (eg, medication, infection, fava beans) causes hemolysis.
- Evaluation includes a complete blood count and reticulocyte count, bilirubin levels, serum aminotransferases, and lactate dehydrogenase.
- Treatment includes early treatment of infection if detected and blood transfusion for severe anemia.

HEREDITARY SPHEROCYTOSIS

- Hereditary spherocytosis results from an erythrocyte membrane defect creating small stiff RBCs, which result in increased rate of destruction by the spleen and a compensatory increase in RBC production.
- Complications include aplastic or megaloblastic crises, cholecystitis or cholelithiasis, splenomegaly and hemolysis with jaundice.
- Treatment includes blood transfusions and splenectomy in severe cases.

For further reading in Tintinalli's *Emergency Medicine: A Comprehensive Study Guide*, 6th ed., see Chapter 231, "Sickle Cell Disease and Other Hereditary Hemolytic Anemias," by Jean Williams-Johnson and Eric Williams.

139 TRANSFUSION THERAPY

T. Paul Tran

EPIDEMIOLOGY

- Approximately 12 million packed red blood cells (PRBCs) are transfused in the United States each year. This number changes over time, reflecting the broader trends in US patient population, aging, practice guidelines, and perceived safety of blood products.

PATHOPHYSIOLOGY

- The two common goals in transfusion therapy are volume expansion and improved oxygen-carrying capacity.
- In shock, volume expansion takes priority over oxygen-carrying capacity.
- Less common goals in transfusion therapy include correction of bleeding diathesis via replacement of clotting factors or platelet.

WHOLE BLOOD

- The total blood volume of a 70-kg adult is approximately 75 mL/kg or 2.5 L/m² (5 L). A unit of whole blood contains 500 mL of blood.
- Although whole blood is the ideal blood product in acute hemorrhage, it is seldom performed in modern hospitals. The two main goals in transfusion, volume expansion and improved oxygen-carrying capacity, can be achieved more efficiently by using individual blood components.

PACKED RED BLOOD CELLS

- PRBCs are used primarily to increase oxygen-carrying capacity.
- One unit of PRBCs has a volume of 250 mL and raises the hemoglobin by 1 gram/dL (adult), or the hematocrit by 3%. One PRBC is usually transfused over 1 to 2 hours, but can be transfused faster if patient is in shock.
- Major indications for PRBC transfusion include (1) acute blood loss greater than 25% to 30% blood volume (1500 mL) in otherwise healthy adults and (2) acute blood loss greater than 2 L in surgical patients. Crystalloid is usually infused concurrently with PRBC to achieve volume expansion.
- Transfusion with PRBCs is also indicated in patients with chronic anemia (ie, slow blood loss conditions) and are symptomatic and in patients with underlying cardiopulmonary disease and hemoglobin levels less than 6 grams/dL.
- A "type and screen" (involving ABO and Rh blood group typing, antibody screen) can be performed in about 30 minutes. Type and screen should be ordered if the anticipated likelihood of a transfusion is low (<1%).
- A "type and cross" (ABO/Rh blood typing, antibody screen, patient's blood, and donor blood are tested for compatibility) can be performed in approximately 1 hour. Type and cross should be ordered if the anticipated likelihood of a transfusion is high (>10%).
- RBCs are available as leukocyte poor, frozen, or washed. Leukocyte-poor RBCs have up to 85% of the leukocytes removed and are indicated for transplant recipients or candidates, and for patients with a history of febrile nonhemolytic transfusion reactions.
- Frozen RBCs are saved rare blood types and have reduced antigen loads. They are used in patients who are at risks for alloimmunization.
- Washed RBCs are for patients who have hypersensitive reactions to plasma, for neonatal transfusions, and for those with paroxysmal nocturnal hemoglobinuria.

PLATELETS

- Thrombocytopenia is a risk factor for spontaneous hemorrhage and transfusion of platelet is indicated for thrombocytopenic patients who are actively bleeding or at risk for significant bleeding (eg, intracranial bleeding).
- Spontaneous bleeding is rare for platelet counts >50,000/μL, but significantly increased for platelet counts <10,000/μL. Prophylactic platelet transfusion is indicated for platelet counts <10,000/μL.
- One unit of platelet contains 3 to 6 × 10^{11} platelets in a volume of 250 to 350 mL. It can raise the platelet count by 5000 to 10,000/μL.
- Dosing is usually 1 unit/10 kg (approximately 6 units for an adult). ABO- and Rh-compatible platelets are preferable.
- Transfused platelets survive 3 to 5 days. The platelet count should be checked 1 and 24 hours after infusion.
- Major indications for prophylactic platelet transfusions include (1) an absolute platelet count <10,000/μL, (2) active bleeding with platelet counts between 10,000 and 50,000/μL, (3) patients with platelet counts <50,000/μL who are undergoing invasive procedures (eg, thoracentesis, paracentesis).

FRESH FROZEN PLASMA

- Fresh frozen plasma (FFP) is indicated in (1) patients who are bleeding or at risk for significant bleeding from an acquired coagulopathy condition (eg, massive transfusion or antithrombotic intoxication), (2) patients who have an acquired coagulopathy condition and are undergoing an invasive procedure, (3) patients who have thrombotic thrombocytopenic purpura (TTP) and are undergoing plasma exchange, (4) patients who have antithrombin III deficiency but antithrombin III concentrate is not available, and (5) patients who have congenital isolated factor deficiencies but specific virally safe products are not available.
- Coagulopathy is defined as prolongation of prothrombin time (PT) or partial thromboplastin time (PTT) 1.5 times of standards, or a coagulation factor assay <25% of normal.
- One bag of FFP contains 200 to 250 mL, 1 U/mL of each coagulation factor, and 1 to 2 milligrams/mL of fibrinogen. Typical starting dose is 8 to 10 mL/kg, or two to four bags. One unit of FFP will increase most coagulation factors by 3% to 5%.
- FFP should be ABO compatible.

CRYOPRECIPITATE

- Cryoprecipitate is derived from FFP; one bag contains 80 to 100 U factor VIIIC, 80 U von Willebrand's factor, 200 to 300 milligrams fibrinogen, 40 to 60 U factor XIII, and variable amounts of fibronectin.
- The usual dose is two to four bags per 10-kg body weight (limit to 20 bags for a typical adult); ABO compatible bags are preferable.
- Indications for cryoprecipitate therapy include (1) fibrinogen level less than 100 milligrams/dL, in association with disseminated intravascular coagulation or congenital fibrinogen deficiency; (2) von Willebrand's disease with active bleeding when desmopressin is not effective or factor VIII concentrate containing von Willebrand's factor is not available; (3) hemophilia A when virally inactivated factor VIII concentrates are not available; (4) use as fibrin glue surgical adhesives; and (5) fibronectin replacement.

INTRAVENOUS IMMUNOGLOBULINS

- Indications for intravenous immunoglobulins include the treatment of primary and secondary immunodeficiency and treatment of immune or inflammatory disorders, such as immune thrombocytopenia and Kawasaki's syndrome.
- Adverse reactions include anaphylaxis, febrile reactions, headache, and renal failure.
- There have been some documented cases of patients developing a positive serology to hepatitis C after intravenous immunoglobulin therapy.

ANTITHROMBIN III

- Antithrombin III (ATIII) is a serum protein that inhibits coagulation factors, thrombin, and activated factors IX, X, XI, and XII.
- Deficiency can be congenital or acquired.
- ATIII is mainly used for prophylaxis of thrombosis or to treat thromboembolism in patients with hereditary ATIII deficiency.

SPECIFIC FACTOR REPLACEMENT THERAPY

- Table 139-1 outlines therapy for congenital coagulation factor deficiencies.

COMPLICATIONS OF TRANSFUSIONS

- Adverse reactions occur in up to 20% of transfusions and are usually mild.

TABLE 139-1 Replacement Therapy for Congenital Factor Deficiencies

COAGULATION FACTOR	ANNUAL INCIDENCE	REPLACEMENT THERAPY
Factor I (fibrinogen)	Rare (1-2/million)	Whole blood, FFP, cryoprecipitate, fibrinogen concentrates
Factor II (prothrombin)	Rare (1-2/million)	FFP, factor II concentrate, prothrombin complex concentrate
Factor V (proaccelerin, labile factor)	Rare (1/million)	Whole blood, FFP
Factor VII (proconvertin, stable factor)	Rare (0.5/million)	FFP, prothrombin complex concentrate, purified factor VIIa, recombinant factor VIIa
Factor VIII (antihemophilic factor A, antihemophilic globulin, "classic hemophilia")	1-2/10,000 male births	Factor VIII concentrates (cryoprecipitate or FFP if not available); DDAVP for mild hemophilia
von Willebrand's disease	Up to 1 in 100 persons	DDAVP for mild von Willebrand's disease (except types 2B or 3); factor VIII concentrates (Alphanate, Humate-P); cryoprecipitate
Factor IX (antihemophilic factor B, plasma thromboplastin component, Christmas factor)	1/30,000 male births	Factor IX concentrates
Factor X (Stuart–Prower factor)	Rare (1-2/million)	Whole blood, FFP, factor X concentrate, prothrombin complex concentrate
Factor XI (plasma thromboplastin antecedent, hemophilia C, Rosenthal syndrome)	1/10,000 in Ashkenazi Jews; 1/100,000 in general population	FFP, cryoprecipitate, factor XI concentrate
Factor XII (Hageman factor)	Rare (1/million)	Replacement not required
Factor XIII (fibrin stabilizing factor, Laki–Lorand factor)	Rare (1/5 million)	FFP, cryoprecipitate, factor X concentrate

Abbreviations: DDAVP = desmopressin, FFP = fresh frozen plasma.

TABLE 139-2 Selected Acute Transfusion Reactions: Recognition, Management, and Evaluation

REACTION TYPE	SIGNS AND SYMPTOMS	EVALUATION	MANAGEMENT
Febrile nonhemolytic transfusion reactions (FNHTR)	Mild fever (<1.5°C rise), chills, urticaria	Can restart infusion at slower rate and observe closely after ascertaining that a hemolytic reaction AIHR is not occurring Can be difficult to initially distinguish FNHTR from AIHR Consider possibility of bacterial infection	Stop transfusion, check temperature, HR, BP, RR, O_2 saturation, verify patient ID; administer acetaminophen for fever, antihistamine for mild urticaria Usually mild but can be life threatening in patients with tenuous cardiopulmonary status
Acute intravascular hemolytic reaction (AIHR) vs bacterial infection	Fever, back pain, hematuria (hemoglobinuria), chills, sense of "doom," flushing, dyspnea, tachycardia, shock, renal failure, syncope, DIC Transfusion of blood contaminated with bacteria tends to precipitate a severe acute reaction with rapid onset of hyper- or hypotension, rigors, and cardiovascular collapse	Stop transfusion, start IV hydration to maintain diuresis; give diuretics if anuria or oliguria (<100 mL/h), take blood cultures, start broad-spectrum antibiotics if suspicious bacterial infection, treat DIC Start cardiorespiratory support (airway, BP support with fluid, pressors) as indicated	Save the blood unit, notify blood bank, retype and crossmatch, direct and indirect Coombs tests, CBC, creatinine, PT, aPTT, haptoglobin, indirect bilirubin, LDH, plasma-free hemoglobin, UA Examination of the blood (discoloration, odor, Gram stain) may rapidly confirm the diagnosis of bacteria-contaminated blood. Etiologic agents include *Staphylococcus epidermidis, Staphylococcus aureus, Bacillus cereus,* group B streptococci, *Escherichia coli, Pseudomonas* species, and other gram-negative organisms
Allergic reaction/ anaphylaxis	Rapid onset, urticarial rash, pruritus, dyspnea, nausea, vomiting, syncope, headache, bronchospasm, angioedema, abdominal pain, hypotension	For mild symptoms that resolve with antihistamines, no further workup is necessary; blood bank should be notified For severe allergic reaction or anaphylaxis, stabilize and admit patients to ICU, notify blood bank	Stop transfusion and assess patient. If allergic reaction is mild, can treat with antihistamines; if symptoms resolve, can restart transfusion If allergic reaction severe, start cardiopulmonary support and treatment as in anaphylaxis (airway and ventilatory support, volume expansion with crystalloid, epinephrine, antihistamines, β-agonist nebulized treatment, steroid)
Fluid overload	Dyspnea, tachycardia, hypertension, headache, jugular venous distention, pulmonary rales, hypoxia, hypotension if volume overload severe	Stop transfusion (or decrease rate to 1 mL/kg/h if very mild symptoms), start diuretics (furosemide)	Perform EKG, chest radiograph, monitor CVP, urine output, blood gas
Transfusion-related acute lung injury (TRALI)	Dyspnea, nonproductive cough, acute respiratory distress syndrome (ARDS), hypotension, fever/chills, monocytopenia/neutropenia	Chest radiograph (bilateral nodular infiltrates, batwing pattern)	Stop transfusion, consult hematology, treat as ARDS
Massive transfusion	Bleeding, hypothermia, citrate toxicity, hypocalcaemia, or hypomagnesaemia	Warm all blood and fluid used in massive transfusion; monitor temperature, coagulation parameters, acid-base balance, serum potassium and calcium	Whole blood, FFP, cryoprecipitate, and platelet transfusion as clinically indicated; blood warmers for hypothermia, replacement therapy for symptomatic hypocalcaemia or hypomagnesaemia

Abbreviations: aPTT = activated partial thromboplastin time, CBC = complete blood count, CXR = chest radiograph, IV = intravenous, LDH = lactate dehydrogenase, PT = prothrombin time.

- Transfusion reactions can be immediate or delayed.
- Table 139-2 summarizes the types of immediate reactions as well as methods of recognition, management, and evaluation.

DELAYED TRANSFUSION REACTIONS

- Delayed hemolytic reactions can occur 7 to 10 days after transfusion.
- Infection may result from transfusion. There is a small risk of transmission of HIV, hepatitis B and C, cytomegalovirus, parvovirus, and human T-cell lymphotropic viruses I and II.
- Other rare but reported pathogens include Epstein-Barr virus, syphilis, malaria, babesiosis, toxoplasmosis, and trypanosomiasis.
- Hypothermia may occur from rapid transfusions of refrigerated blood.

- Noncardiogenic pulmonary edema may be caused by incompatible passively transferred leukocyte antibodies, and usually occurs within 4 hours of transfusion.
- Clinical findings of noncardiogenic pulmonary edema are respiratory distress, fever, chills, tachycardia, and patchy infiltrates on chest radiograph without cardiomegaly. There is no evidence of fluid overload.
- Electrolyte imbalance may occur. Citrate is part of the preservative solution and chelates calcium. Significant hypocalcemia even with massive transfusion is rare because patients with normal hepatic function readily metabolize citrate into bicarbonate.
- Hypokalemia can occur with large transfusions due to the metabolism of citrate to bicarbonate, leading to alkalosis, which drives potassium ions into the intracellular space.
- Hyperkalemia can occur in patients with renal failure or in neonates.
- Graft-versus-host disease, fatal in greater than 90% of cases, occurs when nonirradiated lymphocytes are inadvertently transfused into an immunocompromised patient.
- Table 139-3 summarizes the types of delayed transfusion reactions as well as methods of recognition, management, and evaluation.

EMERGENCY TRANSFUSIONS

- Use of type O or type-specific incompletely crossmatched blood may be life-saving but carries the risk of life-threatening transfusion reactions. Its use should be limited to the early resuscitation of patients with severe hemorrhage without adequate response to crystalloid infusion.
- Before transfusing, blood should be obtained for baseline laboratory tests and type and crossmatching. Rh-negative blood is preferable if it is not fully crossmatched.

MASSIVE TRANSFUSION

- Massive transfusion is the approximate replacement of a patient's total blood volume within a 24-hour period.
- Complications include bleeding, citrate toxicity, and hypothermia.
- Bleeding may result from thrombocytopenia, platelet dysfunction, disseminated intravascular coagulation, or coagulation factor deficiencies.
- Patients receiving more than 5 U of whole blood, those with liver disease, and neonates are at risk for hypocalcemia from citrate toxicity.
- The QT interval is not a reliable indicator in this setting; an ionized calcium level is the preferred tool to assess possible symptomatic hypocalcemia.
- Hypocalcemia should be treated with 5 to 10 mL of IV calcium gluconate infused slowly.
- Physicians should be aware of the possibility of hypothermia when administering 3 U or more of blood rapidly.

TABLE 139-3 Delayed Transfusion Complications

REACTION TYPE	SIGNS AND SYMPTOMS	EVALUATION	MANAGEMENT
Delayed hemolytic transfusion reaction	Hemolytic reaction occurring 4-8 days after transfusion; falling hemoglobin concentration, jaundice, fever, hemoglobinuria/renal failure (rare)	CBC, LDH, direct Coombs' test, renal panel, serum bilirubin, haptoglobin, urinalysis	Notify blood bank, retype and cross using pre- and post-transfusion samples; specific treatment generally is not necessary
Transfusion associated graft vs. host disease	Rash, fever, diarrhea, weakness, prostration 3-4 weeks after transfusion	Clinical suspicion and evaluation. This rare complication occurs when nonirradiated lymphocytes are inadvertently transfused into an immunocompromised patient	Fatal in more than 90% of cases; notify blood bank and get hematology consultation
Post-transfusion purpura	Bleeding, purpura 1-8 weeks after transfusion	Thrombocytopenia; this rare complication occurs when patient's alloantibody against platelet antigens in transfused blood causes destruction of own antigen-negative platelets	Plasma exchange; emergent platelet transfusion only if active bleeding; notify blood bank and get hematology consultation
Infectious disease transmission	Insidious symptoms of an infection	Risks of infectious disease transmission are low, the following only serves as rough estimates: 1:1,000,000 for hepatitis A, 1:30,000-250,000 for hepatitis B, 1:30,000 -150,000 for hepatitis C; 1:200,000-2,000,000 for HIV	Infectious disease and hematology consultation

BLOOD ADMINISTRATION

- The correct identification of the patient and the unit to be transfused should always be ensured.
- An 18-gauge or larger IV catheter is preferred to prevent hemolysis and to permit rapid infusion. Micropore filters should be used to filter out microaggregates of platelets, fibrin, and leukocytes.
- Normal saline solution is the only crystalloid compatible with PRBCs. Warmed saline solution (39°C-43°C or 102.2°F-109.4°F) may be given concurrently or a blood warmer used to prevent hypothermia. Blood will hemolyze if warmed to greater than 40°C (104°F).
- Rapid transfusion may be facilitated by the use of pressure infusion devices.
- Patients at risk for hypervolemia should receive each unit over 3 to 4 hours.

For further reading in *Tintinalli's Emergency Medicine: A Comprehensive Study Guide*, 7th ed., see Chapter 233, "Transfusion Therapy," by Clinton J. Coil and Sally A. Santen.

140 ANTICOAGULANTS, ANTIPLATELET AGENTS, AND FIBRINOLYTICS

Jessica L. Smith

ANTITHROMBOTIC AGENTS

ORAL ANTICOAGULANTS

- Oral anticoagulants inhibit acute thrombus formation and propagation, and also reduce the risk of embolism from an existing thrombus.
- Warfarin inhibits synthesis of vitamin K–dependent clotting factors and antithrombotic proteins C and S. Dosing is guided by the international normalized ratio (INR), which is derived from the prothrombin time (PT).
- The therapeutic range of INR is between 2 and 3. Mechanical heart valves require an INR of 2.5 to 3.5.
- Drug interactions, certain foods, and certain disease states interfere with warfarin absorption or metabolism, which may be clinically significant.
- Warfarin is contraindicated in pregnancy secondary to teratogenicity.
- Full anticoagulation occurs about 3 to 4 days after initiating therapy.
- During the first 24 to 36 hours, a transient hypercoagulable state occurs; therefore, a parenteral anticoagulant should be used until an adequate INR is achieved for 2 days.
- Dabigatran is the only available oral direct thrombin inhibitor in the United States. It requires no monitoring, no reversal agent is available, and long-term safety has not been established.

PARENTERAL ANTICOAGULANTS

- Unfractionated heparin (UFH) inhibits multiple steps in the coagulation cascade.
- An IV bolus of 60 to 80 U/kg is followed by IV infusion at 12 to 18 U/kg/h.
- Dosing is guided by the partial thromboplastin time (PTT); the desired therapeutic range is 1.5 to 2.5 times the normal value.
- Low-molecular-weight heparins (LMWH) (enoxaparin, dalteparin, and ardeparin) are derivatives of heparin.
- Advantages of LMWH over UFH include longer half-life and decreased binding to plasma proteins, endothelial cells, and macrophages.
- LMWH is a much more predictable anticoagulant with fixed dose-response relationships. LMWH (eg, lovenox 1 milligram/kg every 12 hours) can be administered subcutaneously (SC) once to twice daily, and does not require monitoring, except in patients with renal failure and obesity.
- LMWH may be used safely in pregnancy.
- UFH or LMWH is indicated for deep venous thrombosis (DVT) prophylaxis and treatment, pulmonary embolism (PE), unstable angina, and acute myocardial infarction (AMI).
- Only enoxaparin is approved for outpatient management of DVT.

DIRECT THROMBIN INHIBITORS (BIVALIRUDIN, LEPIRUDIN, ARGATROBAN)

- Hirudin, a protein derived from leeches, is now prepared using recombinant technology.
- Hirudin and its analogues inhibit both circulating and clot-bound thrombin.
- These are currently approved for use in patients with heparin-induced thrombocytopenia and as anticoagulants during percutaneous coronary intervention.

ANTIPLATELET AGENTS

- Aspirin is an irreversible inhibitor of cyclooxygenase, an enzyme that inhibits platelet aggregation.
- The recommended antiplatelet dose is usually 81 to 162 milligrams daily.
- Side effects of aspirin are usually gastrointestinal (GI); active GI bleeding is a contraindication. Patients with

guaiac-positive stool and no active bleeding can be treated and carefully monitored.

- Nonsteroidal anti-inflammatory drugs (NSAIDs) reversibly inhibit cyclooxygenase; platelet inhibition usually lasts less than 24 hours.
- **Ticlopidine** 250 milligrams PO twice daily and clopidogrel 75 milligrams PO daily inhibit platelet aggregation.
- These agents should be used for acute coronary syndromes in patients who cannot take aspirin.
- Glycoprotein IIb/IIIa inhibitors (abciximab, eptifibatide, and tirofiban) inhibit platelet aggregation, prevent thrombosis, and may augment fibrinolysis.
- These agents can improve outcomes in select patients with unstable angina and non–ST elevation MI; they should be used in consultation with an interventional cardiologist.

FIBRINOLYTIC AGENTS

- Fibrinolytic agents convert plasminogen to plasmin, which dissolves the fibrin in a thrombus.
- Streptokinase (SK) and anistreplase (APSAC) are antigenic, and treatment should not occur within 6 months of prior therapy, or 12 months of streptococcal infection.
- Tissue plasminogen activator (tPA) is theoretically more "clot specific" than SK or APSAC.
- Reteplase and tenecteplase are modified tPA, designed to improve efficacy and safety.
- Although the side effect profiles of fibrinolytics are similar, bolus-dosing (APSAC, reteplase, and tenecteplase) results in significantly fewer medication errors.

INDICATIONS FOR ANTITHROMBOTIC THERAPY

ACUTE MYOCARDIAL INFARCTION

- If angioplasty within 90 minutes of arrival to the emergency department is unavailable, fibrinolytic therapy should be initiated within 30 minutes. In the absence of contraindications (Table 140-1), use fibrinolytics if the patient is within 12 hours of symptom onset, and has either ST-segment elevation in two or more contiguous leads or new-onset left bundle-branch block.
- Angioplasty is preferred in patients with cardiogenic shock.
- Timely initiation of therapy is more important than the specific agent utilized.
- Aspirin should be administered immediately. In patients with aspirin allergy, clopidogrel or ticlopidine should be used instead.

TABLE 140-1 General Contraindications to Fibrinolytic Therapy

Absolute
Active or recent (<14 d) internal bleeding
Ischemic stroke* within the past 2-6 mo
Any prior hemorrhagic stroke
Intracranial or intraspinal surgery or trauma within the past 2 mo
Intracranial or intraspinal neoplasm, aneurysm, or arteriovenous malformation
Known severe bleeding diathesis
Current anticoagulant treatment (eg, warfarin with INR >1.7 or heparin with increased aPTT)
Uncontrolled hypertension (ie, blood pressure >185/100 mm Hg)
Suspected aortic dissection or pericarditis
Pregnancy
Relative†
Active peptic ulcer disease
Cardiopulmonary resuscitation for longer than 10 min
Hemorrhagic ophthalmic conditions
Puncture of noncompressible vessel within the past 10 d
Advanced age >75 y old
Significant trauma or major surgery within the past 2 wk to 2 mo
Advanced renal or hepatic disease

aPTT = activated partial thromboplastin time, INR = international normalized ratio.

*For ischemic stroke, additional contraindications include symptoms greater than 3 hours, severe hemispheric stroke, platelets below 100/mL, and glucose below 50 or above 400 milligrams/dL.

†Concurrent menses is not a contraindication

PULMONARY EMBOLISM OR DEEP VENOUS THROMBOSIS

- Treatment of PE or DVT can be initiated with either UFH or LMWH.
- LMWH is as effective as UFH, with fewer side effects, and allows for outpatient management of select patients.
- Select patients may benefit from fibrinolytic therapy.

ISCHEMIC STROKE

- tPA may benefit select stroke patients if administered within 3 hours of symptom onset; there is an increased risk of conversion to hemorrhagic stroke.
- Fibrinolytic agents should not be given to patients with uncontrolled hypertension, signs of hemorrhagic stroke, rapidly improving symptoms, or patients with contraindications.

COMPLICATIONS OF ANTICOAGULATION AND ANTITHROMBOTIC THERAPY

- Emergency treatments of bleeding complications of antithrombotic therapy are listed in Table 140-2.

TABLE 140-2 Emergency Treatment of Bleeding Complications of Antithrombotic Therapy

AGENT	MANAGEMENT
Heparin	
Minor bleeding	Immediate cessation of heparin administration. Supratherapeutic aPTT not always present. Anticoagulation effect lasts up to 3 h from last IV dose. Observation with serial aPTT may be sufficient.
Major bleeding	Protamine, 1 milligram/100 units of total amount of IV administered within the past 3 h. Protamine is given slowly IV over 1-3 min to a maximum of 50 milligrams over any 10-min period. Protamine has an anaphylaxis risk. Protamine does not completely reverse low-molecular-weight heparin. Enoxaparin: Protamine 1 milligram IV for every 1 milligram of enoxaparin given in the previous 8 h. If 8-12 h since last enoxaparin dose, give protamine 0.5 milligram IV for every 1 milligram of enoxaparin given. Dalteparin and tinzaparin: Protamine 1 milligram IV per every 100 international units of dalteparin or tinzaparin given. If aPTT (measured 2-4 h after the protamine infusion) remains prolonged, a second dose of protamine 0.5 milligram IV per 100 international units or dalteparin or tinzaparin.
Antiplatelet agents	
Aspirin	Cessation of aspirin administration. Platelet transfusion to increase count by 50,000/mm^3 (typically requires at least 6 units of random donor platelets). Aspirin-induced platelet inhibition may last for 7 d, so repeat platelet transfusions are sometimes required.
Other antiplatelet agents	Platelet transfusion to increase count by 50,000/mm^3 (typically requires at least 6 units of random donor platelets) NSAID-induced platelet inhibition typically lasts <1 d. Clopidogrel-induced platelet inhibition may last up to 7 d.
Fibrinolytics	
Minor external bleeding	Manual pressure
Significant internal bleeding	Immediate cessation of fibrinolytic agent, antiplatelet agent, and/or heparin. Reversal of heparin with protamine as above. Typed and cross-matched blood ordered with verification of aPTT, complete blood count, thrombin clotting time, and fibrinogen level. Volume replacement with crystalloid and packed red blood cells as needed.
Major bleeding or hemodynamic compromise	All measures listed for significant internal bleeding. Cryoprecipitate, 10 units IV, and recheck fibrinogen level; if fibrinogen level <100 milligrams/dL, repeat cryoprecipitate. If bleeding persists after cryoprecipitate or despite fibrinogen level >100 milligrams/dL, administer FFP, 2 units IV. If bleeding continues after FFP, administer an antifibrinolytic such as ε-aminocaproic acid, 5 grams IV over 60 min followed by 1 gram/h continuous IV infusion for 8 h or until bleeding stops, or tranexamic acid, 10 milligrams/kg IV every 6-8 h. Consider transfusion of 10 units of random donor platelets.
Intracranial hemorrhage	All measures listed for significant internal and major bleeding with hemodynamic compromise. Immediate neurosurgery consultation.

Abbreviations: aPTT = activated partial thromboplastin time; FFP = fresh frozen plasma.

For further reading in Tintinalli's *Emergency Medicine: A Comprehensive Study Guide*, 7th ed., see Chapter 234, "Anticoagulants, Antiplatelet Agents, and Fibrinolytics," by David E. Slattery and Charles V. Pollack, Jr.

141 EMERGENCY COMPLICATIONS OF MALIGNANCY

Ross J. Fleischman

BONE METASTASES AND PATHOLOGIC FRACTURES

EPIDEMIOLOGY

- Breast, lung, and prostate cancers are the most common causes of bony metastases, which may cause pain, pathologic fractures, and spinal cord compression.

CLINICAL FEATURES AND DIAGNOSIS

- Approximately 90% of patients with malignant spinal cord compression will have back pain.

- Patients with spinal cord compression may also exhibit muscular weakness, radicular pain, and bowel or bladder dysfunction (late findings).
- Obtain plain radiographs to assess for fractures or bony involvement. Plain radiographs may show a moth-eaten appearance, periosteal reaction, or poorly demarcated areas of increased density (osteoblastic activity).
- Follow with CAT scan or magnetic resonance imaging (MRI) scan to further delineate lesions.

EMERGENCY DEPARTMENT CARE AND DISPOSITION

- Treat pain with opioid analgesics.
- Most pathologic fractures require surgical intervention.
- Painful bone metastases are treated with radiotherapy.

SPINAL CORD COMPRESSION

EPIDEMIOLOGY

- Up to one in five patients with vertebral metastases and 3% to 6% of all cancer patients will develop spinal cord compression.
- The thoracic spine is involved in 70% of cases.

PATHOPHYSIOLOGY

- Neurologic symptoms occur when the spinal cord or nerve roots are compressed or directly infiltrated by tumor.

CLINICAL FEATURES

- Back pain is progressive and usually worse when supine.
- Proximal motor weakness usually occurs before sensory changes because of compression of the anterior portion of the cord from the vertebral bodies.
- Intrinsic involvement of the spinal cord usually presents with unilateral weakness.
- Sensory changes (hyperesthesia or anesthesia) and bladder or bowel retention or incontinence are late findings.
- Physical examination may reveal vertebral percussion tenderness, decreased rectal tone, saddle anesthesia, lower extremity hyporeflexia, and absent anal "wink."

DIAGNOSIS AND DIFFERENTIAL

- Plain radiographs or CT scan can identify vertebral involvement, but should be followed by a gadolinium-enhanced MRI scan of the whole spine.

EMERGENCY DEPARTMENT CARE AND DISPOSITION

- Consider administering **dexamethasone** 10 milligrams IV followed by 4 milligrams IV or PO every 6 hours if imaging will be delayed.
- **Emergent radiation therapy** is generally the first-line treatment.
- **Surgery** may be necessary for rapidly progressive symptoms, unstable vertebral column, and overall status and prognosis compatible with surgery.

AIRWAY OBSTRUCTION

PATHOPHYSIOLOGY

- Patients with respiratory tract tumors may experience acute airway compromise due to edema, bleeding, infection, or loss of protective mechanisms.

CLINICAL FEATURES

- Presenting symptoms and signs include dyspnea, tachypnea, wheezing, and stridor (an ominous sign).

DIAGNOSIS AND DIFFERENTIAL

- Imaging involves plain radiographs, CT scan, and/or endoscopic visualization.

EMERGENCY DEPARTMENT CARE AND DISPOSITION

- Temporizing measures include supplemental humidified oxygen, upright patient positioning, and possibly administration of a helium–oxygen mixture.
- If intubation is required, an "awake look" with a fiberoptic bronchoscope with a 5-0 or 6-0 endotracheal tube is preferred.
- An emergency surgical airway, such as cricothyroidotomy, transtracheal jet ventilation, or tracheotomy, may be needed.
- Consult with an oncologist or surgeon for definitive management.

MALIGNANT PERICARDIAL EFFUSION AND TAMPONADE

EPIDEMIOLOGY

- Pericardial effusions are seen in up to 15% of patients with cancer but are often asymptomatic.

PATHOPHYSIOLOGY

- Common causes include carcinomas of the breast and lung, lymphoma, leukemia, and malignant melanoma. They can also be caused by therapeutic irradiation and chemotherapy.
- Symptoms depend on the rate of accumulation and distensibility of the pericardial sac.
- Sudden or large (>500 mL) effusions may compress the heart, preventing cardiac filling and reducing cardiac output (cardiac tamponade).

CLINICAL FEATURES

- Patients may present with chest heaviness, dyspnea, cough, and syncope.
- Physical examinations findings include tachycardia, narrowed pulse pressure, hypotension, distended neck vein, muffled heart tones, and pulsus paradoxus.

DIAGNOSIS AND DIFFERENTIAL

- Obtain an echocardiogram to evaluate the size of the effusion and the presence of tamponade.
- Chest radiograph may demonstrate an enlarged cardiac silhouette or pleural effusion.
- ECG may show sinus tachycardia, low QRS amplitude, and electrical alternans.
- Cardiomyopathy related to chemotherapy, such as doxorubin, and radiation therapy may have similar findings.

EMERGENCY DEPARTMENT CARE AND DISPOSITION

- **Oxygen**, volume expansion with **crystalloid**, and **dopamine**, up to 20 micrograms/kg/min IV, can be temporizing measures for cardiac tamponade.
- Emergent ultrasound-guided **pericardiocentesis** may be required to relieve cardiac tamponade in an unstable patient. For a more stable patient with a symptomatic effusion, consult a cardiologist for intervention, which may include pericardial window or placement of a pericardial catheter.
- Consult the patient's oncologist, as malignant effusion without symptoms or tamponade may not require treatment.

SUPERIOR VENA CAVA SYNDROME

PATHOPHYSIOLOGY

- Superior vena cava (SVC) syndrome most commonly occurs due to external compression by a malignant mass such as lymphoma (70%) or lung cancer (20%). Less common causes include thrombosis and benign masses.

CLINICAL FEATURES

- The most common symptoms are gradual onset of dyspnea, chest pain, cough, distended neck veins, and face or arm swelling.

DIAGNOSIS AND DIFFERENTIAL

- Obtain a CT of the chest with IV contrast.
- Chest radiograph may show a mediastinal mass.

EMERGENCY DEPARTMENT CARE AND DISPOSITION

- Patients with neurologic symptoms require urgent treatment including supplemental **oxygen** and **elevation of the head and upper body**.
- **Dexamethasone** 20 milligrams IV or **methylprednisolone** 125 to 250 milligrams IV may benefit patients with increased intracranial pressure or lymphoma.
- In patients without neurologic symptoms, SVC syndrome usually does not cause rapid deterioration and can await consultation regarding chemotherapy, radiation, or intravascular stenting.
- Patients with intravascular thrombosis may require anticoagulation, fibrinolysis, or catheter removal.

HYPERCALCEMIA OF MALIGNANCY

EPIDEMIOLOGY

- Hypercalcemia is seen in 10% to 30% of patients with advanced cancer.
- Hypercalcemia is most commonly seen with breast and lung cancer, lymphoma, and multiple myeloma.

PATHOPHYSIOLOGY

- Hypercalcemia is most often caused by a parathyroid hormone–related peptide secreted by the cancer cells. This hormone stimulates osteoclastic activity and promotes renal reabsorption of calcium.

CLINICAL FEATURES

- The symptoms are nonspecific and include polydipsia, polyuria, generalized weakness, lethargy, anorexia, nausea, constipation, abdominal pain, volume depletion, and altered mentation.

DIAGNOSIS AND DIFFERENTIAL

- Clinical signs and symptoms are related to the rate of rise and occur above 12 milligrams/dL (ionized >5.5 milligrams/dL).
- Measure ionized calcium or correct total serum calcium for albumin level: Corrected Ca = {0.8 × (4 – Pt's Albumin [grams/dL])} + Serum Ca (milligrams/dL).
- ECG may show shortened QT interval, ST depression, and atrioventricular blocks.
- Medications (diuretics), granulomatous disorders, primary hyperparathyroidism, and other endocrine disorders can also cause hypercalcemia.

EMERGENCY DEPARTMENT CARE AND DISPOSITION

- Treat initially with an infusion of **normal saline**.
- Further treatment should be discussed with the patient's oncologist.
- Bisphosphonates such as **zoledronic acid** 4 milligrams IV over 15 minutes or **pamidronate** 60 to 90 milligrams IV over 4 to 24 hours can prevent bone resorption, but should be given slowly to prevent the formation of calcium–bisphosphonate precipitants.
- **Calcitonin** 4 international units/kg SC or IM causes a more rapid decrease in calcium levels.
- **Glucocorticoids** may be helpful in lymphoma and multiple myeloma.
- Consider **hemodialysis** for patients with profound mental status changes, renal failure, or those who cannot tolerate a normal saline infusion.
- Furosemide is no longer recommended unless needed to prevent volume overload in patients with impaired cardiac or renal function.

SYNDROME OF INAPPROPRIATE SECRETION OF ANTIDIURETIC HORMONE

EPIDEMIOLOGY

- Inappropriate ADH secretion is most commonly associated with bronchogenic lung cancer, but is also caused by chemotherapy and medications.

PATHOPHYSIOLOGY

- Antidiuretic hormone (ADH, vasopressin) normally acts on the collecting tubule of the kidneys to increase water absorption during hypovolemia.
- In SIADH, excess ADH is secreted by ectopic tumor cells or through abnormal secretory stimulation of or cytotoxicity to the paraventricular and supraoptic neurons.

CLINICAL FEATURES

- Symptoms include anorexia, nausea, headache, altered mentation, and seizures.
- Mild hyponatremia (>125 mEq/L) is usually asymptomatic.

DIAGNOSIS AND DIFFERENTIAL

- SIADH should be suspected in patients with cancer who present with normovolemic hyponatremia.
- Lab abnormalities include serum osmolality <280 mOsm/L, urine osmolality >100 mOsm/L, and urine sodium >20mEq/L. The differential diagnosis includes hypothyroidism, renal failure, cirrhosis, adrenal crisis, and hypo/hypervolemia.

EMERGENCY DEPARTMENT CARE AND DISPOSITION

- Mild hyponatremia >125 mEq/L is treated with a **water restriction** of 500 mL/d and close follow-up.
- More severe hyponatremia is treated with **furosemide**, 0.5 to 1 milligram/kg PO with normal saline infusion to maintain volume.
- **Demeclocycine** 300 to 600 milligrams PO twice daily may increase water excretion.
- **Three percent hypertonic saline** is reserved for severe hyponatremia <120 mEq/L with seizures or coma. Titrate an infusion of 25 to 100 mL/h to a correction of 0.5 to 1 mEq/h with a maximum of 12-mEq/L change per day.

ADRENAL CRISIS

PATHOPHYSIOLOGY

- Adrenal crisis occurs when the adrenal glands decrease hormone production because of long-term exogenous steroid administration and are then unable to produce adequate hormones if those exogenous steroids are discontinued or to meet the additional steroid requirements imposed by physiologic stress.
- Destruction of the adrenal glands by malignancy may also impair steroid production.
- Mineralocorticoid (aldosterone) deficiency impairs sodium conservation (hyponatremia), potassium secretion (hyperkalemia), and proton secretion (acidosis).

- Glucocorticoid (cortisol) deficiency impairs metabolism of carbohydrate, lipid, protein, and water (hypoglycemia and hypotension).
- In secondary adrenal insufficiency, the hypothalamic-pituitary axis malfunctions. Production of cortisol is impaired due to a low level of adrenocorticotropic hormone, but aldosterone production is still appropriate.

CLINICAL FEATURES

- Symptoms include weakness, nausea, and hypotension unresponsive to fluids.

DIAGNOSIS AND DIFFERENTIAL

- Laboratory abnormalities may include hypoglycemia, hyponatremia, hyperkalemia, and low bicarbonate.
- Consider septic, cardiogenic, and hypovolemic shock in the differential diagnosis.

EMERGENCY DEPARTMENT CARE AND DISPOSITION

- Empirically administer stress-dose **hydrocortisone** 100 to 150 milligrams IV, **methylprednisolone** 20 to 30 milligrams IV, or **dexamethasone** 4 milligrams IV, **isotonic IV crystalloids,** and supportive care.
- Check for hypoglycemia with a capillary blood glucose.
- Draw a serum cortisol level before treatment if time permits.

TUMOR LYSIS SYNDROME

PATHOPHYSIOLOGY

- Tumor lysis syndrome occurs when dying tumor cells release massive quantities of potassium, phosphate, and uric acid.
- Calcium binds to phosphate, causing hypocalcemia.
- Uric acid and calcium phosphate deposit in the kidneys, causing renal failure.

CLINICAL FEATURES

- Tumor lysis syndrome usually occurs 1 to 3 days after chemotherapy for acute leukemia or lymphoma.
- Patients may present with fatigue, lethargy, nausea, vomiting, and cloudy urine.
- Hypocalcemia may cause neuromuscular irritability, muscular spasms, seizures, and altered mentation.
- Acute renal failure exacerbates hyperkalemia, which together with hypocalcemia may cause serious cardiac arrhythmias.

DIAGNOSIS AND DIFFERENTIAL

- Obtain a 12-lead ECG, basic electrolyte levels, complete blood count, uric acid, and phosphorus.

EMERGENCY DEPARTMENT CARE AND DISPOSITION

- Aggressive **infusion of isotonic fluids** reverses volume depletion and helps to prevent renal deposition of uric acid and calcium phosphate crystals.
- Hyperkalemia is the most immediate life threat. Treat hyperkalemia with **insulin, glucose, bicarbonate** (if acidotic)**, albuterol,** and **kayexalate** (see Chapter 6 for regimens).
- **Calcium gluconate** 1 gram IV = 10 mL of 10% solution should be given for ventricular arrhythmias or widened QRS complexes. **Otherwise, avoid calcium administration**, as it may worsen calcium phosphate precipitation in the kidney.
- Hyperuricemia may be treated with **rasburicase** 0.2 milligram/kg IV.
- Hyperphosphatemia is managed with IV **insulin** and **glucose**. Phosphate binders have a limited effect.
- Consider **hemodialysis** for potassium levels above 6.0 mEq/L, uric acid levels above 10.0 milligrams/dL, phosphate levels above 10 milligrams/dL, creatinine levels above 10 milligrams/dL, symptomatic hypocalcemia, or volume overload.
- Admit the patient to an intensive care unit.

NEUTROPENIC FEVER

CLINICAL FEATURES

- Neutrophil counts typically reach a nadir 5 to 10 days after chemotherapy and rebound 5 days later.
- Febrile neutropenia is defined by temperatures above 38°C for an hour or a single temperature above 38.3°C with an absolute neutrophil count (ANC) below 1000 cells/mm^3.
- Patient with neutropenic fever can deteriorate rapidly and should be assessed and given empiric antibiotics promptly when indicated.

DIAGNOSIS AND DIFFERENTIAL

- Febrile neutropenic patients often lack localizing signs and symptoms because of an attenuated immune response.
- Meticulously examine all skin surfaces, mucosal areas, and vascular access sites in which the patient may have an occult infection.

- Digital rectal examination is often withheld until after initial antibiotic administration because of the fear of inducing bacteremia.
- Obtain complete blood count with differential, blood cultures through all lumens of indwelling catheters as well as a peripheral site, urinalysis, urine culture, chest radiograph, electrolytes, and renal and liver function tests.
- Additional studies based on symptoms may include stool culture (diarrhea), sputum culture (cough), lumbar puncture (headache, stiff neck, altered mental status), wound culture (drainage), and CT or ultrasound (abdominal pain).
- A chest radiograph may appear normal in neutropenic patients with pneumonia since neutrophils are required for an infiltrate to appear.

EMERGENCY DEPARTMENT CARE AND DISPOSITION

- Give **empiric antibiotics** (Table 141-1) and admit to the hospital for an ANC below <500/mm^3. For neutrophil counts between 500 and 1000, the decision for antibiotics and admission is based on the patient's presentation and should be made with the oncologist.
- Add **vancomycin**, 1 gram IV, for severe mucositis, catheter site infection, recent use of fluoroquinolone prophylaxis, hypotension, residence in an institution with methicillin-resistant *Staphylococcus aureus* (MRSA), or known colonization with other resistant gram-positive organisms.

HYPERVISCOSITY SYNDROME

PATHOPHYSIOLOGY

- Hyperviscosity syndrome refers to impaired blood flow due to abnormal elevations of paraproteins or blood cells.
- It is most common in patients with acute leukemia, polycythemia, and dysproteinemias (Waldenström macroglobulinemia and myeloma).
- The hyperviscosity causes sludging, stasis, impaired microcirculation, and tissue hypoperfusion.

CLINICAL FEATURES

- Initial symptoms include fatigue, abdominal pain, headache, blurry vision, dyspnea, fever, or altered mental status. Thrombosis or bleeding may occur.

TABLE 141-1 Suggestions for Initial Empiric Antibiotic Therapy in Febrile Neutropenia

CIRCUMSTANCE	DRUG AND ADULT DOSAGE	COMMENTS
Outpatient	Ciprofloxacin, 500 milligrams PO every 8 h *and* Amoxicillin/clavulanate, 500 milligrams PO every 8 h	Useful for low-risk patients with daily assessments by a medical provider for the initial 3 d.
Monotherapy	Cefepime, 2 grams IV every 8 h *or* Ceftazidime, 2 grams IV every 8 h *or* Imipenem/cilastatin, 1 gram IV every 8 h *or* Meropenem, 1 gram IV every 8 h *or* Piperacillin/tazobactam, 4.5 grams IV every 6 h	Monotherapy with these broad-spectrum agents appears to be as good as dual-drug therapy in most circumstances.
Dual therapy	One of the monotherapy agents *plus* Gentamicin, 1.7 milligrams/kg IV every 8 h *or* Tobramycin, 1.7 milligrams/kg IV every 8 h *or* Amikacin, 5 milligrams/kg IV every 8 h	Potential advances include synergistic effects against some gram-negative bacteria and reduced emergence of drug resistance. Increased risk for adverse effects, including nephrotoxicity, ototoxicity, and hypokalemia.
Risk factors for severe gram-positive infection (see text)	Vancomycin, 1 gram IV every 12 h *plus* Cefepime, 2 grams IV every 8 h *or* Ceftazidime, 2 grams IV every 8 h *or* Imipenem/cilastatin, 1 gram IV every 8 h *or* Meropenem, 1 gram IV every 8 h	Vancomycin is not usually necessary for initial empiric antibiotic therapy if it is available for subsequent treatment modifications. Vancomycin may be incorporated into initial therapeutic regimens of high-risk patients in institutions with increased gram-positive infection rates.

- Fundoscopic examination findings may include retinal hemorrhages, exudates, and "sausage-linked" vessels.
- Symptoms are worsened by dehydration.

DIAGNOSIS AND DIFFERENTIAL

- Hematocrits above 60% and WBC counts above 100,000/mm^3 often cause hyperviscosity syndromes.
- Elevated serum viscosity (>5 cP), rouleaux formation (red cells stacked like coins), or abnormal protein electrophoresis (IgM >4 grams/dL) support the diagnosis.

EMERGENCY DEPARTMENT CARE AND DISPOSITION

- Administer intravenous **isotonic fluids** and consult a hematologist regarding **plasmapheresis or leukopheresis**.
- A temporizing measure in patients with coma is 1000 mL **phlebotomy** with simultaneous infusion of 2 to 3 L isotonic fluids.
- Red cell transfusion is not recommended, as it may increase blood viscosity.

THROMBOEMBOLISM

EPIDEMIOLOGY

- Thromboembolism is the second leading cause of death in cancer patients.
- Symptomatic deep vein thrombosis occurs in approximately 15% of all patients with cancer and up to 50% of those with advanced malignancies.

PATHOPHYSIOLOGY

- Malignancy is a hypercoagulable state. Neoplastic cells and chemotherapy can cause intimal injury. Obstructive tumors often cause venous stasis, which is exacerbated by decreased mobility.
- Angiogenesis inhibitors such as thalidomide, sunitinib, and bevacizumab are associated with thrombosis.

EMERGENCY DEPARTMENT CARE AND DISPOSITION

- See Chapter 27 for the diagnosis and management of deep vein thrombosis and pulmonary embolism.
- Cancer patients, even those with brain metastases, do not appear at increased risk for anticoagulant-related bleeding complications.

NAUSEA AND VOMITING

PATHOPHYSIOLOGY

- Chemotherapy commonly causes nausea and vomiting.

CLINICAL FEATURES

- Patients present with a history of recent chemotherapy and may show signs of dehydration.

DIAGNOSIS AND DIFFERENTIAL

- Other causes of nausea and vomiting include radiation enteritis, bowel obstruction, infection or tumor infiltration, and increased intracranial pressure.

EMERGENCY DEPARTMENT CARE AND DISPOSITION

- Rehydrate patients with isotonic crystalloids and treat electrolyte abnormalities as needed.
- Administer antiemetics (Table 141-2).

TABLE 141-2 Antiemetic Agents for Chemotherapy-Induced Vomiting

CLASS AND AGENT	ADULT DOSE	COMMENTS
Dopamine receptor antagonists		
Metoclopramide	10 milligrams IV or IM	Dose-related extrapyramidal side effects
Promethazine	25 milligrams IV or IM	IV use common but not approved by FDA
Serotonin antagonists		
Dolasetron	100 milligrams (or 1.8 milligrams/kg) IV over 5 min	Constipation, headaches (all)
Granisetron	10 micrograms/kg IV over 5 min	
Ondansetron	32 milligrams (or 0.15 milligram/kg) IV over 15 min	
Corticosteroids		
Dexamethasone	20 milligrams IV	Mechanism unknown, no immunosuppression
Benzodiazepines		
Lorazepam	1-2 milligrams IV	Sedation, anxiolysis
Histamine receptor antagonists		
Diphenhydramine	50 milligrams IV or IM	Minor therapeutic effect

Abbreviation: FDA = U.S. Food and Drug Administration.

EXTRAVASATION OF CHEMOTHERAPEUTIC AGENTS

CLINICAL FEATURES

- Extravasation may cause pain, erythema, and swelling, usually within hours of the infusion.

EMERGENCY DEPARTMENT CARE AND DISPOSITION

- If irritation develops during infusion through a peripheral line, stop the infusion and attempt aspiration through the line.
- Consult an oncologist to discuss the use of antidotes for extravasation of anthracyclines, vinca alkaloids, mitomycin, cisplatin, mechlorethamine, and paclitaxel.

For further reading in Tintinalli's *Emergency Medicine: A Comprehensive Study Guide*, 7th ed., see Chapter 235, "Emergency Complications of Malignancy," by Paul Blackburn.

Section 16
NEUROLOGY

142 HEADACHE AND FACIAL PAIN

Steven Go

EPIDEMIOLOGY

- Approximately 3.8% of patients presenting to the ED have a serious cause of their headache.

PATHOPHYSIOLOGY

- The vast majority of subarachnoid hemorrhages (SAH) are caused by a ruptured cerebral aneurysm.
- Temporal arteritis is a systemic panarteritis.
- Migraine headaches are caused by a trigger, with resultant dysfunction of brainstem pathways that modulate sensory input, followed by disordered activity of blood vessels.

CLINICAL FEATURES

- Headaches are divided into *primary* headaches and those due to secondary causes. Secondary causes require further evaluation for the etiology.

SUBARACHNOID HEMORRHAGE

- SAH (see Chapter 143) classically presents as the severe, sudden onset at maximal intensity of "the worst headache of my life," precipitated by exertional activities in 20% of cases.
- The headache may be associated with nausea and vomiting, photophobia, and stroke symptoms.
- The neurological examination is normal in 50% of cases.

MENINGITIS

- Meningitis (see Chapter 150) can cause a headache of rapid onset, generally associated with fever, meningismus, and photophobia.
- Immunocompromised patients can experience a more insidious onset with opportunistic infections, without fever or meningismus.

INTRAPARENCHYMAL HEMORRHAGE AND ISCHEMIC STROKE

- These two entities can present with headaches, approximately 50% (intracranial hemorrhage) and <25% (ischemic stroke). Other neurological signs and symptoms are often present.

SUBDURAL HEMATOMA

- Subdural hematoma should be suspected when headaches occur in the setting of remote trauma, usually in at-risk patients (alcoholics, elders, and those on anticoagulants).

BRAIN TUMOR

- Brain tumor headaches may be bilateral, unilateral, constant, or intermittent. The headache may be worse in the morning, associated with nausea and vomiting, and positional in a minority of cases.
- Only 8% have neurological examination abnormalities.

CEREBRAL VENOUS THROMBOSIS

- Cerebral venous thrombosis (CVT) is a rare condition that presents with headache, vomiting, and seizures in patients with a hypercoagulable state (oral contraceptives, postpartum, perioperative, various clotting factor deficiencies, mutations, or polycythemia).
- Papilledema can be present, and neurological findings can wax and wane.

TEMPORAL ARTERITIS

- Temporal arteritis most commonly presents with headache (60-90%), which is most often unilateral

TABLE 142-1	Criteria for Diagnosis of Temporal Arteritis*
Age >50 y	
New-onset localized headache	
Temporal artery tenderness or decreased pulse	
Erythrocyte sedimentation rate >50 mm/h	
Abnormal arterial biopsy findings	

*Three of the five criteria must be met.

frontotemporal (can be bilateral), severe, and throbbing. Associated symptoms may include jaw claudication, polymyalgia rheumatica, upper respiratory infection symptoms, and vision changes.
- It usually occurs in patients >50 years old and more commonly in women (Table 142-1).
- The involved temporal artery can be tender or non-pulsatile, or have a diminished pulse, but can also be normal.

OPHTHALMIC DISORDERS

- Ophthalmic disorders can present with severe headache and are commonly associated with nausea and vomiting (eg, acute glaucoma).

HYPERTENSIVE HEADACHES

- Hypertensive headaches typically become more severe as the diastolic blood pressure rises, and improve with reduction of blood pressure.
- Care must be taken to consider other causes of hypertension, such as stroke, pheochromocytoma, preeclampsia, or any other cause of life-threatening headache.
- Distinction must be made from a true hypertensive emergency, in which there is other organ system involvement.

SINUSITIS

- Sinusitis can result in pain in various sites depending on the particular sinuses that are infected. For maxillary sinusitis (the most common sinusitis) the pain is in the anterior face. The other sinuses include frontal (forehead), ethmoid (behind/between eyes), and sphenoid (diffuse). Headache typically varies with head position.
- Patients with four or more of the following symptoms and signs: colored nasal discharge, maxillary toothache, poor response to decongestants, visible purulent nasal discharge, or abnormal transillumination, have a high likelihood of sinusitis, whereas sinusitis is unlikely if less than two of these findings are present.

BENIGN INTRACRANIAL HYPERTENSION

- Benign intracranial hypertension (pseudotumor cerebri) occurs most commonly in young women of childbearing age who are not necessarily obese. These chronic headaches are associated with thyroid disease and the use of oral contraceptives, vitamin A, and tetracycline. Associated symptoms include nausea, vomiting, and various visual disturbances, including visual field defects.
- Papilledema with a normal level of consciousness is a hallmark of the disease.

CERVICAL ARTERY DISSECTION

- Cervical artery dissection can be either traumatic or atraumatic and typically occurs in patients <40 years of age.
- Internal carotid artery dissection causes unilateral anterior headache, usually around the eye or frontal area, commonly associated with neck pain. Most patients will have or develop neurologic signs such as transient ischemic attack (TIA), stroke, Horner syndrome, monocular blindness, or cranial nerve abnormalities.
- Vertebral artery dissection causes occipital or posterior neck pain, commonly associated with signs of brain stem TIA or stroke.

POST-LUMBAR PUNCTURE HEADACHE

- This occurs in 10% to 36% of patients within 24 to 48 hours of a lumbar puncture (LP). Headache worsens with upright position and improves with recumbency.

MIGRAINE HEADACHES

- Headaches generally have a gradual onset, last 4 to 72 hours, and are typically unilateral, pulsating, and worsened by physical activity. Nausea and vomiting, photophobia, and phonophobia are frequently present.
- Other neurological symptoms such as visual auras, hemiparesthesias, hemiparesis, and aphasia can be present, but other causes of headache must be excluded if these findings are present.
- If four of the five "POUND" criteria (*p*ulsatile quality, *d*uration 4-72 hours, *u*nilateral location, *n*ausea or vomiting, *d*isabling intensity) are present, the likelihood ratio (LR) is 24 for a migraine diagnosis.

CLUSTER HEADACHES

- Cluster headaches present with severe, unilateral orbital, supraorbital, or temporal pain lasting 15 to 180 minutes, frequently associated with lacrimation, nasal congestion, rhinorrhea, and conjunctival injection.

- Symptoms tend to occur daily for weeks before remitting for weeks to years.

DIAGNOSIS AND DIFFERENTIAL

- Noncontrast CT scan of the brain is the initial imaging modality of choice to detect dangerous causes of headache. Latest generation CT scanners have a very high sensitivity for SAH (98%) within 12 hours of symptom onset, but this diminishes rapidly with time (80% after 12 hours).
- LP is indicated in suspected meningitis and to detect SAH if the initial noncontrast CT scan of the brain is negative.
- Imaging of the brain is not necessary prior to LP if there is no papilledema and if the level of consciousness and neurological examination (including lack of cerebellar findings) are completely normal.
- Xanthochromia in cerebrospinal fluid (CSF) is useful to exclude SAH if the LP is done >12 hours after symptom onset and if the local laboratory uses a spectrophotometric test to detect it. However, most laboratories in the United States use visual inspection only.
- CT angiography of the vasculature of the brain and neck is useful in selected cases to detect the presence of an aneurysm or cervical artery dissection.
- MRI has only limited applications in the ED for acute evaluation of headache. It is no more sensitive than CT for acute SAH.
- Most laboratory studies are unhelpful in determining the etiology of headache in the ED. However, various CSF studies such as cell count and differential, glucose, protein, Gram's stain, latex antigen studies, and various cultures are useful in determining the etiology of meningitis (see Chapter 150 for details). In addition, while nonspecific, an elevated erythrocyte sedimentation rate (ESR) and C-reactive protein (CRP) are useful in detecting temporal arteritis.

EMERGENCY DEPARTMENT CARE AND DISPOSITION

- In SAH, the chances of rebleeding can be reduced by maintaining the patient's pre-bleed blood pressure (or MAP <130 mm Hg if baseline blood pressure is unknown). This is best done by administering an IV titratable antihypertensive, such as labetalol (typical adult starting dose is 10-20 milligrams over 1-2 minutes IVP; continuous infusion dosage generally starts at 2 milligrams/min, titrated to effect). Nimodipine (60 milligrams orally every 4 hours) may produce modest improvements in outcome by decreasing vasospasm. Emergent neurosurgical consultation is indicated.
- Patients suspected of having meningitis should receive prompt empiric antibiotic therapy. Antibiotic therapy should not be delayed for LP or imaging (see Chapter 150 for details).
- Patients suspected of having temporal arteritis should be empirically treated with prednisone 40 to 60 milligrams PO daily, and urgent specialty consultation is indicated.
- Medications effective in the treatment of the patient with migraine headache include dihydroergotamine (DHE), sumatriptan, dopamine-antagonist antiemetics (metoclopramide, chlorpromazine, prochlorperazine), and ketorolac. Current guidelines recommend opiates only if migraine-specific therapy fails.
- Cluster headaches will resolve with the administration of high-flow oxygen in 70% of patients. Dihydroergotamine mesylate, NSAIDs, and sumatriptan also may be effective.
- Improvement of a presumed primary headache with treatment does not necessarily exclude an important secondary cause for the headache.
- Indications for admission for headache include presence of life-threatening cause of headache or failure to achieve adequate symptom control in the ED.

CRANIAL AND FACIAL PAIN DISORDERS

TEMPOROMANDIBULAR DISORDER

- Temporomandibular disorder (TMD) causes pain at the temporomandibular joint, surrounding muscles, and ligaments. Patients often will complain of joint pain and noise with movement, locking of the jaw, limited jaw movements, and bruxism.
- ED treatment of TMD consists of NSAIDs and narcotic analgesics. Radiographs are of little value in the ED.
- Follow-up should be made with a dentist or oral surgeon.

TRIGEMINAL NEURALGIA

- Trigeminal neuralgia (Tic Douloureux) presents as an intermittent, seconds-long, "electric shock"-like pain in a unilateral trigeminal nerve distribution.
- Initial treatment may include carbamazepine (100 milligrams PO twice daily), which has been shown to be very effective.
- Referral to a neurologist should be made for intractable cases.

For further reading in Tintinalli's *Emergency Medicine: A Comprehensive Study Guide*, 7th ed., see Chapter 159, "Headache and Facial Pain," by Christopher J. Denny and Michael J. Schull.

143 STROKE, TRANSIENT ISCHEMIC ATTACK, AND CERVICAL ARTERY DISSECTION

Steven Go

EPIDEMIOLOGY

- Ischemic strokes (87%) are more common than hemorrhagic strokes (intracerebral [10%] and nontraumatic subarachnoid hemorrhage [3%]). See Table 143-1.
- Cervical artery dissection (CAD) causes 10% to 25% of strokes in young and middle-aged patients.

PATHOPHYSIOLOGY

- Stroke may be defined as any disease process that interrupts blood flow to the brain. Ischemic strokes result from thrombotic, embolic, or low flow states. Hemorrhagic strokes are secondary to intracerebral hemorrhage (ICH) or subarachnoid hemorrhage (SAH).
- A transient ischemic attack (TIA) is a transient neurologic deficit that typically lasts less than 1 to 2 hours, but duration can no longer be used to discriminate between TIA and stroke; they are best thought of as similar disease processes on a continuum.
- CAD can be associated with neck trauma, major or trivial (chiropractic manipulation), family history of arterial disease, genetic factors, recent upper respiratory illness, connective tissue disease, and history of migraine.
- The vast majority of SAH are caused by a ruptured cerebral aneurysm.

CLINICAL FEATURES

- Specific findings in stroke patients depend on the regions of the brain that are compromised and how severe the insult is (Table 143-2). Stroke presentation

TABLE 143-1 Stroke Classification

STROKE TYPE	MECHANISM	MAJOR CAUSES	CLINICAL NOTES
Ischemic			
Thrombotic	Narrowing of a damaged vascular lumen by an in situ process—usually clot formation	Atherosclerosis Vasculitis Arterial dissection Polycythemia Hypercoagulable state Infection (human immunodeficiency virus infection, syphilis, trichinosis, tuberculosis, aspergillosis)	Symptoms often have gradual onset and may wax and wane. Common cause of transient ischemic attack.
Embolic	Obstruction of a normal vascular lumen by intravascular material from a remote source	Valvular vegetations Mural thrombi Paradoxical emboli Cardiac tumors (myxomas) Arterial-arterial emboli from proximal source Fat emboli Particulate emboli (intravenous drug use) Septic emboli	Typically sudden in onset. Account for 20% of ischemic strokes.
Hypoperfusion	Low–blood flow state leading to hypoperfusion of the brain	Cardiac failure resulting in systemic hypotension	Diffuse injury pattern in watershed regions. Symptoms may wax and wane with hemodynamic factors.
Hemorrhagic			
Intracerebral	Intraparenchymal hemorrhage from previously weakened arterioles	Hypertension Amyloidosis Iatrogenic anticoagulation Vascular malformations Cocaine use	Intracranial pressure rise causes local neuronal damage. Secondary vasoconstriction mediated by blood breakdown products or neuronal mechanisms (diaschisis) can cause remote perfusion changes. Risks include advanced age, history of stroke, tobacco or alcohol use. More common in Asians and blacks.
Nontraumatic subarachnoid	Hemorrhage into subarachnoid space	Berry aneurysm rupture Vascular malformation rupture	May be preceded by a sentinel headache ("warning leak").

TABLE 143-2	Symptoms of Stroke
Traditional symptoms	Sudden numbness or weakness of face, arm, or leg—especially unilateral Sudden confusion or aphasia Sudden memory deficit or spatial orientation or perception difficulties Sudden visual deficit or diplopia Sudden dizziness, gait disturbance, or ataxia Sudden severe headache with no known cause
Nontraditional symptoms	Loss of consciousness or syncope Shortness of breath Sudden pain in the face, chest, arms, or legs Seizure Falls or accidents Sudden hiccups Sudden nausea Sudden fatigue Sudden palpitations Altered mental status

can vary considerably from classically described syndromes.

- Anterior cerebral artery strokes typically cause contralateral leg weakness and sensory changes.
- Middle cerebral artery strokes classically present with hemiparesis (arm > leg) and sensory loss. Weakness in the lower half of the face (variable) and ipsilateral gaze preference may occur. Aphasia (receptive and/or expressive) is often present if the dominant hemisphere (usually left) is affected, while contralateral hemineglect suggests nondominant hemisphere involvement.
- Posterior circulation strokes can present very subtly with findings such as unilateral headache, visual field defects, dizziness, vertigo, diplopia, dysphagia, ataxia, cranial nerve deficits, or bilateral limb weakness. Signs and symptoms can occur alone or in various combinations.
- Occlusion of the basilar artery causes severe quadriplegia, coma, and the locked-in syndrome.
- Cerebellar strokes present similarly to other posterior stroke syndromes, but can deteriorate quickly if a hematoma or edema is present.
- CAD can involve both the anterior and posterior arterial systems. The most common symptoms with an internal carotid dissection are unilateral head pain (50-67%), neck pain (25%), or face pain (10%). Vertebral artery dissections commonly present with headache (69%) and posterior neck pain (46%), which can be unilateral or bilateral. Signs and symptoms of CAD can be transient as well as persistent.
- Intracranial hemorrhages may present with any of the anatomic syndromes discussed above.
- SAH classically presents with sudden onset of a "thunderclap" headache at its most severe. It occurs 20% of the time during activity associated with elevated blood pressures such as sexual intercourse, weight lifting, defecation, or coughing. Vomiting, photophobia, nuchal irritation, low-grade fever, and altered mental status all may occur. Focal findings can occur depending on the location of the aneurysm. A recent history suggestive of a warning leak may be obtained in many patients.
- Symptoms may resolve spontaneously as blood diffuses in the SAH space; therefore, the clinician should not be misled by improving clinical condition when the history is strongly suggestive of SAH.

DIAGNOSIS AND DIFFERENTIAL

- The differential for stroke-like symptoms is found in Table 143-3.

TABLE 143-3 Differential Diagnoses of Consequence for Acute Stroke Symptoms

STROKE MIMIC	DISTINGUISHING CLINICAL FEATURES
Seizures/postictal paralysis (Todd paralysis)	Transient paralysis following a seizure, which typically disappears quickly; can be confused with transient ischemic attack. Seizures can be secondary to a cerebrovascular accident.
Syncope	No persistent or associated neurologic symptoms.
Brain neoplasm or abscess	Focal neurologic findings, signs of infection, detectable by imaging.
Epidural/subdural hematoma	History of trauma, alcoholism, anticoagulant use, bleeding disorder; detectable by imaging.
Subarachnoid hemorrhage	Sudden onset of severe headache.
Hypoglycemia	Can be detected by bedside glucose measurement, history of diabetes mellitus.
Hyponatremia	History of diuretic use, neoplasm, excessive free water intake.
Hypertensive encephalopathy	Gradual onset; global cerebral dysfunction, headache, delirium, hypertension, cerebral edema.
Meningitis/encephalitis	Fever, immunocompromise may be present, meningismus, detectable on lumbar puncture.
Hyperosmotic coma	Extremely high glucose levels, history of diabetes mellitus.
Wernicke encephalopathy	History of alcoholism or malnutrition; triad of ataxia, ophthalmoplegia, and confusion.

(*Continued*)

TABLE 143-3 Differential Diagnoses of Consequence for Acute Stroke Symptoms (Continued)

STROKE MIMIC	DISTINGUISHING CLINICAL FEATURES
Labyrinthitis	Predominantly vestibular symptoms; patient should have no other focal findings; can be confused with cerebellar stroke.
Drug toxicity (lithium, phenytoin, carbamazepine)	Can be detected by particular toxidromes and elevated blood levels. Phenytoin and carbamazepine toxicity may present with ataxia, vertigo, nausea, and abnormal reflexes.
Bell's palsy	Neurologic deficit confined to isolated peripheral seventh nerve palsy; often associated with younger age.
Complicated migraine	History of similar episodes, preceding aura, headache.
Ménière disease	History of recurrent episodes dominated by vertigo symptoms, tinnitus, deafness.
Demyelinating disease (multiple sclerosis)	Gradual onset. Patient may have a history of multiple episodes of neurologic findings in multifocal anatomic distributions.
Conversion disorder	No cranial nerve findings, nonanatomic distribution of findings (eg, midline sensory loss), inconsistent history or examination findings.

- It is critical that an accurate determination of the time the patient was last known to be at their neurological baseline be made.
- Eligibility for thrombolytic therapy should be determined if stroke is the primary working diagnosis (Tables 143-4 and 143-5).
- A National Institutes of Health Stroke Scale (NIHSS) score should be quickly calculated upon presentation (Table 143-6).
- An emergent noncontrast CT scan (best interpreted by a neuroradiologist) should be rapidly performed within 25 minutes of arrival to determine whether hemorrhage or a stroke mimic is present. Most acute ischemic strokes will not be visualized in the early hours of a stroke.
- MRI, MRA, and CT angiography may be of value in detecting particular disease entities (eg, CAD, tumor, circle of Willis aneurysms), but their exact role is currently unclear.
- Modern CTs are thought to be 98% sensitive to detect SAH within 12 hours of symptom onset; however, some studies have found sensitivity as low as 85.7% when a third-generation CT is performed greater than 6 hours after headache onset.

TABLE 143-4 American Heart Association/American Stroke Association 2007 Criteria for IV Recombinant Tissue Plasminogen Activator (rtPA) in Acute Ischemic Stroke

Indications	
Measurable diagnosis of acute ischemic stroke	Use of NIHSS recommended. Stroke symptoms should not be clearing, minor, or isolated. Caution is advised before giving rtPA to persons with severe stroke (NIHSS score of >22), because they have increased risk of intracerebral hemorrhage; however, they are at high risk of death, regardless.
Age ≥18 y	No clear upper age limit.
Time of symptom onset ≤3 h	Must be *well established* (2009 AHA/ASA Scientific Advisory suggests time window may be extended to 3 to 4.5 h if ECASS criteria are met).
Exclusion Criteria	
Symptoms consistent with subarachnoid hemorrhage	
Seizure with postictal residual neurologic impairments	
Previous head trauma or stroke within preceding 3 mo	
Previous myocardial infarction within preceding 3 mo*	
Previous GI or urinary tract hemorrhage within preceding 21 d	
Major surgery within preceding 14 d	
Prior intracranial hemorrhage	
Pretreatment systolic blood pressure >185 mm Hg *or* diastolic blood pressure >110 mm Hg despite therapy (Table 143-7)	
Evidence of active bleeding or acute major fracture	
Blood glucose level <50 milligrams/dL (2.7 mmol/L)	
International normalized ratio >1.7 (oral anticoagulant use in and of itself is not a contraindication to rtPA)	
Use of heparin within preceding 48 h *and* a prolonged activated partial thromboplastin time	
Platelet count <100,000/mm^3	
Head CT shows multilobar infarction (hypodensity of more than one-third cerebral hemisphere) or hemorrhage or tumor	
Failure of the patient or responsible party to understand the risks and benefits of, and alternatives to, the proposed treatment after a full discussion	

Abbreviation: NIHSS = National Institutes of Health Stroke Scale.
*Rationale for this criterion was a statement indicating that myocardial rupture can result if rtPA is given within a few days of acute myocardial infarction.

- If SAH is suspected and the CT is negative, many authorities agree that a lumbar puncture is indicated.
- Cerebrospinal fluid (CSF) xanthochromia does not develop until 12 hours after symptom onset, and

TABLE 143-5 Additional Exclusion Criteria for IV Recombinant Tissue Plasminogen Activator (rtPA) in Acute Ischemic Stroke When Given 3 to 4.5 Hours After Symptom Onset

Age >80 y
Severe stroke as assessed clinically (NIHSS score >25)
Combination of previous stroke and diabetes mellitus
Blood glucose <50 milligrams/dL or >400 milligrams/dL
Oral anticoagulant treatment

Abbreviation: NIHSS = National Institutes of Health Stroke Scale.

TABLE 143-6 National Institutes of Health Stroke Scale (NIHSS)

INSTRUCTIONS	SCALE DEFINITION
1a. Level of consciousness (LOC)* The investigator must choose a response if a full evaluation is prevented by such obstacles as an endotracheal tube, language barrier, or orotracheal trauma/bandages. A 3 is scored only if the patient makes no movement (other than reflexive posturing) in response to noxious stimulation.	0 = Alert; keenly responsive. 1 = Not alert, but arousable by minor stimulation to obey, answer, or respond. 2 = Not alert; requires repeated stimulation to attend, or is obtunded and requires strong or painful stimulation to make movements (not stereotyped). 3 = Responds only with reflex motor or autonomic effects or is totally unresponsive, flaccid, and areflexic.
1b. LOC questions The patient is asked the month and his or her age. The answer must be correct—there is no partial credit for being close. Aphasic and stuporous patients who do not comprehend the questions are given a score of 2. Patients unable to speak because of endotracheal intubation, orotracheal trauma, severe dysarthria from any cause, language barrier, or any other problem not secondary to aphasia are given a score of 1. It is important that only the initial answer be graded and that the examiner not "help" the patient with verbal or nonverbal cues.	0 = Answers both questions correctly. 1 = Answers one question correctly. 2 = Answers neither question correctly.
1c. LOC commands The patient is asked to open and close the eyes and then to grip and release the nonparetic hand. Substitute another one-step command if the hands cannot be used. Credit is given if an unequivocal attempt is made but not completed due to weakness. If the patient does not respond to command, the task should be demonstrated to him or her (pantomime) and the result scored (ie, follows no, one, or two commands). Patients with trauma, amputation, or other physical impediments should be given suitable one-step commands. Only the first attempt is scored.	0 = Performs both tasks correctly. 1 = Performs one task correctly. 2 = Performs neither task correctly.
2. Best gaze Only horizontal eye movements are tested. Voluntary or reflexive (oculocephalic) eye movements are scored, but caloric testing is not done. If the patient has a conjugate deviation of the eyes that can be overcome by voluntary or reflexive activity, the score is 1. If a patient has an isolated peripheral nerve paresis (cranial nerve III, IV, or VI), the score is 1. Gaze is testable in all aphasic patients. Patients with ocular trauma, bandages, preexisting blindness, or other disorder of visual acuity or fields should be tested with reflexive movements, and a choice made by the investigator. Establishing eye contact and then moving about the patient from side to side will occasionally clarify the presence of a partial gaze palsy.	0 = Normal. 1 = Partial gaze palsy; gaze is abnormal in one or both eyes, but forced deviation or total gaze paresis is not present. 2 = Forced deviation, or total gaze paresis not overcome by the oculocephalic maneuver.
3. Visual Visual fields (upper and lower quadrants) are tested by confrontation, using finger counting or visual threat, as appropriate. Patients may be encouraged, but if they look at the side of the moving fingers appropriately, this can be scored as normal. If there is unilateral blindness or enucleation, visual fields in the remaining eye are scored. Score 1 only if a clear-cut asymmetry, including quadrantanopia, is found. If the patient is blind from any cause, score 3. Double simultaneous stimulation is performed at this point. If there is extinction, patient receives a score of 1, and the results are used to respond to item 11.	0 = No vision loss. 1 = Partial hemianopia. 2 = Complete hemianopia. 3 = Bilateral hemianopia (blind including cortical blindness).
4. Facial palsy* Ask—or use pantomime to encourage—the patient to show teeth or raise eyebrows and close eyes. Score symmetry of grimace in response to noxious stimuli in the poorly responsive or noncomprehending patient. If facial trauma/bandages, orotracheal tube, tape, or other physical barriers obscure the face, these should be removed to the extent possible.	0 = Normal symmetric movements. 1 = Minor paralysis (flattened nasolabial fold, asymmetry on smiling). 2 = Partial paralysis (total or near-total paralysis of lower face). 3 = Complete paralysis of one or both sides (absence of facial movement in the upper and lower face).

(*Continued*)

TABLE 143-6 National Institutes of Health Stroke Scale (NIHSS) (Continued)

INSTRUCTIONS	SCALE DEFINITION
5. Motor arm The limb is placed in the appropriate position: extend the arms (palms down) 90 degrees (if sitting) or 45 degrees (if supine). Drift is scored if the arm falls before 10 s. The aphasic patient is encouraged using urgency in the voice and pantomime, but not noxious stimulation. Each limb is tested in turn, beginning with the nonparetic arm. Only in the case of amputation or joint fusion at the shoulder, the examiner should record the score as untestable (UN) and clearly write the explanation for this choice. 5a. Left arm 5b. Right arm	0 = No drift; limb holds 90 (or 45) degrees for full 10 s. 1 = Drift; limb holds 90 (or 45) degrees, but drifts down before full 10 s; does not hit bed or other support. 2 = Some effort against gravity; limb cannot get to or maintain (if cued) 90 (or 45) degrees, drifts down to bed, but has some effort against gravity. 3 = No effort against gravity; limb falls. 4 = No movement.
6. Motor leg The limb is placed in the appropriate position: hold the leg at 30 degrees (the patient is always tested supine). Drift is scored if the leg falls before 5 s. The aphasic patient is encouraged using urgency in the voice and pantomime, but not noxious stimulation. Each limb is tested in turn, beginning with the nonparetic leg. Only in the case of amputation or joint fusion at the hip, the examiner should record the score as untestable (UN) and clearly write the explanation for this choice. 6a. Left leg 6b. Right leg	0 = No drift; leg holds 30-degree position for full 5 s. 1 = Drift; leg falls by the end of the 5-s period but does not hit bed. 2 = Some effort against gravity; leg falls to bed by 5 s, but has some effort against gravity. 3 = No effort against gravity; leg falls to bed immediately. 4 = No movement.
7. Limb ataxia* This item is aimed at finding evidence of a unilateral cerebellar lesion. Test with the patient's eyes open. In case of visual defect, ensure that testing is done in the intact visual field. The finger-nose-finger and heel-shin tests are performed on both sides, and ataxia is scored only if present out of proportion to weakness. Ataxia is absent in the patient who cannot understand or is paralyzed. Only in the case of amputation or joint fusion, the examiner should record the score as untestable (UN) and clearly write the explanation for this choice. In case of blindness, test by having the patient touch the nose from an extended arm position.	0 = Absent. 1 = Present in one limb. 2 = Present in two limbs.
8. Sensory[†] Sensation or grimace to pinprick when tested, or withdrawal from a noxious stimulus in the obtunded or aphasic patient. Only sensory loss attributed to stroke is scored as abnormal, and the examiner should test as many body areas [arms (not hands), legs, trunk, face] as needed to check accurately for hemisensory loss. A score of 2, "severe or total sensory loss," should be given only when a severe or total loss of sensation can be clearly demonstrated. Stuporous and aphasic patients will therefore probably score 1 or 0. The patient with brain stem stroke who has bilateral loss of sensation is scored 2. If the patient does not respond and is quadriplegic, score 2. Patients in a coma (item 1a score = 3) are automatically given a 2 on this item.	0 = Normal; no sensory loss. 1 = Mild-to-moderate sensory loss; patient feels pinprick is less sharp or is dull on affected side, or there is loss of superficial pain with pinprick, but patient is aware of being touched. 2 = Severe to total sensory loss; patient is not aware of being touched on face, arm, and leg.
9. Best language A great deal of information about comprehension is obtained during the preceding sections of the examination. For this scale item, the patient is asked to describe what is happening in the test picture, to name the items on the test naming sheet, and to read from the test list of sentences. Comprehension is judged from responses here as well as responses to all of the commands in the preceding general neurologic examination. If vision loss interferes with the tests, ask the patient to identify objects placed in the hand, repeat, and produce speech. The intubated patient should be asked to write. The patient in a coma (item 1a score = 3) automatically scores 3 on this item. The examiner must choose a score for the patient with stupor or limited cooperation, but a score of 3 should be used only if the patient is mute and follows no one-step commands.	0 = No aphasia; normal. 1 = Mild-to-moderate aphasia; some obvious loss of fluency or facility of comprehension, without significant limitation on ideas expressed or form of expression. However, reduction of speech and/or comprehension makes conversation about provided materials difficult or impossible. For example, in conversation about provided materials, examiner can identify picture or naming card content from patient's response. 2 = Severe aphasia; all communication is through fragmentary expression; great need for inference, questioning, and guessing by listener. Range of information that can be exchanged is limited; listener carries burden of communication. Examiner cannot identify materials provided from patient's response. 3 = Mute, global aphasia; no usable speech or auditory comprehension.

(*Continued*)

TABLE 143-6 National Institutes of Health Stroke Scale (NIHSS) (Continued)

INSTRUCTIONS	SCALE DEFINITION
10. Dysarthria* If the patient is thought to be normal, an adequate sample of speech must be obtained by asking the patient to read or repeat words from the test list. If the patient has severe aphasia, the clarity of articulation of spontaneous speech can be rated. Only if the patient is intubated or has other physical barriers to producing speech, the examiner should record the score as untestable (UN) and clearly write an explanation for this choice. Do not tell the patient why he or she is being tested.	0 = Normal. 1 = Mild-to-moderate dysarthria; patient slurs at least some words and, at worst, can be understood with some difficulty. 2 = Severe dysarthria; patient's speech is so slurred as to be unintelligible in the absence of or out of proportion to any dysphasia, or is mute/anarthric.
11. Extinction and inattention Sufficient information to identify neglect may be obtained during the prior testing. If the patient has a severe vision loss preventing visual double simultaneous stimulation and the responses to cutaneous stimuli are normal, the score is 0. If the patient has aphasia but does appear to attend to both sides, the score is 0. The presence of visual spatial neglect or anosognosia may also be taken as evidence of abnormality. Since the abnormality is scored only if present, the item is never scored as untestable.	0 = No abnormality. 1 = Visual, tactile, auditory, spatial, or personal inattention or extinction to bilateral simultaneous stimulation in one of the sensory modalities. 2 = Profound hemi-inattention or extinction in more than one modality; patient does not recognize own hand or orients to only one side of space.

*Item deleted from modified NIHSS.
†Scale for item 8 is compressed to two elements (0 = Normal; 1 = Abnormal) for modified NIHSS.

the threshold number of RBCs needed in the CSF to be considered diagnostic of SAH is still unclear. Xanthochromia is best excluded by spectrometric means.

- A normal head CT, no xanthochromia, and zero or few RBCs ($<5 \times 10^6$ RBCs/L) are generally considered to exclude an SAH.
- Other diagnostic tests that may be useful in certain patients to rule out stroke mimics or concurrent conditions include a complete blood count, ECG, pulse oximetry, electrolyte and coagulation studies, cardiac enzyme levels, toxicology screen, blood alcohol level, echocardiogram, and carotid duplex scanning.

EMERGENCY DEPARTMENT CARE AND DISPOSITION

- Rapid assessment and stabilization of any airway, breathing, and circulation abnormalities is paramount.
- Routine supplemental oxygen is not indicated, but O_2 saturation should be kept ≥94%.
- IV access should be established while the patient is placed on a cardiac monitor.
- A rapid bedside glucose determination should be done and any hypoglycemia normalized.
- The patient should be kept NPO, on strict bedrest, and aspiration and fall precautions instituted.
- Once the patient's condition is stabilized, the patient should be sent for a noncontrast head CT scan.
- If a patient is not a candidate for thrombolysis, then permissive hypertension is in order (ie, no intervention unless systolic blood pressure [SBP] >220 mm Hg or diastolic blood pressure [DBP] >120 mm Hg). If blood pressure control is needed, a titratable intravenous antihypertensive should be used, such as labetalol (typical starting dose is 10-20 milligrams over 1-2 minutes IVP; continuous infusion dosage generally starts at 2 milligrams/min, titrated to effect) with a target MAP reduction of 10% to 25%. Extreme caution should be taken to avoid overcorrection.
- If a patient is a candidate for recombinant tissue plasminogen activator (rtPA), the target blood pressures are SBP ≤ 185 mm Hg and DBP ≤ 110 mm Hg prior to administration of rtPA (see Table 143-7).
- IV rtPA has been approved for treatment of acute ischemic stroke ≤3 hours of symptom onset.
- The American Heart Association/American Stroke Association recommends expansion of the rtPA treatment window to 4.5 hours, but this indication is still awaiting approval by the U.S. FDA at the time of this writing and is considered "off-label."
- A careful review of rtPA inclusion and exclusion criteria must be meticulously performed prior to administration of rtPA (Table 143-4).
- If the therapeutic window is to be extended to 3 to 4.5 hours, then the additional European Cooperative Acute Stroke Study 3 (ECASS III) exclusion criteria should be used (Table 143-5).
- Informed consent must be obtained from the patient or their designee prior to thrombolytic therapy.
- The risk of symptomatic intracerebral hemorrhage (SIH) is 6.4% (45% mortality) when rtPA is given within ≤3 hours of symptom onset and 7.9% (NINDS definition) between 3 and 4.5 hours.

TABLE 143-7 Approach to Management of Arterial Hypertension Before Potential Administration of Recombinant Tissue Plasminogen Activator (rtPA)

If the patient is a candidate for rtPA therapy, the target arterial blood pressures are: **systolic blood pressure ≤185 mm Hg and diastolic blood pressure ≤110 mm Hg**

DRUG	COMMENTS
Labetalol, 10-20 milligrams IV over 1-2 min, may repeat ×1	Use with caution in patients with severe asthma, severe chronic obstructive pulmonary disease, congestive heart failure, diabetes mellitus, myasthenia gravis, concurrent calcium channel blocker use, hepatic insufficiency. May cause dizziness and nausea. Pregnancy category C (D in second and third trimesters).
or	
Nitroglycerin paste, 1-2 in. to skin	Contraindicated in patients with hypersensitivity to organic nitrates, concurrent use of phosphodiesterase 5 inhibitors (sildenafil, tadalafil, or vardenafil), or angle-closure glaucoma. Increases intracranial pressure. Commonly causes headache. Pregnancy category C.
or	
Nicardipine infusion, 5 milligrams/h, titrate up by 2.5 milligrams/h at 5- to 15-min intervals; maximum dose, 15 milligrams/h; when desired blood pressure attained, reduce to 3 milligrams/h	Use with caution in patients with myocardial ischemia, concurrent use of fentanyl (hypotension), congestive heart failure, hypertrophic cardiomyopathy, portal hypertension, renal insufficiency, hepatic insufficiency (may need to adjust starting dose). Contraindicated in patients with severe aortic stenosis. Can cause headache, flushing, dizziness, nausea, reflex tachycardia. Pregnancy category C.

If the target arterial blood pressures for rtPA administration cannot be reached with these initial measures, then *the patient is no longer a candidate for rtPA therapy*.

- The total dose of rtPA is 0.9 milligrams/kg IV, with a maximum dose of 90 milligrams; 10% of the dose is administered as a bolus, with the remaining amount infused over 60 minutes.
- No aspirin or heparin should be administered in the initial 24 hours after treatment with rtPA. Aspirin (325 milligrams orally) is indicated within 24 to 48 hours if the patient is not at risk for aspiration.
- Intracerebral bleeding should be suspected as the cause of any neurologic worsening.

TABLE 143-8 Management of Blood Pressure during and after Administration of Recombinant Tissue Plasminogen Activator (rtPA)

Blood Pressure Monitoring Frequencies

Time after start of rtPA infusion	Frequency of blood pressure monitoring
0-3 h	Every 15 min
3-9 h	Every 30 min
9-24 h	Every 60 min

Drug Treatment of Hypertension during and after Administration of rtPA

If systolic blood pressure is 180-230 mm Hg *or* Diastolic blood pressure is 105-120 mm Hg	Labetalol, 10 milligrams IV over 1-2 min. The dose may be repeated every 10-20 min up to a total dose of 300 milligrams. *or* Labetalol, 10 milligrams IV followed by infusion at 2-8 milligrams/min.
If systolic blood pressure is >230 mm Hg *or* Diastolic blood pressure is 121-140 mm Hg	Labetalol, 10 milligrams IV over 1-2 min. The dose may be repeated every 10-20 min up to a total dose of 300 milligrams. *or* Labetalol, 10 milligrams IV followed by infusion at 2-8 milligrams/min. *or* Nicardipine infusion, 5 milligrams/h, titrate up by 2.5 milligrams/h at 5- to 15-min intervals; maximum dose 15 milligrams/h.
If blood pressure is not controlled by above measures	Consider sodium nitroprusside infusion (0.5-10 microgram/kg/min). Continuous arterial monitoring advised; use with caution in patients with hepatic or renal insufficiency. Increases intracranial pressure. Pregnancy category C.

- Patients who receive rtPA should have their blood pressure monitored closely and treated if necessary (see Table 143-8).
- For TIA patients, aspirin (325 milligrams orally) plus dipyridamole (400 milligrams orally) is recommended. Antiplatelet therapy is contraindicated for hemorrhagic stroke.
- Heparin or warfarin in the acute treatment of TIA or stroke in the ED is not indicated, even in the presence of atrial fibrillation. A possible exception exists for a weight-based heparin protocol in CAD, but this remains controversial.
- If an ischemic stroke patient presents outside the rtPA therapeutic time window, then aggressive supportive

care should be given in the ED (aspiration prevention, normalization of glucose level, fall precautions, and treatment for comorbidities).

- For patients with evidence of increased intracranial pressure (ICP), head elevation to 30°, analgesia, and sedation are indicated. If more aggressive ICP reduction is indicated, mannitol (0.25-1.0 gram/kg IV), intubation with neuromuscular blockade with mild hyperventilation, and invasive monitoring of ICP may be required.
- In SAH, the chances of rebleeding can be reduced by maintaining the patient's prebleed blood pressure (or MAP <130 mm Hg if baseline blood pressure is unknown). An IV titratable antihypertensive such as labetalol (typical adult starting dose is 10-20 milligrams over 1-2 minutes IVP; continuous infusion dosage generally starts at 2 milligrams/min, titrated to effect) should be used. Nimodipine (60 milligrams orally every 4 hours) may produce modest improvements in outcome by decreasing vasospasm.
- Emergent neurosurgical consultation is indicated in SAH patients. Pain medications and antiemetics should be used as needed.
- Seizure prophylaxis for SAH is controversial and should be discussed with the specialist who will manage the patient after they leave the ED.
- Evidence for the management of blood pressure when spontaneous ICH is present remains controversial. Current guidelines are listed in Table 143-9.
- Emergent consultation with a neurologist may be helpful in difficult stroke cases where thrombolytics are a consideration; however, therapy should not be unduly delayed while waiting for a response.

TABLE 143-9 Suggested Guidelines for Treating Elevated Blood Pressure in Spontaneous Intracranial Hemorrhage

CLINICAL CIRCUMSTANCES	MANAGEMENT
SBP >200 mm Hg or MAP >150 mm Hg	Consider aggressive reduction of blood pressure with continuous IV infusion.
SBP >180 mm Hg or MAP >130 mm Hg and evidence or suspicion of elevated ICP	Consider monitoring ICP and reducing blood pressure using intermittent or continuous IV medications to keep cerebral perfusion pressure >60-80 mm Hg.
SBP >180 mm Hg or MAP >130 mm Hg and no evidence or suspicion of elevated ICP	Consider a modest reduction of blood pressure (eg, MAP of 110 mm Hg or target blood pressure of 160/90 mm Hg) using intermittent or continuous IV medications.

Abbreviations: ICP = intracranial pressure, MAP = mean arterial pressure, SBP = systolic blood pressure.

TABLE 143-10 ABCD² Score to Predict Very Early Stroke Risk after Transient Ischemic Attack

CRITERIA	POINTS
Age ≥60 y	0 = Absent 1 = Present
Blood pressure ≥140/90 mm Hg	0 = Absent 1 = Present
Clinical features	0 = Absent 1 = Speech impairment without unilateral weakness 2 = Unilateral weakness (with or without speech impairment)
Duration	0 = Absent 1 = 10-59 min 2 = ≥60 min
Diabetes	0 = Absent 1 = Present

- Early neurosurgical consultation is indicated for patients with ICH with evidence of increased ICP or in other conditions where surgical intervention may be indicated (eg, cerebellar stroke).
- All patients with acute ischemic stroke or ICH should be admitted, even if they are not candidates for interventional therapy.
- Admission to specialized stroke units is associated with improved outcomes; therefore, transfer to a designated stroke center may be indicated if the patient presents to a non-stroke center.
- The ABCD² scoring system may be used to predict stroke risk in TIA patients (see Table 143-10).
- Using the ABCD², the 2-day risks of subsequent stroke are 1% (ABCD² score 0-3); 4.1% (4-5); and 8.1% (6-7).
- Because of the proven efficacy of early carotid endarterectomy, many stroke experts recommend admission for most TIA patients for inpatient evaluation and observation. In select low-risk, asymptomatic patients, next-day follow-up and evaluation with a specialist may be appropriate, but responsible adults to observe the patient in a favorable social situation must be available and very explicit return precautions given.
- All CAD and SAH patients should be admitted with appropriate specialty consultation.

For further reading in Tintinalli's *Emergency Medicine: A Comprehensive Study Guide*, 7th ed., see Chapter 160, "Spontaneous Subarachnoid and Intracerebral Hemorrhage," by Jeffrey L. Hackman, Melissa D. Johnson, and O. John Ma, and Chapter 161, "Stroke, Transient Ischemic Attack, and Cervical Artery Dissection," by Steven Go and Daniel J. Worman.

144 ALTERED MENTAL STATUS AND COMA

C. Crawford Mechem

DELIRIUM

EPIDEMIOLOGY

- One quarter of ED patients aged 70 years or older have impaired mental status or delirium.
- On admission, 10% to 25% of elderly patients have delirium.

PATHOPHYSIOLOGY

- Pathologic mechanisms producing delirium are thought to involve widespread neuronal or neurotransmitter dysfunction.
- The four general causes are primary intracranial disease, systemic diseases secondarily affecting the central nervous system (CNS), exogenous toxins, and drug withdrawal.

CLINICAL FEATURES

- Delirium generally develops over days, with fluctuating symptoms (Table 144-1).
- Attention, perception, thinking, and memory are altered.
- Alertness is reduced, manifested by difficulty maintaining attention and concentration.
- The patient may fluctuate rapidly between hypoactive and hyperactive states.
- The sleep-wake cycle may be disrupted, with somnolence by day and agitation at night.
- Tremor, asterixis, tachycardia, sweating, hypertension, and emotional outbursts may be present.
- Hallucinations tend to be visual, although auditory hallucinations can also occur.

TABLE 144-1 Features of Delirium, Dementia, and Psychiatric Disorder

CHARACTERISTIC	DELIRIUM	DEMENTIA	PSYCHIATRIC DISORDER
Onset	Over days	Insidious	Sudden
Course over 24 h	Fluctuating	Stable	Stable
Consciousness	Reduced or hyperalert	Alert	Alert
Attention	Disordered	Normal	May be disordered
Cognition	Disordered	Impaired	May be impaired
Orientation	Impaired	Often impaired	May be impaired
Hallucinations	Visual and/or auditory	Often absent	Usually auditory
Delusions	Transient, poorly organized	Usually absent	Sustained
Movements	Asterixis, tremor may be present	Often absent	Absent

DIAGNOSIS AND DIFFERENTIAL

- Both historical and physical examination findings are needed to confirm the diagnosis.
- The acute onset of attention deficits and cognitive abnormalities fluctuating in severity throughout the day and worsening at night ("sundowning") is virtually diagnostic.
- Diagnostic testing is directed at identifying an underlying process and should include serum electrolytes, hepatic and renal studies, urinalysis, CBC, and a chest radiograph.
- A head CT scan should be performed if a mass lesion is suspected, followed by lumbar puncture if meningitis or subarachnoid hemorrhage is a consideration.
- The differential diagnosis of delirium in the elderly is listed in Table 144-2.

TABLE 144-2 Important Medical Causes of Delirium in Elderly Patients

Infectious	Pneumonia Urinary tract infection Meningitis or encephalitis Sepsis
Metabolic/toxic	Hypoglycemia Alcohol ingestion Electrolyte abnormalities Hepatic encephalopathy Thyroid disorders Alcohol or drug withdrawal
Neurologic	Stroke or transient ischemic attack Seizure or postictal state Subarachnoid hemorrhage Intracranial hemorrhage Central nervous system mass lesion Subdural hematoma
Cardiopulmonary	Congestive heart failure Myocardial infarction Pulmonary embolism Hypoxia or CO_2 narcosis
Drug-related	Anticholinergic drugs Alcohol or drug withdrawal Sedatives-hypnotics Narcotic analgesics Polypharmacy

EMERGENCY DEPARTMENT CARE AND DISPOSITION

- Treatment is directed at the underlying cause.
- Sedation is often necessary to relieve agitation. Haloperidol, 5 to 10 milligrams PO, IV, or IM, is a frequent first choice. The dose should be reduced to 1 to 2 milligrams in the elderly.
- Lorazepam, 0.5 to 2 milligrams PO, IV, or IM, may be used in conjunction with haloperidol, with the dose dictated by the patient's age and weight.
- Unless a readily reversible cause is identified and corrected and there is a return to baseline, most patients should be admitted for further evaluation and treatment.

DEMENTIA

PATHOPHYSIOLOGY

- Most cases in the United States are due to Alzheimer's disease. The pathophysiology involves a reduction in neurons in the cerebral cortex, increased amyloid deposition, and the production of neurofibrillary tangles and plaques.
- Vascular dementia accounts for the next largest number of cases and is a cerebrovascular disease with multiple infarctions.

CLINICAL FEATURES

- Impairment of memory, particularly recent memory, is gradual and progressive. Remote memories are often preserved. Alzheimer's disease is often associated with memory impairment and disorientation with preservation of motor and speech abilities.
- Symptoms are progressive and include problems naming objects, forgetting items, trouble reading, decreased performance in social situations, disorientation, difficulty with self-care tasks, personality changes, depression, anxiety, and speech difficulties.
- Patients with vascular dementia often show similar symptoms, but may also have abnormalities of deep tendon reflexes, gait abnormalities, or weakness of an extremity.

DIAGNOSIS AND DIFFERENTIAL

- The history of memory problems in Alzheimer's disease is usually one of slow onset and progression. If specific dates of worsening are noted, the possibility of vascular dementia increases.
- Physical examination may be helpful in identifying associated causes and should include a detailed mental status examination.
- Diagnostic testing may include a CBC, metabolic profile, urinalysis, thyroid function tests, serum vitamin B_{12} level, and serologic testing for syphilis in patients at risk. Other tests may include an ESR, serum folate level, HIV testing, and chest radiograph.
- Cranial CT or MRI should be considered at some point in the diagnostic evaluation.
- A lumbar puncture should be performed if the diagnosis is not readily apparent.
- The differential includes delirium, depression, infection, inflammatory processes, malignancy, toxins, trauma, metabolic disturbances, and normal-pressure hydrocephalus. Normal-pressure hydrocephalus should be considered in the setting of urinary incontinence and gait disturbance. Head CT will reveal excessively large ventricles.

EMERGENCY DEPARTMENT CARE AND DISPOSITION

- All types of dementia may be amenable to environmental or psychosocial interventions.
- Due to adverse effects, antipsychotic drugs should be reserved for patients with persistent psychotic features or those with extreme disruptive or dangerous behaviors.
- Treatment of vascular dementia is directed at risk factors, including hypertension.
- If normal-pressure hydrocephalus is suspected, a trial of lumbar puncture with cerebrospinal fluid (CSF) drainage may be considered.
- Most patients with a new diagnosis of dementia will require admission for further evaluation and management. However, patients with long-standing symptoms, consistent caregivers, and reliable follow-up may be discharged for outpatient evaluation after life-threatening conditions have been excluded.

COMA

- Coma is a state of reduced alertness and responsiveness from which the patient cannot be aroused. The Glasgow Coma Scale is widely used as a scoring system in patients with altered mental status (Table 144-3).

PATHOPHYSIOLOGY

- Coma may be due to a systemic disease that affects the CNS secondarily or a primary CNS process. Both cerebral hemispheres or the brain stem must be involved.
- Examples of systemic disease secondarily resulting in coma are hypoxia and hypoglycemia, in which substrates needed for neuronal function are lacking.

TABLE 144-3 Glasgow Coma Scale

COMPONENT	SCORE	ADULT	CHILD <5 YR	CHILD >5 YR
Motor	6	Follows commands	Normal spontaneous movements	Follows commands
	5	Localizes pain	Localizes to supraocular pain (>9 mo)	
	4	Withdraws to pain	Withdraws from nail bed pressure	
	3	Flexion	Flexion to supraocular pain	
	2	Extension	Extension to supraocular pain	
	1	None	None	
Verbal	5	Oriented	Age-appropriate speech/vocalizations	Oriented
	4	Confused speech	Less than usual ability; irritable cry	Confused
	3	Inappropriate words	Cries to pain	Inappropriate words
	2	Incomprehensible	Moans to pain	Incomprehensible
	1	None	No response to pain	
Eye opening	4	Spontaneous	Spontaneous	
	3	To command	To voice	
	2	To pain	To pain	
	1	None	None	

- In primary CNS causes, coma may result from bilateral cortical dysfunction, localized brain stem pathology, or elevated intracranial pressure with decreased cerebral perfusion.
- Brain stem disorders include hemorrhage and herniation syndromes.
- Uncal herniation results from an expanding mass that causes the medial temporal lobe to shift and compress the brain stem. The ipsilateral pupil will be fixed and dilated. Hemiparesis ipsilateral to the mass may develop from compression of descending motor tracts in the opposite cerebral peduncle.
- Central herniation syndrome is characterized by progressive loss of consciousness, loss of brain stem reflexes, decorticate posturing, and irregular respirations.

CLINICAL FEATURES

- Clinical features vary with the depth of coma and the cause.
- Pupillary and other cranial nerve findings, hemiparesis, and response to stimulation can often assign the cause to diffuse CNS dysfunction (toxic-metabolic coma) or focal CNS dysfunction (structural coma).
- Diffuse CNS dysfunction can result from toxic and metabolic conditions. Physical findings do not point to a specific region of brain dysfunction. If present, movements and muscle stretch reflexes are symmetric. Pupillary response is generally preserved. The pupils are small but reactive, and extraocular movements, if present, are symmetric.
- Structural coma may be further subdivided into hemispheric (supratentorial) or posterior fossa (infratentorial) coma.
- Coma from hemispheric lesions or supratentorial masses may present with progressive hemiparesis or asymmetric muscle tone and reflexes. Coma without lateralizing signs may result from decreased cerebral perfusion secondary to increased ICP. In severe cases, hypertension and bradycardia (the Cushing reflex) may develop.
- Coma from infratentorial or posterior fossa lesions, such as an expanding cerebellar hemorrhage, may cause abrupt coma, abnormal extensor posturing, loss of pupillary reflexes, and loss of extraocular movements. Brain stem compression with loss of brain stem reflexes may develop rapidly. Another infratentorial cause of coma, pontine hemorrhage, may present with pinpoint-sized pupils.
- Pseudocoma or psychogenic coma may generally be distinguished from true coma by good history taking and observation of responses to stimulation. Pupillary responses, extraocular movements, muscle tone, and reflexes are intact. The patient may resist manual eye opening. The patient may consistently look away from the examiner, and nystagmus will be demonstrated with caloric vestibular testing.

DIAGNOSIS AND DIFFERENTIAL

- Assessment is directed at rapidly determining if the CNS dysfunction is from diffuse impairment or from a local, and perhaps surgically treatable, lesion.

- History, physical examination, lab tests, and neuroimaging will usually identify the cause.
- Abrupt coma suggests an acute CNS process such as stroke or seizures, whereas gradual onset suggests a progressive CNS lesion or a metabolic process such as hyperglycemia.
- General examination may reveal signs of trauma or suggest other diagnostic possibilities, such as a toxidrome.
- Asymmetric muscle tone or reflexes, or asymmetric findings on examination of cranial nerves through papillary examination, assessment of corneal reflexes, and testing of oculovestibular reflexes suggest a focal lesion.
- CT is the initial neuroimaging of choice.
- Lumbar puncture should be considered if CT findings are unremarkable and CNS bleeding or infection is suspected.
- Basilar artery thrombosis should be suspected in a comatose patient with a "normal" head CT, in which the only finding may be a hyperdense basilar artery. MRI or cerebral angiography is needed to make the diagnosis.
- If nonconvulsive status epilepticus or subtle status epilepticus is suspected, urgent electroencephalography should be performed and neurologic consultation sought.
- In the pediatric patient, toxic ingestions, infections, and child abuse have a greater frequency and should be actively investigated.
- The differential diagnosis includes generalized disease processes that also affect the brain, as well as primary CNS disorders (Table 144-4).

TABLE 144-4 Differential Diagnosis of Coma

Coma from causes affecting the brain diffusely
Encephalopathies
Hypoxic encephalopathy
Metabolic encephalopathy
Hypoglycemia
Hyperosmolar state (eg, hyperglycemia)
Electrolyte abnormalities (eg, hypernatremia or hyponatremia, hypercalcemia)
Organ system failure
Hepatic encephalopathy
Uremia/renal failure
Endocrine (eg, Addison disease, hypothyroidism, etc.)
Hypoxia
CO_2 narcosis
Hypertensive encephalopathy
Toxins
Drug reactions (eg, neuroleptic malignant syndrome)
Environmental causes—hypothermia, hyperthermia
Deficiency state—Wernicke's encephalopathy
Sepsis
Coma from primary CNS disease or trauma
Direct CNS trauma
Diffuse axonal injury
Subdural hematoma
Epidural hematoma
Vascular disease
Intraparenchymal hemorrhage (hemispheric, basal ganglia, brain stem, cerebellar)
Subarachnoid hemorrhage
Infarction
Hemispheric, brain stem
CNS infections
Neoplasms
Seizures
Nonconvulsive status epilepticus
Postictal state

Abbreviation: CNS = central nervous system.

EMERGENCY DEPARTMENT CARE AND DISPOSITION

- Treatment involves identification of the etiology and initiation of specific therapy.
- Stabilization of airway, ventilation, and circulation is the top priority.
- Readily reversible causes such as hypoglycemia, hypoxia, and opiate overdose should be sought. In the setting of hypoglycemia, thiamine should be administered before glucose in patients with a suspected history of alcohol abuse or malnutrition.
- Naloxone administration is prudent because signs of opiate overdose may be absent.
- If increased ICP is suspected, steps should be taken to reduce it or minimize further rise.
- In intubated patients, paralysis and sedation should be used to prevent the patient from "bucking" the ventilator.
- The head should be elevated 30 degrees and at midline to aid in venous drainage.
- Mannitol, 0.5 to 1.0 gram/kg IV, may transiently reduce ICP.
- In cases of brain edema associated with tumor, dexamethasone, 10 milligrams IV, reduces edema over several hours.

- Hyperventilation can reduce cerebral blood volume and transiently lower ICP. Current recommendations are to avoid excessive hyperventilation (partial pressure of arterial carbon dioxide ≤35 mm Hg) during the first 24 hours after brain injury.
- Patients with readily reversible causes of coma, such as insulin-induced hypoglycemia, may be discharged if treatment is initiated, the patient returns to baseline mental status, the cause of the episode is clear, and the patient has reliable home care and follow-up.
- In all other cases, admission is warranted for further evaluation and treatment.

For further reading in Tintinalli's *Emergency Medicine: A Comprehensive Study Guide*, 7th ed., see Chapter 162, "Altered Mental Status and Coma," by J. Stephen Huff.

145 ATAXIA AND GAIT DISTURBANCES

Ross J. Fleischman

PATHOPHYSIOLOGY

- Ataxia is the failure to produce smooth, intentional movements.
- Ataxia and gait disturbances are not diseases in themselves, but are symptoms of systemic or nervous system conditions.

CLINICAL FEATURES

- Orthostatic vital sign changes and abnormalities beyond the neurologic examination point to systemic illness.
- Key symptoms of serious problems beyond the sensory and motor systems include headache, nausea, fever, and decreased level of alertness.
- Nystagmus suggests an intracranial cause.
- Cerebellar lesions (motor ataxia) are suggested by dysmetria (undershoot or overshoot on finger-to-nose testing) and dysdiadochokinesia (clumsy rapid alternating movements when flipping palms on thighs). Overshoot when sliding one heel down the opposite shin is a sign of cerebellar disease while a wavering course suggests a deficit of proprioception.
- Vibration and position sense in the toes test the posterior columns, which degenerate in tabes dorsalis (neurosyphilis) and vitamin B_{12} deficiency.
- Ask the patient to stand with arms at sides. Instability with the eyes open suggests a cerebellar lesion. Worsening instability with eye closure (a positive Romberg sign) suggests that the patient is relying on visual input for balance caused by a sensory ataxia including posterior column disease or vestibular dysfunction.
- Observing the patient rise from a chair and walk, including tandem walking (heel to toe), is critical, as this may expose subtle weakness and ataxia.
- Motor ataxia is characterized by broad-based, unsteady steps.
- Peroneal muscle weakness causes foot drop, known as an *equine* gait.
- Sensory ataxia with loss of proprioception may be notable for abrupt movements and slapping of the feet with each impact.
- A *senile* gait which is slow, broad based, and shortened may be seen with normal aging, neurodegenerative disease such as Parkinson's, and normal pressure hydrocephalus. Parkinson's disease may also manifest with a festinating gait, which is narrow based, with small shuffling steps that become more rapid.

DIAGNOSIS AND DIFFERENTIAL

- Attempt to classify the problem as a systemic versus nervous system disorder (Table 145-1).
- The extent of ED evaluation will depend on the acuity and severity of symptoms, with patients who have become unable to walk over hours to days requiring extensive evaluation.
- An abrupt onset of gait disturbance and a severe headache may reflect intracranial hemorrhage and should be evaluated by non-contrast CT.
- CT scan is less sensitive than MRI for lesions of the posterior fossa, and is insensitive for acute ischemia.
- A lumbar puncture should be performed if central nervous system infection is suspected.
- Vitamin B_{12} deficiency should be considered in patients with loss of position sense in the second toe or a positive Romberg test, caused by degeneration of the posterior columns. A serum cyanocobalamin level and complete blood count are the initial steps in evaluation, although neurologic manifestations often precede macrocytic anemia.
- Tabes dorsalis (neurosyphilis) causes similar symptoms of posterior column disease and can be screened for by the VDRL or RPR tests.
- Normal pressure hydrocephalus should be suspected in an elderly patient with a broad-based, shuffling gait, urinary incontinence, and dementia. Non-contrast CT scan will show ventricular dilatation out of proportion to sulcal atrophy.

TABLE 145-1	Common Etiologies of Acute Ataxia and Gait Disturbances
Systemic conditions	
Intoxications with diminished alertness	
Ethanol	
Sedative-hypnotics	
Intoxications with relatively preserved alertness (diminished alertness at higher levels)	
Phenytoin	
Carbamazepine	
Valproic acid	
Heavy metals—lead, organic mercurials	
Other metabolic disorders	
Hyponatremia	
Inborn errors of metabolism	
Wernicke's disease	
Disorders predominantly of the nervous system	
Conditions affecting predominantly one region of the central nervous system	
Cerebellum	
Hemorrhage	
Infarction	
Degenerative changes	
Abscess	
Cortex	
Frontal tumor, hemorrhage, or trauma	
Hydrocephalus	
Subcortical	
Thalamic infarction or hemorrhage	
Parkinson's disease	
Normal pressure hydrocephalus	
Spinal cord	
Cervical spondylosis	
Posterior column disorders	
Conditions affecting predominantly the peripheral nervous system	
Peripheral neuropathy	
Vestibulopathy	

EMERGENCY DEPARTMENT CARE AND DISPOSITION

- Administer thiamine 100 milligrams IV to alcoholics and other malnourished individuals who might have Wernicke's encephalopathy, which is suggested by findings of ataxia, altered mental status (confusion and impairment of short-term memory), and ophthalmoplegia.
- Patients with an acute inability to walk or who cannot be cared for at home may require admission for further evaluation.

For further reading in Tintinalli's *Emergency Medicine: A Comprehensive Study Guide*, 7th ed., see Chapter 163, "Ataxia and Gait Disturbances," by J. Stephen Huff.

146 VERTIGO AND DIZZINESS

Steven Go

EPIDEMIOLOGY

- The estimated percentage of ED visits attributed to the complaint of "dizziness" is approximately 4%.
- A cross-sectional analysis of older adolescents and adult visits to US ED's found that the most common causes included otologic/vestibular (32.9%), cardiovascular (21.1%), respiratory (11.5%), neurologic (11.2%), metabolic (11.0%), injury/poisoning (10.6%), psychiatric (7.2%), digestive (7.0%), genitourinary (5.1%), and infectious (2.9%). "Dangerous" disorders were diagnosed in 15% and were especially common in patients >50 years of age.

PATHOPHYSIOLOGY

- Vertigo results from the mismatch of the perception of movement by the visual, vestibular, and proprioceptive symptoms when none actually exists.
- The visual system provides spatial orientation; the vestibular system provides the body's orientation with respect to gravity, while the proprioceptive system helps relate body movements and indicates the position of the head relative to the body.

CLINICAL FEATURES

- Vertigo presents as a sensation of movement when none exists. Patients often say that the "room is spinning," but other descriptions may include rocking, tilting, somersaulting, and descending in an elevator.
- Vertigo is classically separated into two general types: peripheral and central (Table 146-1).
- Peripheral vertigo (involving vestibular apparatus and the eighth cranial nerve) usually has a sudden onset and intense symptoms.

TABLE 146-1 Differentiating Peripheral from Central Vertigo

	PERIPHERAL	CENTRAL
Onset	Sudden	Sudden or slow
Severity of vertigo	Intense spinning	Ill defined, less intense
Pattern	Paroxysmal, intermittent	Constant
Aggravated by position/movement	Yes	Variable
Associated nausea/diaphoresis	Frequent	Variable
Nystagmus	Rotatory-vertical, horizontal	Vertical
Fatigue of symptoms/signs	Yes	No
Hearing loss/tinnitus	May occur	Does not occur
Abnormal tympanic membrane	May occur	Does not occur
Central nervous system symptoms/signs	Absent	Usually present

- Central vertigo (involving brain stem and cerebellum) can present abruptly or gradually, but usually has more ill-defined, less severe symptoms.
- In general, causes of peripheral vertigo tend not to be life-threatening, whereas central vertigo are often more serious; however, this is not true in all cases and significant overlap of presentations can exist.

DIAGNOSIS AND DIFFERENTIAL

- The etiology for vertigo is found in Table 146-2.
- Initially, focus the history on whether true vertigo actually exists because it is often confused with "lightheadedness" or near syncope/syncope, which has its own differential and workup.
- The initial episode should be described in detail by the patient, including speed of onset, severity, associated symptoms (especially involving loss of consciousness or the cranial nerves with special emphasis on aural symptoms), and temporal pattern (Table 146-3). Risk factors for stroke (age, hypertension, cardiovascular disease) and coagulopathy should be investigated.
- Physical examination should include eye, ear, neurologic, and vestibular examinations, with particular focus on the cranial nerves and cerebellum.
- Note the type (horizontal, vertical, rotatory) and direction of the fast component of any nystagmus. Isolated vertical nystagmus (without a rotary component) usually indicates a brain stem abnormality.
- If benign paroxysmal positional vertigo (BPPV, see below) is suspected, a Dix-Hallpike position test may be useful.

TABLE 146-2 An Etiologic Classification of Vertigo

Vestibular/otologic	Benign paroxysmal positional vertigo Traumatic: following head injury Infection: labyrinthitis, vestibular neuronitis, Ramsay Hunt syndrome
Syndrome	Ménière syndrome Neoplastic Vascular Otosclerosis Paget disease Toxic or drug-induced: aminoglycosides
Neurologic	Vertebrobasilar insufficiency Lateral Wallenberg syndrome Anterior inferior cerebellar artery syndrome Neoplastic: cerebellopontine angle tumors Cerebellar disorders: hemorrhage, degeneration Basal ganglion diseases Multiple sclerosis Infections: neurosyphilis, tuberculosis Epilepsy Migraine headaches Cerebrovascular disease
General	Hematologic: anemia, polycythemia, hyperviscosity syndrome Toxic: alcohol Chronic renal failure Metabolic: thyroid disease, hypoglycemia

- Based on history and physical examination, tentatively classify the vertigo as peripheral or central to help narrow the differential and direct the workup.
- Suggested ancillary testing for various specific vertigo-associated conditions are summarized in Table 146-4.
- In general, laboratory investigations are not indicated in true vertiginous patients unless a specific cause for central vertigo is being investigated.
- With regards to imaging, obtain an emergent noncontrast head CT in elders, patients who have signs/symptoms of central vertigo (especially cranial nerve or cerebellar findings), hypertension, cardiovascular disease, other stroke risks, coagulopathy (eg, taking warfarin), headache, or for intractable or persistent (>72 hours) symptoms. If vertebrobasilar insufficiency

TABLE 146-3 Temporal Patterns Seen in Vertigo

PATTERN	CONDITIONS
Seconds	Benign paroxysmal positional vertigo, postural hypotension
Minutes	Transient ischemic attacks
Hours	Ménière disease
Days	Viral labyrinthitis
Constant	Nonspecific dizziness

TABLE 146-4 Ancillary Testing of Vertigo and Dizziness

CONDITION	SUGGESTED TESTS
Bacterial labyrinthitis	CBC, blood cultures, CT scan or MRI for possible abscess, lumbar puncture if meningitis suspected
Vertigo associated with closed head injury	CT scan or MRI
Near-syncope	ECG, Holter monitor, CBC, glucose, electrolytes, renal function, table tilt testing
Cardiac dysrhythmias	ECG, Holter monitor
Suspected valvular heart disease	ECG, echocardiography
Nonspecific dizziness; disequilibrium of aging	CBC, electrolytes, glucose, renal function tests
Thyrotoxicosis	Thyroid stimulating hormone, triiodothyronine, thyroxine
Cerebellar hemorrhage, infarction, or tumor	CT or MRI
Vertebral artery dissection	Cerebral angiogram to include neck vessels or MRA
Vertebrobasilar insufficiency	ECG, cardiac monitoring, echocardiogram, carotid Doppler, MRI, MRA

Abbreviations: CBC = complete blood count, MRA = magnetic resonance angiography.

(VBI) is a consideration, MRI with MRA (or CT angiogram) and duplex US of the carotids are indicated.

DISORDERS CAUSING PERIPHERAL VERTIGO

- BPPV is thought to be caused by loose otoliths that enter the posterior semicircular canal and cause the inappropriate sensation of motion. BPPV occurs most often in women over age 50 years. Cranial nerve or central nervous system (CNS) findings are absent. Findings suggestive of BPPV are listed in Table 146-5.

TABLE 146-5 Supportive Findings in Benign Paroxysmal Positional Vertigo

Latency period of <30 s between the provocative head position and onset of nystagmus.
The intensity of nystagmus increases to a peak before slowly resolving.
Duration of vertigo and nystagmus ranges from 5-40 s.
If nystagmus is produced in one direction by placing the head down, then the nystagmus reverses direction when the head is returned to the sitting position.
Repeated head positioning causes both the vertigo and accompanying nystagmus to fatigue and subside.

- The Dix-Hallpike position test can confirm BPPV. In this test, the patient begins seated with the head turned 45 degrees to the right. The patient is then rapidly lowered to a supine position with the head hanging over the edge of the bed an additional 30 to 45 degrees. Patients with BPPV will exhibit a short-lived nystagmus with the rapid component toward the affected ear. The patient is then returned to the sitting position and the maneuver is repeated with the head turned to the left. The side that is symptomatic serves as the starting point for the curative Epley maneuver.
- Ménière disease is characterized by recurrent bouts of sudden onset of (usually) unilateral roaring tinnitus and a sense of fullness and diminished hearing in the affected ear. Because the diagnosis requires multiple episodes of attacks with progressive hearing loss, Ménière syndrome cannot be diagnosed on the first presentation of vertigo. It can be confirmed by glycerol testing and by vestibular-evoked myogenic potentials.
- A perilymph fistula presents with sudden onset of vertigo during activities that can cause barotrauma such as flying, scuba diving, heavy lifting, and coughing. Infection can also cause a perilymph fistula, and the diagnosis is confirmed by nystagmus elicited by pneumatic otoscopy (Hennebert sign).
- Vestibular neuronitis is characterized by the sudden onset of severe vertigo sometimes associated with unilateral tinnitus and hearing loss. It is thought to be viral in nature, lasts several days to weeks, and does not recur.
- Vestibular ganglionitis causes vertigo when a neurotrophic virus such as varicella zoster reactivates. The most well-known variant, Ramsay Hunt syndrome (Herpes zoster oticus), is characterized by deafness, vertigo, and facial nerve palsy, associated with vesicles inside the external auditory canal.
- Labyrinthitis, although commonly viral, also can be due to bacterial infection from otitis media, meningitis, and mastoiditis and presents with sudden vertigo with hearing loss and middle ear findings.
- Ototoxicity may induce vertigo and hearing loss. Common offenders causing peripheral toxicity include salicylates, aminoglycosides, and cytotoxic agents. Anticonvulsants, antidepressants, neuroleptics, hydrocarbons, alcohol, and phencyclidine may cause centrally mediated vertigo.
- Tumors of the eighth cranial nerve and cerebellopontine angle, such as meningioma, acoustic neuroma, and acoustic schwannoma, also may present as vertigo with hearing loss. These tumors may be associated with ipsilateral facial weakness, impaired corneal reflexes, and cerebellar signs.

- Vertigo may occur after a closed head injury (especially a basilar skull fracture) and tends to resolve over weeks. Vertigo can also occur as a complication of cochlear implantation surgery.

DISORDERS CAUSING CENTRAL VERTIGO

- Cerebellar hemorrhage or infarction causes moderate vertigo and can be associated with nausea and vomiting. Cerebellar findings such as truncal ataxia, abnormal Romberg testing, and abnormal tandem gait are usually present. A sixth cranial nerve palsy or conjugate eye deviation away from the side of the hemorrhage can occur.
- Lateral medullary infarction of the brain stem (Wallenberg syndrome) causes vertigo and ipsilateral facial numbness, loss of the corneal reflex, Horner syndrome, dysphagia, and dysphonia secondary to pharyngeal and laryngeal paralysis. Contralateral loss of pain and temperature sensation in the trunk and extremities also occurs. Sixth, seventh, and eighth cranial nerve findings can also occur.
- VBI may result in sudden vertigo due to a brain stem transient ischemic attack that typically lasts minutes to up to 24 hours. Associated diplopia, dysphagia, dysarthria, blindness, and bilateral long tract signs (eg, clonus, muscle spasticity) and syncope may also be present. Unlike other causes of central vertigo, VBI may be induced by movement of the head due to decreased vertebral artery blood flow.
- Veterbral artery dissection (VAD) can be caused by sudden rotation of the head (motor vehicle crash, chiropractic adjustments, sneezing) and presents with central vertigo. Associated symptoms may include vertigo, headache, and unilateral Horner syndrome.
- Miscellaneous causes of central vertigo include multiple sclerosis, neoplasms, and basilar migraine.

OTHER CONDITIONS

- Disequilibrium of aging is a condition that presents with vague dizziness and gait unsteadiness in the elderly. It is associated with age-related degradation of hearing, balance, proprioception, and vision. Symptoms are worsened by dim lighting, nighttime hours, unfamiliar surroundings, and the use of medications with anticholinergic effects and benzodiazepines.
- Psychiatric dizziness presents as part of a known psychiatric disorder that is not associated with known vestibular disorders. This is often chronic and is frequently associated with anxiety disorders. This is a diagnosis of exclusion.

EMERGENCY DEPARTMENT CARE AND DISPOSITION

- In peripheral vertigo, first-line therapies include the antihistamines, such as diphenhydramine or meclizine, and antiemetics. Second-line drugs for treatment failures include antidopaminergic agents such as metoclopramide or promethazine. Transdermal scopolamine is not useful acutely due to its prolonged onset of action (4-8 hours), but may be used as a discharge medication. Benzodiazepines prevent the process of vestibular rehabilitation and should be used sparingly.
- Antivertigo medications can have undesirable anticholinergic side effects such as drowsiness and urinary retention; therefore, these drugs should not be used in combination.
- Treat patients with BPPV with the Epley maneuver to move the otoliths out of the semicircular canal; this may have curative effects in the ED. If the Epley maneuver is not completely successful, instruct the patient in vestibular rehabilitation exercises.
- Treat Ramsay Hunt syndrome (Herpes zoster oticus) with antiviral therapy and symptomatic treatment within 72 hours of vesicle appearance.
- Bacterial labyrinthitis requires appropriate antimicrobials and ENT consultation and admission.
- Most patients with peripheral vertigo may be discharged home with follow-up for further testing to their PCP or ENT specialist. Patients with tumors should receive neurosurgical consultation. Admit patients with intractable symptoms.
- Patients with central vertigo require imaging studies and specialty referral. Posterior fossa hemorrhage requires immediate neurosurgical consultation. Patients with tumors should also have urgent neurosurgical consultation. Emergent causes of central vertigo such as ischemic cerebrovascular incidents and VAD require neurologic consultation in the ED. Urgent causes such as suspected multiple sclerosis may be referred for outpatient neurologic consultation.

For further reading in Tintinalli's *Emergency Medicine: A Comprehensive Study Guide*, 7th ed., see Chapter 164, "Vertigo and Dizziness," by Brian Goldman.

147 SEIZURES AND STATUS EPILEPTICUS IN ADULTS

C. Crawford Mechem

PATHOPHYSIOLOGY

- A seizure is an episode of abnormal neurologic function caused by inappropriate electrical discharge of brain neurons.
- Epilepsy is a clinical condition in which an individual is subject to recurrent seizures. The term is ordinarily not applied to seizures caused by reversible conditions.
- Primary or idiopathic seizures are those without a clear cause.
- Secondary or symptomatic seizures are the result of another identifiable condition.
- Seizures may be classified in two major groups: generalized and partial (focal) (Table 147-1).
- Generalized seizures are caused by simultaneous activation of the entire cerebral cortex.
- Partial seizures are due to electrical discharges in a localized, structural lesion of the cerebral cortex. The discharges may remain localized or can generalize.
- Complex partial seizures are often due to focal discharges in the temporal lobe.

CLINICAL FEATURES

- Generalized seizures often begin with abrupt loss of consciousness without warning. The patient may then become rigid, with extension of the trunk and extremities, and fall to the ground. Apnea, cyanosis, urinary incontinence, and vomiting may be seen.
- As the rigid (tonic) phase subsides, symmetric rhythmic (clonic) jerking of the trunk and extremities develops. After the attack, the patient is flaccid and unconscious.
- A typical generalized seizure episode lasts from 60 to 90 seconds. Consciousness returns gradually, and postictal confusion and fatigue may persist for several hours.

TABLE 147-1 Classification of Seizures

Generalized seizures (consciousness always lost)
Tonic-clonic seizures (grand mal)
Absence seizures (petit mal)
Others (myoclonic, tonic, clonic, or atonic seizures)
Partial (focal) seizures
Simple partial (no alteration of consciousness)
Complex partial (consciousness impaired)
Partial seizures (simple or complex) with secondary generalization
Unclassified (due to inadequate information)

- Absence seizures are brief, usually lasting only a few seconds. Patients appear confused or withdrawn and do not respond to voice or other stimulation. Postural tone is maintained, and patients usually remain continent. There is no postictal period.
- Simple partial seizures remain localized and consciousness is not affected.
- Unilateral tonic or clonic movements limited to one extremity suggest a focus in the motor cortex.
- Visual symptoms, such as flashing lights, often result from an occipital focus, while olfactory or gustatory hallucinations may arise from the medial temporal lobe.
- Symptoms of complex partial seizures may include automatisms, visceral symptoms, hallucinations, memory disturbances, distorted perception, and affective disorders.
- Automatisms are typically simple, repetitive, purposeless movements such as lip smacking, fiddling with clothing or buttons, or repeating short phrases.
- Visceral symptoms include sensation of butterflies rising up from the epigastrium.
- Hallucinations may be olfactory, gustatory, visual, or auditory.
- There may be complex distortions of visual perception, time, and memory.
- Affective symptoms include fear, paranoia, depression, or elation.
- Eclampsia refers to the combination of seizures, hypertension, edema, and proteinuria in pregnant women beyond 20 weeks' gestation or up to 3 weeks postpartum.
- Status epilepticus is continuous seizure activity for more than 5 minutes.
- Nonconvulsive status epilepticus is characterized by coma, fluctuating mental status, or confusion with minimal or imperceptible convulsive activity. It is confirmed by EEG.
- Epilepsia partialis continua is focal tonic-clonic seizure activity with normal alertness and responsiveness. The distal leg and arm are most commonly affected.

DIAGNOSIS AND DIFFERENTIAL

- The first step in diagnosis is determining if the episode was indeed a true seizure. A careful history should be obtained from the patient and witnesses.
- Important historical information includes the rapidity of onset, presence of a preceding aura, progression of motor activity, whether the activity was local or generalized, and whether the patient became incontinent.
- Determine the duration of the episode and postictal behavior.

- If the patient has a known seizure disorder, investigate the regular pattern of seizures, medications taken, dosage changes, and the possibility of noncompliance.
- Investigate contributing factors such as sleep deprivation, alcohol or substance abuse or withdrawal, infection, or electrolyte disturbances.
- In patients with first-time seizures, a more detailed history should include recent or remote head trauma or headaches, current pregnancy or recent delivery, systemic illness (especially cancer), coagulopathy or anticoagulation, or drug or alcohol ingestion or withdrawal. In patients who have traveled to, or who are natives of, developing world countries, neurocysticercosis, a central nervous system (CNS) infection with the larval stage of the tapeworm *Taenia solium*, should be considered.
- Common causes of secondary seizures are listed in Table 147-2.
- The physical examination should include a search for any injuries or complications resulting from the seizure, such as posterior shoulder dislocation, oral trauma, and aspiration.
- Perform a directed neurologic examination, including level of consciousness and mentation. A transient, focal deficit (usually unilateral) following a focal seizure is referred to as Todd paralysis and should resolve within 48 hours. If the symptoms cannot be attributed to a benign cause, further urgent evaluation is warranted.
- In an adult with a first seizure or when the history is unclear, laboratory tests may include a bedside glucose, basic metabolic panel, calcium, magnesium, a pregnancy test, and toxicology studies.
- Obtain assays for anticonvulsant drug levels when applicable.
- In an adult with a history of seizures who presents after a typical, unremarkable seizure and has a normal physical examination, a bedside glucose level and an anticonvulsant drug level are usually all that are indicated.
- The blood prolactin level may be elevated for 15 to 60 minutes immediately after a seizure and may help distinguish a true seizure from a pseudoseizure.
- Obtain a noncontrast head CT for patients with a first seizure or a change in established seizure pattern to identify an acute intracranial process.
- Because important processes, such as tumors or vascular anomalies, may not be evident on noncontrast studies, a follow-up contrast CT or MRI may be arranged, often in coordination with the consulting neurologist.
- Lumbar puncture is indicated if the patient is febrile or immunocompromised, or if subarachnoid hemorrhage is suspected in the presence of a normal noncontrast head CT.
- EEG can be considered to evaluate patients with persistent, unexplained altered mental status to exclude nonconvulsive status epilepticus or other processes or to detect ongoing status epilepticus after paralysis for endotracheal intubation and induction of general anesthesia.
- The differential diagnosis of seizures includes syncope, pseudoseizures, migraine headache, hyperventilation syndrome, movement disorders, and narcolepsy/cataplexy.

TABLE 147-2 Common Causes of Secondary Seizures

Trauma (recent or remote)
Intracranial hemorrhage (subdural, epidural, subarachnoid, intraparenchymal)
Structural CNS abnormalities
Vascular lesion (aneurysm, arteriovenous malformation)
Mass lesions (primary or metastatic neoplasms)
Degenerative neurologic diseases
Congenital brain abnormalities
Infection (meningitis, encephalitis, abscess)
Metabolic disturbances
Hypo- or hyperglycemia
Hypo- or hypernatremia
Hyperosmolar states
Uremia
Hepatic failure
Hypocalcemia, hypomagnesemia (rare)
Toxins and drugs (many)
Cocaine, lidocaine
Antidepressants
Theophylline
Alcohol withdrawal
Drug withdrawal
Eclampsia of pregnancy (may occur up to 8 weeks postpartum)
Hypertensive encephalopathy
Anoxic-ischemic injury (cardiac arrest, severe hypoxemia)

EMERGENCY DEPARTMENT CARE AND DISPOSITION

- Usually little is required during the course of a seizure other than to protect the patient from injury and prevent aspiration.
- IV anticonvulsants are not indicated during the course of an uncomplicated seizure.

- Once the seizure subsides, a clear airway should be ensured. Suction and airway adjuncts should be readily available.
- In a patient with a known seizure disorder, if anticonvulsant levels are low, supplemental doses may be administered and the regular regimen restarted or adjusted.
- Lorazepam (2-4 milligrams IV) is the initial agent of choice to control a seizure until more specific agents can be given. IV diazepam (5-10 milligrams IV) is an acceptable alternative.
- Oral loading of phenytoin (18 milligrams/kg PO as a single dose or divided into three doses given every 2 hours) will achieve therapeutic levels in 2 to 24 hours.
- IV phenytoin, 10 to 20 milligrams/kg at an IV rate of 25 milligrams/minute, achieves anticonvulsant effects in 1 to 2 hours.
- The dose of fosphenytoin is 10 to 20 milligrams phenytoin equivalent/kg at a maximum IV rate of 150 milligrams/min.
- In the known or suspected noncompliant patient, obtain a serum anticonvulsant level before administering a supplemental dose.
- If anticonvulsant levels are adequate and the patient has had a single attack, specific treatment may not be needed if the pattern falls within the patient's expected range.
- Identify precipitants or conditions that have lowered the seizure threshold. If none is found, a change in or adjustment of medication may be needed. Make this decision in consultation with the patient's primary physician or neurologist.
- Treat patients with secondary seizures due to a neurologic condition due to the risk of recurrence.
- There are no fixed guidelines regarding initiation of anticonvulsant therapy in the patient with a first seizure. The decision depends on the risk of recurrent seizures weighed against the risk-benefit ratio of anticonvulsant therapy.
- The goal of treatment for status epilepticus is seizure control within 30 minutes of onset (Fig. 147-1). Refractory status epilepticus is defined as persistent seizure activity despite the IV administration of adequate amounts of two antiepileptic agents, generally a benzodiazepine and phenytoin.
- Neuromuscular blocking agents, such as vecuronium, may be helpful. These drugs will abolish tonic-clonic movements and may facilitate ventilation, but they have no effect on abnormal neuronal activity. Therefore, EEG monitoring and other pharmacologic interventions are mandatory (Fig. 147-1).
- A large-bore IV line should be established and bedside glucose determination made. IV glucose should be given to hypoglycemic patients.

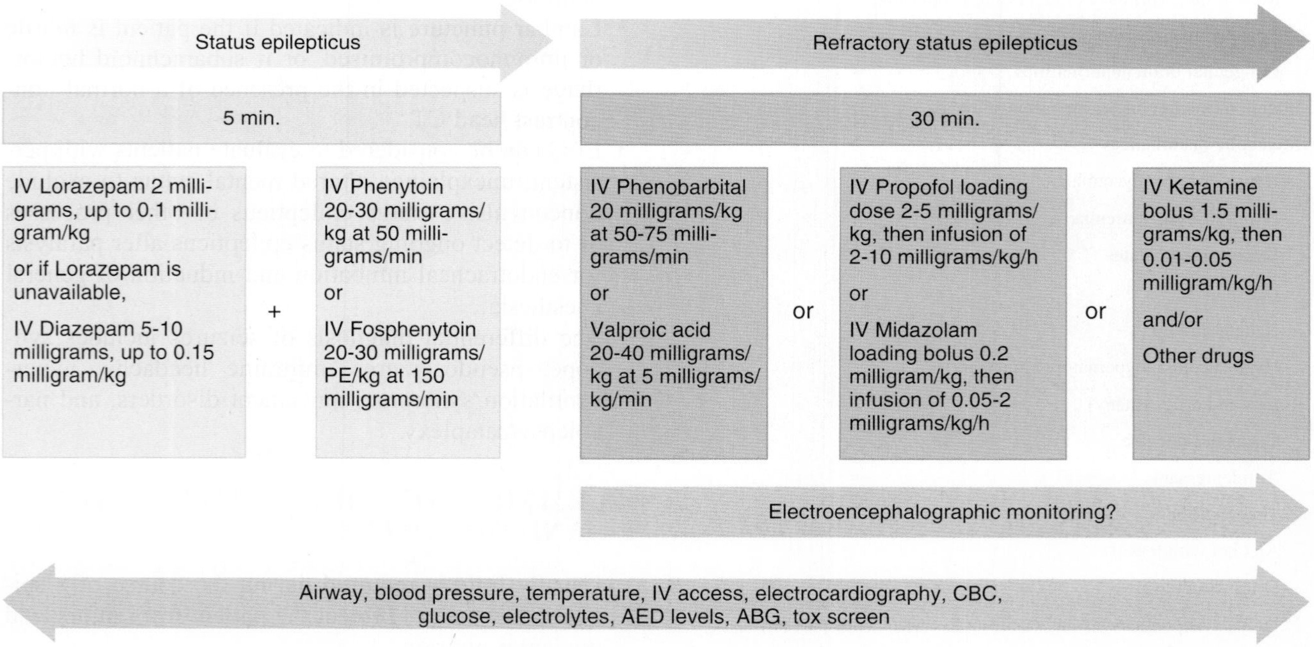

FIG. 147-1. Guidelines for management of status epilepticus. ABG = arterial blood gases; AED = antiepileptic drug; CBC = complete blood count; PE = phenytoin equivalent.

- If toxic ingestion is suspected, perform GI decontamination, if appropriate.
- If bacterial meningitis is suspected, administer empiric antibiotic therapy.
- Patients with a new-onset seizure may be discharged for further outpatient evaluation if they return to baseline and life-threatening conditions have been excluded. Disposition is ideally made in consultation with a neurologist or primary care physician.
- Instruct discharged patients to take precautions to minimize the risks for injury from further seizures. Driving is prohibited until cleared by the neurologist or primary care physician, and driving privileges should conform to state laws.
- Indications for admission following a new-onset seizure include persistent altered mental status, CNS infection or mass, eclampsia, underlying metabolic derangements not readily corrected in the ED, associated head trauma, absence of reliable caretakers at home, and inability to arrange a close follow-up appointment for further evaluation and therapy adjustment.

For further reading in Tintinalli's *Emergency Medicine: A Comprehensive Study Guide*, 7th ed., see Chapter 165, "Seizures and Status Epilepticus in Adults," by Derrick D. Lung, Christina L. Catlett, and Judith E. Tintinalli.

148 ACUTE PERIPHERAL NEUROLOGIC LESIONS

Jeffrey L. Hackman

- History and physical examination findings can help distinguish central from peripheral nervous system disorders (Table 148-1).

TABLE 148-1 Differentiating Central from Peripheral Nervous System Disorders

	CENTRAL	PERIPHERAL
History	Cognitive changes Sudden weakness Nausea, vomiting Headache	Weakness confined to one limb Weakness with pain associated Posture- or movement-dependent pain Weakness after prolonged period in one position
Physical examination		
Reflexes	Brisk reflexes (hyperreflexia) Babinski sign Hoffman sign	Hypoactive reflexes Areflexia
Motor	Asymmetric weakness of ipsilateral upper and lower extremity Facial droop Slurred speech	Symmetric proximal weakness
Sensory	Asymmetric sensory loss in ipsilateral upper and lower extremity	Reproduction of symptoms with movement (compressive neuropathy) All sensory modalities involved
Coordination	Discoordination without weakness	Loss of proprioception

NEUROMUSCULAR JUNCTION DISORDERS

BOTULISM

- Botulism is caused by *Clostridium botulinum* toxin and occurs in three forms: foodborne, wound, and infantile.
- In the United States, the principal source is improperly preserved canned foods.
- In infantile botulism, organisms arise from ingested spores, often in honey, and produce a systemically absorbed toxin.
- Wound botulism should be considered in patients with a wound or a history of injection drug use.
- Clinical features appear 6 to 48 hours following ingestion and may be preceded by nausea, vomiting, abdominal cramps, and diarrhea or constipation.
- Descending, symmetric paralysis is the classic finding.
- The cranial nerves and bulbar muscles are affected first, causing diplopia, dysarthria, and dysphagia.
- Dilated nonreactive pupils help distinguish botulism from myasthenia gravis, which does not affect the pupil.
- Infants present with constipation, poor feeding, lethargy, and weak cry.
- Treatment includes respiratory support, botulinum antitoxin, immunoglobulin, and admission.

TICK PARALYSIS

- Tick paralysis or tick toxicosis is caused by a neurotoxin of multiple tick species.
- Symptoms appear 2 to 6 days after tick attachment.
- Classic symptoms are ataxia and progressive lower than upper extremity weakness.
- Treatment includes removing the tick, local wound care, and supportive care.

ACUTE PERIPHERAL NEUROPATHIES

GUILLAIN–BARRÉ SYNDROME

- Guillain–Barré syndrome usually follows a viral or febrile illness, especially *Campylobacter jejuni* infection, or vaccination.
- The classic pattern includes ascending symmetric weakness or paralysis and loss of deep tendon reflexes.
- Respiratory failure and autonomic dysfunction may occur.
- The Miller Fisher syndrome variant is associated with *C. jejuni* infection and is characterized by ophthalmoplegia, ataxia, and hyporeflexia.
- Cerebrospinal fluid analysis typically show high protein (>45 milligrams/dL) and white cell counts <10 cells/mm^3.
- Treatment includes respiratory support, immunoglobulin and/or plasmapheresis, admission to a monitored or critical care setting, and neurologic consultation.

FOCAL NEUROPATHIES

MEDIAN NEUROPATHY

- Carpal tunnel syndrome is the most common form of any focal mononeuropathy.
- Pain, paresthesias, and numbness in the median nerve distribution are caused by compression of the median nerve at the wrist.
- Tinel sign (performed by tapping the volar surface of the wrist over the median nerve) and Phalen (performed by compressing the opposing dorsal surfaces of the hand with the wrists flexed together) maneuver can confirm the diagnosis, followed by outpatient electrodiagnostic testing.
- ED treatment is conservative, with reduction of aggravating factors, splinting with the wrist in neutral position, pain control, and follow-up with a primary care physician or hand specialist.

ULNAR MONONEUROPATHY

- Cubital tunnel syndrome is the most common ulnar mononeuroapthy.
- Classic symptoms include tingling in the fifth and lateral fourth fingers.
- The diagnosis is suggested either by tapping on the cubital tunnel at the elbow, positive elbow flexion sign, or Froment sign. A positive elbow flexion sign is seen when symptoms recur within 3 minutes when the elbow is held in flexion with the wrist in extension. Froment sign may be noted during resistance testing when the thumb intraphalangeal joint flexes to compensate for weakness of the adductor pollicis brevis.
- ED treatment is conservative, with reduction of aggravating factors, long arm posterior splint or arm sling to rest the elbow, anti-inflammatories, and surgical referral.
- If the nerve compression is acute due to fracture or hematoma, immediate surgical consultation is indicated.

OTHER ENTRAPMENT NEUROPATHIES

- Other common nerve entrapments include deep peroneal (causing foot drop and numbness between the first and second toes) and meralgia paresthetica (entrapment of the lateral femoral cutaneous nerve).
- Meralgia paresthetica may follow weight loss and pelvic or gynecologic surgery, and causes anterolateral thigh numbness and pain.
- These and other entrapments often cause numbness and/or weakness, often respond to conservative management, and may ultimately require referral to a specialist for decompression.

MONONEURITIS MULTIPLEX

- Mononeuritis multiplex is the dysfunction of multiple peripheral nerves separated both temporally and anatomically.
- Signs and symptoms include weakness, paresthesias, numbness, aches, and spasms of sharp pain.
- Diabetes is the most common cause, but it is also associated with other systemic diseases (Table 148-2).

PLEXOPATHIES

BRACHIAL PLEXOPATHY

- Brachial plexopathies typically cause weakness, then pain, and paresthesias in the distribution of the affected nerves.
- Common causes include trauma (penetrating, humeral neck fracture, or dislocation), shoulder dislocation, neoplasm (Pancoast tumor), radiation, or surgery.

LUMBAR PLEXOPATHY

- Plexopathy of the lumbar portion of the plexus causes weakness of hip adduction and flexion and knee extension, decreased sensation at the top and inner thigh, and decreased patellar reflexes.
- Lesions of the sacral portion of the plexus cause inability to abduct the thigh, weakness of hip extension and knee flexion, and decreased sensation of the back of the thigh and below the knee.

TABLE 148-2 Etiologies of Mononeuritis Multiplex
Diabetes mellitus
Vasculitides
Polyarteritis nodosa
Wegener granulomatosis
Temporal arteritis
Infectious
Lyme disease
Human immunodeficiency virus
Leprosy
Hepatitis
Neoplasm
Paraneoplastic syndrome
Intraneural neoplastic infiltration
Connective tissue disorders
Systemic lupus erythematosus
Sjögren syndrome
Rheumatoid arthritis
Sarcoidosis
Lead poisoning
Polycythemia vera
Cryoglobulinemia

- The most common causes are radiation, diabetic amyotrophy, aortic aneurysm, retroperitoneal hemorrhage, or compression from arteriovenous malformations.
- Imaging may be useful to determine the etiology.
- Treatment is directed at the underlying cause.

HIV-ASSOCIATED PERIPHERAL NEUROLOGIC DISEASE

- HIV infection and its complications and treatments cause a variety of peripheral nerve disorders.
- The most common, drug-induced, and HIV neuropathies are chronic and do not cause acute symptoms.
- Patients with HIV have a high rate of mononeuritis multiplex and a myopathy resembling polymyositis.
- In early infection, they are more prone to Guillain–Barré syndrome.
- In the latter stages of AIDS, they may develop cytomegalovirus (CMV) radiculitis, with acute weakness, primarily lower extremity involvement, and variable bowel or bladder dysfunction.
- Primarily, lower extremity weakness and hyporeflexia, as well as sensory deficits, are seen. Rectal tone may be decreased.
- MRI (indicated to exclude mass lesion) shows swelling and clumping of the cauda equina.
- Admission is required for CMV radiculitis; treatment, which should precede definitive diagnosis, consists of ganciclovir.

DIABETIC PERIPHERAL NEUROPATHY

- Half of patients with diabetes have symptoms of neuropathy; 15% require treatment for their symptoms.
- The most common manifestation of diabetic peripheral neuropathy is a distal symmetric polyneuropathy with a typical stocking and glove distribution.
- Non-healing wounds resulting from impaired sensation due to diabetic peripheral neuropathy are the most common cause of nontraumatic amputation.
- Glycemic control and neuropathy are correlated.
- ED treatment is focused on management of symptoms.

For further reading in Tintinalli's *Emergency Medicine: A Comprehensive Study Guide*, 7th ed., see Chapter166, "Acute Peripheral Neurologic Lesions," by Phillip Andrus and Andy Jagoda.

149 CHRONIC NEUROLOGIC DISORDERS

Sarah Andrus Gaines

AMYOTROPHIC LATERAL SCLEROSIS

EPIDEMIOLOGY

- The typical time of onset for amyotrophic lateral sclerosis (ALS) is over age 50 years.

PATHOPHYSIOLOGY

- ALS is caused by upper and lower motor neuron degeneration without other central nervous dysfunction.

CLINICAL FEATURES

- Upper motor neuron dysfunction causes limb spasticity, hyperreflexia, and emotional lability.
- Lower neuron dysfunction causes limb muscle weakness, atrophy, fasciculations, dysarthria, dysphagia, and difficulty in mastication.

- Symptoms are often asymmetric.
- Patients may initially have cervical or back pain consistent with an acute compressive radiculopathy.
- Respiratory muscle weakness causes progressive respiratory depression.

DIAGNOSIS AND DIFFERENTIAL

- The diagnosis is clinical and is often previously established.
- Electromyography (EMG) is the most useful test.
- Other illnesses that should be considered include myasthenia gravis (MG), diabetes, thyroid dysfunction, vitamin B_{12} deficiency, lead toxicity, vasculitis, and central nervous system (CNS) or spinal cord tumors.

EMERGENCY DEPARTMENT CARE AND DISPOSITION

- Emergency care is required for acute respiratory failure, aspiration pneumonia, choking episodes, or trauma from falls.
- The treatment goal is to optimize pulmonary function through the use of nebulizer treatments, steroids, antibiotics, or endotracheal intubation.
- Admit patients with impending respiratory failure, pneumonia, inability to handle secretions, and worsening disease process that may require long-term care.

MYASTHENIA GRAVIS

EPIDEMIOLOGY

- Peak age of onset for myasthenia gravis (MG) is in the second or third decade of life for females and in the fifth or eighth decade for males.

PATHOPHYSIOLOGY

- MG is an autoimmune disease caused by antibody destruction of the acetylcholine receptors at the neuromuscular junction, which results in muscle weakness.
- The thymus is abnormal in 75% of patients and thymectomy resolves or improves symptoms in most patients, especially in those with a thymoma.

CLINICAL FEATURES

- Most MG patients have generalized weakness, specifically of the proximal extremities, neck extensors, and facial or bulbar muscles. There is usually no deficit in sensory, reflex, and cerebellar function.
- Ptosis and diplopia are the most common symptoms. Symptoms usually worsen as the day progresses or with muscle use (eg, prolonged chewing or reading) and improve with rest. Ten percent of patients have ocular muscle weakness only.
- Myasthenic crisis is a life-threatening condition involving extreme weakness of the respiratory muscles that may progress to respiratory failure.

DIAGNOSIS AND DIFFERENTIAL

- The diagnosis is confirmed through administration of edrophonium (Tensilon test), electromyogram, and serum testing for acetylcholine receptor antibodies.
- The differential diagnosis includes Lambert–Eaton syndrome, drug-induced disorders (eg, penicillamines, aminoglycosides, and procainamide), ALS, botulism, thyroid disorders, and other CNS disorders (eg, intracranial mass lesions, stroke).

EMERGENCY DEPARTMENT CARE AND DISPOSITION

- Implement supplemental oxygen and aggressive airway management with myasthenic crisis.
- Avoid depolarizing and nondepolarizing paralytic agents. Etomidate, fentanyl, or propofol can be used.
- If the Tensilon test is positive, then administer pyridostigmine (60-90 milligrams PO or 2-3 milligrams IV every 4 hours), with an onset of 15 to 30 minutes and duration for 3 to 5 hours. An alternative is neostigmine (0.5 milligram IV), which will be effective within 30 minutes and last for 4 hours.
- Steroids, immunosuppressive medications, and plasmapheresis may be used in consultation with a neurologist.
- Several drugs should be used with caution in patients with MG (Table 149-1).
- Consult a neurologist for disposition and admission.

MULTIPLE SCLEROSIS

EPIDEMIOLOGY

- Three clinical courses are seen in multiple sclerosis (MS): relapsing and remitting (up to 90% of cases); relapsing and progressive; or chronically progressive.
- Peak age of onset is the third decade of life. Females are two to three times more likely to contract MS than are males.

TABLE 149-1	Drugs That Should Be Avoided in Myasthenia Gravis
Steroids	Adrenocorticotropic hormone,* methylprednisolone,* prednisone*
Anticonvulsants	Phenytoin, ethosuximide, trimethadione, paraldehyde, magnesium sulfate, barbiturates; lithium
Antimalarials	Chloroquine,* quinine*
IV fluids	Na lactate solution
Antibiotics	Aminoglycosides, fluoroquinolones,* neomycin,* streptomycin,* kanamycin,* gentamicin, tobramycin, dihydrostreptomycin,* amikacin, polymyxin A, polymyxin B, sulfonamides, viomycin, colistimethate,* lincomycin, clindamycin, tetracycline, oxytetracycline, rolitetracycline, macrolides, metronidazole
Psychotropics	Chlorpromazine,* lithium carbonate,* amitriptyline, droperidol, haloperidol, imipramine
Antirheumatics	D-Penicillamine, colchicine, chloroquine
Cardiovascular	Quinidine,* procainamide,* β-blockers (propranolol, oxprenolol, practolol, pindolol, sotalol), lidocaine, trimethaphan; magnesium; calcium channel blockers (verapamil)
Local anesthetics	Lidocaine,* procaine,*
Analgesics	Narcotics (morphine, hydromorphone, codeine, Pantopon, meperidine)
Endocrine	Thyroid replacement*
Eyedrops	Timolol,* echothiophate
Others	Amantadine, diphenhydramine, emetine, diuretics, muscle relaxants, central nervous system depressants, respiratory depressants, sedatives, procaine,* phenothiazines
Neuromuscular blocking agents	Tubocurarine, pancuronium, gallamine, dimethyl tubocurarine, succinylcholine, decamethonium

Note: See also discussion on eMedicine from WebMD by Aashit K. Shah, MD, available at: http://emedicine.medscape.com/article/793136-treatment.

*Case reports implicate drugs in exacerbations of myasthenia gravis.

PATHOPHYSIOLOGY

- Although the etiology of MS is unknown, it involves multifocal areas of CNS demyelination, causing motor, sensory, visual, and cerebellar dysfunction.

CLINICAL FEATURES

- Deficits associated with MS are described as a heaviness, weakness, stiffness, or numbness of an extremity or clumsiness. Lower extremity symptoms are usually more severe.
- Lhermitte's sign is an electric shock–like sensation, a vibration, or dysesthetic pain going down into the arms or legs from neck flexion.
- Physical examination may reveal decreased strength, increased tone, hyperreflexia, clonus, decreased proprioception, reduced pain and temperature, and a positive Babinski reflex.
- Increases in body temperature, associated with exercise, hot baths, or fever, may worsen symptoms.
- Optic neuritis, usually causing unilateral loss of central vision, is the first presenting symptom in up to 30% of cases and may cause an afferent papillary defect (Marcus Gunn pupil).
- Acute bilateral internuclear ophthalmoplegia (INO), which causes abnormal adduction and horizontal nystagmus, is highly suggestive of MS.
- Retrobulbar or extraocular muscle pain usually precedes vision loss. Fundoscopy is usually normal, but the disc may appear pale.
- Rarely, acute transverse myelitis may occur. Cerebellar lesions may cause intention tremor or ataxia. Brain stem lesions may cause vertigo.
- Cognitive and emotional problems are common (eg, mood disorders or dementia).
- Dysautonomia causes vesicourethral, gastrointestinal tract, and sexual dysfunction.

DIAGNOSIS AND DIFFERENTIAL

- The diagnosis of MS is clinical and is suggested by two or more episodes, lasting days to weeks, causing dysfunction that implicates different sites in the white matter.
- MRI of the brain may demonstrate various abnormalities, including discrete lesions in the supratentorial white matter or periventricular areas.
- Cerebrospinal fluid (CSF) protein and gamma-globulin levels are often elevated.
- The differential diagnosis includes systemic lupus erythematosus, Lyme disease, neurosyphilis, and HIV disease.

EMERGENCY DEPARTMENT CARE AND DISPOSITION

- Treat severe motor or cerebellar dysfunction with steroids: high-dose pulsed intravenous methylprednisolone (250 milligrams IV every 6 hours), followed by a PO prednisone taper.
- Fever must be reduced to minimize symptoms. Perform a careful search for a source of infection. Evaluate for acute UTI or pyelonephritis; postvoid residuals >100 mL require intermittent catheterization.
- Respiratory infections and distress must be aggressively managed.
- Admission is required for those at risk for further complications, respiratory compromise, depression

with suicidal ideation, and those requiring IV antibiotics or steroids.

LAMBERT–EATON MYASTHENIC SYNDROME

- Lambert–Eaton myasthenic syndrome is an autoimmune disorder that causes fluctuating proximal limb muscle weakness and fatigue.
- Lambert–Eaton syndrome is seen mostly in older men with lung cancer.
- Strength is improved with sustained activity.
- Patients complain of myalgias, stiffness, paresthesias, metallic tastes, and autonomic symptoms (eg, impotence and dry mouth). Eye movements are unaffected.
- The EMG is abnormal and serum tests are specific for antibodies to voltage-gated calcium channels.
- Treatment of the underlying neoplasm greatly improves symptoms.
- Pyridostigmine and immunosuppressive drugs may reduce symptom severity.

PARKINSON'S DISEASE

EPIDEMIOLOGY

- The average age of onset for Parkinson's disease (PD) is 55 to 60 years of age.

PATHOPHYSIOLOGY

- The etiology of PD is unknown, but patients have reduced functional dopaminergic receptors in the substantia nigra.

CLINICAL FEATURES

- PD presents with four classic signs (mnemonic "TRAP"): resting tremor, cogwheel rigidity, akinesia or bradykinesia, and impaired posture and equilibrium.
- Other signs include facial and postural changes, voice and speech abnormalities, depression, and muscle fatigue.
- Initially, most complain of a unilateral resting arm tremor, described as pill rolling, or a general feeling of stiffness or slowness, which may have been present for years.

DIAGNOSIS AND DIFFERENTIAL

- The diagnosis is clinical and is most often previously established. No laboratory test or neuroimaging study is pathognomonic.
- Parkinsonism can result from street drugs, toxins, neuroleptic drugs, hydrocephalus, head trauma, and other rare neurologic disorders.

EMERGENCY DEPARTMENT CARE AND DISPOSITION

- PD patients may be on medications that increase central dopamine (eg, levodopa, carbidopa, and amantadine), anticholinergics (eg, benztropine), and dopamine receptor agonists (eg, bromocriptine).
- Medication toxicity includes psychiatric or sleep disturbances, cardiac dysrhythmias, orthostatic hypotension, dyskinesias, and dystonia.
- With significant motor or psychiatric disturbances (eg, hallucinations or frank psychosis) or decreased drug efficacy, a "drug holiday" for 1 week should be initiated in consultation with a neurologist.

POLIOMYELITIS AND POSTPOLIO SYNDROME

EPIDEMIOLOGY

- Poliomyelitis leads to paralysis in less than 5% of infected patients.

PATHOPHYSIOLOGY

- Poliomyelitis is caused by an enterovirus that causes paralysis via motor neuron destruction and muscle denervation and atrophy.
- In developed countries, transmission is oral to oral; however, transmission is fecal to oral in developing countries.

CLINICAL FEATURES

- Most symptomatic patients have only a mild viral syndrome and no paralysis. Symptoms include fever, malaise, headache, sore throat, and gastrointestinal symptoms.
- Spinal polio results in asymmetric proximal limb weakness and flaccidity, absent tendon reflexes, and fasciculation. Maximal paralysis occurs within 5 days.
- Other sequelae include bulbar polio (speech and swallowing dysfunction) and encephalitis.
- Postpolio syndrome is the recurrence of motor symptoms after a latent period of several decades.
- Symptoms of postpolio syndrome may include muscle fatigue, joint pain, or weakness of new and previously affected muscle groups. Patients may have new bulbar, respiratory, or sleep difficulties.

DIAGNOSIS AND DIFFERENTIAL

- Consider the diagnosis of polio in patients with an acute febrile illness, aseptic meningitis, and asymmetric flaccid paralysis.
- CSF may reveal a pleocytosis (mostly neutrophils) and positive cultures for poliovirus.
- Throat and rectal swabs are higher yield tests than CSF.
- The diagnosis of postpolio syndrome is based on a prior history of paralytic polio with recovery and new symptoms.
- The differential diagnosis includes Guillain–Barré syndrome, peripheral neuropathies (eg, mononucleosis, Lyme disease, and porphyria), abnormal electrolyte levels, toxins, inflammatory myopathies, and other viruses (eg, coxsackievirus, mumps, echovirus, and various enteroviruses).

EMERGENCY DEPARTMENT CARE AND DISPOSITION

- Treatment is supportive.
- Lamotrigine may improve quality of life.
- Disposition should be made in consultation with a neurologist.

For further reading in Tintinalli's *Emergency Medicine: A Comprehensive Study Guide*, 7th ed., see Chapter 167, "Chronic Neurologic Disorders," by Edward P. Sloan, Daniel A. Handel, and Sarah Andrus Gaines.

150 CENTRAL NERVOUS SYSTEM AND SPINAL INFECTIONS

O. John Ma

■ MENINGITIS

EPIDEMIOLOGY

- The median age of illness has risen to 39 years. The overall incidence of bacterial meningitis has declined.
- Changes in epidemiology have mirrored vaccination practices in adults and children against *Haemophilus influenzae*, *Staphylococcus pneumoniae*, and *Neisseria meningitidis*.
- There is an increasing prevalence of ceftriaxone- and penicillin-resistant *S. pneumoniae* strains in the community.
- Military barracks and college dormitories are environments in which clusters of *N. meningitidis* cases occur.

PATHOPHYSIOLOGY

- Infection begins with entrance of bacteria into the subarachnoid space, usually by upper airway inoculation, and is followed by dissemination into the bloodstream and invasion across the blood-brain barrier. Direct inoculation is also possible from infection of parameningeal structures (eg, otitis media, brain abscess, and sinusitis), neurosurgery, and traumatic or congenital communications with the exterior.
- The brain becomes edematous through several mechanisms: (1) There is reduced cerebrospinal fluid (CSF) drainage through interference with flow and absorption by arachnoid granulations. The increased quantity of CSF results in periventricular edema and hydrocephalus. (2) There is disruption of the blood-brain barrier, which allows entry of protein and water. These mechanisms lead to ischemia as intracranial pressure exceeds cerebral perfusion pressure.

CLINICAL FEATURES

- In classic and fulminant cases of bacterial meningitis, the patient presents with fever, headache, neck stiffness, photophobia, and altered mental status. Seizures may occur in nearly 25% of cases.
- The presenting picture, however, may be more nonspecific, particularly in the very young and elderly. Confusion and fever may be symptoms of meningeal irritation in the elderly.
- Inquire about recent antibiotic use, which may cloud the clinical picture in a less florid case. Other key historical data include living conditions (eg, military barracks, college dormitories), trauma, immunocompetence, immunization status, and recent neurosurgical procedures.
- Assess for meningeal irritation with resistance to passive neck flexion, Brudzinski's sign (flexion of hips and knees in response to passive neck flexion), or Kernig's sign (contraction of hamstrings in response to knee extension while hip is flexed).
- Examine the skin for the purpuric rash characteristic of meningococcemia. Percuss paranasal sinuses and examine ears for evidence of primary infection at those sites.
- Document focal neurologic deficits, which are present in 25% of cases.

DIAGNOSIS AND DIFFERENTIAL

- When the diagnosis of bacterial meningitis is entertained, performing a lumbar puncture (LP) is mandatory. At a minimum, send CSF for Gram's stain and culture, cell count, protein, and glucose. Typical CSF

TABLE 150-1 Typical Spinal Fluid Results for Meningeal Processes

PARAMETER (NORMAL)	BACTERIAL	VIRAL	NEOPLASTIC	FUNGAL
Opening pressure (<170 mm cerebrospinal fluid)	>300 mm	<300 mm	200 mm	300 mm
White blood cell count (<5 mononuclear)	>1000/mm³	<1000/mm³	<500/mm³	<500/mm³
% Polymorphonuclear cells (0)	>80%	1%-50%	1%-50%	1%-50%
Glucose (>40 milligrams/dL)	<40 milligrams/dL	>40 milligrams/dL	<40 milligrams/dL	<40 milligrams/dL
Protein (<50 milligrams/dL)	>200 milligrams/dL	<200 milligrams/dL	>200 milligrams/dL	>200 milligrams/dL
Gram's stain (–)	+	–	–	–
Cytology (–)	–	–	+	+

results for meningeal processes are listed in Table 150-1.

- Additional CSF studies to be considered are latex agglutination or counterimmune electrophoresis for bacterial antigens in potentially partially treated bacterial cases, India ink or serum cryptococcal antigen in immunocompromised patients, acid-fast stain and culture for mycobacteria in tuberculous meningitis, Borrelia antibodies for possible Lyme disease, and viral cultures in suspected viral meningitis.
- Other laboratory tests should include a complete blood count, blood cultures, basic metabolic panel, and coagulation studies.
- LP can be performed safely if intracranial mass lesions and coagulopathy are unlikely based on clinical grounds. Table 150-2 reviews suggested criteria for obtaining computed tomography (CT) of the head prior to LP when meningitis is suspected.
- The differential diagnosis includes subarachnoid hemorrhage, meningeal neoplasm, brain abscess, viral encephalitis, cerebral toxoplasmosis, and other infectious meningitides.

TABLE 150-2 Some Suggested Criteria for Obtaining Head CT before Lumbar Puncture for Suspected Meningitis

Altered mental status or deteriorating level of consciousness
Focal neurologic deficit
Seizure
Papilledema
Immunocompromised state
Malignancy
History of focal central nervous system disease (stroke, focal infection, tumor)
Concern for CNS mass lesion
Age >60 y

EMERGENCY DEPARTMENT CARE AND DISPOSITION

- Upon presentation of the patient with suspected bacterial meningitis, perform the LP expeditiously. Initiate empiric antibiotic therapy as preparations for LP are made. Antibiotic therapy administered up to 2 hours prior to LP will not decrease the diagnostic sensitivity if CSF bacterial antigen assays are obtained along with CSF cultures.
- However, if the patient meets any of the criteria in Table 150-2, order a head CT scan prior to LP in order to determine the possible risks for transtentorial or tonsillar herniation associated with LP. In these cases, empiric antibiotic therapy must be initiated prior to CT. Always initiate antibiotic therapy in the ED and never delay its administration for neuroimaging or LP.
- Empiric treatment for bacterial meningitis is based on the likelihood of certain pathogens and risk factors (Table 150-3).
- Steroid therapy (dexamethasone 10 milligrams IV 15 minutes prior to antibiotic administration) has proven to be beneficial in adults. Its precise role in the ED, where emergency physicians rarely manage known cases of bacterial meningitis and appropriately administer antibiotics prior to confirmed diagnosis, remains unclear.
- Avoid hypotonic fluids. Monitor serum sodium levels to detect the syndrome of inappropriate antidiuretic hormone or cerebral salt wasting. Treat hyperpyrexia with acetaminophen. Correct coagulopathy using specific replacement therapies.
- Treat seizures with standard modalities. Treat increased intracranial pressure with head elevation and mannitol.
- Manage viral meningitis, without evidence of encephalitis, on an outpatient basis provided the patient is nontoxic in appearance, can tolerate oral fluids, and has reliable follow-up within 24 hours.

TABLE 150-3 Guidelines for Empirical Treatment of Bacterial Meningitis in Adults* or with No Organisms on Gram's Stain

PATIENT CATEGORY	POTENTIAL PATHOGENS	EMPIRICAL THERAPY
Age		
18-50 y	*Streptococcus pneumoniae, Neisseria meningitidis*	Ceftriaxone, 2 grams IV every 12 h, plus vancomycin, 15 milligrams/kg IV every 8-12 h (or rifampin if *S. pneumoniae* resistance possible)
>50 y	*S. pneumoniae, N. meningitidis, Listeria monocytogenes,* aerobic gram-negative bacilli	Ceftriaxone, 2 grams IV every 12 h, plus ampicillin, 2 grams IV every 4 h, plus vancomycin, 15 milligrams/kg IV every 8-12 h (or rifampin if *S. pneumoniae* resistance possible)
Special Circumstances		
CSF leak with history of closed head trauma	*S. pneumoniae, Haemophilus influenzae,* group B streptococcus	Ceftriaxone, 2 grams IV every 12 h, plus vancomycin, 15 milligrams/kg IV
History of recent penetrating head injury, neurosurgery, CSF shunt	*Staphylococcus aureus, S. epidermidis,* diphtheroids, aerobic gram-negative bacilli	Vancomycin, 25 milligrams/kg IV load (maximum infusion rate, 500 milligrams per hour), plus ceftazidime, 2 grams IV every 8 h
Penicillin or cephalosporin allergy	*S. pneumoniae, N. meningitidis, L. monocytogenes,* aerobic gram-negative bacilli	Vancomycin 30-60 milligrams/kg IV/d in 2-3 divided doses, plus moxifloxacin 400 milligrams IV once daily, plus trimethoprim-sulfamethoxazole 10-20 milligrams/kg (of the trimethroprim component) IV per day divided every 6-12 h

Note: See also http://www.hopkins-abxguide.org, accessed August 1, 2012.
Abbreviation: CSF = cerebrospinal fluid.
*For pediatric meningitis treatment, see Chapter 68, Fever and Serious Bacterial Illness.

However, it remains a diagnosis of exclusion; unless the diagnosis of viral meningitis is obvious, admission is warranted.

ENCEPHALITIS

EPIDEMIOLOGY

- Viral encephalitis is a viral infection of brain parenchyma producing an inflammatory response. It is distinct from, although often coexists with, viral meningitis.
- In North America, viruses that cause encephalitis are the arboviruses (including the West Nile virus), herpes simplex virus (HSV), herpes zoster virus (HZV), Epstein–Barr virus, cytomegalovirus (CMV), and rabies.
- Arboviruses can account for up to 50% of cases during epidemic outbreaks. The most common arboviral encephalitides in the United States are the La Crosse encephalitis, St. Louis equine encephalitis, western equine encephalitis, eastern equine encephalitis, and West Nile virus.
- Herpes simplex virus type 1 (HSV-1) is typically seen in older children and adults as a reactivation disease. Herpes simplex virus type 2 (HSV-2) is seen in neonates as a result of perinatal transmission.

PATHOPHYSIOLOGY

- Mosquitoes and ticks transmit arboviruses. The bite of an infected animal transmits rabies. Impaired immune status plays a role in herpes zoster and CMV encephalitis.
- Neurologic dysfunction and damage are caused by disruption of neural cell functions by the virus and by the effects of the host's inflammatory responses. Gray matter is predominantly affected, resulting in cognitive and psychiatric signs, lethargy, and seizures.

CLINICAL FEATURES

- Encephalitis should be considered in patients presenting with any or all of the following features: new psychiatric symptoms, cognitive deficits (aphasia, amnestic syndrome, acute confusional state), seizures, and movement disorders. Headache, photophobia, fever, and meningeal irritation may be present.

- Assessment for neurologic findings and cognitive deficits is crucial. Motor and sensory deficits are not typical.
- Encephalitides may show special regional trophism. HSV involves limbic structures of the temporal and frontal lobes, with prominent psychiatric features, memory disturbance, and aphasia. Some arboviruses predominantly affect the basal ganglia, causing chorea-athetosis and parkinsonism. Involvement of the brain stem nuclei leads to hydrophobic choking characteristic of rabies encephalitis.
- Symptoms of West Nile virus infection include fever, headache, muscle weakness, and lymphadenopathy.
- Most infections are mild and last only a few days. More severe symptoms and signs consist of high fever, neck stiffness, altered mental status, tremors, and seizures.
- In rare cases (mostly involving the elderly), the infection can lead to encephalitis and death.

DIAGNOSIS AND DIFFERENTIAL

- Findings on CT or magnetic resonance imaging (MRI) and LP aid in the ED diagnosis of encephalitis.
- Neuroimaging, particularly MRI, not only excludes other potential lesions, such as brain abscess, but may display findings highly suggestive of HSV encephalitis if the medial temporal and inferior frontal gray matter is involved.
- Findings of aseptic meningitis are typically found on CSF examination.
- For the West Nile virus, the most widely used screening test is the IgM ELISA for detecting acute antibodies.
- The differential diagnosis includes brain abscess; Lyme disease; subacute subarachnoid hemorrhage; bacterial, tuberculous, fungal, or neoplastic meningitis; bacterial endocarditis; postinfectious encephalomyelitis; toxic or metabolic encephalopathies; and primary psychiatric disorders.

EMERGENCY DEPARTMENT CARE AND DISPOSITION

- Admit the patient suspected of suffering from viral encephalitis. Treat patients with suspected HSV or HZV encephalitis with acyclovir 10 milligrams/kg IV every 8 hours. Treat patients with suspected CMV encephalitis with ganciclovir 5 milligrams/kg IV every 12 hours.
- Manage potential complications of encephalitis—seizures, disorders of sodium metabolism, increased intracranial pressure, and systemic consequences of a comatose state—with standard methods.
- There is no specific treatment for the West Nile virus infection. In more severe cases, intensive supportive therapy is indicated. The primary prevention step is advocating the use of insect repellant containing DEET when people go outdoors during dawn or dusk.

BRAIN ABSCESS

EPIDEMIOLOGY

- The incidence of brain abscess has progressively declined over the past century, reflecting the effect of antibiotics on predisposing conditions, such as otitis media.

PATHOPHYSIOLOGY

- A brain abscess is a focal pyogenic infection. It is composed of a central pus-filled cavity, ringed by a layer of granulation tissue and an outer fibrous capsule.
- Three known routes are available for organisms to reach the brain: hematogenously (33%); from contiguous infection of the middle ear, sinus, or teeth (33%); or by direct implantation after neurosurgery or penetrating trauma (10%). The route is unknown in 20% of cases.

CLINICAL FEATURES

- Since patients typically are not acutely toxic, the presenting features of brain abscess are nonspecific. Presenting signs and symptoms include headache, neck stiffness, fever, vomiting, confusion, or obtundation. The presentation may be dominated by the origin of the infection (eg, ear or sinus pain).
- Meningeal signs and focal neurologic findings, such as hemiparesis, seizures, and papilledema, are present in less than half the cases.

DIAGNOSIS AND DIFFERENTIAL

- Brain abscess can be diagnosed by a CT scan of the head with contrast, which demonstrates one or several thin, smoothly contoured rings of enhancement surrounding a low-density center and in turn surrounded by white matter edema.

- LP is contraindicated if a brain abscess is suspected or after the diagnosis has been established. Routine laboratory studies are usually nonspecific. Blood cultures should be obtained.
- The differential diagnosis includes cerebrovascular disease, meningitis, brain neoplasm, subacute cerebral hemorrhage, and other focal brain infections, such as toxoplasmosis.

EMERGENCY DEPARTMENT CARE AND DISPOSITION

- Decisions on antibiotic therapy for brain abscess are dependent on the likely source of the infection (Table 150-4).
- Neurosurgical consultation and admission are warranted since many cases will require surgery for diagnosis, bacteriology, and definitive treatment.

For further reading in Tintinalli's *Emergency Medicine: A Comprehensive Study Guide*, 7th ed., see Chapter 168, "Central Nervous System and Spinal Infections," by Keith E. Loring and Judith E. Tintinalli.

TABLE 150-4 Guidelines for Empiric Treatment of Brain Abscess Based on Presumed Source

PRESUMED SOURCE	PRIMARY EMPIRIC THERAPY	ALTERNATIVE THERAPY
Otogenic	Cefotaxime, 2 grams IV every 6 h, plus metronidazole, 500 milligrams IV every 6 h	Cefepime, 2 grams IV every 8 h, plus metronidazole, 500 milligrams IV every 6 h
Sinogenic or odontogenic	Cefotaxime, 2 grams IV every 6 h, plus metronidazole, 500 milligrams IV every 6 h	Clindamycin, 600 milligrams IV every 8 h, plus metronidazole, 500 milligrams IV every 6 h
Penetrating trauma or neurosurgical procedures	Vancomycin, 15 milligrams/kg IV every 12 h (maximum, 1 gram/dose; monitor serum levels), plus ceftazidime, 2 grams IV every 8 h	Nafcillin, 2 grams IV every 4 h, plus ceftazidime, 2 grams IV every 8 h
Hematogenous	Cefotaxime, 2 grams IV every 6 h, plus metronidazole, 500 milligrams IV every 6 h	No recommendation
No obvious source	Cefotaxime, 2 grams IV every 6 h, plus metronidazole, 500 milligrams IV every 6 h	No recommendation

Note: See also http://www.hopkins-abxguide.org, accessed August 2012.

Section 17

EYES, EARS, NOSE, THROAT, AND ORAL SURGERY

151 OCULAR EMERGENCIES

Steven Go

OCULAR INFECTIONS/ACUTE OCULAR INFLAMAITION

PRESEPTAL (PERIORBITAL) CELLULITIS

- Preseptal cellulitis occurs mostly in patients <10 years old, is commonly associated with upper respiratory infection (URI), eyelid problems, and trauma, and is usually caused by *Staphylococcus aureus, Staphylococcus epidermidis,* and *Streptococcus* species.
- Preseptal cellulitis presents with warm, indurated, and erythematous eyelids, without decreased visual acuity, restriction of ocular motility, proptosis, painful eye movement, or impairment of pupillary function.
- Emergency department (ED) care in patients >5 years old includes oral amoxicillin-clavulanate (22.5 milligrams/kg/dose up to 875 milligrams twice daily), warm packs, and close follow-up with an ophthalmologist.
- For toxic-appearing patients, severe cases, patients with significant comorbidities, or children <5 years, hospital admission for parenteral broad-spectrum antibiotics (eg, ceftriaxone [50-75 milligrams/kg daily] and vancomycin [15 milligrams/kg every 12 hours]) may be required.
- Young children also require an ophthalmology consultant and may require a septic workup because concurrent bacteremia and meningitis can be present.

POSTSEPTAL (ORBITAL) CELLULITIS

- Postseptal cellulitis most frequently spreads from sinusitis (most commonly ethmoid), and predisposing factors also include preseptal cellulitis, trauma, foreign body, bacteremia, and ocular surgery. Infection is usually polymicrobial, with *S. aureus, Streptococcus pneumoniae*, and anaerobes being the most common. Atypical organisms can occur in the unimmunized (*Haemophilus influenzae*) and immunocompromised (mucormycosis in diabetics).
- Postseptal cellulitis should be suspected whenever signs and symptoms of periorbital cellulitis presents with fever, painful ocular motility, proptosis, decreased visual acuity, limited extraocular movements (EOMs), chemosis, or pupillary abnormalities. Cranial nerve (CN) abnormalities indicate associated cavernous sinus thrombosis.
- Emergent diagnosis with orbital and sinus thin-slice computed tomography (CT) scan without contrast is required. If this study is negative, a CT scan with contrast should be done, which may reveal a subperiosteal abscess.
- Emergent ophthalmologic consultation and hospital admission for broad-spectrum intravenous antibiotics (with aerobic and anaerobic coverage) are required. In rare cases, emergent lateral canthotomy may be indicated for elevated intraocular pressure or optic neuropathy.

STYE (EXTERNAL HORDEOLUM)

- A stye is an acute infection (usually *S. aureus*) of an oil gland at the lid margin.
- ED care of a stye includes warm compresses and erythromycin ointment for 7 to 10 days. Lid hygiene with baby shampoo may also be helpful.

CHALAZION

- A chalazion is an acute or chronic noninfectious inflammation of the meibomian gland. Acute cases tend to be painful and often cannot be differentiated from an internal hordeolum, while chronic cases are usually painless.
- For an acute chalazion, ED care is the same as for a stye, plus a 14- to 21-day regimen of doxycycline (100 milligrams twice daily in adults, 2.2 milligrams/kg/dose twice daily in children) for refractory cases.
- Persistent chalazia should be referred to an ophthalmologist for incision, curettage, and biopsy.

CONJUNCTIVITIS

- Bacterial conjunctivitis presents with eyelash matting, mucopurulent discharge, and conjunctival inflammation without corneal lesions. Typical pathogens are *Staphylococcus* and *Streptococcus* species. A slit lamp examination with fluorescein should be done to exclude other important disease entities (eg, herpes keratitis).
- Bacterial conjunctivitis is treated with topical antibiotic drops (Table 151-1).
- Contact lens wears should receive ciprofloxacin, ofloxacin, or tobramycin topical antibiotic coverage for *Pseudomonas*. The worn contact lenses should be discarded and use of new contact lenses should not be resumed until the infection has completely cleared.
- Childhood conjunctivitis pathogens may include *H. influenzae* and *Moraxella catarrhalis*, so if initial treatment is unsuccessful, a change in antibiotics is warranted.
- A severe purulent discharge with a hyperacute onset (within 12-24 hours) should prompt an emergent consult with an ophthalmologist for an aggressive workup of possible gonococcal conjunctivitis. Initial ED treatment involves *Neisseria gonorrhoeae* culture, parenteral antibiotics, and saline irrigation to remove the discharge.
- Viral conjunctivitis presents as a monocular or binocular watery discharge, chemosis, and conjunctival inflammation most commonly caused by adenovirus.
- Viral conjunctivitis is often associated with viral respiratory symptoms and a palpable preauricular node. Conjunctival follicles are present.
- Fluorescein staining may reveal occasional superficial punctate keratitis, but should otherwise be clear.
- Treatment of viral conjunctivitis consists of cool compresses, naphazoline/pheniramine as needed for conjunctival congestion, and ophthalmology follow-up in 7 to 14 days.
- Epidemic keratoconjunctivitis is a severe, epidemic, highly contagious type of adenovirus conjunctivitis. It is often preceded with flu-like symptoms (including nausea and vomiting), and often involves marked injection of the conjunctiva, sometimes with frank hemorrhage. Slit lamp examination reveals diffuse superficial keratitis without ulceration. Treatment is supportive as described above, but symptoms may persist for 2 or 3 weeks. The virus survives on inanimate objects for 5 weeks and is not killed by alcohol-based hand gels; therefore, proper anti-infective precautions should be taken.
- Allergic conjunctivitis presents as a monocular or binocular pruritus, watery discharge, and chemosis with a history of allergies.

TABLE 151-1 Common Ophthalmic Medications Used in the Emergency Department

DRUG	INDICATION	DOSE
Cyclopentolate*	Short-term mydriasis and cycloplegia for examination	0.5% in children, one drop; 1% in adults, one drop; onset 30 min, duration ≤24 h
Tropicamide*	Short-term mydriasis and cycloplegia for examination	1-2 drops of 0.5% or 1% solution, onset 20 min; duration of action 6 h
Homatropine*	Intermediate-term pupil dilation, cycloplegia, treatment of iritis	1-2 drops of 2% solution; onset 30 min; duration of action 2-4 d; for iritis 1-2 drops twice a day
Naphazoline and pheniramine*	Conjunctival congestion/itching	One drop 3-4 times a day
Olopatadine	Allergic conjunctivitis	0.1% solution, one drop twice daily, onset of action 30-60 min, duration 12 h
Tetracaine ophthalmic solution	Anesthetic for eye examination, foreign body removal	0.5% solution, 1-2 drops; onset of action 1 min, duration 30 min
Proparacaine ophthalmic solution	Anesthetic for eye examination foreign body removal	0.5% solution, 1-2 drops; onset of action 20 s, duration 15 min
Erythromycin ophthalmic ointment	Conjunctivitis. Do not use for corneal abrasion if a contact lens wearer	½ in. applied to lower eyelid 2-4 times a day
Ciprofloxacin	Conjunctivitis, corneal abrasion if a contact lens wearer	Solution: 1-2 drops when awake every 2 h for 2 d; ointment, ½ in. applied to lower eyelid 3 times a day for 2 d
Tobramycin	Conjunctivitis, corneal abrasions if a contact lens wearer	0.3% solution, 1-2 drops every 4 h; 0.3% ointment, ½ in. applied to lower lid 2-3 times a day
Gentamicin	Conjunctivitis, corneal abrasion if a contact lens wearer	0.3% solution, instill 1-2 drops every 4 h; 0.3% ointment, ½ in. applied to lower lid 2-3 times a day

*Agents that affect pupillary dilation or serve as a conjunctival decongestant should be avoided in patients with glaucoma.

- There should be no lesions with fluorescein staining, and preauricular nodes should be absent. Conjunctival papillae are seen on slit lamp examination.
- Treatment of allergic conjunctivitis consists of elimination of the inciting agent, cool compresses, artificial tears, and naphazoline/pheniramine. Diphenhydramine and topical fluorometholone may be helpful in severe cases.

HERPES SIMPLEX VIRUS

- Herpes simplex virus (HSV) infection can involve eyelids, conjunctiva, and cornea.
- The classic dendrite of herpes keratitis appears as a linear branching, epithelial defect with terminal bulbs that stain brightly with fluorescein dye during slit lamp examination. However, variant presentations abound, including "geographic ulcer," neurotrophic ulceration, and isolated uveitis. Decreased corneal sensation may be a clue to the diagnosis.
- ED care depends on the site of infection: eyelid involvement may be treated with oral acyclovir, while conjunctival involvement requires topical antivirals (eg, trifluridine) five times daily with or without topical erythromycin ointment and warm soaks.
- If the cornea is involved, the trifluorothymidine dosage is increased to nine times daily plus vidarabine ointment.
- Steroids should not be prescribed, and telephone consult with an ophthalmologist to arrange 24- to 48-hour follow-up is probably prudent.
- Neonatal HSV conjunctivitis requires an emergent ophthalmology consult, parenteral antivirals, and a septic workup.

HERPES ZOSTER OPHTHALMICUS

- Herpes zoster ophthalmicus (HZO) is shingles with a trigeminal distribution, ocular involvement, and frequently, a concurrent iritis.
- The presence or eventual development of HZO should be suspected in any patient whose shingles involve the tip of the nose (Hutchinson sign).
- A "pseudo-dendrite" (a poorly staining mucous corneal plaque without epithelial erosion) may be seen. Iritis may also be seen.
- ED care for cutaneous lesions includes oral acyclovir therapy (for lesions <1 week old), along with erythromycin ointment with cool compresses.
- Conjunctivitis is treated with ophthalmic ointment, while iritis without corneal involvement may be treated with topical steroids and cycloplegics.
- Ophthalmologic consultation is advised for iritis, corneal lesions, or involvement of the orbit, optic nerve, or CNs. Hospitalization and parenteral acyclovir may be required.

CORNEAL ULCER

- These infections of the corneal stroma present with pain, redness, and photophobia. Etiologies include desiccation, trauma, direct invasion, and contact lens use, typically in association with *Pseudomonas aeruginosa* (see Fig. 151-1).
- Additional organisms associated with corneal ulcer include the bacteria *Strep. pneumoniae*, *Staphylococcus* species, *Moraxella* species; the viruses herpes simplex and varicella zoster; and the fungi *Candida*, *Aspergillus*, *Penicillium*, and *Cephalosporium*.
- Slit lamp examination reveals a staining corneal defect with a surrounding white hazy infiltrate, or heaped-up edges. If an associated iritis is present, a hypopyon may be seen.
- ED care includes hourly topical ofloxacin or ciprofloxacin drops.
- Topical cycloplegia helps relieve pain, but patching is contraindicated. An ophthalmologist should evaluate the patient within 12 to 24 hours.

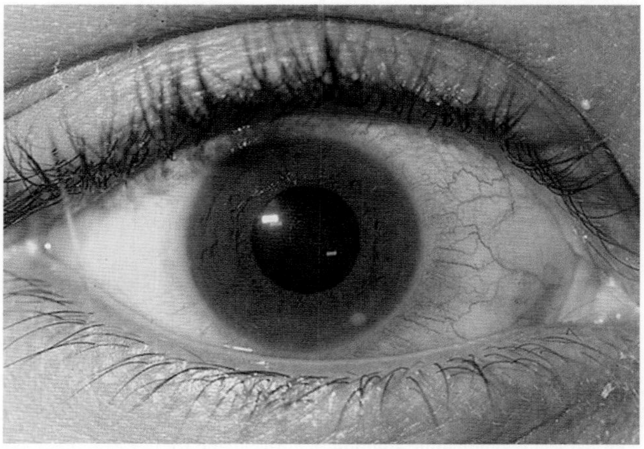

FIG. 151-1. Corneal ulcer. An elliptical ulcer at 5 o'clock near the periphery is seen. This location is atypical for a bacterial ulcer. The patient presented with painful red eyes and normal uncorrected vision, but was a new wearer of soft contact lenses. Bilateral corneal ulcers were diagnosed, which cleared after treatment with topical ciprofloxacin. The impressive ciliary flush is pathognomonic for corneal (versus conjunctival) pathology. (Photo contributed by Kevin J. Knoop, MD, MS. Knoop KJ, Stack LB, Storrow AB, Thurman RJ: *The Atlas of Emergency Medicine*, 3rd ed: http://www.accessmedicine.com. © The McGraw Hill Companies, Inc. All rights reserved.)

UVEITIS/IRITIS

- Iritis is inflammation of the anterior uveal tract (iris and ciliary body) that has many causes (Table 151-2). It presents with red eye, photophobia, and decreased vision.
- Consensual photophobia, perilimbal flush, and a miotic poorly reactive pupil are characteristic of the diagnosis. Slit lamp examination reveals WBCs in the anterior chamber, usually with associated flare, and a hypopyon can eventually occur. Fluorescein examination should be done because possible etiologies may be detected (corneal abrasion, ulcer, or dendrite).
- Once iritis is diagnosed, an appropriate ED workup for a systemic etiology should be undertaken (Table 151-2).
- Treatment is directed toward the underlying cause if found, and symptomatic treatment with homatropine or tropicamide (Table 151-1) is helpful. Steroid drops can be of value, but should only be given if directed by the ophthalmologist.
- Ophthalmology consultation is appropriate with follow up in 24 to 48 hours.

ENDOPHTHALMITIS

- Endophthalmitis is inflammation involving the deep structures of the globe, most commonly postsurgical or from penetrating trauma, although hematologic spread is possible. Pathogens include *Staphylococcus, Streptococcus, Haemophilus,* and *Bacillus.*
- Patients present with headache, eye pain, photophobia, ocular discharge, and vision loss. Examination reveals lid edema and erythema, conjunctival injection and chemosis, hypopyon, and evidence of uveitis.
- Emergency ophthalmology consultation and admission are warranted. Treatment includes intraocular and systemic antibiotics. Steroids intravitreally or orally may be used by the ophthalmologist, and admission is warranted except for postoperative cases.

TABLE 151-2 Differential Diagnosis of Iritis

Systemic diseases	Malignancies
Juvenile rheumatoid arthritis	Leukemia
Ankylosing spondylitis	Lymphoma
Ulcerative colitis	Malignant melanoma
Reiter syndrome	Trauma/environmental
Behçet syndrome	Corneal foreign body
Sarcoidosis	Post-traumatic (blunt trauma)
Infectious	Ultraviolet keratitis
Tuberculosis	
Lyme disease	
Herpes simplex	
Toxoplasmosis	
Varicella zoster	
Syphilis	
Adenovirus	

VITREOUS HEMORRHAGE

- Traction to vitreous attachments from trauma or neovascularization can cause hemorrhage into or behind the vitreous.
- Such bleeds are associated with diabetic retinopathy, sickle-cell disease, retinal detachment, central retinal vein occlusion, lupus, vitreous detachment in the elderly, and shaken baby syndrome. It is seen rarely in subarachnoid hemorrhage.
- Patients present with sudden, painless vision loss with black spots, cobwebs, or hazy vision. Examination reveals a poor view of the posterior segment due to hemorrhage.
- An emergent ophthalmology consult is warranted and ocular US may be used to rule out retinal detachment.

OCULAR TRAUMA

SUBCONJUNCTIVAL HEMORRHAGE

- Disruption of conjunctival blood vessels may occur from trauma, sneezing, gagging, or the Valsalva maneuver, and will resolve spontaneously within 2 weeks.
- When a dense, circumferential bloody chemosis is present, globe rupture must be excluded.

CONJUNCTIVAL ABRASION, LACERATION, AND FOREIGN BODY

- These corneal lesions present primarily with a foreign body sensation without vision loss. They may be impossible to see without fluorescein slit lamp examination.
- In the presence of abrasions or lacerations, an intraocular foreign body should be excluded. A Seidel's test should be performed, but it can be falsely negative if a small laceration has spontaneously closed.
- Foreign bodies can usually be removed with a moistened cotton applicator.
- Superficial conjunctival lesions are treated with erythromycin ointment for 2 or 3 days.

Corneal Abrasion

- Trauma may cause superficial or deep corneal abrasions that present with tearing, photophobia, blepharospasm, and severe pain, which are relieved by a topical anesthetic.
- Instilled fluorescein will reveal dye uptake at the site of the defect. When multiple linear abrasions or punctate keratitis are present, an ocular foreign body underneath the upper lid must be excluded.
- ED care includes administration of a cycloplegic (contraindicated in narrow anterior chamber angle patients) and topical antibiotics may be prescribed (Table 151-3).
- Contact lens abrasions are treated with ciprofloxacin, ofloxacin, or tobramycin drops to cover *Pseudomonas*.
- Tetanus status should probably be updated on all patients with corneal abrasions, especially when organic or soil-based materials are involved.
- Recent studies suggest that patching does not facilitate abrasion healing and is also absolutely contraindicated in dirty abrasions and contact lens abrasions.
- Once the diagnosis of a simple abrasion is made, NSAID ophthalmic drops should be considered for pain control. Opioid analgesia may also be necessary for severe pain.
- Topical anesthetics for home use are strictly contraindicated.
- Intraocular foreign bodies should be suspected if a history compatible with penetrating injury is present.
- Ophthalmology follow-up is advised within 24 hours for all corneal abrasions.

Corneal Laceration

- The presentation of corneal lacerations can vary from obvious (misshapen lens, shallow anterior chamber, and hyphema) to occult (spontaneous closure, negative Seidel's test, and grossly normal anatomy).
- Pain out of proportion to examination and decreased visual acuity associated with a high-risk mechanism (including the use of high-speed machinery) should raise suspicion of this injury.

TABLE 151-3 Suggested Ophthalmic Antibiotics for Corneal Abrasions

SITUATION	ANTIBIOTIC
Not related to contact lens wear	Erythromycin ophthalmic ointment three to four times a day
Related to contact lens wear	Ciprofloxacin, ofloxacin, or tobramycin ointment three to four times a day
Organic source	Erythromycin ointment three to four times a day

- CT of orbit should be obtained, but the sensitivity for this injury is only 56% to 68%.
- ED consultation with an ophthalmologist should be obtained.

Ultraviolet Keratitis

- Ultraviolet (UV) keratitis results from excess UV exposure, typically from tanning booths, welding flashes, or prolonged sun exposure.
- Severe pain and photophobia develop 6 to 12 hours after exposure. Conjunctival hyperemia and superficial punctate keratitis are seen.
- ED care is the same as for superficial corneal abrasions.

Corneal Foreign Bodies

- Corneal foreign bodies can result from numerous mechanisms. They may present with associated iritis and presence of hyphema suggests the presence of globe perforation.
- Superficial corneal foreign bodies may be removed with a fine needle tip, eye spud, or eye burr after applying a topical anesthetic. The resultant corneal defect should be treated as a corneal abrasion.
- Deep corneal stoma foreign bodies or those in the central visual axis require ophthalmology consultation for removal.
- Rust rings are associated with metallic foreign bodies and may be removed with an eye burr, although emergent removal is not required.
- Residual rust, central visual axis lesions, or deep stromal involvement requires ophthalmologic follow-up within 24 hours.

LID LACERATIONS

- Damage to the eye and nasolacrimal system must be excluded in all eyelid and adnexal lacerations.
- Less than 1 mm lid edge lacerations do not require repair.
- Visible orbital fat is a clue to a penetrated ocular septum.
- Any full-thickness laceration raises the possibility of corneal laceration and globe rupture.
- Fluorescein instilled into the tear layer that appears in an adjacent laceration confirms injury to the nasolacrimal system.
- Suspected or proven nasolacrimal injuries, lid margin lacerations, levator mechanism lacerations, ptosis, and all through-and-through lid lacerations require ophthalmology consultation for repair.

BLUNT TRAUMA

- In blunt trauma, the integrity of the globe must be immediately assessed, as well as the visual acuity.
- Signs such as an abnormal anterior chamber depth, an irregular pupil, or blindness indicate a ruptured globe until proven otherwise. Therefore, if any of these signs are present, the examination should be terminated and the eye shielded, and an emergent ophthalmology referral is indicated.
- If the globe appears intact, a complete examination (including a slit lamp examination with fluorescein) should be done and CT scan of facial bones be obtained.
- Traumatic iritis in the absence of a corneal injury can be treated with topical prednisolone acetate and cyclopentolate in conjunction with an ophthalmologist.
- The care of the blunt trauma eye patient should be discussed with an ophthalmologist, and the patient should follow up with them within 48 hours even if no significant injuries are initially found.

HYPHEMA

- A hyphema is blood in the anterior chamber, and it can occur spontaneously (sickle-cell or coagulopathy patients) or following trauma (Fig. 151-2).
- Rebleeding can occur 3 to 5 days following the initial injury and is associated with a high complication rate.
- ED care includes placing the patient upright to allow the blood to settle inferiorly, and placement of a protective eye shield. Pupillary dilatation (to avoid stretching a presumed leaking iris vessel) may be indicated, but should be done in conjunction with an ophthalmologist.

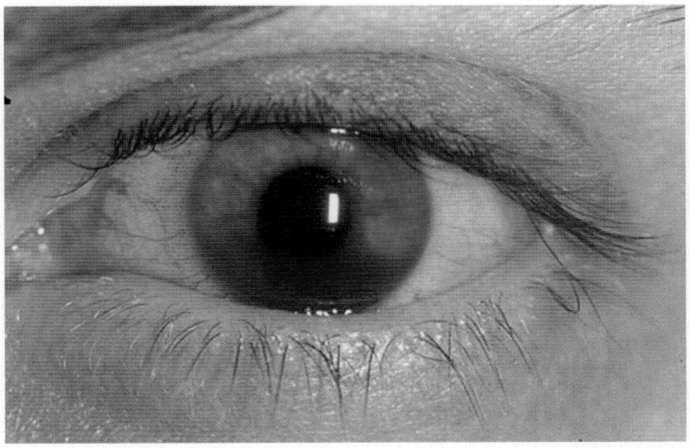

FIG. 151-2. Hyphema. This hyphema is just beginning to layer out reflecting its acute nature. (Photo contributed by Lawrence B. Stack, MD. Knoop KJ, Stack LB, Storrow AB, Thurman RJ: *The Atlas of Emergency Medicine*, 3rd ed: http://www.accessmedicine.com. © The McGraw Hill Companies, Inc. All rights reserved.)

- After ruptured globe has been excluded, intraocular pressure should be measured and controlled (see the Acute Angle Closure Glaucoma section below).
- Sickle-cell patients should not receive carbonic anhydrase inhibitors, which can cause RBC sickling within the anterior chamber and thereby increase intraocular pressure.
- In every hyphema, emergent evaluation at the bedside by an ophthalmologist is indicated.

BLOWOUT FRACTURES

- The inferior and medial wall (lamina papyracea) of the orbit may be fractured from blunt trauma.
- One-third of blowout fractures are associated with ocular trauma.
- Physical examination signs include evidence of inferior rectus entrapment (diplopia on upward gaze), paresthesia of the infraorbital nerve, and subcutaneous emphysema, especially when sneezing or blowing the nose.
- CT of the orbit with thin cuts is the radiographic test of choice to define the lesion.
- ED care includes excluding associated ocular traumatic lesions and oral antibiotics (typically cephalexin).
- All blowout fractures (with or without entrapment) require referral to an appropriate specialist within the next 3 to 10 days. Even if the initial eye examination is normal, the patient should receive an outpatient fully dilated examination to rule out any associated retinal injuries.

RUPTURED GLOBE

- Ruptured globe can result from both blunt and penetrating trauma. Any projectile injury can penetrate the eye and any puncture or laceration of the eyelid or periorbital area should raise suspicion of this injury.
- High-risk mechanisms include hammering metal on metal, use of high-speed machinery, and explosion-related injuries.
- Associated eye pain may range in severity, and visual acuity may or may not be affected.
- Suggestive findings include a severe subconjunctival hemorrhage, irregular or teardrop-shaped pupil, afferent pupillary defect, shallow or deep anterior chamber compared with the other eye, hyphema, limitation of extraocular motility, extrusion of globe contents, lens dislocation, or a significant reduction in visual acuity. However, examination may be virtually normal as well with very small wounds.
- Fluorescein streaming (Seidel's test) is pathognomonic, although it may be absent.
- Once a globe injury is suspected, any further manipulation or examination of the eye must be avoided at all costs, including measurement of intraocular pressure.

- ED care includes placing the patient upright and NPO (nothing by mouth), placing a protective metallic eye shield, administration of intravenous broad-spectrum antibiotics, analgesia, sedation, and antiemetic therapy. Tetanus status should be updated if necessary.
- A CT of the orbit with thin cuts is the test of choice to screen for an intraocular foreign body. US may assist in the diagnosis, but care must be taken not to apply pressure to the eye. MR is contraindicated with metallic foreign bodies.
- Whether or not ruptured globe is a contraindication to the use of succinylcholine remains a controversial topic.
- An ophthalmologist should be called immediately if a globe rupture or a penetrating injury is strongly suspected.

RETROBULBAR HEMATOMA

- Blunt trauma can cause blood to collect within the retrobulbar space, which can raise the intraocular pressure, causing decreased blood flow.
- Patients present with pain, decreased vision, and proptosis.
- Diagnosis is confirmed by CT scan of the orbit, and intraocular pressure should be measured if ruptured globe not present.
- Intraocular pressure >40 mm Hg should prompt consideration of emergent lateral canthotomy.
- Emergent ophthalmology consultation should be obtained, but should not delay canthotomy.

CHEMICAL OCULAR INJURY

- Acid and alkali burns are managed similarly. The eye should be immediately flushed in the prehospital setting, and sterile normal saline or Ringer's lactate Morgan Lens® irrigation should be continued in the ED immediately upon arrival (even before visual acuities or patient registration) until the pH is normal (7.0-7.4).
- Once the pH is normal, the fornices should be swept to remove residual particles and any necrotic conjunctiva. The pH should be rechecked in 10 minutes to ensure that no additional corrosive is leaching out from the tissues.
- After irrigation, a full slit lamp examination should be done to evaluate the cornea and detect iritis. Intraocular pressure should be measured.
- An attempt to identify the substance should be made to research its pH.
- A cycloplegic and narcotic pain medication should be prescribed. Tetanus status should be updated.
- Chemosis indicates the existence of "chemical conjunctivitis" and requires the use of erythromycin ointment.
- Ophthalmology consultation is appropriate for all but the most minor burns. An ophthalmologist should evaluate the patient in the ED if there are signs of a severe injury, such as a pronounced chemosis, conjunctival blanching, corneal edema, defect, or opacification, or increased intraocular pressure.

CYANOACRYLATE (SUPER GLUE/ CRAZY GLUE) EXPOSURE

- Cyanoacrylate glue easily adheres to the eyelids and corneal surface. Corneal injuries can occur from the hard particles that form.
- Initial manual removal is facilitated by heavy application of erythromycin ointment, with special care taken not to damage underlying structures.
- After the easily removable pieces are removed, the patient should be discharged with erythromycin ointment to be applied five times a day in order to soften the remaining glue.
- Complete removal of the residual glue can be accomplished by the ophthalmologist at a follow-up visit within 24 hours.

■ ACUTE VISUAL REDUCTION OR LOSS

ACUTE ANGLE CLOSURE GLAUCOMA

- Acute angle closure glaucoma presents with eye pain, headache, cloudy vision, colored halos around lights, cloudy or steamy appearance of the cornea (see Fig. 151-3), conjunctival injection, a fixed, mid-dilated

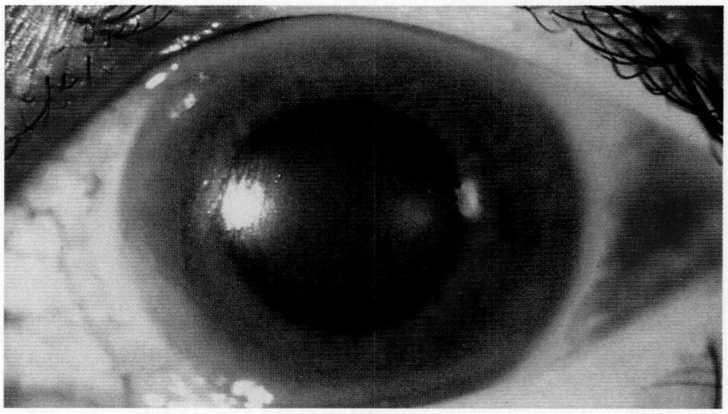

FIG. 151-3. Acute angle-closure glaucoma: Note the cloudy/steamy appearance of the cornea and the midposition dilated pupil. Conjunctival injection is usually more prominent than in this case. (Reproduced with permission from Knoop K, Stack L, Storrow A: Atlas of Emergency Medicine, 2nd ed. © 2002, McGraw-Hill, New York.)

TABLE 151-4 Treatment of Acute Glaucoma

TREATMENT/ASSESSMENT	EFFECT
Topical β-blocker (timolol 0.5%), one drop	Blocks production of aqueous humor
Topical α-agonist (apraclonidine 1%), one drop	Blocks production of aqueous humor
Carbonic anhydrase inhibitor (acetazolamide) 500 milligrams IV or PO	Blocks production of aqueous humor
Mannitol, 1-2 grams/kg IV	Reduces volume of aqueous humor
Recheck intraocular pressure hourly	May determine need for alternative treatments
Topical pilocarpine 1-2%, one drop every 15 min for two doses, once intraocular pressure is below 40 mm Hg, then 4 times daily	Facilitates outflow of aqueous humor

pupil, and increased intraocular pressure of 40 to 70 mm Hg (normal range: 10-20 mm Hg) (Fig. 151-3). Nausea and vomiting are also common.
- Sudden attacks in patients with narrow anterior chamber angles can be precipitated by pupillary dilation in movie theaters, while reading, and after administration of dilatory agents or inhaled anticholinergics.
- The diagnosis is confirmed by measuring the intraocular pressure as diagnosis by manual palpation is unreliable.
- ED care is designed to decrease the intraocular pressure. Immediate medications to administer include timolol, apraclonidine, and prednisolone acetate (Table 151-4).
- If intraocular pressure is greater than 50 mm Hg or if vision loss is severe, then acetazolamide 500 milligrams IV should be considered.
- If intraocular pressure does not decrease and vision does not improve in 1 hour, IV mannitol should be given.
- Pilocarpine 1% to 2% in the affected eye and pilocarpine 0.5% in the contralateral eye may be administered once intraocular pressure is less than 40 mm Hg as long as the patient has a natural lens in place.
- Symptoms of pain and nausea should be treated, and the intraocular pressure monitored hourly. All cases require emergent in-person ophthalmologic consultation, but treatment should not be delayed for consultation. All subsequent treatment and disposition decisions should be made in conjunction with the ophthalmologist at the bedside.

OPTIC NEURITIS

- Inflammation of the optic nerve can be caused by infection, demyelination, and autoimmune disorders. It is famously associated with multiple sclerosis.
- Optic neuritis may present with various degrees of vision loss (often with poor color perception), pain during extraocular movement, visual field cuts, and an afferent pupillary defect.
- Swelling of the optic disc may be seen in anterior optic neuritis (30%).
- Diagnosis can be made with the red desaturation test (after staring at a bright red object with the normal eye only, the object may subsequently appear pink or light red in the affected eye).
- ED treatment with IV steroids is controversial and should be discussed with an ophthalmologist. A neurology consult may also be helpful.

CENTRAL RETINAL ARTERY OCCLUSION

- Central retinal artery occlusion may be caused by embolus, thrombosis, giant-cell arteritis, vasculitis, sickle-cell disease, vasospasm (migraine) glaucoma, hypercoagulable states, low retinal blood flow, and trauma.
- It is often preceded by amaurosis fugax.
- The vision loss is painless, with complete or near-complete vision loss, unless only a single arterial branch is affected.
- An afferent pupillary defect is often present and funduscopy classically reveals a pale fundus with narrowed arterioles with segmented flow ("boxcars"), with a bright red macula ("cherry red spot").
- Classic ED care includes ocular massage (digital pressure for 15 seconds, followed by sudden release) and topical timolol or IV acetazolamide; however, evidence-based treatment is lacking. Emergent ophthalmology consultation is indicated.

CENTRAL RETINAL VEIN OCCLUSION

- Thrombosis of the central retinal vein causes painless, rapid monocular vision loss. It is associated with numerous medical conditions including diabetes, hypertension, CVD, CAD, dyslipidemia, hypercoagulable states, vasculitis, glaucoma, thyroid disease, and orbital tumors.
- Funduscopy classically reveals diffuse retinal hemorrhages, cotton wool spots, and optic disc edema ("blood-and-thunder"). The contralateral optic nerve and fundus are usually normal.
- Predisposing drugs (eg, oral contraceptives, diuretics) should be discontinued.
- No specific treatment is available, and ophthalmology and neurology consultation should be obtained.

FLASHING LIGHTS (PHOTOPSIAS) AND FLOATERS/RETINAL DETACHMENT

- Monocular symptoms indicate involvement of the symptomatic eye, whereas binocular symptoms suggest an intracranial etiology.
- As the vitreous ages, it contracts and tugs on the retinal, causing flashes of light to be perceived. Floaters occur when the vitreous separates completely and are generally benign.
- The separating vitreous can traumatize the retina as it separates, which can create a retinal hole and subsequent detachment (rhegmatogenous type).
- Exudative retinal detachments occur when fluid accumulates behind the retina without a tear, while tractional detachments are caused when acquired fibrocellular bands in the vitreous detach the retina (associated with diabetic retinopathy, sickle-cell disease, and trauma).
- Symptoms of retinal detachment include flashing lights, floaters, a dark curtain or veil in the field of vision, and diminished visual acuity.
- Ultrasound may be useful in the diagnosis (Figure 151-4).
- If retinal tear or detachment is suspected, a dilated indirect retinal examination by an ophthalmologist is mandatory within 24 hours because direct ophthalmoscopy can potentially miss most retinal injuries.

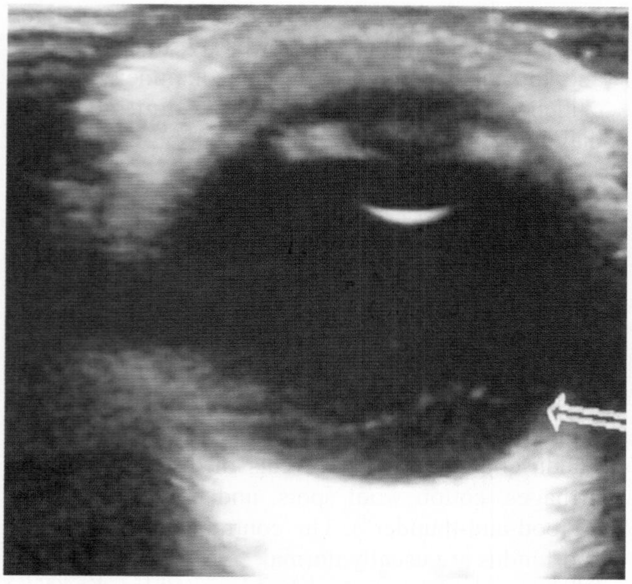

FIG. 151-4. Retinal detachment is seen as a hyperechoic membrane in the posterior aspect of the globe (*arrow*).

GIANT CELL ARTERITIS (TEMPORAL ARTERITIS)

- Giant cell arteritis is a systemic vasculitis that can cause ischemic optic neuropathy. Patients are usually >50 years old, female, and often have polymyalgia rheumatica.
- Symptoms and signs include headache, jaw claudication, myalgias, fatigue, fever, anorexia, temporal artery tenderness, and often neurologic findings (including transient ischemic attack [TIA] and stroke).
- An afferent pupillary defect is often present.
- C-reactive protein and erythrocyte sedimentation rate are usually elevated (70-110 seconds).
- ED care includes IV steroids and ophthalmologic consultation.
- Steroids should not be delayed for temporal artery biopsy, as they may be sight saving and biopsy results will still be positive for 7 days.

BELL'S PALSY

- Bell's palsy is a paralysis of peripheral nerve VII which can lead to exposure keratitis, which is treated with viscous topic wetting agents and eyelid taping.
- It must not be confused with a Genu VII Bell's palsy, which is a CVA. The differentiating feature is the presence of a CN VI paresis on the affected side, and that eye cannot abduct.
- Treatment for Bell's palsy is controversial, but current evidence suggests that antivirals *with* steroids provide benefit. A Genu VII Bell's palsy should be treated as a CVA.

DIABETIC/HYPERTENSIVE CRANIAL NERVE PALSIES

- Over time, diabetes and hypertension can cause a vascular-related CN III palsy.
- Examination reveals ptosis with decreased EOMs (except for abduction). The pupillary reflex is **normal**.
- Diplopia (especially with looking in the direction of the other eye) is a common finding.
- CT scan is required in the ED to rule out an intracranial lesion.
- Assuming glucose and blood pressure do not require acute treatment, the patient may be managed with follow-up with ophthalmology and/or neurology.

POSTERIOR COMMUNICATING ARTERY ANEURYSM

- This presents as an acute CN III palsy with ipsilateral pupillary dilatation, commonly associated with headache.
- ED care includes blood pressure management, emergent CT or MR angiogram, and neurosurgical consultation.

HORNER'S SYNDROME

- The classic triad of ipsilateral ptosis, miosis (pupillary constriction), and anhydrosis (absence of sweating) is present.
- It is associated with CVA, tumors (classically, Pancoast), internal carotid dissection, herpes zoster, and trauma. Childhood etiologies include neuroblastoma, lymphoma, and metastatic disease.
- A CXR, CT scan of the brain and neck, as well as a CT or MR angiogram of the neck and cerebral arteries are indicated.
- Specific treatment is determined by the etiology of the Horner's syndrome.

PAPILLEDEMA

- Papilledema is defined as bilateral edema of the head of the optic nerve due to increased intraocular pressure (ICP). It may be seen in any disease process that raises ICP.
- Examination reveals a blurred disc margin with a diminished or absent cup, with an elevated nerve head (Fig. 151-5).
- When the classic findings are unilateral, it is not from increased ICP and is referred to as optic nerve edema (noninflammatory) or papillitis (inflammatory).
- Vision is generally preserved in true papilledema, whereas papillitis results in decreased visual acuity (eg, optic neuritis).

BENIGN INTRACRANIAL HYPERTENSION (PSEUDOTUMOR CEREBRI)

- Benign intracranial hypertension (BIH) consists of increased ICP and papilledema with normal mental status, CSF, and neuroimaging, and occurs most commonly in young women of childbearing age who are not necessarily obese.
- BIH presents with headache, nausea, vomiting, visual field deficits, and blurred vision. It is sometimes associated with a CN VI deficit, with resultant horizontal diplopia on lateral gaze.
- A CT of the head should be obtained to rule out intracranial pathology.

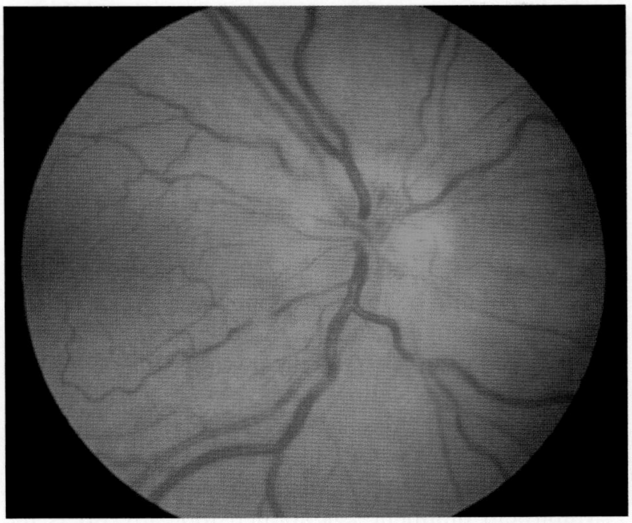

FIG. 151-5. Optic nerve head edema. Vascular congestion, elevation of the nerve head, and blurred disk margins are characteristically seen in papilledema, papillitis, and compressive lesions of the optic nerve. (Reproduced with permission from Knoop K, Stack L, Storrow A: *Atlas of Emergency Medicine, 2nd ed.* © 2002, McGraw-Hill, New York.)

- A lumbar puncture should be performed to measure ICP and to rule out CSF abnormalities.
- A neurosurgery consult should be obtained for management recommendations, which typically include acetazolamide and visual field monitoring.

OCULAR ULTRASONOGRAPHY

- Ocular ultrasonography may be helpful in the diagnosis of retinal detachment (Fig. 151-4), retrobulbar hematoma, globe preformation, lens dislocation, vitreous hemorrhage, and intraocular foreign body.
- Caution must be used when a globe rupture is suspected, and copious gel must be applied to the closed eye to avoid touching the eyelid with the transducer.
- The duration of ocular ultrasonography must be strictly limited due to concerns of mechanical energy (exposure limits that are roughly 50% for that of fetal ultrasonography).
- Ocular ultrasonography is limited by patient cooperation, orbital emphysema, and various artifacts.

For further reading in Tintinalli's *Emergency Medicine: A Comprehensive Study Guide*, 7th ed., see Chapter 236, "Eye Emergencies," by Richard A. Walker and Srikar Adhikari.

152 FACE AND JAW EMERGENCIES

Jeffrey G. Norvell

FACIAL INFECTIONS

IMPETIGO

- Impetigo is a superficial epidermal infection that can be divided into bullous and nonbullous presentations.
- Bullous impetigo is caused by *Staphylococcus aureus,* and it presents as vesicles that rapidly enlarge to form bullae with clear yellow fluid.
- Nonbullous impetigo is caused by *Streptococcus pyogenes* and *Staph. aureus,* and it presents as vesicles that break and form the characteristic honey crusts.
- Mupirocin ointment 2% applied topically tid is the treatment of choice for localized infections.
- Oral antibiotics are indicated for more diffuse infections and for infections that do not respond to topical therapy (Tables 152-1 and 152-2).

TABLE 152-1 Antibiotic Therapy for Facial Infections

Cellulitis	Oral therapy: clindamycin; or cephalosporins are alternatives Suspected MRSA: trimethoprim-sulfamethoxazole, clindamycin, doxycycline, or minocycline Parenteral therapy: vancomycin, clindamycin Total duration 7-14 d
Erysipelas	Oral therapy: penicillin Methicillin-sensitive *Staphylococcus aureus* suspected: amoxicillin/clavulanate, cephalexin, dicloxacillin Bullous erysipelas: trimethoprim-sulfamethoxazole, clindamycin, doxycycline, or minocycline Parenteral therapy: vancomycin, nafcillin, clindamycin Total duration 7-14 d
Impetigo	Topical: mupirocin or retapamulin ointment alone or with oral therapy Oral therapy: dicloxacillin, amoxicillin/clavulanate, cephalexin MRSA suspected: clindamycin or trimethoprim-sulfamethoxazole Total duration: 7 d
Suppurative parotitis	Parental therapy: nafcillin, or ampicillin- sulbactam; if penicillin allergic, clindamycin or the combination of cephalexin with metronidazole, or vancomycin with metronidazole Hospital-acquired or nursing home patients: include vancomycin Total duration: 10-14 d
Masticator space infection	Parenteral therapy: IV clindamycin is recommended; alternatives include ampicillin-sulbactam, cefoxitin, or the combination of penicillin with metronidazole Oral therapy: clindamycin or amoxicillin-clavulanate Total duration: 10-14 d

Abbreviation: MRSA = methicillin-resistant *Staphylococcus aureus.*

TABLE 152-2 Antibiotic Doses for Facial Infections

ANTIBIOTIC	DOSAGE
Topical antibiotics	
Mupirocin ointment	2%, apply to lesions 3 times per day
Retapamulin ointment	1%, apply to lesions 2 times per day
Oral antibiotics	
Amoxicillin/clavulanate	875/125 milligrams 2 times per day
Cephalexin	500 milligrams 4 times per day
Clindamycin	300-450 milligrams 3 times per day
Dicloxacillin	500 milligrams 4 times per day
Doxycycline	100 milligrams 2 times per day
Metronidazole	500 milligrams every 8 h
Minocycline	100 milligrams 2 times per day
Penicillin V	500 milligrams 4 times per day
Trimethoprim-sulfamethoxazole	1-2 double-strength tablets 2 times per day
Parenteral antibiotics	
Ampicillin-sulbactam	1.5-3.0 grams every 6 h
Piperacillin-tazobactam	3.375 grams every 6 h
Clindamycin	600 milligrams every 8 h
Cefazolin	1 gram every 8 h
Metronidazole	1-gram loading dose, then 500 milligrams every 8 h
Nafcillin	1-2 grams every 4 h
Penicillin G	2-3 million units every 6 h
Vancomycin	1 gram every 12 h

ERYSIPELAS

- Erysipelas is a superficial form of cellulitis involving the epidermis, upper levels of the dermis, and the lymphatic system.
- Most common on the lower extremities, but also described on the face.
- Erysipelas is most commonly caused by *Strep. pyogenes* and rarely *Staph. aureus*. *Staphylococcus aureus* is commonly found in bullous erysipelas.
- Clinical features include a painful, red, raised, puffy appearance with a sharply defined, palpable border.
- The diagnosis is clinical.
- Patients are usually treated with oral antibiotics. Hospitalization and parenteral antibiotics should be considered for failed outpatient therapy, immunocompromise, or evidence of systemic illness. Antibiotic recommendations are listed in Tables 152-1 and 152-2.

CELLULITIS

- Cellulitis is a soft tissue infection that involves the skin and subcutaneous tissues.

- Risk factors for cellulitis include violation of the skin barrier, immunosuppression, systemic disease (eg, diabetes), vascular compromise, and foreign bodies.
- The pathogen usually is *Strep. pyogenes* or *Staph. aureus*, with an increasing predominance of methicillin-resistant *Staph. aureus*. Less commonly, cellulitis may represent extension from a deeper facial infection.
- Cellulitis is characterized by erythema, edema, pain, warmth, and loss of function. A well-defined, palpable border is absent.
- The diagnosis of cellulitis is clinical.
- Laboratories and blood cultures may be needed for severe illness, immunocompromise, or significant comorbidities. Ultrasound and computed tomography may be used to evaluate for abscess.
- Most patients can be treated with oral antibiotics (Tables 152-1 and 152-2).
- Consider hospitalization and parenteral antibiotics for signs of systemic illness, failed outpatient therapy, or significant comorbidities (Tables 152-1 and 152-2).

SALIVARY GLAND DISORDERS

VIRAL PAROTITIS

- **Mumps**, a paramyxovirus infection, is the most common cause of viral parotitis in children under age 15 years.
- Other viral etiologies include influenza, parainfluenza, coxsackie viruses, echoviruses, lymphocytic choriomeningitis virus, and HIV.
- The virus is spread by airborne droplets.
- Symptoms begin after an incubation period of 2 to 3 weeks and consist of fever, malaise, headache, myalgias, arthralgias, and anorexia.
- Prodromal symptoms continue for 3 to 5 days and are followed by parotid gland enlargement.
- Bilateral parotid enlargement occurs in 75% of cases and lasts up to 5 days. The gland is tense and painful, but erythema and warmth are absent and no pus can be expressed from Stensen's duct.
- Diagnosis is clinical. Viral serology can be obtained, but it will not affect acute management.
- Treatment is supportive and consists of analgesics and antipyretics.
- The patient is contagious for approximately 9 days after the onset of parotid gland swelling.
- Epididymo-orchitis is the most common extra-salivary gland involvement in postpubertal males, affecting 20% to 30% of patients. It can precede or follow parotitis.
- Oophoritis occurs in only 5% of females.
- Other systemic complications include pancreatitis, aseptic meningitis, hearing loss, myocarditis, arthritis, hemolytic anemia, and thrombocytopenia.

SUPPURATIVE PAROTITIS

- Suppurative parotitis is a serious bacterial infection that occurs in patients with diminished salivary flow.
- Retrograde transmission of oral bacteria leads to infection.
- Factors and conditions that lead to decreased salivary flow include recent anesthesia, dehydration, prematurity, advanced age, sialolithiasis, medications (eg, diuretics, β-blockers, antihistamines, phenothiazines, tricyclic antidepressants), and certain disorders (eg, diabetes, HIV, hypothyroidism, Sjögren's syndrome).
- Suppurative parotitis is usually caused by *Staph. aureus* and less often by *Streptococcus pneumoniae*, *Strep. pyogenes*, and *Haemophilus influenzae*. Anaerobes such as *Bacteroides* species, *Peptostreptococcus*, and *Fusobacterium* are found in 43% of isolates.
- Clinical features may include rapid onset, fever, trismus, erythema, and pain over the parotid gland.
- In contrast to mumps, pus may be expressed from the Stensen's duct.
- The diagnosis is clinical. Ultrasound or CT may be ordered if abscess is suspected.
- Treatment consists of hydration, local massage, heat, sialogogues (eg, lemon drops, orange juice), and oral antibiotics (Tables 152-1 and 152-2).
- Hospitalization and parenteral antibiotics (Tables 152-1 and 152-2) should be considered for trismus, inability to tolerate oral intake, immunocompromise, or failure of outpatient therapy.

SIALOLITHIASIS

- Sialolithiasis is the development of stones is a stagnant salivary duct.
- Eighty percent of salivary calculi occur in the submandibular duct and most of the remainder in the parotid duct.
- Patients present with unilateral pain, swelling, and tenderness of the involved gland that is exacerbated by meals.
- Diagnosis is clinical. The stone may be palpable and the gland will be firm.
- CT is usually only ordered if abscess is in the differential diagnosis.
- Treatment initially consists of analgesics, massage, and sialogogues. If concurrent infection is suspected, treatment with antibiotics is indicated.
- Palpable stones can be milked from the duct.
- Persistently retained calculi can be removed electively by an otolaryngologist.

MASTICATOR SPACE ABSCESS

- The masticator space consists of four contiguous potential spaces bounded by the muscles of mastication.

These spaces include the masseteric, pterygomandibular, superficial temporal, and deep temporal spaces.
- Infections in these spaces, commonly associated with an odontogenic source, are polymicrobial. Typical organisms include species of *Streptococcus*, *Peptostreptococcus*, *Bacteroides*, *Prevotella*, *Porphyromonas*, *Fusobacterium*, *Actinomyces*, *Veillonella*, and anaerobic spirochetes.
- Abscesses in these spaces result in swelling over the buccal, submandibular, or sublingual areas. Patients may also have fever, pain, erythema, and trismus.
- Contrast-enhanced CT can help differentiate cellulitis from abscess, and if an abscess is present, its extent can be detailed.
- Since these spaces ultimately communicate with the tissue planes that extend into the mediastinum, early treatment is imperative.
- Airway compromise is rare, but it should be considered.
- Emergency department treatment includes stabilization, antibiotics (Tables 152-1 and 152-2), otolaryngology consult, and hospitalization.

MANDIBLE DISORDERS

TEMPOROMANDIBULAR JOINT DYSFUNCTION

- The temporomandibular joint (TMJ) combines a hinge and gliding movement. Anatomic internal derangement or systemic disease can cause dysfunction of this joint.
- Patients present with dull pain in the region of the TMJ or pain localized over one of the muscles of mastication. Tenderness to palpation over the condylar head may be present when opening and closing the mouth and range of motion may be limited.
- The diagnosis is usually clinical. For patients with trauma, imaging with CT or panoramic tomorgraphy (Panorex) may be warranted.
- Treatment for nontraumatic conditions consists of warm compresses, soft diet, analgesics, NSAIDs, and referral to a dental specialist.
- An oral-maxillofacial surgeon manages fractures.

MANDIBLE DISLOCATION

- The mandible can be dislocated in an anterior, posterior, lateral, or superior direction.
- Anterior dislocation is most common.
- Patients with acute mandible dislocations present with severe pain, difficulty swallowing, and malocclusion.
- In anterior dislocations, pain is localized anterior to the tragus and a history of extreme mouth opening is typical.

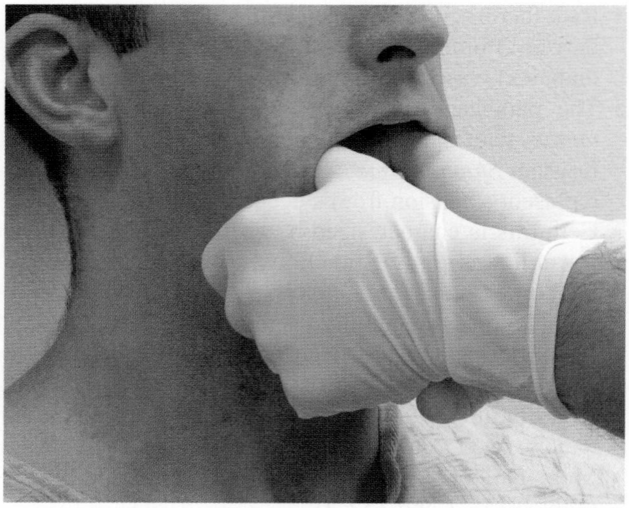

FIG. 152-1. Reduction of dislocated mandible technique in a seated patient. The thumbs are placed over the molars, and pressure is applied downward and backward.

- All other mandibular dislocations require significant trauma.
- The diagnosis of a nontraumatic anterior dislocation is made clinically.
- In other dislocations or if there is a history of trauma, imaging with mandibular radiographs, Panorex, or CT is needed.
- Reduction may be attempted in closed anterior dislocations without fracture. Reduction may be facilitated with analgesia, muscle relaxants, or procedural sedation.
- One technique to reduce anterior dislocations involves the patient in the sitting position and the provider applies downward and posterior pressure to the patient's lower molars as shown in Fig. 152-1. Tape a few layers of gauze over the provider's gloved thumbs for protection.
- Patients with open or nonreducible dislocations, associated fractures, or nerve injury should be emergently referred to an oral-maxillofacial surgeon.
- After successful reduction, patients are placed on a soft diet and instructed not to open their mouths more than 2 cm for 2 weeks.

For further reading in Tintinalli's *Emergency Medicine: A Comprehensive Study Guide*, 7th ed., see Chapter 238, "Face and Jaw Emergencies," by Corey R. Heitz.

153 EAR, NOSE, AND SINUS EMERGENCIES

Medley O. Gatewood

OTOLOGIC EMERGENCIES

OTALGIA

- Primary otalgia, caused by auricular and periauricular disease, may occur from trauma, infection, foreign body, cerumen impaction, cholesteatoma, and neoplasm.
- Referred otalgia may occur with dental disease, oropharyngeal and retropharyngeal processes, nasal cavity pathology, and disorders of the throat and neck.
- Ascertaining the cause of otalgia requires careful history and physical examination, with further management and treatment guided by the diagnosis.

TINNITUS

- Tinnitus is the perception of sound without external stimuli. It may be constant, pulsatile, high or low pitched, hissing, clicking, or ringing in nature.
- Objective tinnitus can be heard by the examiner, whereas the more common subjective tinnitus cannot.
- Causes of tinnitus include sensorineural hearing loss, hypertension, conductive hearing loss, head trauma, medications, temporomandibular joint disorders, depression, acoustic neuromas, multiple sclerosis, benign intracranial hypertension, Ménière's disease, Cogan's syndrome, arteriovenous malformations, arterial bruits, enlarged eustachian tube, palatomyoclonus, and stapedial muscle spasm.
- Common medications resulting in tinnitus include aspirin, nonsteroidal anti-inflammatory drugs, aminoglycosides, loop diuretics, and chemotherapeutics.
- Pharmacologic treatment with antidepressant medications may alleviate tinnitus in which no correctable cause can be found.

SUDDEN HEARING LOSS

- Causes of sudden hearing loss are varied and may be idiopathic (most common), infectious (mumps, Epstein–Barr virus, herpes, cytomegalovirus (CMV), syphilis, and labyrinthitis), vascular/hematologic (leukemia, sickle-cell disease, polycythemia, Berger's disease, and cerebral aneurysm), metabolic (diabetes, hyperlipidemia), rheumatologic (temporal arteritis, Wegener's granulomatosis), conductive causes (otitis externa, otitis media [OM], ruptured tympanic membrane [TM], neoplasm, and osteonecrosis), Ménière's disease, Cogan's syndrome, acoustic neuroma, cochlear rupture, and ototoxic medications.
- Indictors of poor prognosis include severe hearing loss on presentation and the presence of vertigo.
- If the cause is not readily determined by history and physical examination, otolaryngologic consultation is necessary.

OTITIS EXTERNA

Pathophysiology

- The most common organisms implicated in otitis externa are *Pseudomonas aeruginosa,* Enterobacteriaceae, and *Proteus* species, and *Staphylococcus aureus,* with *P. aeruginosa* being the most common organism causing malignant otitis externa.
- Otomycosis (fungal otitis externa) is found in tropical climates and the immunocompromised or subsequent to long-term antibiotic therapy.
- *Aspergillus* and *Candida* are the most common fungal pathogens.
- Risk factors for the development of otitis externa include swimming, trauma of the external canal, and any process that elevates the pH of the canal.

Clinical Features

- Otitis externa is characterized by pruritus, pain, and tenderness of the external ear.
- Erythema and edema of the external auditory canal (EAC), otorrhea, crusting, and hearing impairment may also be present.
- Pain is elicited with movement of the pinna or tragus.

Emergency Department Care and Disposition

- The treatment of otitis externa includes analgesics, cleaning the EAC, acidifying agents, topical antimicrobials, and occasionally topical steroid preparations.
- Ofloxacin otic five drops twice daily, acetic acid/hydrocortisone otic five drops 3 times daily (do not use with perforated TM), and ciprofloxacin/hydrocortisone otic three drops twice daily are commonly used for 7 days to treat otitis externa.
- If significant swelling of the external canal is present, a wick or piece of gauze may be inserted into the canal to allow passage of topical medications.

MALIGNANT OTITIS EXTERNA

- Malignant otitis externa is a potentially life-threatening infection of the EAC with variable extension to the skull base.

- In greater than 90% of cases, it is caused by *P. aeruginosa*.
- Elderly, diabetic, and immunocompromised patients are most commonly affected.
- Diagnosis of malignant otitis externa requires a high index of suspicion.
- Computed tomography (CT) is necessary to determine the extent and stage of the disease.
- Emergent otolaryngologic (ENT) consultation, tobramycin 2 milligrams/kg IV and piperacillin 3 to 4 grams IV, or ceftriaxone 1 gram IV, or ciprofloxacin 400 milligrams IV, and admission to the hospital are mandatory.

OTITIS MEDIA

Epidemiology

- Although adults may present with OM, its incidence and prevalence peak in the preschool years and then decrease with increasing age.

Pathophysiology

- The most common bacterial pathogens in acute OM are *Streptococcus pneumoniae, Haemophilus influenzae,* and *Moraxella catarrhalis.*
- The predominant organisms involved in chronic OM are *S. aureus, P. aeruginosa,* and anaerobic bacteria.

Clinical Features

- Patients with OM present with otalgia, with or without fever; occasionally, hearing loss and otorrhea are present.
- The TM may be retracted or bulging and will have impaired mobility on pneumatic otoscopy.
- The TM may appear red as a result of inflammation or may be yellow or white due to middle ear secretions.
- Complications of OM include TM perforation, conductive hearing loss, acute serous labyrinthitis, facial nerve paralysis, acute mastoiditis, lateral sinus thrombosis, cholesteatoma, and intracranial complications (meningitis, brain abscess, extradural abscess, and subdural empyema).

Emergency Department Care and Disposition

- A 10-day course of amoxicillin 250 to 500 milligrams PO 3 times daily for 7 to 10 days is the preferred initial treatment for OM. Alternative agents include azithromycin 500 milligrams PO daily for 1 day and then 250 milligrams PO daily for 4 days, or cefuroxime 500 milligrams PO twice daily for 10 days.
- Cefuroxime or amoxicillin/clavulanate may be given for OM unresponsive to first-line therapy after 72 hours.
- Antibiotic coverage should be extended to 3 weeks for patients with OM with effusion.
- TM perforation and conductive hearing loss are most often self-limiting and often require no specific intervention.

ACUTE MASTOIDITIS

- Acute mastoiditis occurs as infection spreads from the middle ear to the mastoid air cells.
- Patients present with otalgia, fever, and postauricular erythema, swelling, and tenderness.
- Protrusion of the auricle with obliteration of the postauricular crease may be present.
- CT will delineate the extent of bony involvement.
- Emergent ENT consultation, vancomycin 1 to 2 grams IV or ceftriaxone 1 gram IV, and admission to the hospital are necessary. Surgical drainage ultimately may be required.

LATERAL SINUS THROMBOSIS

- This condition arises from extension of infection and inflammation into the lateral and sigmoid sinuses.
- Headache is common, and papilledema, sixth nerve palsy, and vertigo may be present.
- Diagnosis may be made with CT, although magnetic resonance imaging or angiography may be necessary.
- Therapy consists of emergent ENT consultation, combination therapy with nafcillin 2 grams IV, ceftriaxone 1 gram IV, and metronidazole 500 milligrams IV, and hospital admission.

BULLOUS MYRINGITIS

- Bullous myringitis is a painful condition of the ear characterized by bulla on the TM and deep EAC.
- Numerous pathogens have been implicated including viruses, *Mycoplasma pneumoniae,* and *Chlamydia psittaci.*
- The diagnosis is made by clinical examination.
- The treatment consists of pain control and warm compresses. Antibiotics can be given for concomitant OM.

TRAUMA TO THE EAR

- A hematoma can develop from any type of trauma to the ear.
- Improper treatment of ear hematomas can result in stimulation of the perichondrium and development of asymmetric cartilage formation. The resultant deformed auricle has been termed *cauliflower ear.*

- Immediate incision and drainage of the hematoma with a compressive dressing is necessary to prevent reaccumulation of the hematoma.
- Thermal injury to the auricle may be caused by excessive heat or cold.
- Superficial injury of either type is treated with cleaning, topical non–sulfa-containing antibiotic ointment, and a light dressing.
- Frostbite is treated with rapid rewarming by using saline-soaked gauze at 38°C to 40°C.
- The rewarming process may be very painful and analgesics will be necessary.
- Any second- or third-degree burn requires immediate ENT or burn center consultation.

FOREIGN BODIES IN THE EAR

- Signs of infection or TM perforation should be sought on examination.
- Live insects should be immobilized with **2% lidocaine** solution distilled into the ear canal before removal.
- Foreign bodies may be removed with forceps and direct visualization or with the aid of a hooked probe or suction catheter.
- Irrigation is often useful for small objects; however, organic material may absorb water and swell.
- ENT consultation is required for cases of foreign body with TM perforation or if the object cannot be safely removed.

TYMPANIC MEMBRANE PERFORATION

- TM perforations can result from middle ear infections, barotrauma, blunt/penetrating/acoustic trauma, or (rarely) lightning strikes.
- Acute pain and hearing loss are usually noted, with or without bloody otorrhea. Vertigo and tinnitus, when present, are usually transient.
- As most TM perforations heal spontaneously, antibiotics are not necessary unless there is persistent foreign material in the canal or middle ear.

NASAL EMERGENCIES AND SINUSITIS

EPISTAXIS

- Epistaxis is classified as anterior or posterior.
- Posterior epistaxis is suggested if an anterior source is not visualized, if bleeding occurs from both nares, or if blood is seen draining into the posterior pharynx after anterior sources have been controlled.
- Have patients blow their nose to dislodge any clots. Instill 0.05% **oxymetazoline** two sprays/nostril or 0.25% phenylephrine two sprays/nostril. Apply direct external pressure for 15 minutes while leaning forward in the "sniffing" position. Repeat if necessary.
- If this approach fails, and an anterior source of bleeding is visualized, proceed to chemical cautery with silver nitrate after hemostasis is achieved with cotton swabs or pledgets soaked in a 1:1 mixture of a 4% lidocaine and 0.05% oxymetazoline inserted into the nasal cavity. If no source is identified, proceed to packing.
- Anterior nasal packing may be performed with dehydrated nasal sponges, anterior epistaxis balloons (Fig. 153-1), thrombogenic foams and gels, or gauze. If packing or local cautery fails to control anterior bleeding, ENT consultation is necessary.
- Posterior epistaxis may be treated with a dehydrated posterior sponge pack or an inflatable balloon posterior tamponade device. All patients with posterior packs require ENT consultation for hospital admission.
- All patients with nasal packs should be started on antibiotic prophylaxis with amoxicillin/clavulanate 500/125 milligrams PO three times daily to prevent toxic shock syndrome.
- Treatment of elevated blood pressure during an acute episode of epistaxis is generally not advised except in consultation with an otolaryngologist for cases of persistent epistaxis not uncontrolled by the above measures.

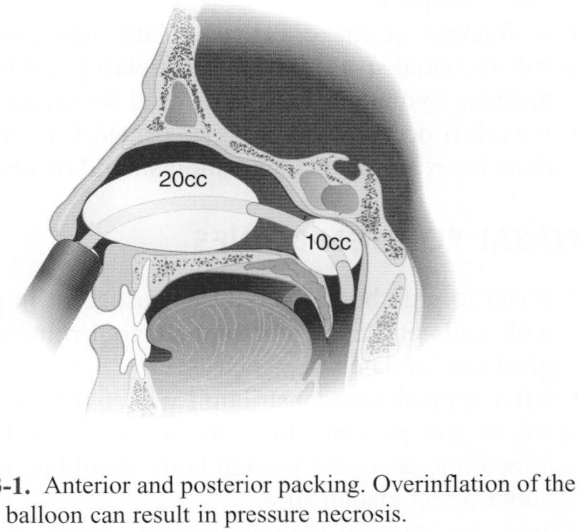

FIG. 153-1. Anterior and posterior packing. Overinflation of the posterior balloon can result in pressure necrosis.

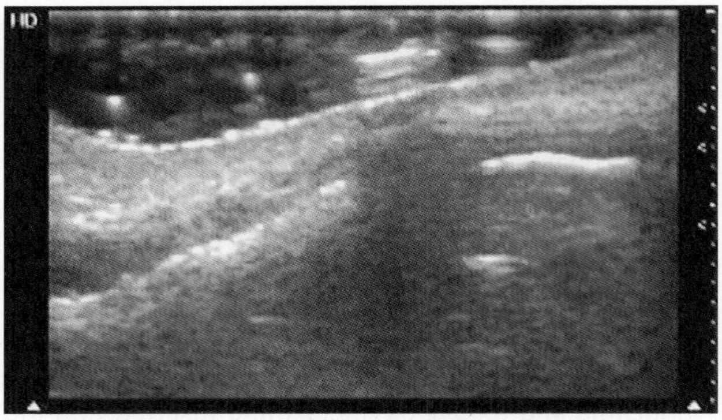

FIG. 153-2. US still image of nasal fracture demonstrating cortical disruption. A large gap is seen between bone fragments. (Reproduced with permission from Ma OJ, Mateer JR, Blaivas M: *Emergency Ultrasound, 2nd ed.* © 2008, McGraw-Hill, New York.)

NASAL FRACTURES

- Nasal fractures are the most common facial fracture.
- Nasal fracture is a clinical diagnosis suggested by the injury mechanism, swelling, tenderness, crepitance, gross deformity, and periorbital ecchymosis.
- Radiographic diagnosis usually is not necessary in the ED; ultrasound is an alternative to plain radiography (Fig. 153-2).
- Intermittent ice application, analgesics, and over-the-counter decongestants are the normal treatment.
- ENT follow-up within 6 to 10 days for reexamination and possible fracture reduction is prudent.
- The nose should be examined for a septal hematoma. If left untreated, a septal hematoma may result in abscess formation or necrosis of the nasal septum.
- The treatment of septal hematoma is local incision and drainage with subsequent placement of an anterior nasal pack.
- A fracture of the cribriform plate may violate the subarachnoid space and cause cerebrospinal fluid rhinorrhea. Symptoms may be delayed for several weeks.
- If a cribriform plate injury is suspected, CT and immediate neurosurgical consultation should be obtained.

NASAL FOREIGN BODIES

- Nasal foreign bodies should be suspected in patients with unilateral nasal obstruction, foul rhinorrhea, or persistent unilateral epistaxis.
- After topical vasoconstriction with 0.05% oxymetazoline and possibly local anesthesia with 4% nebulized lidocaine, the foreign body should be removed under direct visualization.
- Tools for removal include forceps, suction catheters, hooked probes, and balloon-tipped catheters. ENT consultation is required for any unsuccessful removal.

SINUSITIS AND RHINOSINUSITIS

Epidemiology

- Rhinosinusitis affects one in seven adults in the United States, resulting in approximately 31 million patients being diagnosed annually.
- The primary cause is viral illness; bacterial infections account for only 2% to 10% of acute rhinosinusitis cases.

Pathophysiology

- Sinusitis is inflammation of the mucosal lining of the paranasal sinuses (maxillary, frontal, ethmoid, and frontal).
- Rhinosinusitis is sinusitis also involving the nasal cavity, almost always involves rhinitis, and is extremely common. It can be classified as acute, subacute, or chronic.

Clinical Features

- Symptoms include nasal congestion or blockage, facial pain or pressure, hyposmia, nasal discharge, tooth pain, fever, and sinus pressure with head/body movement.
- There may be pain and tenderness with sinus percussion, mucosal swelling, facial swelling, and redness.

Diagnosis and Differential

- The diagnosis of uncomplicated acute rhinosinusitis is clinical, and imaging is not necessary in nontoxic, uncomplicated rhinosinusitis patients.
- In 2012 the Infectious Disease Society of America recommend using the following criteria to diagnose bacterial sinusitis: bacterial rather than viral rhinosinusitis should be diagnosed when *any* of the following three criteria are met: (1) persistent symptoms lasting at least 10 days, without improvement; (2) severe symptoms or high fever and purulent nasal discharge or facial pain for 3 to 4 days at illness onset; or (3) acutely worsening symptoms after 5 to 6 days of a previously improving upper respiratory infection.
- CT scans are helpful in evaluating toxic patients and possible intracranial extension. Patients with chronic rhinosinusitis or recurrent acute rhinosinusitis warrant bacterial cultures and a sinus CT, preferably as an outpatient.

Emergency Department Care and Disposition

- Treatment for acute uncomplicated disease is generally supportive.

- Nasal irrigation with or without nasal decongestants (0.05% **oxymetazoline** two sprays/nostril twice daily or 0.25% **phenylephrine** two sprays/nostril four times daily) is first-line therapy. Decongestants' use is to be limited to ≤3 days.
- Empirical antibiotic therapy should be started as soon as acute bacterial rhinosinusitis is diagnosed clinically; amoxicillin-clavulanate orally, 22.5 milligrams/kg/dose up to 850 milligrams, twice daily, is recommended for both children and adults. Amoxicillin alone, macrolides, and trimethoprim-sulfamethoxazole are not recommended.
- Doxycycline (2.2 milligrams/kg/dose up to 100 milligrams, twice daily) is an alternative. Levofloxacin and gatifloxacin are alternatives.
- Complications include meningitis, cavernous sinus thrombosis, intracranial abscess and empyema, orbital cellulitis, and osteomyelitis. Patients with these deeper complications usually appear systemically ill or have focal neurologic findings.

For further reading in Tintinalli's *Emergency Medicine: A Comprehensive Study Guide*, 7th ed., see Chapter 237, "Common Disorders of the External, Middle, and Inner Ear," by Mark Silverberg and Michael Lucchesi, and Chapter 239, "Epistaxis, Nasal Fractures, and Rhinosinusitis," by Shane M Summers and Tareg Bey.

154 ORAL AND DENTAL EMERGENCIES

Steven Go

OROFACIAL PAIN

- Normal adult anatomy includes 32 permanent teeth (Fig. 154-1), and general tooth anatomy is shown in Fig. 154-2.
- The differential diagnosis for orofacial pain is listed in Table 154-1.

PAIN OF ODONTOGENIC ORIGIN

Tooth Eruption and Pericoronitis

- Eruption of the primary teeth in infants and children may be associated with pain, irritability, and drooling, but fever and diarrhea should *not* be attributed to teething.

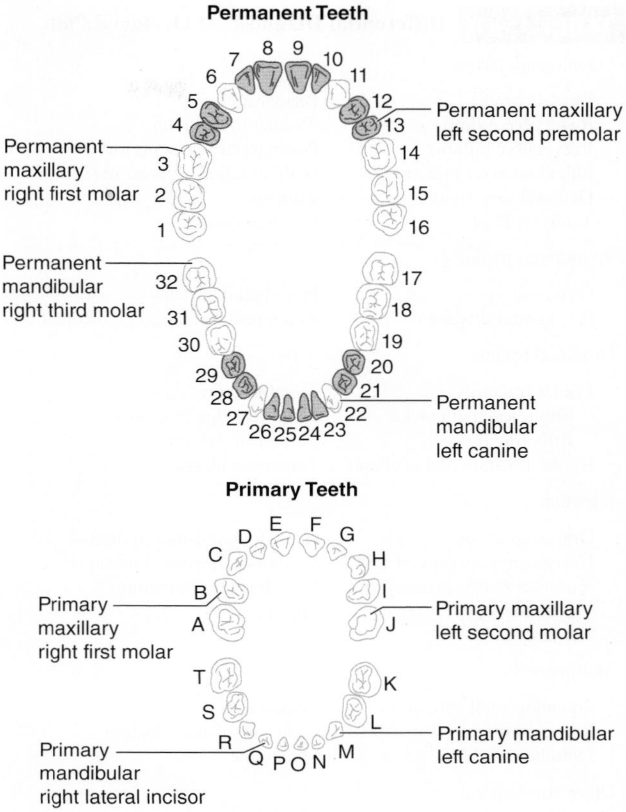

FIG. 154-1. Identification of teeth.

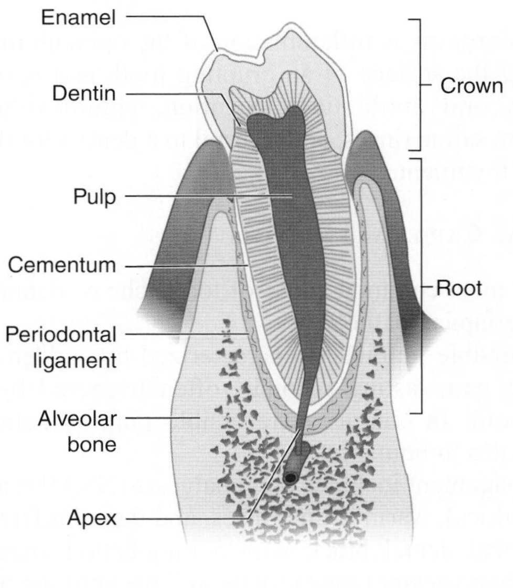

FIG. 154-2. The dental anatomic unit and attachment apparatus.

TABLE 154-1 Differential Diagnosis of Orofacial Pain

Odontogenic origin	
Dental caries	Pericoronitis
Reversible pulpitis	Postrestorative pain
Irreversible pulpitis	Postextraction discomfort
Pulpal necrosis and abscess	Postextraction alveolar osteitis
Dentinal sensitivity	Bruxism
Tooth eruption	Cervical erosion
Periodontal pathology	
Gingivitis	Periodontal abscess
Periodontal disease	Acute necrotizing gingivostomatitis
Orofacial trauma	
Dental fractures	Facial fractures
Subtle enamel cracks	Alveolar ridge fractures
Ellis fractures	Soft tissue lacerations
Dental luxation and avulsion	Traumatic ulcers
Infection	
Oral candidiasis	Hand-foot-and-mouth disease
Herpes simplex types 1 and 2	Sexually transmitted diseases
Varicella zoster, primary and secondary	Mycobacterial infections
Herpangina	Mumps
Malignancies	
Squamous cell carcinoma	Leukemia
Kaposi sarcoma	Graft-versus-host disease
Lymphoma	Melanoma
Other etiologies	
Cranial neuralgias	Vesiculoulcerative disease
Stomatitis and mucositis	Lichen planus
Uremia	Cicatricial pemphigoid
Vitamin deficiency	Pemphigus vulgaris
Other	Erythema multiforme
Benign migratory glossitis	Crohn disease
Pyogenic granuloma	Behçet syndrome

- Pericoronitis is inflammation of the operculum overlying the surface of an erupting tooth and is treated with oral antibiotics, irrigation, chlorhexidine or warm saline rinses, and referral to a dentist for definitive treatment.

Dental Caries and Pulpitis

- The most common cause of toothache or dental pain is periapical pathology.
- Reversible pulpitis is characterized by sudden, transient pain lasting seconds, often triggered by heat or cold. In contrast, irreversible pulpitis pain lasts minutes to hours.
- Management includes oral analgesia (NSAIDs and/or narcotics), warm saline rinses, and dental referral.
- A local dental block with a long-acting anesthetic (ie, bupivacaine) may provide relieve until the patient can see a dentist the following day.
- Although antibiotics are prescribed frequently in reversible pulpitis, evidence for their efficacy is lacking. Likewise, antibiotics do not improve symptoms in irreversible pulpitis in the absence of clear signs of infection.

Periradicular Periodontitis

- Periradicular periodontitis represents extension of pulp disease into adjacent tissues, which can result in a parulis (swelling of gingiva with fistula next to the tooth).
- Fluctuant oral abscesses require local incision and drainage, oral antibiotics effective against mouth flora, oral analgesia, chlorhexidine or warm saline rinses, and close follow-up.

Complicaions of Odontogenic Infections

- Odontogenic infections can spread readily to the facial spaces.
- **Ludwig's angina** is a cellulitis involving the submandibular spaces and the sublingual space that can spread to the neck and mediastinum, causing airway compromise, overwhelming infection, and death.
- Treatment of Ludwig's angina includes intravenous broad-spectrum antibiotics and emergent surgical consultation for consideration of surgical intervention.
- If dental infections spread to the infraorbital space, a cavernous sinus thrombosis may result.
- **Cavernous sinus thrombosis** may produce limitation of lateral gaze, meningeal signs, sepsis, and coma.
- Treatment of cavernous sinus thrombosis includes intravenous broad-spectrum antibiotics.
- Administration of heparin and corticosteroids should be considered for cavernous sinus thrombosis, but a paucity of prospective data exists supporting their efficacy. Surgery is not indicated.

Postextraction Pain and Postextraction Alveolar Osteitis (Dry Socket)

- Periosteitis causes pain within 24 to 48 hours of a tooth extraction; it responds well to analgesics. Postoperative edema can be managed with ice packs, elevation, NSAIDs, and oral narcotics. Trismus can also occur but usually decreases after 24 hours unless an infection develops.
- Postextraction alveolar osteitis ("dry socket") occurs when the clot from the socket is displaced, typically on postoperative day 2 or 3. It presents with severe pain with foul odor and taste. Dental radiographs should be taken to rule out retained root tip or foreign body.

- Treatment of postextraction alveolar osteitis consists of saline irrigation and packing of the socket with eugenol-impregnated gauze. Smoking should be avoided. Antibiotic therapy is indicated in most cases, with 24-hour dental follow-up.

Postextraction Bleeding

- Most cases can be stopped with direct pressure with folded gauze for 20 minutes, application of absorbable gelatin sponge, gentle suturing, or injection with lidocaine with epinephrine. If these sequential measures fail, then an oral maxillofacial surgery consult is appropriate.

Postrestorative Pain

- NSAIDs and/or oral narcotics with dental referral are appropriate for pain after restorative procedures.

PERIODONTAL PATHOLOGY

Periodontal Abscess

- Periodontal abscesses are treated similarly to other oral abscesses.

Acute Necrotizing Ulcerative Gingivitis (ANUG)

- ANUG ("Vincent disease" or "trench mouth") is the only periodontal disease in which bacteria invade non-necrotic tissue.
- ANUG presents with pain, ulcerated or "punched-out" interdental papillae, gingival bleeding, fever, malaise, and fetid breath. It occurs mainly in patients with lowered resistance due to HIV, malnourishment, and stress.
- Treatment of ANUG consists of oral metronidazole and chlorhexidine mouth rinses and addressing predisposing conditions. Symptomatic improvement can be expected <24 hours.

FACIAL NEURALGIAS

- Trigeminal neuralgia is discussed in Chapter 142, Headache and Facial Pain.

SOFT TISSUE LESIONS OF THE ORAL CAVITY

ORAL CANDIDIASIS

- Oral candidiasis lesions consist of removable white, curd-like plaques on an erythematous mucosal base. Risk factors include extremes of age, immunocompromised states, use of intraoral prosthetic devices, concurrent antibiotic use, and malnutrition.
- Treatment of oral candidiasis is with oral antifungal agents such as clotrimazole troches or nystatin oral suspension, or fluconazole (see Chapter 94, Human Immunodeficiency Virus Infection and Acquired Immunodeficiency Syndrome).

APTHOUS STOMATITIS

- Aphthous stomatitis is a common pattern of mucosal ulceration triggered by cell-mediated immunity. The painful lesions typically resolve in 48 hours when treated with topical steroids, although some larger, deeper lesions (Aphthous major) may take weeks to heal.

HERPES SIMPLEX

- Herpes gingivostomatitis causes painful ulcerations of the gingiva and mucosal surfaces. Fever, lymphadenopathy, and tingling often precede the eruption of numerous vesicles, which then rupture and form ulcerative lesions.
- If acyclovir or valacyclovir is initiated during the prodromal phrase of herpes gingivostomatitis, the clinical duration and severity may be attenuated (see Chapter 93, Disseminated Viral Infections).

VARICELLA ZOSTER

- Herpes zoster occurs in the trigeminal nerve distribution 15% to 20% of the time.
- Painful paresthesias precede the appearance of a painful vesicular eruption that does not cross the midline. The lesions last 7 to 10 days (see Chapter 93, Disseminated Viral Infections).
- Isolated intraoral lesions occur uncommonly.
- If the ophthalmic branch of the trigeminal nerve is involved, it represents an ophthalmology emergency (see Chapter 151, Ocular Emergencies).

HERPANGINA AND HAND-FOOT-AND-MOUTH DISEASE

- Herpangina and hand-foot-and-mouth disease are both caused by infection with coxsackievirus A species.
- Herpangina is a typically seasonal (summer/autumn) infection that presents with high fever, sore throat, headache, and malaise, followed by eruption of oral vesicles, which rupture to form painful, shallow ulcers on the soft palate, uvula, and tonsillar pillars. Unlike herpes infection, the gingiva is spared.

- Hand-foot-and-mouth disease causes vesicles to initially form on the soft palate, gingiva, tongue, and buccal mucosa. The vesicles then rupture, leaving painful ulcers surrounded by red halos. Lesions may also appear on the buttocks, palms, and soles.
- Treatment of herpangina and hand-foot-and-mouth disease is supportive and consists of hydration and acetaminophen or ibuprofen.

TRAUMATIC ULCERS AND PYOGENIC GRANULOMA

- Traumatic ulcers result from direct trauma to the oral mucosa by ill-fitting dental appliances, hot foods, or traumatic oral hygiene. Improvement results from removal of the inciting factor and supportive care.
- A pyogenic granuloma is a benign connective tissue tumor that can result from chronic trauma to the gingiva. One form can occur during pregnancy (pregnancy tumor) and should be removed if it does not resolve spontaneously 2 to 3 months postpartum.

MEDICATION-RELATED SOFT TISSUE ABNORMALITIES

- Gingival hyperplasia is a common side effect of many medications, most notably phenytoin, cyclosporine, and calcium channel blockers, especially nifedipine.
- Other well-known oral lesions from medications include stomatitis and ulcerations secondary to chemotherapeutic agents and xerostomia-induced mucosal abnormalities from anticholinergics, antidepressants, and antihistamines.

SEXUALLY TRANSMITTED DISEASES

- Oral-genital contact can result in STD-related lesions.
- Gonorrhea can cause pharyngitis, with or without pustules or exudates, while human papillomavirus (HPV) can cause oral condyloma. The primary syphilis chancre can appear in the mouth as well.
- Treatment is similar to that of genital lesions from these organisms (see Chapter 89, Sexually Transmitted Diseases).

LESIONS OF THE TONGUE

- Benign migratory glossitis ("geographic tongue") is a common benign finding marked by multiple circumscribed zones of erythema found predominantly on the tip and lateral borders of the tongue. The lesions wax and wane with stress and menstrual cycle. It is usually asymptomatic, but topical oral steroids may provide relief for symptomatic cases.
- Strawberry tongue appears as red spots on a white-coated background. It is associated with several conditions, including Kawasaki's disease and *Streptococcus pyogenes* infection. If it is due to the latter, it responds to antibiotics effective against group A streptococci.

ORAL CANCER

- Leukoplakia is a white patch that cannot be scraped off and is not secondary to another condition. It is the most common precursor for oral cancer, although most lesions are benign.
- Erythroplakia is a red patch that cannot be classified as secondary to any other disease, and it has a greater potential for cancer than leukoplakia.
- Symptoms and signs of oral cancer include pain, paresthesias, persistent ulcers, bleeding, lesion rigidity, induration, lymphadenopathy, and functional impairment.
- Risk factors for oral cancer include tobacco (including chewing tobacco) use, alcoholism, sun exposure, general malnutrition, chronic iron deficiency anemia, candidiasis, immunosuppressive states, and various viruses (eg, HIV, HPV, herpes).
- The most common site for oral cancer is the tongue (50%), with the floor of the mouth accounting for 35% of cancers.
- Lesions that do not resolve with palliative treatment in 10 to 14 days should be referred for biopsy.

OROFACIAL TRAUMA

DENTOALVEOLAR TRAUMA

Dental Fractures

- The Ellis classification of dental fractures is shown in Fig. 154-3.
- Ellis class 1 fractures involve only the enamel of the tooth. These injuries may be smoothed with an emery board or referred to a dentist for cosmetic repair.
- Ellis class 2 fractures (70% of tooth fractures) involve the creamy yellow dentin underneath the white enamel. The patient complains of air and temperature sensitivity. The exposed dentin must be thoroughly dried and promptly covered with a temporary dental dressing such as zinc oxide/eugenol paste with dental referral <24 hours.
- Ellis class 3 fractures are tooth-threatening fractures that involve the pulp and can be identified by a red blush of the dentin or a visible drop of blood after wiping the tooth.

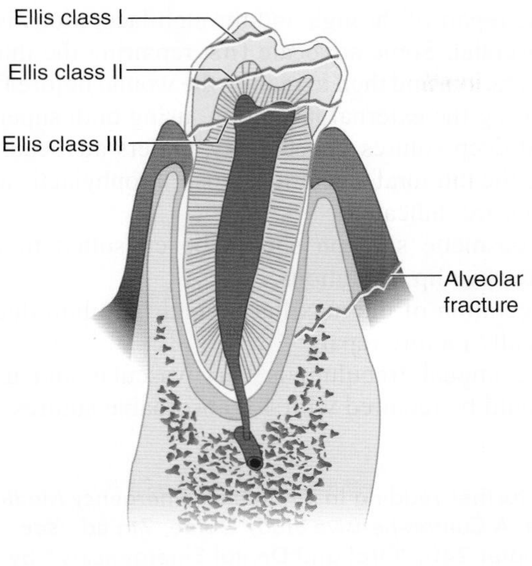

FIG. 154-3. Ellis classification for fractures of teeth.

- Ideally, a dentist should evaluate the patient with an Ellis class 3 fracture immediately. If a dentist is not immediately available, the tooth may be temporarily covered with a dental dressing such as zinc oxide/eugenol paste until the patient is seen within 24 hours. Oral analgesics may be needed, but topical anesthetics are contraindicated. The use of prophylactic antibiotics is controversial.
- In patients under the age of 12 years, the protective dentinal layer is thin. A visible blush of pulp under this thin dentinal layer thus indicates that the pulp is at risk, and should be treated like an Ellis class 3 fracture.

Concussions, Luxations, and Avulsions

- Concussion injuries involve tenderness to percussion with no mobility.
- Dental trauma with tenderness to percussion and mobility without evidence of dislodgment is called subluxation, which has a higher incidence of future pulp necrosis.
- Management of concussion injuries and subluxation includes NSAIDs, soft diet, and referral to a dentist.
- Extrusive luxation occurs when a tooth is partially avulsed from alveolar bone. Treatment involves gentle repositioning of the tooth to its original location and splinting with zinc oxide periodontal dressing (Fig. 154-4) with dental referral <24 hours.
- When the tooth is laterally displaced with a fracture of the alveolar bone, the condition is called lateral luxation.

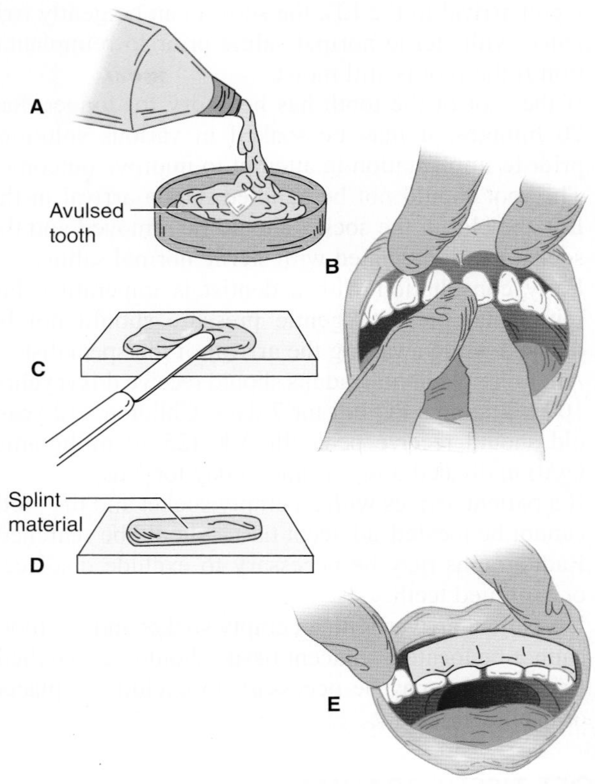

FIG. 154-4. Reimplantation and stabilization of an avulsed tooth. **A.** Tooth is rinsed. **B.** Tooth is placed back into socket. **C.** Splint material is mixed thoroughly. **D.** Splint material is shaped and made ready for application. **E.** Packing is molded over reimplanted tooth and two adjacent teeth to each side.

- Although manual relocation is possible, the treatment of lateral luxation is best done in consultation with a dentist in the emergency department (ED), especially if the alveolar fracture is significant.
- An intrusive luxation occurs when the tooth is forced below the gingiva and often has a poor outcome. Treatment is similar to that of subluxations.
- Dental avulsion is a dental emergency in which a tooth has been completely removed from the socket.
- Primary teeth in children should not be replaced because of potential damage to the permanent teeth. Intruded primary teeth should be left alone.
- Permanent teeth that have been avulsed for less than 3 hours must be immediately reimplanted in an attempt to save the periodontal ligament fibers.
- If reimplantation at the scene is not possible due to risk of aspiration, the tooth should be rinsed and placed in a nutrient solution, such as Hank's solution, sterile saline, milk, or saliva and the tooth transported immediately with the patient to the ED.

- Upon arrival in the ED, the socket can be gently irrigated with sterile normal saline prior to reimplantation if the root is still moist.
- If the root of the tooth has been dry for longer than 20 minutes, it may be soaked in various solutions prior to implantation in attempt to improve outcome.
- The root should not be handled. Upon arrival in the ED, the clot in the socket should be removed and the socket gently irrigated with sterile normal saline.
- Early consultation with a dentist is imperative, but reimplantation with gentle pressure should not be delayed while awaiting the arrival of the specialist.
- After reimplantation, adults should receive doxycycline 100 milligrams PO bid for 7 days. Children <12 years old should receive penicillin VK (25-50 milligrams/kg/d) in divided doses 4 times a day for 7 days.
- If a patient arrives with an empty socket and the tooth cannot be located, adjacent tissue should be searched. Radiographs may be necessary to exclude displaced or aspirated teeth.
- If a patient arrives with an empty socket and the tooth cannot be located, adjacent tissue should be searched. Radiographs may be necessary to exclude displaced or aspirated teeth.

SOFT TISSUE TRAUMA

- Stabilization of dental injuries and an aggressive search for retained foreign bodies should take place before repair of lacerations.
- Most intraoral mucosal lacerations will heal by themselves; however, they should be repaired if they are gaping or if flaps are present. Treatment consists of achieving good anesthesia, debridement, irrigation, and close approximation (rather than a tight tissue seal) with 5-0 absorbable sutures. Antibiotics are only prescribed for the largest lacerations, and 48-hour follow-up is indicated.
- Tongue lacerations that gape widely, actively bleed, are flap shaped, or involve muscle should be closed. Lacerations may be repaired with 4-0 absorbable sutures. Extreme care must be taken to precisely repair the edges of dorsal lacerations because malapproximation will result in clefts in the tongue that will require revision. Extensive lesions or those in uncooperative patients may require operative repair.
- Lip lacerations are potentially complex because of the possible involvement of the vermilion border (the transition between lip tissue and the skin of the face), which must be aligned precisely with 6-0 nonabsorbable sutures to avoid a noticeable cosmetic defect.
- Violated deep muscle layers and intraoral lesions must be closed as well. Prophylactic penicillin VK or clindamycin should be prescribed.
- The repair of through and through lacerations is controversial. Some advocate first repairing the intraoral laceration, and then irrigating the wound before finally closing the external laceration, using both superficial and deep sutures if necessary. Others advocate leaving the intraoral lacerations open. Prophylactic antibiotics are indicated.
- A cosmetic surgeon should be consulted to repair extensive lip lacerations.
- Laceration of the maxillary labial frenulum does not usually require repair.
- The lingual frenulum is very vascular and usually should be repaired with 4-0 absorbable sutures.

For further reading in Tintinalli's *Emergency Medicine: A Comprehensive Study Guide*, 7th ed., see Chapter 240, "Oral and Dental Emergencies," by Ronald W. Beaudreau.

155 INFECTIONS AND DISORDERS OF THE NECK AND UPPER AIRWAY

Aaron Barksdale

- This chapter covers common causes of pharyngitis, including those disorders that threaten the integrity of the airway; however, Epstein–Barr virus as a cause of pharyngitis is covered in more detail in Chapter 93, Disseminated Viral Infections.

PHARYNGITIS/TONSILLITIS

PATHOPHYSIOLOGY

- Pharyngitis/tonsillitis is typically due to an infectious etiology, most commonly viral (also see Chapter 71, Stridor and Drooling, for discussion of disease spectrum in children). Other infectious causes include bacteria, fungi, and parasites.
- Group A β-hemolytic *Streptococcus* (GABHS) is the most common bacterial cause, up to 15% of pharyngitis in adults and 15% to 30 % in children.
- Certain virulent strains of GABHS may lead to acute rheumatic fever in children.
- Other bacterial causes include group C and G streptococci, *Haemophilus influenzae*, *Mycoplasma pneumoniae*, *Chlamydia pneumoniae*, *Neisseria gonorrhoeae*, and *Corynebacterium diphtheriae*.
- Transmission of most cases of pharyngitis is via person-to-person contact with droplets of saliva.

CLINICAL FEATURES

- Acute viral pharyngitis is often associated with rhinorrhea and may display a petechial or vesicular pattern on the soft palate and tonsils.
- Viral pharyngitis typically lacks tonsillar exudates and cervical adenopathy, except for infectious mononucleosis (see Chapter 93), influenza, and acute retroviral syndrome.
- GABHS typically presents with the sudden onset of sore throat, odynophagia, chills, and fever, and lacks cough, rhinorrhea, or conjunctivitis.
- Diphtheria (*C. diphtheriae*) often displays a grayish membrane adhered to the tonsillar or pharyngeal surface.

DIAGNOSIS AND DIFFERENTIAL

- The Centor criteria for GABHS pharyngitis are (1) tonsillar exudate, (2) tender anterior cervical adenopathy, (3) fever, and (4) absence of cough.
- In patients with two or fewer criteria, most authorities recommend acquiring a rapid antigen test.
- In those with three or more criteria, some authorities recommend empiric treatment (such as the American Academy of Family Practice), while the American Academy of Pediatrics recommends rapid antigen testing in this group, using the results to determine treatment.
- Most rapid streptococcal antigen detection tests report sensitivities around 90%.
- Throat cultures following negative rapid tests should be considered, particularly in children and those with increased Centor scores.

EMERGENCY DEPARTMENT CARE AND DISPOSITION

- Nonbacterial causes should be treated with antipyretics, analgesics, and IV fluids if dehydrated.
- Penicillin remains the antibiotic of choice for treatment of GABHS pharyngitis. A single dose of benzathine penicillin G 1.2 million units IM or penicillin VK 500 milligrams PO three to four times a day for 10 days may be used.
- In penicillin-allergic patients, a macrolide or clindamycin may be used.
- A single dose of PO or IM dexamethasone may be considered in moderate to severe cases, which may shorten the duration of pain.
- Treatment with antibiotics is recommended in patients with GABHS to help prevent suppurative sequelae, including cervical lymphadenitis, peritonsillar abscess, retropharyngeal abscess, and sinusitis.
- Antibiotic treatment of GABHS can help prevent acute rheumatic fever and does not have any effect on the development of poststreptococcal glomerulonephritis.

PERITONSILLAR ABSCESS

PATHOPHYSIOLOGY

- Peritonsillar abscess (PTA) is commonly a polymicrobial infection that develops between the tonsillar capsule and the superior constrictor and palatopharyngeus muscles.
- Risk factors include prior PTA, smoking, periodontal disease, chronic tonsillitis, and repeat courses of antibiotics.
- Most commonly occurs in young adults in the winter and spring months.

CLINICAL FEATURES

- Patients may appear ill and often present with fever, malaise, sore throat, odynophagia, varying degrees of trismus, dysphagia, drooling, and potentially a muffled voice ("hot potato voice").
- The involved tonsil is often displaced medially and inferiorly, causing deflection of the uvula to the contralateral side (see Fig. 155-1).

DIAGNOSIS AND DIFFERENTIAL

- The differential diagnosis includes tonsillitis, peritonsillar cellulitis, infectious mononucleosis, retropharyngeal abscess, neoplasm, and internal carotid artery aneurysm.

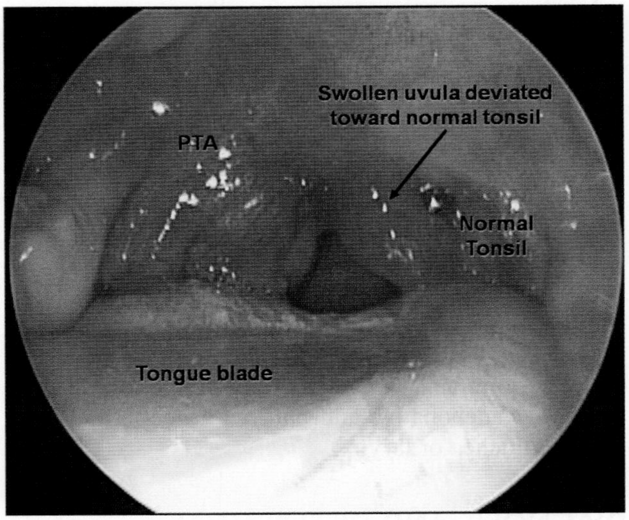

FIG. 155-1. Right peritonsillar abscess (PTA) displacing right tonsil medially and the uvula toward the normal left tonsil. Abscess is between the right tonsil and the superior constrictor muscle.

- Diagnosis is typically made through the history and physical examination.
- When diagnosis is in question, needle aspiration, CT, or ultrasound may help provide confirmation.

EMERGENCY DEPARTMENT CARE AND DISPOSITION

- Needle aspiration of purulent material (18 or 20 gauge) is both diagnostic and therapeutic for PTA and will effectively treat more than 90% of these patients.
- Needle penetration should not exceed 1 cm, in order to avoid carotid artery puncture (lateral and posterior to tonsil).
- Experienced clinicians may perform incision and drainage (I&D) after local anesthesia.
- More severe cases may require otolaryngology consultation.
- Following adequate drainage or aspiration, antibiotic therapy is recommended. Penicillin VK 500 milligrams PO four times daily or clindamycin 300 to 450 milligrams three times daily for 10 days can be used.

ADULT EPIGLOTTITIS (SUPRAGLOTTITIS)

PATHOPHYSIOLOGY

- This is an infectious process that typically causes inflammation of the epiglottis, but may involve the entire supraglottic region.
- The majority of cases are now seen in adults, as a result of the conjugate vaccine for *H. influenzae* type b.
- Most cases are caused by *Streptococcus* and *Staphylococcus* species, but may also be the result of viruses or fungi.

CLINICAL FEATURES

- Patients typically present with a 1- to 2-day history of worsening dysphagia, odynophagia, and dyspnea (worse when supine).
- Patients classically position themselves in an upright, leaning-forward position, and may display drooling and inspiratory stridor.
- Other symptoms include anxiety, fever, tachycardia, cervical adenopathy, and pain with gentle palpation of the trachea or larynx.

DIAGNOSIS AND DIFFERENTIAL

- Diagnosis is made through history and physical examination, radiographs, and/or fiber-optic laryngoscopy.

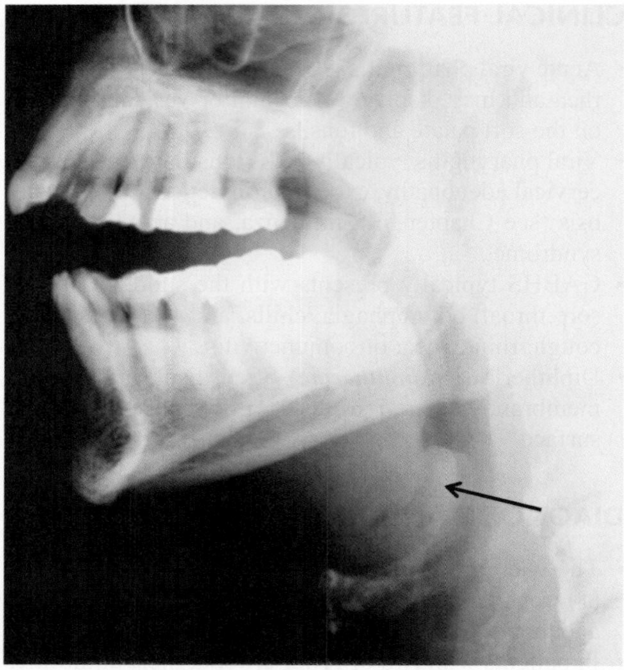

FIG. 155-2. Acute epiglottitis. Arrow points to thickened epiglottis resembling a thumb print on a soft tissue lateral radiograph.

- Lateral soft-tissue neck radiographs may show an edematous epiglottis ("thumbprint sign") with loss of the vallecula (see Fig. 155-2).
- Direct fiber-optic laryngoscopy classically reveals a cherry red epiglottis.
- Differential diagnosis includes pharyngitis, infectious mononucleosis, croup, deep space neck abscess, diphtheria, pertussis, laryngeal trauma, foreign body aspiration, and laryngospasm.

EMERGENCY DEPARTMENT CARE AND DISPOSITION

- Patients with suspected epiglottitis require emergent otolaryngology consultation, and the emergency physician must be prepared to establish a definitive airway.
- Patients should remain in the upright position and avoid agitation.
- Initial airway management consists of supplemental humidified oxygen and comfortable patient positioning. Heliox can be given as a temporizing measure.
- Endotracheal intubation may be difficult secondary to anatomic distortion, and is preferably performed by awake fiber-optic intubation in the operating room.
- The physician must be prepared to perform a surgical airway, cricothyrotomy or needle cricothyrotomy.

- Ceftriaxone 2 grams IV is the recommended first-line antibiotic. Steroids (methylprednisolone, 125 milligrams IV) may reduce airway inflammation and edema.

RETROPHARYNGEAL ABSCESS

PATHOPHYSIOLOGY

- Retropharyngeal abscess is most common in children less than 5 years old, but also occurs in adults.
- In children, the abscess typically consists of suppurative changes within a lymph node.
- In adults, a retropharyngeal abscess is more likely to extend into the mediastinum.
- The infection is usually polymicrobial, but common aerobic species include *Streptococcus viridans* and *Streptococcus pyogenes*. *Bacteroides* and *Peptostreptococcu*s are the most commonly isolated anaerobes.

CLINICAL FEATURES

- Patients commonly present with fever, sore throat, torticollis, and dysphagia. Additional symptoms include neck pain and stiffness, muffled voice, cervical lymphadenopathy, and respiratory distress.
- Stridor and neck edema is more common in children.
- In contrast to epiglottitis, these patients tend to prefer a supine position with the neck in slight extension to minimize compression of the upper airway. Sitting them up may worsen their dyspnea.

DIAGNOSIS AND DIFFERENTIAL

- An intravenous contrast-enhanced CT of the neck is the gold standard and differentiates cellulitis from an abscess (Fig. 155-3).
- Differential diagnosis includes retropharyngeal space tumor, foreign body, aneurysm, hematoma, edema, and lymphadenopathy.

EMERGENCY DEPARTMENT CARE AND DISPOSITION

- All patients require an immediate otolaryngologist consultation and airway management as indicated.
- IV hydration and antibiotics should be initiated in the ED.
- Clindamycin 600 to 900 milligrams (10 milligrams/kg) IV or ampicillin/sulbactam 3 grams (50-75 milligrams/kg) IV.

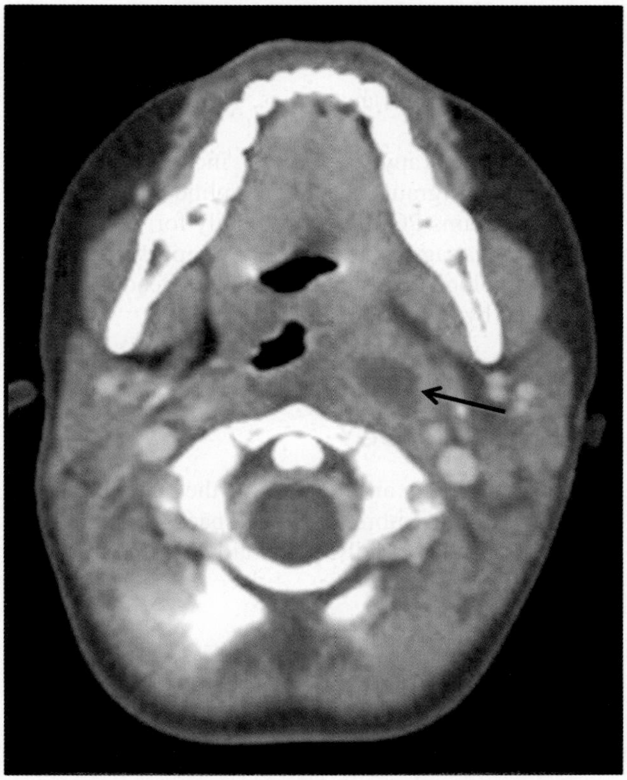

FIG. 155-3. Contrasted CT of a left retropharyngeal abscess (*arrow*).

ODONTOGENIC ABSCESS

PATHOPHYSIOLOGY

- Odontogenic infections are typically the result of an infected tooth or following tooth extraction. They are usually polymicrobial, consisting of oral aerobes and anaerobes.

CLINICAL FEATURES

- Patients often present with pain, fever, and potential swelling and suppurative changes in the adjacent gingival, buccal, sublingual, or submandibular spaces.
- Abscesses may extend into the prevertebral, parapharyngeal, and retropharyngeal spaces, resulting in a neck mass, trismus, dysphagia, or dyspnea.

DIAGNOSIS AND DIFFERENTIAL

- A contrast-enhanced CT scan should be acquired when there is concern for a deep neck space abscess.

EMERGENCY DEPARTMENT CARE AND DISPOSITION

- Treatment includes analgesics, I&D of abscess, and antibiotics.
- Antibiotic therapy in adults includes penicillin VK 500 milligrams PO qid or clindamycin 300 to 450 milligrams PO three times daily for 7 to 10 days.
- Airway management should be performed and otolaryngologic consultation should be obtained as indicated by severity of illness.

LUDWIG ANGINA

PATHOPHYSIOLOGY

- Ludwig angina is an infection of the submandibular, sublingual, and submandibular spaces bilaterally. It often progresses rapidly, potentially leading to airway compromise.

CLINICAL FEATURES

- Patients present with trismus, dysphagia, and odynophagia.
- Clinical examination will reveal diffuse edema of the entire upper neck and floor of the mouth.

EMERGENCY DEPARTMENT CARE AND DISPOSITION

- All patients require emergent otolaryngology consultation.
- Initial management should focus on providing a definitive airway, often acquired by awake fiber-optic intubation or tracheostomy.

NECK MASSES

PATHOPHYSIOLOGY

- Neck masses may arise from congenital, infectious, or neoplastic origin.
- Squamous cell carcinoma is the most common malignancy of the upper airway and is usually associated with a significant tobacco and/or alcohol history.
- In adults >40 years old, a neck mass is likely malignant if it has been present for greater than 6 weeks.

CLINCAL FEATURES

- Patients may present with dysphagia, odynophagia, or secondary infections.
- Patients with malignant masses may report experiencing night sweats, weight loss, and malaise.
- Branchial cleft cysts can present at any age and typically appear as fluctuant, painless masses located anterior to the sternocleidomastoid muscle.
- Thyroglossal duct cysts usually occur in children and present as an asymptomatic midline subhyoid neck mass.

DIAGNOSIS AND DIFFERENTIAL

- Indeterminate masses should undergo CT with IV contrast.

EMERGENCY DEPARTMENT CARE AND DISPOSITION

- Patients may require airway management and/or IV hydration.
- Stable patients who can tolerate oral intake can be referred to an otolaryngologist on an outpatient basis.

POSTTONSILLECTOMY BLEEDING

PATHOPHYSIOLOGY

- Hemorrhage is a result of sloughing of fibrinous debris from the tonsillar bed and typically occurs between postoperative days 5 and 10.
- The incidence of bleeding is significantly higher in the third decade of life.

CLINICAL FEATURES

- Bleeding can be severe and sometimes fatal.

EMERGENCY DEPARTMENT CARE AND DISPOSITION

- Active bleeding requires immediate otolaryngologist consultation.
- Patients should be placed on a monitor, pulse oximetry, and IV access established. They should also be kept in an upright position and remain NPO.
- In patients with significant bleeding, obtain a CBC, coagulation studies, and type and cross.
- Gauze moistened with thrombin or epinephrine (1:10,000) and 1% lidocaine should be applied with direct pressure to the bleeding area. A suture should be placed through the gauze and taped to the face to prevent airway compromise from accidental displacement.
- Establish definitive airway if bleeding is compromising patients' ability to protect their airway.

LARYNGEAL TRAUMA

PATHOPHYSIOLOGY

- Laryngeal injuries may be the result of blunt or penetrating trauma.
- "Clothesline injury" is the result of blunt trauma that occurs when a moving victim's neck strikes a stationary object. This results in damage to the thyroid cartilage and potential laryngotracheal separation.
- With high-impact mechanisms, asphyxiation often occurs at the scene.

CLINICAL FEATURES

- Patients may present with hoarseness, dyspnea, dysphagia, stridor, hemoptysis, and in severe cases aphonia and/or apnea.
- Physical examination may reveal anterior neck tenderness, laryngeal swelling, tracheal displacement, or subcutaneous emphysema.
- Minor laryngeal injuries may progress, due to edema and expanding hematomas, and close observation is needed.
- A high level of suspicion for cervical spine injury is appropriate.

DIAGNOSIS AND DIFFERENTIAL

- Fiber-optic laryngoscopy, with patient in an upright position, can be used to evaluate the integrity of the laryngeal airway and should be done prior to obtaining a CT.
- Those patients with an intact airway should undergo CT to further delineate the degree of injury.

EMERGENCY DEPARTMENT CARE AND DISPOSITION

- Emergent otolaryngologic consultation is warranted.
- In patients with a compromised laryngeal airway (ecchymosis and/or edema), but the tracheal lumen can be visualized, an attempt at endotracheal intubation is appropriate.
- In unstable patients with massive laryngeal trauma or complete obliteration of the laryngeal airway, immediate tracheostomy should be performed. Do not attempt a cricothyrotomy in these patients.

ANGIOEDEMA OF THE UPPER AIRWAY

PATHOPHYSIOLOGY

- Angioedema is a non-pruritic, non-pitting swelling of the subcutaneous and deep dermal (mucosa) layers of the skin.
- Causes of angioedema include (1) C1-esterase inhibitor deficiency (hereditary or acquired), (2) IgE-mediated type 1 allergic reaction, (3) adverse reaction to angiotensin-converting enzyme (ACE) inhibitor therapy, and (4) idiopathic reaction.
- The incidence of ACE inhibitor–related angioedema is up to 2.2% and is more common in African Americans.
- The majority of ACE inhibitor–induced angioedema occurs within a month of initiating treatment, but can occur years later.

CLINICAL FEATURES

- Angioedema may involve the face, lips, eyelids, tongue, and larynx, and can progress rapidly.
- Patients with airway involvement can present with "throat tightness," dyspnea, cough, hoarseness, and stridor.

EMERGENCY DEPARTMENT CARE AND DISPOSITION

- Patients with potential for airway compromise should receive 0.3 milligram (0.01 milligram/kg) of epinephrine 1:1000, administered IM in the lateral thigh. If the patient is responding to treatment, this can be repeated every 5 to 10 minutes.
- Additional medications that should be administered include diphenhydramine 50 milligrams (1 milligram/kg) IV, and methylprednisolone 125 milligrams (2 milligrams/kg) IV.
- Patients with hereditary angioedema (C1-esterase inhibitor deficiency) and ACE inhibitor–induced angioedema typically do not respond to the treatments above.
- Currently approved medications for treatment of acute hereditary angioedema (HAE) in the United States are Berinert (human C1-esterase inhibitor) 20 units/kg IV, and Ecallantide (kallikrein inhibitor) 30 milligrams subcutaneously in three 10-milligram injections.
- Fiber-optic laryngoscopy can help assess the extent of laryngeal edema.
- In those with airway compromise or progressing symptoms, a definitive airway needs to be established. This is best performed by awake fiber-optic intubation or potentially a surgical airway (cricothyrotomy) if the edema is too severe.

For further reading in Tintinalli's *Emergency Medicine: A Comprehensive Study Guide,* 7th ed., see Chapter 241, "Infections and Disorders of the Neck and Upper Airway," by Rupali N. Shah, Trinitia Y. Cannon, and Carol G. Shores.

Section 18
SKIN DISORDERS

156 DERMATOLOGIC EMERGENCIES

Daniel A. Handel

ERYTHEMA MULTIFORME

EPIDEMIOLOGY

- The highest incidence is in young adults (20-40 years of age), with males affected twice as often as females.

PATHOPHYSIOLOGY

- Erythema multiforme (EM) is an acute inflammatory skin disease that ranges from a mild papular eruption (EM minor) to a severe vesiculobullous form with mucous membrane involvement and systemic toxicity (Stevens–Johnson syndrome).
- EM is usually due to infection, drugs (antibiotics and anticonvulsants), malignancy, rheumatologic disorders, or pregnancy.
- No cause is found in 50% of cases.

CLINICAL FEATURES

- Symptoms include malaise, arthralgias, myalgias, fever, diffuse pruritus, and a generalized burning sensation that may be noted days prior to skin abnormalities.
- Signs noted on examination primarily involve the skin and mucosal surfaces, including erythematous papules (which appear first) and maculopapules, target lesion (evolves in 24-48 hours), urticarial plaques, vesicles, bullae, vesiculobullous lesions, and mucosal (oral, conjunctival, respiratory, and genitourinary) erosions.
- The target lesion is highly characteristic of EM. The erythematous papules appear symmetrically on the dorsum of the hands and feet, and the extensor surfaces of the extremities.
- Ocular involvement occurs in approximately 9% of patients with EM minor and in almost 70% of patients with Stevens–Johnson syndrome.
- Patients are at risk for significant fluid and electrolyte deficiencies as well as secondary infection.
- Recurrence is noted, especially involving cases in which infection or medication is involved.

DIAGNOSIS AND DIFFERENTIAL

- The diagnosis of EM is based on the simultaneous presence of lesions with multiple morphologies at times with mucous membrane involvement.
- The differential diagnosis includes herpetic infections, vasculitis, toxic epidermal necrolysis (TEN), primary blistering disorders, Kawasaki's disease, and toxic-infectious erythemas.

EMERGENCY DEPARTMENT CARE AND DISPOSITION

- Patients with localized papular disease without systemic manifestations and mucous membrane involvement may be managed on an outpatient basis with dermatologic consultation. Systemic steroid bursts as well as oral antihistamines can be used but are unproven to change outcomes and duration of symptoms.
- Diphenhydramine and lidocaine rinses are useful for stomatitis; cool Burrow's solution compresses are applied to blistered regions.
- Inpatient therapy in a critical care setting with immediate dermatologic consultation is advised for patients with extensive disease or systemic toxicity.
- Intensive management of potential fluid, electrolyte, infectious, nutritional, and thermoregulatory issues, as well as parenteral analgesics and antihistamines are required for patients with severe cases.

TOXIC EPIDERMAL NECROLYSIS

PATHOPHYSIOLOGY

- TEN is an explosive dermatosis characterized by tender erythema, bullae formation, and subsequent exfoliation.

- The most common cause of TEN is medications; other etiologies include chemicals, infections (eg, HIV), malignancy, or immunologic factors.
- Sulfa-based drugs, penicillin, anticonvulsants, and nonsteroidal anti-inflammatory drugs (NSAIDs) are the most frequent medication triggers for TEN.

CLINICAL FEATURES

- Patients may complain of malaise, anorexia, myalgias, arthralgias, fever, painful skin, and symptoms of upper respiratory infection. These symptoms may be present for 1 to 2 weeks prior to the development of skin abnormalities.
- Physical examination findings include a warm and tender erythema, flaccid bullae, positive Nikolsky's sign, erosions with exfoliation, mucous membrane (oral, conjunctival, respiratory, and genitourinary) lesions, and systemic toxicity.
- Nikolsky's sign is positive when the superficial layers of skin slip free from the lower layers with a slight rubbing pressure; large areas of the skin will blister and peel away, leaving wet, red, painful areas.
- Infection, hypovolemia, and electrolyte disorders are typical causes of death, an end result in as many as 25% to 35% of cases.
- Predictors of poor prognosis include advanced age, extensive disease, leukopenia, azotemia, and thrombocytopenia.

DIAGNOSIS AND DIFFERENTIAL

- Diagnosis of TEN is confirmed by skin biopsy.
- The differential diagnosis includes toxic-infectious erythemas, exfoliative drug eruptions, primary blistering disorders, Kawasaki's disease, and Stevens–Johnson syndrome.

EMERGENCY DEPARTMENT CARE AND DISPOSITION

- Patients with TEN are best cared for in a critical care setting such as a burn unit.
- Attention to adequate cardiorespiratory function is essential; correction of fluid, electrolyte, and infectious complications are early treatment considerations.
- Immediate dermatologic consultation is required.

EXFOLIATIVE DERMATITIS

EPIDEMIOLOGY

- Males are affected twice as often as females, and most patients are over the age of 40 years.

PATHOPHYSIOLOGY

- Exfoliative dermatitis, a cutaneous reaction to a drug, chemical, or underlying systemic disease state, occurs when most or all of the skin is involved with a scaling erythema, leading subsequently to exfoliation.
- The underlying mechanism is largely unknown.
- Etiologies responsible for exfoliative dermatitis include (in decreasing order of incidence) generalized flares of preexisting skin disease (eg, psoriasis, atopic and seborrheic dermatitides, lichen planus, and pemphigus foliaceus), contact dermatitis, malignancy, and medications or chemicals.

CLINICAL FEATURES

- Patients may present with acute, acute-on-chronic, or chronic disease.
- The acute-onset form is encountered most often in cases involving medications, contact allergens, or malignancy, while the chronic variety usually is related to an underlying cutaneous disease.
- Patients may complain of pain, pruritus, tightening of the skin, a chilling sensation of the skin, fever, nausea, vomiting, weight loss, and fatigue.
- The physical examination may show generalized warmth and erythroderma, scaling with desiccation, and exfoliation of the skin, as well as fever and other signs of systemic toxicity.
- The process usually begins on the face and upper trunk with progression to other skin surfaces.
- Chronic findings include dystrophic nails, thinning of body hair, alopecia, and hypo- or hyperpigmentation.
- Acute complicating factors include fluid and electrolyte losses, secondary infection, and excessive heat loss with hypothermia.
- High-output congestive heart failure (CHF) may be noted due to extensive cutaneous vasodilation in poorly compensated individuals.

DIAGNOSIS AND DIFFERENTIAL

- Diffuse erythema with desiccation or exfoliation must be considered exfoliative dermatitis until proven otherwise.
- Diagnosis of exfoliative dermatitis is confirmed by skin biopsy.
- The differential diagnosis includes acute generalized exanthematous pustulosis, TEN, primary blistering disorders, Kawasaki's disease, and the toxic-infectious erythemas.

EMERGENCY DEPARTMENT CARE AND DISPOSITION

- Correct hypothermia and hypovolemia with appropriate correction of any life-threatening abnormality.
- After resuscitation has been completed, treatment of secondary infection, correction of electrolyte disorders, and management of CHF are clinical issues to address.
- For patients with a new presentation or a significant recurrence of exfoliative dermatitis, admission with dermatologic consultation is advised. Systemic steroids are commonly given after consultation.
- For patients with chronic disease with mild recurrence who are not systemically ill, outpatient treatment with prompt dermatologic follow-up is reasonable.

TOXIC-INFECTIOUS ERYTHEMAS

PATHOPHYSIOLOGY

- Toxic-infectious erythemas include toxic shock syndrome (TSS), streptococcal toxic shock syndrome (STSS), and staphylococcal scalded-skin syndrome (SSSS).
- TSS is a multisystem illness presenting with fever, shock, and erythroderma followed by desquamation associated with toxigenic *Staphylococcus aureus*.
- The causative agent of STSS is *Streptococcus pyogenes* (group A strep).
- SSSS is divided into three stages: (1) initial (erythroderma), (2) exfoliative, and (3) desquamation (recovery).
- In SSSS, exotoxins released by bacteria cause acantholysis and intraepidermal cleavage of the skin.
- SSSS occurs primarily in infants, young children, and the immunocompromised.

CLINICAL FEATURES

- The manifestations of TSS range from a mild, trivial disease to a rapidly progressive, potentially fatal, multisystem illness.
- The dermatologic hallmark of TSS is a nonpruritic, blanching macular erythroderma.
- The clinical presentation of STSS is similar to that of TSS; in fact, similar criteria may be used for the diagnosis.
- STSS presents with fever, hypotension, and skin infections.
- The majority of cases of STSS are associated with soft tissue infections; cellulitis, myositis, and fasciitis were the most common presenting diagnoses.
- In SSSS, there is a sudden appearance of a tender, diffuse erythroderma. The involved skin may have a sandpaper texture similar to the rash of scarlet fever.
- The exfoliative stage of SSSS begins on the second day of the illness with a wrinkling and peeling of the previously erythematous skin; Nikolsky's sign is found. Large, flaccid, fluid-filled bullae and vesicles then appear. These lesions easily rupture and are shed in large sheets; the underlying tissue resembles scalded skin and rapidly desiccates.
- During the exfoliative phase of SSSS, the patient is often febrile and irritable. After 3 to 5 days of illness, the involved skin desquamates, leaving normal skin in 7 to 10 days.

DIAGNOSIS AND DIFFERENTIAL

- The diagnosis of TSS requires fever, hypotension, rash, desquamation, and the involvement of three or more systems (Table 156-1).
- For TSS and STSS, fever and hypotension with associated erythroderma should suggest the diagnosis.
- Infants and toddlers with fever and diffuse erythroderma suggest SSSS.

TABLE 156-1 Case Definition of Toxic Shock Syndrome

An illness with the following clinical manifestations:
Fever: temperature $\geq$38.9°C ($\geq$102.0°F)
Rash: diffuse macular erythroderma
Desquamation: 1-2 wk after onset of illness, particularly on the palms and soles
Hypotension: systolic blood pressure $\leq$90 mm Hg for adults or less than fifth percentile by age for children aged <16 y; orthostatic drop in diastolic blood pressure $\geq$15 mm Hg from lying to sitting, orthostatic syncope, or orthostatic dizziness
Multisystem involvement (three or more of the following):
GI: vomiting or diarrhea at onset of illness
Muscular: severe myalgia or creatine phosphokinase level at least twice the upper limit of normal
Mucous membrane: vaginal, oropharyngeal, or conjunctival hyperemia
Renal: blood urea nitrogen or creatinine level at least twice the upper limit of normal for laboratory, or urinary sediment with pyuria ($\geq$5 leukocytes per high-power field) in the absence of urinary tract infection
Hepatic: total bilirubin, alanine aminotransferase enzyme, or aspartate aminotransferase enzyme levels at least twice the upper limit of normal for laboratory
Hematologic: platelet count <100,000/mm^3
Central nervous system: disorientation or alterations in consciousness without focal neurologic signs when fever and hypotension are absent
Laboratory criteria: negative results on the following tests, if obtained:
Blood, throat, or cerebrospinal fluid cultures (blood culture may be positive for *Staphylococcus aureus*)
Rise in titer to Rocky Mountain spotted fever, leptospirosis, or measles
Case classification:
Probable: a case in which five of the six clinical findings described above are present
Confirmed: a case in which all six of the clinical findings described above are present, including desquamation, unless the patient dies before desquamation occurs

Reproduced with permission from Toxic-Shock Syndrome (TSS): 1997 Case Definition. Centers for Disease Control and Prevention. Available at: http://www.cdc.gov/ncphi/disss/nndss/casedef/toxicsscurrent.htm.

EMERGENCY DEPARTMENT CARE AND DISPOSITION

- Management of patients with TSS and STSS is dictated by the severity of their illness. If the patient presents in extremis, airway control, ventilatory status, and hemodynamic status should be addressed emergently.
- Patients must be checked for evidence of organ system dysfunction. The vast majority of patients with TSS require hospital admission; the patient who is critically ill is best managed in the intensive care setting.
- Management of the patient with SSSS includes fluid resuscitation and correction of electrolyte abnormalities, as well as identification and treatment of the source of the toxigenic Staphylococcus with the appropriate antistaphylococcal antibiotic, including nafcillin, oxacillin, and clindamycin.
- The newborn may be treated with topical sulfadiazine or its equivalent.
- Corticosteroids are not recommended.

DISSEMINATED GONOCOCCAL INFECTION

PATHOPHYSIOLOGY

- Generally 0.5% to 3.0% of patients with mucosal lesions develop disseminated disease.
- The incidence is higher for those in late pregnancy, immediate postpartum period, or within 1 week of onset of menses.

CLINICAL FEATURES

- Fever, arthralgias, and multiple papular, vesicular, or pustular skin lesions are noted.
- Rash develops on dorsal aspects of ankles and feet.
- Lesions are initially small red papules or maculopapules; they either resolve or evolve into vesicles with purulent fluid and central necrosis.

DIAGNOSIS AND DIFFERENTIAL

- Diagnosis is made in sexually active persons with tenosynovitis, arthralgias, and appropriate dermatologic symptoms.
- Gram's stain of lesion fluid may show *Neisseria gonorrhoeae*. Blood cultures may be positive.

EMERGENCY DEPARTMENT CARE AND DISPOSITION

- Parenteral **ceftriaxone**, **cefotaxime**, **ceftizoxime**, or **spectinomycin** should be administered for 7 days.
- Fluoroqinolones are no longer recommended.

MENINGOCOCCEMIA

PATHOPHYSIOLOGY

- Meningococcemia is a potentially fatal infectious illness caused by *Neisseria meningitidis*.
- It has a wide clinical spectrum, including pharyngitis, meningitis, and bacteremia.
- Illness typically affects patients under 20 years of age. Epidemics are seen with very virulent strains.

CLINICAL FEATURES

- Infection develops usually within 3 to 4 days (range 2-10 days) after exposure and presents with severe headache, fever, altered mental status, nausea, vomiting, myalgias, arthralgia, and neck stiffness.
- Dermatologic manifestations include petechiae, urticaria, hemorrhagic vesicles, and macules.

DIAGNOSIS AND DIFFERENTIAL

- Diagnosis relies on clinical suspicion based on presentation of an ill-appearing patient with petechial rash and associated symptoms.
- Cerebrospinal fluid cultures may be positive.
- The differential diagnosis includes Rocky Mountain spotted fever, TSS, gonococcemia, bacterial endocarditis, vasculitis, viral and bacterial infection, and disseminated intravascular coagulation.

EMERGENCY DEPARTMENT CARE AND DISPOSITION

- **Ceftriaxone** 2 grams IV and **vancomycin** 1 gram IV should be administered empirically as soon as the disease is suspected.
- Hospital admission is necessary.

PEMPHIGUS VULGARIS

PATHOPHYSIOLOGY

- Pemphigus vulgaris (PV) is a generalized mucocutaneous autoimmune blistering eruption characterized by intraepidermal acantholytic blistering.

CLINICAL FEATURES

- The primary lesions of PV are vesicles or bullae that vary in diameter from less than 1 cm to several centimeters, commonly first affecting the head, trunk, and mucous membranes.
- The blisters are usually clear and tense, originating from normal skin or atop an erythematous or

urticarial plaque. Within 2 to 3 days, the bullae become turbid and flaccid with rupture soon following, producing painful, denuded areas. These erosions are slow to heal and prone to secondary infection.
- Nikolsky's sign is positive in PV and absent in other autoimmune blistering diseases. Mucous membranes are affected in most patients.

DIAGNOSIS AND DIFFERENTIAL

- Diagnosis is suspected with the appearance of the blistering lesions and confirmed by skin biopsy and immunofluorescence testing.
- The differential diagnosis of PV includes all of those diseases that can present with primary skin blistering, including TEN, EM, other autoimmune blistering diseases, burns, severe contact dermatitis, bullous diabeticorum, and friction blisters.

EMERGENCY DEPARTMENT CARE AND DISPOSITION

- Patients with PV should be hospitalized with early dermatologic consultant; begin high-dose parenteral steroids and other immunosuppressive drugs to prevent mortality.
- Close observation and rapid treatment with appropriate antibiotics for secondary infection of erosions is imperative.

For further reading in Tintinalli's *Emergency Medicine: A Comprehensive Study Guide*, 7th ed., see Chapter 245, "Serious Generalized Skin Disorders," by J. Jeremy Thomas, Andrew D. Perron, and William J. Brady.

157 OTHER DERMATOLOGIC DISORDERS

Daniel A. Handel

HERPES ZOSTER INFECTION

CLINICAL FEATURES

- Herpes zoster results from activation of latent varicella zoster virus.
- Pain or dysesthesia precedes the eruption by 3 to 5 days.
- Eruptions can occur anywhere on the body. Thoracic dermatomes are involved in greater than 50% of cases, cranial or trigeminal regions in 20%, lumbar 15%, and sacral 5%.
- Erythematous papules progress to clusters of vesicles with an erythematous base.
- Lesions involving the nose should lead to significant concern for ophthalmic involvement and development of keratitis, which can lead to blindness.

DIAGNOSIS AND DIFFERENTIAL

- A Tzanck prep and viral culture can confirm a diagnosis typically made on history and physical examination.
- The differential diagnosis includes herpes simplex, erysipelas, impetigo, and contact dermatitis.

EMERGENCY DEPARTMENT CARE AND DISPOSITION

- Antivirals such as **acyclovir**, **famciclovir**, or **valacyclovir** are beneficial if administered within 24 to 72 hours after the eruption of the lesions.
- **Aluminum acetate solution** or **petroleum jelly compresses** provide symptomatic treatment.

TINEA INFECTIONS

CLINICAL FEATURES

- Tinea pedis is a fungal infection of the feet, also known as athlete's foot.
- Tinea manuum, a dermatophyte infection of the hand, is often unilateral and frequently associated with tinea pedis.
- The most common form of tinea pedis is the interdigital presentation, manifested by maceration and scaling in the web spaces between the toes. Ulcerations may be present in severe cases with secondary infection.
- The second type of tinea pedis is characterized by chronic, dry scaling with minimal inflammation on the palmar or plantar surfaces. It often extends to the medial and lateral aspects of the feet, but not the dorsal surface. Maceration between the toes is common.
- The third type of fungal infection (bullous tinea pedis) presents as an acute, painful, pruritic vesicular eruption on the palms or soles. Erythema is a prominent feature, while the nails and web spaces are usually spared.
- Tinea cruris, a fungal infection of the groin commonly called jock itch, is very common in males. Erythema with a peripheral annular, scaly edge is seen. The rash extends onto the inner thighs and the buttocks and spares the penis and scrotum—a feature that is important in distinguishing tinea cruris from other eruptions in the groin.

DIAGNOSIS AND DIFFERENTIAL

- Identification of fungal elements on a KOH preparation or with fungal culture may be required if the diagnosis is uncertain. Typically, the diagnosis is made clinically.

EMERGENCY DEPARTMENT CARE AND DISPOSITION

- Nonbullous tinea pedis and tinea manuum can be treated with topical antifungal agents, such as **clotrimazole**, **miconazole**, **ketoconazole**, or **econazole,** twice daily until 1 week after clearing has occurred.
- Nail infections also should be treated with oral antifungal agents (**itraconazole**, **fluconazole**, or **terbinafine**) as well.
- Bullous tinea pedis often does not respond to topical treatment; oral antifungal treatment is necessary.
- Treatment of tinea cruris is with antifungal creams such as **clotrimazole**, **ketoconazole**, or **econazole**. Antifungal powders should be used on a daily basis to prevent recurrences.
- Follow-up with a dermatologist if eruption does not resolve in 4 to 6 weeks.

CANDIDA INTERTRIGO

- Candidal infections of the skin favor moist, occluded areas of the body.
- Superficial candidal infections are commonly seen in the diaper area, the vulva and groin of women, the glans penis (balanitis) in uncircumcised males, and the inframammary and pannus folds of obese patients.
- Antibiotic therapy, systemic corticosteroid therapy, urinary or fecal incontinence, immunocompromised states, and obesity are predisposing factors.
- The typical presentation of candida intertrigo is erythema and maceration with surrounding small erythematous papules or pustules. The satellite pustules are a characteristic finding in differentiating between candida intertrigo and other inflammatory disorders affecting the skin folds.
- KOH preparation of the pustules may demonstrate short hyphae and spores.
- Apply stringent solutions like **aluminum acetate** to help dry weepy eruptions.
- After drying, apply topical antifungals such as **clotrimazole**, **ketoconazole**, or **econazole.**

HUMAN SCABIES

CLINICAL FEATURES

- Human scabies is an infestation of the skin by *Sarcoptes scabiei.* Scabies is transmitted by close physical contact or linens and clothing.
- Scabetic mites burrow into the stratum corneum. The time from infestation to clinical symptoms is 4 to 6 weeks.
- The eruptions are very pruritic. Hands, feet, elbows, knees, umbilicus, groin, and genitals may be involved.
- Excoriations and pruritic papules may be the only visible clues.
- In crusted scabies, hyperkeratosis develops on the hands and feet, with nails frequently affected.

DIAGNOSIS AND DIFFERENTIAL

- Diagnosis is based on high clinical suspicion and positive scabies preparation.

EMERGENCY DEPARTMENT CARE AND DISPOSITION

- Topical scabicides are applied from the neck down to the feet. **Permethrin 5% cream** and **lindane 1% lotion** are equally effective.
- Lindane is neurotoxic in infants, children, and pregnant women.
- **Ivermectin**, 200 micrograms/kg PO once, is an alternative to permethrin cream but should be avoided in pregnant and lactating women.
- Oral antihistamines and topical corticosteroids help relieve symptoms.

PEDICULOSIS

CLINICAL FEATURES

- Pediculosis capitis is an infestation of the hair and scalp with the mite *Pediculus capitis*, and occurs most commonly in school-aged children.
- The louse is spread via close personal contact, clothing, and bed linens. Itching can be mild or intense.
- Excoriation may be seen in the posterior neck and occiput.
- *Pediculus corporis* (body lice) is less commonly seen. It typically occurs in overcrowded conditions with poor hygiene.
- Bites are typically not felt by individuals, but red urticarial papules are left. Areas not covered by clothing are typically spared.
- *Pthirus pubis* is pubic lice and is sexually transmitted.

DIAGNOSIS AND DIFFERENTIAL

- Diagnosis of pediculosis capitis is made by visualization of lice and nits (eggs firmly attached to hair shafts) on physical examination.

EMERGENCY DEPARTMENT CARE AND DISPOSITION

- **Permethrin cream, 1% or 5%,** is first-line therapy for head lice. It should be applied to the scalp overnight. Alternatively, pyrethrin cream can be applied for 10 minutes then rinsed out.
- A repeat treatment is recommended in 1 to 2 weeks.
- Treatment for pediculosis pubis and corporis is the same as for scabies above.

CONTACT DERMATITIS

CLINICAL FEATURES

- Contact dermatitis may be a primary irritant reaction or an allergic-mediated event.
- Agents capable of causing an aerosolized reaction include rhus (poison ivy and oak) when the plant has been burned.
- Allergic contact dermatitis resulting from an aerosolized allergen presents with erythema or scaling, at times accompanied by blistering. The involvement is diffuse with upper and lower eyelids affected.

DIAGNOSIS AND DIFFERENTIAL

- Direct application of the allergen produces similar findings on the most sensitive skin areas, such as the eyelids.

EMERGENCY DEPARTMENT CARE AND DISPOSITION

- Corticosteroids (topical or oral, depending on the severity) are often required. Only low-potency topical corticosteroids (**hydrocortisone 2.5%**) should be used on the face; cream or ointment should be used initially. Alternatively, medium- to high-potency topical corticosteroids can be used on the face for no more than 3 to 5 days.
- Extensive and severe periocular involvement requires oral prednisone.
- Oral antihistamines are also useful in reducing pruritus.

PHOTOSENSITIVITY

CLINICAL FEATURES

- Patients with sunburn have an inflammatory response to ultraviolet radiation and may present with minimal discomfort or extreme pain with extensive blistering.
- A tender, warm erythema is seen in sun-exposed areas. Vesiculation may occur, representing a second-degree burn injury.
- Exogenous photosensitivity results from either the topical application or the ingestion of an agent that increases the skin's sensitivity to ultraviolet light.
- Topically applied furocoumarins—lime juice, various fragrances, figs, celery, and parsnips—are the most common group of agents causing photoeruptions. Other topical photosensitizers include Para-Aminobenzoic Acid (PABA) esters and topical psoralens.
- The exogenous photoeruption is similar to a severe sunburn reaction, often with blistering.

DIAGNOSIS AND DIFFERENTIAL

- Sunburn should be suspected in a patient who has frequented the outdoors with significant ultraviolet light exposure.
- The diagnosis of exogenous photosensitivity is based on identifying the offending agent.
- A linear appearance to the rash suggests an externally applied substance.

EMERGENCY DEPARTMENT CARE AND DISPOSITION

- Sunburns are treated symptomatically with tepid baths, oral analgesics, and burn wound care.
- Initial management of exogenous photosensitivity is similar to the sunburn reaction, including the avoidance of the sun until the eruption has cleared. Any causative agent should be discontinued if possible.

PSORIASIS

- Psoriasis vulgaris presents with erythema, scales, and fissures as discrete plaques located on palms and soles.
- In pustular psoriasis erythema, some scaling and numerous pustules are seen on the palms and soles.
- The diagnosis is usually made clinically. Biopsy may be helpful.
- Treatment options include petroleum jelly, topical steroids, tar preparations, and vitamin D formulations.

For further reading in Tintinalli's *Emergency Medicine: A Comprehensive Study Guide*, 7th ed., see Chapter 246, "Disorders of the Face and Scalp," by Dean S. Morrell and Emily J. Schwartz; Chapter 247, "Disorders of the Hands, Feet, and Extremities," by Craig N. Burkhart and Dean S. Morrell; Chapter 248, "Disorders of the Groin and Skinfolds," by Dean S. Morrell and Kelly Nelson; and Chapter 249, "Skin Disorders Common on the Trunk," by Mark R. Hess and Suzanne P. Hess.

Section 19
TRAUMA

158 TRAUMA IN ADULTS

Jonathan S. Ilgen

CLINICAL FEATURES

- Trauma patients who present with obviously abnormal vital signs must prompt a thorough search for the specific underlying injuries.
- Nonspecific signs such as tachycardia, tachypnea, or mild alterations in consciousness must similarly be presumed to signify serious injury until proven otherwise. These findings should be aggressively evaluated and treated.
- Even without significant physical examination findings, the mechanism of trauma may suggest potential injury patterns that should be pursued diligently.

DIAGNOSIS AND DIFFERENTIAL

- Obtain the history from the patient, witnesses, or paramedics, and include the mechanism of injury, sites of injury, blood loss at the scene, degree of damage to any vehicles, and descriptions of weapons used.
- Patterns of injuries, and expected physiologic responses to these injuries, can be ascertained by collecting history regarding the circumstances of the event (eg, single vehicle crash, fall from height, smoke inhalation, environmental exposures), ingestion of intoxicants, preexisting medical conditions, and medications.
- The primary survey (ABCDE), including a complete set of vital signs, is characterized by the orderly identification and immediate treatment of life-threatening conditions.
- Assess airway patency and breathing by examining for a gag reflex, pooling of secretions, airway obstruction, tracheal deviation, presence and quality of breath sounds, flail chest, chest or neck crepitus, sucking chest wounds, and fractures of the sternum.
- In the appropriate clinical setting, ensure cervical spine immobilization during the airway assessment.
- Problems such as tension pneumothorax, pneumothorax, hemothorax, and malpositioned endotracheal tube should be remedied before proceeding further in the primary survey.
- Circulatory status is evaluated via vital signs, level of consciousness, skin color, and the presence and magnitude of peripheral pulses. Sites of obvious bleeding, indications of shock, and signs of cardiac tamponade (Beck's triad of hypotension, jugular venous distention, and muffled heart sounds) should be identified.
- The primary survey concludes with a brief neurologic examination for disability using the Glasgow Coma Scale (GCS), pupil size and reactivity, and motor function assessment. The GCS assessment can be insensitive in patients with normal or near-normal scores, and a GCS score of 15 does not exclude the presence of traumatic brain injury.
- The patient is then completely exposed in order to identify other injuries.
- The focused assessment with sonography for trauma (FAST) examination is a screening tool that should be used to identify causes of shock immediately after the primary survey. Among patients with hypotension, diagnostic peritoneal lavage (DPL) is an alternative method of identifying intraperitoneal blood in lieu of a FAST examination. If a patient is hemodynamically stable, definitive imaging can be performed with a CT scan of the abdomen and pelvis with IV contrast.
- The secondary survey is a rapid but thorough head-to-toe examination aimed toward the identification of all injuries and thereby set priorities for care. Resuscitation and frequent monitoring of vital signs continue throughout this process. Do not start the secondary survey until basic functions under the primary survey have been corrected and resuscitation has been initiated.
- Assess for evidence of significant head injury (eg, skull and facial fractures) and recheck the pupils. Complete the neck, chest, and abdominal examinations and assess the stability of the pelvis.
- Evaluate the genitourinary system by external inspection and rectal examination. If there is blood at the urethral meatus or a displaced prostate on rectal examination, perform a retrograde urethrogram to evaluate for urethral injury. Otherwise, place a Foley catheter and check the urine for blood. Order a pregnancy test for female patients of childbearing age.

- Vaginal blood on a bimanual examination raises concern for a vaginal laceration from a pelvic fracture, and is an indication for a speculum examination.
- Check the extremities for soft tissue injury, fractures, and pulses.
- Complete a more thorough neurologic examination, carefully checking motor and sensory function.
- After the secondary survey, laboratory and imaging studies (plain radiographs and CT scans) should be considered. In younger patients in whom the clinical indication for CT scan may be equivocal, avoid the use of ionizing radiation if possible.
- Certain conditions, such as injuries to the esophagus, diaphragm, and small bowel, often remain undiagnosed even after thorough serial examinations and imaging. Prolonged observation for delayed presentations may be required in the appropriate clinical settings.
- The most frequently missed injuries are orthopedic. A tertiary survey has been recommended in patients with multisystem trauma within the first 24 hours to lessen the risk of missed injuries.

EMERGENCY DEPARTMENT CARE AND DISPOSITION

- Confirm airway patency at the outset of the primary survey.
- A jaw thrust may initially help in opening the airway; suctioning may remove foreign material, blood, loose tissue, or avulsed teeth.
- Endotracheal intubation via a rapid sequence technique is indicated for airway management. Whenever possible, use of a two-person spinal stabilization technique is suggested in which one provider provides in-line immobilization of the cervical spine while the other manages the airway.
- Endotracheal intubation is indicated in comatose patients (GCS <8) to protect the airway and prevent secondary brain injury from hypoxemia.
- In cases of extensive facial trauma or when endotracheal intubation is not possible, cricothyrotomy or another advanced airway technique should be employed to secure the airway. Avoid nasal airway insertion in patients with suspected basilar skull fractures.
- Treat clinically suspected tension pneumothorax immediately with needle decompression followed by tube thoracostomy. Treat large or open pneumothoraces identified during the primary survey with a tube thoracostomy.
- The presence of a flail chest may mandate endotracheal intubation to ventilate patients adequately.
- Reassess hypotensive patients without an obvious indication for surgery after infusion of 2 L of warm crystalloid solution (LR or normal saline). If there is no marked improvement, type O blood should be transfused (O-negative for females of childbearing age).
- If patients require >10 units of packed red blood cells (PRBCs), they should receive PRBCs in a 1:1 ratio with fresh frozen plasma. Both acidosis and hypothermia contribute to coagulopathy and should be corrected as soon as possible.
- In patients with penetrating abdominal trauma who are in shock, early operative intervention results in better outcomes.
- Manage severe external hemorrhage with compression at the bleeding site.
- Tamponade of severe epistaxis may be achieved with balloon compression devices or nasal packing.

For further reading in Tintinalli's *Emergency Medicine: A Comprehensive Study Guide*, 7th ed., see Chapter 250, "Trauma in Adults," by Patrick H. Brunett and Peter A. Cameron.

159 TRAUMA IN CHILDREN

Matthew Hansen

EPIDEMIOLOGY

- Trauma is the most common cause of death and disability in children 1 year of age and older; motor vehicle crash is the leading mechanism of injury in these children.
- Head injury is the most frequent cause of death.

PATHOPHYSIOLOGY

- Differences in anatomy, physiology, and psychology mandate modifications to trauma evaluation and management in children.

CLINICAL FEATURES

- Airway management in children can be challenging due to anatomic differences including a large occiput, large tongue, and cephalad location of the larynx.
- Infants younger than 6 months are nose breathers, and facial trauma may cause respiratory distress. Tachypnea is often the first sign of dyspnea.

- Children with compensated shock from hemorrhage have normal blood pressure and tachycardia. Other signs of shock include prolonged cap refill, cool extremities, weak peripheral pulses, and altered mental status. Hypotension is a pre-arrest finding.
- Age-dependent adaptation of the traditional Glasgow Coma Scale (GCS) score should be used.
- The ratio of surface area to mass is greater in children, increasing risk of hypothermia.

DIAGNOSIS AND DIFFERENTIAL

- Infants and neonates are at the highest risk of intracranial injury, especially those with altered mental status, >1 minute loss of consciousness, vomiting, and/or seizures. Noncontrast computed tomography (CT) is the imaging modality of choice for head trauma.
- Scalp injuries, particularly in neonates, may result in significant blood loss and shock.
- The increased flexibility of the spine in preadolescent children is responsible for the relatively lower incidence of spinal fracture in this group. As a result, children with spinal cord injuries frequently do not have fractures and have symptoms concerning for spinal cord injury without radiographic abnormality (SCIWORA).
- "Clearing the cervical spine" in children is challenging as there is little evidence to guide practice. Multisystem trauma or head trauma are general indications for neck immobilization and cervical spine imaging. Due to the low incidence of spine fractures in younger children and the need to lower ionizing radiation, plain radiographs of the cervical spine remain a useful tool (Table 159-1).
- In blunt chest trauma, considerable force may be transmitted to intrathoracic structures, causing serious injury with a paucity of external signs. Rib fractures require a significant mechanism of injury.
- The physical examination in children has been shown to be unreliable in determining the severity of injury in up to 45% of pediatric trauma patients.

TABLE 159-1 Considerations for Cervical Spine Imaging in Children
Moderate- or high-risk head injury
Multiple trauma
Signs or symptoms of spinal injury
Direct mechanism for spinal injury
Altered mental status or focal neurologic findings
Distracting painful injury
Agitation with possible mechanism for spinal injury

- CT imaging of the abdomen is indicated in patients with a suspicious mechanism of injury, tenderness, seatbelt sign, distention, or vomiting.
- Identification of a pelvic fracture, particularly an anterior ring fracture, should prompt investigation for associated urethral or bladder injury.
- Suspect nonaccidental trauma (child abuse) when evaluating pediatric trauma patients, especially when the described mechanism of injury is inconsistent with the injuries sustained in infants and neonates.
- Other markers for child abuse include the presence of an injury not consistent with the child's developmental status such as bruising in nonambulatory children.

EMERGENCY DEPARTMENT CARE AND DISPOSITION

- Complete an organized primary and secondary survey for all pediatric patients with significant mechanism of injury. Many problems are managed in a fashion similar to that used in adult patients.
- Initially administer all patients with 100% oxygen. With difficult bagging, consider two-person mask technique and placement of an oral airway.
- Orotracheal intubation is indicated for airway management. The following formula is used to estimate endotracheal tube size: size = 4 + (age/4). Cuffed or uncuffed endotracheal tubes can be used. However, the appropriate cuffed tube size is ½ size smaller than what is calculated using the formula above.
- Rapid sequence intubation using pretreatment with 100% oxygen, appropriate sedation, and paralysis is indicated for a patient with an unstable airway.
- Obtain intraosseous cannulation in unstable patients if intravenous access cannot be promptly established.
- Administer resuscitative fluids in 20 mL/kg boluses of isotonic crystalloid. If there is no response to 2 to 3 boluses, then infuse 10 mL/kg boluses of packed red blood cells.
- Resuscitate burn patients according to a standard burn formula, such as the Parkland formula.
- For pain control, fentanyl 1 microgram/kg or morphine 0.05 to 0.1 milligram/kg are appropriate.
- If a head-injured patient has signs of impending herniation, the $Paco_2$ should be maintained at 30 to 35 mm Hg, blood pressure optimized with IV fluids, the head of the bed elevated to 30 degrees, the head and neck positioned at neutral, and mannitol 1 gram/kg administered.
- Spinal immobilization must be achieved in infants and younger children with allowance for their relatively larger head by placement of padding behind the shoulders.

- Admit children with skull fractures, intracranial hemorrhage, spinal trauma, significant chest trauma, abdominal trauma with internal organ injury, significant burns, or other concerning injuries. Guidelines for referral to a pediatric trauma center are **mechanisms of injury:** injury from motor vehicle, fall from a height, motor vehicle collision with prolonged extrication, and motor vehicle collision with death of another vehicle occupant; and **anatomic injury:** multiple severe trauma, more than three long-bone fractures, spinal fractures or spinal cord injury, amputations, severe head or facial trauma, and penetrating head, chest, or abdominal trauma.
- Social service consultation and reporting to child protective services are indicated if there is any suspicion of nonaccidental trauma.

For further reading in Tintinalli's *Emergency Medicine: A Comprehensive Study Guide*, 7th ed., see Chapter 251, "Trauma in Children," by William E. Hauda II.

160 GERIATRIC TRAUMA

O. John Ma

EPIDEMIOLOGY

- While persons over 65 years of age represent 12% of the population, they account for 36% of all ambulance transports, 25% of hospitalizations, and 25% of total trauma costs.
- Approximately 28% of deaths due to accidental causes involve persons 65 years and older.

PATHOPHYSIOLOGY

- Chronologic age is the actual number of years the individual has lived. Physiologic age describes the actual functional capacity of the patients' organ systems in a physiologic sense.
- Comorbid disease states such as diabetes mellitus, coronary artery disease, renal disease, arthritis, and pulmonary disease can decrease the physiologic reserve of certain patients, which makes it more difficult for them to recover from a traumatic injury.
- Physiologic reserve describes the various levels of functioning of the patients' organ systems that allow them to compensate for traumatic derangement.
- Falls are the most common cause of injury in patients over 65 years of age. Falls are reported as the underlying cause of 9500 deaths each year in patients over the age of 65 years. In the >85-year-old age group, 20% of fatal falls occur in nursing homes.
- Motor vehicle crashes rank as the second leading mechanism of injury that brings elderly patients to a trauma center in the United States and are the most common mechanism for fatal incidents in elderly persons through 80 years of age.

CLINICAL FEATURES

- Following injury, elderly patients have higher admission rates, longer hospital stays, increased long-term morbidity, and higher mortality rates despite lower injury severity.
- The clinician should not be led into a false sense of security by "normal" vital signs. In one study of 15 patients initially considered to be hemodynamically "stable," 8 had cardiac outputs less than 3.5 L/min and none had an adequate response to volume loading. Of seven patients with a normal cardiac output, five had inadequate oxygen delivery.
- There is progressive stiffening of the myocardium with age that results in a decreased effectiveness of the pumping mechanism. A normal tachycardic response to pain, hypovolemia, or anxiety may be absent or blunted in the elderly trauma patient. Medications such as β-blockers may mask tachycardia and hinder the evaluation of the elderly patient.
- Elderly patients suffer a much lower incidence of epidural hematomas than the general population; however, there is a higher incidence of subdural hematomas. As the brain mass decreases with advancing age, there is greater stretching and tension of the bridging veins that pass from the brain to the dural sinuses.
- The incidence of cervical spine injury has been found to be twice as great in geriatric patients as in a younger cohort of blunt trauma patients. Odontoid fractures were particularly common in geriatric patients, accounting for 20% of geriatric cervical spine fractures compared with 5% of non-geriatric fractures.
- Severe thoracic injuries, such as hemopneumothorax, pulmonary contusion, flail chest, and cardiac contusion, can quickly lead to decompensation in elderly individuals whose baseline oxygenation status may already be diminished.

- Reduction in pulmonary compliance, total lung surface area, and mucociliary clearance of foreign material and bacteria result in an increased risk for elderly patients to develop nosocomial gram-negative pneumonia.
- Hip fracture is the single most common diagnosis that leads to hospitalization in all age groups in the United States.
- Hip fractures occur primarily in four areas: intertrochanteric, transcervical, subcapital, and subtrochanteric. Intertrochanteric fractures are the most common, followed by transcervical fractures. Emergency physicians must be aware that pelvic and long bone fractures are not infrequently the sole etiology for hypovolemia in elderly patients.
- The incidence of humeral head and surgical neck fractures in elderly patients are increased by falls on the outstretched hand or elbow.

DIAGNOSIS AND DIFFERENTIAL

- The base deficit and lactate levels provide good initial measures of shock, and serial measurements can guide resuscitation decisions. The base deficit and lactate levels both correlate with systemic hypoperfusion that may be "occult" in patients, and admission levels of these markers correlate with ICU length of stay, hospital length of stay, and mortality.
- For older patients, the adhesions associated with previous abdominal surgical procedures increase the risk of performing diagnostic peritoneal lavage.
- It is important to ensure adequate hydration and baseline assessment of renal function prior to the contrast load for the CT scan. Some patients may be volume depleted due to medications, such as diuretics. This hypovolemia coupled with contrast administration may exacerbate any underlying renal pathology.
- For unstable patients, and especially those with multiple scars on the abdominal wall from previous procedures, the focused assessment with sonography for trauma (FAST) examination is the ideal diagnostic study to detect free intraperitoneal fluid.

EMERGENCY DEPARTMENT CARE AND DISPOSITION

- Prompt endotracheal intubation and use of mechanical ventilation should be considered in patients with more severe injuries, respiratory rates greater than 40 breaths per minute, or when the Pao_2 is <60 mm Hg or $Paco_2$ >50 mm Hg.
- Early invasive monitoring has been advocated to help physicians assess the elderly's hemodynamic status. One study demonstrated that by reducing the time to invasive monitoring in elderly trauma patients from 5.5 to 2.2 hours, and thus recognizing and appropriately treating occult shock, the survival rate of their patients increased from 7% to 53%. Survival was improved because of enhanced oxygen delivery through the use of adequate volume loading and inotropic support.
- During the initial resuscitative phase, crystalloid, while the primary option, should be administered judiciously since elderly patients with diminished cardiac compliance are more susceptible to volume overload. Strong consideration should be made for early and more liberal use of packed red blood cell transfusion. Depending on the type of injury and severity of blood loss, switching to blood transfusion after 1 to 2 L of crystalloid resuscitation should be considered.
- Despite the multitude of options, there is as yet no true panacea for reversing anticoagulation in the patient with intracranial bleeding. Full reversal with FFP may require administration of up to 4 L of FFP, contributing to fluid overload in some elderly trauma patients. Hematoma expansion appears to occur largely within the first several hours following injury, making sole administration of vitamin K, with its slow onset of action, inadequate.
- Among geriatric trauma patients who are hospitalized, the mortality rate has been reported to be between 15% and 30%. These figures far exceed the mortality rate of 4% to 8% found in younger patients. In general, multiple organ failure and sepsis cause more deaths in elderly patients than in younger trauma victims.
- Age >75 years, Glasgow Coma Scale score ≤7, presence of shock upon admission, severe head injury, and the development of sepsis are associated with worse outcome and higher mortality figures.
- Data demonstrate that immediately after discharge one-third of trauma survivors return to independent living, one-third return to dependent status but living at home, and one-third require nursing home facilities.

For further reading in Tintinalli's *Emergency Medicine: A Comprehensive Study Guide*, 7th ed., see Chapter 252, "Geriatric Trauma," by O. John Ma, Jennifer H. Edwards, and Stephen W. Meldon.

161 TRAUMA IN PREGNANCY

Nicole M. DeIorio

EPIDEMIOLOGY

- Trauma is the leading cause of nonobstetric morbidity and mortality in pregnant women.
- Motor vehicle crash is the most common mechanism of blunt abdominal trauma in pregnant patients, followed by falls and assault.
- A significant percentage of trauma in pregnancy results from intimate partner violence.

PATHOPHYSIOLOGY

- Abruption may be seen in patients with only minor abdominal trauma.
- Physiologic changes of pregnancy make determination of injury severity problematic.
- Heart rate increases 10 to 20 beats per minute in the second trimester, while systolic and diastolic blood pressures drop 10 to 15 mm Hg.
- Pregnant patients exhibit a physiologic anemia due to a disproportionate increase in blood volume (up to 45%) compared to red cell mass.
- Tachycardia, hypotension, and anemia may be due to blood loss or simply normal physiologic changes.
- Due to the hypervolemic state, a patient may lose 30% to 35% of her blood volume before manifesting signs of shock.

CLINICAL FEATURES

- The uterus is shielded by the bony pelvis until 12 weeks' gestation. At 20 weeks, it reaches the level of the umbilicus and blood flow increases, making severe maternal hemorrhage from uterine trauma more likely.
- The uterus can compress the inferior vena cava when the patient is supine, leading to the "supine hypotension syndrome."
- Decreased intestinal motility is associated with gastroesophageal reflux, predisposing the patient to vomiting and aspiration.
- The bladder moves into the abdomen in the third trimester, increasing its susceptibility to injury.
- Fetal injuries are more likely to be seen in the third trimester, often associated with pelvic fractures or penetrating trauma in the mother.
- Uterine rupture is rare, but is associated with a fetal mortality rate of close to 100%.
- More common complications of trauma include preterm labor and abruptio placentae.
- Maternal death is the most common cause of fetal death.
- Abruptio placentae is also a common cause of fetal death, with a 50% to 80% mortality rate.
- Abruption presents with abdominal pain, vaginal bleeding, uterine contractions, and signs of disseminated intravascular coagulation.
- Fetal-maternal hemorrhage must be considered in cases of significant trauma and may result in Rh-isoimmunization of Rh-negative women.

DIAGNOSIS AND DIFFERENTIAL

- Maternal stability and survival offer the best chance for fetal well being, so do not withhold critical interventions or diagnostic procedures out of concern for potential adverse effects on the fetus.
- In addition to the standard trauma evaluation, direct special attention to the gravid abdomen, looking for evidence of injury, tenderness, or uterine contractions.
- If abdominal or pelvic trauma is suspected, perform a sterile speculum examination, looking for genital trauma, vaginal bleeding, or ruptured amniotic membranes.
- Fluid with a pH of 7 in the vaginal canal suggests amniotic rupture, as does a branch-like pattern, or "ferning," on drying of vaginal fluid on a microscope slide.
- Shield the uterus from ionizing radiation when possible, and limit radiographs to those that will significantly impact the patient's care.
- Adverse fetal effects from ionizing radiation are negligible with doses <5 rad, which is an exposure far greater than that received from most trauma radiographs.
- Abdominal and pelvic computed tomography (CT) scanning, pelvic angiography, and pelvic fluoroscopy result in the highest doses of radiation to the fetus.
- Radiation exposure may be decreased by reducing the number of CT cuts obtained.
- Bedside ultrasonography is a highly sensitive and specific radiation-free abdominal imaging alternative. In addition to assessing for free intraperitoneal fluid, ultrasonography can also identify fetal heart rate, gestational age, fetal activity or demise, placental location, and amniotic fluid volume. Ultrasound may miss uterine rupture, however.
- MRI has not been associated with adverse fetal outcomes.
- Diagnostic peritoneal lavage remains a valid modality for evaluating the pregnant abdominal trauma patient, but has been replaced primarily by ultrasound. An open supraumbilical technique should be used.

- Auscultation of fetal heart tones for determining fetal viability and identifying fetal distress should be performed early in the evaluation; a normal rate is 120 to 160 beats per minute.
- Fetal bradycardia is most likely to be caused from hypoxia due to maternal hypotension, respiratory compromise, or placental abruption.
- Fetal tachycardia is most likely due to hypoxia or hypovolemia.
- In the setting of blunt abdominal trauma, external fetal monitoring is indicated for all patients beyond 20 weeks' gestation. A minimum of 4 to 6 hours is the generally accepted initial period of monitoring, which should be extended up to 24 hours in the case of documented uterine irritability. This should be performed even in those women who do not have an obvious abdominal injury.
- Fetal tachycardia, lack of beat-to-beat or long-term variability, or late decelerations on tocodynamometry signify fetal distress and may be indications for emergent cesarean section if the pregnancy is beyond the viable gestational age.

EMERGENCY DEPARTMENT CARE AND DISPOSITION

- As is the case with all trauma patients, initial priorities are the ABCs of resuscitation directed to the mother. Coordinate care with surgical and obstetric consultants.
- Provide all pregnant trauma patients supplemental oxygen.
- Initiate large-bore, peripheral IV lines with crystalloid infusions.
- Avoid placement of IV lines in the femoral region and lower extremity if possible due to compression of the inferior vena cava by the uterus and possible pooling in the pelvic veins.
- For patients beyond 20 weeks' gestation who must remain supine, a wedge may be placed under the right hip, tilting the patient 30 degrees to the left, thus reducing the likelihood of supine hypotension syndrome. Otherwise, keep the patient in a left lateral decubitus position whenever possible.
- Perform early gastric intubation to reduce the risk of aspiration.
- Vasopressors can have deleterious effects on uterine perfusion and should be avoided.
- Administer tetanus prophylaxis when indicated since it is not contraindicated in pregnancy.
- Administer Rho-D immune globulin to all nonsensitized Rh-negative pregnant patients following abdominal trauma.
- Tocolytics have a variety of side effects, including fetal and maternal tachycardia. Only administer them in consultation with an obstetrician.
- Indications for emergent laparotomy in the pregnant patient remain the same as in the nonpregnant patient.
- The decision to admit or discharge a pregnant trauma patient is based on the nature and severity of the presenting injuries and is often made after consultation with surgical and obstetric consultants.
- Admit patients who display evidence of fetal distress or increased uterine irritability during initial observation.
- Instruct patients who are discharged to seek medical attention immediately if they develop abdominal pain or cramps, vaginal bleeding, leakage of fluid, or perception of decreased fetal activity.

For further reading in Tintinalli's *Emergency Medicine: A Comprehensive Study Guide*, 7th ed., see Chapter 253, "Trauma in Pregnancy," by Nicole M. Delorio.

162 HEAD TRAUMA IN ADULTS AND CHILDREN

O. John Ma

EPIDEMIOLOGY

- The vast majority (80%) of traumatic brain injuries (TBIs) in the United States are mild.
- Approximately 40% of patients with moderate TBI have an abnormal finding on CT and 8% require neurosurgical intervention.
- Elderly individuals, children, and alcoholics are at greater risk for TBI.

PATHOPHYSIOLOGY

- Direct injury is caused immediately by the forces of an object striking the head or by penetrating injury.
- Indirect injuries are from acceleration/deceleration forces that result in the movement of the brain inside the skull.
- Secondary insults that may worsen the clinical outcome of TBI patients include cerebral edema, hypoxemia, hypotension, anemia, and elevated intracranial pressure (ICP).
- Cerebral perfusion pressure (CPP) is the difference between the mean arterial pressure (MAP) and the ICP.

Elevation of the ICP and/or hypotension results in a depressed CPP and leads to further brain injury.

- Rapid rises in the ICP can lead to the "Cushing reflex," which is characterized by hypertension, bradycardia, and respiratory irregularities. The Cushing reflex is seen uncommonly and usually occurs in children.

CLINICAL FEATURES

- TBI is classified as mild, moderate, or severe based on the Glasgow Coma Scale (GCS, see Table 162-1) score.

TABLE 162-1 Glasgow Coma Scale for All Age Groups

	4 Y TO ADULT	CHILD <4 Y	INFANT
Eye opening			
4	Spontaneous	Spontaneous	Spontaneous
3	To speech	To speech	To speech
2	To pain	To pain	To pain
1	No response	No response	No response
Verbal response			
5	Alert and oriented	Oriented, social, speaks, interacts	Coos, babbles
4	Disoriented conversation	Confused speech, disoriented, consolable, aware	Irritable cry
3	Speaking but nonsensical	Inappropriate words, inconsolable, unaware	Cries to pain
2	Moans or unintelligible sounds	Incomprehensible, agitated, restless, unaware	Moans to pain
1	No response	No response	No response
Motor response			
6	Follows commands	Normal, spontaneous movements	Normal, spontaneous movements
5	Localizes pain	Localizes pain	Withdraws to touch
4	Moves or withdraws to pain	Withdraws to pain	Withdraws to pain
3	Decorticate flexion	Decorticate flexion	Decorticate flexion
2	Decerebrate extension	Decerebrate extension	Decerebrate extension
1	No response	No response	No response
3-15			

Note: In intubated patients, the Glasgow Coma Scale verbal component is scored as a 1 and the total score is marked with a "T" (or tube) denoting intubation (eg, 8T).

- Mild TBIs include patients with a GCS score ≥14. Patients may be asymptomatic with only a history of head trauma, or may be confused and amnestic of the event. They may have experienced a brief loss of consciousness and complain of a diffuse headache, nausea, and vomiting. Patients at high risk in this subgroup include those with a skull fracture, large subgaleal swelling, focal neurologic findings, coagulopathy, age >60 years, or drug/alcohol intoxication.
- Moderate TBIs include patients with a GCS score of 9 to 13.
- Severe TBI (GCS score <9) mortality approaches 40%. The immediate clinical priority in these patients is to prevent secondary brain injury, identify other life-threatening injuries, and identify treatable neurosurgical conditions.
- Prehospital medical personnel often may provide critical parts of the history, including mechanism and time of injury, presence and length of unconsciousness, initial mental status, seizure activity, vomiting, verbalization, and movement of extremities. For an unresponsive patient, contact family and friends to gather key information, including past medical history, medications (especially anticoagulants), and recent use of alcohol or drugs.
- Clinically important features of the neurologic examination that should be addressed include assessing the mental status and GCS score; pupils for size, reactivity, and anisocoria; cranial nerve function; motor, sensory, and brain stem function; and noting any development of decorticate or decerebrate posturing.
- Infants with TBI demonstrate a global diminished level of responsiveness. Pupillary or facial asymmetry, extremity motor function abnormality, or a decreased sucking reflex may be found. Signs of increased intracranial pressure in infants include decreased arousal, lethargy, seizure, vomiting, apnea, and bradycardia.
- Signs or symptoms of TBI in the older child include headache, nausea, vomiting, diminished level of consciousness, motor weakness, visual changes, hypertension, bradycardia, and respiratory arrest.

SPECIFIC INJURIES

Skull Fractures

- Depressed skull fractures are classified as open or closed, depending on the integrity of the overlying scalp.
- Although basilar skull fractures can occur at any point in the base of the skull, the typical location is in the petrous portion of the temporal bone. Findings associated with a basilar skull fracture include

hemotympanum, cerebrospinal fluid (CSF) otorrhea or rhinorrhea, periorbital ecchymosis ("raccoon eyes"), and retroauricular ecchymosis (Battle's sign).
- In children, linear skull fractures that result from a fall from a small height (<4 ft) generally are not associated with the development of clinically significant intracranial lesions. Significant intracranial injuries in children often occur after falls from more extreme heights or higher impact collisions.

Cerebral Contusion and Intracerebral Hemorrhage

- Common locations for contusions are the frontal poles, the subfrontal cortex, and the temporal lobes.
- Contusions may occur directly under the site of impact or on the contralateral side (contrecoup lesion). The contused area is usually hemorrhagic with surrounding edema, and occasionally associated with subarachnoid hemorrhage.
- Neurologic dysfunction may be profound and prolonged, with patients demonstrating mental confusion, obtundation, or coma. Focal neurologic deficits are usually present.

Traumatic Subarachnoid Hemorrhage

- This condition results from the disruption of subarachnoid vessels and presents with blood in the CSF. Patients may complain of diffuse headache, nausea, or photophobia.
- Traumatic subarachnoid hemorrhage may be the most common CT abnormality in patients with moderate or severe TBI. Some cases may be missed if the CT scan is obtained less than 6 hours after injury.

Epidural Hematoma

- An epidural hematoma results from an acute collection of blood between the inner table of the skull and the dura mater. It is typically associated with a skull fracture that lacerates a meningeal artery, most commonly the middle meningeal artery.
- Underlying injury to the brain may not necessarily be severe.
- In the classic scenario, the patient experiences loss of consciousness after a head injury. The patient may present to the ED with clear mentation, signifying the "lucid interval," and then begin to develop mental status deterioration in the ED. A fixed and dilated pupil on the side of the lesion with contralateral hemiparesis is a classic late finding.
- The high-pressure arterial bleeding of an epidural hematoma can lead to herniation within hours of injury.
- An epidural hematoma appears biconvex on CT scan.

Subdural Hematoma

- A subdural hematoma (SDH), which is a collection of venous blood between the dura mater and the arachnoid, results from tears of the bridging veins that extend from the subarachnoid space to the dural venous sinuses.
- A common mechanism is sudden acceleration–deceleration. Patients with brain atrophy, such as in alcoholics or the elderly, are more susceptible to an SDH.
- In infants, SDH is strongly associated with nonaccidental trauma. In acute SDH, patients present within 14 days of the injury, and most become symptomatic within 24 hours of injury.
- After 2 weeks, patients are defined as having a chronic SDH.
- Symptoms may range from a headache to lethargy or coma. It is important to distinguish between acute and chronic SDHs by history, physical examination, and CT scan.
- An acute SDH appears as a hyperdense, crescent-shaped lesion that crosses suture lines.

Herniation

- Diffusely or focally increased ICP can result in herniation of the brain at several locations.
- Transtentorial (uncal) herniation occurs when an SDH or temporal lobe mass forces the ipsilateral uncus of the temporal lobe through the tentorial hiatus into the space between the cerebral peduncle and the tentorium. This results in compression of the oculomotor nerve and parasympathetic paralysis of the ipsilateral pupil, causing it to become fixed and dilated. When the cerebral peduncle is further compressed, it results in contralateral motor paralysis. The increased ICP and brain stem compression result in progressive deterioration in the level of consciousness. Occasionally, the contralateral cerebral peduncle is forced against the free edge of the tentorium on the opposite side, resulting in paralysis ipsilateral to the lesion—a false localizing sign.
- Central transtentorial herniation occurs with midline lesions in the frontal or occipital lobes, or in the vertex. Bilateral pinpoint pupils, bilateral Babinski signs, and increased muscle tone are found initially, which eventually develop into fixed midpoint pupils, prolonged hyperventilation, and decorticate posturing.
- Cerebellotonsillar herniation through the foramen magnum occurs much less frequently. Medullary compression causes flaccid paralysis, bradycardia, respiratory arrest, and sudden death.

Penetrating Injuries

- Gunshot wounds and penetrating sharp objects can result in penetrating injury to the brain. The degree of neurologic injury will depend on the energy of the missile, whether the trajectory involves a single or multiple lobes or hemispheres of the brain, the amount of scatter of bone and metallic fragments, and whether a mass lesion is present.

Shaken Baby Syndrome

- This potential life-threatening head injury in children <2 years is caused by rapid acceleration and rotation of the head. Shearing injuries of the brain or intracranial vessels and cervical spine injuries may result. Almost half of children found with this syndrome exhibit no external signs of trauma, so clinical vigilance must remain high.

DIAGNOSIS AND DIFFERENTIAL

- Tables 162-2 and 162-3 provide evidence-based indications for obtaining a CT scan of the head after injury.
- Approximately 8% of patients suffering a severe TBI will have an associated cervical spine fracture. Obtain imaging studies of the cervical spine on all trauma patients who present with altered mental status, neck pain, intoxication, neurologic deficit, or severe distracting injury, or if the mechanism of injury is deemed serious enough to potentially produce cervical spine injury.
- Laboratory work should include type and crossmatching, complete blood count, basic metabolic panel, arterial blood gas analysis, directed toxicologic studies, and coagulation studies.

TABLE 162-2 New Orleans and Canadian CT Clinical Decision Rules

NEW ORLEANS CRITERIA—GCS 15*	CANADIAN CT HEAD RULE—GCS 13-15*
Headache	GCS <15 at 2 h
Vomiting	Suspected open or depressed skull fracture
Age >60 y	Any sign of basal skull fracture
Intoxication	More than one episode of vomiting
Persistent antegrade amnesia	Retrograde amnesia >30 min
Evidence of trauma above the clavicles	Dangerous mechanism (fall >3 ft or struck as pedestrian)
Seizure	Age ≥65 y
Identification of patients who have an intracranial lesion on CT	
100% sensitive, 5% specific	83% sensitive, 38% specific
Identification of patients who will need neurosurgical intervention	
100% sensitive, 5% specific	100% sensitive, 37% specific

Abbreviation: GCS = Glasgow Coma Scale.
*Presence of any one finding indicates need for CT scan.

TABLE 162-3 Summary of Indications for CT Scanning for Adults with Mild Traumatic Brain Injury (TBI)

Mild TBI even if no loss of consciousness if one or more of the following is present:
Glasgow Coma Scale score <15
Focal neurologic findings
Vomiting more than two times
Moderate to severe headache
Age >65 y
Physical signs of basilar skull fracture
Coagulopathy
Dangerous mechanism of injury (eg, fall >4 ft)
Mild TBI with loss of consciousness or amnesia if one or more of the following is present:
Drug or alcohol intoxication
Physical evidence above the clavicles
Persistent amnesia
Post-traumatic seizures

EMERGENCY DEPARTMENT CARE AND DISPOSITION

- Initiate standard protocols for evaluation and stabilization of trauma patients. Search carefully for other significant injuries.
- Administer 100% oxygen, and secure cardiac monitoring and two IV lines. For patients with severe TBI, endotracheal intubation (via rapid sequence intubation) to protect the airway and prevent hypoxemia is the top priority. Provide cervical spine immobilization, and use an adequate sedation/induction agent when securing the airway.
- Hypotension is associated with increased mortality rates. Restoration of an adequate blood pressure is vital to maintain cerebral perfusion. Resuscitation with IV crystalloid fluid to an MAP ≥80 mm Hg is indicated; if aggressive fluid resuscitation is not effective, then add vasopressors to maintain an MAP ≥80 mm Hg.
- Obtain immediate neurosurgical consultation after a head CT scan demonstrating intracranial injury has

been identified. Patients with new neurologic deficits from an acute epidural or SDH require emergent neurosurgical treatment.

- All patients who demonstrate signs of increased ICP should have the head of their bed elevated 30 degrees (provided that the patient is not hypotensive), adequate sedation, and maintenance of adequate arterial oxygenation. If the patient is not hypotensive, consider administering mannitol, 0.25 to 1.0 gram/kg IV bolus.
- Hyperventilation is not recommended as a prophylactic intervention to lower ICP because of its potential to cause cerebral ischemia. Reserve hyperventilation as a last resort for lowering ICP; if used, implement it as a temporary measure and monitor the P_{CO_2} closely to maintain a range of 30 to 35 mm Hg.
- Patients with signs of impending brain herniation may need emergency decompression by trephination ("burr holes") when all other methods to control the elevated ICP have failed. CT scan prior to attempting trephination is recommended to localize the lesion and direct the decompression site.
- Treat seizures immediately with benzodiazepines, such as lorazepam, and fosphenytoin at a loading dose of 18 to 20 milligrams PE/kg IV.
- Use of prophylactic anticonvulsants remains controversial, and its administration should be in consultation with the neurosurgeon.
- Admit patients with a basilar skull fracture or penetrating injuries (gunshot wound or stab wound) to the neurosurgical service, and start them on prophylactic antibiotic therapy (eg, ceftriaxone 1 gram every 12 hours).
- Discharge patients who have an initial GCS score of 15 that is maintained during an observation period and who have normal serial neurologic examinations and a normal CT scan.
- Those who have an abnormal CT scan require neurosurgical consultation and admission.
- Patients who have an initial GCS score of 14 and a normal CT scan should be observed in the ED. If their GCS score improves to 15 and they remain symptom free and neurologically intact after serial examinations, they can be discharged home.
- Discharge patients home with a reliable companion who can observe them for at least 24 hours, carry out appropriate discharge instructions, and follow the head injury sheet instructions.

For further reading in Tintinalli's *Emergency Medicine: A Comprehensive Study Guide*, 7th ed., see Chapter 254, "Head Trauma in Adults and Children," by David W. Wright and Lisa H. Merck.

163 SPINE AND SPINAL CORD TRAUMA

Todd Ellingson

EPIDEMIOLOGY

- The incidence of spinal cord injuries (SCIs) has been estimated at 40 cases per million population at risk. The mean age is 40 years with a male-to-female predominance of 4 to 1.
- Forty-two percent of SCIs are related to motor vehicle crashes, 27% to falls, and 15% to acts of violence.

PATHOPHYSIOLOGY

- Three main vertebral columns provide stability to the spine.
- The anterior column is made up of the anterior wall of the vertebral body, the anterior annulus, and the anterior longitudinal ligament.
- The middle column consists of the posterior wall of the vertebral body, the posterior annulus fibrosus, and the posterior longitudinal ligament.
- The posterior column includes the bony complex of the posterior vertebral arch and the posterior ligamentous complex.
- For a vertebral injury to be considered unstable, disruption of two or more of these columns must be present.
- While >25% compression from the third to seventh cervical vertebrae is considered unstable, the same status for the thoracic and lumbar vertebrae occurs with >50% compression.
- Damage to the spinal cord results in two phases of injury. Initially, a direct mechanical injury may result in hemorrhage, edema, and ischemia. Within hours, a secondary tissue degeneration phase begins with release of membrane-destabilizing enzymes and inflammatory mediators, which induces lipid peroxidation and hydrolysis.
- There are three main spinal cord tracts. The corticospinal tract fibers decussate in the lower medulla and descend through the lateral aspect of the spinal cord. Damage to the corticospinal tract (upper motor neurons) results in ipsilateral muscle weakness, spasticity, increased deep tendon reflexes, and Babinski's sign.
- The spinothalamic tracts transmit pain and temperature sensation and decussate shortly after entering the vertebral column. Injury to the spinothalamic tract causes contralateral loss of pain and temperature sensation.

- The dorsal (or posterior) columns transmit vibration and proprioception sensation. The neurons in this tract do not synapse until they reach the medulla, where they then decussate. Injury to a dorsal column will cause ipsilateral loss of vibration and proprioception sensation.
- Light touch is transmitted through both the spinothalamic and dorsal tracts. Light touch is not lost unless there is damage to both of these tracts.

CLINICAL FEATURES

- Not all patients with SCI have neurologic deficits on initial presentation. Many unstable spinal fractures may present without spinal cord or nerve root trauma.
- Symptomatic patients may complain of paresthesias, dysesthesias, weakness, or other sensory disturbances with or without specific physical examination findings. More severely injured patients may have an obvious neurologic deficit on physical examination.
- Spinal cord injuries or lesions are considered incomplete if sensory, motor, or both are partially present below the neurologic level of injury. Complete lesions include total absence of both below the injury.
- Incomplete lesions have some level of recovery, while complete lesions have minimal chance of recovery.
- Spinal shock is the temporary loss or depression of spinal reflex activity below a complete or incomplete injury. It may cause incomplete injuries to appear complete and may persist for days to weeks.
- Patients may present with neurogenic shock, in which hypotension and relative bradycardia are commonly seen due to loss of sympathetic tone.
- Hypovolemic shock must be considered the cause of the hypotension until proven otherwise. Patients with neurogenic shock generally have pink, warm extremities, and adequate urine output.

DIAGNOSIS AND DIFFERENTIAL

- The mechanism of injury is helpful in predicting the potential type of cervical injury along with its subsequent stability (Table 163-1).
- Any neurologic complaints, even if transitory, must raise suspicion for an SCI. Palpation of the entire spine will identify any potential areas of injury.
- A complete neurologic examination should include motor strength and tone (corticospinal tract), pain and temperature sensation (spinothalamic tract), proprioception and vibration sensation (dorsal columns), and reflexes. Each sensory dermatome should be evaluated (Fig. 163-1).

TABLE 163-1 Cervical Spine Injuries

Flexion
Anterior subluxation (hyperflexion sprain) (stable)*
Bilateral interfacetal dislocation (unstable)
Simple wedge (compression) fracture (usually stable)
Spinous process avulsion (clay-shoveler's) fracture (stable)
Flexion teardrop fracture (unstable)
Flexion-rotation
Unilateral interfacetal dislocation (stable)
Pillar fracture
Fracture of lateral mass (can be unstable)
Vertical compression
Jefferson burst fracture of atlas (potentially unstable)
Burst (bursting, dispersion, axial-loading) fracture (unstable)
Hyperextension
Hyperextension dislocation (unstable)
Avulsion fracture of anterior arch of atlas (stable)
Extension teardrop fracture (unstable)
Fracture of posterior arch of atlas (stable)
Laminar fracture (usually stable)
Traumatic spondylolisthesis (hangman's fracture) (unstable)
Lateral flexion
Uncinate process fracture (usually stable)
Injuries caused by diverse or poorly understood mechanisms
Occipital condyle fractures (can be unstable)
Occipitoatlantal dissociation (highly unstable)
Dens fractures (type II and III are unstable)

*Usual occurrence. Overall stability is dependent on integrity of the other ligamentous structures.

- Incomplete injuries or lesions of the spinal cord with different involvment of these tracts result in various spinal cord syndromes (Table 163-2).
- Preserved anogenital reflexes, such as bulbocavernosius reflex, the cremaster reflex, and contraction of anal musculature ("anal wink"), denote an incomplete spinal cord lesion.
- NEXUS criteria and Canadian Cervical Spine Rule for Radiograpy both seek to identify "low-risk" patients not requiring cervical spine imaging (Table 163-3 and Table 163-4).
- CT is more sensitive and specific than plain radiography for cervical spine trauma and has become the current trend in most trauma centers for initial imaging.
- For the cervical spine plain radiography, a minimum of three views (lateral, odontoid, and anteroposterior) are necessary.

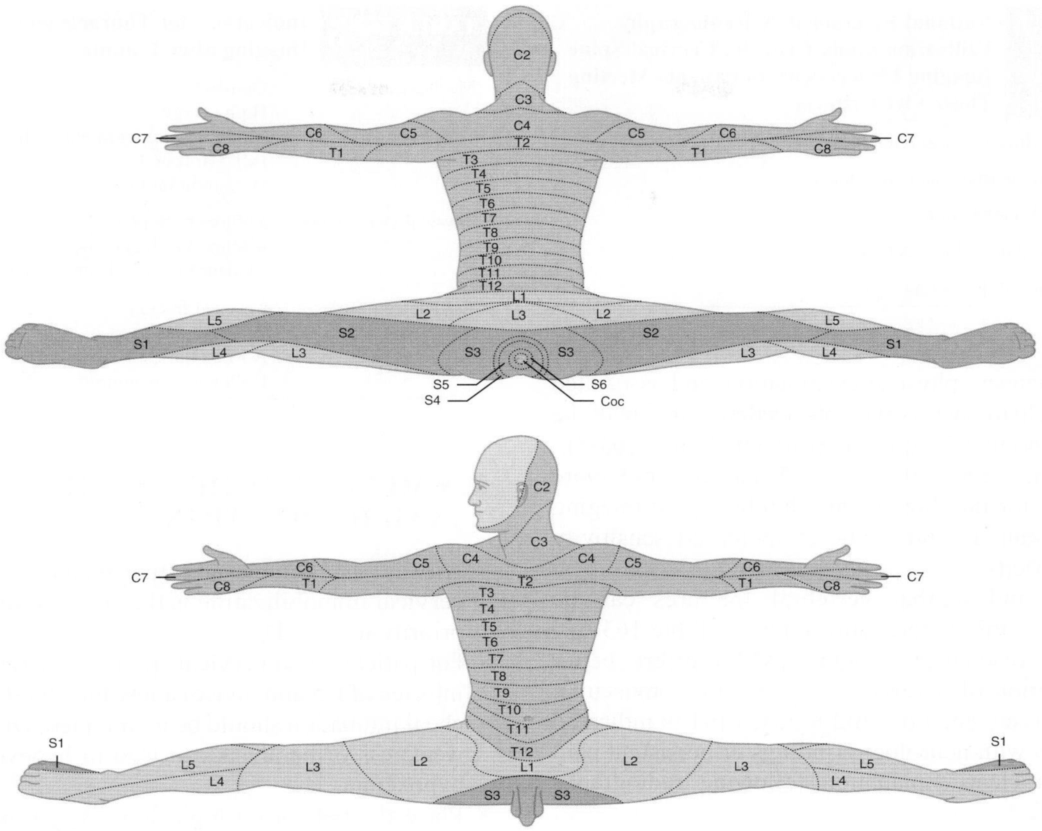

FIG. 163-1. Dermatomes for sensory examination.

- Since occult fractures and ligamentous injuries may be missed on plain radiographs, clinical clearance of the cervical spine must be performed after a negative cervical spine series on alert and oriented patients without distracting injuries.
- Flexion and extension views may reveal ligamentous injury in a patient who cannot be clinically cleared. A step-off of 3.7 mm or an angulation of greater than 11 degrees indicates cervical instability. Patients with persistent pain, including those with normal flexion/extension radiographs, can then be placed in a hard collar to follow up with a spine specialist in 3 to 5 days.
- Ten percent of patients with spine fracture in one segment will have a second fracture in another. Therefore, determination of spinal column injury at one level mandates radiographic evaluation of the entire spine.

TABLE 163-2 Incomplete Spinal Cord Syndromes

SYNDROME	ETIOLOGY	SYMPTOMS	PROGNOSIS*
Anterior cord	Direct anterior cord compression Flexion of cervical spine Thrombosis of anterior spinal artery	Complete paralysis below the lesion with loss of pain and temperature sensation Preservation of proprioception and vibratory function	Poor
Central cord	Hyperextension injuries Disruption of blood flow to the spinal cord Cervical spinal stenosis	Quadriparesis—greater in the upper extremities than the lower extremities. Some loss of pain and temperature sensation, also greater in the upper extremities	Good
Brown-Séquard	Transverse hemisection of the spinal cord Unilateral cord compression	Ipsilateral spastic paresis, loss of proprioception and vibratory sensation, and contralateral loss of pain and temperature sensation	Good
Cauda equina	Peripheral nerve injury	Variable motor and sensory loss in the lower extremities, sciatica, bowel/bladder dysfunction, and "saddle anesthesia"	Good

*Outcome improves when the effects of secondary injury are prevented or reversed.

TABLE 163-3	National Emergency X-Radiography Utilization Study Criteria: Cervical Spine Imaging Unnecessary in Patients Meeting These Five Criteria
Absence of midline cervical tenderness	
Normal level of alertness and consciousness	
No evidence of intoxication	
Absence of focal neurologic deficit	
Absence of painful distracting injury	

- The mechanism, physical examination, and associated injuries help to identify patients needing imaging of the thoracic and lumbar spine after trauma (Table 163-5).
- As with the cervical spine, CT has become more important for the thoracic and lumbar spine imaging at most trauma centers due to increased sensitivity and specificity.
- Thoracic and lumbar vertebral fractures can be divided into minor and major injuries (Table 163-6).
- Magnetic resonance imaging (MRI) offers better determination of neurologic, ligamentous, muscular, and soft tissue anatomy and injury. MRI is indicated in patients with neurologic findings or persistent pain without a clear explanation following radiographs and/or CT.
- Spinal cord injury without radiographic abnormality (SCIWORA) is an entity that is most commonly seen in the pediatric population.

TABLE 163-4 Canadian Cervical Spine Rule for Radiography: Cervical Spine Imaging Unnecessary in Patients Meeting These Three Criteria

QUESTION OR ASSESSMENT	DEFINITIONS
There are no high-risk factors that mandate radiography.	High-risk factors include: Age 65 years or older A dangerous mechanism of injury (fall from a height of >3 ft; an axial loading injury; high-speed motor vehicle crash, rollover, or ejection; motorized recreational vehicle or bicycle collision) The presence of paresthesias in the extremities
There are low-risk factors that allow a safe assessment of range of motion.	Low-risk factors include: Simple rear-end motor vehicle crashes Patient able to sit up in the ED Patient ambulatory at any time Delayed onset of neck pain Absence of midline cervical tenderness
The patient is able to actively rotate his/her neck.	Can rotate 45 degrees to the left and to the right

TABLE 163-5 Indications for Thoracic and Lumbar Imaging after Trauma

Mechanism	Gunshot High energy Motor vehicle crash with rollover or ejection Fall >10 ft or 3 m Pedestrian hit by car
Physical examination	Midline back pain Midline focal tenderness Evidence of spinal cord or nerve root deficit
Associated injuries	Cervical fracture Rib fractures Aortic injuries Hollow viscus injuries

EMERGENCY DEPARTMENT CARE AND DISPOSITION

- Airway assessment and management with in-line cervical immobilization is the first and most pressing priority in the ED.
- For patients with cervical spine injury (especially for injuries of C5 and above) a low threshold for endotracheal intubation should be maintained. Diaphragmatic weakness or paralysis can lead to hypoventilation or hypoxemia.
- Place the patient on high-flow oxygen and establish two large-bore IVs.
- Fluid resuscitation facilitates spinal cord resuscitation; control obvious bleeding and rapidly assess other life-threatening injuries.
- While maintaining in-line spinal immobilization that prevents secondary injury to the spine and preserves residual spinal cord function, logroll the patient to identify any obvious fractures or associated injuries.
- Remove the patient off of a hard backboard in order to prevent skin breakdown and pressure sores. Standard hospital mattresses provide adequate spinal support.
- Treat neurogenic shock with oxygen, IV fluids, and positive inotropic pressors as necessary.
- The use of methylprednisolone remains an option for blunt spinal cord trauma with neurologic deficits; however, the current evidence suggesting harmful

TABLE 163-6 Thoracic and Lumbar Spine Fractures

MINOR INJURIES	MAJOR INJURIES
Transverse process fracture	Compression (wedge) fractures
Spinous process fracture	Burst fractures
Pars interarticularis fractures	Flexion-distraction ("seat-belt") injuries
	Fracture-dislocation (translation) injuries

TABLE 163-7 The National Acute Spinal Cord Injury Study Protocol

Indications	Blunt trauma Neurologic deficit referable to the spinal cord Treatment can be started within 8 h of injury
Treatment	Methylprednisolone, 30 milligrams/kg bolus, is administered IV over 15 min Followed by a 45-min pause Methylprednisolone, 5.4 milligrams/kg/h, is then infused for 23 h

side effects of the medication may outweigh potential benefit. Consultation with a spinal surgeon prior to administration is recommended. Indications for use and administration guidelines can be found in Table 163-7.

- Methylprednisolone therapy has not been proven to be beneficial in penetrating spinal cord injury.
- Patients with penetrating spinal injuries should receive empiric antibiotics in the ED.
- Patients with progressive neurologic deterioration require operative intervention. Most injuries that do not progress are treated nonoperatively.
- Admit any patient with a significant injury to the spine or spinal cord to the hospital.

For further reading in Tintinalli's *Emergency Medicine: A Comprehensive Study Guide*, 7th ed., see Chapter 255, "Spine and Spinal Cord Trauma," by Bonny J. Baron, Kevin J. McSherry, James L. Larson, Jr., and Thomas M. Scalea.

164 TRAUMA TO THE FACE

Jonathan S. Ilgen

CLINICAL FEATURES

- After maxillofacial trauma has been identified during the primary survey, the clinician should first consider the potential need for endotracheal intubation, as mechanical disruption or massive hemorrhage can rapidly lead to airway compromise. Severe facial injuries are associated with injuries to the brain, orbits, cervical spine, and lungs.
- Table 164-1 lists the important history and physical examination issues in facial trauma.

TABLE 164-1 Important Clinical Issues in Facial Trauma

History
How is your vision? Do any parts of your face feel numb? Does your bite feel normal?
Inspection
Lateral view for dish face with Le Fort III fractures. Frontal view for donkey face with Le Fort II or III fractures. Bird's eye view for exophthalmos with retrobulbar hematoma. Worm's view for endophthalmos with blow-out fractures or flattening of malar prominence with zygomatic arch fractures. Raccoon eyes (bilateral orbital ecchymosis) and Battle's sign (mastoid ecchymosis) typically develop over several hours, suggesting basilar skull fracture.
Palpation
Palpating the entire face will detect the majority of fractures. Intraoral palpation of the zygomatic arch, palpating lateral to posterior maxillary molars to distinguish bony from soft tissue injury. Assess for Le Fort fractures by gently rocking the hard palate with one hand while stabilizing the forehead with the other.
Eye
Examine early before swelling of lids, or use retractors. Document visual acuity. Systematically examine the eye from front to back. Specifically, the pupil for teardrop sign pointing to globe rupture, hyphema, and swinging flashlight test for afferent papillary defect. Fat through eyelid wound indicates septal perforation. Check intraocular pressure for evidence of orbital compartment syndrome only in absence of globe injury.
Nose
Crepitus over any facial sinus suggests sinus fracture. Septal hematoma appears as blue, boggy swelling on nasal septum.
Ears
Examine for: Auricular hematoma. Cerebrospinal fluid leak. Hemotympanum.
Oral
Jaw deviation due to mandible dislocation or condyle fracture. Malocclusion occurs in mandible, zygomatic, and Le Fort fractures. Missing or injured tooth. Lacerations and mucosal ecchymosis suggest mandible fracture. Place finger in external ear while the patient gently opens and closes jaw to detect condyle fractures. Tongue blade test: Patient without fracture can bite down on a tongue blade enough to break blade twisted by examiner.

DIAGNOSIS AND DIFFERENTIAL

- Maxillofacial injuries can be diagnosed clinically as described above and with radiographs.
- Plain radiographs are helpful when computed tomography (CT) is not available or to screen for injuries in low-risk patients.
- Maxillofacial CT is frequently required to make definitive diagnoses and guide surgical management.

EMERGENCY DEPARTMENT CARE AND DISPOSITION

- Focus initial management on airway control. A chin lift or jaw thrust without neck extension often restores airway patency.
- While rapid sequence intubation is the preferred method of airway management in trauma, always plan for a difficult airway in patients with facial injuries. To prevent a "can't intubate, can't oxygenate" scenario, do not administer paralytics unless a patient can be hand ventilated effectively or alternative airway plans (such as airway adjuncts or cricothyroidotomy) are in place.
- Awake intubation with sedation and local airway anesthesia may allow the emergency physician to assess the feasibility of orotracheal intubation while preserving the patient's airway reflexes.
- When endotracheal intubation is required, the oral route is preferred because of concern for nasocranial intubation or severe epistaxis with nasotracheal intubation.
- In severe mandible fractures, loss of bony support may result in posterior displacement of the tongue. To prevent airway obstruction, pull the tongue forward with a gauze pad, towel clips, or a suture passed through the tip.
- Hemorrhage may be controlled with direct pressure. Avoid blind clamping because of the risk of damaging the facial nerve or parotid duct.
- Reduction of significantly displaced nasal fractures and Le Fort injuries is rarely needed to stop arterial bleeding. If bleeding persists, either operative ligation or arterial embolization may be necessary.
- Severe epistaxis requires direct pressure or nasal packing. Posterior epistaxis can be controlled with nasal tampons, dual balloon devices, or Foley catheter placement, again being careful to avoid intracranial placement in the setting of severe midface fractures.
- All patients with sinus fractures should receive oral or intravenous antibiotics, such as second-generation cephalosporins, clindamycin, or amoxicillin-clavulanate.
- Frontal sinus fractures are uncommon and increase the immediate risk of traumatic brain injury, additional facial fractures, and cervical spine injury. Fractures that involve both the anterior and posterior tables for the frontal sinus require operative intervention to prevent pneumocephalus, cerebrospinal fluid (CSF) leak, and infection. Depressed fractures also require operative repair.
- Patients with isolated fractures of the anterior wall of the frontal sinus may be treated on an outpatient basis.
- Naso-orbito-ethmoid fractures often have associated injury to the lacrimal duct, dural tears, and traumatic brain injury. These fractures require consultation with facial surgery and neurosurgery.
- Blowout fractures are the most common orbital fracture and occur when a blunt object strikes the globe, fracturing the medial or inferior orbital wall. Suggestive physical examination findings include enophthalmos, infraorbital anesthesia, diplopia on upward gaze, and a step-off deformity on palpation of the infraorbital rim.
- The oculomotor and ophthalmic divisions of the trigeminal nerve course through the superior orbital fissure. An orbital fracture involving this canal leads to the superior orbital fissure syndrome, characterized by paralysis of extraocular motions, ptosis, and periorbital anesthesia. When the orbital apex is involved, the patient may develop these symptoms and blindness. The swinging light test and visual acuity determination are crucial in making this diagnosis.
- Orbital blowout fractures require surgery if they result in extraocular muscle or oculomotor nerve entrapment, or significant enophthalmos. Patients with superior orbital fissure syndrome or orbital apex injuries also require emergent ophthalmologic consultation. The remainder of isolated orbital fractures can be managed on an outpatient basis with oral antibiotics, decongestants, and instructions to avoid nose blowing until the defect has healed or has been repaired.
- Zygoma fractures occur in two major patterns: tripod fractures and isolated zygomatic arch fractures.
- Tripod fractures cause disruption of the infraorbital rim, diastasis of the zygomaticofrontal suture, and disruption of the zygomaticotemporal junction. These fractures require admission for open reduction and internal fixation.
- Patients with isolated fractures of the zygomatic arch can have elective outpatient repair.
- Midface fractures are high-energy injuries and are often seen in victims of multisystem trauma. Patients frequently require endotracheal intubation for airway control.
- Visual acuity should be tested, especially with Le Fort III fractures, where the incidence of blindness is high.
- Both Le Fort II and III injuries can result in CSF leaks.
- Le Fort injuries require admission for the management of significant associated injuries, IV antibiotics, and surgical repair.
- Mandible fractures are often diagnosed in the setting of malocclusion or pain with attempted movement. A careful intraoral examination is important to exclude small breaks in the mucosa seen with open fractures, sublingual hematomas, and dental or alveolar ridge fractures.

- Patients with open mandible fractures require admission and IV antibiotics.
- Many patients with closed fractures may be managed on an outpatient basis. A Barton bandage—an elastic bandage wrapped around the jaw and head—may be worn for comfort.

For further reading in Tintinalli's *Emergency Medicine: A Comprehensive Study Guide*, 7th ed., see Chapter 256, "Trauma to the Face," by John Bailitz.

165 TRAUMA TO THE NECK

Katrina A. Leone

PATHOPHYSIOLOGY

- The neck contains a high concentration of vascular, aerodigestive, and spinal structures in a relatively confined space.
- The platysma is the most superficial structure beneath the skin. Penetrating injuries that violate the platysma require evaluation for deep structure injuries.
- Beneath the platysma is the deep cervical fascia that creates a series of tight fascial compartments. A tamponade effect within these compartments limits the potential for external bleeding from vascular injuries, but can result in airway compression and compromise.

CLINICAL FEATURES

- All signs and symptoms associated with neck trauma require diagnostic evaluation, but hard signs are more often associated with significant injury than soft signs (Table 165-1).

TABLE 165-1 Signs and Symptoms of Neck Injury

HARD SIGNS	SOFT SIGNS
Hypotension in ED	Hypotension in field
Active arterial bleeding	History of arterial bleeding
Diminished carotid pulse	Unexplained bradycardia (without central nervous system injury)
Expanding hematoma	Nonexpanding large hematoma
Thrill/bruit	Apical capping on chest radiograph
Lateralizing signs	Stridor
Hemothorax >1000 mL	Hoarseness
Air or bubbling in wound	Vocal cord paralysis
Hemoptysis	Subcutaneous emphysema
Hematemesis	Seventh cranial nerve injury
Tracheal deviation	

- Blunt and penetrating laryngeal or pharyngeal trauma can cause dysphonia, stridor, hemoptysis, hematemesis, dysphagia, neck emphysema, and dyspnea progressing to respiratory arrest.
- Patients may present with signs of shock (diaphoresis, tachycardia, and hypotension) after experiencing significant blood loss.
- Neurologic injury demonstrated by subjective complaints of pain and paresthesias, or more objective findings of hemiplegia, quadriplegia, and coma, may be observed.
- Signs of esophageal injury include dysphagia and hematemesis.
- Strangulation is a unique mechanism of blunt neck injury caused by hanging, ligature application, or manual neck compression.
- The clinical presentation of strangulation depends upon the duration and amount of force applied to the neck. Cardiac arrest, cervical spine fractures, cerebral anoxia, arotid artery injuries, and hyoid bone and laryngeal fractures are possible. Increased venous pressure above the location of a ligature causes facial and conjunctival petechial hemorrhages.

DIAGNOSIS AND DIFFERENTIAL

- The Roon and Christensen anatomic classification divides the neck into three zones (Table 165-2).
- At-risk structures located in zone I are the proximal vertebral and carotid arteries, thoracic vessels, superior mediastinum, lungs, esophagus, trachea, thoracic duct, and spinal cord.
- At-risk structures located in zone II are the mid-carotid and vertebral arteries, jugular veins, esophagus, trachea, larynx, and spinal cord.
- At-risk structures located in zone III are the distal carotid and vertebral arteries, pharynx, and spinal cord.
- Plain radiographs of the neck can identify the presence of penetrating foreign bodies, and a chest radiograph is warranted to assess for associated thoracic cavity injuries.
- Helical CT angiography is the most commonly utilized diagnostic study for vascular injuries of the neck. It has a reported sensitivity of 90% to 100% and specificity of 98.6% to 100% for significant carotid and vertebral artery injuries, but is limited in detecting low zone I and high zone III injuries.

TABLE 165-2 Zones of the Neck

Zone I	Clavicles to the cricoid cartilage
Zone II	Cricoid cartilage to the angle of the mandible
Zone III	Angle of the mandible to the base of the skull

- Proximal and distal surgical control of bleeding vessels is also more difficult in zones I and III, so conventional angiography may be preferred with injuries to these areas.
- Blunt and penetrating esophageal injuries are often initially asymptomatic. Delayed diagnosis and treatment results in significant morbidity and mortality from deep space infections and mediastinitis.
- CT is the initial diagnostic study to assess for esophageal injuries, but if this is nondiagnostic or suspicion of injury is high, esophagography and esophagoscopy should be performed. This combination of studies has a sensitivity of detecting injury that is nearly 100%.
- Patients with any symptoms suggestive of laryngotracheal injury require laryngoscopy and bronchoscopy.

EMERGENCY DEPARTMENT CARE AND DISPOSITION

- Initiate standard trauma protocols for evaluation and stabilization of trauma patients. Quickly establish high-flow oxygen, cardiac and respiratory monitoring, and IV access.
- Immobilize and assess the cervical spine, as clinically appropriate.
- Any patient with acute respiratory distress, expanding hematoma on the neck, massive subcutaneous emphysema, tracheal shift, impending respiratory arrest, or severe alteration in mental status requires the establishment of a definitive airway with endotracheal intubation or cricothyrotomy.
- Evaluate the integrity of the larynx before intubation attempts as intubation of a fractured larynx may result in complete transection or creation of a false passage. Tracheostomy may be the best option for airway control in these patients.
- Initiate volume resuscitation with crystalloid followed by blood products as needed.
- Probing of neck wounds in the ED is never indicated; full exploration should occur in the operating room where the capacity for proximal and distal vascular control is optimal.
- Direct pressure can often control active hemorrhage.
- Blind clamping of blood vessels is contraindicated due to the complex vital anatomy compressed into a relatively small space and the danger of causing further injury with a misguided surgical instrument.
- Injuries in proximity to the base of the neck predispose patients to simultaneous injury to the chest. Assess the chest for injuries such as pneumothorax and hemothorax.
- Minor penetrating wounds that do not violate the platysma muscle require standard meticulous wound care and closure. Observe these patients for several hours in the ED. If asymptomatic and hemodynamically stable after 4 to 6 hours, these patients may be discharged home with close follow-up.
- Wounds that violate the platysma muscle mandate surgical consultation. Admit these patients for surgical exploration or diagnostic evaluation for deep structure injury.
- Patients with blunt neck trauma initially may present with subtle signs of injury and may develop significant symptoms on a delayed basis. After a period of observation, asymptomatic patients may be discharged with close follow-up, although a low threshold for admission should be maintained.

For further reading in Tintinalli's *Emergency Medicine: A Comprehensive Study Guide*, 7th ed., see Chapter 257, "Trauma to the Neck," by Bonny J. Baron.

166 CARDIOTHORACIC INJURIES

Ross J. Fleischman

EPIDEMIOLOGY

- Blunt chest trauma accounts for 25% of civilian trauma deaths.

CLINICAL FEATURES

- Follow the Advanced Trauma Life Support primary survey for the initial assessment and management of airway, breathing, circulation, and disability.
- Patients in respiratory distress need endotracheal intubation. Maintaining good oxygenation is especially important in head-injured patients.
- Recognize tension pneumothorax and treat with needle thoracostomy (decompression) during the primary survey without waiting for radiologic confirmation.
- Subclavian venous catheterization should be done on the side of suspected injury if needed.
- In patients with cardiac arrest due to chest trauma, closed chest compressions are generally ineffective and may cause further damage, so it should only be undertaken while preparing for ED thoracotomy. An exception would be the patient whose cardiac arrest might be due to a direct blow to the heart with resulting arrhythmia (commotio cordis).

- Evaluate for tension pneumothorax in any patient who suddenly decompensates while on mechanical ventilation.
- Administer IV crystalloid fluids judiciously to avoid causing pulmonary edema. Consider early administration of blood products for patients needing resuscitation.

CHEST WALL INJURIES

CLINICAL FEATURES AND DIAGNOSIS

- Examine for tracheal deviation, unequal chest rise, unequal breath sounds, and subcutaneous emphysema (suggestive of pneumothorax).
- Flail chest occurs when multiple fractures of a section of ribs allow them to move paradoxically to the motion of breathing.
- Fractures of the first and second ribs require a large force and raise high suspicion for other major injuries.
- Multiple lower rib fractures raise suspicion for hepatic or splenic injuries.
- Up to 50% of simple rib fractures are not seen on chest radiograph. The goal of diagnostic imaging is to exclude other significant thoracic injuries.

EMERGENCY DEPARTMENT CARE AND DISPOSITION

- Assume that patients with subcutaneous emphysema have a pneumothorax even if not seen on chest radiograph. Insert a chest tube prior to endotracheal intubation or aeromedical transport.
- Penetrating wounds should never be probed deeply.
- Mark puncture wound sites with a paper clip prior to chest radiograph.
- Cover open chest wounds with sterile petroleum gauze taped on three sides to allow air to exit but not enter. Place a chest tube at another site and not through the wound.
- Even simple rib fractures may lead to splinting, ventilatory compromise, and pneumonia. Patients being discharged should receive nonsteroidal as well as opioid analgesics. Teach them to breathe deeply and perform incentive spirometry exercises.
- Consider admitting patients with multiple rib fractures, medical comorbidities, or older age until they are stabilized on a regimen of pain control and pulmonary toilet. Intercostal nerve blocks and epidural anesthesia may be considered. Attempts to stabilize the chest wall with tape or binding are not recommended.
- Intubation and positive pressure ventilation will stabilize a flail segment, so patients with respiratory compromise should be intubated, as should those with shock, severe head injury, preexisting pulmonary disease, fracture of eight or more ribs, other associated injuries, and age >65 years. Surgical fixation should be considered.
- Assess patients with sternal fractures for cardiac injury, as described in the section on blunt cardiac trauma.

LUNG INJURIES

CLINICAL FEATURES AND DIAGNOSIS

- Patients with a tension pneumothorax may have dyspnea, tachycardia, hypotension, distended neck veins, and tracheal deviation along with unequal chest rise, percussion, and breath sounds.
- Supine chest radiograph is an insensitive screening tool (52%) for pneumothorax and for hemothoraces of less than 200 mL; up to 1000 mL may appear as only diffuse haziness. Lung collapse from intubation of a mainstem bronchus can have a similar appearance. Upright and expiratory views are more sensitive.
- A small stab wound may develop a delayed pneumothorax. Repeat a chest radiograph after 4 to 6 hours of observation before discharging an asymptomatic patient.
- Ultrasound is very sensitive for detecting pneumothorax and may be useful for diagnosing pneumothorax, hemothorax, cardiac tamponade, and intra-abdominal hemorrhage in a patient with chest trauma. Use a high-frequency linear probe to look for loss of the sliding pleura sign and absence of comet tail artifacts. A hemothorax will show fluid in the dependent portion of the pleural cavity.
- CT is highly sensitive for hemothorax and pneumothorax in the stable patient.
- Pulmonary contusions are direct injuries to the lung parenchyma without laceration. Hypoxia ensues as bruised lung tissue is compromised by bleeding and edema.
- Seventy percent of pulmonary contusions are not visible on initial radiograph, but may appear as patchy opacities over the first 6 hours. Radiographic findings of fat embolism and aspiration pneumonia are similar, but usually appear 12 to 24 hours after injury. CT is more sensitive than radiographs.

EMERGENCY DEPARTMENT CARE AND DISPOSITION

- Recognize and treat tension pneumothorax immediately without waiting for radiographs. Insert a 14-gauge, 4.5-cm over-the-needle catheter in the second intercostal space at the midclavicular line. A rush of air is confirmatory. Leave the catheter in until a chest tube is inserted.

- A small pneumothorax may be treated with observation without a chest tube.
- For larger pneumothoraces without hemopneumothorax, a 24- to 28-F (8.0- to 9.3-mm) chest tube should be inserted. If blood is suspected in the chest, a 32- to 40-F (10.7- to 13.4-mm) tube should be inserted.
- Insert a chest tube in all patients with pneumothorax or presumed pneumothorax (subcutaneous emphysema) who will be intubated or transported by air.
- Treat patients with hemothoraces larger than 200 to 300 mL or with ongoing bleeding with tube thoracostomy. Surgical exploration should be strongly considered for an immediate return of 1000 mL of blood or ongoing bleeding of 150 to 200 mL/h for 2 to 4 hours. A large blood return can be collected in a heparinized autotransfusion device.
- Always confirm chest tube placement with a chest radiograph.
- Initial management of pulmonary contusions includes pain control to prevent hypoventilation, avoidance of unnecessary fluids to prevent pulmonary edema, and pulmonary toilet. Positive pressure ventilation by mask may be used in a patient with normal mental status who requires limited respiratory support.
- Patients with a contusion of greater than 25% of lung tissue will likely require intubation, but should not be intubated obligatorily. If intubated, positive end expiratory pressure should be used.
- Diuretics can be used for pulmonary contusion if the patient is thought to be volume overloaded from excessive IV fluids. Steroids are not recommended. Admit patients to a setting where they can be closely monitored for expected deterioration.

TRACHEOBRONCHIAL INJURIES

CLINICAL FEATURES AND DIAGNOSIS

- Major deceleration injuries can result in injuries to the trachea and large airways, usually within 2 cm of the carina or at the origin of lobar bronchi.
- Signs of tracheobronchial injury include hemoptysis, subcutaneous emphysema in the neck, a crunching sound with the cardiac cycle (Hamman's sign), and a massive continued air leak through a chest tube.
- Mediastinal air, large pneumothorax, and a round appearance of the endotracheal tube balloon on plain radiograph or CT suggest tracheobronchial injuries.

EMERGENCY DEPARTMENT CARE AND DISPOSITION

- Obtain bronchoscopy in a major trauma patient with mediastinal air or other signs of tracheobronchial injury.

DIAPHRAGMATIC INJURIES

CLINICAL FEATURES AND DIAGNOSIS

- All penetrating injuries between the nipples and the umbilicus may injure the diaphragm. Left-sided injuries are more commonly diagnosed because the liver may prevent herniation of abdominal contents into the chest.
- Small lacerations can be asymptomatic and allow herniation of abdominal contents into the chest weeks to months later.
- Auscultate for bowel sounds in the chest.
- The diagnosis is obvious if the chest radiograph reveals abdominal contents or coiling of a gastric tube within the chest.
- A normal chest radiograph, CT, or upper GI series with contrast does not exclude diaphragmatic injury.

EMERGENCY DEPARTMENT CARE AND DISPOSITION

- Laparotomy or laparoscopy remain the gold standards to exclude diaphragmatic injuries.
- All diaphragmatic lacerations require surgical repair.

PENETRATING INJURIES TO THE HEART

CLINICAL FEATURES AND DIAGNOSIS

- Suspect cardiac injury in any patient with penetrating trauma to the "cardiac box" bordered by the clavicles, xiphoid process, and nipples.
- The right ventricle is the most commonly injured portion of the heart.
- Accumulation of blood in the pericardium compresses the heart, preventing filling during diastole. Beck's triad of hypotension, distended neck veins, and muffled heart tones may be seen. The diagnosis of cardiac tamponade is confirmed by bedside ultrasound.

EMERGENCY DEPARTMENT CARE AND DISPOSITION

- Cardiac tamponade can be temporized in the ED by pericardiocentesis prior to definitive operative management. Pericardiocentesis is technically difficult and may result in further injury; therefore, it should only be attempted for a patient in shock with confirmed cardiac tamponade. Stable patients should have a pericardial window or thoracotomy in the operating room.
- Patients in shock who do not respond to adequate fluid resuscitation and who are suspected of having a cardiac injury should undergo emergent thoracotomy.

- Patients with penetrating injuries who showed signs of life in the field but subsequently became pulseless may be candidates for ED thoracotomy. ED thoracotomy is a high-risk procedure for bloodborne pathogen exposure to staff. Potential interventions include open cardiac massage, relieving cardiac tamponade, cross-clamping the descending aorta, or repairing a myocardial laceration with staples or sutures.

BLUNT INJURIES TO THE HEART

CLINICAL FEATURES AND DIAGNOSIS

- Blunt cardiac injury can lead to death from damage to cardiac structures, coronary artery injury and thrombosis, and contusion of the myocardium resulting in impaired contractility and arrhythmias.
- A patient with cardiac injury may present with chest pain, tachycardia unexplained by hemorrhage, or arrhythmias.
- If a patient with myocardial rupture survives to ED arrival, a "splashing mill wheel" murmur may be heard. The diagnosis is confirmed by echocardiogram and treated surgically.
- ECG changes consistent with ischemia suggest coronary artery dissection or thrombosis, which are evaluated and treated by cardiac catheterization and stenting. A direct blow to the chest such as when a young athlete is struck by a hard ball can induce ventricular fibrillation cardiac arrest even without myocardial injury (commotio cordis).

EMERGENCY DEPARTMENT CARE AND DISPOSITION

- Antiarrhythmic and inotropic medications should be administered, according to Advanced Cardiac Life Support algorithms.
- Bedside echocardiogram by the emergency provider should be performed as a first screen for cardiac tamponade and grossly impaired contractility.
- Patients with hypotension not explained by another cause, arrhythmias, and impaired contractility should undergo further evaluation by formal echocardiography and cardiac enzymes. Transesophageal echocardiogram is three times more sensitive than transthoracic echo for blunt myocardial injury.
- A normal initial echocardiogram does not rule out subsequent development of complications.
- Admit patients with arrhythmias, abnormal ECG, or cardiac markers for serial cardiac enzymes and ECGs.
- Admit patients with an abnormal initial ECG but no other findings of myocardial injury to a monitored setting.
- Patients with normal vital signs, normal ECG, no underlying cardiac disease, and age under 55 years may be discharged home after 4 to 6 hours of normal cardiac monitoring.

PERICARDIAL INFLAMMATION SYNDROME

- Patients may develop chest pain, fever, and a friction rub 2 to 4 weeks after cardiac trauma or surgery. ECG may show the diffuse ST-segment elevation of pericarditis. Pericardial and pleural effusions may be seen on echocardiography and chest radiograph.
- Treat with nonsteroidal anti-inflammatory medications, such as indomethacin 25 to 50 milligrams by mouth every 6 hours.

TRAUMA TO THE GREAT VESSELS

CLINICAL FEATURES AND DIAGNOSIS

- Injury to the great vessels may be caused by penetrating trauma or rapid deceleration injury.
- Trauma to the major thoracic vessels is usually lethal, with 90% of those sustaining blunt aortic injury dying at the scene.
- The most common site of blunt aortic injury is between the left subclavian artery and the ligamentum arteriosum. Injury to the subclavian and innominate arteries can be related to shoulder belts and fractures of the first and second ribs and proximal clavicle and can cause a unilateral radial pulse deficit.
- Assess patients for subtle findings, including unequal bilateral blood pressures, diminished lower extremity pulses, chest bruits, and new murmurs.
- Descending aortic injuries may cause paraplegia, mesenteric ischemia, anuria, and lower extremity ischemia if they affect flow to the relevant arteries.
- Table 166-1 lists radiographic findings of great vessel injury. Chest radiograph has poor sensitivity for injury to the great vessels.
- All stable patients with a mechanism concerning for great vessel injury should undergo CT angiogram with IV contrast. Conventional aortography may be used to assess injuries and guide operative planning.
- Transesophageal echocardiogram is highly sensitive for aortic intimal lesions and can be done at the bedside of an unstable patient. It is contraindicated in airway compromise or suspected cervical spine injury.
- With gunshot wounds, a discrepancy between the number of presumed entrance and exit wounds and bullets seen on imaging should make the provider consider entry into a vessel with embolization to another part of the body. Fuzzy appearance of a projectile on radiograph suggests an intravascular missile vibrating with blood flow.

TABLE 166-1 Radiographic Findings Suggestive of a Great Vessel Injury

Fractures	
	Sternum
	Scapula
	Multiple ribs
	Clavicle in multisystem-injured patients
	First rib
Mediastinal clues	
	Obliteration of the aortic knob contour
	Widening of the mediastinum
	Depression of the left mainstem bronchus >140 degrees from trachea
	Loss of paravertebral pleural stripe
	Calcium layering at aortic knob
	Abnormal general appearance of mediastinum
	Deviation of nasogastric tube to the right at T4
	Lateral displacement of the trachea
Lateral chest x-ray	
	Anterior displacement of the trachea
	Loss of the aortic/pulmonary window
Other findings	
	Apical pleural hematoma (cap)
	Massive left hemothorax
	Obvious diaphragmatic injury

EMERGENCY DEPARTMENT CARE AND DISPOSITION

- A patient with no signs of life in the field requires no further resuscitative efforts. If the patient lost vital signs immediately prior to hospital arrival, then consider ED thoracotomy.
- Patients with severe shock, radiographic evidence of a rapidly expanding hematoma, or large chest tube output should have emergent surgery or intravascular stenting.
- Patients with multiple injuries, advanced age, or uncontrolled medical comorbidities may require stabilization before delayed repair.
- Administer narcotic pain medications and sedatives to control hypertension in order to decrease shear stress on the vessel wall.
- A short-acting beta-blocker, such as esmolol 50 to 300 micrograms/kg/min, may be titrated to a systolic blood pressure of 100 to 120 mm Hg and a heart rate above 60 beats/min. If bradycardia prevents further dosing of a beta-blocker, an arterial dilator such as sodium nitroprusside 0.25 to 10 micrograms/kg/min IV may be infused.

ESOPHAGEAL AND THORACIC DUCT INJURIES

CLINICAL FEATURES AND DIAGNOSIS

- Penetrating, and occasionally blunt, trauma may cause injury to the thoracic esophagus.
- If suspected, evaluate the patient by esophagram with water-soluble contrast. While water-soluble contrast is less likely to cause mediastinitis, a negative study should be followed by the use of barium contrast, which has a higher sensitivity for injury.
- Flexible esophagoscopy is an alternative modality.
- Injuries to the area of the left proximal subclavian vein may result in chylothorax, which usually is discovered as a delayed right-sided pleural effusion.

EMERGENCY DEPARTMENT CARE AND DISPOSITION

- Esophageal injuries require emergent surgical repair in order to prevent mediastinitis.
- Initial treatment of chylothorax is with chest tube drainage and observation.

For further reading in Tintinalli's *Emergency Medicine: A Comprehensive Study Guide*, 7th ed., see Chapter 258, "Pulmonary Trauma," by Patrick H. Brunett, Lalena M. Yarris, and Arif Alper Cevik, and Chapter 259, "Cardiac Trauma," by Christopher Ross and Theresa M. Schwab.

167 ABDOMINAL TRAUMA

O. John Ma

EPIDEMIOLOGY

- The most common mechanism of blunt abdominal trauma in the United States is a motor vehicle crash.

PATHOPHYSIOLOGY

- The injury pattern of blunt abdominal trauma is often diffuse. Blunt injuries involve a compression or crushing mechanism by direct energy transmission. If the compressive, sheering, or stretching forces exceed the tolerance limits of the organ tissue, then tissue disruption occurs.

- Injury also can result from movement of organs within the body. Some organs are rigidly fixed, whereas others are mobile. Typical examples in the abdomen include mesenteric or small bowel injuries, particularly at the ligament of Treitz or at the junction of the distal small bowel and right colon.
- Falls from a height produce solid organ injuries less commonly and hollow visceral injuries more commonly. Retroperitoneal injuries associated with significant blood loss occurs from falls because force is transmitted up the axial skeleton.
- Gunshot wounds may injure the victim by having the bullet directly injure the organ or secondarily from missiles, such as bone and bullet fragments, or from energy transmission from the bullet.

CLINICAL FEATURES

SOLID VISCERAL INJURIES

- Injury to the solid organs causes morbidity and mortality primarily as a result of acute blood loss.
- The spleen is the most frequently injured organ in blunt abdominal trauma and is commonly associated with other intra-abdominal injuries. Kehr's sign, representing referred left shoulder pain, is a classic finding in splenic rupture. Lower left rib fractures should heighten clinical suspicion for splenic injury.
- The liver also is commonly injured in both blunt and penetrating injuries.
- Tachycardia, hypotension, and acute abdominal tenderness are the primary physical examination findings associated with intra-abdominal injury.
- Some patients with solid organ injury occasionally may present with minimal symptoms and nonspecific findings on physical examination. This is commonly associated with younger patients and those with distracting injuries, head injury, and/or intoxication.
- A single physical examination and set of vital signs are insensitive for diagnosing abdominal injuries. Serial physical examinations on an awake, alert, and reliable patient are important for identifying intra-abdominal injuries.

HOLLOW VISCERAL INJURIES

- These injuries produce symptoms by the combination of blood loss and peritoneal contamination. Perforation of the stomach, small bowel, or colon is accompanied by blood loss from a concomitant mesenteric injury.
- Gastrointestinal contamination will produce peritoneal signs over a period of time. Patients with head injury, distracting injuries, or intoxication may not exhibit peritoneal signs initially.
- Small bowel and colon injuries are most frequently the result of penetrating trauma. However, a deceleration injury can cause a bucket-handle tear of the mesentery or a blowout injury of the antimesenteric border.
- Suppurative peritonitis may develop from small bowel and colonic injuries. Inflammation may take 6 to 8 hours to develop.

RETROPERITONEAL INJURIES

- Duodenal injuries are most often associated with high-speed vertical or horizontal decelerating trauma. Duodenal injuries may range in severity from an intramural hematoma to an extensive crush or laceration.
- Clinical signs of duodenal injury are often slow to develop. Patients may present with abdominal pain, fever, nausea, and vomiting, although these may take hours to become clinically obvious.
- Duodenal rupture is usually contained within the retroperitoneum with blunt trauma.
- Pancreatic injury often accompanies rapid deceleration injury or a severe crush injury. The classic case is a blow to the midepigastrium from a steering wheel or the handlebar of a bicycle.
- Leakage of activated enzymes from the pancreas can produce retroperitoneal autodigestion, which may become superinfected with bacteria and produce a retroperitoneal abscess.

DIAPHRAGMATIC INJURIES

- Presentation of diaphragm injuries is often insidious. Only occasionally is the diagnosis obvious when bowel sounds can be auscultated in the thoracic cavity.
- On chest radiograph, herniation of abdominal contents into the thoracic cavity or a nasogastric tube coiled in the thorax confirms the diagnosis. In most cases, however, the only finding on chest radiograph is blurring of the diaphragm or an effusion.
- CT is usually needed to diagnose a diaphragmatic injury. Occasionally, cavitary endoscopy or laparotomy is necessary to make the definitive diagnosis.

DIAGNOSIS AND DIFFERENTIAL

PLAIN RADIOGRAPHS

- A chest radiograph is helpful in evaluating for herniated abdominal contents in the thoracic cavity and for evidence of free air under the diaphragm.
- An AP pelvis radiograph is important for identifying pelvic fractures, which can produce significant blood loss and be associated with intra-abdominal visceral injury.

ULTRASONOGRAPHY

- The focused assessment with sonography for trauma (FAST) examination is an accurate screening tool for abdominal trauma. The underlying premise behind the use of the FAST examination is that most clinically significant injuries will be associated with the presence of free fluid accumulating in dependent areas.
- Advantages of the FAST examination are that it is accurate, rapid, noninvasive, repeatable, portable, and involves no contrast material or radiation exposure to the patient. There is limited risk for patients who are pregnant, are coagulopathic, or have had previous abdominal surgery.
- A major feature of the FAST examination is its ability to rapidly evaluate for free pericardial and pleural fluid along with a pneumothorax. It is also very useful when caring for the trauma patient who is pregnant.
- A FAST-inclusive trauma protocol has been found to significantly decrease time to operative care in patients with suspected torso trauma, with improved resource use and lower medical charges.
- Disadvantages include the inability to determine the exact etiology of the free intraperitoneal fluid and the operator-dependent nature of the examination. CT is the preferred diagnostic imaging study for evaluating the retroperitoneum.
- Other disadvantages of the FAST examination are the difficulty in interpreting the views in patients who are obese and have subcutaneous air or excessive bowel gas, and the inability to distinguish intraperitoneal hemorrhage from ascites.

COMPUTED TOMOGRAPHY

- With the increasing sensitivity and availability of CT scanners, CT has become the gold standard for the diagnosis of abdominal injury. Only CT can make the diagnosis of organ-specific abdominal injury.
- A triple-contrast helical CT scan can quickly discern either contrast extravasation or the presence of air or fluid. The accuracy of triple-contrast CT as a single diagnostic study is reported to be 97% to 100% following penetrating trauma.
- Advantages of CT include its ability to precisely locate intra-abdominal lesions preoperatively, to evaluate the retroperitoneum, and to identify injuries that may be managed nonoperatively, as well as its noninvasiveness.
- The disadvantages of CT are its expense, radiation exposure, need to transport the trauma patient to the radiology suite, and the need for contrast materials.

DIAGNOSTIC PERITONEAL LAVAGE

- Diagnostic peritoneal lavage (DPL) remains a good screening test for evaluating abdominal trauma if ultrasonography is not available. Its advantages include its relative speed with which it can be performed and low complication rate (1%).
- Drawbacks include its invasiveness, the potential for iatrogenic injury, its misapplication for evaluation of retroperitoneal injuries, and its lack of specificity.
- Laparotomy based solely on a positive DPL results in a nontherapeutic laparotomy approximately 30% of the time. Minor injury can produce hemoperitoneum sufficient to render DPL positive.
- In penetrating trauma, DPL should be performed when it is not clear that exploratory laparotomy is indicated. DPL is useful in evaluating patients sustaining stab wounds where local wound exploration indicates that the superficial muscle fascia has been violated. Also, it may be useful in confirming a negative physical examination when tangential or lower chest wounds are involved.
- In blunt abdominal trauma, the DPL is considered positive if more than 10 mL of gross blood is aspirated immediately, the red blood cell count is >100,000 cells/μL, the white blood cell count is >500 cells/μL, bile is present, or vegetable matter is present.
- The only absolute contraindication to DPL is when surgical management is clearly indicated, in which case the DPL would delay patient transport to the operating room.
- Relative contraindications include patients with advanced hepatic dysfunction, severe coagulopathies, previous abdominal surgeries, or a gravid uterus.

EMERGENCY DEPARTMENT CARE AND DISPOSITION

- Administer 100% oxygen and secure cardiac monitoring and two large-bore IV lines.
- For hypotensive abdominal trauma patients, resuscitate with IV crystalloid fluid. Consider transfusion with O-negative or type-specific packed red blood cells in addition to crystalloid resuscitation.

TABLE 167-1 Indications for Laparotomy

	BLUNT	PENETRATING
Absolute	Anterior abdominal injury with hypotension Abdominal wall disruption Peritonitis Free air under diaphragm on chest radiograph Positive FAST or DPL in hemodynamically unstable patient CT-diagnosed injury requiring surgery (ie, pancreatic transection, duodenal rupture, diaphragm injury)	Injury to abdomen, back, and flank with hypotension Abdominal tenderness GI evisceration High suspicion for transabdominal trajectory after gunshot wound CT-diagnosed injury requiring surgery (ie, ureter or pancreas)
Relative	Positive FAST or DPL in hemodynamically stable patient Solid visceral injury in stable patient Hemoperitoneum on CT without clear source	Positive local wound exploration after stab wound

Abbreviations: DPL = diagnostic peritoneal lavage, FAST = focused assessment with sonography for trauma.

- Order laboratory work for abdominal trauma patients based on the mechanism of injury (blunt versus penetrating); it may include type and crossmatching, complete blood count, electrolytes, arterial blood gas, directed toxicologic studies, coagulation studies, hepatic enzymes, and lipase.
- Table 167-1 lists the indications for exploratory laparotomy.
- If organ evisceration is present, then cover it with a moist, sterile dressing prior to surgery.
- The evolution of nonoperative therapy has been greatly advanced by the evolution of CT. CT not only can make the diagnosis of solid visceral injury but can also often rule out other injuries requiring surgery.
- For the hemodynamically stable blunt trauma patient with a positive FAST examination, further evaluation with CT may be warranted prior to admission.
- For an equivocal stab wound to the abdomen, surgical consultation for local wound exploration is indicated. If the wound exploration demonstrates no violation of the anterior fascia, the patient can be discharged home safely.
- Local wound exploration is only appropriate for anterior abdominal stab wounds and not for those in the flank or back.

For further reading in Tintinalli's *Emergency Medicine: A Comprehensive Study Guide*, 7th ed., see Chapter 260, "Abdominal Trauma," by Thomas M. Scalea, Sharon Boswell, Bonny J. Baron, and O. John Ma.

168 PENETRATING TRAUMA TO THE FLANK AND BUTTOCK

Christine Sullivan

PENETRATING TRAUMA TO THE FLANK

PATHOPHYSIOLOGY

- The flank is the area between the anterior and posterior axillary lines, from the sixth rib to the iliac crest.
- Any intraperitoneal or retroperitoneal structure may be injured. Missile pathways are unpredictable, and the appearance of stab wounds can be misleading.

CLINICAL FEATURES

- Patients may present with hemorrhagic shock, peritonitis, evisceration, or an innocuous-appearing wound with stable vital signs.
- Gross blood on digital rectal examination indicates bowel injury.
- Blood at the urethral meatus or hematuria suggests genitourinary injury.

DIAGNOSIS AND DIFFERENTIAL

- Wound exploration is of limited value.
- CT is the diagnostic study of choice in hemodynamically stable patients. Double-contrast (PO and IV) studies, with the addition of rectal contrast when there is suspicion of rectal or sigmoid colon injury, is recommended.

EMERGENCY DEPARTMENT CARE AND DISPOSITION

- Follow standard resuscitation protocols, including immediate surgical consultation.
- Emergent laparotomy is indicated when patients are hemodynamically unstable and have peritonitis, and in patients with most flank gunshot wounds. Many stab wounds can be managed conservatively.
- Give broad-spectrum antibiotics (eg, piperacillin-tazobactam 3.375 grams IV) if the patient has peritonitis.
- In stable patients, utilize CT to determine the need for operation and to detect occult injuries. CT can often determine the exact depth of stab wounds. High-risk stab wounds (penetration beyond the deep fascia) require surgical consultation and admission.
- Admit all patients for observation with the exception of those sustaining low-risk stab wounds (superficial to deep fascia). Patients with low-risk stab wounds

whose diagnostic evaluation reveals no injury can be discharged if stable after observation for several hours.

PENETRATING BUTTOCK INJURIES

PATHOPHYSIOLOGY

- Operative intervention is rarely required for stab wounds to the buttock.

CLINICAL FEATURES

- Approximately 30% of patients with gunshot wounds to the buttock require surgical intervention. An entrance wound above the level of the greater trochanters or a transpelvic or transabdominal bullet trajectory predicts the need for laparotomy.
- Gross hematuria is associated with the need for surgery.
- Perform a rectal examination for gross blood.
- Evaluate the lower extremities for vascular or neurologic injury, including special attention for sciatic and femoral nerve injury.

DIAGNOSIS AND DIFFERENTIAL

- Wound exploration is of limited value except in very superficial stab wounds to detect gross foreign bodies.
- Hemodynamically stable patients should undergo CT with oral, intravenous, and rectal contrast.
- Proctosigmoidoscopy can be performed if blood is noted on rectal examination or if the missile pathway suggests possible rectal injury.
- A cystourethrogram (either as a separate study or in conjunction with CT scanning) can be performed in patients with hematuria or wounds near the genitourinary tract.
- CT angiography or traditional angiography and venography may be indicated if pelvic hematoma is found on CT.
- Plain abdominal or pelvic radiographs can help determine missile pathway and detect fractures.

EMERGENCY DEPARTMENT CARE AND DISPOSITION

- Follow standard resuscitation protocols, including immediate surgical consultation.
- Emergent laparotomy is indicated when patients are hemodynamically unstable, have peritonitis, or have an intrapelvic or transabdominal bullet path.
- Give broad-spectrum antibiotics (eg, piperacillin-tazobactam 3.375 grams IV) if the patient has symptoms concerning for peritonitis.
- If no immediate indication for laparotomy is found, utilize CT to determine the need for operation and to detect occult injuries.
- Admit all patients for observation with the exception of those sustaining very superficial stab wounds whose diagnostic evaluation reveals no significant injury.

For further reading in Tintinalli's *Emergency Medicine: A Comprehensive Study Guide*, 7th ed., see Chapter 261, "Penetrating Trauma to the Flank and Buttocks," by Alasdair K.T. Conn.

169 GENITOURINARY TRAUMA

Matthew C. Gratton

EPIDEMIOLOGY

- Falls, assaults, motor vehicle crashes, and sports injuries are the most common causes of blunt genitourinary (GU) injury while gunshot and stab wounds are the most common causes of penetrating injury.
- GU injuries frequently occur in the setting of multiple trauma, and so a thorough evaluation is necessary to avoid missing significant injuries.

CLINICAL FEATURES

- Patients with any abdominal trauma, including penetrating trauma in the vicinity of GU structures, are at risk.
- High-velocity deceleration predisposes to renal pedicle injuries, including lacerations and thromboses of the renal artery and vein.
- Fractures of the lower ribs or lower thoracic or lumbar vertebrae are often associated with renal injuries, while pelvic fractures and straddle injuries are associated with bladder or urethral injuries.
- Flank ecchymoses, tenderness, mass, or penetrating injury raises concern for renal injury.
- The perineum should be inspected for blood or lacerations, which may denote an open pelvic fracture.
- The presence of a penile, scrotal, or perineal hematoma or blood at the penile meatus suggests urethral injury.
- If blood at the meatus is present, then do not attempt to insert a urethral catheter due to the concern for converting a partial urethral laceration into a complete transection.

- Perform a rectal examination, assessing sphincter tone, checking for blood, and determining the position of the prostate.
- A high-riding prostate or one that feels boggy suggests injury to the membranous urethra.
- Examine the scrotum in male patients for ecchymoses, lacerations, or testicular disruption.
- Inspect the vaginal introitus in female patients for lacerations and hematomas, which may be associated with pelvic fractures. If there is evidence of injury in this area, or if injury is suspected, a bimanual examination should be performed. If blood is present, a speculum examination is warranted to check for vaginal lacerations.

DIAGNOSIS AND DIFFERENTIAL

- Urinalysis is important, but there is no direct relationship between the degree of hematuria and the severity of renal injury.
- There is some evidence that gross hematuria or microscopic hematuria in patients with a systolic blood pressure <90 mm Hg are associated with more significant injury.
- In hemodynamically stable patients, isolated microscopic hematuria rarely represents significant injury. However, a renal pedicle or vascular injury from rapid deceleration may be an exception.
- In stable children, renal injury is unlikely if the urine contains <50 RBCs/hpf.
- Analysis of the first-voided urine may help localize the injury. Initial hematuria suggests injury to the urethra or prostate, while terminal hematuria is associated with bladder neck trauma. Continuous hematuria may be due to injury to the bladder, ureter, or kidney.
- An IV contrast-enhanced abdominopelvic CT is the imaging "gold standard" for the stable trauma patient with suspected kidney injury.
- A "one shot" intraoperative IV urogram is recommended by some for the unstable patient, although this is controversial.
- A retrograde cystogram (plain radiograph or CT) is the "gold standard" for demonstrating bladder injury, as is a retrograde urethrogram for demonstrating urethral injury.
- Indications for imaging in suspected renal trauma patients are listed in Table 169-1.

EMERGENCY DEPARTMENT CARE AND DISPOSITION

- Take a standardized approach to all multiple trauma patients to identify and treat life-threatening injuries (primary survey) and then perform a thorough secondary survey, including a GU examination to avoid missing subtle injuries.
- Patients with isolated microscopic hematuria and no other injuries may be discharged with repeat urinalysis in 1 to 2 weeks.

TABLE 169-1 Indications for Imaging in Patients with Suspected Renal Trauma

BLUNT TRAUMA	PENETRATING TRAUMA
Gross hematuria	Any degree of hematuria
Adult with blood pressure <90 mm Hg and any degree of hematuria	
Child with >50 red blood cells per high power field	
High index of suspicion for renal trauma	
Deceleration injuries (especially vertical) even with no hematuria	
Suspected other associated intra-abdominal or intrapelvic injuries (multiple trauma patient)	

MANAGEMENT OF SPECIFIC INJURIES

KIDNEY

- Renal injuries are present in 8% to 10% of patients with abdominal trauma, and 80% of those with renal injury have additional visceral or skeletal injuries.
- Most renal injuries are handled nonoperatively, but indications for exploration and intervention include life-threatening bleeding from the kidney; expanding, pulsatile, or noncontained hematoma (thought to be from a renal avulsion); renal avulsion injury; and renal pelvis or ureteral injuries.
- Renal contusions and lacerations not involving the collecting system are managed nonoperatively. In the absence of other injuries, patients with renal contusions may be discharged with repeat urinalysis in 1 to 2 weeks.
- Admit patients with renal lacerations, pedicle injuries, or lacerations involving the collecting system. Many of these patients have associated injuries requiring surgical repair.
- Urinary extravasation alone is not an indication for operative repair as it resolves spontaneously in the majority of cases. Extravasation from a renal pelvis or ureteral injury does require repair.
- In the case of isolated renal injury with no indication for operative repair, patients need frequent reassessment

and should be put on bed rest, kept well hydrated, and have frequent hematocrit determinations and urinalyses until hematuria clears.
- Some gunshot and stab wounds to the kidney can be treated nonoperatively with the absolute indications for exploration mentioned above. Many with renal injuries will have other injuries that mandate exploration.

URETER

- Ureteral injuries are the rarest of the GU injuries and usually result from penetrating trauma or are complications due to instrumentation.
- The absence of hematuria does not rule out injury.
- Ureteral injuries are managed operatively, including simple stenting in some cases.

BLADDER

- Bladder injury occurs in about 2% of blunt abdominal trauma and 80% are associated with pelvic fractures.
- Gross hematuria is present in about 95% of patients with significant injury.
- Intraperitoneal rupture usually results from a burst injury of a full bladder and always requires surgical exploration and repair.
- Extraperitoneal rupture is more common, is often associated with a pelvic ring fracture, and can usually be managed by bladder catheter drainage alone.
- Symptoms and signs of bladder rupture include lower abdominal pain and tenderness, gross hematuria, lower abdominal bruising, abdominal swelling from urinary ascites, perineal or scrotal edema from urinary extravasation, and inability to void.
- Penetrating bladder injuries are managed operatively.

URETHRA

- Urethral injuries in males can involve the posterior (prostatic and membranous) urethra and/or the anterior (bulbous and penile) urethra.
- Posterior injuries are typically related to major blunt force trauma and are associated with pelvic fractures. Treatment is via suprapubic bladder drainage followed in several weeks by surgical repair.
- A urinary catheter should not be placed if there is suspicion of a posterior urethral injury without first obtaining a retrograde urethrogram since the catheter could convert a partial to a complete disruption.
- Anterior injuries result from direct trauma or instrumentation and are usually managed conservatively, with or without a urethral catheter.
- Penetrating injuries to the anterior urethra usually require operative repair.
- In females, urethral injuries are often associated with pelvic fractures and commonly present with vaginal bleeding.

TESTICLES AND SCROTUM

- Blunt testicular injuries should be evaluated with color Doppler ultrasonography to determine the extent of injury and determine if a rupture is present.
- Contusions may be managed conservatively with nonsteroidal anti-inflammatory drugs, ice, elevation, scrotal support, and urologic follow-up.
- Testicular rupture or penetrating trauma requires operative repair to improve outcome.
- Scrotal skin avulsion is managed by housing the testicle in the remaining scrotal skin, which will usually return to normal size in several months.

PENIS

- Injuries range from small contusions to degloving injuries or amputations.
- Simple skin lacerations can be directly repaired but deeper lacerations and/or penetrating injuries require operative exploration and repair.
- Amputations require microvascular reimplantation if the amputated segment is viable.
- A fractured penis, due to traumatic rupture of the corpus cavernosum, is managed by immediate surgical drainage of blood clot and repair of the torn tunica albuginea and any associated urethral injuries.
- Penile skin avulsion is managed with split-thickness skin grafting after debridement.
- Zipper injury to the penis results when the penile skin is trapped in the trouser zipper. Mineral oil and lidocaine infiltration are useful in freeing the penile skin from the zipper. Wire-cutting or bone-cutting pliers are used to cut the median bar (diamond) of the zipper, causing the zipper to fall apart.
- Contusions to the perineum or penis are treated conservatively with cold packs, rest, and elevation.
- If the patient is unable to void, catheter drainage may be required.

For further reading in Tintinalli's *Emergency Medicine: A Comprehensive Study Guide*, 7th ed., see Chapter 262, "Genitourinary Trauma," by John McManus, Matthew C. Gratton, and Peter J. Cuenca.

170 PENETRATING TRAUMA TO THE EXTREMITIES

Amy M. Stubbs

EPIDEMIOLOGY

- More than 50% of penetrating traumatic injuries involve the extremities. This accounts for up to 82% of vascular injuries to the extremities.
- Penetrating injuries to the extremities result in amputation in <5% of cases.
- Injuries to major nerves are the most likely to lead to long-term disability.
- Gunshots and stab wounds account for the majority of penetrating extremity injuries.

PATHOPHYSIOLOGY

- Injuries from stab wounds may be predicted based on the anatomy of the area.
- Tissue damage from a missile or blast injury is variable and dependent upon multiple factors.

CLINICAL FEATURES

- After the primary and secondary surveys are completed, including appropriate resuscitation, perform a thorough history, including the events surrounding the injury, type of weapon used, and any prior injuries to the affected limb.
- A detailed examination should be performed on the affected extremity, quickly noting any "hard" signs of vascular injury that require immediate intervention. "Soft" signs of arterial injury should be noted as well (Table 170-1).
- Wound characteristics, bony deformities, soft tissue defects, and location of pain should be evaluated and noted.

TABLE 170-1 Clinical Manifestations of Extremity Vascular Trauma

Hard signs
Absent or diminished distal pulses
Obvious arterial bleeding
Large expanding or pulsatile hematoma
Audible bruit
Palpable thrill
Distal ischemia (pain, pallor, paralysis, paresthesias, coolness)
Soft signs
Small, stable hematoma
Injury to anatomically related nerve
Unexplained hypotension
History of hemorrhage
Proximity of injury to major vascular structures
Complex fracture

- Examine range of motion, strength and sensation, adjacent joints, and the surrounding compartments; concerns for compartment syndrome, open joint, and arterial or nerve injury warrant emergent consultation with the appropriate specialist.

DIAGNOSIS AND DIFFERENTIAL

- Diagnosis of significant extremity injuries may require imaging and measurement of ankle-brachial indices (ABIs).
- Plain radiographs of the affected limb and the joint above and below the injury are useful to diagnose bone and joint injuries, retained foreign bodies, and embolized bullet fragments.
- Although traditional angiography is considered the gold standard for identifying vascular injuries, multidetector CT (MDCT) angiography is rapid, noninvasive, sensitive, and specific for vascular injuries, as well as fractures and foreign bodies.
- Duplex ultrasonography is rapid, safe, and accurate for the detection of vascular injury. It can also assist in identifying foreign bodies and may be the preferred imaging modality in some cases.
- ABIs are performed by measuring the systolic blood pressure in all four extremities with the patient supine, using a manual blood pressure cuff and Doppler. An ABI is then calculated by dividing the ankle systolic blood pressure by the greater of the two systolic upper extremity systolic blood pressures.
- An ABI ≥1.0 = normal, 0.5 to 0.9 = injury to a single arterial segment, <0.5 = severe arterial injury or injury to multiple segments of the artery.
- ABIs have variable sensitivity and specificity for arterial injury, and may be affected by underlying conditions such as peripheral vascular disease and hypothermia.
- ABIs are not reliable for detecting intimal flaps or psuedoaneurysms.

EMERGENCY DEPARTMENT CARE AND DISPOSITION

- For patients with "hard" signs of arterial injury, immediate surgical intervention or expedient vascular imaging is required.
- Vascular imaging in patients with "soft" signs of arterial injury is controversial. Most can be managed conservatively with admission for 24-hour observation and serial examinations, as incidence of significant injury in this group is low. Rapidly initiate intervention and/or imaging if signs of vascular compromise develop.
- Control bleeding with direct pressure. Do not clamp or ligate blood vessels in the ED.

- Open fractures or joints should be evaluated by an orthopedic surgeon. Fractures due to penetrating injury require surgical debridement and parenteral antibiotics (cephalosporin ± aminoglycoside).
- General principles of wound management including irrigation, debridement, and tetanus prophylaxis apply. Copious irrigation with saline or tap water at high pressure is a key component.
- Primary closure of low-risk wounds may be considered. Delayed primary closure (72-96 hours post injury) may be appropriate in some cases.
- Prophylactic antibiotics are generally not indicated. Consider immunocompromised patients to have high-risk wounds.
- If considering wound exploration for foreign body removal, the clinician should take into account size, location, material, and risk/benefit ratio to the patient.
- Patients with no signs of significant injury, minimal tissue damage, and an unremarkable examination after an observation period may be safely discharged.

For further reading in Tintinalli's *Emergency Medicine: A Comprehensive Study Guide*, 7th ed., see Chapter 263, "Penetrating Trauma to the Extremities," by Roberta Capp and Richard D. Zane.

Section 20
INJURIES TO BONES AND JOINTS

171 INITIAL EVALUATION AND MANAGEMENT OF ORTHOPEDIC INJURIES

Michael P. Kefer

PATHOPHYSIOLOGY

- Bone fracture results in severing of the microscopic vessels crossing the fracture line, which cuts off the blood supply to the involved fracture edges. Callus formation ensues and becomes progressively more mineralized.
- Necrotic edges of the fracture are gradually resorbed by osteoclasts. This explains why some occult fractures are not immediately detected on radiographs, but then appear several days later after this resorption process is well established.
- Remodeling deposits new bone along the lines of stress. This process often lasts years.

CLINICAL FEATURES

- Knowing the mechanism of injury and listening carefully to the patient's symptoms is important in diagnosing fracture or dislocation.
- Pain may be referred to an area distant from the injury (eg, hip injury presenting as knee pain).
- The physical examination includes (1) inspection for deformity, edema, or discoloration; (2) assessment of active and passive range of motion of joints proximal and distal to the injury; (3) palpation for tenderness or deformity; and (4) assessment of neurovascular status distal to the injury.
- Careful palpation can prevent missing a crucial diagnosis due to referred pain.
- Radiologic evaluation is based on the history and physical examination, not simply on where the patient reports pain.
- Radiographs of all long bone fractures should include the joints proximal and distal to the fracture to evaluate for coexistent injury.
- A negative radiograph does not exclude a fracture. This commonly occurs with scaphoid, radial head, or metatarsal shaft fractures.
- Diagnosis in the ED is often clinical and is not confirmed until 7 to 10 days after the injury, when enough bone resorption has occurred at the fracture site to detect a lucency on the radiograph.
- An accurate description of the fracture to the orthopedic consultant is crucial and should include the following details:
  - Closed versus open: whether overlying skin is intact (closed) or not (open).
  - Location: midshaft, junction of proximal and middle or middle and distal thirds, or distance from the bone end, or intra-articular. Anatomic bony reference points should be used when applicable. For example, a humerus fracture just above the condyles is described as supracondylar, as opposed to distal humerus.
  - Orientation of fracture line (Fig. 171-1).
  - Displacement: amount and direction of distal fragment is offset from proximal fragment.
  - Separation: amount two fragments have been pulled apart; unlike displacement, alignment is maintained.
  - Shortening: reduction in bone length due to impaction or overriding fragments.
  - Angulation: degree and direction of the angle formed by the distal fragment.
  - Rotational deformity: degree distal fragment is twisted on the axis of normal bone; usually detected by physical examination and not seen on the radiograph.
  - Associated disruption of proper joint alignment is described as fracture-dislocation (joint surfaces have no contact) or fracture-subluxation (joint surfaces still in partial contact).
- Fractures involving the growth plate of long bones in pediatric patients are described by the Salter–Harris classification (Figs. 171-2 and 171-3, and Table 171-1). Note type I and V may be radiographically undetectable.

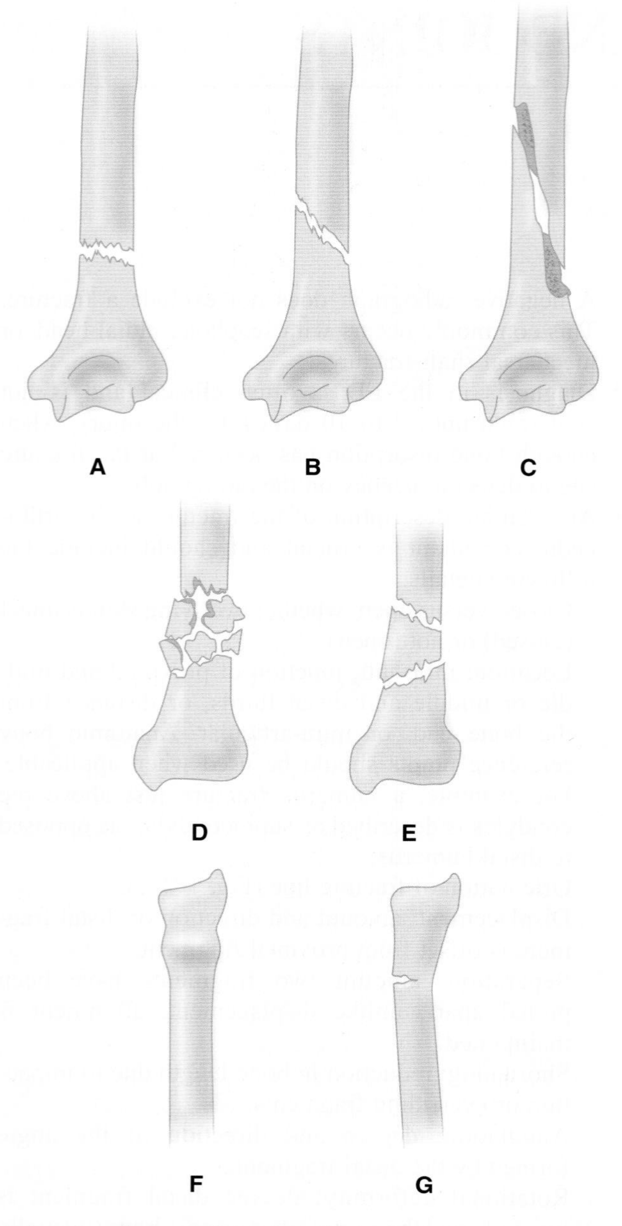

FIG. 171-1. Fracture line orientation. **A.** Transverse. **B.** Oblique. **C.** Spiral. **D.** Comminuted. **E.** Segmental. **F.** Torus. **G.** Greenstick.

- Complications from neurovascular deficit may be immediate or delayed. Compartment syndrome that presents with the five classic signs of pain, pallor, paresthesias, pulselessness, and paralysis is well advanced.
- Long-term complications of fracture include malunion, nonunion, avascular necrosis, arthritis, and osteomyelitis.

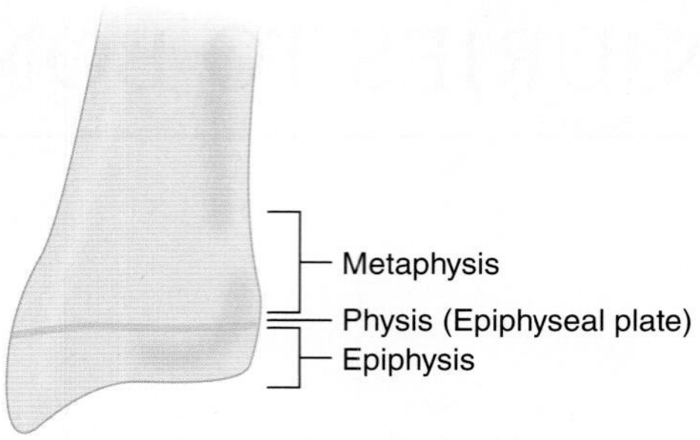

FIG. 171-2. Epiphyseal anatomy in the growing child.

EMERGENCY DEPARTMENT CARE AND DISPOSITION

- Control swelling with cold packs and elevation. Remove objects such as rings or watches that may constrict the injury before swelling progresses.
- Provide pain control.
- Prompt reduction of fracture deformity with steady, longitudinal traction is indicated to (1) alleviate pain; (2) relieve tension on associated neurovascular structures; (3) minimize the risk of converting a closed fracture to an open fracture when a sharp, bony fragment tents overlying skin; and (4) restore circulation to a pulseless distal extremity (the most time critical).

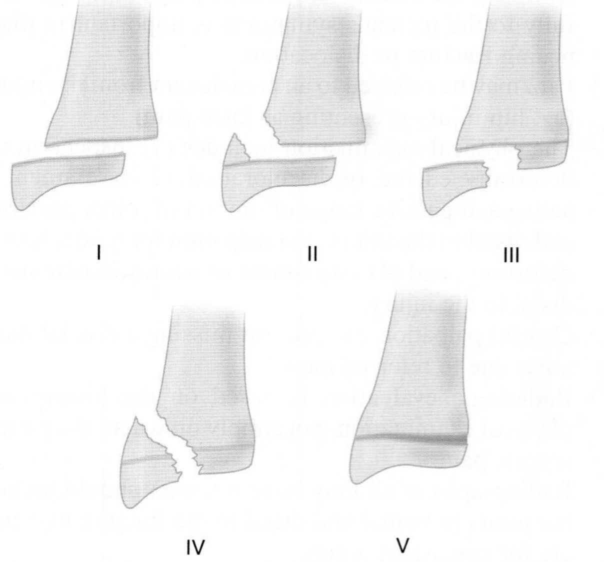

FIG. 171-3. Epiphyseal plate fractures based on the classification of Salter and Harris.

TABLE 171-1 Description of Salter–Harris Fractures

SALTER TYPE	WHAT IS BROKEN OFF
I	The entire epiphysis.
II	The entire epiphysis *along with* a portion of the metaphysis.
III	A portion of the epiphysis.
IV	A portion of the epiphysis *along with* a portion of the metaphysis.
V	Compression injury of the epiphyseal plate. Nothing is "broken off."

- Open fractures require immediate prophylactic antibiotics, irrigation, and debridement, to prevent osteomyelitis.
- Immobilize the fracture or relocated joint. Fiberglass or plaster splinting material is commonly used.
- The chemical reaction causing the splint material to set is exothermic and begins upon contact with water. The amount of heat liberated is directly proportional to water temperature. To avoid burns, use water slightly warmer than room temperature.
- Splints should be long enough to immobilize the joint above and below the fracture.
- Crutches should be prescribed for the patient with a lower extremity injury that requires prevention of weight bearing. The pressure of the crutch pads is borne by the sides of the thorax, not the axilla, to avoid injury to the brachial plexus.

For further reading in Tintinalli's *Emergency Medicine: A Comprehensive Study Guide*, 7th ed., see Chapter 264, "Initial Evaluation and Management of Orthopedic Injuries," by Jeffrey S. Menkes.

172 HAND AND WRIST INJURIES

Michael P. Kefer

ANATOMY AND EXAMINATION

- The intrinsic muscles of the hand originate and insert within the hand. These are the thenar and hypothenar muscle groups, adductor pollicis, the interossei, and the lumbricals.
- Thenar muscles abduct, oppose, and flex the thumb and are innervated by the median nerve.

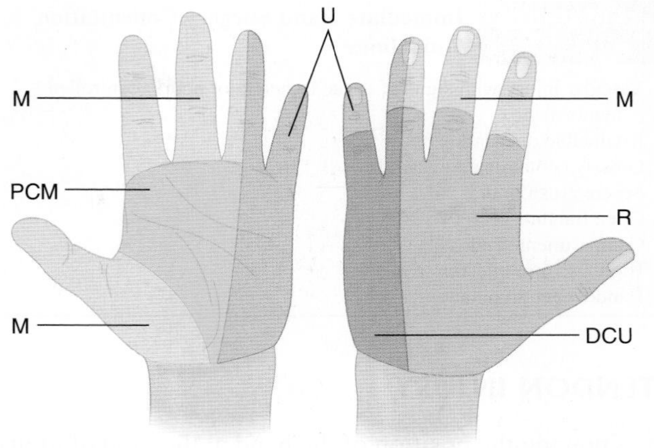

FIG. 172-1. The cutaneous nerve supply in the hand. DCU = dorsal branch of ulnar nerve; M = median; PCM = palmar branch of median nerve; R = radial; U = ulnar.

- Hypothenar muscles abduct, oppose, and flex the little finger and are innervated by the ulnar nerve.
- Adductor pollicis adducts the thumb and is innervated by the ulnar nerve.
- Interosseous muscles adduct and abduct the fingers and are innervated by the ulnar nerve.
- Lumbricals flex and extend the digits. The two radial lumbricals are innervated by the median nerve. The two ulnar lumbricals are innervated by the ulnar nerve.
- Flexor digitorum superficialis inserts into the middle phalanges and flexes all the joints it crosses. Function is tested when the patient flexes the proximal interphalangeal (PIP) joint while the other fingers are held in extension.
- Flexor digitorum profundus inserts at the base of the distal phalanges and flexes the distal interphalangeal (DIP) joint as well as all the other joints flexed by flexor digitorum superficialis. Function is tested when the patient flexes the DIP joint while the PIP and metacarpal phalangeal (MCP) joints are held in extension.
- Extensor digitorum extends all the digits. Function is tested by having the patient hold the hand in the "stop traffic" position. This also tests radial nerve motor function.
- None of the intrinsic muscles of the hand are innervated by the radial nerve.
- Figure 172-1 shows sensory innervation of the hand. This is best screened by testing two-point discrimination.

HAND INJURIES

- Injuries requiring hand surgery consult are listed in Tables 172-1 and 172-2.

TABLE 172-1 Immediate Hand Surgery Consultation Guidelines

Vascular injury with signs of tissue ischemia or poorly controlled hemorrhage
Irreducible dislocations
Grossly contaminated wounds
Severe crush injury
Open fracture
Compartment syndrome
High pressure injection injury
Hand/finger amputation

TENDON INJURY

- Knowing the position of the hand at the time of injury predicts where, along its course, a tendon is injured.
- Extensor tendon repair can often be performed by the emergency physician.
- Flexor tendon repair should be performed by the hand surgeon.
- It is common for the emergency care of tendon lacerations to consist of closing the skin and splinting until definitive repair by the hand surgeon.

MALLET FINGER

- This injury results from rupture of the extensor tendon at the base of the distal phalanx.
- On examination, the DIP joint is flexed at 40 degrees.
- Splint the DIP joint in slight hyperextension and refer to a hand specialist.

BOUTONNIÈRE DEFORMITY

- This results from injury at the dorsal surface of the PIP joint that disrupts the extensor hood.
- Lateral bands of the extensor mechanism become flexors of the PIP joint and hyperextensors of the DIP joint.
- Splint the PIP joint in extension and refer.

DISTAL INTERPHALANGEAL JOINT DISLOCATION

- This is uncommon due to firm attachment of skin and fibrous tissue to underlying bone.
- Dislocation is usually dorsal.

TABLE 172-2 Delayed Hand Surgery Consultation Guidelines

Extensor/flexor tendon laceration (if not repaired in ED)
Flexor digitorum profundus rupture (closed)
Nerve injury (proximal to mid middle phalanx)
Closed fractures
Dislocations
Ligamentous injuries with instability

- Reduction is performed under digital block anesthesia. The dislocated phalanx is distracted, slightly hyperextended, and then repositioned.
- Splint the joint in full extension.
- Inability to reduce the joint may be from an entrapped volar plate, profundus tendon, or avulsion fracture.

PROXIMAL INTERPHALANGEAL JOINT DISLOCATION

- Dislocation is usually dorsal and results from rupture of the volar plate. Volar dislocation is rare.
- Lateral dislocation results from rupture of the collateral ligaments.
- Reduction is the same method as described above for DIP joint dislocation.
- An irreducible joint from an entrapped volar plate may require surgical reduction.
- Splint the joint in 30-degree flexion after reduction and refer.

METACARPOPHALANGEAL JOINT DISLOCATION

- Dislocation is usually dorsal and requires surgical reduction due to volar plate entrapment.
- Closed reduction is attempted with the wrist flexed and pressure applied to the proximal phalanx in a distal and volar direction.
- Splint the joint in 70- to 90-degree flexion.

THUMB DISLOCATION

- Interphalangeal (IP) and MCP joint dislocations usually involve volar plate rupture.
- Reduction of the IP joint is as described above for DIP joint dislocation.
- Reduction of the MCP joint is by flexing and abducting the metacarpal and applying pressure directed distally to the base of the proximal phalanx.
- Apply a thumb spica splint after reduction.

THUMB ULNAR COLLATERAL LIGAMENT RUPTURE

- Also known as gamekeeper's or skier's thumb, this results from forced radial abduction at the MCP joint.
- This is the most critical of collateral ligament injuries due to affect on pincer function.
- Ligament integrity is tested with the MCP joint in both full extension and 30-degree flexion. Complete rupture is diagnosed when abduction stress on the proximal phalanx causes more than 40 degrees of radial angulation relative to the metacarpal.
- Splint in thumb spica and refer.

DISTAL PHALANX FRACTURES

- Tuft fracture is the most common. If associated with subungual hematoma, drainage is recommended. Treat with a volar or hairpin splint.
- Transverse fracture with displacement is always associated with nail bed laceration, which may require repair.
- Avulsion fracture of the base results in a mallet finger (see above).

MIDDLE AND PROXIMAL PHALANX FRACTURES

- Fracture of the base or neck that is nondisplaced and stable can be treated with buddy taping.
- Transverse or spiral midshaft fracture or intra-articular fracture often requires surgical fixation. Place a gutter splint with flexion of the MCP joint at 90 degrees, the PIP joint at 20 degrees, and the DIP joint at 10 degrees and refer.

METACARPAL FRACTURES

- Fracture of the fourth or fifth metacarpal neck, often called a boxer's fracture, is the most common. Angulation more than 20 degrees in the ring finger, 40 degrees in the fifth finger, or 15 degrees in the middle or index finger should be reduced.
- Treat with a gutter splint with the wrist extended 20 degrees and the MCP joint flexed 90 degrees and refer.
- First metacarpal base fractures with intra-articular involvement (Bennett and Rolando fractures) should be immobilized in a thumb spica splint and referred for surgical repair.

COMPARTMENT SYNDROME

- Crush injury to the hand is especially at risk for compartment syndrome, which is a surgical emergency.
- The patient will complain of pain that is out of proportion to examination findings.
- Examination reveals the hand in a resting position is extended at the MCP joint and slightly flexed at the PIP joint. There is pain with passive stretch of the involved compartment and tense edema.

HIGH PRESSURE INJECTION INJURY

- This injury, which is a surgical emergency, occurs when substances in a high-pressure device, such as grease, paint, or hydraulic fluid, are injected into the hand.
- Oil-based paint causes the most severe tissue reaction and can result in ischemia, leading to amputation.
- Radiographs of the hand and forearm are indicated to evaluate for radiopaque substances and subcutaneous air.

WRIST INJURIES

SCAPHOLUNATE DISSOCIATION

- This injury presents with wrist pain at the scapholunate joint.
- Posteroanterior (PA) radiograph demonstrates a space more than 3 mm between the scaphoid and lunate and the cortical ring sign of the subluxed scaphoid.
- Treat this injury with a radial gutter splint and refer for ligament repair.

LUNATE AND PERILUNATE DISLOCATION

- In both injuries, a lateral wrist radiograph reveals the dislocation, as the normal alignment of the radius-lunate-capitate (the "3 C's" sign) is lost.
- With a lunate dislocation, the lunate dislocates volar to the radius, but the remainder of the carpus aligns with the radius. On PA radiograph, the lunate has a triangular shape, referred to as the "piece of pie" sign. Lateral radiograph reveals the lunate to be displaced and tilted volar, which has been described as the "spilled teacup sign."
- With a perilunate dislocation, the lunate remains aligned with the radius, but the capitate and the remainder of the carpus are dislocated, usually dorsal to the lunate.
- Emergent hand surgery consult for closed reduction or surgical repair is indicated.

CARPAL BONE FRACTURES

- Management is summarized in Table 172-3.
- The scaphoid is the most common carpal fractured.
- Fracture of the scaphoid, lunate, or capitate can cause avascular necrosis of the bone.
- Scaphoid and lunate fractures are often not detected on plain wrist radiograph, so diagnosis and treatment should be based on examination findings alone.

COLLES, SMITH, AND BARTON FRACTURES

- These fractures involve the distal radius at the metaphysis (Table 172-4).
- Most of these fractures can be treated with closed reduction and a sugar tong splint.

TABLE 172-3 Summary of Carpal Bone Fractures and ED Management

CARPAL BONE	MECHANISM OF INJURY	EXAMINATION	INITIAL ED MANAGEMENT
Scaphoid	Fall on outstretched hand	Snuffbox tenderness. Pain with radial deviation and flexion	Short arm, thumb spica, in dorsiflexion with radial deviation
Triquetrum	Avulsion fracture—twisting of hand against resistance or hyperextension Body fracture—direct trauma	Tenderness at the dorsum of the wrist, distal to the ulnar styloid	Short arm, sugar tong splint
Lunate	Fall on outstretched hand	Tenderness at shallow indentation of the mid-dorsum of the wrist, ulnar and distal to Lister tubercle	Short arm, thumb spica splint
Trapezium	Direct blow to thumb; force to wrist while dorsiflexed and radially deviated	Painful thumb movement and weak pinch strength Snuffbox tenderness	Short arm thumb spica splint
Pisiform	Fall directed on the hypothenar eminence	Tender pisiform, prominent at the base of the hypothenar eminence	Short arm, volar splint in 30 degrees of flexion and ulnar deviation
Hamate	Interrupted swing of a golf club, bat, or racquet	Tenderness at the hook of the hamate, just distal and radial to the pisiform	Short arm, volar wrist splint with fourth and fifth metacarpal joints in flexion
Capitate	Forceful dorsiflexion of the hand with radial impact	Tenderness over the capitate just proximal to the third metacarpal	Short arm, volar wrist splint
Trapezoid	Axial load onto the index metacarpal	Tenderness over the radial aspect of the base of the index metacarpal	Short arm thumb spica splint

RADIAL STYLOID FRACTURE

- Radial styloid fracture can produce carpal instability with scapholunate dissociation as major carpal ligaments insert here.
- Splint the wrist in mild flexion and ulnar deviation and refer.

ULNAR STYLOID FRACTURE

- Ulnar styloid fracture may result in radial ulnar joint instability.

TABLE 172-4 Radiographic Appearance of Distal Radius Fractures

Colles fracture
Dorsal angulation of the plane of the distal radius
Distal radius fragment is displaced proximally and dorsally
Radial displacement of the carpus
Ulnar styloid may be fractured
Smith fracture
Volar angulation of the plane of the distal radius
Distal radius fragment is displaced proximally and volarly
Radial displacement of the carpus
The fracture line extends obliquely from the dorsal surface to the volar surface
1-2 cm proximal to the articular surface
Barton fracture
Volar and proximal displacement of a large fragment of radial articular surface
Volar displacement of the carpus
Radial styloid may be fractured

- Place an ulnar gutter splint with the wrist in neutral and slight ulnar deviation and refer.

For further reading in Tintinalli's *Emergency Medicine: A Comprehensive Study Guide*, 7th ed., see Chapter 265, "Injuries to the Hand and Digits," by Moira Davenport, and Dean G. Sotereanos, and Chapter 266, "Wrist Injuries," by Robert Escarza, Maurice F. Loeffel III, and Dennis T. Uehara.

173 INJURIES TO THE ELBOW AND FOREARM

Sandra L. Najarian

BICEPS AND TRICEPS TENDON RUPTURES

PATHOPHYSIOLOGY

- Tendon ruptures are often the result of microtrauma and overuse. Steroids can contribute to the breakdown of the tendon.

CLINICAL FEATURES

- The most common type is rupture of the proximal long head of the bicep, and usually occurs after a sudden or prolonged contraction of the bicep against resistance.

- Patients often describe a "snap" or "pop" and complain of pain in the anterior shoulder.
- Swelling, tenderness, and crepitus over the bicipital groove can be seen on examination as well as a midarm "ball" when the elbow is flexed.
- Distal biceps ruptures are less common; weakness in flexion and supination of the forearm is more apparent than in proximal ruptures. Patients have pain, swelling, and a palpable defect in the antecubital fossa.
- Triceps ruptures are rare and almost always occur distally, resulting from a direct blow to the olecranon or from a fall on an outstretched hand causing a forceful flexion of the extended forearm.
- Patients with triceps ruptures present with pain, swelling, tenderness in the posterior elbow just proximal to the olecranon, and weakness with forearm extension.
- A modified Thompson's test can be used to assess triceps function. With the arm supported, elbow flexed at 90 degrees, and forearm hanging in a relaxed position, squeezing the triceps muscle should produce extension of the forearm unless a complete tear is present.

DIAGNOSIS AND DIFFERENTIAL

- Diagnosis is clinical, and radiographs should be obtained to exclude an associated avulsion fracture.

EMERGENCY DEPARTMENT CARE AND DISPOSITION

- Treatment includes sling, ice, analgesics, and referral to an orthopedic surgeon for definitive management.

EPICONDYLITIS

PATHOPHYSIOLOGY

- Repetitive movements involving the muscle groups originating on the lateral and medial epicondyles of the distal humerus result in an overuse syndrome.

CLINICAL FEATURES

- Lateral epicondylitis ("tennis elbow") presents with pain over the lateral elbow and tenderness with forced extension and supination of the forearm against resistance.
- Medical epicondylitis ("golfer's elbow") presents with pain over the medial elbow and tenderness with forced flexion and pronation of the forearm, wrist, and digits. It may be associated with an ulnar neuropathy.

EMERGENCY DEPARTMENT CARE AND DISPOSITION

- Conservative treatment is indicated, which includes rest, ice, anti-inflammatory medications, and immobilization with a counterforce brace.

ELBOW DISLOCATIONS

CLINICAL FEATURES

- Most elbow dislocations are posterolateral (90%) and often occur from a fall on the outstretched hand.
- The patient holds the elbow in 45 degrees of flexion, and significant swelling often obscures the olecranon, which is displaced posteriorly.
- Neurovascular injury occurs in 8% to 21% of cases; the ulnar nerve and brachial artery are the most frequently injured structures (Table 173-1).
- Absence of radial pulse before reduction, the presence of other systemic injuries (especially to the head, chest, and abdomen), and open dislocations are often associated with arterial injury.

DIAGNOSIS AND DIFFERENTIAL

- Radiographs of the elbow confirm the diagnosis.
- The ulna and the radius are displaced posteriorly on the lateral view and displaced medial or lateral on the AP view, but still maintain their normal relationship to each other.
- Associated fractures, especially of the radial head and coronoid process, can render the elbow joint unstable and complicate treatment.

TABLE 173-1 Sensory and Motor Function Testing of the Radial, Median, and Ulnar Nerves

	RADIAL	MEDIAN	ULNAR
Test for sensory function	Dorsum of the thumb index web space	Two-point discrimination over the tip of the index finger	Two-point discrimination over the little finger
Test for motor function	Extend both wrist and fingers against resistance	"OK" sign with thumb and index finger; abduction of the thumb (recurrent branch)	Abduct index finger against resistance

EMERGENCY DEPARTMENT CARE AND DISPOSITION

- After adequate sedation, closed reduction is indicated. Apply gentle traction on the wrist and forearm while an assistant applies countertraction on the upper arm. With the other hand on the proximal forearm, correct for medial and lateral displacement and apply downward pressure to disengage the coronoid process from olecranon fossa.
- Apply a long arm posterior splint to immobilize the elbow in slightly less than 90 degrees of flexion.
- Assess neurovascular status, obtain postreduction films, and arrange for urgent orthopedic follow-up.
- Patients with instability in extension, neurovascular compromise, or open dislocations require immediate orthopedic consultation.

ELBOW FRACTURES

PATHOPHYSIOLOGY

- Radial head fractures are the most common fracture of the elbow and result from a fall on the outstretched hand. Associated injuries around the elbow and even the wrist (Essex-Lopresti lesion) are common.
- Intercondylar fractures result from a force directed against the posterior elbow, driving the olecranon against the humeral surface.
- Ninety-five percent of supracondylar fractures are extra-articular and are commonly seen in children as the result of a fall on the outstretched hand with the elbow in full extension.
- Olecranon fractures often result from direct trauma or forced hyperextension of the elbow.
- Articular surface, epicondylar, and condylar fractures are rare.

CLINICAL FEATURES

- Radial head fractures produce lateral elbow pain and tenderness and an inability to fully extend the elbow.
- Patients with intercondylar and supracondylar fractures will have significant swelling, tenderness, and limited range of motion.
- Supracondylar fractures may resemble a posterior elbow dislocation.
- The anterior interosseus nerve, a motor branch of the median nerve, has the highest incidence of injury in supracondylar fractures. Anterior interosseus nerve function is demonstrated by flexing the index finger distal interphalangeal joint and thumb interphalangeal joint, forming the "OK" sign.

TABLE 173-2	Complications of Supracondylar Fractures
Early complications	Neurologic Radial nerve Median nerve (anterior interosseous branch) Ulnar Vascular Volkmann ischemic contracture (compartment syndrome of the forearm)
Late complications	Nonunion Malunion Myositis ossificans Loss of motion

- The most serious complication (Table 173-2) of supracondylar fractures is Volkmann's ischemic contracture.
- Pain with passive extension of the fingers, forearm tenderness, and refusal to open the hand are signs of impending Volkmann's ischemia.
- Acute vascular injuries such as decreased or absent radial pulse are usually secondary to transient vasospasm and are not necessarily a sign of ischemia unless accompanied by the clinical signs described above.
- Patients with olecranon fractures present with posterior elbow swelling and tenderness, limited mobility, and weak triceps function.
- Ulnar nerve injury is common in olecranon fractures.

DIAGNOSIS AND DIFFERENTIAL

- Fracture lines may not be visible on AP and lateral radiographs.
- The presence of abnormal fat pads (any posterior effusion or a very prominent anterior fat pad called the "sail sign") and/or the disruption of the radiocapitellar line (a line drawn from the center of the radial shaft transects the radial head and capitellum in all views) may be the only evidence of injury.

EMERGENCY DEPARTMENT CARE AND DISPOSITION

- Immobilization in a long arm posterior splint and orthopedic referral are appropriate for nondisplaced fractures.
- Nondisplaced radial head fractures with no restrictions in range of motion may be treated with sling immobilization and follow-up with orthopedics in 1 week.
- Emergent orthopedic consultation is warranted for all displaced fractures, open fractures, and fractures with evidence of neurovascular compromise.

FOREARM FRACTURES

PATHOPHYSIOLOGY

- Both bone forearm fractures usually occur from significant trauma, such as a motor vehicle crash or fall from height.
- Isolated ulnar fractures ("nightstick fractures") usually occur from a direct blow to the forearm.
- Radius fractures usually result from direct trauma or from a fall on an outstretched hand.

CLINICAL FEATURES

- Both bone forearm fractures present with swelling, tenderness, and deformity.
- Isolated ulnar or radius fractures present with localized swelling and tenderness.
- Monteggia fracture-dislocation, a fracture of the proximal ulna shaft with radial head dislocation, presents with significant pain and swelling over the elbow.
- Galeazzi fracture-dislocation, a fracture of the distal radius with an associated distal radioulnar joint dislocation, presents with localized swelling and tenderness over the distal radius and wrist.
- Neurovascular function must be carefully assessed in all forearm fractures. Paralysis of the posterior interosseus nerve (deep branch of the radial nerve) can occur in Monteggia fracture-dislocation. Injury to the ulnar and anterior interosseus nerve can occur in Galeazzi fracture-dislocation.

DIAGNOSIS AND DIFFERENTIAL

- AP and lateral radiographs are diagnostic. The amount of displacement, angulation, and shortening needs to be evaluated, and any rotational deformity should be noted.
- Isolated ulna fractures are unstable if the proximal third of the ulna is involved, displacement is greater than 50%, or angulation is greater than 10%.
- In a Monteggia fracture-dislocation, the radial head dislocation is in the same direction as the apex of the ulna fracture.
- In a Galeazzi fracture-dislocation, an increase in the distal radioulnar joint space may be seen on the AP view, and the ulna is displaced dorsally on the lateral view.

EMERGENCY DEPARTMENT CARE AND DISPOSITION

- Nondisplaced fractures are treated with long arm splint immobilization and referral to orthopedics.
- Closed reduction is often adequate for both bone fractures in children.
- Urgent orthopedic referral for open reduction and internal fixation is necessary for all displaced fractures in adults and Monteggia and Galeazzi fracture-dislocations.

For further reading in Tintinalli's *Emergency Medicine: A Comprehensive Study Guide*, 7th ed., see Chapter 267, "Injuries to the Elbow and Forearm," by Jason H. Bredenkamp, Brian P. Jokhy, and Dennis T. Uehara.

174 SHOULDER AND HUMERUS INJURIES

Sandra L. Najarian

STERNOCLAVICULAR JOINT SPRAINS AND DISLOCATION

PATHOPHYSIOLOGY

- The sternoclavicular joint is the most frequently moved, nonaxial joint of the body. Sprains are more common than dislocations or fractures.
- Injuries result from direct trauma or forceful rolling of the shoulder forward or backward.
- Anterior dislocations are more common than posterior dislocations.
- Posterior dislocations can be associated with life-threatening injuries to mediastinal contents.

CLINICAL FEATURES

- Patients with simple sprains have pain and tenderness localized to the joint, whereas patients with dislocations have severe pain that is exacerbated by arm motion and lying supine.
- The medial clavicle is visibly prominent and palpable anterior to the sternum in anterior dislocations.
- The medial clavicle is less visible and often not palpable in posterior dislocations.
- Symptoms of hoarseness, dysphagia, dyspnea, upper extremity paresthesias, or weakness may indicate life-threatening injuries to mediastinal contents, such as pneumothorax or compression or laceration of surrounding great vessels, trachea, and esophagus.

DIAGNOSIS AND DIFFERENTIAL

- CT is the imaging test of choice, and IV contrast may be needed to detect injury to adjacent mediastinal structures.

- Consider septic arthritis in the nontraumatic patient, especially in injection drug users.

EMERGENCY DEPARTMENT CARE AND DISPOSITION

- Treatment for sprains and uncomplicated anterior dislocations includes arm sling, ice, analgesics, and orthopedic referral. Attempted closed reduction is not necessary.
- All posterior dislocations require urgent orthopedic consultation for operative reduction.

CLAVICLE AND SCAPULA FRACTURES

PATHOPHYSIOLOGY

- A direct blow to the shoulder or fall on an outstretched hand is the most common mechanism for fracture.
- The middle third of the clavicle is involved in 80% of clavicle fractures.
- Associated injuries to the adjacent lung and neurovascular structures rarely occur with clavicle fractures.
- Scapula fractures have a high incidence (>75%) of associated injuries to the thoracic cage, ipsilateral lung, and shoulder girdle. The scapula is well protected and requires a significant force to break.
- Rib fractures are the most common injury associated with scapula fracture.

CLINICAL FEATURES

- Patients with clavicle fracture have localized tenderness, swelling, and deformity overlying the clavicle.
- Patients with scapula fractures have localized tenderness over the scapula, hold the ipsilateral arm in adduction, and resist any arm movement.

DIAGNOSIS AND DIFFERENTIAL

- Routine radiographs can miss clavicle and scapula fractures.
- CT can confirm the diagnosis of scapula fracture as well as identify any associated pathology.

EMERGENCY DEPARTMENT CARE AND DISPOSITION

- Treatment includes sling immobilization, ice, analgesics, and early range of motion exercises.
- Orthopedic consultation is warranted for clavicle fractures that are open, have neurovascular compromise, or have persistent skin tenting or interposition of soft tissue.
- The presence of scapular fracture mandates an investigation for associated intrathoracic injuries.
- Displaced glenoid articular fractures, angulated glenoid neck fractures, and certain acromial and coracoid fractures may require surgical intervention.

ACROMIOCLAVICULAR JOINT INJURIES

CLINICAL FEATURES

- Injuries range from mild sprain to complete disruption of all ligaments that attach the scapula and clavicle.
- The mechanism of injury is usually from direct trauma to the shoulder with arm adducted, such as a sports-related injury.
- Patients typically present with tenderness and deformity at the acromioclavicular joint. The classification of injuries and their physical findings are outlined in Table 174-1.

DIAGNOSIS AND DIFFERENTIAL

- Diagnosis is often clinical.
- Stress radiographs are low yield and not recommended.

EMERGENCY DEPARTMENT CARE AND DISPOSITION

- Treatment for Type I and II injuries includes sling immobilization, ice, analgesics, and early range of motion exercises at 7 to 14 days.
- Treatment for Type III injuries is controversial, but the trend favors conservative management with sling immobilization.
- Type IV, V, and VI injuries are severe and require urgent orthopedic consultation for surgical repair.

GLENOHUMERAL JOINT DISLOCATION

CLINICAL FEATURES

- The most common major joint dislocation is the glenohumeral joint dislocation.
- The majority of glenohumeral joint dislocations are anterior.
- The axillary nerve is the most common neurovascular structure injured in anterior dislocations and is tested by pinprick sensation over the skin of the lateral deltoid muscle.

TABLE 174-1 Classification and Physical Findings in Acromioclavicular Joint Injuries

TYPE	INJURY	RADIOGRAPH	EXAMINATION
I	Sprained acromioclavicular ligaments	Normal	Tenderness over acromioclavicular joint
II	Acromioclavicular ligaments ruptured; coracoclavicular ligaments sprained	Slight widening of acromioclavicular joint; clavicle elevated 25%-50% above acromion; may be slight widening of the coracoclavicular interspace	Tenderness and mild step-off deformity of acromioclavicular joint
III	Acromioclavicular ligaments ruptured; coracoclavicular ligaments ruptured; deltoid and trapezius muscles detached	Acromioclavicular joint dislocated 100%; coracoclavicular interspace widened 25%-100%	Distal end of clavicle prominent; shoulder droops
IV	Rupture of all supporting structures; clavicle displaced posteriorly in or through the trapezius	May appear similar to Type II and III; axillary radiograph required to visualize posterior dislocation	Possible posterior displacement of clavicle
V	Rupture of all supporting structures (more severe form of Type III injury)	Acromioclavicular joint dislocated; generally 200%-300% disparity of coracoclavicular interspace compared to normal shoulder	More pain; gross deformity of clavicle
VI	Acromioclavicular ligaments disrupted; coracoclavicular ligaments may be disrupted; deltoid and trapezius muscles disrupted	Acromioclavicular joint dislocated; clavicle displaced inferiorly	Severe swelling; multiple associated injuries

- Table 174-2 describes the various mechanisms of injury, physical findings, and associated injuries with each type of glenohumeral joint dislocation.

DIAGNOSIS AND DIFFERENTIAL

- AP and scapular "Y" view radiographs confirm the type of dislocation and identify any associated fractures.
- The presence of minor fractures, such as a Hill–Sachs lesion or Bankart fracture, does not change ED management.
- Consider omitting pre-reduction radiographs in patients with a history of recurrent shoulder dislocation who present with signs and symptoms of a recurrence in the absence of trauma.

EMERGENCY DEPARTMENT CARE AND DISPOSITION

- Main reduction techniques include traction, leverage, and scapular manipulation.
- Procedural sedation is recommended; however, an intra-articular injection of 10 to 20 mL of 1% lidocaine can facilitate reduction and may obviate the need for sedation.
- Assess neurovascular status and provide sling immobilization after reduction.
- Post-reduction radiographs are useful for confirmation and documentation of successful reduction.
- Urgent orthopedic follow-up is necessary. Shoulder dislocations associated with proximal humerus fractures often mandate orthopedic consultation for surgical repair.

HUMERUS FRACTURES

CLINICAL FEATURES

- Proximal humerus fractures typically occur in elderly patients with osteoporosis after a fall on an outstretched hand.
- Humeral shaft fractures typically occur in active young men and elderly women after direct or indirect trauma to the humeral shaft.
- Patients with proximal humerus fractures present with pain, swelling, ecchymosis, and tenderness over the shoulder with the arm held in adduction.
- Patients with humeral shaft fractures present with localized pain, swelling, tenderness, and abnormal mobility. Shortening of the upper extremity is present in displaced shaft fractures.
- The axillary nerve and the radial nerve are the most commonly injured nerves in proximal humerus and humeral shaft fractures, respectively.

DIAGNOSIS AND DIFFERENTIAL

- Radiographs are confirmatory.
- The Neer classification system divides the proximal humerus into four "parts" (the articular surface of the humeral head, the greater tubercle, the lesser tubercle, and the diaphysis of the humerus) and is used to guide treatment.

TABLE 174-2 Classification and Physical Findings in Dislocations of the Glenohumeral Joint

TYPE	DESCRIPTION/MECHANISM OF INJURY	ASSOCIATED INJURIES
Anterior	Patient presentation: Arm is held in abduction and slight external rotation with shoulder appearing "squared off." Mechanism of injury: Indirect blow with arm in abduction, extension, and external rotation.	Axillary nerve palsy Fracture of the greater tuberosity Fracture of the humeral neck Disruption of the glenoid rim (Bankart lesion) Axillary artery disruption
Subcoracoid	Humeral head is displaced anterior to the glenoid and inferior to the coracoid.	
Subglenoid	Humeral head lies inferior and anterior to the glenoid fossa.	
Subclavicular	Humeral head is displaced medial to the coracoid below the clavicle.	
Intrathoracic	Humeral head lies between the ribs and thoracic cavity.	
Posterior	Patient presentation:	Fractures of the posterior glenoid rim
Subacromial	Arm is adducted and internally rotated.	Fractures of the humeral head (reversed fractures of the Hill-Sachs deformity)
Subglenoid	Anterior shoulder is flat and the posterior aspect full.	
Subspinous	Coracoid process is prominent.	Fractures of the humeral shaft
	Patient will not allow external rotation or abduction because of severe pain.	Fractures of the lesser tuberosity
	Mechanism of injury:	
	Indirect force that produces forceful internal rotation and adduction.	
Inferior (luxatio erecta)	Patient presentation:	Severe soft tissue injuries
	Patient is in severe pain.	Fractures of the proximal humerus
	Humerus is fully abducted.	Rotator cuff tear
	The elbow is flexed.	Neurovascular compression injuries
	Patient's hand is on or behind the head.	
	Humeral head can be palpated on the lateral chest wall.	
	Mechanism of injury:	
	Neck of the humerus is levered against the acromion and inferior capsule tears.	
	Humeral head is forced out inferiorly.	

EMERGENCY DEPARTMENT CARE AND DISPOSITION

- Proximal humerus fractures that are nondisplaced or one-part fractures (displaced less than 1 cm or angulated less than 45 degrees) require sling immobilization, ice, analgesics, and orthopedic referral.
- Humeral shaft fractures that are nondisplaced require a coaptation splint (sugar tong), hanging cast, or functional bracing.
- Multipart proximal humerus fractures, significantly displaced or angulated shaft fractures, open fractures, or any fracture with neurovascular injuries require immediate orthopedic consultation.

For further reading in Tintinalli's *Emergency Medicine: A Comprehensive Study Guide*, 7th ed., see Chapter 268, "Shoulder and Humerus Injuries," by John P. Rudzinski, Laura M. Pittman, Dennis T. Uehara.

175 PELVIS, HIP, AND FEMUR INJURIES

Jeffrey G. Norvell

PELVIS FRACTURES

EPIDEMIOLOGY

- Pelvic fractures are associated with high morbidity and mortality rates because of the immense forces needed to fracture the bony pelvis; concomitant abdominal, chest, and head injuries; and the potential of severe hemorrhage.
- Most pelvic fractures are the result of motor vehicle crashes or falls from height.

CLINICAL FEATURES

- Pelvic fractures should be considered in all patients with serious blunt trauma.

- In patients who are awake and alert, the physical examination is very sensitive for the diagnosis of pelvic fractures.
- Signs and symptoms of pelvic injuries vary from local pain and tenderness to pelvic instability and severe shock.
- Examine the patient for pain, pelvic instability, deformities, lacerations, ecchymoses, and hematomas.
- Rectal examination may reveal rectal injury or a displaced prostate.
- Blood at the urethral meatus may suggest urethral injury.
- A pelvic examination may be necessary to detect lacerations that would suggest an open fracture.
- Avoid excessive movement of unstable pelvic fractures as this could cause further injury.
- Hypotension may be secondary to abdominal or thoracic injuries, or blood loss from disrupted pelvic bones or vessels.

DIAGNOSIS AND DIFFERENTIAL

- An anteroposterior (AP) pelvic radiograph is often used to evaluate for bony injury.
- Other radiographic views include lateral views, AP views of either hemipelvis, internal and external oblique views of the hemipelvis, or inlet and outlet views of the pelvis.
- In an unstable trauma patient, a pelvic radiograph can be used to quickly identify a pelvic fracture and allow for emergent stabilization maneuvers.
- Routine pelvic radiographs are probably not needed in stable trauma patients who will undergo emergent CT scan of the abdomen and pelvis.
- CT is superior to pelvic radiographs for identifying pelvic fractures and evaluating pelvic ring instability. Contrast extravasation on CT scan is 80% to 90% sensitive for the identification of arterial bleeding.
- Consider CT in patients with a high suspicion for pelvic fractures and negative radiographs, or in patients with fractures on radiographs to evaluate for additional injuries.
- Pelvic fractures include those that involve a break in the pelvic ring, fractures of a single bone without a break in the pelvic ring, and acetabular fractures.
- The Young–Burgess classification system for pelvic ring fractures is shown in Table 175-1. This system differentiates fracture patterns based on mechanism of injury and direction of force. The incidence of complications is correlated with fracture pattern.
- Single bone fractures are described in Table 175-2.

EMERGENCY DEPARTMENT CARE AND DISPOSITION

- Due to pelvic bleeding and associated injuries, patients with pelvic fractures may need resuscitation with crystalloid, blood, and blood products.
- Most bleeding in pelvic fractures is due to low-pressure venous bleeding and bleeding from the bone edges. Arterial bleeding occurs in 10% to 15% of patients with pelvic fractures.
- The pelvis can be stabilized with a bedsheet or other pelvic-binding device to reduce pelvic volume and to stabilize fracture ends. The simplest technique is the application of a folded bedsheet tightly wrapped around the pelvis and upper legs and secured by towel clips.
- In hemodynamically unstable patients, evaluate for other locations of bleeding such as the thorax and peritoneal cavity using a chest radiograph and the focused assessment with sonography for trauma (FAST), respectively.
- After excluding other sources for bleeding, treatment for ongoing hemodynamic instability in patients with pelvic fractures includes angiography with embolization and external fixation.
- Angiographic embolization is effective at controlling arterial bleeding, and external fixation is thought to be effective at controlling venous bleeding.
- Hemorrhage refractory to resuscitation is more likely arterial than venous in origin; angiography with possible embolization should be pursued.
- Pelvic ring fractures require orthopedic consultation and hospital admission.
- With the exception of lateral compression type I and anteroposterior compression type I injuries, all pelvic ring fractures require open reduction and internal fixation.
- The management and complications of pelvic ring fractures are described in Table 175-1.
- The treatment and disposition of avulsion and single bone fractures are described in Table 175-2.

ACETABULAR FRACTURES

- Acetabular fractures are usually secondary to a motor vehicle crash.
- If an acetabular fracture is suspected, it can be evaluated with an AP view, a 45-degree iliac oblique view, and a 45-degree obturator oblique view, together known as Judet views.
- CT is more sensitive than radiography in detecting acetabular injury. Also, CT gives additional information about the severity of fracture that is useful in preoperative planning.
- The most common complication is a sciatic nerve injury.

TABLE 175-1 Young-Burgess Classification System and Incidence of Complications

CATEGORY	CHARACTERISTICS	SEVERE HEMORRHAGE (%)	BLADDER RUPTURE (%)	URETHRAL INJURY (%)
Lateral compression fractures	Transverse fracture of pubic rami, ipsilateral or contralateral to posterior injury.			
Type I	I—Sacral compression on side of impact, transverse fractures of pubic rami. *Treatment is bed rest, pain control, followed by protected weightbearing.*	0.5	4.0	2.0
Type II	II—Crescent (iliac wing) fracture on side of impact.	36.0	7.0	0.0
Type III	III—LC-I or LC-II injury on side of impact; contralateral open-book (APC) injury.	60.0	20.0	20.0
APC fractures	Symphyseal diastasis and/or longitudinal rami fractures.			
Type I	I—Slight widening of pubic symphysis and/or anterior SI joint; stretched but intact anterior SI, sacrotuberous, and sacrospinous ligaments; intact posterior SI ligaments. *Treatment is bed rest, pain control, followed by protected weightbearing.*	1.0	8.0	12.0
Type II	II—Widened anterior SI joint; disrupted anterior SI, sacrotuberous, and sacrospinous ligaments; intact posterior SI ligaments. *Treatment is open reduction and internal fixation.*	28.0	11.0	23.0
Type III	III—Complete SI joint disruption with lateral displacement; disrupted anterior SI, sacrotuberous, and sacrospinous ligaments; disrupted posterior SI ligaments. *Treatment is open reduction and internal fixation.*	53.0	14.0	36.0
VS fractures	Symphyseal diastasis or vertical displacement anteriorly and posteriorly, usually through SI joint, occasionally through the iliac wing and/or sacrum; may have a fracture of the ipsilateral transverse process of L5. *Treatment is open reduction and internal fixation.*	75.0	15.0	25.0
Mixed patterns	Combination of other injury patterns, LC/VS being the most common.	58.0	16.0	21.0

Abbreviations: APC = anteroposterior compression, LC = lateral compression, SI = sacroiliac, VS = vertical shear.

- Early orthopedic consultation and hospital admission are indicated for patients with acetabular fractures.
- Early reduction and internal fixation is indicated for displaced fractures.

HIP FRACTURES

EPIDEMIOLOGY

- The vast majority of hip fractures occur in older patients with osteoporosis or other bony pathology secondary to systemic disease.

CLINICAL FEATURES

- The affected leg is classically shortened and externally rotated.
- Patients with a hip fracture will typically have pain at the site of injury, but may also report knee pain or groin pain.
- After performing a primary survey and stabilizing the patient, examine the patient for pain, shortening, rotation, deformities, pelvic instability, and neurovascular status.
- If no significant abnormalities are detected, carefully evaluate range of motion.
- The demographics and clinical features of hip fractures are shown in Table 175-3.

DIAGNOSIS AND DIFFERENTIAL

- The threshold for imaging in elderly patients should be low.
- Radiographic evaluation of the hip includes AP and lateral views. Other radiograph views that may be helpful are an AP view of the pelvis and Judet views. Radiographs of the femur and knee may be indicated.
- Significant pain with weightbearing or inability to bear weight should raise suspicion of occult fracture.

TABLE 175-2 Avulsion and Single Bone Fractures

FRACTURE	DESCRIPTION/MECHANISM OF INJURY	TREATMENT	DISPOSITION AND FOLLOW-UP
Iliac wing (Duverney) fracture	Direct trauma, usually lateral to medial	Analgesics, non-weightbearing until hip abductors pain-free, usually nonoperative	Discharge with orthopedic follow-up in 1-2 wk; admit for open fracture or concerning abdominal examination
Single ramus of pubis or ischium	Fall or direct trauma in elderly; exercise-induced stress fracture in young or in pregnant women	Analgesics, crutches	Discharge with PCP or orthopedic follow-up in 1-2 wk
Ischium body	External trauma or from fall in sitting position; least common pelvic fracture	Analgesics, bed rest, donut-ring cushion, crutches	Discharge with orthopedic follow-up in 1-2 wk
Sacral fracture	Transverse fractures from direct anteroposterior trauma; upper transverse fractures from fall in flexed position	Analgesics, bed rest, surgery may be needed for displaced fractures or neurologic injury	Discharge with orthopedic follow-up 1-2 wk; orthopedic consultation for displaced fractures or neurologic deficits
Coccyx fracture	Fall in sitting position; more common in women	Analgesics, bed rest, stool softeners, sitz baths, donut-ring cushion	PCP or orthopedic follow-up in 2-3 wk; surgical excision of fracture fragment if chronic pain
Anterior superior iliac spine	Forceful sartorius muscle contraction (eg, adolescent sprinters)	Analgesics, bed rest for 3-4 wk with hip flexed and abducted, crutches	Discharge with orthopedic follow-up in 1-2 wk
Anterior inferior iliac spine	Forceful rectus femoris muscle contraction (eg, adolescent soccer players)	Analgesics, bed rest for 3-4 wk with hip flexed, crutches	Discharge with orthopedic follow-up in 1-2 wk
Ischial tuberosity	Forceful contraction of hamstrings	Analgesics, bed rest for 3-4 wk in extension, external rotation, crutches	Discharge with orthopedic follow-up in 1-2 wk

Abbreviation: PCP = primary care physician.

- MRI is very sensitive (near 100%) for identifying occult hip fractures.
- CT may be helpful in identifying fractures not seen on radiographs, but it is not as sensitive as MRI for occult fractures.
- Bone scanning may also be used for the detection of occult fractures.

EMERGENCY DEPARTMENT CARE AND DISPOSITION

- The treatment of hip fractures is listed in Table 175-4.
- If clinical suspicion of an occult fracture is high, obtain CT or MRI imaging in the ED. Alternatively, arrange urgent follow-up for imaging and the patient should remain non-weightbearing.

TABLE 175-3 Proximal Femur Fractures: Demographics and Clinical Features

FRACTURE	INCIDENCE/DEMOGRAPHICS	MECHANISM	CLINICAL FINDINGS
Femoral head	Isolated fracture rare; seen in 6%-16% of hip dislocations; usually result of high-energy trauma; dashboard to flexed knee most common	Superior aspect or impaction fracture in anterior dislocation; inferior aspect in posterior dislocation	Limb shortened and externally rotated (anterior dislocation); shortened, flexed, and internally rotated (posterior dislocation)
Femoral neck	Common in older patients with osteoporosis; rarely seen in younger patients	Low-impact falls or torsion in elderly; high-energy trauma or stress fractures in young	Ranges from pain with weightbearing to inability to ambulate; limb may be shortened and externally rotated
Greater trochanteric	Uncommon; older patients or adolescents	Direct trauma (older patients); avulsion due to contraction of gluteus medius (young patients)	Ambulatory; pain with palpation or abduction
Lesser trochanteric	Uncommon; adolescents (85%) > adults	Avulsion due to forceful contraction of iliopsoas (adolescents); avulsion of pathologic bone (older adults)	Usually ambulatory; pain with flexion or rotation
Intertrochanteric	Common in older patients with osteoporosis; rare in younger patients	Falls; high-energy trauma	Severe pain; swelling; limb shortened and externally rotated
Subtrochanteric	Similar to intertrochanteric; 15% of hip fractures	Falls; high-energy trauma; may also be pathologic	Severe pain; ecchymosis; limb shortened, abducted, and externally rotated

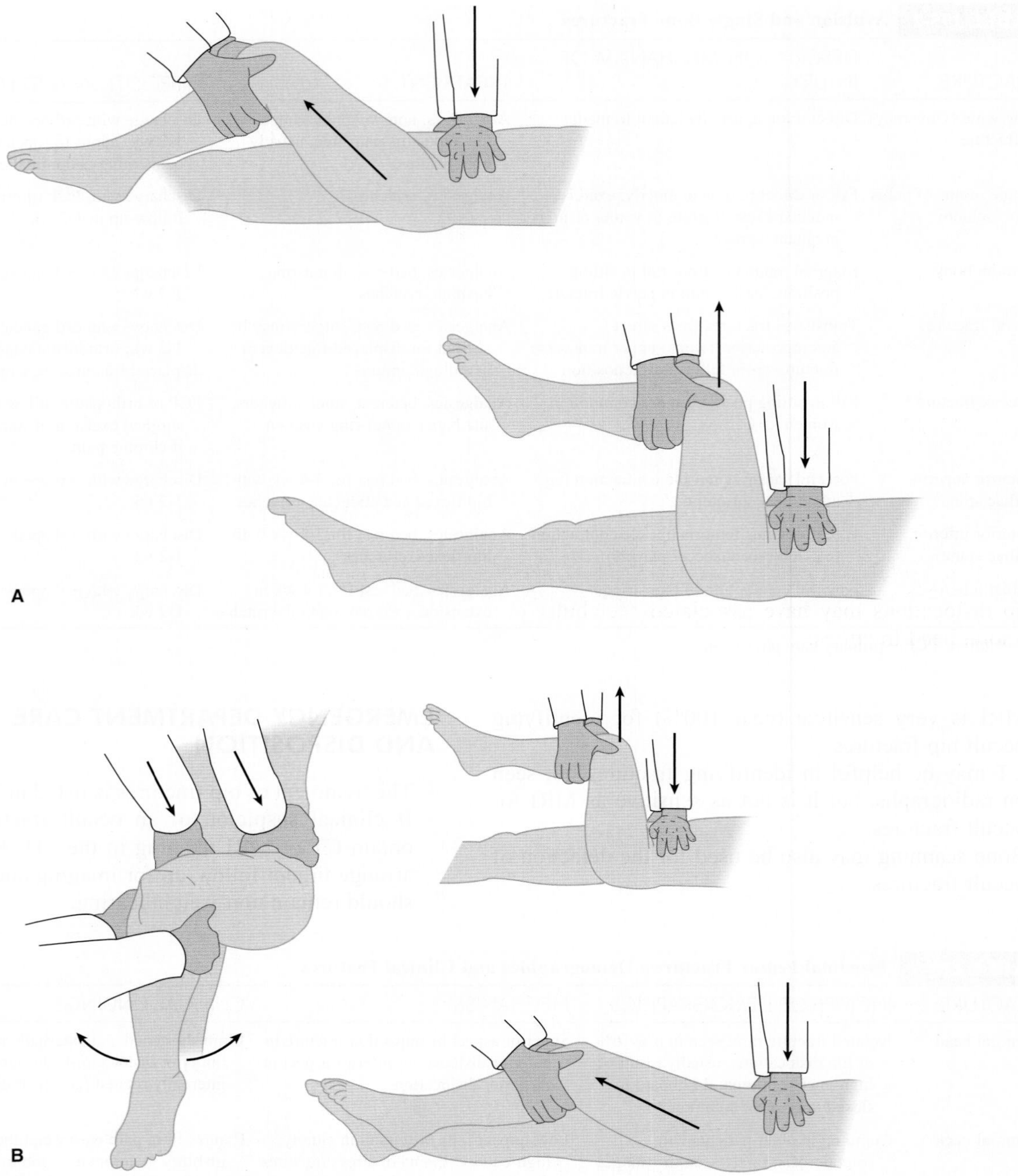

FIG. 175-1. **A** and **B.** Allis maneuver for reduction of posterior hip dislocation.

- Traction devices may be used for immobilization of subtrochanteric fractures. However, if there is concern for neurovascular injury, traction should not be applied.
- Traction is contraindicated in femoral neck fractures.

HIP DISLOCATIONS

- Hip dislocations are true orthopedic emergencies and commonly result from a high-speed motor vehicle crash.
- Ninety percent of dislocations are posterior. Ten percent of dislocations are anterior.

TABLE 175-4 Proximal Femur Fractures: Treatment Issues

FRACTURE	ED MANAGEMENT	DISPOSITION AND FOLLOW-UP	COMPLICATIONS
Femoral head	Immediate orthopedic consultation; emergent closed reduction of dislocation; ORIF if closed unsuccessfully	Admission to orthopedic or trauma service	AVN; post-traumatic arthritis; sciatic nerve injury; heterotopic ossification
Femoral neck	Orthopedic consultation; ranges from nonoperative to total hip arthroplasty	Admission to orthopedic service	AVN; infection; DVT and/or pulmonary embolus
Greater trochanteric	Analgesics; protected weightbearing	Orthopedic follow-up 1-2 wk; possible ORIF if displacement >1 cm	Nonunion rare
Lesser trochanteric	Analgesics; weightbearing as tolerated; evaluate for possible pathologic fracture	Orthopedic or PCP follow-up in 1-2 wk; admit or urgent follow-up for pathologic fracture	Nonunion rare
Intertrochanteric	Orthopedic consultation	Admit for eventual ORIF; may need preoperative testing and clearance by PCP or hospitalist	DVT and/or pulmonary embolism; infection
Subtrochanteric	Orthopedic consultation; Hare® or Sager® splint	Admit for ORIF	DVT and/or pulmonary embolism; infection; malunion (shortened limb); nonunion

Abbreviations: AVN = avascular necrosis, DVT = deep venous thrombosis, ORIF = open reduction and internal fixation, PCP = primary care physician.

- Hip dislocations may have associated acetabular or femoral head fractures.
- Assess neurovascular status.
- Radiographs of the hip and pelvis will evaluate for hip dislocation. Further assessment of the femur and acetabulum may be done with Judet views or CT.
- Reduce hip dislocations within 6 hours in order to decrease the incidence of avascular necrosis.
- One of the most common techniques for hip reduction is described in Fig. 175-1.
- Order post-reduction radiographs or CT to confirm reduction and evaluate for injuries not apparent on initial radiographs.

FEMORAL SHAFT FRACTURES

- Fractures of the femoral shaft occur most commonly in younger patients secondary to high-energy trauma.
- Pathologic fractures may occur due to malignancies.
- Clinical features include pain, swelling, deformity, and shortening.
- Assess the patient for neurovascular status, signs of an open fracture, and other injuries.
- Obtain radiographs to evaluate for fractures.
- ED treatment includes splinting the extremity with a traction splint unless the patient has a sciatic nerve injury or open fracture with grossly contaminated, exposed bone.
- Obtain urgent orthopedic consultation.
- Open fractures require broad-spectrum antibiotics.

For further reading in Tintinalli's *Emergency Medicine: A Comprehensive Study Guide*, 7th ed., see Chapter 269, "Pelvis Injuries," by Mark T. Steele and Jeffrey G. Norvell, and Chapter 270, "Hip and Femur Injuries," by Mark T. Steele and Amy M. Stubbs.

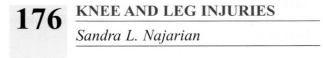

176 KNEE AND LEG INJURIES

Sandra L. Najarian

FRACTURES

CLINICAL FEATURES

- Patients with patellar fractures present with localized tenderness, swelling, and often, a disrupted extensor mechanism (inability to extend the knee or perform a straight leg raise against gravity).
- Transverse fractures are the most common type of patellar fracture; other types include comminuted, non-displaced, vertical, and avulsion-type.
- Patients with femoral condyle fractures present with pain, swelling, deformity, rotation, shortening, and an inability to ambulate.
- Popliteal artery injury, deep peroneal nerve injury, ipsilateral hip dislocation or fracture, and quadriceps mechanism injury can be associated with femoral condyle fractures.

- The tibia is the most commonly fractured long bone.
- Patients with tibial spine fractures present with diffuse knee swelling and tenderness, inability to extend the knee, and a positive Lachman's test.
- Anterior tibial spine fractures are 10 times more common than posterior tibial spine fractures.
- Patients with tibial tuberosity fractures present with tenderness over the proximal anterior tibia and pain with passive or active extension.
- Patients with tibial plateau fractures have pain, swelling, and limited range of motion.
- Ligamentous instability can be present in up to one-third of tibial plateau fractures. Injuries to the anterior cruciate and medial collateral ligament are associated with lateral plateau fractures; injuries to the posterior cruciate and lateral collateral ligaments occur with medial plateau fractures.
- Patients with tibial shaft fractures present with pain, swelling, and crepitance.
- Distal tibial fractures involving the articular surface (tibial plafond or pilon fracture) present with pain, swelling, and tenderness about the ankle.
- A thorough neurovascular examination is necessary as the risk of compartment syndrome is high in tibial shaft and tibial plafond fractures.
- In patients with tibial plafond fractures, a search for other injuries associated with an axial-loading mechanism, such as vertebral body fractures of the lumbar spine, is indicated.
- Proximal fibular fractures may be associated with ankle injuries (Maisonneuve fracture).
- Patients with isolated fibular fracture may be able to bear weight.

DIAGNOSIS AND DIFFERENTIAL

- Use the Ottawa Knee Rules (Table 176-1) or the Pittsburgh Knee Rules (Fig. 176-1) to determine if radiography is needed for knee injuries. These rules have been validated in both children and adults.
- In suspected tibial and fibular injuries, radiographs of the ankle and knee may be necessary to exclude associated fractures.

TABLE 176-1	Ottawa Knee Rules: Radiograph If One Criterion Is Met
Patient age >55 y (rules have been validated for children 2-16 y of age)	
Tenderness at the head of the fibula	
Isolated tenderness of the patella	
Inability to flex knee to 90 degrees	
Inability to transfer weight for four steps both immediately after the injury and in the ED	

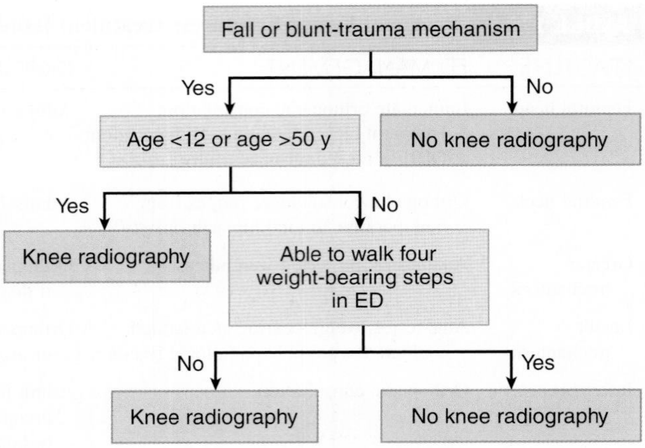

FIG. 176-1. Pittsburgh Knee Rules for radiography. (Reproduced with permission from Seaberg DC, Yealy DM, Lukens T, et al.: Multicenter comparison of two clinical decision rules for the use of radiography in acute, high-risk knee injuries. *Ann Emerg Med* 32:8;1998. Copyright Elsevier.)

EMERGENCY DEPARTMENT CARE AND DISPOSITION

- Table 176-2 describes the mechanism and treatment for the various knee fractures.
- Emergency orthopedic consultation is necessary for the majority of tibial fractures. Open fractures, vascular compromise, and compartment syndrome are indications for emergent operative repair.
- Patients with tibial fractures may be placed in long-leg immobilization and discharged home if they have a low-energy mechanism, have their pain well controlled, and are not at risk for compartment syndrome.
- Proximal fibular fractures associated with ankle injuries require surgical intervention and urgent orthopedic consult.
- Treatment for isolated fibular fractures includes splinting, ice, elevation, and orthopedic or primary care physician follow-up. Patients with less pain may only need knee immobilizer or elastic wrap for immobilization and are encouraged to bear weight as tolerated.

DISLOCATIONS

PATHOPHYSIOLOGY

- Knee dislocations are a result of high-energy mechanisms, such as falls, motor vehicle crashes, and sporting accidents.
- Patellar dislocations are more common in women and result from a twisting injury on an extended knee.

TABLE 176-2 Mechanism of Knee Injury and Treatment

FRACTURE	MECHANISM	TREATMENT
Patella	Direct blow (ie, fall, motor vehicle crash) or forceful contraction of quadriceps muscle	Nondisplaced fracture with intact extensor mechanism: knee immobilizer, rest, ice, analgesia Displaced >3 mm or with disruption of extensor mechanism: above treatment plus early referral for ORIF Severely comminuted fracture: surgical debridement of small fragments and suturing of quadriceps and patellar tendons Open fracture: irrigation and antistaphylococcal antibiotics in the ED; debridement and irrigation in the operating room
Femoral condyles	Fall with axial load or a blow to the distal femur	Incomplete or nondisplaced fractures in any age group or stable impacted fractures in the elderly: long leg splinting and orthopedic referral Displaced fractures or fractures with any degree of joint incongruity: splinting and orthopedic consult for ORIF
Tibial spines and tuberosity	Force directed against flexed proximal tibia in an anterior or posterior direction (ie, motor vehicle crash, sporting injury)	Incomplete or nondisplaced fractures: immobilization in full extension (knee immobilizer) and orthopedic referral in 2-7 d Complete or displaced fracture: early orthopedic referral, often requires ORIF
Tibial tubercle	Sudden force to flexed knee with quadriceps contracted	Incomplete or small avulsion fracture: immobilization Complete avulsion: ORIF
Tibial plateau	Valgus or varus forces combined with axial load that drives the femoral condyle into the tibia (ie, fall, leg hit by car bumper)	Nondisplaced, unilateral fracture: knee immobilizer with non-weightbearing and orthopedic referral in 2-7 d Depression of articular surface: early orthopedic consult for ORIF

Abbreviation: ORIF = open reduction internal fixation.

CLINICAL FEATURES

- Knee dislocations result in significant ligamentous and capsular disruption.
- Anterior dislocation is the most common knee dislocation (40%), followed by posterior dislocations (33%), lateral dislocations (18%), medial dislocations (4%), and rotary dislocations.
- Spontaneous reduction occurs in 50% patients with knee dislocation.
- Multidirectional instability of the knee should raise suspicion for a spontaneously reduced knee dislocation.
- A high incidence of associated injuries to the popliteal artery and peroneal nerve, as well as ligaments and meniscus, exists with knee dislocations.
- Patellar dislocations present with pain and deformity over the knee as the patella is displaced over the lateral condyle.
- Tearing of the medial joint capsule can occur with patellar dislocations.

DIAGNOSIS AND DIFFERENTIAL

- Radiographs are warranted to rule out associated fractures.
- Some recommend arteriography for all patients with confirmed knee dislocations.

EMERGENCY DEPARTMENT CARE AND DISPOSITION

- For knee dislocations, early reduction is essential along with documentation of pre- and post-reduction neurovascular status.
- Immediate orthopedic and vascular surgery consultation is warranted for all confirmed and suspected knee dislocations, and admission is mandatory for observation of neurovascular status. Normal distal pulses do not rule out a popliteal injury.
- For patellar dislocations, closed reduction under procedural sedation is indicated. Flexing the hip and hyperextending the knee while sliding the patella back into place will reduce the patella dislocation.
- Place patients with patellar dislocations in knee immobilization and refer them to orthopedics or primary care for follow-up in 1 to 2 weeks. Patients may bear weight as tolerated, take NSAIDs, and perform isometric quadriceps strengthening exercises.

TENDON INJURIES

PATHOPHYSIOLOGY

- Quadriceps and patellar tendon ruptures result from a forceful contraction on the quadriceps muscle or falling on a flexed knee.

- Patients younger than 40 years old with a history of patellar tendonitis or steroid injections are at risk for patellar tendon rupture.
- Quadriceps rupture is most commonly seen in patients over 40 years of age.
- The Achilles tendon is the strongest and largest tendon in the body.
- Achilles tendon rupture occurs when an eccentric force is suddenly applied to the dorsiflexed foot. It is most frequently ruptured at a point 2 to 6 cm above the calcaneous where the vascular supply is weakest.
- Middle-aged males with subpar athletic conditioning and patients with history of prior steroid or prior quinolone use are at risk for Achilles tendon rupture.

CLINICAL FEATURES

- Patients with quadriceps or patellar tendon rupture have pain and swelling about the knee and will not be able to extend the knee against resistance. A palpable defect is present above or below the knee depending on which tendon is involved.
- Patients with an Achilles tendon rupture have severe pain and are unable to perform toe walk, run, or climb stairs. A positive Thompson test (with the patient lying prone and knee flexed at 90 degrees, the foot fails to plantar flex when the calf is squeezed) is diagnostic.

DIAGNOSIS AND DIFFERENTIAL

- The diagnosis is largely clinical.
- A high riding patella may be seen on the lateral radiograph of the knee with patellar tendon rupture.
- Ultrasound or MRI of the Achilles tendon may be useful when the diagnosis is not clear.

EMERGENCY DEPARTMENT CARE AND DISPOSITION

- Treatment of patellar or quadriceps tendon rupture includes knee immobilization and orthopedic consultation for surgical repair, usually within the first 7 to 10 days after the injury.
- Treatment of an Achilles tendon rupture includes splinting in plantar flexion, non-weightbearing, and referral to orthopedics for possible surgical repair.

LIGAMENTOUS AND MENISCAL INJURIES

CLINICAL FEATURES

- Most ligamentous injuries present with hemarthrosis, although serious ligamentous injuries may present with little pain and no hemarthrosis due to disruption of the capsule.
- Disruption of the anterior cruciate ligament accounts for 75% of all hemarthroses.
- Patients with anterior cruciate ligament tears often describe a "pop" and significant swelling over the next several hours after injury.
- Lachman's test is the most sensitive test for ACL injuries. The anterior drawer and pivot shift test are also useful for diagnosis.
- Posterior cruciate ligament injuries are less common than ACL injuries and may result in a positive posterior drawer test (55% sensitivity); the composite history and examination findings, however, are more accurate for diagnosis.
- Medical and lateral collateral ligament injuries are diagnosed with abduction (valgus) and adduction (varus) stress testing in 30-degree flexion. Laxity greater than 1 cm without a firm end point compared with the other knee is diagnostic for a complete medial or lateral collateral ligament rupture.
- Stress testing for collateral ligaments should be repeated with the knee fully extended. If laxity is detected, then injury has occurred to the cruciate ligaments and posterior capsule.
- Peroneal nerve injuries can occur in lateral injuries.
- Cutting, squatting, and twisting maneuvers can cause injury to the meniscus.
- Meniscal injuries often occur in combination with ligamentous injuries.
- The medial meniscus is injured more commonly than the lateral meniscus.
- Symptoms of meniscal injury include painful locking of the knee; a popping, clicking, or snapping sensation; a sense of instability with activity or joint swelling after activity.
- McMurray's test and other tests for meniscal injury are not sensitive.

DIAGNOSIS AND DIFFERENTIAL

- Radiographs are usually normal or show a joint effusion in ligamentous or meniscal injuries.
- An avulsion fracture at the site of the lateral capsular ligament on the lateral tibial condyle (Segond fracture) is associated with anterior cruciate ligament rupture.
- Outpatient MRI or arthroscopy provides definitive diagnosis.

EMERGENCY DEPARTMENT CARE AND DISPOSITION

- Treatment for ligamentous and mensical injuries includes knee immobilization, ice, elevation, analgesics, and orthopedic referral.

OVERUSE INJURIES

CLINICAL FEATURES

- Patellar tendonitis or "jumper's knee" presents with pain over the patellar tendon worsened by running up hills or standing from a seated position. Patients have point tenderness over the distal aspect of the patella and proximal patellar tendon.
- Patients with shin splints and stress fractures present with activity-induced anterior leg pain initially relieved by rest, but eventually progresses to constant pain. Patients typically describe a change or sudden increase in their training pattern.

DIAGNOSIS AND DIFFERENTIAL

- The diagnosis is clinical. Radiographs are usually normal. If a stress fracture is suspected, an outpatient bone scan or MRI can confirm the diagnosis.

EMERGENCY DEPARTMENT CARE AND DISPOSITION

- Treatment for patellar tendonitis includes heat, NSAIDs, and quadriceps-strengthening exercises. Steroid injections should be avoided.
- Discontinuation of the activity is the treatment for both shin splints and stress fractures.

For further reading in Tintinalli's *Emergency Medicine: A Comprehensive Study Guide*, 7th ed., see Chapter 271, "Knee Injuries," by Jeffrey N. Glaspy and Mark T. Steele, and Chapter 272, "Leg Injuries," by Paul R. Haller.

177 ANKLE AND FOOT INJURIES

Sarah Andrus Gaines

ANKLE INJURIES

PATHOPHYSIOLOGY

- Ankle joint injuries are due to abnormal movement of the talus within the mortise and the resultant stress on the malleoli and ligaments.
- Injuries resulting in disruption of both sides of the joint (malleoli fracture plus ruptured ligament, fracture of both malleoli, or disruption of both ligaments) are unstable.

ANKLE SPRAINS

CLINICAL FEATURES

- Sprains result from abnormal motion of the talus within the mortise, leading to stretching or disruption of the ligaments.
- Typically, the patient is able to bear weight immediately after the injury, with subsequent increase in pain and swelling as the patient continues to ambulate.
- Physical examination reveals tenderness and swelling over the involved ligament with a corresponding lack of tenderness over the bony prominences of the ankle.
- The lateral ankle is injured more frequently, with the anterior talofibular ligament being the most commonly injured ligament.
- Isolated sprain of the medial deltoid ligament is rare, and an associated fibular fracture (Maisonneuve fracture) or syndesmotic ligament injury may be present.
- Joint stability, either on physical examination or radiographically, is the primary determinant of a treatment plan for a sprain.

DIAGNOSIS AND DIFFERENTIAL

- To exclude other injuries, evaluation of the injured ankle begins with examination of the joints above and below the injury.
- Palpate the Achilles tendon for tenderness or a defect, and perform the Thompson test (squeezing the calf while observing for resultant plantar flexion).
- Palpate the proximal fibula for tenderness resulting from a Maisonneuve fracture or fibulotibialis ligament tear.
- Squeeze the fibula toward the tibia to evaluate for syndesmotic ligament injury.
- Palpate the calcaneus, tarsals, and the base of the fifth metatarsal to evaluate for foot fractures causing ankle pain that may not readily be apparent on standard ankle radiograph.
- Palpate the posterior aspects of the medial and lateral malleoli from 6 cm proximally to the distal tips. If tenderness is isolated to the posterior aspect of the lateral malleolus, then a peroneal tendon subluxation may be present.
- The Ottawa Ankle Rules are simple guidelines that have been extensively validated in numerous clinical trials (Fig. 177-1). When applied properly, they can help the emergency physician identify a subset of patients who can be safely treated without undergoing radiographic studies.

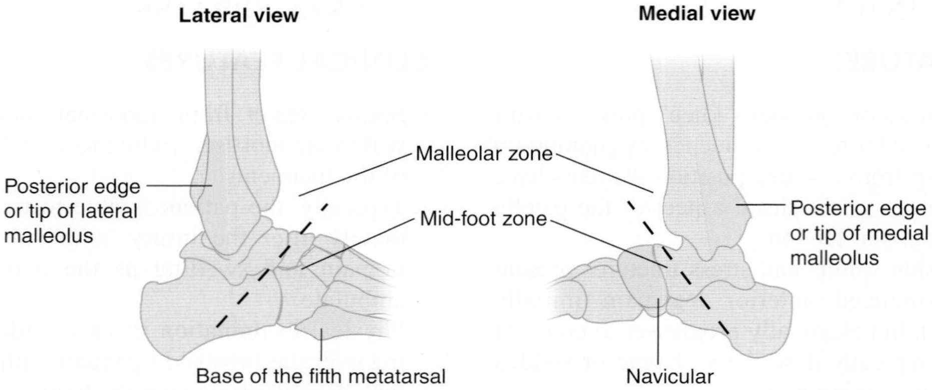

FIG. 177-1. Ottawa Ankle Rules for ankle and midfoot injuries. Ankle radiographs are required only if there is any pain in the malleolar zone or midfoot zone along with bony tenderness in any of these four locations or the inability to bear weight both immediately and in the ED.

- Any asymmetry in the gap between the talar dome and the malleoli on the talus radiographic view suggests joint instability.

EMERGENCY DEPARTMENT CARE AND DISPOSITION

- Treatment for the patient with a stable joint and able to bear weight is analgesics, protection, rest, ice, compression, and elevation (PRICE) for 48 to 72 hours; motion and strength exercises within 48 to 72 hours; and 1-week follow-up if the pain persists. An elastic bandage or ankle brace can be used.
- For patients who have a stable joint and are unable to bear weight, treatment consists of an ankle brace and a 1-week follow-up for repeat examination. Some injuries may require orthopedic consultations and operative repair.
- Patients with unstable joints require a posterior splint and referral to an orthopedist for definitive care.

ANKLE FRACTURES

- Ankle fractures are classified as unimalleolar, bimalleolar, and trimalleolar. Bi-and trimalleolar fractures require open reduction-internal fixation (ORIF).
- ED care includes posterior splinting, elevation, ice application, and initiating orthopedic consultation.
- Unimalleolar fractures are usually treated with non-weight posterior splinting and orthopedic follow-up. Minimally displaced, small (<3 mm) avulsion fractures of the fibula are treated like ankle sprains.
- Open fractures require wet sterile dressing coverage, splinting, and administration of tetanus toxoid, as necessary, and a first-generation cephalosporin (eg, cefazolin) and immediate orthopedic consultation.
- If gross contamination is noted, then add tetanus immunoglobulin and an aminoglycoside to the treatment regimen.

ANKLE DISLOCATIONS

- Posterior dislocations are the most common and occur with a backward force on the plantarflexed foot, usually resulting in rupture of the tibiofibular ligaments or a lateral malleolus fracture.
- If vascular compromise is present, indicated by absent pulses, a dusky foot, or skin tenting, immediate reduction by the emergency physician is warranted.
- Reduction is performed by grasping the heel and foot and applying downward traction with analgesia and sedation as indicated.
- Follow successful reduction by performing splinting, post-reduction neurovascular examination, radiographic evaluation, and immediate orthopedic consultation in the ED.

FOOT INJURIES

PATHOPHYSIOLOGY

- The foot is divided into the hindfoot, midfoot, and forefoot. The Chopart joint separates the hind- and midfoot and the Lisfranc joint separates the mid- and forefoot. Foot injuries most commonly result from direct or twisting forces, with twisting-type mechanisms resulting in more minor avulsion-type injuries.

- The first metatarsal bears twice the weight of any other metatarsal, necessitating a more conservative approach to fracture management.
- The base of the second metatarsal is an important component of the Lisfranc complex and any sign of injury warrants caution.
- Major fractures of the talus and subtalar dislocations are at risk for avascular necrosis because of the tenuous blood supply of the foot.

Hindfoot Injuries

- Small avulsion fractures of the talus are treated with posterior splinting and orthopedic follow-up.
- Major fractures of the talar neck and body and subtalar dislocations require immediate orthopedic consultation.
- Calcaneal injuries require a large force and associated injuries are common. Compression fractures of the calcaneus require the measurement of the Boehler angle (formed by the intersection of a line connecting the posterior tuberosity and apex of the posterior facet and a line from the posterior facet to the apex of the anterior facet, on the lateral radiograph view). An angle <25 degrees increases the likelihood of a fracture. Treatment consists of posterior splinting, elevation, analgesics, and orthopedic consultation.

Midfoot Injuries

- Pain with torsion of the midfoot is suspicious for a Lisfranc injury as are injuries about the tarsometatarsal joint.
- Lisfranc joint injuries are often associated with a fracture, especially at the base of the second metatarsal.
- On radiograph, a gap >1 mm between the bases of the first and second metatarsals is considered unstable.
- Lisfranc joint injuries require CT and orthopedic consultation.
- Isolated navicular, cuboid, and cuneiform injuries are rare and treated conservatively.

Forefoot Injuries

- Treat nondisplaced metatarsal shaft fractures with a posterior splint or orthopedic shoe, with the exception of keeping fractures of the first metatarsal non-weightbearing.
- Fractures with at least 3-4 mm displacement require surgical reduction.
- Treat pseudo-Jones avulsion fractures with a walking cast.
- Treat the true Jones fracture (metaphyseal-diaphyseal junction fracture) with a non-weightbearing cast and orthopedic follow-up for potential surgery.
- Treat nondisplaced phalangeal fractures with buddy taping and a stiff-soled cast shoe.
- Treat displaced phalangeal fractures and dislocations with digital block, reduction by manual traction, and buddy taping.

CRUSH INJURY AND COMPARTMENT SYNDROME

- A crushed foot that becomes tensely swollen and is associated with complaints of pain out of proportion to physical examination findings suggests the possibility of compartment syndrome.
- Typically, pain is not relieved by elevation of the foot and is increased with passive dorsiflexion of the great toe.
- Distal neurovascular examination may yield normal results.
- Diagnosis is made by measurement of intracompartmental pressure.

For further reading in Tintinalli's *Emergency Medicine: A Comprehensive Study Guide*, 7th ed., see Chapter 273, "Ankle Injuries," by Daniel A. Handel and Sarah Andrus Gaines, and Chapter 274, "Foot Injuries," by Sarah Andrus Gaines, Daniel A. Handel, and Peter N. Ramsey.

178 COMPARTMENT SYNDROME

Sandra L. Najarian

PATHOPHYSIOLOGY

- Compartment syndromes result from elevated pressures within a confined muscle compartment that result in functional and circulatory impairment of that limb.
- External compressive forces on a compartment, such as a tight dressing or cast, or an increase in volume within a compartment, usually from hemorrhage and/or edema, are the mechanisms by which compartment syndrome occurs.
- The most common compartments affected are in the leg and forearm.
- Tissue perfusion is defined as the difference between arterial pressure and the pressure of venous return, and perfusion diminishes as tissue pressure increases.
- Normal tissue pressure is <10 mm Hg.
- The exact pressure elevation at which cell death occurs is unclear.

- Traditionally, compartment pressures between 30 and 50 mm Hg are detrimental to nerve and muscle if pressures remain elevated for several hours.
- The "delta pressure" is the diastolic pressure minus the measured intracompartmental pressure. It is thought to be a better predictor of the potential for irreversible muscle damage.
- Hypotensive patients do not tolerate elevated compartment pressures as well as normotensive patients.

CLINICAL FEATURES

- Severe and difficult-to-control pain, pain out of proportion to examination, and pain with passive stretch are the hallmarks of this syndrome.
- Nerve dysfunction often accompanies the pain and manifests as burning or dysesthesias in the sensory distribution of the nerve.
- On clinical examination, the compartment is swollen, firm, and tender to palpation, but the affected limb will maintain color, temperature, and a detectable pulse until late in the course of the disease process.
- Untreated compartment syndrome results in muscle necrosis and permanent muscle contracture (Volkmann's ischemia).

DIAGNOSIS AND DIFFERENTIAL

- A high index of suspicion based on mechanism of injury is essential to making the diagnosis, especially in unconscious or obtunded patients.
- If the diagnosis is in question after the clinical examination, then direct measurement of the compartment is indicated.
- Several commercial devices are available to measure compartment pressures.
- A "delta pressure" $\leq$30 mm Hg is most commonly used to diagnose acute compartment syndrome.

EMERGENCY DEPARTMENT CARE AND DISPOSITION

- Surgical fasciotomy is indicated once the diagnosis is confirmed.
- Administer oxygen, remove restrictive casts or dressings, correct hypotension, and elevate affected limb to the level of the heart while arranging for definitive management.
- Functional outcomes are favorable when diagnosis and treatment of compartment syndrome occurs within 6 hours of onset.

For further reading in Tintinalli's *Emergency Medicine: A Comprehensive Study Guide*, 7th ed., see Chapter 275, "Compartment Syndrome," by Paul R. Haller.

Section 21
MUSCULOSKELETAL DISORDERS

179 NECK AND THORACOLUMBAR PAIN

Amy M. Stubbs

EPIDEMIOLOGY

- Neck and back pain are common complaints and account for approximately 2% of all physician office visits.
- Myelopathy is the most common cause of spastic paraparesis in patients >55 years old.
- In the majority of atraumatic neck and back pain cases, no specific cause can be identified.
- Patients <18 years old or >50 years old with back pain are more likely to have serious underlying pathology.

PATHOPHYSIOLOGY

- Nontraumatic neck and back pain are often due to nonspecific musculoskeletal causes.
- Radiculopathy is caused by compression of a single spinal nerve root.
- Myelopathy is seen with spinal cord dysfunction, which may be caused by a lesion, stenosis, or compression.
- Knowledge of spinal anatomy, specific dermatomes, and spinal nerve innervations may guide the examiner to a particular cause or location of pathology.

CLINICAL FEATURES

- Neck pain patients can be classified into two groups: (1) those with pain from joint or muscular components, and (2) those with signs of radiculopathy or myelopathy. Symptoms and historical features of these groups are summarized in Table 179-1.
- Back pain can be divided into groups based on duration of symptoms: acute (<6 weeks), subacute (between 6 and 12 weeks), and chronic (>12 weeks).
- A positive straight leg raise test causes radicular pain of the affected leg radiating to below the knee (see Fig. 179-1).
- Signs and symptoms of radiculopathy include sensory abnormalities (paresthesias or numbness), motor

TABLE 179-1 Historical Clues to Differentiate Muscular Neck Pain from Nerve Root or Spinal Cord Related Pain

GROUP 1: CERVICAL PROBLEMS ARISING MAINLY FROM NECK JOINTS AND ASSOCIATED LIGAMENTS AND MUSCLES	GROUP 2: CERVICAL PROBLEMS INVOLVING THE CERVICAL NERVE ROOTS OR THE SPINAL CORD
Patients complain of pain and stiffness.	Patients complain of significant root pain, typically sharp, intense, and may be described as "burning."
Pain is a deep, dull aching sensation and often episodic.	Pain may radiate to the trapezial and periscapular areas or down the arm.
Patients have a history of excessive or unaccustomed activity or of sustaining an awkward posture.	Patients complain of numbness and motor weakness in a myotomal distribution.
There is no history of specific injury.	Headache may occur if the upper cervical roots are involved.
Ligament and muscle pain are localized and asymmetric.	Symptoms often become more severe with neck hyperextension (especially when the head is toward the affected extremity).
Pain from upper cervical segments is referred toward the head, and pain from lower segments, to the upper limb girdle.	Patients may experience gradual onset of shocklike sensations spreading down spine to extremities.
Symptoms are aggravated by neck movement and relieved by rest.	Most common myelopathy at the level of the fifth cervical vertebra and affects shoulder abduction (deltoid) and external rotation (infraspinous).

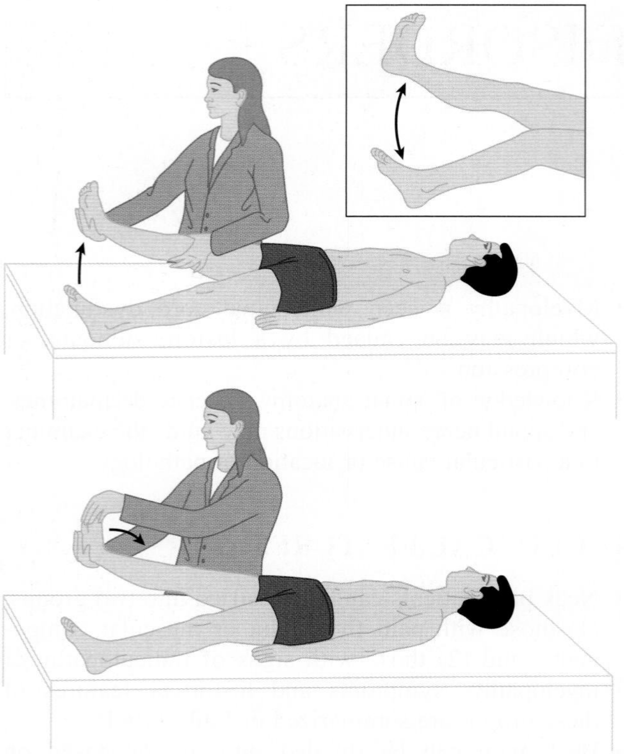

FIG. 179-1. Straight leg raise testing. Instructions for the straight leg raising test. 1. Ask the patient to lie as straight as possible on a table in the supine position. 2. With one hand placed above the knee of the leg being examined, exert enough firm pressure to keep the knee fully extended. Ask the patient to relax. 3. With the other hand cupped under the heel, slowly raise the straight limb. Tell the patient "If this bothers you, let me know, and I will stop." 4. Monitor for any movement of the pelvis before complaints are elicited. True sciatic tension should elicit complaints before the hamstrings are stretched enough to move the pelvis. 5. Estimate the degree of leg elevation that elicits complaint from the patient. Then determine the most distal area of discomfort: back, hip, thigh, knee, or below the knee. 6. While holding the leg at the limit of straight leg raising, dorsiflex the ankle. Note whether this aggravates the pain. Internal rotation of the limb can also increase the tension on the sciatic nerve roots.

weakness, and diminished reflexes in a dermatomal distribution.

- Signs and symptoms of cervical and lumbar radiculopathy are summarized in Table 179-2 and Fig. 179-2.
- Thoracic nerve root compression may result in pain that radiates to the chest or abdomen.
- Insidious onset of pain, impaired fine motor movements, gait disturbances, hyperreflexia or clonus, and sexual or bladder dysfunction may be seen with myelopathy. A positive Babinski sign may also be observed.
- Urinary retention, with or without overflow incontinence, is the most common finding in cauda equina syndrome. Other common findings include diminished rectal tone and saddle anesthesia (numbness over the buttocks, upper posterior thighs, and perineal regions).
- Specific physical examination findings that are characteristic of spinal pathology are summarized in Table 179-3.
- Many patients with neck and back pain complain of localized stiffness and decreased range of motion. Often the pain is worsened with certain movements or positions.
- Pain in conjunction with systemic complaints such as fever, night sweats, or weight loss is concerning for malignancy, infection, or rheumatologic disease. Night pain or unremitting pain is also suggestive of serious pathology.
- Pain from disc herniation is often exaggerated by coughing, valsalva, or sitting.
- Pain from spinal stenosis is characterized by bilateral sciatic pain exacerbated by walking, standing, or back extension. It may be relieved by rest or flexion of the spine.

DIFFERENTIAL AND DIAGNOSIS

- The majority of patients with nontraumatic neck and back pain do not require imaging or laboratory tests.
- For patients with history of recent trauma and cervical spine pain, the National Emergency X-Radiography Utilization Study (NEXUS) criteria are useful to determine the need for imaging (see Chapter 163 for further reading on spinal trauma).
- Plain radiographs of the spine have low sensitivity but may be of use in some subsets of patients. Three views of the cervical spine may be useful in patients with chronic neck pain with or without history of trauma, neck pain, and history of malignancy or prior neck surgery, or those with neck pain and known spinal disorders. Anterior-posterior and lateral radiographs of the thoracic and/or lumbar spine should be considered if suspicion exists for tumor, infection, or fracture.
- Abnormal plain radiographs or neurologic deficits on examination should prompt further imaging.
- Flexion-extension films of the cervical spine may help identify spinal instability.
- CT scanning is valuable in diagnosing bony pathology, but insensitive for nerve root or spinal cord disorders.
- **MRI is the test of choice for patients with neck or back pain and neurologic deficits.**
- CT myelography is an alternative when MRI is contraindicated.
- If serious pathology (eg, malignancy, infection) is suspected, a complete blood count (CBC), erythrocyte sedimentation rate (ESR), and urinalysis should be ordered. ESR has a sensitivity of 90% to 98% for infectious causes of spinal pain.

TABLE 179-2 Signs and Symptoms of Cervical Radiculopathy

DISK SPACE	CERVICAL ROOT	PAIN COMPLAINT	SENSORY ABNORMALITY	MOTOR WEAKNESS	ALTERED REFLEX
C1-C2	C2	Neck, scalp	Scalp		
C4-C5	C5	Neck, shoulder, upper arm	Shoulder	Infraspinatus, deltoid, biceps	Reduced biceps reflex
C5-C6	C6	Neck, shoulder, upper medial, scapular area, proximal forearm, thumb, index finger	Thumb and index finger, lateral forearm	Deltoid, biceps, pronator teres, wrist extensors	Reduced biceps and brachioradialis reflex
C6-C7	C7	Neck, posterior arm, dorsum proximal forearm, chest, medial third of scapula, middle finger	Middle finger, forearm	Triceps, pronator teres	Reduced triceps reflex
C7-T1	C8	Neck, posterior arm, ulnar side of forearm, medial inferior scapular border, medial hand, ring, and little fingers	Ring and little fingers	Triceps, flexor carpi ulnaris, hand intrinsics	Reduced triceps reflex

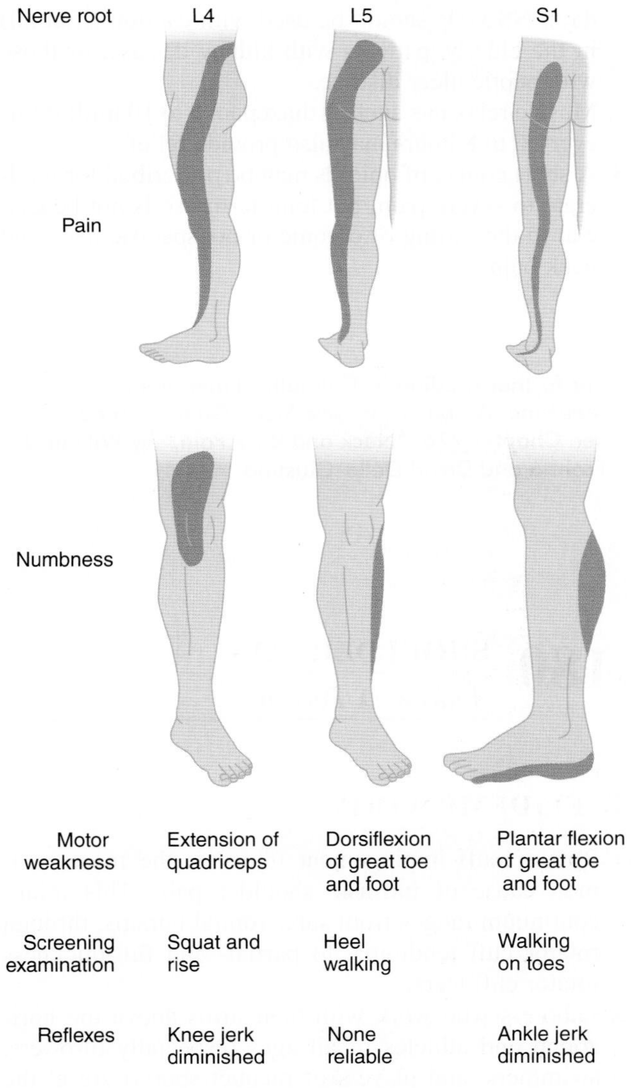

FIG. 179-2. Testing for lumbar nerve root compromise.

- Bowel or bladder incontinence in conjunction with back pain should raise concern for epidural compression. A post-void residual (determined by catheterization or bedside ultrasound) of >100 mL suggests incomplete bladder emptying (and therefore suggests that any incontinence is overflow incontinence).
- Mechanical disorders may result in acute or chronic neck pain; the majority of cases arise from motor vehicle collisions, falls, sports injuries, and work-related injuries. (See Chapter 163 for further discussion of spinal injuries.)
- Cervical disc herniation, spondylosis, or spinal stenosis may result in radiculopathy or myleopathy. Herniation and spondylosis are most common at levels C5-C6 and C6-C7.
- The risk of cervical myelopathy increases if the spinal canal diamter is reduced to <13 mm; this may occur from congenital narrowing, osteophyte formation, or buckling of the ligamentum flavum.
- The differential diagnosis for nontraumatic neck pain includes metastatic cancer, myofascial pain syndrome, temporal arteritis, and ischemic heart disease.
- Thoracic compression fractures are seen in the elderly, and in patients with osteoporosis.
- Patients with sciatica generally complain more of radicular symptoms than back pain.
- Ninety-five percent of lumbar disc herniations occur at the L4-L5 or L5-S1 levels.
- Spinal cord compression, cauda equina syndrome, and conus medullaris syndrome comprise epidural compression syndromes and may initially present in a similar fashion (weakness, sensory changes, and autonomic dysfunction).
- Epidural compression may be caused by malignancy, abscess, or massive midline disc herniation.

TABLE 179-3 Examination Findings Associated with Spinal Pathology

SIGN	TECHNIQUE	SIGNIFICANCE
Spurling	Gentle pressure applied to the patient's head during extension and lateral rotation	May reproduce radicular pain with radiation into the ipsilateral upper extremity
Abduction relief	Patient places hand of affected upper extremity on top of head to obtain relief from pain	Indicates soft disc protrusion causing radicular pain
Lhermitte	Neck flexion	Elicits electric shock sensation in spine and extremities from cord compression
Hoffman	Flick tip of middle finger while hand is relaxed in neutral position	Flexion of thumb and index finger indicates upper motor neuron lesion
Straight leg raise	Lift affected leg to 70 degrees with patient lying flat	Pain radiating below knee in affected leg indicates disc herniation (L4-L5 or L5-S1)
Crossed straight leg raise test	Leg opposite affected leg lifted to 70 degrees with patient lying flat	Pain radiating down affected leg is specific (but not sensitive) for disc herniation

Compression due to hemorrhage or hematoma should also be considered in patients at risk for coagulopathy.
- Spinal infections such as discitis, osteomyelitis, and epidural abscess should also be considered, especially in the setting of immunocompromise or intravenous drug abuse. The ESR will typically be elevated. MRI is preferred for diagnosis.
- Transverse myelitis, ruptured aortic aneurysm, pancreatitis, posterior lower lobe pneumonia, herpetic neuralgia, and renal colic or infarct should be included in the differential for back pain.

EMERGENCY DEPARTMENT CARE AND DISPOSITION

- Patients with neck or back pain accompanied by significant or progressive neurologic deficits require emergent imaging (ideally MRI), and admission to the appropriate service.
- For suspected epidural compression, dexamethasone 10 milligrams IV should be given prior to imaging.
- For patients with suspected spinal infection, broad-spectrum intravenous antibiotics, such as piperacillin-tazobactam (3.375 grams) and vancomycin (1 gram), should be given unless directed otherwise by consultants.
- Patients with nonspecific neck and back pain or a stable, mild radiculopathy may be managed conservatively and discharged with pain medication, explicit return precautions for worsening symptoms, and instructions to return to routine activity. Those who fail conservative management may require MRI and surgical referral.
- Pain management options include acetaminophen (650-975 milligrams every 4-6 hours) alone or in combination with nonsteroidal anti-inflammatory drugs (NSAIDs) such as ibuprofen (800 milligrams twice a day) or naproxen (250-500 milligrams twice a day). NSAIDs should be used with caution (if at all) in the elderly, patients with kidney disease, or those with peptic ulcer disease.
- Muscle relaxants such as diazepam 5 to 10 milligrams every 6 to 8 hours may also provide relief.
- A short course of opioids may be prescribed for moderate to severe pain, but long-term use is not beneficial in the setting of chronic or nonspecific neck and back pain.

For further reading in Tintinalli's *Emergency Medicine: A Comprehensive Study Guide*, 7th ed., see Chapter 276, "Neck and Back Pain," by William J. Frohna and David Della-Giustina.

180 SHOULDER PAIN

Andrew D. Perron

EPIDEMIOLOGY

- Rotator cuff impingement injury is the most common cause of intrinsic shoulder pain. This injury continuum ranges from subacromial bursitis, through rotator cuff tendinitis, to partial- and full-thickness rotator cuff tears.
- Laborers who work with their arms above the horizontal and athletes of all ages (especially throwers, swimmers, and players of racquet sports) are at the highest risk for shoulder overuse syndromes.

- Adhesive capsulitis ("frozen shoulder") is most common in postmenopausal, diabetic women younger than 70 years. It is rarely associated with rotator cuff tears and is frequently associated with prior immobilization, trauma, or cervical disc disease.

PATHOPHYSIOLOGY

- The muscles of the rotator cuff (supraspinatus, infraspinatus, teres minor, and subscapularis) are dynamic stabilizers of the glenohumeral joint and provide much of the power for shoulder movement.
- The muscles of the rotator cuff must function within the coracoacromial arch, between the humeral head and the coracoid, acromion, and acromioclavicular ligament. They also function beneath the deltoid muscle and subacromial bursa. The rotator cuff is therefore prone to compression and impingement.
- The biceps tendon inserts on the glenoid labrum after passing between the subscapularis and supraspinatus tendons, and assists with rotator cuff function. The long head of the biceps can become impinged due to its location.
- The biceps tendon can rupture or become subluxed or dislocated out of the bicipital groove of the humerus.
- Activities that cause repeated compression of these structures can cause impingement syndromes.
- The supraspinatus muscle or its tendon is the most commonly injured rotator cuff structure.
- Calcific tendinitis, associated with reversible calcium hydroxyapatite deposition within one or more rotator cuff tendons, is most common in the supraspinatus tendon.
- Adhesive capsulitis is associated with idiopathic fibrosis and scarring of the shoulder joint capsule.

CLINICAL FEATURES

- Subacromial bursitis is commonly associated with positive impingement tests and tenderness at the lateral proximal humerus or in the subacromial space.
- Rotator cuff tendinitis is more common between ages 25 and 40 years and is associated with signs of impingement, tenderness of the rotator cuff, and rotator cuff muscular weakness (Fig. 180-1).
- Decreased range of motion, crepitus, weakness, or atrophy of shoulder muscles may accompany various causes of shoulder pain, especially the more severe impingement syndromes.
- Neer's test involves compressing the rotator cuff and subacromial bursa as the examiner forcibly but smoothly fully forward flexes the straightened arm. Pain is associated with a positive test.

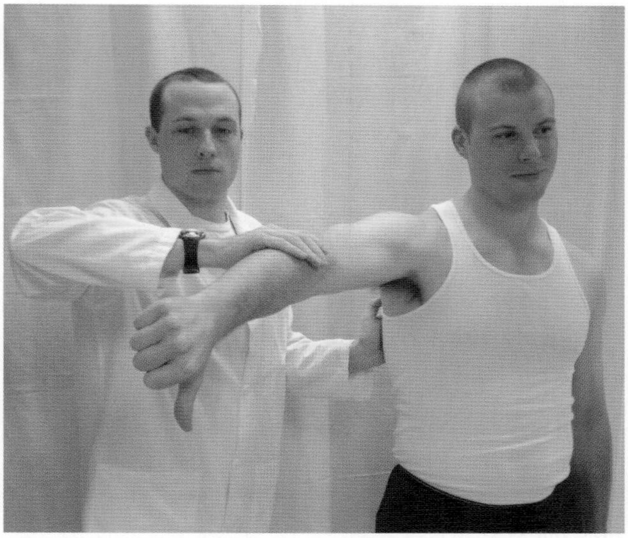

FIG. 180-1. The "empty beer can" position (aka supraspinatus load test) isolates the supraspinatus tendon. Pain indicates tendon irritation and weakness can indicate a rotator cuff tear.

- Hawkins' test involves inward rotation of an arm previously placed in 90 degrees of abduction and 90 degrees of elbow flexion. Inward rotation of the arm across the front of the body compresses the rotator cuff and bursa between the coracoacromial ligament and the humeral head. Pain is associated with a positive test (Fig. 180-2).
- Speed's and Yergason's tests are used to identify biceps tendon pathology.

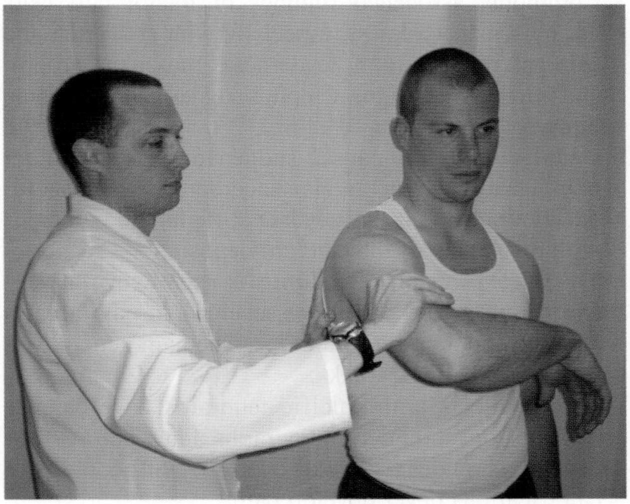

FIG. 180-2. Hawkins' impingement test. The examiner positions the patient's shoulder at 90 degrees of abduction and 90 degrees of elbow flexion. The examiner then rotates the shoulder internally and brings the patient's arm across the front of the patient.

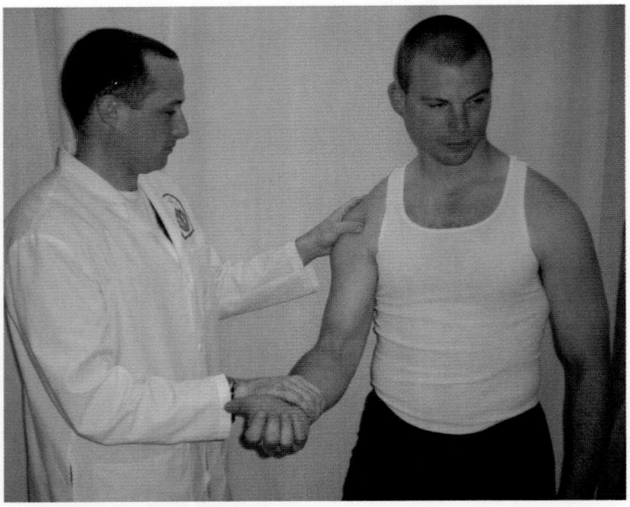

FIG. 180-3. Yergason's test is used to identify bicipital tendonitis. With the patient's elbow flexed at 90 degrees, the examiner palpates the bicipital groove as the patient attempts forearm supination against resistance. Pain or instability at the proximal bicipital groove indicates biceps tendonitis or tendon subluxation.

- A positive Speed's test finds pain in the anterior shoulder with resisted forward flexion of the shoulder when the elbow is extended and forearm supinated.
- A positive Yergason's test finds pain in the anterior shoulder with the elbow flexed to 90 degrees when forearm supination is resisted (Fig. 180-3).
- Acute injuries to the rotator cuff generally involve acute traumatic forced hyperabduction or hyperextension of the shoulder.
- Rotator cuff tears may be partial or full thickness.
- Commonly associated findings of rotator cuff tears are muscular weakness, especially with abduction and external rotation, cuff tenderness, muscular atrophy, and impingement signs. Crepitus suggests more chronic injury.
- Calcific tendinitis causes sudden onset of shoulder pain, usually at rest, and is exacerbated by any shoulder motion. It is usually worse at night and coincides with resorption of the calcium deposit.
- The onset of calcific tendinitis is usually over a very short time period and more severe than pain associated with rotator cuff tendinitis. The pain generally is self-limited after 2 weeks.
- Some patients with calcific tendinitis have calcific deposits on shoulder radiographs long before they develop shoulder pain, and over 60% of people with calcifications never develop pain.
- Adhesive capsulitis often follows periods of immobilization of the shoulder, and causes diffuse aching, especially at night, and limited passive and active range of motion. Pain is reproduced at the limits of motion, but not by palpation.
- Primary osteoarthritis is associated with degenerative disease in other joints. Osteoarthritis of the shoulder is rare, as it is not a weight-bearing joint.
- Osteoarthritis is often present in multiple joints, but is especially likely in a previously injured shoulder.
- Osteoarthritis causes pain with activity, and is relieved with rest.

DIAGNOSIS AND DIFFERENTIAL

- The most specific radiographic sign for large rotator cuff tears is a narrowing of the acromiohumeral space (<7 mm).
- Radiographs are rarely diagnostic, but help detect abnormal calcifications with calcific bursitis, osteophytes, or other arthritic changes, or subtle glenohumeral dislocations, which can be mistaken for adhesive capsulitis.
- Extrinsic causes of shoulder pain should be considered in the differential diagnosis, and these include acute cardiac, pulmonary, aortic, and abdominal pathology.
- Cervical spine radiculopathy, brachial plexus disorders, Pancoast's tumor, and axillary artery thrombosis must be considered in the evaluation of shoulder pain.

EMERGENCY DEPARTMENT CARE AND DISPOSITION

- Reduction of pain and inflammation is the goal of emergency department care. This usually involves nonsteroidal anti-inflammatory drugs, "relative rest," cryotherapy (icing), and immobilization. "Relative rest" means avoidance of painful activities.
- Gentle range-of-motion exercises should begin as soon as pain allows.
- A potential complication of local steroid injection is tendon rupture.

For further reading in Tintinalli's *Emergency Medicine: A Comprehensive Study Guide*, 7th ed., see Chapter 277, "Shoulder Pain," by David Della Giustina and Benjamin Harrison.

181 HIP AND KNEE PAIN

Jeffrey L. Hackman

DIAGNOSIS OF KNEE AND HIP DISEASES AND SYNDROMES

- Most knee and hip diseases and syndromes are diagnosed or suggested by a focused history and physical examination (see Table 181-1).

REGIONAL NERVE ENTRAPMENT SYNDROMES

MERALGIA PARESTHETICA

- Compressive inflammation of the lateral femoral cutaneous nerve is the most common lower extremity nerve entrapment syndrome.
- Symptoms include pain in the hip, thigh, or groin, burning or tingling paresthesias, and hypersensitivity to light touch.
- Tapping over the anterior superior iliac spine may reproduce the pain.
- Treatment involves removing the source of irritation (eg, obesity, pregnancy, tight pants belt) and NSAIDs.

OBTURATOR NERVE ENTRAPMENT

- The nerve is most commonly entrapped by pelvic fractures, causing pain in the groin and down the inner thigh.
- Other causes include fascial bands at the distal obturator canal in athletes, pelvic masses, and pelvic hematomas.

TABLE 181-1 Suggested Clues for the Differential Diagnosis of Hip and Knee Pain

Determine the location of the pain to narrow down the potential diagnosis.
Determine the activities that bring on the pain.
The knee "giving out" or "buckling" generally is due to pain and reflex muscle inhibition rather than an acute neurologic emergency. This complaint may also represent patellar subluxation or ligamentous injury and joint instability.
Poor conditioning or quadriceps weakness generally causes anterior knee pain of the patellofemoral syndrome; therapy should address this weakness.
Locking of the knee suggests a meniscal injury, which may be chronic.
A popping sensation or sound at the onset of pain is reliable for a ligamentous injury.
A recurrent effusion after activity suggests a meniscal injury.
Pain at the joint line suggests a meniscal injury.

ILIOINGUINAL NERVE ENTRAPMENT

- Hypertrophy of the abdominal wall musculature or pregnancy may cause entrapment.
- Pain and hypoesthesia may be exacerbated by hyperextension of the hip.

PIRIFORMIS SYNDROME

- Irritation of the sciatic nerve by the piriformis muscle causes pain in the buttocks and hamstring muscles.
- Pain is exacerbated by sitting, climbing stairs, or squatting.

PSOAS ABSCESS

- Abscess of the psoas muscle may present with abdominal pain radiating to the hip or flank, fever, and limp.
- *Staphylococcus aureus* is the most common pathogen (80%).
- The diagnosis is made by CT.
- Treatment includes antibiotics and surgical drainage.

BURSAL SYNDROMES OF THE HIP AND KNEE

- Hip and knee bursae may cause localized pain due to inflammation, infection, rheumatologic disorders (psoriatic arthritis, rheumatoid arthritis, ankylosing spondylitis), or crystalline disease (gout, pseudogout).
- Infection may be difficult to distinguish from noninfectious inflammation.
- Table 181-2 describes characteristics of the bursal syndromes.
- Figure 181-1 shows bursal swelling of the left knee.
- Treatment is directed at the underlying cause.
- NSAIDs, rest, heat, and time are the basis of treatment for inflammatory conditions.
- Steroid injections into readily accessible bursa may be useful, but only if infection has been definitively excluded.
- Care should be taken to avoid injecting steroids into tendons.
- Infections should be treated with antibiotics.
- Immunocompromised patients with suspected infections should be admitted for IV antibiotics and orthopedic surgery consultation.

MYOFASCIAL SYNDROMES/OVERUSE SYNDROMES

- Overuse syndromes are caused by repetitive microtrauma that outpaces the body's ability to heal.

TABLE 181-2 Characteristics of Bursal Syndromes of the Hip and Knee

	LOCATION OF PAIN	ASSOCIATED SYMPTOMS	COMMON POPULATIONS
Trochanteric bursitis	Posterolateral hip	Pain with walking and climbing stairs	Female runners, older women
Iliopsoas bursitis	Groin	Pain with hip extension, tenderness over the middle third of the inguinal ligament	
Ischial or ischiogluteal bursitis	Ischial prominence	Pain with sitting on a hard surface for long periods	Sedentary people
Iliopectineal bursitis	Anterior hip, pelvis/groin	Pain improves with the hip flexed and externally rotated	
Pes anserine bursitis	Anterior medial knee		Obese women, runners, others with overuse
Prepatellar bursitis	Anterior to the patella	Significant swelling of the bursa	People who repetitively kneel on hard surfaces

- Table 181-3 describes characteristics of various overuse syndromes.
- Treatment includes NSAIDs, heat, and rest, followed by gradual resumption of activities, physical therapy, and strengthening where appropriate.

BONE/ARTICULAR DERANGEMENTS

OSTEONECROSIS/AVASCULAR NECROSIS

- Bone infarction caused by a lack of blood supply may be an idiopathic or primary disorder, secondary to a systemic condition, or following trauma.
- Osteonecrosis may cause pain from the buttock to the knee.

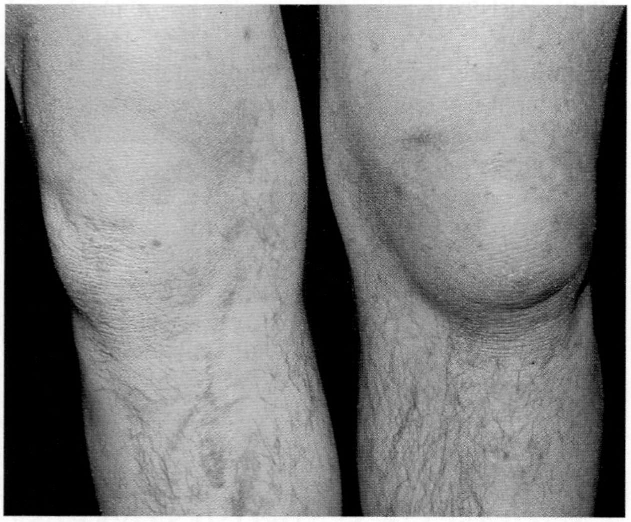

FIG. 181-1. Prepatellar bursitis of the left knee. (Reproduced with permission from Knoop K, Stack L, Storrow A, Thurman RJ: *Atlas of Emergency Medicine*, 3rd ed. © 2010, McGraw-Hill, New York.)

- Plain radiographs may establish the diagnosis, but CT or MRI is more helpful early in the disease process.
- Traumatic causes of avascular necrosis of the femoral head include femoral neck fracture, hip dislocation, and occult or minor trauma.
- Nontraumatic necrosis may be idiopathic; other causes include sickle-cell disease, collagen vascular diseases, alcohol abuse, renal transplant, systemic lupus erythematosus, dysbarism, chronic pancreatitis, exogenous steroid administration, Cushing disease, caisson disease, Gaucher disease, and renal osteodystrophy.

OSTEOMYELITIS

- Bony destruction is caused by bacterial or fungal infection.
- The infection comes from contiguous structures in about 80% of cases; hematogenous spread is responsible for the remainder of cases.
- See Table 181-4 for risk factors, likely organisms, and empiric treatments.

PAGET DISEASE

- Paget disease, or osteitis deformans, is a familial disorder resulting in enlarged, deformed bones due to overactive breakdown and reformation.
- The hip joint is affected in 50% of patients.
- ED treatment is symptomatic.
- Surgery may be required for complications.
- Long-term medications to reduce the rate of bone turnover (eg, calcitonin and alendronate) may help control the disease.

OSTEITIS PUBIS

- Osteitis pubis occurs following pregnancy, in athletes due to overuse of the adductors and gracilis muscles, and after bladder and prostate surgery.

TABLE 181-3 Characteristics of Myofascial/Overuse Syndromes

	LOCATION OF PAIN	ASSOCIATED SYMPTOMS	COMMON POPULATIONS
Snapping hip syndrome	Posterior lateral hip	Snapping sound and popping sensation with hip flexion/extension	Athletes, young women
Fascia lata syndrome	Lateral thigh/anterior groin		Athletes
Patellofemoral syndrome	Anterior knee	Pain exacerbated by prolonged knee flexion	Females
Iliotibial band syndrome	Lateral knee	Localized tenderness over lateral epicondyles	Distance runners, cyclists
Popliteus tendinitis	Posterior lateral knee	Pain exacerbated by running downhill	Athletes
Patellar tendinitis	Anterior superior knee	Pain exacerbated by running uphill	Jumpers
Infrapatellar fat pad syndrome	Anterior inferior knee	Commonly associated with patellar tendinitis	
Quadriceps tendinitis	Anterior superior knee		Athletes on hard playing surfaces
Semimembranous tendinitis	Posteromedial knee		Younger patients (athletes and overuse), older patients (degenerative changes)

- Pain in the region of the pubis starts gradually and may become very severe, causing a characteristic "duck waddling gait."
- Symptoms may resolve over several months with rest and NSAIDs.

MYOSITIS OSSIFICANS

- Myositis ossificans or heterotopic calcification is the post-traumatic deposition of bone in abnormal sites.
- Symptoms include pain and a palpable mass, which may limit motion.

TABLE 181-4 Risk Factors, Likely Infecting Organism, and Recommended Initial Empiric Antibiotic Therapy for Osteomyelitis

RISK FACTOR	LIKELY INFECTING ORGANISM	RECOMMENDED INITIAL EMPIRIC ANTIBIOTIC THERAPY*
Elderly, hematogenous spread	*Staphylococcus aureus*, including MRSA, gram-negative bacteria	Vancomycin, 1 gram IV, *plus* piperacillin-tazobactam, 3.375 grams IV or imipenem, 500 milligrams IV
Sickle cell disease	*Salmonella,* gram-negative bacteria, (*S. aureus* becoming more common)	Ciprofloxacin, 400 milligrams, consider vancomycin, 1 gram IV
Diabetes mellitus, or vascular insufficiency	Polymicrobial: *S. aureus*, *Streptococcus agalactiae*, and *Streptococcus pyogenes* plus coliforms and anaerobes	Vancomycin, 1 gram IV, *plus* piperacillin-tazobactam, 3.375 grams IV, or imipenem, 500 milligrams IV
Injection drug user	*S. aureus* including MRSA, and *Pseudomonas*	Vancomycin, 1 gram IV
Developing nations	*Mycobacterium tuberculosis*	See Chapter 70, Tuberculosis
Newborn	*S. aureus* including MRSA, gram-negative bacteria, Group B *Streptococcus*	Vancomycin, 15 milligrams/kg load, then reduce dose, *plus* ceftazidime, 30 milligrams/kg IV every 12 h
Children	*S. aureus* including MRSA	Vancomycin, 10 milligrams/kg every 6 h, *plus* ceftazidime, 50 milligrams/kg every 8 h
Postoperative with or without retained orthopedic hardware	*S. aureus* and coagulase-negative staphylococci	Vancomycin, 1 gram IV
Human bite	Streptococci or anaerobic bacteria	Piperacillin-tazobactam, 3.375 grams IV, or imipenem, 500 milligrams IV
Animal bite	*Pasteurella multocida*, *Eikenella corrodens*	Cefuroxime, 500 milligrams IV if known *P. multocida*, piperacillin-tazobactam, 3.375 grams IV or imipenem, 500 milligrams IV

Abbreviation: MRSA = methicillin-resistant *Staphylococcus aureus.*
*All patients require bone biopsy and debridement of infected/dead bone.

- Plain radiographs show an irregularly shaped mass near a joint or in a fascial plane.

For further reading in Tintinalli's *Emergency Medicine: A Comprehensive Study Guide*, 7th ed., see Chapter 278, "Hip and Knee Pain," by Kelly P. O'Keefe and Tracy G. Sanson.

182 ACUTE DISORDERS OF THE JOINTS AND BURSAE

Matthew C. DeLaney

CLINICAL FEATURES

- Identifying the disorder as monoarticular or polyarticular can help narrow the differential diagnosis (Table 182-1).
- Disorders with a migratory distribution include gonococcal arthritis, acute rheumatic fever, Lyme disease, viral arthritis, and systemic lupus erythematosus.
- The most concerning diagnosis is septic arthritis, and all decision making should involve confirming or excluding this diagnosis.
- Obtaining and examining synovial fluid is the most important aspect of the workup of an affected joint. The clinician should be familiar with standard approaches to joint aspiration (Figs. 182-1 to 182-3).

TABLE 182-1 Classification of Arthritis by Number of Affected Joints

NUMBER OF JOINTS	DIFFERENTIAL CONSIDERATIONS
1 = Monoarthritis	Trauma-induced arthritis Nongonococcal septic arthritis Gonococcal septic arthritis Crystal-induced (gout, pseudogout) Osteoarthritis (acute) Lyme disease Avascular necrosis Tumor
2-3 = Oligoarthritis	Lyme disease Reactive arthritis (Reiter syndrome) Ankylosing spondylitis Gonococcal arthritis Rheumatic fever
>3 = Polyarthritis	Rheumatoid arthritis Systemic lupus erythematosus Viral arthritis Osteoarthritis (chronic) Serum sickness Serum sickness–like reactions

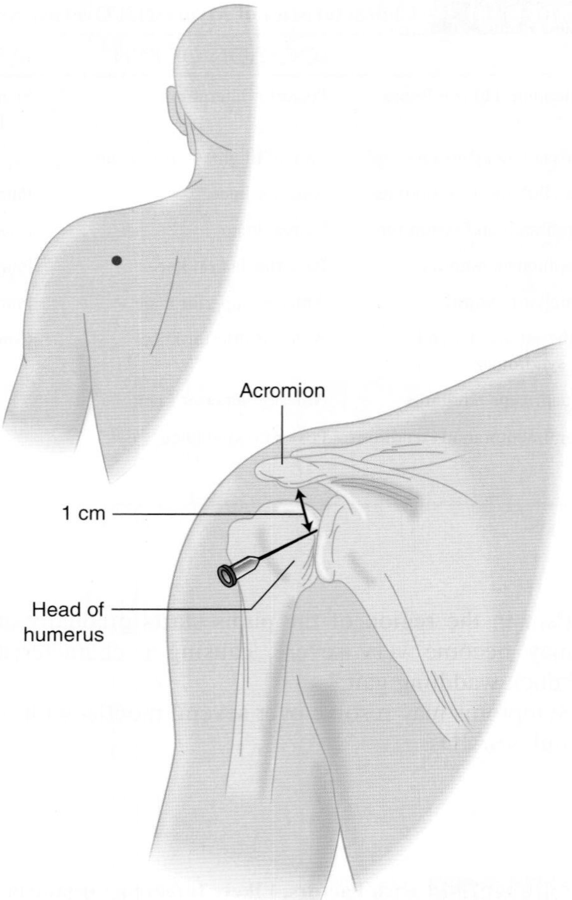

FIG. 182-1. Arthrocentesis of the shoulder, posterior approach.

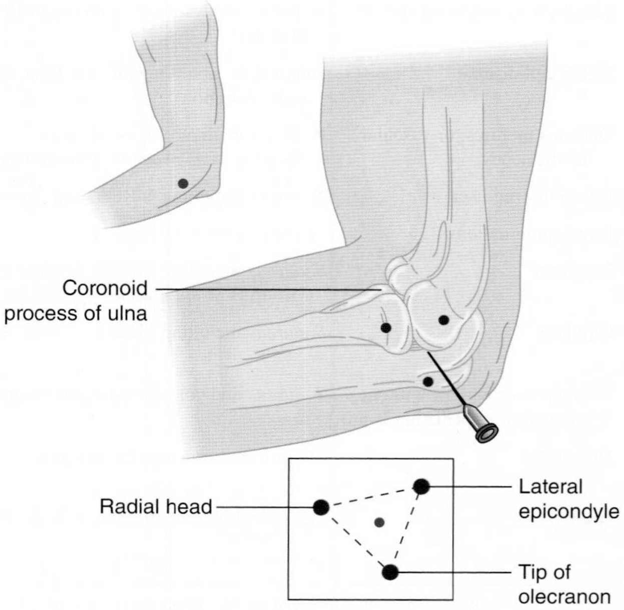

FIG. 182-2. Arthrocentesis of the elbow.

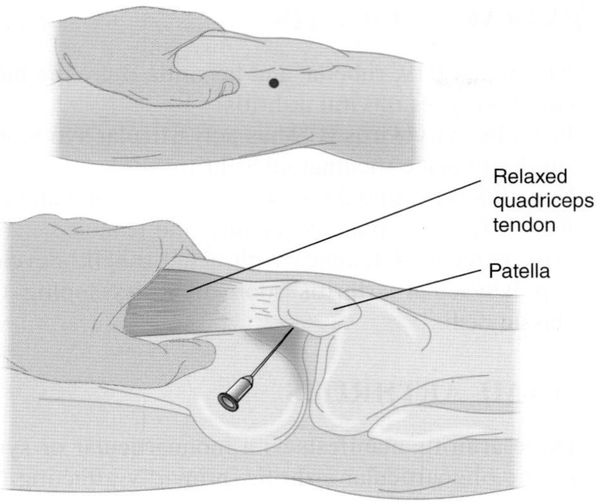

FIG. 182-3. Arthrocentesis of the knee, lateral approach.

SEPTIC ARTHRITIS

- In an acutely tender, warm joint with restricted range of motion, bacterial non-gonococcal septic arthritis is the most concerning diagnosis and must be ruled out.
- Resistance to movement and a limited range of motion are notable findings. Constitutional symptoms (eg, chills and rigors) may be absent.
- The peripheral white blood cell count lacks sensitivity and specificity in both adults and children with septic arthritis.
- The erythrocyte sedimentation rate has a sensitivity of 96% using a cutoff of 30 mm/h, but has a poor specificity.
- In septic arthritis, synovial fluid analysis usually reveals cloudy yellow fluid with a white blood cell count greater than 25,000 WBC/mL, and cultures that are positive more than 50% of the time (Table 182-2).
- Patients with ongoing concern for septic arthritis after clinical evaluation require admission to the hospital for parenteral antibiotics and orthopedic consultation for possible surgical drainage.
- Antibiotic coverage, typically involving vancomycin and a third-generation cephalosporin, should target staphylococcal and streptococcal species, including methicillin-resistant *Staphylococcus* organisms.
- Specific patient demographics can help guide empiric antibiotic therapy in septic arthritis (Table 182-3).

GONOCOCCAL ARTHRITIS

- Gonococcal arthritis is the most common cause of septic arthritis in adolescents and young adults, and typically features a prodromal phase of fever, chills, and migratory arthralgias or tenosynovitis followed by a monarthritis.
- Vesiculopustular lesions may be present distal to the involved joint.
- Synovial fluid cultures are often negative. Cultures of the posterior pharynx, urethra, cervix, and rectum may increase the yield of isolating the organism.

CRYSTAL-INDUCED SYNOVITIS

- Gout, caused by uric acid crystal deposition, is the most common cause of inflammatory joint disease in men over the age of 40 years, and typically affects the great toe or knee.
- Gout or pseudogout may be precipitated by trauma, surgery, significant illness, or a change in medication.

TABLE 182-2 Examination of Synovial Fluid

	NORMAL	NONINFLAMMATORY	INFLAMMATORY	SEPTIC
Clarity	Transparent	Transparent	Cloudy	Cloudy
Color	Clear	Yellow	Yellow	Yellow
WBC*/microliter	<200	<200-2000	200-50,000	>25,000
PMNs (%)*	<25	<25	>50	>90
Culture	Negative	Negative	Negative	>50% positive
Crystals	None	None	Multiple or none	None†
Associated conditions	—	Osteoarthritis, trauma, rheumatic fever	Gout, pseudogout, spondyloarthropathies, rheumatoid arthritis, Lyme disease, systemic lupus erythematosus	Nongonococcal or gonococcal septic arthritis

*The white blood cell count (WBC) and percent polymorphonuclear leukocytes (PMNs) are affected by a number of factors, including disease progression, infecting organism, and host immune status. The joint aspirate WBC and PMNs should be considered part of a continuum for each disease, particularly nongonococcal septic arthritis, and should be correlated with other clinical information.
†Crystal-induced arthritis may coexist with septic arthritis; therefore, the presence of crystals does not rule out infection.

TABLE 182-3 Commonly Encountered Organisms in Septic Arthritis in Adolescents and Adults*

PATIENT/ CONDITION	EXPECTED ORGANISMS	ANTIBIOTIC CONSIDERATIONS
Older children and healthy adults, or patients with risk factors for *Neisseria gonorrhoeae*	*Staphylococcus*, *N. gonorrhoeae*, *Streptococcus*, gram-negative bacteria	Vancomycin, 15 milligrams/kg IV load–if Gram stain reveals gram-positive organisms in clusters; ceftriaxone, 1 gram IV, or imipenem, 500 milligrams IV, should be used/added if either gram-negative organisms are present or no organisms present on Gram stain and *N. gonorrhoeae* suspected (also culture urethra, cervix, or anal canal as indicated).
Adults with comorbid disease (rheumatoid arthritis, human immunodeficiency virus, cancer) or injection drug users	*Staphylococcus*, gram-negative bacilli	Vancomycin, 15 milligrams/kg IV load, plus ceftriaxone, 1 gram IV, or ciprofloxacin, 400 milligrams IV; imipenem, 500 milligrams IV, may be used as an alternative agent.
Sickle-cell patients	*Salmonella* (increasingly *Staphylococcus*)	Vancomycin, 15 milligrams/kg IV load, plus ciprofloxacin, 400 milligrams IV; imipenem, 500 milligrams IV, may be used as an alternative agent.

*Recommendations differ from the 2006 British Society of Rheumatology treatment guidelines primarily due to the current need to empirically treat methicillin-resistant *Staphylococcus aureus*, which has been shown to be an increasing cause of bacterial arthritis, the most common in some regions.

- Identifying crystals in synovial fluid through a polarizing microscope is an important aspect of diagnosing both gout and pseudogout.
- Uric acid (gout) crystals appear needle shaped and blue with negative birefringence, while calcium pyrophosphate (pseudogout) crystals are rhomboid shaped and yellow with positive birefringence.
- Up to 30% of patients with acute gout will have normal serum uric acid levels making this test of little utility in diagnosing gout.
- Acute treatment for patients with adequate renal function is with nonsteroidal anti-inflammatory drugs (NSAIDs) such as ibuprofen or indomethacin. Opioid analgesia may also be required.
- Colchicine can be prescribed at 0.6 milligram/h orally until efficacy ensues or the patient experiences the intolerable side effects of vomiting or diarrhea.

VIRAL ARTHRITIS

- Parvovirus B19, rubella, and hepatitis B are the most common types of viral arthritis.
- In adults, parvovirus B19 has polyarticular symptoms similar to acute rheumatoid arthritis.
- Hepatitis B commonly involves the knee joint and can feature fevers, lymphadenopathy, and jaundice.
- Fifty percent of females with acute rubella develop a polyarticular arthritis soon after developing the classic rash.

LYME ARTHRITIS

- Lyme arthritis manifests as a monoarticular or symmetric oligoarticular arthritis, primarily affecting the large joints.
- Lyme arthritis occurs weeks to years after a primary, Stage I infection of Lyme disease.
- History of a tick bite or erythema migrans rash is often absent.
- Synovial fluid cultures are usually negative and treatment is often based on clinical suspicion.
- Treatment of Lyme arthritis consists of 3 to 4 weeks of doxycycline, penicillin, amoxicillin, or ceftriaxone.

TRAUMATIC HEMARTHROSIS

- Hemarthrosis has a high association with intraarticular fracture and ligamentous injury.
- Spontaneous hemarthrosis should prompt an investigation for a coagulopathy.

RHEUMATOID ARTHRITIS

- Rheumatoid arthritis is a chronic, progressive, polyarticular synovial joint disease that affects women more frequently than men.
- This disease is associated with stiffness after periods of inactivity, or "morning stiffness."
- Articular involvement is noted for symmetric, painful, tender joints, with sparing of the distal interphalangeal joints.
- Acute exacerbations are managed with NSAIDs and brief courses of corticosteroids. Disease-modifying antirheumatic agents are used for long-term therapy.

OSTEOARTHRITIS

- Osteoarthritis is notable for chronic, polyarticular exacerbations that lack the constitutional symptoms of rheumatoid arthritis.
- The distal interphalangeal joint space is commonly involved.

- Radiographs may show joint space narrowing.
- Acute pain is treated with NSAIDs and resting the affected joint.

REITER'S SYNDROME

- Reiter's syndrome is a seronegative spondyloarthropathy that manifests as an acute, asymmetric oligoarthritis with a predilection for the lower extremities that may be preceded 2 to 6 weeks earlier by an infectious illness, usually urethritis (*Ureaplasma* or *Chlamydia*) or enteritis (*Salmonella* or *Shigella*).
- The classic triad of urethritis, conjunctivitis, and arthritis is not mandatory for diagnosis.
- NSAIDs should be used for analgesia. Antibiotics have no proven benefit.

ANKYLOSING SPONDYLITIS

- Ankylosing spondylitis is a seronegative spondyloarthropathy primarily affecting the spine and pelvis that is characterized by morning stiffness in individuals <40 years old, with symptoms lasting more than 3 months.
- Classic radiographic findings include sacroiliitis and squaring of the vertebral bodies (eg, bamboo spine).
- Joint pain should be treated symptomatically with NSAIDs.

TABLE 182-4 Characteristics of Bursal Fluid in Patients with Septic and Nonseptic Olecranon and Prepatellar Bursitis

	SEPTIC	TRAUMATIC AND IDIOPATHIC	CRYSTAL INDUCED
Appearance	Purulent; may be straw colored or serosanguineous	Straw colored, serosanguineous, or bloody	Straw colored to bloody
Leukocytes/microliter	1500-300,000; mean, 75,000, typically >30,000	50-11,000; mean 1100, typically <28,000	1000-6000; mean, 2900
Differential count	Predominantly polymorphonuclear leukocytes	Predominantly mononuclear	Highly variable
Ratio bursal fluid to serum glucose	<50% in 90% of cases	>50%, 70%-80% in 98% of cases	Unknown
Gram stain	Positive in 70%	Negative	Negative
Crystals present	No*	No	Yes
Culture results	Positive	Negative	Negative

*The presence of crystals does not rule out infection.

BURSITIS

- Bursitis is an inflammatory process involving any bursae. It can be caused by infection, trauma, rheumatologic disorders, or crystal deposition, or be idiopathic in nature.
- Commonly affected bursae include the prepatellar bursa (eg, carpet layer's knee) and the olecranon bursa.
- Septic and aseptic bursitis cannot reliably be differentiated by physical examination alone, so aspiration of bursal fluid is required for cell count and differential, Gram's stain, and culture.
- Septic bursal fluid characteristically is purulent in appearance, with greater than 30,000 white blood cells/mL and is usually culture positive (Table 182-4).
- Treatment entails resting the affected joint, analgesics, and antistaphylococcal antibiotics for 10 to 14 days if there is evidence of infection.

For further reading in Tintinalli's *Emergency Medicine: A Comprehensive Study Guide*, 7th ed., see Chapter 281, "Acute Disorders of the Joints and Bursae," by John H. Burton.

183 EMERGENCIES IN SYSTEMIC RHEUMATIC DISEASES

Michael P. Kefer

EPIDEMIOLOGY

- Morbidity and mortality in rheumatic disease usually involves multiple organ systems and results from the disease, its complications, and/or its treatment (Table 183-1).

AIRWAY

- Relapsing polychondritis presents with the abrupt onset of pain, redness, and swelling of the ears or nose. The tracheobronchial cartilage is involved in approximately 50% of cases. Hoarseness and throat tenderness over the cartilage are noted. Repeated attacks can lead to airway collapse.
- Rheumatoid arthritis (RA) may involve the cricoarytenoid joints causing pain with speaking, hoarseness, or stridor. The cricoarytenoid joints may fix in a closed position, which may mandate emergent tracheostomy. Anticipate difficult endotracheal intubation from temporomandibular joint dysfunction, atlantoaxial instability, or cervical ankylosis.

TABLE 183-1 Common Features and Complications of Systemic Rheumatic Diseases

DISORDER	COMMON CLINICAL FEATURES AND COMPLICATIONS
Anti-phospholipid syndrome	Multiple and recurrent venous and arterial thromboses, recurrent abortions. Secondary form is associated with SLE, RA, systemic sclerosis, and Sjögren's syndrome. Thrombophlebitis and DVT, pulmonary embolism, thrombocytopenia, hemolytic anemia, livedo reticularis, stroke, transient ischemic attack, eye vascular complications. Coronary, renal, mesenteric and stroke, ARDS.
Ankylosing spondylitis	Chronic inflammatory disease of the axial skeleton, with progressive stiffness of the spine. Young adults (peak at 20 and 30 years). Back pain (improves with exercise), buttock, hip, or shoulder pain, systemic complaints (fever, malaise, fatigue, weight loss, myalgias), uveitis, restrictive pulmonary failure due to costovertebral rigidity, renal impairment, fracture of the ankylosed spine, acute spinal cord compression.
Adult still disease	Inflammatory disorder. Systemic complaints (fever, malaise, fatigue, weight loss, myalgia), arthritis, myalgia, evanescent rash, pharyngitis, lymphadenopathy, splenomegaly, anemia, thrombocytopenia. Pericarditis, myocarditis, pleurisy, ARDS, arrhythmias, heart and liver failure.
Behçet's disease	Chronic, relapsing, inflammatory disease. Systemic vasculitis involving arteries and veins of all sizes (carotid, pulmonary, aortic, and inferior extremities vessels are most commonly involved, with aneurysm, dissection, rupture, or thrombosis). Systemic complaints (fever, malaise, fatigue, weight loss, myalgia), recurrent painful skin and mucosal lesions; asymmetric, nondeforming arthritis of the medium and large joints; thrombophlebitis and DVT; ocular complications. Neuropsychiatric manifestations. Pericarditis, myocarditis, bowel perforation.
Churg-Strauss syndrome	Vasculitis with a multisystemic involvement. Systemic complaints (fever, malaise, fatigue, weight loss, myalgia), allergic rhinitis, recurrent sinusitis, asthma, and peripheral blood eosinophilia. Systemic hypertension, pericarditis, abdominal pain, peripheral neuropathy; skin lesions, AMI, bowel perforation.
Dermatomyositis/ polymyositis	Idiopathic inflammatory myopathies. Muscle weakness, myalgia, and muscle tenderness. Elevated serum CK. Systemic complaints (fever, malaise, fatigue, weight loss, myalgia), Raynaud phenomenon, nonerosive inflammatory polyarthritis, esophageal dysfunction, respiratory failure, aspiration lung infections, conduction disturbances.
Giant cell arteritis (temporal arteritis)	Chronic vasculitis of large and medium-sized vessels. Elderly (mean age at diagnosis: 70 years). Localized headache of new onset, tenderness of the temporal artery, and biopsy revealing a necrotizing arteritis. Temporal artery may be normal on clinical examination. Gradual onset, systemic complaints, jaw or tongue claudication, eye complaints, and visual loss. Aortic regurgitation and aortic arch syndrome. Neurologic complications due to carotid and vertebrobasilar vasculitis.
Henoch-Schönlein purpura	Systemic vasculitis associated with IgA deposition, generally in children. Palpable purpura (in patients with neither thrombocytopenia nor coagulopathy), arthritis/arthralgia, abdominal pain, GI bleeding, and renal impairment (adult).
Microscopic polyangiitis	Small-vessel systemic vasculitis, characterized by rapidly progressive glomerulonephritis and pulmonary involvement. Lung complications differentiate microscopic polyangiitis from polyarteritis nodosa. Systemic complaints (fever, malaise, fatigue, weight loss, myalgia), arthralgias, skin lesions, hemoptysis, abdominal pain, renal impairment, systemic hypertension.
Polyarteritis nodosa	Systemic necrotizing vasculitis of the medium-sized muscular arteries. Systemic complaints (fever, malaise, fatigue, weight loss, myalgia), arthralgias, skin lesions, abdominal pain, renal impairment, systemic hypertension, peripheral mononeuropathy typically with both motor and sensory deficits, eye complications, leucocytosis and anemia, stroke, mesenteric ischemia, acute scrotum.
Rheumatoid arthritis	Chronic, systemic, inflammatory disorder. Symmetrical and potentially destructive arthritis. Systemic symptoms (fever, malaise, fatigue, weight loss, myalgia), skin lesions, splenomegaly. Cervical spine involvement, pleuritis, pericarditis, myocarditis, and aortitis. Cricoarytenoid arthritis with potential for airway obstruction. Ocular involvement. Peripheral artery disease, Sjögren's syndrome, vasculitis, and renal impairment. Abdominal pain. Anemia, leucopenia, thrombocytosis, and Felty syndrome. ACS, respiratory failure.
Polymyalgia rheumatica	Immune-mediated condition. Ears (violaceous and erythematous auricula), nose (saddle nose deformity), and other cartilaginous structures inflammation (especially eyes, joints, and respiratory tract). One-third of cases associated with another SRD. Sternoclavicular, costochondral, and manubriosternal arthritis, upper airway involvement, aortic or mitral valvular regurgitation, pericarditis, renal impairment, peripheral neuropathies, ocular complications.
Systemic lupus erythematosus	Systemic autoimmune disease, characterized by relapses and remissions, and affecting virtually every organ. Systemic complaints (fever, malaise, fatigue, weight loss, myalgia), symmetric and polyarticular arthritis (small joints of the hands, the wrists, and the knees), butterfly rash, mucocutaneous manifestations, oral and/or nasal ulcers, Raynaud phenomenon. Neuropsychiatric manifestations, pleurisy, lupus pneumonitis, shrinking or vanishing lung syndrome, and pulmonary hypertension. Libman–Sacks endocarditis, pericarditis, myocarditis, endocarditis. GI unspecific complaints. Renal impairment, leucopenia, mild anemia, and thrombocytopenia. Ocular complications, ACS.
Sjögren's syndrome	Autoimmune disease. May be primary; secondary form is mostly associated with RA, SLE, polymyositis, or dermatomyositis. Systemic symptoms, arthralgia, skin lesions, Raynaud phenomenon. Pulmonary hypertension, pericarditis, neuropsychiatric manifestations, peripheral neuropathy, hepatic abnormalities, renal impairment, hypokalemic respiratory arrest, stroke, pulmonary embolism, transverse myelitis.

(*Continued*)

TABLE 183-1 Common Features and Complications of Systemic Rheumatic Diseases (Continued)

DISORDER	COMMON CLINICAL FEATURES AND COMPLICATIONS
Systemic sclerosis (scleroderma)	Inappropriate and excessive accumulation of collagen in a variety of tissues; widespread vascular lesions with vascular spasm, thickening of the vascular wall and narrowing of the lumen. Systemic complaints (fever, malaise, fatigue, weight loss, myalgia), skin lesions (fingers, hands, and face), carpal tunnel syndrome, Raynaud phenomenon. Renal impairment, GI dysmotility, gastroesophageal reflux (aspiration pneumonitis), chronic esophagitis, and stricture formation. Vascular ectasia in the stomach ("watermelon stomach"). Alveolar hemorrhage, ARDS, arrhythmias, scleroderma renal crisis.
Takayasu arteritis	Chronic vasculitis, young women, predominantly Asians. Systemic complaints (fever, malaise, fatigue, weight loss, myalgia), arthralgias, skin lesions, abdominal pain, and diarrhea. Aorta and its primary branches, and pulmonary artery involvement. Neurologic manifestations, syncope, subclavian steal syndrome, extremities ischemia. Normochromic, normocytic anemia, ACS, bowel ischemia and perforation, stroke.
Wegener's granulomatosis	Multiple organ system vasculitis and necrotizing granulomas. Respiratory tract manifestations in approximately 100% cases, with nose, oral cavity, upper trachea, external and middle ear, and orbits, inflammations. Upper airway and pulmonary manifestations. Constitutional symptoms, arthralgias, glomerulonephritis and small vessel vasculitis (scleritis and episcleritis, palpable purpura or cutaneous nodules, peripheral neuropathy, deafness). Pericarditis, myocarditis. Renal impairment. Anemia, leukocytosis and thrombocytosis, ACS.

Abbreviations: ACS = acute coronary syndrome, AMI = acute myocardial infarction, AH = alveolar hemorrhage, ARDS = adult respiratory distress syndrome, DVT = deep vein thrombosis, GI = gastrointestinal, RA = rheumatoid arthritis, SLE = systemic lupus erythematosus, SRD = systemic rheumatic disease.

RESPIRATORY MUSCLE

- Dermatomyositis and polymyositis may lead to respiratory failure from respiratory muscle involvement in poorly controlled disease.

LUNG

- Pulmonary hemorrhage complicates Goodpasture's disease, systemic lupus erythematosus (SLE), Wegener's granulomatosis, and other vasculitic conditions.
- Pulmonary fibrosis occurs in ankylosing spondylitis, scleroderma, and other conditions.
- Pleural effusion occurs in RA and SLE.

HEART

- Pericarditis occurs in RA and SLE.
- Myocardial infarction may occur from coronary artery involvement in Kawasaki's disease or polyarteritis nodosa.
- Pancarditis occurs in acute rheumatic fever.
- Valvular heart disease occurs in ankylosing spondylitis, relapsing polychondritis, and rheumatic fever. Involvement may extend into the conduction system causing arrhythmias.

NERVOUS SYSTEM

- Patients with rheumatologic involvement of the cervical spine may be at high risk for cervical spine or spinal cord injury from otherwise trivial trauma as occurs with manipulation during endotracheal intubation if not done with extreme caution.
- Destruction of the transverse ligament of C-2, with resultant symptoms of cord compression, may complicate RA.
- Cervical spine inflexibility from ankylosing spondylitis predisposes to injury out of proportion to the mechanism.
- Anterior spinal artery syndrome may result from rheumatologic conditions causing vasculitis, aortic dissection, or thromboembolism.

EYE

- Temporal arteritis is a cause of sudden blindness and should be considered in any patient older than 50 years who presents with new-onset headache, visual change, or jaw claudication.
- Dry eyes (and dry mouth) from Sjögren's syndrome may occur alone or coexist with many rheumatologic conditions.
- In RA, episcleritis is a self-limited, painless injection of the episcleral vessels. Scleritis presents as purple discoloration and marked tenderness of the eye with risk of scleral rupture.

KIDNEY

- Nephritis is a common complication of SLE, Wegener's granulomatosis, and systemic vasculitis.
- Renal insufficiency can result from malignant hypertension as occurs with scleroderma, from rhabdomyolysis in the patient with florid myositis, or from prostaglandin inhibition by nonsteroidal anti-inflammatory drugs used in treatment.

- Nephrotic syndrome in patients with SLE predisposes to renal vein thrombosis.

HYPERTENSION

- Hypertension can complicate any condition that affects the kidneys directly, as in polyarteritis nodosa, scleroderma, or SLE, or indirectly, from nephrotoxic drugs used in treatment.

ADRENAL GLAND

- Glucocorticoids are often used in the treatment of rheumatic conditions. Doses required may result in adrenal suppression. As a result, these patients are at risk for acute adrenal insufficiency.

BLOOD

- Anemia and thrombocytopenia are common.
- Many medications used for treatment are potent immunosuppressants.

For further reading in Tintinalii's *Emergency Medicine: A Comprehensive Study Guide*, 7th ed., see Chapter 279, "Emergencies in Systemic Rheumatic Diseases," by Gemma C. Morabito and Bruno Tartaglino.

184 INFECTIOUS AND NONINFECTIOUS DISORDERS OF THE HAND

Michael P. Kefer

INTRODUCTION

- Rest and elevation are the mainstays of treatment for many inflammatory conditions of the hand. This helps to decrease inflammation, avoid secondary injury, and prevent spread of any existing infection.
- The optimal position for splinting the hand is the position of function: wrist in 15-degree extension, metacarpophalangeal (MCP) joint in 50- to 90-degree flexion, proximal interphalangeal (PIP) joint in 10- to 15-degree flexion, and distal interphalangeal (DIP) joint in 10- to 15-degree flexion.

HAND INFECTIONS

- Hand infections most commonly occur from injury to the dermis. Skin organisms, *Staphylococcus* and *Streptococcus* species, are the most common pathogens.
- Refer to Table 184-1 for recommended antibiotic therapy for the common hand infections described below.

CELLULITIS

- Presents with localized warmth, erythema, and edema.
- Exclude involvement of deeper structures of the hand by demonstrating absence of tenderness on deep palpation and range of motion.
- Treat with antibiotics, splinting in the position of function, elevation, and close follow-up.

FLEXOR TENOSYNOVITIS

- This is a surgical emergency and is diagnosed on examination (Table 184-2).
- Treat with splinting, elevation, IV antibiotics, and hand surgery consult for drainage.

DEEP SPACE INFECTION

- Involves the web or midpalmar space.
- Web space infection presents as dorsal and volar swelling of the web space causing separation of the affected digits.
- Midpalmar space infection occurs from spread of a flexor tenosynovitis or penetrating wound to the palm, causing infection of the radial or ulnar bursa of the hand.
- Treat with splinting, elevation, IV antibiotics, and hand surgery consult for drainage.

CLOSED FIST INJURY

- Essentially a human bite wound to the MCP joint, this results from a punch to the teeth.
- There is high risk of infection spreading along the extensor tendons.
- Wounds penetrating the skin should be explored, irrigated, and allowed to heal by secondary intention.
- When inspecting for extensor tendon injury, it is essential to consider the position of the hand at the time of injury.
- Treat with splinting, elevation, IV antibiotics, and hand surgery consult.
- Extensor tendon repair is delayed until the risk of infection has passed.

PARONYCHIA

- Paronychia is an infection of the lateral nail fold.
- If there is no pus, treat with warm soaks, elevation, and antibiotics if warranted.
- Drainage of a small paronychia is by lifting the nail fold with a needle or number 11 blade (see Fig. 184-1).

TABLE 184-1 Initial Antibiotic Coverage for Common Hand Infections

INFECTION	INITIAL ANTIMICROBIAL AGENT(S)	LIKELY ORGANISMS	COMMENTS
Cellulitis	*For mild to moderate cellulitis:* TMP/SMX double strength, one to two tablets twice per day PO for 7-10 d. *Plus/minus* cephalexin, 500 milligrams PO four times per day for 7-10 d, *or* dicloxacillin, 500 milligrams PO four times daily for 7-10 d. *For severe cellulitis:* Vancomycin, 1 gram IV every 12 h.	*Staphylococcus aureus* (MRSA) *S. pyogenes*	Clindamycin is an option, but increasing MRSA resistance to clindamycin has been reported. Consider vancomycin for injection drug abusers.
Felon/ paronychia	TMP/SMX double strength, one to two tablets twice per day PO for 7-10 d. *Plus/minus* cephalexin, 500 milligrams PO four times per day for 7-10 d, *or* dicloxacillin, 500 milligrams PO four times daily for 7-10 d. *Consider* addition of clindamycin or amoxicillin-clavulanate to TMP/SMX (rather than cephalexin) if anaerobic bacteria are suspected.	*S. aureus* (MRSA), *S. pyogenes*, anaerobes, polymicrobial	Antibiotics indicated for infections with associated localized cellulitis, otherwise drainage alone may be sufficient, culture recommended by hand surgeons.
Flexor tenosynovitis	Ampicillin-sulbactam, 1.5 grams IV every 6 h, *or* cefoxitin, 2 grams IV every 8 h, *or* piperacillin/tazobactam, 3.375 grams IV every 6 h. *Plus:* vancomycin, 1 gram IV every 12 h, if MRSA is prevalent in community.	*S. aureus,* streptococci, anaerobes, gram negatives	Parenteral antibiotics are indicated; consider ceftriaxone for suspected *Neisseria gonorrhoeae*.
Deep space infection	Ampicillin-sulbactam, 1.5 grams IV every 6 h, *or* cefoxitin, 2 grams IV every 8 h, *or* piperacillin/tazobactam, 3.375 grams IV every 6 h. *Plus:* vancomycin, 1 gram IV every 12 h, if MRSA is prevalent in community.	*S. aureus,* streptococci, anaerobes, gram-negatives	Inpatient management.
Animal bites (including human)	If no visible signs of infection: amoxicillin-clavulanate, 875/125 milligrams PO twice daily for 5 d. For signs of infection: ampicillin-sulbactam, 1.5 grams IV every 6 h, *or* cefoxitin, 2 grams IV every 8 h, *or* piperacillin/tazobactam, 3.375 grams every 6 h. For penicillin allergy, use clindamycin plus ciprofloxacin.	*S. aureus,* streptococci, *Eikenella corrodens* (human), *Pasteurella multocida* (cat), anaerobes, and gram-negative bacteria	All animal bite wounds should receive prophylactic oral antibiotics.
Herpetic whitlow	Acyclovir, 400 milligrams PO three times daily for 10 d.	Herpes simplex	No surgical drainage is indicated.

Abbreviations: MRSA = methicillin-resistant *Staphylococcus aureus*, TMP/SMX = trimethoprim-sulfamethoxazole.

- If pus is seen beneath the nail, a portion of the nail may have to be removed and packing placed for adequate drainage. Avoid injury to the nail bed.
- Recheck the wound in 24 to 48 hours, pull the packing, and begin warm soaks.

FELON

- Felon is an infection of the pulp space of the fingertip.
- Drainage is by the lateral approach to protect the neurovascular bundle. The incision should remain within the borders of the DIP joint crease proximally and the base of the phalangeal tuft distally. Incise deep enough across the finger pad to divide the septae at the bony insertions.
- Unless there is a pointing abscess, the radial aspect of the index and middle fingers and the ulnar aspect of the thumb and small finger should be avoided.
- Pack the wound. Splint the hand in the position of function.
- Recheck the wound in 24 to 48 hours, pull the packing, and begin warm soaks.

TABLE 184-2 Kanavel Four Cardinal Signs of Flexor Tenosynovitis

Percussion tenderness	Tenderness over the entire length of the flexor tendon sheath
Uniform swelling	Symmetric finger swelling along the length of the tendon sheath
Intense pain	Intense pain with passive extension
Flexion posture	Flexed posture of the involved digit at rest to minimize pain

HERPETIC WHITLOW

- Herpetic whitlow is a viral infection of the fingertip with intracutaneous vesicles.
- Clinically, this may present similar to a felon, but vesicles are present.
- Treat with immobilization, elevation, and protection with a dry dressing to prevent autoinoculation and transmission. Antiviral agents may shorten the duration.

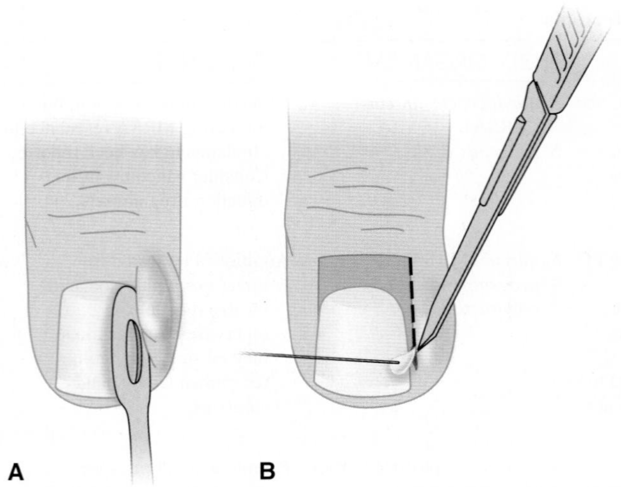

FIG. 184-1. Paronychia. **A.** The eponychial fold is elevated using a flat probe or a number 11 blade to allow the wound to drain. **B.** Alternatively, for more extensive infections, a number 11 blade may be used to incise the area of greatest fluctuance directly into the eponychium. The wound may then be gently probed with a small clamp to ensure drainage.

NONINFECTIOUS DISORDERS

TENDINITIS

- Tendinitis is usually due to overuse.
- Examination reveals tenderness over the involved tendon.
- Treat with immobilization and nonsteroidal anti-inflammatory drugs (NSAIDs).

TRIGGER FINGER

- Results from a tenosynovitis of the flexor sheath of the digit where inflammation or scarring causes stenosis of the sheath.
- Impingement and snap release of the tendon occur as the finger is extended from a flexed position.
- Steroid injection may be effective in early stages. Definitive treatment is surgery.

DEQUERVAIN'S TENOSYNOVITIS

- Involves the extensor pollicis brevis and abductor pollicis tendons.
- Pain occurs at the radial aspect of the wrist and radiates into the forearm.
- The Finkelstein test is diagnostic: the patient grasps the thumb in the fist and deviates the hand ulnarly, reproducing the pain.
- Treat with a thumb spica splint, NSAIDs, and referral.

CARPAL TUNNEL SYNDROME

- Results from compression of the median nerve by the transverse carpal ligament.
- The cause is usually edema from overuse, pregnancy, or congestive heart failure.
- Pain in the median nerve distribution of the hand tends to be worse at night.
- On examination, pain may be reproduced by tapping over the nerve at the wrist (Tinel's sign) or by holding the wrist flexed maximally for about 1 minute (Phalen's sign).
- Treat with a wrist splint and NSAIDs. Advanced cases require surgical decompression.

DUPUYTREN'S CONTRACTURE

- Results from fibrous changes in the subcutaneous tissues of the palm, which may lead to tethering and joint contractures.
- Refer to hand surgery.

GANGLION CYST

- Ganglion cyst is a cystic collection of synovial fluid within a joint or tendon sheath.
- Treat with NSAIDs and referral.

For further reading in Tintinalli's *Emergency Medicine: A Comprehensive Study Guide*, 7th ed., see Chapter 280, "Nontraumatic Disorders of the Hand," by Carl A. Germann and Mark W. Foure.

185 SOFT TISSUE PROBLEMS OF THE FOOT

Robert L. Cloutier

- Depending on the disease, patients with chronic or complicated foot problems generally should be referred to a dermatologist, orthopedist, general surgeon, or podiatrist.

- Tinea pedis and onychomycosis are discussed in Chapter 157, Other Dermatologic Disorders. Puncture wounds of the foot are discussed in Chapter 17, Puncture Wounds and Bites.

CORNS AND CALLUSES

CLINICAL FEATURES

- Calluses represent a dermatologic reaction to focal pressure whether external (ill-fitting shoe) or internal (bunion) creating focal hyperkeratosis.
- Calluses initially grow outward but with continued pressure will grow inward to form corns.
- Hard corns develop over bony protuberances and soft corns in softer areas between toes.
- Corns can be differentiated from calluses by examining the dermal lines. Corns will violate dermal lines; calluses form along, but do not cross, dermal lines.
- Corns may be painful and can be differentiated from warts when incised; warts will bleed and corns will not.

DIAGNOSIS AND DIFFERENTIAL

- Keratotic lesions may be indicative of more severe underlying disease, a mechanical problem, or local disease.
- The differential diagnosis may include syphilis, tinea, psoriasis, lichen planus, rosacea, arsenic poisoning, basal cell nevus syndrome, and malignancy.

EMERGENCY DEPARTMENT CARE AND DISPOSITION

- Treatment involves paring with a number 15 blade; the incision should include removal of the central keratin plug.

PLANTAR WARTS

CLINICAL FEATURES

- Plantar warts are common, contagious, and caused by the human papillomavirus. They may be painful and tend to develop over the bony protuberances of the foot.

DIAGNOSIS AND DIFFERENTIAL

- Diagnosis is clinical and the differential diagnosis may include corns or melanoma.

EMERGENCY DEPARTMENT CARE AND DISPOSITION

- Topical treatment with 15% to 20% salicylic acid is most effective. Warts may require repeated treatments. Nonhealing lesions may represent undiagnosed melanoma and should be referred to a dermatologist or podiatrist.

ONYCHOCRYPTOSIS (INGROWN TOENAIL)

CLINICAL FEATURES

- Onychocryptosis is characterized by increased inflammation or infection of the lateral or medial aspects of the toenail. This occurs when the nail plate penetrates the nail sulcus and subcutaneous tissue; most commonly this involves the great toe.
- Patients with underlying diabetes, arterial insufficiency, cellulitis, ulceration, or necrosis are at risk for amputation if treatment is delayed.

EMERGENCY DEPARTMENT CARE AND DISPOSITION

- ***Toenail is uninfected***: Often, all that is required is a combination of nail elevation (eg, with a wisp of cotton between the nail plate and the skin), daily foot soaks, and avoidance of pressure on the area. A second option is digital block followed by removal of a spicule of the nail, with debridement of the nail groove. Partial removal of the nail will be necessary if there is either granulation tissue or infection (see Fig. 185-1).

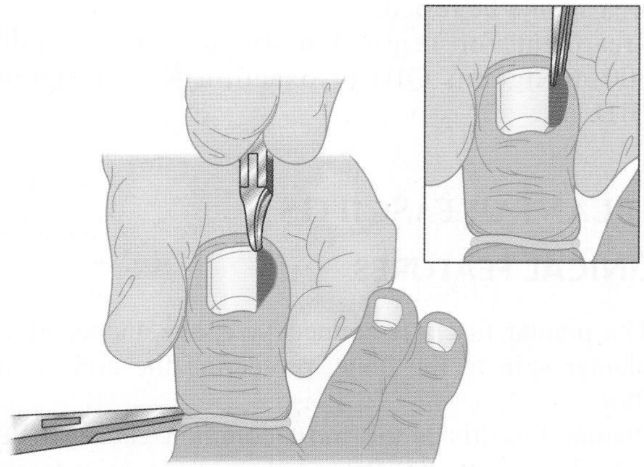

FIG. 185-1. Partial toenail removal (infection present). This method is used for onychocryptosis in the setting of significant granulation tissue or infection.

- ***Toenail is infected:*** After digital block, one-fourth of the nail should be cut longitudinally (including beneath the cuticle) and removed. A non-adherent bulky dressing should be placed and the wound checked in 24 to 48 hours (see Fig. 185-1).

BURSITIS

CLINICAL FEATURES

- Pathologic changes of the foot bursae are subdivided as follows: (1) noninflammatory, (2) inflammatory, (3) suppurative, and (4) calcified.
- Noninflammatory bursae become painful as a result of direct pressure.
- Inflammatory bursae become painful as a result of gout, syphilis, or rheumatoid arthritis.
- Suppurative bursae become painful due to pyogenic organisms from adjacent wounds.

DIAGNOSIS AND DIFFERENTIAL

- Inflammatory bursitis: gout and rheumatoid arthritis.
- Retrocalcaneal bursitis may mimic Achilles tendinitis.
- Suppurative bursitis: pyogenic organisms (ie, *Staphylococcus* spp.) from adjacent wounds.
- Ultrasound (US) and magnetic resonance imaging (MRI) are useful diagnostically but not vital to ED evaluation.

EMERGENCY DEPARTMENT CARE AND DISPOSITION

- Complications include a hygroma, calcified bursae, fistula, and ulcer formation.
- Patients should be non-weightbearing and the affected area should be rested.
- Treatment for septic bursitis includes nafcillin 500 milligrams QID or oxacillin 500 milligrams QID.

PLANTAR FASCIITIS

CLINICAL FEATURES

- The plantar fascia is connective tissue anchoring the plantar skin to the bone, protecting the arch of the foot.
- Plantar fasciitis is the most common cause of heel pain due to overuse. Patients have deep point tenderness, worse on arising and after activity, over the anterior-medial calcaneus at the point of insertion of the plantar fascia.

DIAGNOSIS AND DIFFERENTIAL

- The differential diagnosis may include abnormal joint mechanics, poorly cushioned shoes, Achilles tendon pathology, and rheumatoid disease.
- Diagnosis is clinical, but MRI and US may be useful but are not critical in ED setting.

EMERGENCY DEPARTMENT CARE AND DISPOSITION

- Treatment includes rest, ice, and nonsteroidal anti-inflammatory drugs (NSAIDs). Eighty percent of cases are self-limited.
- Plantar-specific stretches are helpful. Other options to unload the plantar fascia include foot strapping, night-time splints, arch supports, and short-leg walking casts.
- Glucocorticoid injections are not indicated in the ED.

TARSAL TUNNEL SYNDROME

CLINICAL FEATURES

- Tarsal tunnel syndrome involves compression of the posterior tibial nerve as it courses inferior to the medial malleolus causing foot and heel pain.
- Causes include running, restrictive footwear (eg, ski boots, skates), edema of pregnancy, posttraumatic fibrosis, ganglion cysts, osteophytes, and tumors.
- The pain of tarsal tunnel syndrome involves the more medial heel and arch and worsens with activity.
- Pain may also be worse at night at the medial malleolus, the heel, the sole of the foot, and the distal calf.

DIAGNOSIS AND DIFFERENTIAL

- The differential diagnosis may include plantar fasciitis and Achilles tendinitis.
- Tinel's sign is positive; eversion and dorsiflexion of foot worsens symptoms.
- US, computed tomography (CT), and MRI may aid in diagnosis.

EMERGENCY DEPARTMENT CARE AND DISPOSITION

- Treatment includes NSAIDs, rest, and possible orthopedic referral.

DEEP PERONEAL NERVE ENTRAPMENT

CLINICAL FEATURES

- Occurs most frequently where the nerve courses beneath the extensor retinaculum. Recurrent ankle

sprains, soft tissue masses, and restrictive footwear represent the most common causes.
- Symptoms include dorsal and medial foot pain as well as hypesthesia in the web space between the first two toes. Nighttime pain is common.

DIAGNOSIS AND DIFFERENTIAL

- Pain may be exacerbated by palpation of the peroneal nerve at the site of entrapment and with plantar flexion and inversion of the foot.

EMERGENCY DEPARTMENT CARE AND DISPOSITION

- US, CT, or MRI may aid in diagnosis. Treatment includes NSAIDs, rest, and possible orthopedic referral.

GANGLIONS

- A ganglion is a benign synovial cyst, typically 1.5 to 2.5 cm in diameter, attached to a joint capsule or tendon sheath. The anterolateral ankle is a typical site.
- Ganglions may appear suddenly or gradually, enlarge or diminish in size, and may be painful or asymptomatic.
- A firm, usually nontender, cystic lesion is seen on examination. The diagnosis is clinical, but MRI or US can be used if in doubt.
- Initial treatment includes aspiration and injection of glucocorticoids, but most require surgical excision.

TENDON LESIONS

TENOSYNOVITIS AND TENDINITIS

- Tenosynovitis or tendinitis is usually due to overuse and presents with pain over the involved tendon. Treatment includes ice, rest, and NSAIDs.
- The flexor hallicus longus, posterior tibialis, and Achilles tendons are those that are most frequently affected.
- Flexor hallicus longus tenosynovitis typically affects ballet dancers, but is also seen in runners and nonathletes. The presentation is similar to plantar fasciitis and tarsal tunnel syndrome. Management is often surgical.

TENDON LACERATIONS

- Tendon lacerations should be explored and repaired if the ends are visible in the wound.
- Due to the high complication rate, specialty consultation is often necessary. After repair, extensor tendons are immobilized in dorsiflexion and flexor tendons in equinus.

TENDON RUPTURES

- ***Achilles tendon*** rupture presents with pain and a palpable defect in the area of tendon. Patients are unable to stand on tiptoes, and display an absence of plantar flexion with squeezing of the calf (Thompson sign).
- Treatment is generally surgical in younger patients and conservative (casting in equinus) in the elderly.
- ***Anterior tibialis tendon*** rupture results with a palpable defect and mild foot drop. These tendon ruptures are rare, usually not as painful as Achilles ruptures, and occur after the fourth decade of life. Surgical repair is often unnecessary.
- ***Posterior tibialis tendon*** rupture is usually chronic and insidious and presents with a flattened arch and swelling over the medial ankle. It usually occurs after fourth decade with two-thirds of cases being in women. Examination may show weakness on inversion, a palpable defect, and inability to stand on tiptoes. Treatment is either surgical or conservative.
- ***Flexor hallicus longus*** rupture presents with loss of plantar flexion of the great toe. Need for surgery depends on patient occupation and lifestyle.
- ***Disruption of the peroneal retinaculum*** occurs with a direct blow during dorsiflexion, causing localized pain behind the lateral malleolus and clicking while walking as the peroneal tendon is subluxed. The treatment is surgical.

PLANTAR INTERDIGITAL NEUROMA (MORTON'S NEUROMA)

- Neuromas form in plantar digital nerves just proximal to their bifurcations and are thought to occur from entrapment of the plantar digital nerve due to tight-fitting shoes.
- Women between the ages of 25 and 50 years are the most commonly affected patients with the third interspace being the most commonly affected area.
- Patients may present with burning, cramping, or aching over the affected metatarsal head.
- Diagnosis is clinical, but US, MRI, and nerve conduction studies may be helpful.
- Conservative treatment includes wide shoes and glucocorticoid injections, which may be curative. Surgical neurolysis is occasionally required.

COMPARTMENT SYNDROMES OF THE FOOT

CLINICAL FEATURES

- Nine compartments have been identified in the foot.
- Compartment syndromes in the foot are most commonly associated with high-energy crush injuries. Other causes include post-ischemic swelling after arterial injury, ankle fractures, burns, bleeding disorders, and exercise. Chronic compartment syndromes have been noted with overuse.
- At-risk patients include those with increasingly severe pain exacerbated by active and passive motion, coupled with paresthesias and neurovascular deficits.

DIAGNOSIS AND DIFFERENTIAL

- At-risk patients must have compartment pressures checked. Any difference of less than 30 mm Hg between the Stryker STIC device (Stryker Kalamazoo, MI) and diastolic blood pressure is considered positive.

EMERGENCY DEPARTMENT CARE AND DISPOSITION

- Prompt consideration of emergent fasciotomy.

PLANTAR FIBROMATOSIS

- Plantar fibromatosis (Dupuytren contracture of the plantar fascia) involves small, asymptomatic, palpable, slowly growing, firm masses on the non-weight-bearing plantar surface of the foot.
- Onset is usually during adolescence. MRI may be helpful for diagnosis. Toe contractures do not occur, lesions tend to reabsorb spontaneously, and treatment is conservative.

MALIGNANT MELANOMA

- Melanoma of the foot accounts for 15% of all cutaneous melanomas.
- Many present as atypical nonpigmented or pigmented lesions including the nail with a predilection for plantar surfaces.
- Vigilance is key as these lesions often mimic more benign conditions such as fungal infection, plantar warts, and foot ulcers.
- Patients with atypical or nonhealing lesions should be sent for biopsy.

For further reading in Tintinalli's *Emergency Medicine: A Comprehensive Study Guide*, 7th ed., see Chapter 282, "Soft Tissue Problems of the Foot," by Franz R. Melio.

Section 22
PSYCHOSOCIAL DISORDERS

186 CLINICAL FEATURES OF BEHAVIORAL DISORDERS

Lance H. Hoffman

PSYCHIATRIC SYNDROMES (AXIS I DISORDERS)

DEMENTIA, DELIRIUM, AND AMNESTIC DISORDERS

- Dementia is a disorder consisting of a pervasive disturbance in cognition-impairing memory, abstraction, judgment, personality, and higher critical functions such as language in which the onset is typically gradual, and the patient's normal level of consciousness is maintained.
- Metabolic and endocrine disorders, adverse drug effects and interactions, and depression are potentially reversible causes of dementia.
- Delirium is characterized by a global impairment in cognitive functioning that is usually acute in onset with a fluctuating severity of symptoms in which a diminished level of consciousness, inattention, and sensory misperceptions, such as visual hallucinations, are experienced.
- Most causes of delirium are reversible and include infection, electrolyte abnormalities, toxic ingestions, and head injury. Treatment should be directed toward correcting the underlying cause.
- Amnestic patients cannot learn new information or recall previously learned information.
- Causes of amnesia can include brain trauma, stroke, anoxic brain injury, substance abuse, and chronic nutritional deficiencies.

SUBSTANCE-INDUCED DISORDERS

- Intoxication is an exogenous substance-induced syndrome that results in maladaptive behavior and impaired cognitive functioning and psychomotor activity.
- Repeated use of such a substance is defined as substance abuse and may lead to physical or psychological dependence on the substance.
- Substance withdrawal entails a collection of symptoms specific to a substance of abuse that result from the reduction or cessation of use of that substance with symptoms promptly subsiding with continued use of the exogenous substance.

SCHIZOPHRENIA AND OTHER PSYCHOTIC DISORDERS

- Schizophrenia is a chronic disease characterized by functional deterioration; the presence of hallucinations, delusions, disorganized speech or behavior, or catatonic behavior ("positive symptoms"); the presence of blunted affect, emotional withdrawal, lack of spontaneity, anhedonia, or impaired attention ("negative symptoms"); cognitive impairment expressed as loose associations or incoherence; and the relative absence of a mood disorder.
- Schizophreniform disorder is diagnosed when an individual experiences symptoms and demonstrates signs consistent with schizophrenia for less than 6 months.
- A brief psychotic disorder is a psychosis that lasts less than 4 weeks and is a response to a traumatic life experience.

MOOD DISORDERS

- Major depression consists of a persistent dysphoric mood or a pervasive loss of interest and pleasure in usual activities (anhedonia) lasting longer than 2 weeks.
- Associated psychological symptoms of major depression include feelings of guilt over past events, self-reproach, worthlessness, hopelessness, and recurrent thoughts of death or suicide.
- Vegetative symptoms of major depression affecting physiologic functioning include a loss of appetite and weight, sleep disturbances, fatigue, inability to concentrate, and psychomotor agitation or retardation.
- The lifetime risk of suicide in patients with major depression is 15%.
- Bipolar disorder is characterized by recurrent, cyclic episodes of manic and depressive symptoms,

with depressive episodes being more common than manic episodes.

- Manic individuals demonstrate an elated or irritable mood; act energetically and expansively; and demonstrate a decreased need for sleep, poor impulse control, racing thoughts, and pressured speech.

ANXIETY DISORDERS

- Panic disorder consists of recurrent episodes of severe anxiety and sudden, extreme autonomic symptoms that peak quickly.
- Panic disorder is a diagnosis of exclusion because its symptoms can mimic those of life-threatening cardiovascular and pulmonary disorders.
- Post-traumatic stress disorder is an anxiety reaction to a severe, psychosocial stressor, typically perceived as life threatening in which the individual experiences repetitive, intrusive memories of the event.
- Obsessive-compulsive disorder patients experience intrusive thoughts or images that create anxiety (obsessions) and are controlled by the patients by engaging in repetitive behaviors or rituals (compulsions).

PERSONALITY DISORDERS (AXIS II DISORDERS)

- Individuals with a personality disorder exhibit a lifelong pattern of maladaptive behavior that is not limited to periods of illness.
- Ten personality disorders named according to their characteristic maladaptive behavior exist and include paranoid, schizoid, schizotypal, antisocial, borderline, histrionic, narcissistic, avoidant, dependent, and obsessive-compulsive.

For further reading in Tintinalli's *Emergency Medicine: A Comprehensive Study Guide*, 7th ed., see Chapter 284, "Behavioral Disorders: Diagnostic Criteria," by Leslie Zun.

187 EMERGENCY ASSESSMENT AND STABILIZATION OF BEHAVIORAL DISORDERS

Lance H. Hoffman

EPIDEMIOLOGY

- Mental health-related visits to US emergency departments increased 38% to 23.6 per 1000 population in the last two decades.
- Patients who are suicidal, homicidal, or violent or have a rapidly progressive medical condition resulting in abnormal behavior require stabilization.

CLINICAL FEATURES

- Suicidal patients are often forthcoming about their intentions for self-harm; however, the patient's intentions may be more difficult to infer if a nontraumatic suicide attempt has been made or the patient has an altered level of consciousness.
- Risk stratification schemes for suicidal patients should be used (Table 187-1).
- Patients with schizophrenia, substance abuse, and depression are at higher risk of being suicidal.

TABLE 187-1 Evaluation of Suicide Risk in Adults and Adolescents

DEMOGRAPHIC, HEALTH, AND SOCIAL PROFILE	HIGH RISK	LOWER RISK
Gender	Male	Female
Marital status	Separated, divorced, or widowed	Married
Family history	Chaotic, conflictual Family history of suicide	Stable No family history of suicide
Job	Recently unemployed	Employed
Relationships	Recent conflict or loss of a relationship	Stable relationships
School	In disciplinary trouble	No disciplinary problems
Religion	Weak or no suicide taboo	Strong taboo against suicide
Health		
Physical	Acute or chronic, progressive illness Excessive drug or alcohol use	Good health Little or no drug or alcohol use
Mental	Depression (SIG E CAPS + MOOD)* History of schizophrenia or bipolar disorder Panic disorder Antisocial or disruptive behavior Feelings of helplessness or hopelessness Few, weak reasons for living Unstable, inappropriate affect	No depression No psychosis Minimal anxiety Directable, oriented Has hope, optimism Good, strong reasons for living Appropriate affect

(Continued)

TABLE 187-1 Evaluation of Suicide Risk in Adults and Adolescents (Continued)

DEMOGRAPHIC, HEALTH, AND SOCIAL PROFILE	HIGH RISK	LOWER RISK
Suicidal ideation	Frequent, intense, prolonged, pervasive	Infrequent, low intensity, transient
Suicide attempts	Repeated attempts	No prior attempts
	Realistic plan, including access to means	No plan, lacks access to means
	Previous attempt(s) planned	Previous attempt(s) impulsive
	Rescue unlikely	High likelihood of rescue
	Lethal method	Method of low lethality
	Guilt	Embarrassment about suicide ideation
	Unambiguous or continuing wish to die	No previous or continuing wish to die; large appeal component
Relationship with health professional	Lacks insight	Insight
	Poor rapport	Good rapport
Social support	Unsupportive family, friends	Concerned family, friends
	Socially isolated	Socially integrated

*SIG E CAPS + MOOD is a mnemonic for the eight symptoms of depression plus depressed mood, S = sleep disturbance; I = loss of interest in usual pleasurable activities, G = guilt; E = loss of energy, C = inability to concentrate, A = loss of appetite, P = psychomotor slowing, S = suicidal thoughts, MOOD = depressed mood (ie, "Have you felt blue, down, or depressed most of the day for most days in the last 2 weeks?"). Fulfillment of five or more of the eight items from the list of eight symptoms indicates the presence of major depression. Symptoms must be present nearly every day for 2 weeks and must include depressed mood or loss of interest or pleasure in activities. Symptoms must represent a change from previous functioning resulting in social, occupational, or other life impairment, and they cannot be the direct result of substance use, a medical condition, or bereavement.

- A high index of suspicion for depression should be maintained in patients with vague, seemingly unrelated, somatic complaints.
- Medication overdose is the most common type of suicide attempt.
- The language of potentially violent patients may contain profanity, escalate in volume, and be rapid or pressured.
- Mannerisms suggestive of a potentially violent patient include restlessness, pacing in the examination room, clenched fists, acts of violence directed toward inanimate objects in the room, and hypervigilance.

DIAGNOSIS AND DIFFERENTIAL

- Differentiating medical (organic) and psychiatric etiologies is important to appropriately managing the patient demonstrating abnormal behavior.
- Evaluation includes a detailed history of present illness, past medical and psychiatric history, medication history, social history, and a physical examination.
- Important components of the mental status examination are documentation of the patient's physical appearance, affect, orientation, speech pattern, behavior, level of consciousness, attention, language, memory, judgment, thought content, and perceptual abnormalities.
- Multiple clinical features can be associated with organic etiologies of abnormal behavior (Table 187-2).
- A variety of reversible medical conditions might result in the acute onset of a behavioral abnormality including hypoglycemia, hypoxemia, hypertensive encephalopathy, meningitis or encephalitis, head trauma, seizure, intracranial neoplasm, stroke, acute organ system failure, delirium secondary to infection, endocrinopathy (thyroid, parathyroid, or adrenal), and substance intoxication, poisoning, or withdrawal.
- A third-party account of the patient's behavior as it compares with the patient's normal behavior and level of functioning is important to obtain.
- Important historical information includes the presence of previous psychiatric illness, fever, head trauma, infections, ingestion of medications or legal and illegal substances, disorientation or confusion, impaired speech, syncope or loss of consciousness, headaches, and difficulty performing routine tasks.
- All abnormal vital signs should be investigated and corrected before attributing the patient's abnormal behavior to a psychiatric etiology with special attention being devoted to discovering signs of trauma, infection, substance abuse, endocrine disorders, and disorders of the central nervous system.
- Visual hallucinations tend to be more suggestive of a medical etiology, whereas auditory hallucinations tend to support a psychiatric etiology.
- If the patient is unable to draw a clock face correctly with the hands reading a specific time designated by the examiner, then a medical etiology of the behavioral abnormality is likely.

TABLE 187-2 Features Associated with an Organic Cause of Psychosis

Abnormal vital sign values
Disorientation with clouded consciousness
Abnormal mental status examination findings
Recent memory loss
Age >40 y without a previous history of psychiatric disorder
Focal neurologic signs
Visual hallucinations
Psychomotor retardation

- Determining the patient's capillary glucose concentration and oxygen saturation on room air is critical in rapidly excluding hypo- or hyperglycemia and hypoxemia as potential causes of the patient's altered behavior.
- Obtaining a urinalysis to evaluate for urinary tract infections resulting in delirium is important in the elderly individual.
- Additional tests that can be useful depending on the clinical situation include a complete blood count, serum electrolytes, creatinine, hepatic enzymes, T_4 level, TSH, ethanol, urine drug screen, pregnancy test, arterial blood gas analysis, cerebrospinal fluid analysis, electrocardiogram, and computed tomography or magnetic resonance imaging of the brain.
- Salicylate and acetaminophen levels also are useful in the suicidal patient.

EMERGENCY DEPARTMENT CARE AND DISPOSITION

- Emergency psychiatric evaluation should be prioritized in a stepwise fashion (Table 187-3).
- Violent patients should be physically and chemically sedated to avoid self-injury and harm to nearby individuals.
- An algorithmic approach can be used to safely chemically sedate an agitated patient (Fig. 187-1).
- Suicidal and homicidal or violent patients should be disrobed, gowned, and searched for potentially dangerous items.
- The clinician should approach the violent patient with a nonthreatening voice and posture while avoiding excessive eye contact and keeping the room's exit easily accessible.
- Enforceable limits as to what constitutes acceptable behavior by the patient must be set by the clinician.
- After excluding a medical (organic) etiology for the patient's abnormal behavior, patients judged to be at high risk to themselves or others or who

TABLE 187-3 Emergency Psychiatric Assessment Steps

STEP	COMMENT
Safety and stabilization	Contain violent and dangerously psychotic persons to provide a safe environment for staff, patients, family, and visitors while simultaneously attending to airway, breathing, and circulation.
Identification of homicidal, suicidal, or other dangerous behavior	Determine if the patient needs to be forcibly detained for emergency evaluation.
Medical evaluation	Determine the presence of any serious organic medical conditions that might cause or contribute to abnormal behavior or thought processes (eg, hypoglycemia, meningitis, drug withdrawal, or other causes of delirium).
Psychiatric diagnosis and severity assessment	If the behavior change is not due to an underlying medical condition, it is primarily psychiatric or functional, requiring a psychiatric diagnosis and assessment of the severity of the primary psychiatric problems.
Psychiatric consultation	Determine the need for immediate psychiatric consultation.

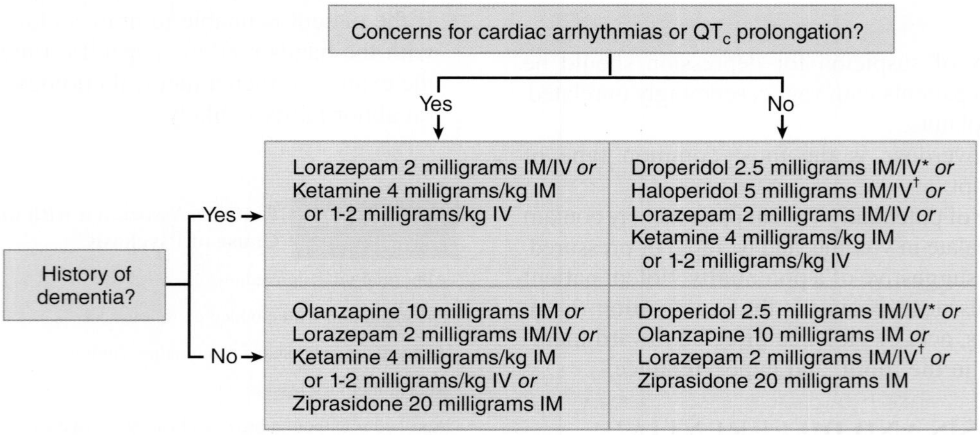

FIG. 187-1. Suggested algorithm for the ED management of patients with acute undifferentiated agitation. *Droperidol dosing may be repeated if clinically indicated. †Consider reduced dosing in the elderly; lorazepam, 1 milligram IM, haloperidol, 2 milligrams IM, and ketamine, 2 milligrams/kg IM.

are unable to effectively care for themselves while alone should be admitted to a psychiatric facility for definitive care.
- Patients whose evaluation demonstrates a medical etiology for their behavioral change should receive appropriate medical therapy specific to the disorder, and hospital admission is necessary if the disorder is not readily reversible, is likely to recur or progress, or if the patient's behavior remains such that independent living would be dangerous.

For further reading in Tintinalli's *Emergency Medicine: A Comprehensive Study Guide*, 7th ed., see Chapter 283, "Behavioral Disorders: Emergency Assessment," by Gregory Larkin and Annette Beautrais, and Chapter 285, "Psychotropic Medications and Rapid Tranquilization," by Marc Martel and Michelle Biros.

188 PANIC AND CONVERSION DISORDERS

Lance H. Hoffman

PANIC DISORDER

EPIDEMIOLOGY

- Panic disorder has a national lifetime prevalence of 3.5%.
- Women are two to three times more likely than men to be afflicted with this disorder.
- Symptoms usually begin in the second to fourth decades of life.

CLINICAL FEATURES

- The patient experiences acute, recurrent episodes of intense anxiety and fear, resulting in a persistent fear regarding the implications of having another such episode.
- Most episodes begin unexpectedly. Symptom severity peaks within 10 minutes of symptom onset and lasts for up to 1 hour.
- Different somatic and cognitive symptoms dominate the panic attacks (Table 188-1).

TABLE 188-1 Symptoms of a Panic Attack

SOMATIC SYMPTOMS	COGNITIVE SYMPTOMS
Palpitations, pounding heart, or tachycardia	Fear of losing control
Sweating	Fear of dying
Sensations of shortness of breath or smothering	Derealization (feeling of unreality) or depersonalization (feeling detached from oneself)
Trembling or shaking	
Feeling of choking	
Chest pain or discomfort	
Nausea or abdominal distress	
Feeling dizzy, unsteady, light-headed, or faint	
Paresthesias	
Chills or hot flashes	

- Tachycardia and mild hypertension are common physical examination findings.

DIAGNOSIS AND DIFFERENTIAL

- Panic disorder is a diagnosis of exclusion because its symptoms and signs mimic those of many potentially life-threatening disorders.
- Multiple medical diagnoses should be considered in the differential for panic disorder (Table 188-2).
- Victims of intimate partner violence or sexual abuse or assault may present similarly to a patient with panic disorder.

EMERGENCY DEPARTMENT CARE AND DISPOSITION

- Life-threatening causes of the patient's symptoms must first be excluded.
- Benzodiazepines are the mainstay of therapy for controlling symptoms acutely. **Alprazolam** 0.25 to 0.5 milligram PO or **lorazepam** 1 to 2 milligrams PO or IV is effective.
- The patient should be questioned specifically about suicidal thoughts and depression because patients with panic disorder and depression have a lifetime suicide risk of 19.5%.
- Referral to a psychiatrist for outpatient cognitive behavioral therapy and pharmacotherapy is warranted if symptoms are controlled and suicidality is lacking. Otherwise, psychiatric consultation for admission is necessary.

CONVERSION DISORDER

EPIDEMIOLOGY

- Conversion disorder is rare, but affects women approximately four times more often than men.

TABLE 188-2 Medical Differential Diagnosis of Panic Attacks

Cardiovascular	Neurologic	Drug withdrawal
Angina	Migraine headache	Alcohol
Myocardial infarction	Ménière disease	Barbiturates
Mitral valve prolapse	Complex partial seizures	Benzodiazepines
Congestive heart failure	Transient ischemic attacks	Opiates
Tachyarrhythmias: premature atrial contractions, supraventricular tachycardia	Drug induced	β Antagonists
Pulmonary	Caffeine	Psychiatric
Hyperventilation	Cocaine	Post-traumatic stress disorder
Asthma	Sympathomimetics	Depressive disorders
Pulmonary embolus	Theophylline	Other anxiety disorders
Endocrine	Thyroid preparations	Psychosocial
Hyperthyroidism	Selective serotonin reuptake inhibitors	Partner violence
Hypoglycemia	Cannabis	Sexual abuse or assault
Hyponatremia	Corticosteroids	Other situational stressors
Pheochromocytoma	β Agonists	
Carcinoid syndrome	Triptans	
Cushing syndrome	Nicotine	
	Yohimbine	
	Hallucinogens	
	Anticholinergics	

CLINICAL FEATURES

- Conversion disorder is a somatoform disorder in which a person unconsciously and acutely produces a symptom suggestive of a physical disorder that results in a change or loss of physical functioning as a response to a stressor or conflict.
- The symptom cannot be explained by a known organic etiology or culturally sanctioned response pattern, and it cannot be limited to pain or sexual dysfunction.
- The symptom typically involves a loss of neurologic functioning.

DIAGNOSIS AND DIFFERENTIAL

- An organic explanation for the patient's symptom must be excluded before the diagnosis of conversion disorder can be made.
- A variety of physical examination maneuvers have been described to assist the clinician in differentiating neurologic symptoms caused by a psychological etiology from an organic etiology (Table 188-3).
- A high index of suspicion must be maintained for organic etiologies that might explain the symptom, including systemic lupus erythematosus, polymyositis, multiple sclerosis, Lyme disease, and drug toxicity.

TABLE 188-3 Testing Techniques for Conversion Disorder

FUNCTION	TECHNIQUE
Sensation	
Yes–no test	Patient closes eyes and responds yes or *no* to touch stimulus. *No* response in numb area favors conversion disorder.
Bowlus and Currier test	Patient extends and then crosses the arms, with thumbs pointed down and palms facing together. Fingers (but not thumbs) are then interlocked, and then the hands are rotated inward toward chest. Sharp stimuli are applied to each finger in turn and the patient is asked to indicate normal or abnormal sensation in each digit. Patients with conversion disorder make mistakes and are inconsistent with responses.
Strength test	Patient closes eyes. Test "strength" by touching finger to be moved. True lack of sensation would not allow patient to ascertain finger to be moved.
Pain	
Gray test	With abdominal pain due to psychological factors, the patient will close eyes during palpation. In pain of organic basis, the patient is more likely to watch the examiner's hand to anticipate pain.
Motor	
Drop test	When a patient with paralysis of nonorganic etiology lifts a thumb, the affected limb will drop more slowly or fall with exaggerated speed as compared with the unaffected limb. In addition, an extremity dropped from above the face will miss it.
Thigh adductor test	Examiner places hands against both inner thighs of the patient who is told to adduct the "good" leg against resistance. With pseudoparalysis, the adductor muscles of "bad" leg will also adduct.
Hoover test	Examiner's hands cup both heels of the patient who is asked to elevate the "good" leg. With pseudoparalysis the "bad" leg will push downward. When the patient is asked to lift the "bad" leg, if there is no downward pressure in the "good" leg, the patient is not trying.
Sternocleido-mastoid test	Contraction of normal sternocleidomastoid muscle causes face to rotate away from side of the contracted muscle. Patient with conversion hemiplegia cannot turn head to the weak side.
Coma	
Corneal reflex	Corneal reflexes remain intact in an awake patient.
Bell phenomenon	Eyes divert upward when lids are opened, whereas eyes remain in neutral position in true coma.
Lid closing	In true coma, lids when opened close rapidly initially and then more slowly as lids descend. Awake patients will have lids stay open, snap shut, or flutter.

(*Continued*)

TABLE 188-3	Testing Techniques for Conversion Disorder (Continued)
FUNCTION	TECHNIQUE
Seizures	
Corneal reflex	Usually intact in pseudoseizure.
Abdominal musculature	Palpation of abdominal musculature reveals lack of contractions with pseudoseizure.
Blindness	
Opticokinetic drum	Rotating drum with alternating black and white stripes or piece of tape with alternating black and white sections pulled laterally in front of a patient's open eyes will produce nystagmus in a patient with intact vision.

EMERGENCY DEPARTMENT CARE AND DISPOSITION

- An organic etiology to the symptom must first be excluded.
- After presenting the normal test results, reassure the patient that a serious medical illness is not present as directly confronting the patient that the symptom has no organic etiology may worsen the symptom.
- The physician should suggest to the patient that the symptom often spontaneously resolves in cases in which the test results are normal.
- Psychiatric or neurologic consultation in the ED is warranted if the symptom does not resolve and precludes discharging the patient home. Otherwise, outpatient psychiatric referral is mandatory as repetitive reassurance may be needed before full function returns.

For further reading in Tintinalli's *Emergency Medicine: A Comprehensive Study Guide,* 7th ed., see Chapter 287, "Panic Disorder," by Linda M. Nicholas and Elizabeth Shumann, and Chapter 288, "Conversion Disorder," by Gregory Moore and Kenneth Jackimczyk.

189 CHILD AND ELDERLY ABUSE

Jonathan Glauser

CHILD ABUSE

- More than 1 million cases of child maltreatment are recorded annually in the United States. Two-thirds of victims of physical abuse are <3 years old.
- Child maltreatment includes physical abuse, sexual abuse, emotional abuse, supervisional neglect, parental substance abuse, and Munchausen syndrome by proxy.

CLINICAL FEATURES

- Children with failure to thrive are generally under the age of 3 years.
  - They may present with skin infections, severe diaper dermatitis, or acute gastroenteritis.
  - Weight tends to be more affected than length, with body mass index under the fifth percentile. Infants may have little subcutaneous tissue, protruding ribs, or occipital alopecia from lying on their back all day.
  - They are wide eyed, wary, and difficult to console.
  - They may have increased muscle tone in their lower extremities.
  - Weight gain in the hospital is thought to be diagnostic of failure to thrive.
- Children over the age of 2 years with environmental neglect are termed psychosocial dwarfs.
  - Their short stature is more prominent than their low weight.
  - They tend to be hyperactive with unintelligible or delayed speech and bizarre and voracious appetite.
- Physical abuse is suggested by a history that is inconsistent with the nature of the injuries.
  - For example, a fall off of a bed should not cause a femur fracture.
  - Children under the age of 6 months cannot induce accidents or ingest drugs or poisons, as another example.
- The history of the event given by the caretaker may keep changing, or may be different from that given by the child.
- The following findings suggest physical abuse:
  1. Bruises over multiple areas.
  2. Bites with an intercanine diameter >3 cm, since these must be inflicted by an adult.
  3. Lacerations of the frenulum or oral mucosa, from force-feeding.
  4. Burns of an entire hand or foot, or burns of the buttocks or genitalia from toilet training punishment.
  5. Cigarette burns, with approximately 5-mm scab-covered injuries.
  6. Spiral fractures caused by twisting of long bones.
  7. Metaphyseal chip fractures.
  8. Periosteal elevation from new bone formation at sites of previous microfractures.
  9. Multiple fractures at different stages of healing.
  10. Fractures at unusual sites such as lateral clavicle, ribs, and sternum.

11. Vomiting, irritability, seizures, change in mental status, or apnea from intracranial hemorrhage (shaken baby syndrome). Retinal hemorrhages on funduscopic examination may be present.
12. Vomiting, abdominal pain, and tenderness with diminished bowel sounds or abdominal distention may be due to a duodenal hematoma, as evidenced by a "double-bubble" sign on abdominal radiographs.

- Munchausen syndrome by proxy is a synonym for medical child abuse. A parent fabricates illness in a child in order to secure prolonged contact with health care providers.
  - Complaints may be numerous, including seizures, bleeding, fever, altered mental status, vomiting, or rash. Agents such as ipecac or warfarin may have been given to precipitate these complaints.
  - Parents typically encourage more diagnostic tests, and are happy if they are positive.
- Sexual abuse is suggested with complaints referable to the anogenital area, such as bleeding, discharge, or the presence of a sexually transmitted disease.
  - Clefts or concavities in the hymen typically present in the 6 o'clock position.

DIAGNOSIS AND DIFFERENTIAL

- Any serious injury in a child under the age of 5 years should be viewed with suspicion.
- Parents and caregivers may appear to be under the influence of drugs or alcohol. They may refuse diagnostic studies.
- Victims of neglect may appear dirty, may be improperly clothed, and may be unimmunized.
- Victims of child abuse may seem overly compliant with painful medical procedures.
  - They may be overly protective of the abusing parent, or appear to be overly affectionate to medical staff.
- A skeletal survey of the long bones may be performed to detect any evidence of physical abuse.
- Laboratory workup may include a CBC and PT/PTT and PFA-100 screen for coagulation abnormalities.
- Careful inspection of the genital area is generally sufficient to establish genital injury.
- Speculum examination in the preadolescent is generally not needed unless perforating vaginal trauma is suspected.
  - Children can be examined in a frog-leg position; stirrups are usually unnecessary.
  - Colposcopy and toluidine blue may detect subtle acute injuries but are generally not available.
  - The diameter of the hymeneal orifice may not be indicative of prior vaginal penetration.
  - Fissures, abrasions, thickened perianal folds, lichenified perianal skin, or decreased anal tone may result from acute or chronic sodomy.
  - Absence of physical findings does not rule out abuse.
- Laboratory testing for sexual abuse should include cultures of the throat, vagina, and rectum for gonorrhea and chlamydia.
  - Rapid antigen assays are **not** considered reliable forensic evidence in prepubescent children.
  - Syphilis testing should be performed if there is clinical suspicion, if there is a high incidence in the community, or if the assailant has a history of syphilis.
  - If there is a reason to suspect HIV and appropriate counseling is available, testing should be done.

EMERGENCY CARE AND DISPOSITION

- Infants suspected of suffering from failure to thrive should be admitted to the hospital.
- Every state requires that suspected cases of child abuse be reported.
- The law protects physicians from legal retaliation by parents.
- Children with suspected Munchausen syndrome by proxy should be admitted for social and psychological evaluation.

■ ELDER ABUSE

- Elder abuse is an act or omission resulting in harm to the health or welfare of an elderly person, and affects 3% of the US elderly population.
  - This may entail neglect, such as deprivation of food, clothing, shelter or medical care, physical or sexual abuse, or abandonment of an elder in a home, hospital, or public location such as a shopping mall.
  - Unique to this age group is financial exploitation: use of pensions or Social Security checks for personal gain, forcible transfer of property, or changing an elderly person's will.

CLINICAL FEATURES

- Physical abuse is the most easily recognized form of elder abuse, although chemical restraint such as intentional overmedication may be subtle.
- Caregiver neglect, defined as failure of a caregiver to provide basic care, goods, and services such as clothing and shelter, accounts for the majority of cases of elder abuse.
- Financial abuse is the second commonest form of abuse, and occurs when family members take control of or steal assets, checks, or pensions for personal gain.
- Emotional abuse entails inflicting anguish, emotional pain, or distress.

  - Verbal threats, social isolation, and harassment can contribute to depression and other mental health problems.
  - Self-neglect includes those behaviors of an elderly person that threaten his or her own safety: failure to provide adequate food, medical care, hygiene, clothing, or shelter.

DIAGNOSIS AND DIFFERENTIAL

- Risk factors for elder abuse may be associated with caregivers/perpetrators or with the elders. Patient characteristics include the following:
  1. Cognitive impairment
  2. Female sex
  3. Physical dependency
  4. Alcohol abuse
  5. Developmental disability, special medical or psychiatric needs
  6. Lack of social support
  7. Limited experience managing finances
- Risk factors for perpetrators of abuse include the following:
  1. History of violence within or outside of the family.
  2. Excessive dependence on the elder for financial support.
  3. History of mental illness or substance abuse.
- To make the diagnosis, potential sufferers of abuse should be interviewed in private.
- Screening questions have been developed for elder abuse, querying whether anyone has touched or hurt them, forced them to do things, taken something of theirs without asking, threatened them, or made them feel afraid.
- Caretakers may give a conflicting report of an injury or illness.
- The patient may appear fearful of his or her companion.
- The caretaker may seem indifferent or angry toward the patient, or may be overly concerned with costs of treatment needed by the patient.
- The following are suggestive on physical examination for abuse:
  1. Bruising or trauma
  2. Poor general appearance and hygiene
  3. Malnutrition and dehydration
  4. Contusions and lacerations to normally protected areas of the body: inner thighs, mastoid, palms, soles, buttocks
  5. Unusual burns or multiple burns in different stages of healing
  6. Rope or restraint marks on ankles or wrists
  7. Spiral fractures of long bones
  8. Midshaft ulnar (nightstick) fractures from attempts to shield blows
  9. Multiple deep/uncared-for ulcers
  10. Poor personal hygiene, inappropriate or soiled clothing

EMERGENCY DEPARTMENT CARE AND DISPOSITION

- Elder abuse is widely underreported and underrecognized. Treatment entails three key components:
  1. Addressing medical and psychosocial needs
  2. Ensuring patient safety
  3. Compliance with local reporting requirements
- Medical problems and injuries may be best managed with hospital admission.
- Elders left in the same position for an extended period of time should be screened for rhabdomyolysis.
- All 50 states have reporting requirements for elder abuse and neglect. Adult protective services should be notified.
- Patients in immediate danger should be hospitalized.
- If neglect is unintentional, education of the caregiver may be all that is needed.
- Requirements for reporting within one's practice area are available at www.nceaaoa.gov

For further reading in Tintinalli's *Emergency Medicine: A Comprehensive Study Guide*, 7th ed., see Chapter 290, "Child Abuse and Neglect," by Carol D. Berkowitz, and Chapter 293, "Abuse of the Elderly and Impaired," by Frederic M. Hustey and Jonathan Glauser.

Section 23

ABUSE AND ASSAULT

190 SEXUAL ASSAULT AND INTIMATE PARTNER VIOLENCE AND ABUSE

Sara Laskey

SEXUAL ASSAULT

- Victims do not always sustain injury.
- The perpetrator is often known to the victim.
- Intimate partner violence and abuse (IPVA) is a pattern of behavior and can include sexual, psychological abuse, intimidation, stalking, threats, and deprivation.
- Occurs in every race, religion, ethnicity, culture, and sexual orientation.

CLINICAL FEATURES

- Elements of a sexual assault history are listed in Table 190-1.
- Risk factors for IPVA include females between 20 and 24 years of age, low income status, and being separated from partner.
- Look for injuries inconsistent with history, injuries in various stages of healing, and delay in reporting of injury.
- Complaints of chronic pain syndromes, gynecologic pain, and psychiatric and substance abuse issues may be initial presentations.
- Patients may appear frightened if the partner is present during history. Partner may exhibit hostile behaviors.
- Patients should be asked about any suicidal or homicidal ideation and get appropriate, immediate evaluation.

PHYSICAL EXAMINATION

- Perform a complete general medical examination.
- Look for defensive injury areas—extremities and hidden injuries—oral cavity, breast, thighs, and buttocks.
- Record all signs of trauma using a body map.
- Note signs of trauma, discharge and/or abrasions found on speculum examination.

TABLE 190-1 Assault History

Who?
Did the assault survivor know the assailant?
Was it a single assailant or multiple assailants?
What were the assailant's identity and race? (Document in the medical records.)
What happened?
Was the patient physically assaulted?
With what (eg, gun, bat, or fist) and where?
Was there actual or attempted vaginal, anal, or oral penetration?
Did ejaculation occur? If so, where?
Was a foreign object used?
Was a condom used?
When?
When did the assault occur?
(Emergency contraception is most effective when started within 72 h of the assault.)
Where?
Where did the assault occur?
(Corroborating evidence may be found based on the location of the assault.)
Suspicion of drug-facilitated rape?
Was there a period of amnesia?
Is there a history of being out drinking and then suddenly feeling very intoxicated?
Is there a history of waking up naked or with genital soreness?
Douche, shower, or change of clothing?
Did the patient douche, shower, or change clothing after the assault? (Performing any of these activities prior to seeking medical attention may decrease the probability of sperm or acid phosphatase recovery, as well as recovery of other bits of trace evidence.)

- Anal examination is required if anal penetration is reported.
- Characteristic injuries include fingernail scratches, bite marks, cigarette burns, rope burns, forearm bruising, and nightstick fractures (Table 190-2).
- Pregnant patients are at higher risk for abdominal injuries.
- Evidence collection is performed only within the first 72 hours after sexual assault.
- Informed consent is required for evidence collection.
- Most hospitals have a prepackaged rape kit and chain of custody must be maintained.
- If >72 hours have elapsed or the patient declines a rape kit, perform a history and physical examination, document injuries, and provide prophylaxis for pregnancy and sexually transmitted infections.

TABLE 190-2 Signs Suggestive of Intimate Partner Violence

FINDINGS	COMMENTS
Injuries characteristic of violence	Fingernail scratches, broken fingernails, bite marks, dental injuries, cigarette burns, bruises suggesting strangulation or restraint, and rope burns or ligature marks may be seen.
Injuries suggesting a defensive posture	Forearm bruises or fractures may be sustained when individuals try to fend off blows to the face or chest.
Injuries during pregnancy	Up to 45% of women report abuse or assault during pregnancy. Preterm labor, placental abruption, direct fetal injury, stillbirth can occur.
Central pattern of injury	Injuries to the head, neck, face, and thorax, and abdominal injuries in pregnant women may suggest violence.
Extent or type of injury inconsistent with the patient's explanation	Multiple injuries may be seen at different anatomic sites inconsistent with the described mechanism of injury. The most common explanation of injury is a "fall." Embarrassment, evasiveness, or lack of concern with the injuries may be noted.
Multiple injuries in various stages of healing	These may be reported as "accidents" or "clumsiness."
Delay between the time of injury and the presentation for treatment	Victims may wait several days before seeking medical care for injuries. Victims may seek care for minor or resolving injuries.
Visits for vague or minor complaints without evidence of physiologic abnormality	This pattern may include frequent ED visits for a variety of injuries or illnesses, including chronic pelvic pain and other chronic pain syndromes.
Suicide attempts	Women who attempt or commit suicide often have a history of intimate partner violence.

DIAGNOSIS AND DIFFERENTIAL

- Sexual assault is a legal determination, not a medical diagnosis.
- The legal definition requires carnal knowledge, non-consent and compulsion, or fear of harm.
- Many experts recommend routine screening for IPVA for all adolescent and adult women who present to the ED. This should be conducted in a safe and private environment.

EMERGENCY DEPARTMENT CARE AND DISPOSITION

SEXUAL ASSAULT

- Obtain pregnancy test.
- Offer emergency contraception: **levonorgesterol** only 1.5 milligrams PO in a single dose or two doses 0.75 milligram PO 12 hours apart, *or* combined **estrogen-progestin,** two doses of **ethinyl estradiol**, 100 micrograms PO, plus **lovenorgestrel**, 0.5 milligram PO, 12 hours apart.

TABLE 190-3 Hotlines for Patients

National Domestic Violence Hotline: 24 h; links caller to help in her (or his) area—emergency shelter, domestic violence shelters, legal advocacy and assistance programs, social services	800-799-SAFE (7233) 800-787-3224 (TTY)
Rape, Abuse, and Incest National Network: 24 h; automatically transfers caller to nearest rape crisis center anywhere in the nation	800-656-HOPE (4673) http://www.rainn.org

STI TREATMENT/PROPHYLAXIS

- Gonorrhea: **ceftriaxone**, 250 milligrams IM, or **ceftixine**, 400 milligrams PO—single dose.
- Chlamydia: **azithromycin**, 1 gram PO, *or* **doxycycline**, 100 milligrams PO twice a day for 7 days (do not use during pregnancy).
- Trichomoniasis and bacterial vaginosis: **metronidazole**, 2 grams PO, in single dose (do not use during first trimester of pregnancy).
- Syphilis: **penicillin G benzathine** 2.4 million IU IM. Use **erythromycin** 500 milligrams PO four times each day for 15 days if penicillin allergy (no prophylaxis).
- Hepatitis: Administer vaccines at the time of examination if not previously vaccinated. Schedule follow-up doses at 1 to 2 months and 4 to 6 months after initial dose.
- HIV: Circumstances should guide prophylaxis. Rates of seroconversion are low. Routine prophylaxis is *not* recommended. See CDC Web site (www.cdc.gov) for recommendations.

INTIMATE PARTNER VIOLENCE AND ABUSE

- Assess for lethal situations, increased frequency or severity of violence, and threat or use of weapons.
- Hospital admission is an option if a safe location cannot be established before discharge.
- National hotlines are available (Table 190-3).

For further reading in Tintinalli's *Emergency Medicine: A comprehensive Study Guide*, 7th ed., see Chapter 291, "Female and Male Sexual Assault," by Sheryl L. Heron and Debra E. Houry, and Chapter 292, "Intimate Partner Violence and Abuse," by Mary Hancock.

Section 24
PRINCIPLES OF IMAGING

191 PRINCIPLES OF EMERGENCY DEPARTMENT USE OF COMPUTED TOMOGRAPHY AND MAGNETIC RESONANCE IMAGING

Clare F. Wallner

COMPUTED TOMOGRAPHY

- Computed tomography (CT) creates a cross-sectional image of a patient by placing a radiograph source and a detector on a gantry that rotates around a patient. An image is displayed after computer reconstruction.
- CT can best be used to differentiate calcified from noncalcified tissue. Major advantages over MRI include availability, speed, and decreased cost.
- Major disadvantages include its associated ionizing radiation, and potential allergies, or renal insult with IV contrast.
- Hounsfield units (HU) or CT numbers quantify the amount of attentuation through tissue. Air is most negative and cortical bone is the most positive.
- The image can be manipulated to differentiate between structures. Window width refers to the range of HU for image processing; densities above the chosen range will be white and those below will be black. A narrow window width will look at a structure with little difference in tissue densities, such as the brain. Window level refers to where the range lies (low with densities close to air, like the lungs, or higher density to visualize bony structres).
- Spiral (helical) scanning allows for continuous image acquisition by rotating the gantry around a moving patient table.
- Multidetector array CT scanners can provide multiple (64, 128, or 256) images at the same time, reducing time and contrast needed. Combined with software improvements, they also allow for multiplanar and 3-D reconstruction.
- Electron beam CT (EBCT) uses a stationary beam and anode to produce a very high resolution, rapidly obtained image. It is most used for cardiovascular imaging, but is limited by large size, higher cost, and limited availability.

GENERAL USES AND LIMITATIONS OF CT

- Head CT is the primary study for screening ED patients for acute intracranial bleeding, trauma, and stroke.
- CT is the imaging study of choice for many disorders of the abdomen, pelvis, retroperitoneum, and thoracic cavity including evaluation of the vasculature.
- Fractures and other bony abnormalities are usually well demonstrated by CT, especially cervical spine, facial, and pelvic fractures.
- Body areas that are poorly visualized with CT include the posterior cranial fossa and the pituitary fossa; the spinal cord cannot be well differentiated from cerebrospinal fluid without contrast (CT myelogram).

USE OF CONTRAST

- Contrast material can be administered by the oral, intravenous, rectal, intra-arterial, intra-articular, or intrathecal route.
- Oral contrast for abdominal CT scanning improves the likelihood of detecting bowel wall abnormalities, including hematoma, edema, mass, or laceration.
- If contrast is to be administered to trauma patients, a water-soluble agent should be used to avoid the extravasation of barium-containing agents.
- Adverse reactions include (1) idiosyncratic anaphylactoid reactions that occurs with increased frequency in those with prior adverse reactions, asthmatics, diabetics, those on beta blockers or metformin, renal or cardiac failure, extremes of age, and those with a history of atopy and (2) allergic reactions, including minor side effects, intermediate reactions such as hypotension or bronchospasm, and severe reactions including laryngeal or bronchial edema, severe bronchospasm, or cardiac dysrhythmias and arrest.
- Pretreatment with steroids and diphenhydramine hours prior to IV contrast can reduce risk of reaction by a factor of 10.
- Contrast-induced nephropathy (CIN) is an increased risk for those with preexisting renal insufficiency, diabetic nephropathy, or those taking nephrotoxic drugs. Hydration may help reduce the risk of CIN.

- Patients who are on metformin may have an accumulation of metformin resulting in potentially fatal lactic acidosis. Metformin should be held for 48 hours after the injection of IV contrast and then restarted after renal function is rechecked.

IONIZING RADIATION

- There is a linear dose–response relationship between exposure to ionizing radiation and the development of solid cancers. One in 100 persons exposed to 100 mSv will develop cancer (whole-body CT scan is an exposure of 10 mSv).
- Children are at greatest risk.
- Alternative imaging modalities should be utilized in the pregnant patient. If CT is necessary, the abdomen and pelvis of pregnant patients should be shielded whenever possible to reduce radiation to the fetus.

MAGNETIC RESONANCE IMAGING

- MRI takes advantage of the fact that the nuclei of hydrogen atoms in water and fat molecules act like spinning magnets. When placed in a strong magnetic field, these "magnets" align with the field, and when a short pulse of a radio wave of specific frequency is applied, the magnets change alignment and then realign with the external magnetic field. The resultant small voltage can be measured and displayed as an image.
- T1 and T2 images are generated by net recovery in different planes and change with different tissues. T1 images clearly delineate different tissues and are considered "anatomy" scans. T2 images reveal bright fluid with most other tissues gray allowing edema to be easily seen. They are considered "pathology" scans.
- The major advantages of MRI over other imaging modalities are (1) it does not use ionizing radiation and no short- or long-term side effects have been demonstrated, (2) it can produce image slices of any orientation through the body, and (3) in many body areas, it produces better contrast resolution and tissue discrimination than radiographs or ultrasound.

MRI SAFETY AND OTHER CONSIDERATIONS

Considered Safe

- There is no known increased risk to pregnant patients, although no definitive evidence of lack of teratogenic or acoustic effects on the fetus. MRI is prefered over imaging involving ionizing radiation in weeks 2 to 20 of pregnancy.
- Many cardiac implanted devices are nonferromagnetic or only weakly ferromagnetic, and are considered safe for MRI. These include most cardiac stents, although additional protection is conferred 6 weeks after placement due to epithilialization. Prosthetic heart valves are also considered safe; although those with stainless steel components may experience strong magnetic forces, they are less than the normal stress from cardiac function and gravity.

Contraindications and Safety

- Internal cardiac pacemakers and transvenous pacers may experience electrical currents or heating and may malfunction.
- Hemodynamic support and monitoring devices, such as pulmonary artery catheters (Swan–Ganz), an intra-aortic balloon pump, or a ventricular assist device, may experience electrical currents or heating and may malfunction.
- Certain (ferromagnetic) aneurysm clips may be affected, causing brain injury.
- Steel slivers in the eye (asymptomatic in some metal workers) may injure the retina.
- Cochlear implants may be damaged or cause injury.
- Other implanted devices (neurostimulators, bone growth stimulators, etc.) may malfunction or cause injury.
- Life-support equipment containing steel is attracted to the magnetic field and could injure the patient and the system.
- Any ferromagnetic object carried into the room can also become a potential missile.
- The examination can take from 30 to 60 minutes, and there must be no motion (except breathing). This may be difficult for patients who are claustrophobic or in pain and unsafe for an unstable patient.

Adverse Effects

- There is an unclear effect on a fetus. Gadolinium does cross the placenta and is relatively contraindicated during pregnancy.
- Loud noise caused by the gradient coils may cause acoustic damage.
- Gadolinium may lead to contrast nephropathy at high doses, although unlikely at standard doses.
- Allergy reactions do occur, but are less common than with iodinated contrast.
- Gadolinium may cause nephrogenic systemic fibrosis in patients with severe renal insufficiency

(GFR <30 mL/min/1.73 m^2), resulting in an FDA warning. Renal impairment due to hepatorenal syndrome or perioperative liver transplant patients may also lead to nephrogenic systemic fibrosis.

APPLICATIONS

- MRI of the brain and spinal cord provides better diagnostic quality images than CT. Intravenous contrast agents (that are less toxic than agents used for CT) are sometimes required.
- MRI has a major role in imaging the musculoskeletal system because it visualizes soft tissue with better resolution than CT and because it is sensitive to marrow and trabecular bone changes. This aids in the detection of osteomyelitis and avascular necrosis.
- MRI is useful in evaluation of other soft tissue musculoskeletal trauma such as muscle or tendon tears, hemorrhage, and edema, and injuries to medium-sized nerves and the brachial plexus.
- MRI can detect metastatic disease with high sensitivity and specificity.
- Because it is fast, readily available, and compatible with life-support equipment, CT is still the imaging technique of choice for suspected head, spine, and abdominal injuries.

MRI SCANNING IN THE EMERGENT SETTING

- In the ED setting, MRI is the imaging modality of choice for (1) evaluation of suspected spinal cord compression of any cause, (2) evaluation of radiographically occult femoral intertrochanteric and femoral neck fractures, and (3) evaluation of posterior cranial fossa pathology.
- Potential uses include (1) evaluation of aortic dissection as well as carotid and vertebral artery dissection, (2) evaluation of appendicitis in pregnancy if ultrasound is unavailable or nondiagnostic, (3) evaluation of pulmonary embolism, (4) evaluation of cerebral venous sinus thrombosis, and (5) evaluation of CVA (higher sensitivity than CT). MR diffusion weighted imaging can detect ischemic injury within minutes and MR perfusion imaging can identify the ischemic penumbra.

For further reading in Tintinalli's *Emergency Medicine: A Compresensive Guide*, 7th ed., see Chapter 299.2, "Computed Tomography," by William Roper and Stephanie Abbuhl, and Chapter 299.3, "Magnetic Resonance Imaging," by Esther K. Choo and Robert F. DeMayo.

192 PRINCIPLES OF EMERGENCY DEPARTMENT ULTRASONOGRAPHY

Catherine Erickson

FUNDAMENTALS

- Ultrasound waves that are completely reflected (eg, bone) appear white and are referred to as hyperechoic.
- A perfect transmitter of ultrasound waves (eg, fluid) appears black and is referred to as anechoic.
- Structures on the left side of the monitor correspond to the marker on the probe. This marker is generally oriented toward the patient's head in sagittal planes and toward the patient's right in transverse planes. Visualize structures in both the long and the short axis.
- Structures toward the top of the monitor correspond to structures closest (more superficial) to the probe. Hash marks on the screen correspond to increasing depths.

ULTRASONOGRAPHY IN THE EMERGENCY DEPARTMENT

PRIMARY INDICATIONS

Ultrasonography in Trauma

- The focused assessment with sonography in trauma (FAST) examination has a sensitivity of 90%, a specificity of 99%, and an accuracy rate of 99% for detecting free intraperitoneal fluid. It is the ideal imaging modality of choice in patients who are too unstable for CT because of its rapid and noninvasive features.
- The standard FAST views include (1) the subxiphoid view for the evaluation of pericardial fluid; (2) Morison's pouch (hepatorenal recess); (3) left subphrenic and splenorenal recess views; and (4) the pouch of Douglas and rectovesicular space.
- In addition, the upper abdominal views are useful in the evaluation of the patient for hemothorax.
- Hemodynamically unstable blunt trauma patients with a positive FAST examination for free intraperitoneal fluid should be taken directly to the operating room for exploratory laparotomy.
- Anteromedial lung windows can be visualized to detect pneumothorax in the extended FAST (EFAST) examination. An absence of the normal "lung sliding" has a sensitivity of 86% to 98% for detecting pneumothorax and is superior to the supine chest radiograph.

Cardiac Ultrasonography

- The major applications for ED cardiac ultrasonography are in the evaluation of pulseless electrical activity, cardiac trauma, and pericardial tamponade. Key sonographic findings are pericardial fluid collections and myocardial wall activity.
- Pericardial effusions appear as echo-free areas within the pericardial sac. A small pericardial effusion (<100 mL)will occupy a dependent position, while a large effusion (>300 mL) will present circumferentially.
- Sonographic localization of the pericardial sac is the best approach for performing pericardiocentesis.

Abdominal Aortic Aneurysms

- Ultrasonography is as accurate as CT in detecting and measuring the diameter of an abdominal aortic aneurysm.
- When the aorta is imaged from the diaphragm to its distal bifurcation (at the level of the umbilicus), it is nearly 100% accurate in the evaluation for an abdominal aortic aneurysm.
- An abdominal aortic diameter >3 cm is abnormal. Transverse images measured horizontally from outside wall to outside wall are the most reliable in determining the true size of the aorta.
- Potential indications for performing a screening aortic ultrasound in the ED include age >50 years with unexplained back, flank, abdominal, or groin pain and in patients with hypotension, syncope, or dizziness.

Evaluation of First-Trimester Pregnancy

- In the ED, ultrasound detection of an intrauterine pregnancy (IUP) greatly reduces the possibility of ectopic pregnancy. The prevalence of spontaneous heterotopic (simultaneous intrauterine and extrauterine pregnancies) is less than 1 in 30,000. However, the incidence greatly increases with fertility assistance.
- First-trimester pregnant patients presenting to the ED with any abdominal or pelvic pain, vaginal bleeding, or risk factors for ectopic pregnancy should have an ultrasound evaluation to confirm the presence of an intrauterine pregnancy.
- The earliest sonographic finding of a pregnancy is the gestational sac. This appears as a round or oval anechoic area within the uterus surrounded by two concentric echogenic rings (double decidual sign).
- The first reliable sign of an IUP is a yolk sac within the gestational sac. Transvaginal ultrasound can detect a yolk sac between 5 and 6 weeks' gestational age.
- An IUP should be detectable on endovaginal scanning if the beta-human chorionic gonadotropin (β-hCG) is >1000 mIU/mL (termed the discriminatory zone).
- Patients with a β-hCG greater than the discriminatory zone and who do not have evidence of an IUP on ultrasound should be presumed to have an ectopic pregnancy until proven otherwise.

Vascular Access

- Ultrasound use in central venous catheter placement decreases failure rates and complications.
- Additionally, in difficult access patients, ultrasound-guided peripheral vascular access decreases time to cannulation and the number of puncture attempts.

URGENT INDICATIONS

Gallbladder Disease

- Ultrasound is the imaging modality of choice in evaluating biliary disease.
- Gallstones appear as echogenic structures with posterior shadowing lying within the gallbladder. They will move with positional changes unless embedded in the gallbladder neck.
- A sonographic Murphy's sign is positive when the point of maximal tenderness to transducer pressure is directly over the visualized gallbladder. This sign, in the presence of gallstones, is reported to have a 92% positive predictive value for cholecystitis.
- Gallbladder wall thickening, defined as proximal gallbladder wall thickness >3 mm, occurs in 50% to 75% of patients with acute cholecystitis. It is not pathognomonic for cholecystitis; it is also seen in patients with ascites and other hypoproteinemic states.

Renal Colic

- The renal sinus appears as an extremely echogenic region within the center of the kidney and includes the collecting system. The renal cortex surrounds the sinus and appears slightly less echogenic than that of the liver or spleen.
- Both longitudinal and transverse images should be obtained of both kidneys. The identification of hydronephrosis, an anechoic fluid collection within the renal sinus, is a marker for renal calculi. One method of grading hydronephrosis is from mild (minimal separation of the sinus) to severe (extensive communicating anechoic regions in the sinus with cortical thinning).
- In patients with flank pain and hematuria, bedside ultrasound has a sensitivity >85% in diagnosing a ureteral stone.
- Ureteral calculi typically lodge at the ureterovesicular junction, the ureteropelvic junction, or the pelvic brim, and are only visualized on ultrasound in 19% of patients with documented kidney stones.

MISCELLANEOUS EMERGENCY DEPARTMENT APPLICATIONS

- Compression ultrasound for the diagnosis of deep venous thrombosis (DVT) has a sensitivity of 95%. The femoralpopliteal region is evaluated for complete vessel collapse to rule out thrombus. Because calf ultrasound is less sensitive, repeat ultrasound should be performed within 1 week when a calf thrombus is suspected.
- Ultrasonography can guide the emergency physician in performing procedures such as thoracentesis and paracentesis.
- Ultrasound evaluation of soft tissues can help to differentiate cutaneous abscesses from cellulitis, confirm need for drainage, and avoid unnecessary procedures. Soft tissue can also be evaluated for radiolucent foreign bodies, such as wood and plastic.

For further reading in Tintinalli's *Emergency Medicine: A Comprehensive Study Guide*, 7th ed., see Chapter 299.4, "Emergency Ultrasonography," by O. John Ma, Robert F. Reardon, and Alfredo Sabbaj.

Section 25
ADMINISTRATION

193 EMERGENCY MEDICAL SERVICES

C. Crawford Mechem

- Emergency medical services (EMS) are the extension of emergency medical care into the prehospital setting.
- The U.S. EMS Systems Act of 1973 set aside large federal grants to develop regional EMS systems. Approximately 300 EMS regions were established around the United States. To receive funding, the Act required that EMS systems address 15 key elements, which have become the foundation for many EMS systems today.
- The Omnibus Budget Reconciliation Act of 1981 eliminated direct federal funding. Instead, federal funds were given to states in the form of block grants for health services. The result was a decrease in overall funding and decreased coordination of EMS systems around the country, a change that has had long-term consequences.

EMS SYSTEM OVERVIEW

- A review of the 15 elements of EMS systems identified by the EMS Systems Act of 1973 provides insight into the current structure of EMS systems and the challenges they face.

MANPOWER

- EMS personnel commonly fall into one of four levels of training based on the U.S. Department of Transportation EMS provider curricula (Table 193-1).

TABLE 193-1 EMS Personnel

PERSONNEL	COMMENT
First responder	First professional or trained layperson to arrive at a medical emergency
EMT-B (Basic)	Oxygen, CPR, AED, extrication, immobilization, hemorrhage control
EMT-I (Intermediate)	EMT-B plus IV insertion, some medication administration, ECG interpretation
EMT-P (Paramedic)	Advanced resuscitation techniques such as intubation

Abbreviation: AED = automated external defibrillator.

TRAINING

- Training includes initial provider training and continuing education.
- As EMS call volume increases, providers often find themselves caring for a disproportionate number of patients with minor medical issues. Skills retention may become an important issue for EMS agencies.

COMMUNICATIONS

- As the nationwide emergency telephone number in the United States, 9-1-1 has greatly facilitated public access to emergency medical care.
- Enhanced equipment that automatically gives answering centers the number and location of the caller is becoming widespread.
- Emergency call takers undergo training to ensure they collect the necessary information, dispatch appropriate resources, and offer pre-arrival medical instructions while the ambulance is en route.
- Ambulance personnel also have the ability to communicate with the destinated hospital, both for notification and for medical direction from physicians.

TRANSPORTATION

- Ambulances are designed to ensure that EMS providers can perform lifesaving interventions while safely transporting the patient.
- Basic life support (BLS) ambulances carry equipment appropriate for EMT-Bs, including oxygen, AEDs, bag-mask ventilation devices, immobilization and splinting equipment, and dressings for wound care and hemorrhage control.
- Advanced life support (ALS) ambulances are equipped for EMT-Ps and carry IV supplies and medications, advanced airway devices, cardiac monitors, and other specialized equipment.

- Air transport should be considered for critically ill patients when the ground transport time is anticipated to be long.

FACILITIES AND CRITICAL-CARE UNITS

- EMS patients are often transported to the closest appropriate hospital or to the hospital of the patient's choice.
- In recent years, the number of specialty hospitals has increased, including pediatric hospitals, trauma centers, spinal cord injury centers, burn centers, stroke centers, cardiac centers, and hospitals with large numbers of critical care beds.
- Because of increasing hospital censuses, boarding of admitted patients in the ED, and general crowding, EDs may request that EMS services divert patients to other hospitals.

PUBLIC SAFETY AGENCIES

- EMS systems should have strong ties with police and fire departments. In addition to providing scene security, public safety agencies can perform first responder services, including CPR and use of AEDs for cardiac arrest victims.
- In turn, EMS personnel often provide medical support to police and fire departments in hazardous circumstances or extended operations.

CONSUMER PARTICIPATION

- Public support is necessary for a good EMS system. One way to accomplish this is to encourage public representation on regional EMS councils to participate in policy making.

ACCESS TO CARE

- EMS systems should ensure that all individuals have access to emergency care regardless of their ability to pay or type of insurance coverage.
- Communities need to ensure that EMS assets can reach patients in a timely fashion, even in remote parts of the country.
- Potential strategies include deploying ambulances throughout the area with one central dispatch center or heavy reliance on air medical services, weather permitting.

PATIENT TRANSFER

- Patients are often transferred from one medical facility to another for a higher level of care.
- The U.S. Emergency Medical Treatment and Active Labor Act (EMTALA) sets forth rules that hospitals participating in the Medicare program must adhere to when considering a patient transfer.
- Under the EMTALA, all patients must receive a medical screening examination and be stabilized before transfer to another facility is considered, and there must be explicit acceptance of the transfer by the receiving hospital.

COORDINATED PATIENT RECORD KEEPING

- EMS records need to be legible, intelligible, readily accessible to hospital providers, and compliant with the U.S. Health Insurance Portability and Accountability Act of 1996 (HIPAA).

PUBLIC INFORMATION AND EDUCATION

- EMS systems have a responsibility to train the public how to access them and use them appropriately.
- EMS agencies can play an important role in public training and education, including CPR, first aid, and disaster preparedness principles.
- Experience has shown that in disaster situations, a public that is adequately prepared and is trained to administer first aid will be in a better position to safely await help.

REVIEW AND EVALUATION

- To ensure that patients receive the highest quality care, EMS agencies must have in place a system for ongoing review and evaluation.
- A continuous quality improvement program, including EMS provider and physician input, should be established to assess system performance and formulate improvements.
- This should involve routine audits of radio or telephone communications, response times, scene times, and patient care records.

DISASTER PLAN

- The EMS system is an integral part of disaster preparedness and should be involved in planning along with other agencies and the medical community.
- EMS agencies must maintain a high level of disaster preparedness.
- This involves having written policies and procedures, stockpiling supplies that may be rapidly depleted in multi-casualty situations, and participating in regional disaster drills with other agencies and hospitals.

MUTUAL AID

- EMS services should develop mutual aid agreements with other jurisdictions so that uninterrupted emergency care is available when local agencies are overwhelmed.
- Working out in advance details such as reimbursement, credentialing, liability, and chain of command at incident scenes will enhance interagency cooperation and response.

CURRENT CHALLENGES AND FUTURE TRENDS

- The 2006 U.S. Institute of Medicine publication, *Emergency Medical Services: At the Crossroads*, detailed many of the challenges EMS faces today. These include fragmentation and lack of interoperability between EMS systems, between EMS and other public safety agencies, and between EMS and the rest of the health care system.
- Cuts in funding and staffing limitations impact the ability of EMS agencies to provide routine care. They also limit agencies' surge capacity, referring to their ability to accommodate a sudden, large increase in demand for services, as in a disaster.
- Research has demonstrated the importance of BLS skills in cardiac arrest and other emergencies. These skills include early use of AEDs and performance of high-quality, uninterrupted CPR.
- Advances in ALS skills are helping to enhance patient outcomes. Obtaining prehospital 12-lead ECGs on patients with chest pain is becoming common. This results in shorter door-to-balloon times in patients with ST-elevation myocardial infarctions.

For further reading in Tintinalli's *Emergency Medicine: A Comprehensive Study Guide*, 7th ed., see Chapter 1, "Emergency Medical Services," by C. Crawford Mechem.

194 EMERGENCY MEDICINE ADMINISTRATION

David M. Cline

NEGLIGENCE AND MEDICAL MALPRACTICE

- Negligence is defined as the omission to do something that a reasonable man, guided by those ordinary considerations that ordinarily regulate human affairs, would do, or the doing of something that a reasonable and prudent man would not do.
- The four components of negligence are duty, breach of duty, damages, and causation. The plaintiff (injured or complaining party) must prove all four elements exist in order to successfully sue for malpractice.
- Duty is considered a contract created by formation of a physician–patient relationship whereby the physician must act in accordance with "standards of care" to protect the patient from unreasonable risk. In general, by contract with the hospital, emergency physicians have a duty to see all patients who present themselves to the emergency department to be seen.
- The standard of care is that which a similarly trained, "reasonable and prudent physician" would exercise under similar circumstances. The emergency physician is not required to exercise the optimally highest degree of skill and care possible, but must use the degree of skill and care ordinarily exercised by physicians within the same specialty.
- Breach of duty occurs if the physician with an established duty fails to act in accordance with these standards of care by commission or omission of a certain act. Emergency physicians are held to a national standard of care for a specialist in emergency medicine.
- Damages encompass any actual loss, injury, or deterioration sustained by the plaintiff due to the breach of duty. A plaintiff must prove that the damage occurred because of the physician's negligence.
- Legal causation theoretically consists of two branches: causation in fact and foreseeability. Causation in fact means that "an event A is the cause of another event B, if and only if B would not have occurred when and as it did but for event A."
- The concept of foreseeability is fulfilled if the patient's damages must be the foreseeable result of the defendant's substandard practice, as compared with the standard of the reasonable physician. A bad result without proof of violation of the standard of care does not constitute negligence.
- Failure to diagnose myocardial infarction represents the largest single category of monetary settlements for emergency medicine physicians. Other high-risk areas for emergency physicians include abdominal pain, wounds, fractures, pediatric fever/meningitis, airway obstruction, central nervous system bleeding, and abdominal aortic aneurysms.
- Table 194-1 lists high-risk conditions or diagnoses that warrant physician caution in when managing.

CONSENT

- Informed consent is considered ideal—the patient knows and understands the risks, benefits, and consequences of

TABLE 194-1	Patient Complaints and Diagnoses Associated with High Risk
Life threatening disorders with time sensitive guideline directed care	
Chest pain/missed acute myocardial infarction	
Wounds (retained foreign body, nerve or tendon damage, poor healing)	
Fractures	
Abdominal pain (including appendicitis and aortic aneurysm)	
Pediatric fever	
Meningitis	
Central nervous system bleed	
Stroke	
Embolism	
Trauma related	
Spinal cord injuries	
Ectopic pregnancy	

accepting or refusing treatment. Specific, informed consent should be sought and obtained by the emergency physician whenever an invasive, risky, or complicated treatment or procedure is proposed. Examples include non-emergent thoracentesis, tube thoracostomies, paracentesis, and incision and drainage of a complex abscess.

- Informed consent requires two conditions: that the patient possesses decision-making capacity and that the patient can make a voluntary choice free of undue influence.
- Table 194-2 lists factors that should be considered when considering patient capacity.
- Elements of informed consent include the following: (a) a concise statement of the patient's medical condition or problem; (b) an understandable statement of the nature and purpose of the proposed test, treatment, or procedure; (c) a description of the risks, consequences, and benefits of the proposed test, treatment, or procedure; (d) a statement regarding any viable alternatives to the test, treatment, or procedure; and (e) a statement regarding the patient's prognosis if the proposed test, treatment, or procedure is not given.
- Express consent entails an awareness of the proposed care and an overt agreement (eg, in oral or written form) to proceed. An example would be the patient who comes to the emergency department, requests assistance for a problem, and signs a registration form authorizing evaluation and treatment of the problem.
- Implied consent is invoked if an emergency exists and the patient is incompetent (eg, a minor, or someone with an altered mental status). Simple procedures such as minor wound suturing, phlebotomy, injections, and peripheral IVs are allowed under express or implied consent. An exception to this is testing for human immunodeficiency virus (HIV), which requires written informed consent.
- Emergency consent bypasses normal consent standards due to the rapid need to treat a clinically ill patient. Implied consent is inferred by the patient's actions but without specific agreement. Emergency consent covers actions such as emergent intubation or placement of central lines in a critical patient when there is no other access.
- Failure to obtain appropriate consent can leave the emergency physician vulnerable to a legal action based on battery (intentional, unauthorized touching).

TABLE 194-2	Factors for Emergency Physicians to Consider When Determining Capacity
Presence of conditions impairing mental function	
Presence of basic mental functioning (awareness, orientation, memory, attention)	
The patient has understanding of specific treatment-related information	
Appreciation of the significance of the information for the patient's situation	
Patient's ability to reason about treatment alternatives in light of values and goals	
Complexity of the decision	

MINORS AND CONSENT

- The law always implies consent for treatment of a child in the event of an emergency. Parental consent is not needed; it is implied.
- All states without a general consent statute for minors have provisions that specifically permit the physician to treat any minor for venereal disease.
- Most states have treatment statutes for minors (usually 16 years or older), which enable them to consent for medical care. Many states also specifically permit treatment of minors for drug or alcohol problems, pregnancy, and psychiatric conditions.
- "Mature minor" statutes vary from state to state but allow a minor (usually between 14 and 18 years of age) to give informed consent when he or she understands the risks and benefits of a treatment. This generally applies to treatments that do not pose a serious risk.
- A parent with sole custody of a child has the legal right to provide consent for medical treatment. Obtain this permission prior to treatment, whenever possible. On a practical basis, however, if a medical necessity exists and a delay could be deleterious, the emergency physician (EP) may need to assume that a parent in possession of a child has the authority to provide consent.

REFUSAL OF CONSENT AND PATIENTS LEAVING AGAINST MEDICAL ADVICE

- On general principle, adult patients may ethically and legally refuse treatment totally or in part. A patient does not require a global decision-making ability to refuse treatment, but rather enough for a given situation, that is, a relative decision-making capacity. Clinical circumstances require the use of the term capacity, whereas competence is a legal term, which can only be determined by a court ruling.

- Multiple components are required for a decision-making capacity. These include understanding the options, awareness of the consequences of each option, and appreciation of the costs and benefits of the options in relation to relatively stable values and preferences.
- Informed refusal should be carefully documented on the chart of a patient who leaves AMA. The following five issues can be problematic and should be addressed in the chart:
  a. Capacity—Document the patient's mental status. Ideally, a patient should be awake and alert, able to carry on a reasonable conversation, and possess the mental ability to discuss the problem and act with self-interest.
  b. Discussion—Use and document clear terms, which a layperson can understand; avoid euphemisms and technical jargon. If death is a possibility, say so.
  c. Offer of alternative treatment—Document whether or not alternative treatments are available and are offered.
  d. Family involvement—Document efforts to involve family or friends in the decision process. If the patient forbids family involvement, document this accordingly.
  e. Patient's signature—The physician is not legally protected if the patient signs a standard AMA form devoid of the other four elements. However, if a patient refuses to sign after an appropriate informed discussion, simply document the refusal to sign.

RESUSCITATION AND DO-NOT-RESUSCITATE ORDERS

- Current standards suggest that when the possibility exists that the brain is viable and there are no compelling medical or legal reasons to act otherwise, resuscitation should be initiated.
- The current medical standard used to terminate resuscitations should be brain death or cardiovascular unresponsiveness. This principle is well founded in the standard references and well supported ethically.
- Medically and ethically, it is important to remember that there is no obligation to deliver treatment that is futile. When a person with a terminal illness is expected to die within a few hours or days, further aggressive diagnostic or therapeutic care would not benefit the patient and would be considered medically futile (and thus an ethical reason to withhold or cease resuscitation).
- It is prudent to stabilize the patient first and then seek further clarification of his or her wishes, either from the patient directly or with the family or physician. Appropriate, ethical reasons to withhold or cease resuscitation include irreversible cessation of cardiac function, brain death, competent patient refusal, or an advance directive such as "do not resuscitate" (DNR).
- Even with a valid DNR order, conditions such as pain, infection, dehydration, and respiratory difficulty should be addressed. A patient with a DNR deserves respectful and compassionate care, which can maximize comfort and possibly improve the remaining quality of life.

PHYSICIAN TELEPHONE ADVICE

- Even brief, seemingly straightforward advice is potentially a high-risk action when given over the telephone. A legally binding relationship (duty—the first element of a negligence tort) is established once advice is given. Since one cannot see the patient and further information may not be forthcoming, an accurate assessment truly cannot be made.
- It is acceptable, however, to give basic first aid advice if one includes a rejoinder to come immediately to the emergency department.
- Medical facilities with formal telephone advise programs should use specific guidelines, track outcomes, provide close follow-up, and complete the calls with a patient reminder to come to the emergency department.

THE EMERGENCY MEDICAL TREATMENT AND ACTIVE LABOR ACT (EMTALA)

- In 1986 Congress enacted the Comprehensive Omnibus Budget Reconciliation Act (COBRA) to combat widespread patient-dumping practices. The Emergency Medical Treatment and Active Labor Act (EMTALA) is the section of COBRA that applies to emergency departments.
- According to EMTALA regulations, a medically unstable patient can be transferred to another facility only if the transferring physician certifies the transfer is medically necessary and the receiving facility agrees to accept the patient.
- A patient with an illness or injury who presents to an emergency department (whose hospital has a Medicare contract) must receive a medical screening examination, regardless of the patient's ability to pay or insurance coverage.
- If the medical screening examination determines that an emergency medical condition exists, the patient must have that condition stabilized. Stabilization

should take prior to transfer to another facility, up to the full capacity of that facility.

- The patient must understand the risks and benefits, and sign informed consent for the transfer.
- EMTALA also applies to patients who are not being transferred, as all ED patients must receive a screening examination and be stabilized according to the standard procedures of the emergency department. The patient's condition may preclude successful stabilization and failure to stabilize the patient alone is not an EMTALA violation. However, the physician and hospital may be subject to an EMTALA investigation if it can be established that standard procedures including specialty consultation were not implemented in the attempt to stabilize the patient.
- EMTALA do's and don'ts are listed in Table 194-3.

MEDICAL ETHICS

- There are five basic principles that should guide ethical decision making in medical practice.
- Veracity is telling the truth. It forms the basis of maintaining an open health care provider–patient relationship and of keeping promises.
- Patient autonomy is based upon a person's right and freedom to make an informed choice about what will and will not be done; it also acknowledges the patient's right to privacy.
- Beneficence is the principle of doing good; it involves promoting the well being of others, and responding to those in need.

TABLE 194-3 EMTALA Do's and Don'ts

EMTALA ***Do's***
1. Treat all patients in the same way.
2. Provide a medical screening examination appropriate to the patient's complaints.
3. Appropriately transfer patients you cannot stabilize.
4. Accept transfers who require specialized services your hospital offers, as long as the specialized services have the capacity for care.
5. Involve on-call specialists when needed to diagnose or stabilize an emergency medical condition.
6. Educate ED, hospital staff, and faculty on the EMTALA rules.
7. See patients quickly and efficiently.
EMTALA ***Don'ts***
1. Substitute triage for a medical screening examination.
2. Discourage or coerce patients away from receiving their screening examinations and stabilization.
3. Allow yourself to be convinced that a specialist does not need to come to the ED.
4. Fail to stabilize within your capabilities.
5. Delay the medical screening examination for preauthorization or registration.

Abbreviation: EMTALA = Emergency Medical Treatment and Active Labor Act.

TABLE 194-4 HIPAA Do's and Don'ts

HIPAA ***Do's***
1. Talk freely with patient's primary physician.
2. Discuss protected health information with consultants and other members of the patient's health care team.
3. Use protected health information for reimbursement and operational issues.
4. Release records to the patient or an authorized representative.*
5. Discuss patient protected health information with family or friends if the patient is in an emergency situation, unable to consent, and the information would be beneficial to the patient.
HIPPA ***Don'ts***
1. Discuss patients or protected health information in public or unsecured areas.
2. Leave computers with access to protected health information logged on and unattended.
3. Discuss protected health information in front of others without permission.
4. Speak loudly when discussing protected health information, particularly in public areas.
5. Look at records for which you have no legitimate purpose as a provider.

Abbreviation: HIPAA = Health Information Portability and Accountability Act of 1996.
*May require the patient to sign an authorization form.

- Nonmaleficence is the principle of "do no harm," which obliges the physician (or other health care provider) to protect others from danger, pain, and suffering. This concept stems from the Hippocratic Oath as well as other ancient medical traditions.
- Justice involves fairness, respect for human equality, and the equitable allocation of scarce resources.

THE HEALTH INSURANCE PORTABILITY AND ACCOUNTABILITY ACT (HIPAA) AND PROTECTED HEALTH INFORMATION

- HIPAA is the most important U.S. law that protects the health care privacy and confidentiality of individuals.
- This legislation required the establishment of standards for the security, exchange, and integrity of electronic health information, and set rules for basic national privacy standards and fair information practices for health care.
- HIPPA allows covered entities to use protected health information (PHI), without authorization, for purposes of treatment, payment, and operations.
- Treatment is the provision, management, and coordination of health care and related services, including consultations and referrals.
- The payment exclusion allows a health care provider to use PHI to obtain payment or be reimbursed for the care provided to an individual.

- Operations include a number of activities, including, but not limited to, quality improvement, employee evaluation and credentialing, auditing programs, and business activity such as planning, development, management, and administration.
- An exception to this rule is that psychotherapy notes often require written consent for their use except for treatment, certain legal matters, and the protection of the public from a serious threat.
- HIPPA do's and don'ts are listed in Table 194-4.

For further reading in Tintinalli's *Emergency Medicine: A Comprehensive Study Guide*, 7th ed.,see Chapter 298, "Legal Issues in Emergency Medicine," by Jonathan E. Siff.

INDEX

A *t* following a page number indicates tabular material, and *f* following a page number indicates a figure.

A

Abciximab, 78*t*
Abdominal aortic aneurysms, 112–113, 113*f*, 143*t*, 653
Abdominal distention, 235
Abdominal pain
  clinical features of, 140–142
  diagnosis and differential of, 142, 142*t*
  differential diagnosis of, 141*f*
  emergency department care and disposition of, 142–143
  epidemiology of, 140
  nonspecific, 267
  pathophysiology of, 140
  pediatric, 265*t*, 265–268
  rebound tenderness, 140–141
  visceral, 140
Abdominal surgery, 225–226
Abdominal trauma, 569
  blunt, 584–586
  chest radiographs of, 586
  clinical features of, 585
  computed tomography of, 586
  diagnosis and differential of, 586
  diagnostic peritoneal lavage of, 586
  diaphragmatic injuries, 585
  emergency department care and disposition of, 586–587
  epidemiology of, 584
  focused assessment with sonography for trauma, 563, 586
  pathophysiology of, 584–585
  retroperitoneal injuries, 585
  stab wounds, 587
  ultrasonography of, 586
Abduction relief sign, 620*t*
ABI. *See* Ankle-brachial index
Abortion, 212, 226–227
Abruptio placentae, 216, 218, 568
Abscess
  anorectal, 173
  Bartholin gland, 327
  brain, 526–527, 527*t*
  cutaneous, 327–328
  intra-abdominal, 182
  local, 64
  lung, 125, 128
  masticator space, 539–540
  odontogenic, 553–554
  ovarian, 226
  periodontal, 547
  peritonsillar, 242*t*, 247–248, 551*f*, 551–552
  pilonidal, 327
  psoas, 623
  retropharyngeal, 242*t*, 247, 553, 553*f*
  scrotal, 197–198
  tubo-ovarian, 143*t*
Absence seizure, 270, 514
Absorbable sutures, 50
Abuse
  child, 234, 565, 645–646
  elder, 646–647
  intimate partner, 649, 649*t*
Acalculous cholecystitis, 159
Accelerated idioventricular rhythm, 16, 16*f*
Acetabular fractures, 605–606
Acetaminophen
  absorption of, 391
  fever treated with, 230
  liver disease caused by, 178
  N-acetylcysteine antidote for, 391–392
  pain management using, 36
  pharmacokinetics of, 391
  toxicity of, 391–392, 392*t*
Acetazolamide, 434
Acetoacetate, 460
Acetone, 460
Acetylcysteine, 365*t*
Achilles tendon
  motor function of, 61*t*
  rupture of, 61, 612, 637
Acid(s), 406–407, 444, 445*t*, 534
Acid–base disorders
  clinical features of, 29
  clinical problem-solving method for, 29–30
  compensatory responses for, 29–30
  diagnosis and differential of, 29
  metabolic acidosis, 29–31, 30*t*, 390
  metabolic alkalosis, 31
  respiratory acidosis, 30–32
  respiratory alkalosis, 32
Acidosis
  clinical features of, 29
  metabolic, 29–31, 30*t*
  respiratory, 30–32
Acquired immunodeficiency syndrome. *See also* Human immunodeficiency virus
  cytomegalovirus radiculitis associated with, 519
  diarrhea associated with, 335
  epidemiology of, 333
  hepatomegaly associated with, 336
  highly active antiretroviral therapy for, 334
  hospitalization for, 337
  indicator conditions for, 334, 334*t*
  pathophysiology of, 333–334
Acromioclavicular joint injuries, 602, 603*t*
ACTH. *See* Adrenocorticotropic hormone
Activated charcoal, 365*t*, 367, 371–372, 377, 382, 393–394
Activated partial thromboplastin time, 79, 469*t*
Activated protein C resistance, 473*t*
Acute airway inflammation, 136
Acute allergic reactions, 34–35
Acute angle-closure glaucoma, 534*f*, 534–535
Acute appendicitis, 143*t*, 163–165
Acute arterial occlusion, 115, 116*t*, 118
Acute bacterial sinusitis, 240
Acute bronchitis, 123–125, 124*t*
Acute chest syndrome, 302, 302*f*, 478*t*
Acute constipation, 151–153, 152*t*
Acute coronary syndromes
  definition of, 82
  diagnosis and differential of, 74–77, 83–84
  emergency department care and disposition of, 77–80, 84–85
  epidemiology of, 73
  as hypertensive emergency, 110
  low probability, 82–85
  pathophysiology of, 73–74
  percutaneous coronary interventions for, 77, 79
  reperfusion for, 77

Acute coronary syndromes (*Cont.*):
- risk stratification for, 83*t*
- treatment of, 84–85

Acute dystonia, 374
Acute gastroenteritis, 260–261
Acute glomerulonephritis, 310–311
Acute hypoxia, 435
Acute infectious diarrhea, 147–148
Acute intravascular hemolytic reaction, 482*t*
Acute ischemic stroke, 111
Acute kidney injury, 184
Acute lung injury, 385, 472*t*, 482*t*
Acute lymphoblastic leukemia, 305
Acute mastoiditis, 542
Acute mitral regurgitation, 82
Acute mountain sickness, 433–435
Acute myocardial infarction
- angioplasty for, 485
- anterior, 76*f*
- antithrombotic therapy for, 485
- cardiogenic shock as cause of, 81–82
- chest pain and, 71, 71*t*–72*t*
- conduction system injuries caused by, 74
- diagnosis and differential of, 74–77
- electrocardiogram findings, 75*f*–77*f*, 77*t*
- emergency department care and disposition of, 77–80
- inferior wall, 74, 75*f*
- inferolateral, 75*f*
- pain caused by, 74
- serum markers of, 72, 73*f*

Acute necrotizing ulcerative gingivitis, 547
Acute otalgia, 238
Acute otitis media, 238*f*, 238–239
Acute pericarditis, 100–101
Acute prostatitis, 201
Acute prosthetic valvular dysfunction, 96
Acute pulmonary edema, 88–90, 95
Acute pyelonephritis, 194
Acute renal failure
- in children, 309–310, 310*t*
- clinical features of, 185
- creatinine evaluations, 184
- diagnosis and differential of, 185–186, 186*t*
- dialysis for, 188, 188*t*
- emergency department care and disposition of, 186–188
- epidemiology of, 184
- hospitalization for, 188
- hyperkalemia affected by, 490
- hypertension caused by, 110
- intrinsic, 184, 186–188
- ischemic, 184
- mortality rates, 184
- nephrotoxins as cause of, 184, 186
- pathophysiology of, 184, 185*t*
- postobstructive, 184
- postrenal, 188, 310*t*
- prerenal, 184, 185*t*, 186–187, 309, 310*t*
- RIFLE classification of, 184

Acute rheumatic fever, 292–293
Acute splenic sequestration crises, 303
Acute sympathetic crisis, 110
Acute tubular necrosis, 184, 186
Acute urinary retention, 196–197
Acyclovir
- eczema herpeticum treated with, 295
- herpes labialis treated with, 295
- herpes simplex infections treated with, 316, 330, 337, 547
- varicella treated with, 331

Addisonian crisis, 144
Addison's disease, 30*t*
Adductor pollicis, 595
Adenosine, 12
Adenovirus, 124*t*
Adhesive capsulitis, 621–622
Adhesive tapes, 52–53
Adhesives, cyanoacrylate, 53, 534
Adrenal crisis, 463–465, 489–490
Adrenal insufficiency, 463–465, 464*t*–465*t*
Adrenocorticotropic hormone, 463
Adult still disease, 630*t*
Advanced life support ambulances, 655
Adynamic ileus, 182
AEIOUS TIPS mnemonic, 274, 275*t*
Aeromonas hydrophila, 62, 346
Afebrile seizures, 273
African sleeping sickness, 355
African tick typhus, 354
African trypanosomiasis, 355
Agitation, 642*f*
AICDs. *See* Automated internal cardiac defibrillators
AIDS dementia complex, 335
Airway inflammation, 136
Airway obstruction, 242–243, 487
Airway support, advanced
- alternative devices for, 7–8
- emergency care and disposition, 6
- initial approach, 6
- noninvasive positive pressure ventilation, 9, 9*t*
- orotracheal intubation, 6–7
- pathophysiology of, 6
- rapid-sequence intubation, 7, 8*t*–9*t*
- rescue devices for, 8
- tongue size classification, 6*f*

Akathisia, 374–375
Albendazole, 356
Albumin, 180, 311
Albuterol, 27
- asthma treated with, 138, 251
- bronchospasm treated with, 35
- chronic obstructive pulmonary disease treated with, 138

Alcohol(s)
- ethanol, 366*t*, 380, 382*t*
- ethylene glycol, 381–383, 383*t*
- isopropanol, 381
- methanol, 381–383
- osmolal gap, 380
- in pregnancy, 215

Alcoholic hepatitis, 176, 179
Alcoholic ketoacidosis, 460
Alcoholic liver disease, 178
Aldosterone, 463
Alkalis, 406–407, 444, 445*t*, 534
Alkalosis
- clinical features of, 29
- metabolic, 31
- respiratory, 32

Allergic keratoconjunctivitis, 529
Allis maneuver, 608*f*
Alpha-blockers, 204
Alprazolam, 643
Alteplase, 78*t*
Altered mental status, 274–275
Alternobaric vertigo, 438
Alveolar osteitis, postextraction, 546–547
Alveolar ventilation per minute, 120
Amanita phalloides, 451
Amanita smithiana, 452
Ambulances, 655
Amebiasis, 356
American Board of Emergency Medicine examinations
- certification, 3–4
- continuous certification, 2–3
- in-training, 3
- qualification, 1–2
- test-taking techniques for, 4–5
- tips for taking of, 5

American Osteopathic Board of Emergency Medicine, 1
American Society of Anesthesiologists' physical classification system, 40
American trypanosomiasis, 355
Amikacin, 491*t*
Amiloride, 180
τ-aminobutyric acid, 377
Amiodarone
- atrial fibrillation treated with, 14
- dilated cardiomyopathy treated with, 97
- in pregnancy, 214
- ventricular fibrillation treated with, 17
- ventricular tachycardia treated with, 17

Ammonia, 416
Amnestic disorders, 639
Amniotic fluid embolism, 218
Amoxicillin
  acute otitis media treated with, 239
  chlamydia treated with, 313
  otitis media treated with, 542
Amoxicillin/clavulanate
  acute otitis media treated with, 239
  bite wound prophylaxis, 66–68
  community-acquired pneumonia treated with, 127
  diverticulitis treated with, 167
  human bite wound prophylaxis, 66–67
  neutropenic fever treated with, 491*t*
  otitis media treated with, 542
  peritonsillar abscess treated with, 248
Amphetamines, 385–386
Amphotericin, 337
Ampicillin/sulbactam
  bowel obstruction treated with, 168
  diverticulitis treated with, 166
  human bite wound prophylaxis, 66
  pelvic inflammatory disease treated with, 224*t*
  posttransplant pneumonia treated with, 358
  spontaneous bacterial peritonitis treated with, 180
Amygdalin, 451
Amylase, 161
Amyotrophic lateral sclerosis, 519–520
Anal canal neoplasms, 174
Anal fissures, 172
Anal fistula, 172–173
Analgesia
  definition of, 40
  nonopioid, 36–37
  opioid, 37
Analgesics, 40–41
Anaphylactoid reactions, 34
Anaphylaxis, 34–35
Anastomotic leaks, 182
Ancylostoma duodenale, 356
Anemia
  autoimmune hemolytic, 307–308
  in children, 307–308
  clinical features of, 466
  diagnosis and differential of, 466
  emergency department care and disposition of, 466–467
  evaluation of, 466–467, 467*t*, 468*f*
  in hemodialysis, 191
  iron deficiency, 307–308
  microcytic, 468*f*
  pathophysiology of, 466
  sickle cell, 304
  treatment of, 305
Anesthesia
  local, 37–38
  nerve blocks for. *See* Nerve blocks
  regional, 37–38, 38
  topical, 38
Anesthetics, local, 37–38
Aneurysms
  abdominal aortic, 112–113, 113*f*, 143*t*, 653
  posterior communicating artery, 537
Angina pectoris, 72*t*
Angioedema, 35, 555
Angioplasty, 485
Angiotensin-converting enzyme inhibitors
  angioedema treated with, 555
  dilated cardiomyopathy treated with, 97
  nonallergic angioedema caused by, 35
Animal bites, 66*t*
Anion gap metabolic acidosis, 29–30, 30*t*
Anistreplase, 485
Ankle
  dislocation of, 614
  fracture of, 614
  injuries of, 613–614
  lacerations of, 61
  sprain of, 613–614
Ankle-brachial index, 117, 117*f*, 591
Ankylosing spondylitis, 629, 630*t*
Annelida, 431
Anogenital reflexes, 574
Anorectal abscess, 173
Anorectal disorders
  in AIDS patients, 336
  anal fissures, 172
  cryptitis, 171–172
  fistula in ano, 172–173
  hemorrhoids, 170–171, 171*f*
  pilonidal sinus, 175
  proctitis, 173
  pruritus ani, 175
Anorectal tumors, 174
Anterior cerebral artery stroke, 498
Anterior cord syndrome, 575*t*
Anterior cruciate ligament tear, 612
Anterior humeral line, 290*f*
Anterior inferior iliac spine fracture, 607*t*
Anterior interosseous nerve, 600
Anterior myocardial infarction, 76*f*
Anterior superior iliac spine fracture, 607*t*
Anterior tibial spine fractures, 610
Anterior tibialis tendon rupture, 637
Anterograde amnesia, 378
Anthraquinones, 152
Anthrax, 350–351
Antibiotic-associated diarrhea, 147, 181–182
Antibiotics. *See also specific antibiotic*
  acute appendicitis treated with, 165
  acute bacterial sinusitis treated with, 240
  acute otitis media treated with, 239
  bacterial tracheitis treated with, 247
  cellulitis treated with, 538*t*
  cholecystitis treated with, 163
  diverticulitis treated with, 166
  epiglottitis treated with, 246
  erysipelas treated with, 538*t*
  facial infections treated with, 538*t*
  group A β-hemolytic *Streptococcus* pharyngitis treated with, 241
  impetigo treated with, 538*t*
  in infants, 229, 229*t*
  necrotizing soft tissue infections treated with, 325
  neutropenic fever treated with, 491*t*
  odontogenic abscess treated with, 554
  pharyngitis treated with, 551
  urologic stone disease treated with, 204
Anticardiolipin antibodies, 473
Anticholinergics, 138, 368*t*, 368–369
Anticoagulants
  acute coronary syndromes treated with, 78*t*
  complications of, 485
  deep vein thrombosis treated with, 107–108
  endogenous, 473
  mechanical valves, 96
  oral, 484
  parenteral, 484
Anticonvulsants, 272
  carbamazepine, 401
  fosphenytoin, 400–401, 516
  phenytoin, 400–401, 516
  second-generation, 402
  valproate, 401–402
Antidepressants
  atypical, 370
  chronic pain treated with, 46
  cyclic, 369–370
Antidiarrheal agents, 147, 263
Antidotes, 365*t*–367*t*
Antiemetics
  indications for, 142–143, 346
  nausea and vomiting treated with, 145, 492*t*
Antiepileptic drugs, 273
Anti-Factor Xa activity, 470*t*
Antihypertensive agents, 398

Antimotility agents, 148, 263
Antiphospholipid antibodies, 470*t*, 473
Antiphospholipid syndrome, 630*t*
Antiplatelet agents
  acute coronary syndromes treated with, 78*t*
  bleeding caused by, 486*t*
  description of, 484–485
Antipsychotics, 374–375
Antiretroviral therapy, 337
Anti-Rh immunoglobulin, 308
Antithrombin, 470*t*
Antithrombotic agents
  anticoagulants, 484
  complications of, 485, 486*t*
  direct thrombin inhibitors, 484
  fibrinolytic agents, 78*t*, 79, 485, 485*t*–486*t*
  indications for, 485
Antivenom Fab, 365*t*
Antiviral agents
  herpes zoster treated with, 560
  influenza treated with, 333
ANUG. *See* Acute necrotizing ulcerative gingivitis
Anxiety, 37
Anxiety disorders, 640
AOBEM. *See* American Osteopathic Board of Emergency Medicine
Aortic aneurysms, abdominal, 112–113, 113*f*, 143*t*, 653
Aortic balloon counterpulsation, 93
Aortic dissection
  chest pain caused by, 72*t*
  description of, 95
  epidemiology of, 113
  as hypertensive emergency, 110
  pathophysiology of, 113–114
Aortic incompetence, 94–95
Aortic injuries, 583
Aortic regurgitation, 91*t*, 95
Aortic stenosis, 91*t*, 94, 94*f*
Aortoenteric fistulas, 112
Apathetic thyrotoxicosis, 462
Apgar score, 219
Aphthous stomatitis, 547
Apnea, 236, 252
Apparent life-threatening events, 237, 237*t*
Appendicitis, acute
  in adults, 143*t*, 163–165
  in children, 267
Arboviral infections, 332
Arboviruses, 525
Arrhythmias
  atrial fibrillation, 13–14, 13*f*
  atrial flutter, 12–13, 13*f*
  AV block. *See* AV block
  bradyarrhythmias, 10–11
  fascicular blocks, 19
  multifocal atrial tachycardia, 14–15, 14*f*
  premature atrial contractions, 9, 10*f*
  premature ventricular contractions, 15–16, 15*f*, 89
  preterminal rhythms, 20
  sinus, 10, 10*f*
  sinus bradycardia, 10–11
  sinus tachycardia, 11
  supraventricular bradyarrhythmias, 10–11
  supraventricular tachyarrhythmias, 11–15
  supraventricular tachycardia, 11–12, 11*f*
  tachyarrhythmias, 11–15
  ventricular, 15–17
Arsenic poisoning, 413–414, 414*t*
Artemether/lumefantrine, 344
Arterial blood gases
  asthma evaluations, 137
  chronic obstructive pulmonary disease evaluations, 137
Arterial gas embolism, 436*t*
Artesunate, 345
Arthritis
  classification of, 626*t*
  clinical features of, 626
  gonococcal, 627
  Lyme, 628
  osteoarthritis, 622, 628–629
  rheumatoid, 628–629, 630*t*
  septic, 627, 628*t*
  viral, 628
Arthrocentesis, 626*f*–627*f*
Artificial urinary sphincters, 206
Ascariasis, 356
Ascaris lumbricoides, 356
Ascending cholangitis, 160
Ascites, 180
Aspiration, 40
Aspiration pneumonia, 125
Aspiration pneumonitis, 125, 127–128
Aspirin
  absorption of, 388–389
  acute coronary syndromes treated with, 78, 78*t*
  bleeding caused by, 486*t*
  description of, 484
  toxicity of, 388–390
Assault, sexual, 648*t*, 648–649
Assisted reproductive technology, 227
Asterixis, 179
Asthma
  beta-adrenergic agonists for, 138
  chest radiographs of, 250
  in children, 250–251
  clinical features of, 136–137, 250
  death caused by, 137
  diagnosis and differential of, 137, 250
  emergency department care and disposition of, 137–139
  epidemiology of, 136, 250
  exacerbations of, 136–137, 250
  pathophysiology of, 136, 250
  in pregnancy, 214–215
  respiratory failure caused by, 250
Asymptomatic bacteriuria, 193, 205
Asystole, 20
Ataxia, 509–510
Atelectasis, 181–182
Atenolol, 78*t*
Atherosclerotic plaques, 83
Atonic seizure, 270
Atopic dermatitis, 299
Atovaquone-proguanil, 344
Atrial fibrillation, 13–14, 14*f*
Atrial flutter, 12–13, 13*f*
Atrioventricular block. *See* AV block
Atrioventricular nodal reentrant tachycardia, 11
Atrophic vaginitis, 222–223
Atropine
  bradycardia treated with, 397
  bronchorrhea treated with, 42
  junctional rhythms treated with, 15
  Mobitz I AV block treated with, 18
  Mobitz type II AV block treated with, 18
  sinus bradycardia treated with, 11
Atypical antidepressants, 370
Auricular block, 40
Autoimmune hemolytic anemia, 307–308
Automated internal cardiac defibrillators, 20
Autonomy, 660
AV block
  first-degree, 18
  second-degree, 18*f*, 18
  third-degree, 18–19, 18*f*
Avascular necrosis of femoral head, 302*f*, 624
Avian influenza, 124*t*
Avulsed teeth, 549*f*, 549–550
Avulsion fractures, 607*t*
Axillary nerve, 602
Azathioprine
  Crohn's disease treated with, 150
  ulcerative colitis treated with, 151
Azithromycin
  acute otitis media treated with, 239
  chancroid treated with, 317
  chlamydia treated with, 313
  community-acquired pneumonia treated with, 127
  otitis media treated with, 542

B

B vitamins, 419
Bacillus anthracis, 350
Back pain
  chronic, 44
  clinical features of, 617–618
  nonspecific, 620
Bacteremia, 229*t*, 230
Bacteria
  acute bronchitis caused by, 123, 124*t*
  gastroenteritis caused by, 264*t*
  pneumonia caused by, 125, 126*t*, 253
Bacterial conjunctivitis, 529
Bacterial endocarditis, 338–339, 339*t*
Bacterial meningitis, 523, 525*t*
Bacterial tracheitis, 242*t*, 246–247
Bacterial vaginosis, 221–222, 649
Bag-valve-mask ventilation
  device for, 6
  dyspnea treated with, 119
Balanoposthitis, 198
Bankart fracture, 603
Barbiturates, 376–377
Bariatric surgery, 183
Barotrauma
  of ascent, 436*t*, 436–437
  of descent, 436*t*, 436–437
Bartholin gland abscess, 327
Barton fracture, 597
Bartonella henselae, 241
Basic life support ambulances, 655
Basilar artery
  occlusion of, 498
  thrombosis of, 508
Basilar skull fractures, 570–571, 573
Beck's triad, 563, 582
Bedbugs, 429
Bee stings, 426–427
Behavioral disorders
  clinical features of, 640–641
  diagnosis and differential of, 641–642
  emergency department care and disposition of, 642–643
  epidemiology of, 640
  suicide risks, 639, 640*t*–641*t*
  types of, 639–640
Behçet disease, 630*t*
Bell phenomenon, 644*t*
Bell's palsy, 499*t*, 536
Beneficence, 660
Benign intracranial hypertension, 495, 537
Benign migratory glossitis, 548
Benign paroxysmal positional vertigo, 511–512, 512*t*
Benign prostatic hypertrophy, 196
Benzodiazepines
  clinical features of, 378
  epidemiology of, 377
  flumazenil reversal of, 41, 180, 275, 378
  overdose of, 377
  pathophysiology of, 378
  in pregnancy, 215
  procedural sedation use of, 41*t*, 42
  seizures treated with, 386
  status epilepticus treated with, 271, 271*t*
Beta-blockers
  acute coronary syndromes treated with, 84
  asthma treated with, 251
  great vessel injury treated with, 584
  narrow-complex supraventricular tachycardia treated with, 12
  toxicity of, 396–397
Bicarbonate
  diabetic ketoacidosis treated with, 283, 456
  metabolic acidosis treated with, 31, 31*t*
Biceps tendon rupture, 598–599, 621
Bifascicular block, 19
Bigeminal rhythms, 15
Bilevel positive airway pressure
  chronic obstructive pulmonary disease treated with, 139
  description of, 9
  hypercapnia treated with, 121
Biliary colic, 159
Biliary obstruction, 361
Biliary tract strictures, 176
Bilious vomiting, 235, 266
BiPAP. *See* Bilevel positive airway pressure
Bipolar disorder, 639–640
Bipyridyl herbicides, 411
Bismuth subsalicylate, 148
Bisphosphonates, 489
Bite(s)
  animal, 66*t*
  antibiotic prophylaxis for, 66–68
  cat, 66*t*, 67–68
  dog, 66*t*, 67
  gila monsters, 430
  human, 65–66, 66*t*, 633*t*
  snakebites, 429–430
  spider, 427
Bivalirudin, 78*t*
Black cohosh, 419*t*
Black widow spider bite, 427
Bladder trauma, 590
Bleeding. *See also* Hemorrhage
  gastrointestinal, 153–154, 265
  peptic ulcers, 154
  posttonsillectomy, 554
  vaginal, 208, 209*t*, 216
  variceal, 154
Bleeding disorders
  circulating inhibitors of coagulation, 473
  clinical features of, 466
  clotting disorders, 473–474
  disseminated intravascular coagulation. *See* Disseminated intravascular coagulation
  in liver disease, 471
  in renal disease, 471–472
Bleeding time, 469*t*
Blood administration, 484
Blowout fractures, 533, 578
Blue spells, 236
Blue toe syndrome, 116*t*
Blunt trauma
  abdominal, 569, 584–586
  cardiac, 583
  chest, 565
  esophageal, 580
  neck, 580
  ocular, 533
Boehler angle, 615
Boerhaave's syndrome, 156
Bone fractures. *See also* Fracture(s)
  clinical features of, 593
  pathophysiology of, 593
Bone metastases, 486–487
Bone sarcomas, 306–307
Bordetella pertussis, 124*t*
Borrelia burgdorferi, 348
Botulism, 345, 517
Boutonnière deformity, 596
Bowel obstruction, 143*t*, 144, 167–168
Bowlus and Currier test, 644*t*
Box jellyfish, 431
Boyle's law, 436
Brachial plexopathy, 518
Brachioradial delay, 94
Bradyarrhythmias, 10–11
Bradycardia
  in children, 21
  fetal, 569
  sinus, 10–11
Brain abscess, 526–527, 527*t*
Brain tumors, 306, 494
Branchial cleft cysts, 554
BRAT diet, 263
Braxton Hicks contractions, 218
Breach of duty, 657
Breast surgery, 182
Breech presentation, 221
Brief psychotic disorder, 639
Bronchial pneumonia, 125
Bronchiolitis, 236, 251–253, 360
Bronchitis, acute, 123–125, 124*t*
Bronchopulmonary dysplasia, 236
Bronchorrhea, 42

Bronchospasms, 35, 138
Brown recluse spider bite, 427
Brown-Séquard syndrome, 575*t*
Brucellosis, 354
Brudzinski's sign, 523
Brugada syndrome, 19, 19*f*
B-type natriuretic peptide, 82, 89–90
Bullous impetigo, 297, 298*f*, 538
Bullous myringitis, 542
Bupivacaine, 37
Buprenorphine, 384
Bupropion, 371
Burns
chemical, 444, 445*t*–446*t*, 534
thermal
American Burn Association classification of, 443*t*
body surface area calculations, 441, 441*f*–442*f*
classification of, 442, 442*t*
clinical features of, 441–442
depth of, 442*t*
diagnosis and differential of, 442, 443*t*
emergency department care and disposition of, 442–444, 443*t*
epidemiology of, 441
escharotomy for, 443
first-degree, 442*t*
fluid resuscitation for, 443, 565
full-thickness, 441
inhalation, 442
Lund and Browder diagram for, 441, 442*f*
pathophysiology of, 441
rule of nines for, 441, 441*f*
second-degree, 442*t*
Bursal syndromes, 623, 624*f*, 624*t*
Bursitis, 629, 636
Buspirone, 379
Butoconazole, 223
Buttocks trauma, 588

C
Caffeine, 393–394
Calcaneal injuries, 615
Calcific aortic stenosis, 94
Calcific tendinitis, 621–622
Calcitonin
chronic pain treated with, 46
hypercalcemia of malignancy treated with, 489
Calcium abnormalities
in children, 286
hypercalcemia, 28, 286, 286*t*
hypocalcemia, 27–28, 273, 286, 286*t*
Calcium channel blockers
mechanism of action, 397
narrow-complex supraventricular tachycardia treated with, 12
toxicity of, 397–398
urologic stone disease treated with, 204
Calcium chloride
as antidote, 365*t*, 397–398
hyperkalemia treated with, 27
hypermagnesemia treated with, 29
Calcium gluconate, 27–28, 490
Calcium oxalate stones, 202
Calcium phosphate stones, 202
Calf vein thrombosis, 108
Calluses, 635
Campylobacter, 264*t*
Candida intertrigo, 561
Candida vaginitis, 221–223
Candidal diaper dermatitis, 299
Candidiasis, oral, 336–337, 547
Capitate, 598*t*
Capnography, 40
Carbamates, 409
Carbamazepine, 401
Carbon monoxide poisoning, 442, 449–450
Carbon tetrachloride, 405
Carbonic anhydrase inhibitors, 389–390, 399
Carboxyhemoglobin, 121, 442, 449–450
Carbuncles, 327–328
Cardiac medications
angiotensin-converting enzyme inhibitors, 399
antihypertensive agents, 398
beta-blockers. *See* Beta-blockers
calcium channel blockers. *See* Calcium channel blockers
digitalis glycosides, 395*t*–396*t*, 395–396
diuretics, 398–399
sympatholytic agents, 399
vasodilators, 399–400
Cardiac pacing, 10
Cardiac syncope, 278
Cardiac tamponade, 101, 191, 487–488, 582
Cardiac transplantation, 359
Cardiac trauma
blunt, 583
penetrating, 582–583
Cardiac ultrasonography, 653
Cardiogenic shock, 81–82, 260
Cardiomegaly, 97, 259*f*
Cardiomyopathy
cardiomegaly and, 97
in children, 260
definition of, 97
dilated, 97
hypertrophic, 98–99, 277
inflammatory, 98
restrictive, 99
Cardiothoracic injuries
chest wall, 581
clinical features of, 580–581
diaphragm, 582
epidemiology of, 580
heart, 582–583
lung injuries, 581–582
tracheobronchial, 582
Cardiovascular disease
abdominal aortic aneurysms, 112–113, 113*f*, 143*t*
acute coronary syndromes. *See* Acute coronary syndromes
acute myocardial infarction. *See* Acute myocardial infarction
aortic dissection. *See* Aortic dissection
cardiomyopathy. *See* Cardiomyopathy
chest pain, 71–73
congestive heart failure, 88*t*, 88–90
deep vein thrombosis. *See* Deep vein thrombosis
hypertension. *See* Hypertension
occlusive arterial disease, 115–118, 116*t*
pulmonary embolism. *See* Pulmonary embolism
syncope, 85*t*, 85–86, 87*f*, 88*t*
valvular disease. *See* Valvular disease
Cardioversion
in children, 22
supraventricular tachycardia treated with, 12
Caregiver neglect, 646
Carisoprodol, 379
Carnett sign, 141
Carotid endarterectomy, 504
Carotid sinus hypersensitivity, 86
Carotid sinus massage, 12
Carpal bone fractures, 597, 598*t*
Carpal tunnel syndrome, 634
Castor bean, 451*t*
Cathartics, 367
Catheter-based thrombectomy, 109
Catheters, urinary, 205–206
Cats
bites from, 66*t*, 67–68
rabies transmission from, 342–343
Cauda equina syndrome, 575*t*
Cauliflower ear, 542
Causalgia, 45*t*
Causation, 657
Caustics, 406–407
Cavernous sinus thrombosis, 546
Cavitary tuberculosis, 130, 130*f*
Cefazolin, 432
Cefepime, 491*t*

Cefotaxime
cholecystitis treated with, 163
epiglottitis treated with, 246
posttransplant pneumonia treated with, 358
spontaneous bacterial peritonitis treated with, 180
Staphylococcus treated with, 432
Cefotetan, 224*t*
Cefoxitin
gonococcal infections, 314
postpartum endometritis treated with, 218
Cefpodoxime
acute bacterial sinusitis treated with, 240
acute otitis media treated with, 239
urologic stone disease treated with, 204
Cefprozil, 240
Ceftazidime
neutropenia treated with, 324
neutropenic fever treated with, 491*t*
wound infections treated with, 65
Ceftizoxime, 314
Ceftriaxone
acute otitis media treated with, 239
bacterial tracheitis treated with, 247
cholecystitis treated with, 163
community-acquired pneumonia treated with, 127
epiglottitis treated with, 246
in infants, 229
shock treated with, 156
spontaneous bacterial peritonitis treated with, 180
Staphylococcus treated with, 432
Cefuroxime
acute bacterial sinusitis treated with, 240
bite wound prophylaxis, 68
epiglottitis treated with, 246
otitis media treated with, 542
Cellulitis
antibiotics for, 538*t*
clinical features of, 325
definition of, 325, 538
description of, 64
diagnosis and differential of, 325–326
emergency department care and disposition of, 326
of hand, 632, 633*t*
postseptal, 528
preseptal, 528
rash associated with, 298–299
risk factors for, 539
treatment of, 538*t*
vaginal cuff, 225–226
Centor criteria, 241
Central cord syndrome, 575*t*
Central cyanosis, 121, 256, 257f
Central diabetes insipidus, 25
Central herniation syndrome, 507
Central nervous system infections
encephalitis. *See* Encephalitis
meningitis. *See* Meningitis
Central nervous system toxoplasmosis, 337
Central nervous system tumors, 306
Central retinal artery occlusion, 535
Central retinal vein occlusion, 535
Central transtentorial herniation, 571
Central venous pressure catheter, 319
Central vertigo, 511, 511*t*, 513
Centruroides-specific antivenin, 428
Cephalexin
bacterial endocarditis treated with, 339
cellulitis treated with, 326
mastitis treated with, 218
Staphylococcus treated with, 432
wound infection prophylaxis using, 64
Cephalic tetanus, 340
Cerebellar hemorrhage, 513
Cerebellar stroke, 498
Cerebellotonsillar herniation, 571
Cerebral arterial gas embolism, 437–438
Cerebral contusion, 571
Cerebral edema
diabetic ketoacidosis as cause of, 282–283, 456
high-altitude, 433–435
Cerebral malaria, 343
Cerebral perfusion pressure, 569
Cerebral venous thrombosis, 494
Cerebrospinal fluid analysis, for meningitis diagnosis, 232, 524*t*
Cervical artery dissection, 495, 497–498
Cervical lymphadenitis, 241
Cervical myelopathy, 619
Cervical radiculopathy, 618, 619*t*
Cervical spine injuries, 574*t*
Chagas disease, 355
Chalazion, 528
Chancroid, 316–317, 317*f*
Chaparral, 419*t*
Charcot triad, 160
Cheek lacerations, 56, 56*f*
Chelation therapy, 404, 413*t*
Chemical burns, 444, 445*t*–446*t*, 534
Chemical pneumonitis, 404–405
Chemotherapeutic agents
extravasation of, 493
nausea and vomiting caused by, 492
Chest pain
causes of, 72, 72*t*
clinical features of, 71
diagnosis and differential of, 71–73
epidemiology of, 71
esophageal causes of, 155–156
ischemic, 71, 74
pathophysiology of, 71
Chest radiographs
abdominal trauma, 586
acute chest syndrome, 302, 302*f*
aortic dissection, 114*f*
asthma, 250
chronic obstructive pulmonary disease, 137*f*
congestive heart failure, 89*f*
cyanosis, 257
dilated cardiomyopathy, 97
foreign bodies, 248
hypertrophic cardiomyopathy, 99
lobar pneumonia, 126*f*
mitral incompetence, 93
pleural effusion, 122*f*
pneumonia, 254, 254*f*
pneumothorax, 132
septic shock, 322
tuberculosis, 130, 130*f*
Chest trauma, 565
Chest wall injuries, 581
Chickenpox. *See* Varicella
Chiggers, 428
Chikungunya, 353
Child abuse, 234, 565, 645–646
Children. *See also* Infants; Neonate(s); Pediatrics
abdominal emergencies, 265–268
abdominal pain in, 265*t*, 265–268
acute glomerulonephritis in, 310–311
acute renal failure in, 309–310, 310*t*
altered mental status, 274–275
anemia in, 307–308
anxiety management in, 37
appendicitis in, 267
asthma in, 250–251
bacteremia in, 230
bacterial tracheitis in, 242*t*, 246–247
bone sarcomas in, 306–307
bronchiolitis in, 251–253
cardiomyopathy in, 260
central nervous system tumors in, 306
cervical lymphadenitis, 241
cervical spine imaging in, 565*t*
congestive heart failure in, 259*f*, 259–260, 260*t*
conjunctivitis in, 529
constipation in, 235–236, 267
croup in, 242*t*, 244–245
cyanide poisoning in, 418*t*
dehydration in, 262, 262*t*, 284–285, 285*t*
diabetes mellitus in, 282–284
diarrhea in, 260–264

Children (*Cont.*):
dysrhythmias in, 22
ear infections in, 238–240
electrolyte disorders in, 285–287
epiglottitis in, 242*t*, 245*f*, 245–246
epilepsy in, 273
fever in, 228–230
head trauma in. *See* Head trauma
headaches in, 275–277, 276*t*–277*t*
heart disease in, 255–260
hematological disorders in, 307–309
hernia in, 168–170
hypertensive emergencies in, 111
hypoglycemia in, 279–281, 280*t*
inborn errors of metabolism in, 279–282, 280*t*
leukemia in, 304–306
maintenance fluids in, 23
malaria in, 344
meningitis in, 228, 229*t*, 231–232, 274
mental status alterations in, 274–275
musculoskeletal disorders in
acute rheumatic fever, 292–293
clavicle fracture, 289
greenstick fractures, 289
juvenile immune arthritis, 291
Legg-Calvé-Perthes disease, 292
Osgood-Schlatter disease, 292
physeal fractures, 287f–288*f*, 287–288
plastic deformities, 289
post-streptococcal reactive arthritis, 292
radial head subluxation, 290–291
slipped capital femoral epiphysis, 291
supracondylar fractures, 289–290, 290*f*
torus fractures, 288–289
transient tenosynovitis of the hip, 293
nephroblastoma in, 306
nephrotic syndrome in, 311
neutropenia in, 324
oncologic emergencies in, 304–307
pain management in, 37
pericarditis in, 260
pharyngitis, 240–241
pneumonia in, 253–255
procedural sedation in, 43
rashes in. *See* Rashes
renal emergencies in, 309–312, 310*t*
resuscitation of, 20–23
retinoblastoma in, 306, 307*f*
salicylate toxicity in, 390
seizures in. *See* Seizures, pediatric
sepsis in, 230–231
septic shock in, 323–324
sickle cell disease in. *See* Sickle cell disease
stomatitis, 240–241
stridor in. *See* Stridor
sudden death in, 277–279
syncope in, 277–279, 278*t*–279*t*
trauma in, 564–566
urinary tract infections in, 230, 268–269
urologic stone disease in, 202
viral croup in, 242*t*, 244–245
vomiting in, 260–264, 263*t*
wheezing in, 249*t*, 249–250
Wilms tumor in, 306
Chlamydia, 313, 649
Chlamydia trachomatis, 193, 223, 268, 313, 317
Chlamydophila pneumoniae, 124*t*, 126*t*
Chloral hydrate, 42, 379
Chloramphenicol, 347
Chlorine, 415–416
Chloroform, 405
Chloroquine, 344
Cholangitis, 159–160
Cholecystitis, 143*t*
acalculous, 159
antibiotics for, 163
clinical features of, 160
complications of, 160*t*
definition of, 159
diagnosis and differential of, 160–161
epidemiology of, 159
jaundice caused by, 176
postoperative, 182
Choledocholithiasis, 159–160
Cholelithiasis, 159
Cholinesterase inhibition, 408*t*
Chopart joint, 614
Chronic constipation, 151–153, 152*t*
Chronic hepatitis, 179–181
Chronic mountain polycythemia, 435
Chronic obstructive pulmonary disease
beta-adrenergic agonists for, 138
clinical features of, 136–137
corticosteroids for, 138
diagnosis and differential of, 137
emergency department care and disposition of, 137–139
epidemiology of, 136
exacerbations of, 138
noninvasive partial pressure ventilation for, 138–139
pathophysiology of, 136
respiratory failure caused by, 137
risk factors for, 136
smoking and, 136
Chronic pain, 44*t*–45*t*, 44–46
Churg-Strauss syndrome, 630*t*
Chvostek's sign, 27
Cicutoxin, 451
Ciguatera poisoning, 346
Ciprofloxacin
bite wound prophylaxis, 66–67
chancroid treated with, 317
Crohn's disease treated with, 150
diverticulitis treated with, 166–167
fistula in ano treated with, 173
human bite wound prophylaxis, 66
infectious diarrhea treated with, 148
neutropenic fever treated with, 491*t*
ophthalmic uses of, 529*t*
ulcerative colitis treated with, 151
urologic stone disease treated with, 204
wound infection prophylaxis using, 64
Circulating inhibitors of coagulation, 473
Cirrhosis, 179–181
Clavicle fracture, 289, 602
Clenched fist injury, 65
Clindamycin
bacterial endocarditis treated with, 339
bacterial vaginosis treated with, 222
bite wound prophylaxis, 66–67
diverticulitis treated with, 167
human bite wound prophylaxis, 66
mastitis treated with, 218
odontogenic abscess treated with, 554
pelvic inflammatory disease treated with, 224*t*
postpartum endometritis treated with, 218
retropharyngeal abscess treated with, 553
shock treated with, 156
Staphylococcus treated with, 432
streptococcal toxic shock syndrome treated with, 320
toxic shock syndrome treated with, 320
Clonidine, 399
Clopidogrel, 78, 78*t*
Closed fist injury, 632
Clostridium botulinum, 345, 517
Clostridium difficile
diagnosis and differential of, 346
diarrhea caused by, 148–149, 182
Clostridium tetani, 339–340
Clotrimazole, 223, 337
Clotting disorders, 473–474
Cluster headache, 277, 495–496
Cnidaria, 431
Coagulation factors
deficiencies of, 466
replacement therapy, 481, 481*t*
Coagulopathy, 480

Cocaine, 215, 385–386
Coccyx fracture, 607*t*
Colchicine, 628
Cold injuries
frostbite, 422
hypothermia, 422–423
nonfreezing, 422
submersion, 440
Cold sores. *See* Herpes labialis
Colic, 233–234
Colles fracture, 597
Colon injuries, 585
Colonoscopy, 183
Colorado tick fever, 349
Columns of Morgagni, 171
Coma, 506–509, 507*t*–508*t*
Comfrey, 419*t*
Community-acquired pneumonia, 125, 127. *See also* Pneumonia
Compartment syndrome, 430, 597, 615–616, 638
Complete abortion, 212
Complex febrile seizures, 272
Complex regional pain syndrome, 44, 45*t*
Compression ultrasound, 654
Computed tomography
abdominal aortic aneurysm findings, 113*f*
abdominal pain, 142
abdominal trauma, 586
acute appendicitis, 165, 165*f*
aortic dissection, 115*f*
contrast-enhanced, 650–651
description of, 650
electron beam, 650
limitations of, 650
multidetector array, 650
pancreatitis, 161, 162*f*
pelvis fractures, 605
urologic stone disease, 203, 203*f*
uses of, 650–651
Computed tomography angiography, 107, 107*f*
Computed tomography coronary angiography, 84
Computed tomography myelography, 618
Computed tomography pulmonary angiography, 107, 107*f*
Concussion injuries, 549
Conduction blocks, 19
Cone snail, 432*t*–433*t*
Congenital adrenal hyperplasia, 279–281, 463–464
Congenital heart disease
cyanosis associated with, 256–258, 257*f*
definition of, 256
diagnosis and differential of, 257
shock presenting with, 258–259
Congestive heart failure
in adults, 88*t*, 88–90, 190
in children, 259*f*, 259–260, 260*t*
Conium spp., 452
Conjunctival abrasion, 531–532
Conjunctivitis, 529–530
Conscious sedation, 36
Consent
description of, 657–658
minors and, 658
refusal of, 658–659
Constipation
in adults, 151–153, 152*t*, 191
in neonates and infants, 235–236, 267
Constrictive pericarditis, 101–102
Contact dermatitis, 562
Contact lenses, 529
Contact vulvovaginitis, 222–223
Continuous certification examination, 2–3
Continuous Osteopathic Learning Assessment, 1
Continuous percutaneous sutures, 51, 51*f*
Continuous positive airway pressure
bronchiolitis treated with, 252
chronic obstructive pulmonary disease treated with, 139
description of, 9
hypercapnia treated with, 121
Contrast venography, of deep vein thrombosis, 105
Contrast-enhanced computed tomography, 650–651
Conversion disorder, 499*t*, 643–645, 644*t*
Convulsive generalized seizure, 270
COPD. *See* Chronic obstructive pulmonary disease
Coprinus atramentarius, 451
Coral snake bite, 430
Cord prolapse, 220
Corneal abrasion, 532, 532*t*
Corneal foreign bodies, 530
Corneal laceration, 532
Corneal reflex, 644*t*–645*t*
Corneal ulcers, 530, 530*f*
Corns, 635
Coronary artery disease, 74
Coronary plaque, 73
Coronavirus, 124*t*
Corticosteroids
anaphylaxis treated with, 35
asthma treated with, 138, 251
chronic obstructive pulmonary disease treated with, 138
contact dermatitis treated with, 562
meningitis treated with, 524
septic shock treated with, 324
Cortinarius orellanus, 452
Cortisol, 463, 490
Costochondritis, 72*t*
Costosternal syndrome, 72*t*
Costovertebral angle tenderness, 193
COX-2 inhibitors, 46, 392–393
Coyotillo, 451*t*
CPAP. *See* Continuous positive airway pressure
Crack cocaine, 385
Creatine kinase, 72, 189, 446
Creatinine phosphokinase, 279
Cricothyrotomy, 7
Crimean–Congo hemorrhagic fever, 354–355
Critical-care units, 656
Critically ill patients, 43
Crohn's disease
clinical features of, 149
definition of, 149
diagnosis and differential of, 149
diarrhea associated with, 149–150
emergency department care and disposition of, 149–150
pathophysiology of, 149
treatment of, 149–150
Crossed straight leg raise test, 620*t*
Croup, viral, 242*t*, 244–245
Crush injury, 615
Crutches, 595
Crying, 233, 234*t*
Cryoprecipitate, 472, 477, 481
Cryptitis, 171–172
Cryptococcosis, 337
Crystal-induced synovitis, 627–628
Cubital tunnel syndrome, 518
Cuff cellulitis, 225–226
Cullen's sign, 112
Cutaneous abscesses, 327–328
Cutaneous anthrax, 351
Cyanide, 365*t*, 416–418, 417*t*
Cyanoacrylate adhesive, 53, 534
Cyanocobalamin, 419, 509
Cyanosis
in adults, 121*t*, 121–122
clinical presentation of, 257*f*
in congenital heart disease, 256–258, 257*f*
in neonates and infants, 236
Cyanotic heart disease, 256–258, 257*t*
Cyclic antidepressants, 369–370
Cyclopentolate, 529*t*
Cycloplegia, 530
Cycloplegics, 532
Cyproheptadine, 372
Cysticercosis, 355
Cystitis, 192

Cytochrome a_3, 416
Cytomegalovirus pneumonia, 357–358
Cytomegalovirus radiculitis, 519
Cytomegalovirus retinitis, 336

D

Dabigatran, 484
Dactylitis, 301
Dalteparin, 108
Dalton's law, 436
Dantrolene, 374
Dapsone, 427
DDAVP, 476
D-dimer testing
  deep vein thrombosis, 104
  hemostasis evaluations, 469*t*
  pulmonary embolism, 106
DDT, 409
DeBakey system, 114
Debridement of wound, 49
Decompression illness, 437
Decompression sickness, 436–438
Deep dermal sutures, 51, 52*f*
Deep peroneal nerve
  block of, 39
  entrapment of, 636–637
  motor function of, 61*t*
Deep space infection, 632, 633*t*
Deep vein thrombosis
  adjunctive therapy for, 108–109
  algorithm for, 104, 105*f*
  ancillary testing for, 104–105, 105*f*
  anticoagulants for, 107–108
  calf veins, 108
  clinical features of, 103
  clotting disorders and, 473
  compression ultrasound of, 654
  contrast venography of, 105
  D-dimer assays for, 104
  diagnosis and differential of, 104
  emergency department care and disposition of, 107–109
  epidemiology of, 102
  heparin for, 107–108
  pathophysiology of, 102–103
  in pregnancy, 214
  signs and symptoms of, 103
  thrombolytic therapy for, 108
  treatment of, 107–109, 485
  venous ultrasonography evaluations, 105, 105*f*
  Wells score for, 104*t*
DEET, 410
Deferoxamine, 365*t*, 404
Defibrillation
  in children, 22
  ventricular fibrillation treated with, 17
Degenerative heart disease, 94
Dehydration
  in children, 284–285, 285*t*
  hyponatremic, 284
  severity of, 262
  signs in, 262*t*
Delayed transfusion reactions, 482–483, 483*t*
Delayed wound closure, 52
Delirium, 505*t*, 505–506, 639
Delta pressure, 616
Demeclocycline, 489
Dementia, 505*t*, 506, 639
Demyelinating disease, 499*t*
Dengue fever, 353
Dental caries, 546
Dental fractures, 548–549, 549*f*
Deoxyhemoglobin, 121
DeQuervain's tenosynovitis, 634
Dermal-epidermal junction, 51, 52*f*
Dermatitis
  atopic, 299
  candidal diaper, 299
  contact, 562
  exfoliative, 557–558
  seborrheic, 299
Dermatomes, 575*f*
Dermatomyositis, 630*t*, 631
Desmopressin, 471
Dexamethasone
  acute mountain sickness treated with, 434
  epiglottitis treated with, 246
  spinal cord compression treated with, 487
  superior vena cava syndrome treated with, 488
  thyroid storm treated with, 462*t*
  viral croup treated with, 244
Dextrose
  as antidote, 366*t*
  for hypoglycemia, 280–281, 281*t*
Diabetes insipidus, 25, 375
Diabetes mellitus
  in children, 282–284
  emergencies associated with
    diabetic ketoacidosis, 213–214, 282–283, 455–456, 457*f*
    foot ulcers, 458–459
    hyperglycemic, hyperglycemic state, 456, 458, 458*f*
    hypoglycemia, 454*t*–455*t*, 454–455
  insulin-dependent, 282
  in pregnancy, 213–214
Diabetic ketoacidosis, 213–214, 282–283, 455–456, 457*f*
Diabetic neuropathy, 45*t*
Diabetic peripheral neuropathy, 519
Diagnostic peritoneal lavage, 563, 568, 586
Dialysis
  acute renal failure treated with, 188, 188*t*
  emergencies in, 190–192
  gastrointestinal complications of, 191
  hematologic complications of, 191
  hemodialysis, 191, 383, 390, 394
  hypertension associated with, 190
  neurologic complications of, 191
  peritoneal, 192
  vascular access complications, 191–192
Dialysis disequilibrium, 191
Diaper dermatitis, 299
Diaper rash, 299
Diaphragmatic injuries, 582, 585
Diarrhea
  acute infectious, 147–148
  in AIDS patients, 335
  antibiotic-associated, 147, 181–182
  antidiarrheal agents for, 147, 263
  antimotility agents for, 148, 263
  in children, 260–264
  clinical features of, 146, 261
  Clostridium difficile-associated, 148–149, 182
  Crohn's disease as cause of, 149–150
  definition of, 146
  diagnosis and differential of, 146–147, 261–262
  dietary causes of, 146
  dietary management of, 263
  emergency department care and disposition of, 147–148, 263
  fluid therapy for, 147
  in infants, 235, 260–264
  in neonates, 235
  pathophysiology of, 146, 261
  stool culture testing for, 146
  traveler's, 147–148
  ulcerative colitis as cause of, 150–151
Diastolic dysfunction, 89
Diazepam
  seizures treated with, 370
  status epilepticus treated with, 271*t*
Dicloxacillin
  bacterial endocarditis treated with, 339
  mastitis treated with, 218
Digital nerve blocks, 38f–39*f*, 38–39
Digitalis glycosides, 395*t*–396*t*, 395–396
Digoxin
  atrial fibrillation treated with, 14
  narrow-complex supraventricular tachycardia treated with, 12
Digoxin immune Fab, 27
Digoxin-specific Fab, 366*t*, 395, 396*t*, 453

Dihydroergotamine, 276
1,25-Dihydroxyhydrocalciferol, 419
Dilated cardiomyopathy, 97
Diltiazem
  atrial fibrillation treated with, 13
  multifocal atrial tachycardia treated with, 15
  narrow-complex supraventricular tachycardia treated with, 12
Dilute Russell viper venom time, 470*t*
Dimercaprol, 414*t*
Diphenhydramine, 35, 492*t*, 650
Diphenoxylate and atropine, 148
Diphyllobothrium latum, 356
Diplopia, 536
Direct Coombs test, 467*t*
Direct thrombin inhibitors, 79, 484
Disaster plan, 656
Disc battery ingestion, 407
Dislocation
  ankle, 614
  distal interphalangeal joint, 596
  elbow, 599–600
  glenohumeral joint, 602–603, 604*t*
  hip, 608–609
  knee, 610–611, 611*t*
  lunate, 597
  mandible, 540, 540*f*
  metacarpophalangeal joint, 596
  patellar, 610–611
  perilunate, 597
  proximal interphalangeal joint, 596
  sternoclavicular joint, 601–602
  thumb, 596
Disseminated gonococcal infection, 559
Disseminated intravascular coagulation
  clinical features of, 472
  diagnosis and differential of, 472
  emergency department care and disposition of, 472
  laboratory abnormalities associated with, 472*t*–473*t*
  pathophysiology of, 472
  in septic shock, 322
  treatment of, 324
Distal interphalangeal joint dislocation, 596
Distal phalanx fracture, 597
Diuretics, 97, 398–399
Diverticulitis, 143*t*, 166–167
Diving injuries
  barotrauma, 436*t*, 436–437
  clinical features of, 436–437
  decompression sickness, 436–438
  overview of, 435–436
  pathophysiology of, 436
Diving reflex, 12, 439
Dix-Hallpike position, 511–512
Dizziness, 510–513, 512*t*
Dogs
  bites from, 66*t*, 67
  rabies transmission from, 342–343
Dolasetron, 492*t*
Domestic violence, 215
Do-not-resuscitation orders, 659
Dopamine
  shock treated with, 231
  sinus bradycardia treated with, 11
Doripenem, 167
Dorsal hand lacerations, 57
Doxycycline
  bite wound prophylaxis, 68
  community-acquired pneumonia treated with, 127
  louse-borne typhus treated with, 354
  Lyme disease treated with, 348–349
  pelvic inflammatory disease treated with, 224*t*
  Rocky Mountain spotted fever treated with, 347–348
  scrub typhus treated with, 354
  sinusitis treated with, 545
  Staphylococcus treated with, 432
  syphilis treated with, 315
Dressings, wound, 68
Dressler's syndrome, 74, 100
Drooling, 242
Droperidol, 43
Drowning, 438–440, 439*t*, 440*t*
Drug(s). *See specific drug*
Drug-induced parkinsonism, 375
Drugs of abuse
  cocaine, 385–386
  hallucinogens, 386–388, 387*t*
  opioids, 383–385
  in pregnancy, 215
Drug-seeking behavior, 46*t*, 46–47
"Dry drowning," 439
Dry socket, 546
Duloxetine, 372
Dumping syndrome, 183
Duodenal injuries, 585
Dupuytren's contracture, 634, 638
Duroziez sign, 95
Duty, 657
Duverney fracture, 607*t*
DVT. *See* Deep vein thrombosis
Dysarthria, 502*t*
Dysautonomia, 521
Dysbarism, 435–438
Dysfunctional uterine bleeding, 208
Dyshemoglobinemias
  methemoglobinemia, 121, 420–421
  sulfhemoglobinemia, 421
Dysmenorrhea, 209
Dyspepsia, 157–158
Dysphagia, 154–155
Dyspnea, 119, 120*t*
Dysrhythmias, 359
  in children, 22
  in infants, 22
  in pregnancy, 214

E

Ear(s)
  barotrauma of, 436*t*
  emergencies of, 541–543
  foreign bodies in, 543
  hematomas of, 542
  infections of, 238–240
  laceration of, 55, 56*f*
  trauma to, 542–543
Echinodermata, 431
Echocardiography
  dilated cardiomyopathy findings, 97
  mitral incompetence findings, 93, 93*f*
  pulmonary embolism findings, 105
  transthoracic, 93
  valvular regurgitation findings, 95
Eclampsia, 217, 514
Ectopic pregnancy, 143*t*, 210–212
Ectopic supraventricular tachycardia, 11
Eczema herpeticum, 295, 295*f*
Edema
  cerebral, 282–283, 433–435
  heat, 426
  pulmonary. *See* Pulmonary edema
Ehrlichiosis, 349
Elbow
  dislocation of, 599–600
  fracture of, 600, 600*t*
Elderly
  abuse of, 646–647
  delirium in, 505*t*
  disequilibrium in, 513
  hip fractures in, 567
  procedural sedation in, 43
  trauma in, 566–567
Electrical alternans, 101
Electrical injuries, 446–448, 447*t*
Electrocardiogram
  accelerated idioventricular rhythm findings, 16, 16*f*
  acute myocardial infarction findings, 75*f*–77*f*, 77*t*
  atrial fibrillation findings, 13–14, 14*f*
  atrial flutter findings, 13, 13*f*
  chest pain evaluations, 72
  chronic obstructive pulmonary disease findings, 137, 138*f*
  hyperkalemia findings, 26*f*
  mitral stenosis findings, 92*f*
  multifocal atrial tachycardia findings, 15, 14*f*
  myocardial infarction findings, 75*f*–77*f*
  pneumothorax findings, 132

Electrocardiogram (*Cont.*):
premature atrial contraction findings, 9, 10*f*
premature ventricular contractions findings, 15, 15*f*
sinus arrhythmia findings, 9, 10*f*
sinus bradycardia findings, 10
sinus tachycardia findings, 11
syncope evaluations, 279
ventricular fibrillation findings, 17, 17*f*
ventricular tachycardia findings, 16–17, 16*f*
Electrocardiography
acute pericarditis findings, 100
hypertrophic cardiomyopathy findings, 99
Electrolyte disorders
in children, 285–287
description of, 23–24
hypercalcemia, 28, 286, 286*t*
hyperkalemia, 26*f*, 26–27, 27*t*, 286, 286*t*, 395–396, 425, 483
hypermagnesemia, 29, 286*t*
hypernatremia, 24–25, 25*t*, 286, 286*t*
hypocalcemia, 27–28, 273, 286, 286*t*
hypokalemia, 25, 26*t*, 286, 286*t*, 483
hypomagnesemia, 28–29, 286, 286*t*
hyponatremia, 24, 24*t*, 273, 285, 286*t*, 388, 489
pediatric, 285–287
Electron beam computed tomography, 650
Embolism
acute arterial occlusion caused by, 116*t*
cerebral arterial gas, 437–438
pulmonary. *See* Pulmonary embolism
Emergence reactions, 42
Emergency consent, 658
Emergency contraception, 649
Emergency delivery, 218–221
Emergency medical services
access to, 656
challenges for, 657
communications used in, 655
critical-care units, 656
disaster plan, 656
facilities, 656
history of, 655
overview of, 655–657
patient transfer, 656
personnel, 655, 655*t*
public information and education purposes of, 656
public safety agencies, 656
recordkeeping, 656
review systems in, 656
training in, 655
transportation methods, 655–656
Emergency Medical Treatment and Active Labor Act, 656, 659–660, 660*t*
Emergency medicine administration
consent, 657–658
do-not-resuscitation orders, 659
informed refusal, 658–659
medical ethics, 660
medical malpractice, 657
minors, 658
negligence, 657
physician telephone advice, 659
resuscitation, 659
Emergency transfusion, 483
EMLA, 38
Emotional abuse, of elderly, 646
Emphysema
mediastinal, 156
pulmonary, 137
Empyema, 128
EMTALA. *See* Emergency Medical Treatment and Active Labor Act
Encephalitides, 525–526
Encephalitis
clinical features of, 525–526
description of, 274
diagnosis and differential of, 526
emergency department care and disposition of, 526
epidemiology of, 525
herpes labialis as cause of, 328–329
pathophysiology of, 525
Endobronchial intubation, 7
Endocarditis, infective, 96, 338–339
Endocrine disorders
adrenal crisis, 463–465
adrenal insufficiency, 463–465, 464*t*–465*t*
diabetes mellitus. *See* Diabetes mellitus
thyroid gland, 461–463
Endometriosis, 209
Endometritis, 218, 227
Endophthalmitis, 531
Endoscopic retrograde cholangiopancreatography, 161
Endoscopy, 43
Endotracheal intubation
in elderly, 567
for hemoptysis, 136
in trauma, 564
Endotracheal tube
in children, 21
in neonates, 21
End-stage renal disease, 190–191
End-tidal CO_2 monitoring, 250
Enemas, 152
Enoxaparin
acute coronary syndromes treated with, 78*t*, 79
deep vein thrombosis treated with, 108
Entamoeba histolytica, 356
Enterobiasis, 356
Enterotoxins, 147
Enteroviruses
acute bronchitis caused by, 124*t*
characteristics of, 293
rashes caused by, 293–294
Entrapment neuropathies, 518
Envenomations
marine, 430–433, 432*t*–433*t*
snakebites, 429–430
Environmental injuries
burns. *See* Burns
carbon monoxide poisoning, 449–450
cold-related. *See* Cold injuries
diving injuries. *See* Diving injuries
drowning, 438–440, 439*t*, 440*t*
electrical injuries, 446–448, 447*t*
heat injuries, 424–426
high-altitude syndromes. *See* High-altitude syndromes
insect bites and stings. *See* Insect bites and stings
lightning, 448*t*, 448–449
Enzyme-linked immunoassay, 336
Ephedra, 419*t*
Epicondylitis, 599
Epidermic keratoconjunctivitis, 529
Epididymitis, 200, 200*f*
Epididymo-orchitis, 539
Epidural compression, 619–620
Epidural hematoma, 566, 571
Epigastric pain, 158–159
Epiglottitis
in adults, 552*f*, 552–553
in children, 242*t*, 245*f*, 245–246
Epilepsia partialis, 514
Epilepsy
definition of, 514
seizures in children with, 273
Epinephrine
anaphylaxis treated with, 34
pulseless electrical activity treated with, 20
sinus bradycardia treated with, 11
ventricular fibrillation treated with, 17
viral croup treated with, 244
Epinephrine autoinjector injury, 65
Episcleritis, 631
Episiotomy, 219
Epistaxis, 543, 578
Epley maneuver, 513
Epstein–Barr virus
infections caused by, 331–332

pharyngitis caused by, 240
treatment of, 358
Eptifibatide, 78*t*
Equine gait, 509
Ertapenem, 166
Erysipelas, 298, 299*f*, 326–327, 538, 538*t*
Erythema infectiosum, 294*f*, 294–295
Erythema multiforme, 556
Erythema toxicum, 299
Erythromycin, 317
Erythromycin ethylsuccinate, 241
Erythroplakia, 548
Escharotomy, 443
Escherichia coli
E. coli 0157:H7, 147
enteroaggregative, 264*t*
enteroinvasive, 264*t*
enteropathogenic, 264*t*
enterotoxigenic, 264*t*
foodborne illnesses caused by, 345–346
Shiga toxin-producing, 264*t*, 345–346
urinary tract infections caused by, 268
Esmolol, 12
Esomeprazole, 154
Esophageal emergencies
blunt trauma, 580
caustic ingestion, 406
chest pain, 155–156
dysphagia, 154–155
perforation, 156
trauma, 580, 584
Esophageal rupture, 72*t*
Esophagitis, 155
Estrogens, 208, 209*t*
Ethambutol, 131*t*
Ethanol, 366*t*, 380, 382*t*
Ethinyl estradiol, 209*t*, 649
Ethylene glycol, 381–383, 383*t*
Etomidate, 8*t*
in critically ill patients, 43
in elderly, 43
procedural sedation use of, 41*t*, 42
Ewing sarcoma, 307, 307*f*
Exanthem subitum. *See* Roseola infantum
Exanthems
bacterial infections that cause, 297f–298*f*, 297–299
cellulitis, 298–299
definition of, 293
description of, 293
diaper, 299
erysipelas, 298, 299*f*
erythema infectiosum, 294*f*, 294–295
fungal, 296–297
Henoch–Schönlein purpura, 300, 300*f*
herpes virus, 295, 295*f*
impetigo, 297, 297*f*
Kawasaki's disease, 300
measles, 294
neonatal, 299
pityriasis rosea, 300–301
roseola infantum, 296, 296*f*
rubella, 294
scarlet fever, 297–298, 298*f*
varicella, 295–296, 296*f*
viral, 293–296
Exercise treadmill testing, 84
Exercise-related syncope, 279
Exfoliative dermatitis, 557–558
Express consent, 658
Extended focused assessment with sonography for trauma, 652
Extensor digitorum, 595
Extensor hallucis longus, 61*t*
Extensor tendon lacerations, 58, 58*f*
External hordeolum, 528
Extracorporeal shock wave lithotripsy, 202, 205
Extrapulmonary tuberculosis, 129–130
Extravasation
chemotherapeutic agents, 493
urinary, 589
Extremity trauma, 591–592
Exudative pleural effusions, 122, 123*t*
Eye(s)
alkali burns of, 444
caustic exposure effects on, 407
inflammation of. *See* Ocular inflammations
ultrasonography of, 537
visual reduction and loss. *See* Visual reduction and loss
Eyelid lacerations, 54, 54*f*, 532

F

Facial infections, 538–539
Facial lacerations, 56, 56*f*
Facial trauma, 564, 577*t*, 577–579
Factitious anemia, 191
Factitious hyponatremia, 24
Factor I, 481*t*
Factor II, 481*t*
Factor IX, 481*t*
Factor level assays, 469*t*
Factor V, 481*t*
Factor V Leiden, 470*t*
Factor VII, 481*t*
Factor VIII, 475, 481*t*
Factor VIII inhibitor, 473
Factor X, 481*t*
Factor XI, 481*t*
Factor XII, 481*t*
Factor XIII, 481*t*
False labor, 218
Famciclovir, 316, 330
Fascicular blocks, 19
Fasting, 261
Fat-soluble vitamins, 418–419
Febrile nonhemolytic transfusion reaction, 482*t*
Febrile seizures, 270–272
Fecal impaction, 152
Feeding difficulties, 235
Felbamate, 402
Felon, 633, 633*t*
Femoral condyle fractures, 609, 611*t*
Femoral head
avascular necrosis of, 302*f*
fracture of, 607*t*
Femoral hernia, 169
Femoral neck fracture, 607*t*
Femoral nerve block, 40
Femoral shaft fractures, 609
Fentanyl
procedural sedation use of, 41*t*, 42
rigid chest syndrome caused by, 42
Ferritin, 467*t*
Fetal heart tones, 569
Fetal hemoglobin, 301
Fever
in children, 228–230, 269
neutropenic, 305*t*, 490–491
pediatric, 228–230
postoperative, 181
Fiber-optic laryngoscopy, 555
Fibrin degradation products, 469*t*
Fibrinogen, 469*t*, 481*t*
Fibrinolytic agents
acute coronary syndromes treated with, 78*t*, 79
description of, 485, 485*t*
Fibroids, 209
Fibromyalgia, 44, 44*t*–45*t*, 72*t*
Fifth disease. *See* Erythema infectiosum
Financial abuse, of elderly, 646
Finger lacerations, 59, 59*f*
Fingertip injuries, 59, 59*f*
Fire coral, 431, 432*t*
Fireworms, 433*t*
First-degree AV block, 17
First-degree burn, 442*t*
Fish, 66*t*
Fishhook removal, 63
Fist injuries, 57, 65, 632
Fistula in ano, 172–173
Fistula test, 438
Flail chest, 581
Flank trauma, 587–588
Flashing lights, 536
Flavivirus, 355
Flea bites, 428
Flexon tendon sheath digital nerve block, 39, 39*f*
Flexor digitorum profundus, 595
Flexor digitorum superficialis, 595

Flexor hallucis longus rupture, 637
Flexor tendon lacerations, 59, 59*f*
Flexor tenosynovitis, 632, 633*t*
Floaters, 536
Fluconazole, 223, 337
Flucytosine, 337
Fluid therapy
  diarrhea managed with, 147
  shock managed with, 33
  thermal burns treated with, 443
  toxic shock syndrome managed with, 319
Fluids
  in children, 22
  daily requirements, 23
  maintenance, 23, 285
  in neonates, 22
  volume overload, 23
  volume status assessments, 23
Flumazenil, 41, 180, 275, 365, 366*t*
Fluoroquinolones
  otitis externa treated with, 239
  pregnancy contraindications, 215
  Staphylococcus treated with, 432
  urinary tract infections treated with, 194–195
Focal neuropathies, 518
Focused assessment with sonography for trauma, 563, 586, 605, 652
Folate, 418*t*
Folic acid, 366*t*
Folliculitis, 327–328
Fomepizole, 366*t*, 382*t*, 382–383
Fondaparinux, 79
Foodborne diseases, 345–347
Foot
  bursitis of, 636
  compartment syndrome of, 638
  crush injury of, 615
  diabetic ulcers of, 458–459
  forefoot, 615
  hindfoot, 615
  injuries of, 614–615
  lacerations of, 60–62
  midfoot, 615
  soft tissue disorders of, 634–638
Forearm
  extensor compartments in, 58*t*
  flexor tendons of, 58*t*
  fractures of, 601
  lacerations of, 57, 57*f*
Forehead lacerations, 53–56
Foreign bodies
  aspiration of, 242*t*, 248
  corneal, 530
  ear, 543
  nasal, 544
  radiopaque, 63
  rectal, 174–175
  soft tissue, 62–63
  stridor caused by aspiration of, 242*t*, 248
  swallowed, 156–157
  urethral, 201
  vaginal, 222–223
Foreseeability, 657
Formaldehyde, 381
Formic acid, 381
Fosphenytoin, 400–401, 516
Fournier's gangrene, 198, 198*f*
Fourth-degree burn, 442*t*
Foxglove, 451*t*
Fracture(s)
  acetabular, 605–606
  ankle, 614
  avulsion, 607*t*
  Barton, 597
  blowout, 533, 578
  carpal bone, 597, 598*t*
  clavicle, 289, 602
  clinical features of, 593
  coccyx, 607*t*
  Colles, 597
  dental, 548–549, 549*f*
  distal phalanx, 597
  elbow, 600, 600*t*
  emergency department care and disposition of, 594–595
  femoral condyle, 609
  femoral shaft, 609
  forearm, 601
  frontal sinus, 578
  hip, 567, 606–608
  humerus, 603–604
  intercondylar, 600
  knee, 609–610
  long-term complications of, 594
  lunate, 597
  mandible, 578–579
  metatarsal, 615
  middle phalanx, 597
  midface, 578
  nasal, 544, 544*f*
  naso-orbito-ethmoid, 578
  odontoid, 566
  olecranon, 600
  open, 592
  patellar, 609, 611*t*
  pathologic, 486–487
  pelvis, 565, 604–605
  penile, 199, 590
  physeal, 287*f*–288*f*, 287–288, 593, 594*f*
  proximal femur, 607*t*, 609*t*
  proximal fibular, 610
  proximal phalanx, 597
  radial head, 600
  radial styloid, 598
  rib, 581, 588, 602
  sacral, 607*t*
  Salter–Harris classification of, 287*f*–288*f*, 287–288, 593, 594*f*, 595*t*
  scaphoid, 597, 598*t*
  scapula, 602
  skull, 570–571, 573
  Smith, 597
  spine, 565, 575
  supracondylar, 289–290, 290*f*, 600, 600*t*
  thoracic vertebral, 576
  torus, 288–289
  tripod, 578
  ulnar styloid, 598
  zygoma, 578
Fracture line, 593, 594*f*
Francisella tularensis, 350
Free fatty acids, 455
Free thyroxine, 461
Fresh frozen plasma, 472, 475, 480, 567
Froment sign, 518
Frontal sinus fractures, 578
Frostbite, 422
Frostnip, 422
Frozen shoulder, 621
Full-thickness burns, 441
Fungal infections
  rashes caused by, 296–297
  tinea, 560–561
Furocoumarins, 562
Furosemide, 27

G

Gabapentin, 402
Gait disturbances, 509–510, 510*t*
Galeazzi fracture-dislocation, 601
Gallbladder disease, 653
Gallstones, 159–161, 653
Gamma-hydroxybutyrate, 384
Ganciclovir, 337
Ganglion cyst, 634
Ganglions, 637
Gastric lavage, 374
Gastritis, 157–159, 381
Gastroenteritis
  acute, 260–261
  bacterial, 264*t*
  viral, 260–261
Gastroesophageal reflux disease
  clinical features of, 155
  exacerbation of, 155
  in neonates and infants, 235, 237
  pathophysiology of, 155
  prevalence of, 155
Gastroesophageal varices, 180

Gastrointestinal bleeding
in adults, 153–154
in children, 265
Gastrointestinal emergencies
abdominal pain. *See* Abdominal pain
acute appendicitis, 143*t,* 163–165
anal fissures, 172
anorectal abscess, 173
anorectal disorders, 170–175
bowel obstruction, 143*t,* 144, 167–168
cholecystitis. *See* Cholecystitis
constipation, 151–153, 152*t,* 191
cryptitis, 171–172
diarrhea. *See* Diarrhea
diverticulitis, 166–167
fistula in ano, 172–173
gastritis, 157–159
hemorrhoids, 170–171, 171*f*
hernia, 168–170, 169*f*–170*f*
nausea and vomiting, 101, 144–146
pancreatitis. *See* Pancreatitis
peptic ulcer disease, 157–159
pilonidal sinus, 175
proctitis, 173
pruritus ani, 175
rectal foreign bodies, 174–175
rectal prolapse, 173–174
swallowed foreign bodies, 156–157
Gastrointestinal reflux, 235
Gastrointestinal surgery, 182–183
Generalized seizures, 270
Genital warts, 318
Genitourinary trauma
bladder, 590
clinical features of, 588–589
diagnosis and differential of, 589
emergency department care and disposition of, 589
epidemiology of, 588
kidneys, 589*t,* 589–590
testes, 590
ureter, 590
urethra, 590
Gentamicin
neutropenic fever treated with, 491*t*
ophthalmic uses of, 529*t*
pelvic inflammatory disease treated with, 224*t*
postpartum endometritis treated with, 218
posttransplant pneumonia treated with, 358
Geographic tongue, 548
GERD. *See* Gastroesophageal reflux disease
Geriatric trauma, 566–567
German measles, 294
Gestational trophoblastic disease, 212
Giant cell arteritis, 536, 630*t*
Giardia lamblia, 261
Gila monsters, 430
Gilbert's syndrome, 176
Gingival hyperplasia, 548
Gingivostomatitis, herpes simplex, 240, 295*f*
Glasgow Coma Scale, 439, 506, 507*t,* 565, 570*t*
Glaucoma, acute angle-closure, 534*f,* 534–535
Glenohumeral joint dislocation, 602–603, 604*t*
Glomerulonephritis, acute, 310–311
Glucagon, 281, 366*t,* 397–398
Glucocorticoids
Crohn's disease treated with, 150
deficiency of, 490
hypercalcemia of malignancy treated with, 489
ulcerative colitis treated with, 151
Glucose, 27
Glucose-6-phosphate dehydrogenase deficiency, 479
Glycerine rectal suppositories, 152
Glycogenolysis, 455
Glycoprotein IIb/IIIa inhibitors
acute coronary syndromes treated with, 78*t,* 80
description of, 485
Glycopyrrolate, 42
Golfer's elbow, 599
Gonococcal arthritis, 627
Gonococcal infections, 313–314, 559
Gonorrhea, 548, 649
Gout, 627–628
Graft-versus-host disease, 361–362
Granisetron, 492*t*
Granular casts, 186
Graves' disease, 462
Great vessel injuries, 583–584, 584*t*
Greater trochanteric fracture, 607*t*
Greenstick fractures, 289
Grey-Turner's sign, 112
Groove sign, 317
Gross hematuria, 195
Group A β-hemolytic *Streptococcus*
acute rheumatic fever secondary to, 292
pharyngitis caused by, 240–241, 550–551
scarlet fever caused by, 297
Guaiac testing, 153
Guanethidine, 462*t*
Guessing, 5
Guillain–Barré syndrome, 518
Gunshot wounds, 572, 583, 585, 591
Gyromitrin, 451

H

H_2 receptor antagonist, 158–159
Haemophilus influenzae, 126*t*
Haemophilus influenzae type b, 228, 231
Hair-thread tourniquet syndrome, 62
Hallucinations, 641
Hallucinogens, 386–388, 387*t*
Halogenated hydrocarbons, 405
Haloperidol, 506
Hamate, 598*t*
Hammon's crunch, 156
Hampton's hump, 106
Hand
anatomy of, 595
cellulitis of, 632, 633*t*
cutaneous nerve supply of, 595*f*
examination of, 595
human bites to, 66, 633*t*
infections of, 632–633
injuries of, 595–597
noninfectious disorders of, 634
splinting of, 632
tendon injury of, 596
Hand surgery, 596*t*
Hand-foot-and-mouth disease, 240, 293, 547–548
Hantavirus, 350
Hawkins' impingement test, 621, 621*f*
Hawthorn, 419*t*
β-hCG, 211
Head tilt–chin lift maneuver, 6
Head trauma
cerebral contusion, 571
diagnosis and differential of, 572, 572*t*
emergency department care and disposition of, 572–573
epidemiology of, 569
epidural hematoma, 566, 571
herniation, 571
intracerebral hemorrhage, 571
pathophysiology of, 569–570
pediatric, seizures in, 273
penetrating, 572
shaken baby syndrome, 572
skull fractures, 570–571
subarachnoid hemorrhage, 571
subdural hematoma, 571
traumatic brain injuries, 569–570
Headaches
in children, 275–277, 276*t*–277*t*
cluster, 277, 495–496
diagnosis and differential of, 276, 496
emergency department care and disposition of, 276–277, 496
epidemiology of, 494
hypertensive, 495
migraine, 276, 494–495

Headaches (*Cont.*):
myofascial, 44*t*–45*t*
ophthalmic disorders caused by, 495
pain associated with, 276
pathophysiology of, 276
post-lumbar puncture, 495
in pregnancy, 215
primary, 276
secondary, 276, 276*t*–277*t*, 494–496
sinusitis as cause of, 495
sleep-related, 306
tension, 44*t*–45*t*, 277
Health Insurance Portability and Accountability Act, 660–661
Hearing loss, sudden, 541
Heart failure, 88*t*, 88–90, 190
Heart murmurs, 91*t*, 255, 256*t*
Heart sounds, 91*t*, 98
Heartburn, 155
Heat cramps, 425
Heat edema, 426
Heat exhaustion, 425
Heat injuries, 424–426
Heat loss, 424
Heat rash, 426
Heat stroke, 424
Heat syncope, 425
Heat tetany, 425–426
Helicobacter pylori, 158–159
Heliox, 138, 244, 251–252
HELLP syndrome, 217
Hematemesis, 144, 153
Hematochezia, 153
Hematological emergencies
anemia. *See* Anemia
bleeding disorders. *See* Bleeding disorders
clotting disorders, 473–474
hemophilias, 474–475, 475*t*–476*t*
sickle cell disease. *See* Sickle cell disease
von Willebrand's disease, 475–477
Hematoma
ear, 542
epidural, 566, 571
retrobulbar, 534
subdural, 494, 571
subungual, 59
wound, 181–182
Hematopoietic stem cell transplantation, 361–362
Hematuria, 195
Hemodialysis
description of, 191
hypercalcemia of malignancy treated with, 489
overdoses treated with, 383, 390, 394
Hemoglobin S, 301
Hemoglobin SS, 301
Hemolysis, 490
Hemolytic-uremic syndrome, 147
Hemophilia, 474–475, 475*t*–476*t*
Hemoptysis, 134–136, 135*f*
Hemorrhage. *See also* Bleeding
cerebellar, 513
gastrointestinal, 153–154
intracerebral, 502, 571
intracranial, 111, 486*t*, 504*t*
intraparenchymal, 494
postpartum, 217
retinal, 435
subarachnoid, 111, 494, 496, 504, 571
subconjunctival, 531
vascular access as cause of, 192
vitreous, 531
Hemorrhagic gastritis, 381
Hemorrhagic stroke, 497, 497*t*
Hemorrhoids, 170–171, 171*f*
Hemostasis
description of, 48
tests of, 469*t*–470*t*
Hemothorax, 581–582
Henoch–Schönlein purpura, 267, 300, 300*f*, 630*t*
Henry's law, 436
Heparin
acute coronary syndromes treated with, 78*t*, 79
in atrial fibrillation, 13
bleeding caused by, 486*t*
deep vein thrombosis treated with, 107–108
low molecular weight
acute coronary syndromes treated with, 79
deep vein thrombosis treated with, 108, 485
description of, 484
pulmonary embolism treated with, 108, 485
types of, 108
in pregnancy, 214
transient ischemic attack treated with, 503
unfractionated
acute coronary syndromes treated with, 79
description of, 484
pulmonary embolism treated with, 108, 485
Heparin-induced thrombocytopenia, 108
Hepatic encephalopathy, 179
Hepatitis
A, 176–178
B, 176–178
C, 176–178
chronic, 179–181
prophylaxis, 649
Hepatomegaly
in AIDS patients, 336
description of, 176, 179
Hepatorenal syndrome, 180
Herbal products, 419–420
Herbicides, 410–411
Hereditary angioedema, 35, 555
Hereditary spherocytosis, 479
Hernia, 168–170, 169*f*–170*f*, 267
Herniation, 571
Herpangina, 240–241, 547
Herpes keratitis, 530
Herpes labialis, 295, 295*f*, 328–329
Herpes simplex infections
cutaneous, 337
genital, 315–316, 316*f*
gingivostomatitis, 240, 295*f*, 547
HSV-1, 328–330, 329*f*, 525
HSV-2, 525
ocular, 530
recurrent, 330
Herpes zoster, 330*f*, 330–331, 547, 560
Herpes zoster ophthalmicus, 331, 336–337, 530
Herpetic whitlow, 295, 633, 633*t*
Hesselbach triangle, 169
HIDA scan, 161
Hidradenitis suppurativa, 327
High pressure injection injury, 597
High-altitude cerebral edema, 433–435
High-altitude pulmonary edema, 433–435
High-altitude retinopathy, 435
High-altitude syndromes
clinical features of, 433–434
diagnosis and differential of, 434
emergency department care and disposition of, 434–435
epidemiology of, 433
pathophysiology of, 433
Highly active antiretroviral therapy, 334
High-pressure-injection injuries, 65
Hill–Sachs lesion, 603
Hindfoot, 615
Hip
bursal syndromes of, 623, 624*f*, 624*t*
dislocation of, 608–609
fracture of, 567, 606–608
Hip pain, 623
HIPAA. *See* Health Insurance Portability and Accountability Act
Hirudin, 484
HIV. *See* Human immunodeficiency virus
Hobo spider bite, 427
Hodgkin's lymphoma, 306

Hoffman sign, 620*t*
Homans' sign, 103
Homatropine, 529*t*
Hookworms, 356
Hoover test, 644*t*
Horizontal mattress sutures, 51–52, 52*f,* 57*f*
Horner's syndrome, 306, 537
Hospitalization
- abdominal pain evaluations, 143
- acquired immunodeficiency syndrome, 337
- electrical injuries, 447*t*
- hypoglycemia, 455*t*
- infective endocarditis, 338

Hounsfield units, 650
Human bites, 65–66, 66*t,* 633*t*
Human diploid cell vaccine, 341–342
Human herpesvirus 6, 296
Human immunodeficiency virus. *See also* Acquired immunodeficiency syndrome
- antiretroviral therapy for, 337
- CD4 counts, 334, 336
- clinical features of, 334–336
- constitutional symptoms of, 334–335
- cutaneous manifestations of, 336
- cytomegalovirus associated with, 335, 337
- diagnosis and differential of, 336–337
- emergency department care and disposition of, 337–338
- enzyme-linked immunoassay for, 336
- epidemiology of, 333
- febrile illnesses associated with, 334–335
- gastrointestinal complications of, 335–336
- *Mycobacterium avium* complex secondary to, 334–335, 337
- needle-stick injuries, 65
- neurologic complications of, 335
- neuropathy associated with, 45*t*
- ophthalmologic manifestations of, 336
- opportunistic infections associated with, 334–335
- pathophysiology of, 333–334
- peripheral neurologic disease, 519
- *Pneumocystis* pneumonia in, 334–335, 337
- post-exposure prophylaxis for, 337–338, 649
- pregnancy and, 215
- pulmonary complications of, 335
- risk factors for, 333
- tuberculosis secondary to, 130

Human immunodeficiency virus encephalopathy, 335
Human papillomaviruses, 318, 548
Human rabies immune globulin, 341
Humerus fractures, 603–604
Hydralazine, 217
Hydrocarbons, 404–406, 445*t*
Hydrocortisone, 151, 281, 461
Hydrofluoric acid, 406–407, 444, 446*t*
Hydrogen sulfide, 416
Hydromorphone, 37
Hydronephrosis, 187*f*
Hydroxocobalamin, 366*t,* 417
β-Hydroxybutyrate, 455–456, 460
τ-Hydroxybutyrate, 379
Hydrozoans, 431
Hyperammonemia, 282
Hyperbaric oxygen therapy
- carbon monoxide poisoning treated with, 450
- cyanide poisoning treated with, 417
- decompression illness treated with, 438

Hyperbilirubinemia, 175, 178
Hypercalcemia
- description of, 28, 286, 286*t*
- of malignancy, 488–489

Hypercapnia, 120–121, 121*t,* 137
Hypercoagulable states, 102, 473*t*
Hypercyanotic spells, 257
Hyperemesis gravidarum, 144, 213
Hyperglycemia, 322
Hyperglycemic, hyperglycemic state, 456, 458, 458*f*
Hyperglycemic, hyperosmolar nonketotic syndrome, 282
Hyperinsulinemia-euglycemia therapy, 397*t,* 397–398
Hyperkalemia, 26*f,* 26–27, 27*t,* 286, 286*t,* 395–396, 425, 483
Hyperleukocytosis, 306
Hypermagnesemia, 29, 286*t*
Hypernatremia, 24–25, 25*t*
Hyperosmolar agents, 152
Hyperphosphatemia, 490
Hyperpronation technique, for radial head subluxation, 291, 291*f*
Hypertension
- benign intracranial, 537
- clinical features of, 109–110
- description of, 109
- diagnosis and differential of, 110
- in dialysis, 190
- emergency department care and disposition of, 110–111
- pathophysiology of, 109
- in pregnancy, 217
- pulmonary, 112
- in rheumatologic diseases, 632

Hypertensive emergencies
- acute renal failure, 110
- aortic dissection, 110
- childhood, 111
- definition of, 109
- preeclampsia, 111
- treatment of, 111

Hypertensive encephalopathy, 110–111
Hypertensive headaches, 495
Hypertensive urgency, 109, 111
Hyperthyroidism, 214, 462
Hypertonic hyponatremia, 24
Hypertrophic cardiomyopathy, 98–99, 277
Hyperuricemia, 490
Hyperventilation, 573
Hyperviscosity syndrome, 491–492
Hypervitaminosis, 418*t*
Hyphema, 533, 533*f*
Hypoaldosteronism, 30*t*
Hypobaric hypoxemia, 433
Hypocalcemia, 27–28, 273, 286, 286*t*
Hypoglycemia
- in children, 279–281, 280*t*
- clinical features of, 454
- diabetes mellitus as cause of, 454*t*–455*t,* 454–455
- diagnosis and differential of, 454
- emergency department care and disposition of, 454–455
- epidemiology of, 454
- hospitalization for, 455*t*
- pathophysiology of, 454
- pediatric seizures caused by, 273
- treatment of, 280–281, 281*t*

Hypokalemia, 25, 26*t,* 286, 286*t,* 483
Hypomagnesemia, 28–29, 286, 286*t*
Hyponatremia, 24, 24*t,* 273, 285, 286*t,* 388, 489
Hyponatremic dehydration, 284
Hypoproteinemia, 311
Hypotension
- description of, 32–34
- in hemodialysis, 191
- intradialytic, 191

Hypothenar muscles, 595
Hypothermia, 422–423
Hypothyroidism, 461
Hypotonic hyponatremia, 24
Hypoventilation, 120
Hypovolemic shock, 285, 574
Hypoxemia, 125, 250, 252, 433
Hypoxia
- acute, 435
- description of, 119–120

Hysteroscopy, 225

I

Iatrogenic pneumothorax, 132–134
Ibuprofen, 230
Ibutilide, 14
Idiopathic thrombocytopenic purpura, 308, 471
Idioventricular rhythm, 20
Ileal conduit, 207
Ileus, 182
Iliac wing fracture, 607*t*
Ilioinguinal nerve entrapment, 623
Iliopectineal bursitis, 624*t*
Iliopsoas bursitis, 624*t*
Imipenem
  diverticulitis treated with, 167
  neutropenia treated with, 324
  posttransplant pneumonia treated with, 358
Imipenem-cilastin, 162
Immersion pulmonary edema, 438
Immune reconstitution illness to *Mycobacterium avium* complex, 335
Immunocompromised patients
  herpes simplex virus 1 in, 329*f*, 329–330
  tuberculosis in, 130
Immunosuppressive agents
  Crohn's disease treated with, 150
  description of, 358–359
"Impact seizures," 273
Impetigo, 297, 297*f*, 538, 538*t*
Implied consent, 658
Inborn errors of metabolism, 279–282, 280*t*
Incarcerated hernia, 169, 267
Incisional hernia, 169
Incomplete abortion, 212
Increased intracranial pressure, 504
Indirect Coombs test, 467*t*
Induced abortion, 226*t*, 226–227
Industrial toxins, 415–418
Inevitable abortion, 212
Infants. *See also* Children; Neonate(s)
  abdominal emergencies, 265–268
  antibiotics in, 229, 229*t*
  apnea in, 252
  bronchiolitis in, 251–253
  crying by, 233, 234*t*
  dehydration in, 262, 262*t*
  diarrhea in, 260–264
  fever in, 228–230, 269
  inguinal hernia in, 170
  intestinal colic in, 233–234
  nonaccidental trauma, 234
  normal vegetative functions in, 233
  pneumonia in, 253–255
  premature, 233
  rashes in. *See* Rashes
  renal emergencies in, 309–312
  respiratory rates in, 233
  seizures in. *See* Seizures, pediatric
  sepsis in, 231*t*
  urinary tract infections in, 230, 268–269
  vomiting in, 260–264, 263*t*
  wheezing in, 249*t*, 249–250
Infections. *See also specific infection*
  ear, 238–240
  facial, 538–539
  hand, 632–633
  odontogenic, 546
  postpartum, 218
  soft tissue. *See* Soft tissue infections
  soft tissue foreign bodies as cause of, 62
  traveler. *See* World traveler infections
  urinary tract. *See* Urinary tract infection
  vascular access, 192
  viral. *See* Viral infections
  world traveler. *See* World traveler infections
  wound. *See* Wound infections
Infectious mononucleosis, 331–332
Infective endocarditis, 96, 338–339
Inferior vena cava, 187*f*
Inferior vena cava filters, 108–109
Inferolateral acute myocardial infarction, 75*f*
Inflammatory bursitis, 636
Inflammatory cardiomyopathy, 98
Influenza
  A, 332–333
  acute bronchitis caused by, 124*t*
  antiviral agents for, 333
  B, 332–333
  clinical features of, 333
  diagnosis and differential of, 333
  emergency department care and disposition of, 333
  pathophysiology of, 333
  rapid viral antigen tests for, 254
Informed consent, 657–658
Infraorbital nerve block, 40
Ingrown toenail, 635*f*, 635–636
Inguinal hernia, 168–170
Inhalational anthrax, 351
Inner ear barotrauma, 436*t*, 437
Innocent murmurs, 255
Inotropic agents, 93
Insect bites and stings
  bedbugs, 429
  bees, 426–427
  chiggers, 428
  fleas, 428
  kissing bugs, 429
  lice, 428
  scabies, 428, 561
  scorpion, 428
  spiders, 427
  wasp, 426–427
Insulin, 283
Insulin-dependent diabetes mellitus, 282
Intercondylar fracture, 600
Interferon gamma release assays, for tuberculosis, 129–130
Intermittent claudication, 116*t*
Interstitial pneumonia, 125
Intertrochanteric fracture, 607*t*
Intestinal colic, 233–234
Intestinal malrotation, 266
Intestinal obstruction, 143*t*, 144, 167–168
Intimate partner violence, 649, 649*t*
Intoxication, 639
Intra-abdominal abscesses, 182
Intracerebral hemorrhage, 502, 571
Intracranial hemorrhage, 111, 486*t*, 504*t*
Intracranial pain, 276
Intradialytic hypotension, 191
In-training examination, 3
Intraocular pressure, 535
Intraparenchymal hemorrhage, 494
Intrauterine pregnancy, 653
Intravenous immunoglobulin, 308, 320, 471
Intravenous pyelogram, 203
Intrinsic renal failure, 184, 186–188
Intubating stylets, 7
Intubation
  endobronchial, 7
  orotracheal, 6–7
  rapid sequence
    in adults, 7–8, 8*t*, 564, 578
    in children, 21, 565
Intussusception, 266, 266*f*
Ionizing radiation, 651
Ipratropium bromide
  asthma treated with, 251
  bronchospasms treated with, 35
Iritis, 531, 531*t*
Iron deficiency anemia, 307–308
Iron toxicity, 402–404
Irreversible pulpitis, 546
Irrigation of wound, 49
Ischemic chest pain, 71, 74
Ischemic renal failure, 184
Ischemic stroke, 303, 485, 494, 497, 497*t*, 503
Ischial bursitis, 624*t*
Ischial tuberosity fracture, 607*t*
Ischiogluteal bursitis, 624*t*
Ischium body fracture, 607*t*
Isoniazid, 130, 131*t*, 337
Isopropanol, 381

Isoproterenol
sinus bradycardia treated with, 11
ventricular tachycardia treated with, 17
Isotonic hyponatremia, 24
Itraconazole, 328

J

Janeway lesions, 338
Jaundice
in adults, 175–176
in neonates and infants, 236–237
Jaw thrust, 6, 564
Jellyfish, 431
Jequirity bean, 451*t*
Jimson weed, 452–453
Jock itch, 560
Jones fracture, 615
Jumper's knee, 613
Junctional rhythms, 15*f,* 15–16
Juniper, 419*t*
Justice, 660
Juvenile immune arthritis, 291

K

Kaposi sarcoma, 336
Kawasaki's disease, 300
Kayexalate. *See* Sodium polystyrene sulfonate
Kehr's sign, 585
Keratitis
herpes, 530
ultraviolet, 435, 532
Kerion, 297
Kerley B lines, 89
Kernig's sign, 523
Ketamine, 8*t*
asthma treated with, 251
bronchorrhea caused by, 42
in children, 43
laryngospasm caused by, 42
procedural sedation use of, 41*t,* 42
propofol and, 41*t,* 43
Ketoacidosis
alcoholic, 460
diabetic, 213–214, 282–283, 455–456, 457*f*
Ketonemia, 455
Ketones, 460
Kidney(s)
acute failure of. *See* Acute renal failure
end-stage renal disease, 190–191
hydronephrosis of, 187*f*
trauma to, 589*t,* 589–590
Kidney-ureter-bladder radiograph, 203
Kissing bugs, 429
Klebsiella pneumoniae, 126*t*
Knee
arthrocentesis of, 627*f*
bursal syndromes of, 623, 624*f,* 624*t*
dislocation of, 610–611, 611*t*
fracture of, 609–610
injuries of, 61, 611–613
ligamentous injuries of, 612
meniscal injuries, 612
overuse injuries of, 613
prepatellar bursitis of, 624*f,* 624*t*
tendon injuries of, 611–612
Knee pain, 623
Koplik's spots, 294
Kussmaul's sign, 99

L

Labetalol, 217, 340
Labor and delivery. *See also* Pregnancy
breech presentation in, 221
emergency, 218–221
normal movements of, 220*f*
preterm, 216–217
Labyrinthitis, 499*t,* 512*t,* 512–513
Lacerations
ankle, 61
cheek, 56, 56*f*
closure of, 49
corneal, 532
dorsal hand, 57
ear, 55, 56*f*
epidemiology of, 53
extensor tendon, 58, 58*f*
eyelid, 54, 54*f*
facial, 56, 56*f*
finger, 59, 59*f*
fingertip, 59, 59*f*
flexor tendon, 59, 59*f*
foot, 60–62
forearm, 57, 57*f*
forehead, 53–56
intraoral mucosal, 550
leg, 60–62
lips, 55, 55*f,* 550
nasal, 54–55
palm, 57
pathophysiology of, 53
scalp, 53–54
stellate, 51*f*
tendon, 637
toe, 62
tongue, 550
wrist, 57
Lachman's test, 612
Lacosamide, 402
Lacrimators, 444, 445*t*
Lactated Ringer's solution, 23
Lactulose, 152, 179
Lambert–Eaton myasthenic syndrome, 522
Lansoprazole, 159
Laparoscopy, 225, 225*t*
Laparotomy, 407, 586, 587*t*
Laryngeal mask airway, 8
Laryngeal trauma, 555
Laryngomalacia, 236, 243
Laryngospasm, 42
Laryngotracheobronchitis. *See* Viral croup
Latent syphilis, 315
Latent tuberculosis, 129
Lateral collateral ligament injuries, 612
Lateral epicondylitis, 599
Lateral luxation, 549
Lateral sinus thrombosis, 542
Le Fort injuries, 578
Lead poisoning, 412*t,* 412–413
Left anterior fascicular block, 19
Left ventricular hypertrophy, 94
Leg lacerations, 60–62
Legal causation, 657
Legg-Calvé-Perthes disease, 292
Legionella pneumophila, 126, 126*t,* 127*f*
Leiomyomas, 209
Leishmaniasis, 355
Leptospira interrogans, 354
Leptospirosis, 354
Lesser trochanteric fracture, 607*t*
Leucovorin, 366*t*
Leukemia
acute lymphoblastic, 305
childhood, 304–306
Leukocoria, 306, 307*f*
Leukocyte esterase reaction, 194
Leukocytosis, 254, 322
Leukoplakia, 548
Levalbuterol, 138
Level of consciousness, 500*t*
Levetiracetam, 402
Levofloxacin
community-acquired pneumonia treated with, 127
diverticulitis treated with, 166
Staphylococcus treated with, 432
urologic stone disease treated with, 204
Levonorgestrel, 649
Lhermitte sign, 521, 620*t*
Lice, 428
Lid lacerations, 54, 54*f,* 532
Lidocaine
cerebral arterial gas embolism treated with, 438
pain management uses of, 37–38
premature ventricular contractions treated with, 16
ventricular fibrillation treated with, 17
Lidocaine, epinephrine, tetracaine, 38
Lightning injuries, 448*t,* 448–449

Limaprost, 422
Limb ataxia, 501*t*
Linezolid, 320
Lipase, 161
Lipid emulsions, 366*t*
Lips
  laceration of, 55, 55*f*, 550
  suturing of, 55, 55*f*
Lisfranc injury, 615
Listeria monocytogenes, 357–358
Lithium, 375–376
Lithotripsy, extracorporeal shock wave, 202, 205
Liver disorders
  hepatitis, 176–178
  jaundice, 175–176
Liver transplantation, 361
Livestock, 66*t*, 68
Lobar pneumonia, 125, 126*f*, 254*f*
Lobelia, 419*t*
Local anesthesia, 37–38
Long-QT syndrome, 19, 278
Loop diuretics, 398
Loperamide, 148, 346
Lorazepam
  nausea and vomiting treated with, 492*t*
  pacing use of, 10
  panic disorder treated with, 643
  seizures treated with, 370, 516
  status epilepticus treated with, 271*t*
  tetanus managed with, 340
Louse-borne typhus, 354
Low molecular weight heparin
  acute coronary syndromes treated with, 79
  deep vein thrombosis treated with, 108, 485
  pulmonary embolism treated with, 108, 485
  types of, 108
Low probability acute coronary syndrome, 82–85
Lower esophageal sphincter, 155, 157
Lower gastrointestinal bleeding, 265*t*
LSD. *See* Lysergic acid diethylamide
Ludwig's angina, 546, 554
Lumbar nerve root compromise, 619*f*
Lumbar plexopathy, 518–519
Lumbar puncture, 271, 322, 515, 523–524
Lumbar radiculopathy, 618
Lumbar spine fractures, 576, 576*t*
Lumbricals, 595
Lunate dislocation, 597
Lunate fracture, 597
Lund and Browder burn diagram, 441, 442*f*
Lung
  abscess of, 125, 128
  injuries of, 581–582
Lung transplantation, 360
Lupus anticoagulant, 473
Lyme arthritis, 628
Lyme disease, 348–349
Lymphadenitis, cervical, 241
Lymphocytic pleocytosis, 329
Lymphogranuloma venereum, 317*f*, 317–318
Lymphoma, 306
Lysergic acid diethylamide, 386–387, 387*t*

M

Magnesium abnormalities
  in children, 286*t*
  hypermagnesemia, 29, 286*t*
  hypomagnesemia, 28–29, 286, 286*t*
Magnesium citrate, 152
Magnesium sulfate
  asthma treated with, 251
  eclampsia treated with, 217
  multifocal atrial tachycardia treated with, 15
  tetanus treated with, 340
  ventricular fibrillation treated with, 17
  ventricular tachycardia treated with, 17
Magnetic resonance imaging
  acute appendicitis, 165
  advantages of, 651
  adverse effects of, 651–652
  applications of, 652
  emergent setting use of, 652
  safety of, 651
Maisonneuve fracture, 610, 613
Major depression, 639
Malaria
  cerebral, 343
  in children, 344
  clinical features of, 343–344
  diagnosis and differential of, 344
  emergency department care and disposition of, 344–345
  epidemiology of, 342
  geographic distribution of, 342, 343*t*
  pathophysiology of, 342–343
  treatment of, 344–345
  in world travelers, 353
Male genital conditions
  acute prostatitis, 201
  epididymitis, 200, 200*f*
  orchitis, 200, 200*f*
  penis, 198*f*, 198–199
  scrotum, 197–198
  testicular torsion, 199–200, 200*f*
  urethra, 201
Malignancy complications
  adrenal crisis, 489–490
  bone metastases, 486–487
  extravasation of chemotherapeutic agents, 493
  hypercalcemia, 488–489
  hyperviscosity syndrome, 491–492
  nausea and vomiting, 492
  spinal cord compression, 487
  superior vena cava syndrome, 488
  syndrome of inappropriate secretion of antidiuretic hormone, 489
  thromboembolism, 492
Malignant melanoma, 638
Malignant otitis externa, 541–542
Mallampati grading system, 7*f*, 40
Mallet finger, 596
Mallory–Weiss tear, 144, 153
Mandible disorders, 540
Mandible fractures, 578–579
Mania, 640
Mannitol, 508
Mantoux method, 130
Marcus Gunn pupil, 521
Marijuana, 387*t*, 388
Marine envenomations, 430–433, 432*t*–433*t*
Massive transfusion, 483
Masticator space infection, 538*t*, 539–540
Mastitis, 218
Mastoiditis, 239, 542
Mattress sutures, 51–52, 52*f*, 57*f*
May-Thurner syndrome, 108
McMurray's test, 612
MDMA, 386–388, 387*t*
Mean corpuscular hemoglobin, 467*t*
Mean corpuscular hemoglobin concentration, 467*t*
Mean corpuscular volume, 467*t*
Measles, 294
Mebendazole, 356
Mechanical ventilation, 567
Meclizine, 145
Meconium, 236
Meconium aspiration, 22–23
Medial collateral ligament injuries, 612
Medial epicondylitis, 599
Median nerve
  motor testing of, 56*t*, 599*t*
  sensory testing of, 57*t*, 599*t*
Median neuropathy, 518
Mediastinal emphysema, 156
Medical ethics, 660
Medical malpractice, 657

Medication. *See specific medication*
Medroxyprogesterone, 209*t*
Mees' lines, 413
Mefloquine, 344
Melena, 153
Membranous laryngotracheobronchitis. *See* Bacterial tracheitis
Ménière's disease, 499*t*, 512
Meningitis
  bacterial, 231, 523, 525*t*
  cerebrospinal fluid studies for, 524*t*
  in children, 228, 229*t*, 231–232, 274
  clinical features of, 232, 523
  corticosteroids for, 524
  diagnosis and differential of, 232, 322
  emergency department care and disposition of, 232, 524–525
  epidemiology of, 231, 523
  headaches caused by, 494
  lumbar puncture for, 322, 523–524, 524*t*
  pathophysiology of, 231, 523
  positive blood cultures for, 232
  tuberculous, 129
  viral, 524–525
Meningococcemia, 559
Meniscal injuries, 612
Mental nerve block, 40
Mental status alterations
  in children, 274–275
  coma, 506–509, 507*t*–508*t*
  delirium, 505*t*, 505–506
  dementia, 505*t*, 506, 639
Meperidine, 37
Meprobamate, 379
Meralgia paresthetica, 518, 623
6-Mercaptopurine
  Crohn's disease treated with, 150
  ulcerative colitis treated with, 151
Mercury poisoning, 414–415, 415*t*
Meropenem, 162
  diverticulitis treated with, 167
  neutropenic fever treated with, 491*t*
  posttransplant pneumonia treated with, 358
Mesalamine
  Crohn's disease treated with, 150
  ulcerative colitis treated with, 151
Mescaline, 387*t*
Mesenteric ischemia, 142, 143*t*
Metabolic acidosis, 29–31, 30*t*, 390
Metabolic alkalosis, 31
Metabolic encephalopathy, 274
Metabolic toxins, 416–418
Metacarpophalangeal joint dislocation, 596
Metalloids, 412–415
Metals, 412–415, 445
Metastases, bone, 486–487
Metatarsal fractures, 615
Methadone, 384
Methamphetamine, 385
Methanol, 381–383
Methemoglobinemia, 121, 416, 420–421
Methicillin-resistant *Staphylococcus aureus,* 64–65, 127, 297, 299, 324–325
Methimazole, 462*t*
Methohexital, 41*t*, 42
Methylene blue, 366*t*, 421
Methylene chloride, 449
Methylenedioxymethamphetamine, 386–388, 387*t*
Methylprednisolone
  anaphylaxis treated with, 35
  asthma treated with, 138
  cardiac transplantation rejection prevented with, 359
  chronic obstructive pulmonary disease treated with, 138
  epiglottitis treated with, 246
  multiple sclerosis treated with, 521
  spinal cord trauma treated with, 576–577
  superior vena cava syndrome treated with, 488
  toxic shock syndrome treated with, 320
  ulcerative colitis treated with, 151
Methylxanthines, 393–394
Metoclopramide, 142–143, 145, 492*t*
Metoprolol
  acute coronary syndromes treated with, 78*t*
  atrial fibrillation treated with, 14
  narrow-complex supraventricular tachycardia treated with, 12
Metronidazole
  bacterial vaginosis treated with, 222
  cholecystitis treated with, 163
  Clostridium difficile-associated diarrhea treated with, 149
  Crohn's disease treated with, 150
  diverticulitis treated with, 166, 167
  fistula in ano treated with, 173
  infectious diarrhea treated with, 148
  posttransplant pneumonia treated with, 358
  shock treated with, 156
  trichomoniasis, 223
  trichomoniasis treated with, 314
  ulcerative colitis treated with, 151
Miconazole, 223
Microcytic anemia, 468*f*
Microscopic hematuria, 195
Microscopic polyangiitis, 630*t*
Midazolam
  anxiety management using, 37, 340
  before ketamine administration, 43
  procedural sedation use of, 41*t*, 42
  status epilepticus treated with, 271*t*
Middle cerebral artery stroke, 498
Middle phalanx fracture, 597
Midface fractures, 578
Migraine headaches, 276, 494–495
Miliary tuberculosis, 129–130
Milk of magnesia, 152
Miller Fisher syndrome, 518
Miller laryngoscope blade, 21
Milrinone, 82
Mineralocorticoid deficiency, 489
Minors, 658
Minute ventilation, 120
Mirizzi's syndrome, 161
Mirtazapine, 371
Missed abortion, 212
Mitral incompetence, 92–93
Mitral regurgitation, 91*t*
Mitral stenosis, 91*t*, 91–92, 92*f*
Mitral valve prolapse, 91*t*, 93–94
Mittelschmerz, 209
Mobitz AV block
  type I, 18, 18*f*, 74
  type II, 18, 18*f*, 74
Mollucsa, 431
Monoamine oxidase inhibitors, 373*t*, 373–374
Monoarthritis, 626*t*
Mononeuritis multiplex, 518, 519*t*
Mononucleosis, infectious, 331–332
Monospot test, 332
Monteggia fracture-dislocation, 601
Moraxella catarrhalis, 126*t*
Morphine sulfate
  abdominal pain managed with, 142
  acute coronary syndromes treated with, 78, 78*t*
  congestive heart failure treated with, 90
  pacing use of, 10
  pain management using, 37
  tetanus treated with, 340
Morton's neuroma, 637
Motor ataxia, 509
Moxifloxacin, 167
Multifocal atrial tachycardia, 14–15, 14*f*
Multiple sclerosis, 499*t*, 520–522
Mumps, 539
Munchausen syndrome by proxy, 646
Mural thrombi, 97
Murmurs, 91*t*, 255, 256*t*
Murphy's sign, 161, 653

Musculoskeletal disorders
acute rheumatic fever, 292–293
clavicle fracture, 289
greenstick fractures, 289
juvenile immune arthritis, 291
Legg-Calvé-Perthes disease, 292
Osgood-Schlatter disease, 292
physeal fractures, 287*f*–288*f*, 287–288
plastic deformities, 289
post-streptococcal reactive arthritis, 292
radial head subluxation, 290–291
slipped capital femoral epiphysis, 291
supracondylar fractures, 289–290, 290*f*
torus fractures, 288–289
transient tenosynovitis of the hip, 293
Mushrooms, 451–453, 452*t*
Myasthenia gravis, 520, 521*t*
Myasthenic crisis, 520
Mycobacterium avium complex, 334–335, 337
Mycobacterium marinum, 346
Mycobacterium tuberculosis, 129
Mycoplasma pneumoniae
bronchitis caused by, 124*t*
pneumonia caused by, 126*t*
Myelopathy, 617
Myocardial infarction
acute. *See* Acute myocardial infarction
non-ST-segment elevation, 74, 83
ST-segment elevation, 74, 83
Myocardial ischemia, 143*t*
Myocarditis, 98, 260
Myoclonic jerks, 379
Myoclonic seizure, 270
Myofascial back pain syndrome, 44*t*–45*t*
Myofascial headache, 44*t*–45*t*
Myofascial neck pain, 44*t*–45*t*
Myofascial syndromes, 623–624, 625*t*
Myoglobin, 72
Myoglobinuria, 189
Myositis ossificans, 625–626
Myxedema coma, 461

N

N-acetylcysteine, 391–392
N-acetyl-p-benzoquinoneimine, 391
Nafcillin, 320
Naloxone, 41, 142, 365, 366*t,* 384, 399, 508
Naphazoline and pheniramine, 529*t*
Naproxen, 392
Narrow-complex supraventricular tachycardia, 12
Nasal emergencies
epistaxis, 543, 578
foreign bodies, 544
fractures, 544, 544*f*
Nasal speculum, 55
Nasogastric tube, 153
Naso-orbito-ethmoid fractures, 578
National Institutes of Health Stroke Scale, 499, 500*t*–502*t*
Native valve endocarditis, 338
Nausea and vomiting
antiemetics for, 145, 492*t*
chemotherapy-induced, 492
description of, 144–146, 191
of pregnancy, 212–213
Near drowning, 439
Necator americanus, 356
Neck
trauma to, 579*t,* 579–580
zones of, 579*t*
Neck masses, 554
Neck pain
clinical features of, 617–618
diagnosis and differential of, 618–620
epidemiology of, 617
muscular, 617*t*
nonspecific, 620
pathophysiology of, 617
Necrotizing enterocolitis, 235, 267
Necrotizing fasciitis, 181–182
Necrotizing soft tissue infections, 325
Needle decompression, 438
Needle-stick injuries, 65
Neer classification system, 603
Neer's test, 621
Negligence, 657
Neisseria gonorrhoeae, 223, 313
Neisseria meningitidis, 523
Neobladder, 207
Neonatal acne, 299
Neonatal emergencies
abdominal distention, 235
apnea, 236
apparent life-threatening events, 237, 237*t*
bronchopulmonary dysplasia, 236
cardiovascular, 236–237
child abuse, 234, 565, 645–646
constipation, 235–236, 267
crying, 233, 234*t*
cyanosis, 236
diarrhea, 235
feeding difficulties, 235
gastrointestinal reflux, 235, 237
gastrointestinal symptoms, 234–25
intestinal colic, 233–234
jaundice, 236–237
nonaccidental trauma, 234
oral thrush, 237
stridor, 236
surgical conditions, 234
vomiting, 235, 263*t*
Neonate(s)
apneic, 23
emergency delivery of, 218–221
encephalitis in, 328
hypoglycemia in, 280
normal vegetative functions in, 233
periodic breathing in, 236
rashes in, 299
respiratory rates in, 233
resuscitation of, 20–23
seizures in, 272
septic shock in, 323
stridor in, 236, 243–244
tetanus in, 340
Neostigmine, 520
Nephritis, 631
Nephroblastoma, 306
Nephrogenic diabetes insipidus, 25, 375
Nephrostomy tubes, 206
Nephrotic syndrome, 311
Nerve blocks
auricular, 40
deep peroneal, 39
digital, 38*f*–39*f,* 38–39
femoral, 40
infraorbital, 40
mental, 40
posterior tibial, 39
radial, 39
saphenous, 39
superficial peroneal, 39
supraorbital, 40
supratrochlear, 40
sural, 39
ulnar, 39
Neurally mediated syncope, 278
Neuroblastoma, 306
Neuroleptic malignant syndrome, 374–375
Neurologic disorders
amyotrophic lateral sclerosis, 519–520
ataxia, 509–510
coma, 506–509, 507*t*–508*t*
delirium, 505*t,* 505–506
dementia, 505*t,* 506, 639
dizziness, 510–513, 512*t*
gait disturbances, 509–510, 510*t*
headaches. *See* Headaches
Lambert–Eaton myasthenic syndrome, 522
mental status alterations, 505–509
multiple sclerosis, 520–522
myasthenia gravis, 520, 521*t*
Parkinson's disease, 522
peripheral neurologic lesions. *See* Peripheral neurologic lesions

poliomyelitis, 522–523
postpolio syndrome, 522–523
vertigo, 510–513, 511*t*–512*t*
Neuromuscular blockade, 340
Neuromuscular junction disorders, 517
Neuromuscular paralytic agents, 8*t*
Neuropathic pain, 44, 45*t*
Neuropathy, organophosphate-induced, 408
Neutropenia, 308–309, 324
Neutropenic fever, 305*t*, 490–491
Niacin, 418*t*, 419
Nicardipine, 110
Nicotine, 393–394
Nifedipine, 422, 435
Nifedipine-XL, 204
Nikolsky sign, 297, 557
Nitrofurantoin, 194, 215
Nitrogen dioxide, 416
Nitrogen narcosis, 438
Nitrogen oxides, 416
Nitroglycerin
acute coronary syndromes treated with, 78, 78*t*
congestive heart failure treated with, 90
transdermal, 78
Nitroprusside, 93, 95
Nitrous oxide, for procedural sedation, 41*t*, 41–42
N,N-diethyl-3-methylbenzamide, 410
Nociceptive pain, 44
Nonabsorbable sutures, 50
Noncardiogenic pulmonary edema, 483
Nonconvulsive generalized seizure, 270
Nondeflating retention balloon, 206
Nondepolarizing neuromuscular agents, 374
Nondraining catheter, 205–206
Non-Hodgkin's lymphoma, 306, 335
Noninvasive positive pressure ventilation, 9, 8*t*, 138–139
Nonmaleficence, 660
Nonopioid analgesia, 36–37
Nonsteroidal anti-inflammatory drugs
overdose of, 392–393
pain management using, 36, 46
toxicity of, 392–393
Non-ST-segment elevation myocardial infarction, 74, 83
Nontraumatic cardiac tamponade, 101
Nonwidened anion gap metabolic acidosis, 29
Norepinephrine, 231
Normal pressure hydrocephalus, 509
Normal saline, 24, 145
Norovirus, 147
Nose
anterior packing of, 543, 543*f*
emergencies of. *See* Nasal emergencies
epistaxis of, 543, 578
foreign bodies of, 544
fractures of, 544, 544*f*
lacerations of, 54–55
packing of, 543*f*
NPPV. *See* Noninvasive positive pressure ventilation
Nuchal cord, 219
Nursemaid's elbow, 290–291
Nutmeg, 419*t*
Nystagmus, 511

O

Obliterative bronchiolitis, 360
Obsessive-compulsive disorder, 640
Obstructive pain, 266
Obstructive uropathy, 187*f*
Obtundation, 321
Obturator nerve entrapment, 623
Occlusive arterial disease, 115–118
Octreotide, 154, 366*t*
Ocular inflammations
chalazion, 528
conjunctivitis, 529–530
corneal ulcers, 530, 530*f*
endophthalmitis, 531
herpes simplex virus, 530
iritis, 531, 531*t*
postseptal cellulitis, 528
preseptal cellulitis, 528
stye, 528
uveitis, 531
vitreous hemorrhage, 531
Ocular trauma
blowout fractures, 533
blunt, 533
chemical-induced, 534
conjunctival abrasion, laceration, and foreign body, 531–532
lid lacerations, 532
retrobulbar hematoma, 534
ruptured globe, 533–534
subconjunctival hemorrhage, 531
Ocular ultrasonography, 537
Odontogenic abscess, 553–554
Odontogenic infections, 546
Odontoid fractures, 566
Ogilvie's syndrome, 168
Oleander, 451*t*
Olecranon bursitis, 629*t*
Olecranon fractures, 600
Oligoarthritis, 626*t*
Olopatadine, 529*t*
Omeprazole, 159
Omnibus Budget Reconciliation Act, 655
Oncologic emergencies
in children, 304–307
leukemia, 304–306
lymphoma, 306
Ondansetron, 142, 145, 263, 394, 434, 492*t*
Onychocryptosis, 635*f*, 635–636
Oophoritis, 539
Ophthalmic medications, 529*t*
Ophthalmologist, 54
Opiates, 383
Opioid(s)
abuse of, 383–385
analgesia using, 37
chronic pain treated with, 46*t*
naloxone for, 41, 142, 365, 366*t*, 384
overdose of, 384
pain treated with, 209, 478
pelvic pain treated with, 209
respiratory depression caused by, 384
side effects of, 37
toxidromes, 364*t*
withdrawal from, 384
Opioid receptors, 383
Optic nerve head edema, 537*f*
Optic neuritis, 535
Opticokinetic drum, 645*t*
Oral cancer, 548
Oral candidiasis, 336–337, 547
Oral lesions, 547–548
Oral rehydration solution, 145, 213, 235, 262, 285
Oral thrush, 237, 336*f*, 336–337
Orbicularis oculi, 55*f*
Orbital blowout fractures, 578
Orbital cellulitis, 528
Orchitis, 200, 200*f*
Organochlorines, 409–410
Organophosphates, 408–409, 409*t*
Orofacial pain, 545–547, 546*t*
Orofacial trauma, 548–550
Orogastric lavage, 367
Orotracheal intubation, 6–7, 565
Orthopedic injuries
clinical features of, 593–594
emergency department care and disposition of, 594–595
fractures. *See* Fracture(s)
pathophysiology of, 593
Orthostatic hypotension, 85
Orthostatic syncope, 86
Orthotopic bladder substitution, 207
Osgood-Schlatter disease, 292
Osler nodes, 338
Osmolal gap, 380
Osmolarity, 24
Osteitis pubis, 624–625

Osteoarthritis, 622, 628–629
Osteomyelitis
  description of, 624, 625*t*
  post-puncture wound, 64
Osteonecrosis, 624
Osteosarcoma, 306–307
Otalgia, 541
Otic barotrauma, 436*t*
Otitis externa, 239–240, 541–542
Otitis media, 542
Otologic emergencies, 541–543
Otomycosis, 541
Ototoxicity, 512
Ottawa Ankle Rules, 613, 614*f*
Ottawa Knee Rules, 610, 610*t*
Ovarian abscess, 226
Ovarian cysts, 209
Ovarian hyperstimulation syndrome, 227
Ovarian torsion, 143, 209
Overuse syndromes, 623–624, 625*t*
Oxacillin, 320
Oxalic acid, 381
Oxcarbazepine, 402
Oxygen saturation, 6
Oxygen supplementation, 425
Oxygen toxicity, 438
Oxymetazoline, 543, 545
Oxytocin, 217, 221

P

Pacemakers, 20
Pacing, cardiac, 10
Packed red blood cell transfusions, 302–303, 466, 480
PACs. *See* Premature atrial contractions
Paget disease, 624
Pain
  acute appendicitis, 163
  acute myocardial infarction, 74
  anxiety and, 37
  back. *See* Back pain
  chest. *See* Chest pain
  chronic, 44*t*–45*t*, 44–46
  clinical features of, 36
  epidemiology of, 36
  epigastric, 158–159
  headache, 276
  hip, 623
  intracranial, 276
  knee, 623
  neuropathic, 44, 45*t*
  nociceptive, 44
  orofacial, 545–547, 546*t*
  pathophysiology of, 36
  pelvic, 209
  postherpetic neuralgia, 331
  propofol administration as cause of, 42
  right left quadrant, 163
  shoulder, 620–622, 621*f*
  urologic stone disease, 202
Pain clinics, 45
Pain crises, 301–302
Pain management
  local anesthetics for, 37–38
  nonopioids for, 36–37
  nonpharmacologic methods of, 36
  opioids for, 37
  pediatric, 37
  wound, 69
Palm lacerations, 57
Pamidronate, 489
Pancolitis, 150
Pancreatic injury, 585
Pancreatitis, 143*t*
  causes of, 159*t*
  clinical features of, 160
  diagnosis and differential of, 160–161
  emergency department care and disposition of, 161–163
  epidemiology of, 159
  imaging of, 161
  surgery as cause of, 182
Panic attack, 643*t*–644*t*
Panic disorder, 640, 643
Pantoprazole, 154
Papillary muscle rupture, 74
Papilledema, 494, 537, 537*f*
Paracentesis, 180
Parainfluenza virus, 124*t*
Paralytic agents, 8*t*
Paralytic ileus, 166–167
Paraphimosis, 198*f*, 199
Paravalvular leaks, 96
Parietal abdominal pain, 140
Parkinsonism, 374–375
Parkinson's disease, 522
Parkland formula, 443
Paronychia, 632–633, 633*t*
Parotitis, 538*t*, 539
Paroxysmal supraventricular tachycardia, 10, 11
Partial seizures, 270
Pasteurella multocida, 67
Pastia's lines, 298
Patella
  dislocation of, 610–611
  fracture of, 609, 611*t*
Patellar tendon rupture, 611–612
Patellar tendonitis, 613
Pathologic fractures, 486–487
Pauciarticular disease, 291
PCP, 386–388, 387*t*
PE. *See* Pulmonary embolism
Peak expiratory flow rate, 137
Pediatric advanced life support, 271
Pediatric emergencies
  child abuse, 234, 565, 645–646
  crying, 233, 234*t*
  intestinal colic, 233–234
  nonaccidental trauma, 234
  types of, 233*t*
Pediatric heart disease
  clinical presentation of, 255–260
  congestive heart failure, 259*f*, 259–260, 260*t*
  cyanosis associated with, 256–258, 257*f*
  description of, 255–260
  murmurs, 256*t*
  shock presenting with, 258–259
Pediatrics. *See also* Children
  abdominal emergencies, 265–268
  abdominal pain, 265*t*, 265–268
  altered mental status, 274–275
  appendicitis, 267
  bronchiolitis, 251–253
  central nervous system tumors in, 306
  dehydration, 262, 262*t*, 284–285, 285*t*
  diabetes mellitus, 282–284
  diarrhea, 260–264
  ear infections, 238–240
  electrolyte disorders, 285–287
  fever, 228–230
  head trauma. *See* Head trauma
  headaches, 275–277, 276*t*–277*t*
  hypoglycemia, 279–281, 280*t*
  inborn errors of metabolism in, 279–282, 280*t*
  meningitis, 228, 229*t*, 231–232, 274
  mental status alterations, 274–275
  musculoskeletal disorders
    acute rheumatic fever, 292–293
    clavicle fracture, 289
    greenstick fractures, 289
    juvenile immune arthritis, 291
    Legg-Calvé-Perthes disease, 292
    Osgood-Schlatter disease, 292
    physeal fractures, 287*f*–288*f*, 287–288
    plastic deformities, 289
    post-streptococcal reactive arthritis, 292
    radial head subluxation, 290–291
    slipped capital femoral epiphysis, 291
    supracondylar fractures, 289–290, 290*f*
    torus fractures, 288–289
    transient tenosynovitis of the hip, 293
  pain management, 37
  pneumonia, 253–255
  procedural sedation, 43
  rashes. *See* Rashes

sepsis, 230–231
septic shock, 323–324
sickle cell disease in. *See* Sickle cell disease
stomatitis, 240–241
stridor. *See* Stridor
sudden death, 277–279
syncope, 277–279, 278*t*–279*t*
trauma, 564–566
urinary tract infections, 230, 268–269, 269*t*
urologic stone disease, 202
vomiting, 260–264
Pediculosis, 561–562
Pediculus capitis, 561
Pelvic inflammatory disease, 143*t,* 223–225
Pelvic pain, 209
Pelvis fractures, 565, 604–605
Pemphigus vulgaris, 559–560
Penetrating trauma
buttocks, 588
extremities, 591–592
flank, 587–588
head, 572
heart, 582–583
Penicillin
amatoxin poisoning treated with, 453
group A β-hemolytic *Streptococcus* pharyngitis treated with, 241
leptospirosis treated with, 354
odontogenic abscess treated with, 554
streptococcal toxic shock syndrome treated with, 320
Penis
entrapment injuries of, 199
fracture of, 199, 590
sexually transmitted infections of, 198*f,* 198–199
zipper injury of, 590
Pennyroyal, 419*t*
Pentobarbital, 41*t,* 42
Pentoxifylline, 422
Peptic ulcer disease, 157–159
Peptic ulcers
bleeding, 154
perforated, 72*t*
Percutaneous coronary interventions, 77, 79, 82
Percutaneous endoscopic gastrostomy tubes, 183
Percutaneous nephrostomy
description of, 188
tubes for, 206
Perforation
esophageal, 156
peptic ulcers, 72*t*
Perianal abscess, 173
Pericardial effusion, 100*f,* 487–488
Pericardial friction rub, 98, 100
Pericardial inflammation syndrome, 583
Pericardial "knock," 101
Pericardiocentesis, 101, 488, 582
Pericarditis
acute, 100–101
chest pain caused by, 72*t*
in children, 260
constrictive, 101–102
in end-stage renal disease, 191
uremic, 191
Pericoronitis, 545–546
Perilunate dislocation, 597
Perilymph fistula, 512
Periodic breathing, 236
Periodontal abscess, 547
Periodontitis, 546
Perionychium, 59*f*
Periosteitis, 546
Peripheral blood smear, 467*t,* 470*t*
Peripheral cyanosis, 121
Peripheral neurologic lesions
acute peripheral neuropathies, 518
botulism, 517
brachial plexopathy, 518
diabetic peripheral neuropathy, 519
entrapment neuropathies, 518
focal neuropathies, 518
Guillain–Barré syndrome, 518
HIV-associated peripheral neurologic disease, 519
lumbar plexopathy, 518–519
median neuropathy, 518
mononeuritis multiplex, 518, 519*t*
neuromuscular junction disorders, 517
tick paralysis, 517
ulnar mononeuropathy, 518
Peripheral neuropathy, 191
Peripheral vertigo, 510, 511*t*
Periradicular periodontitis, 546
Peritoneal dialysis, 192
Peritoneal pain, 266
Peritonitis, 192
Peritonsillar abscess, 242*t,* 247–248, 551*f,* 551–552
Permethrin, 428, 562
Peromyscus maniculatus, 350
Peroneal retinaculum, 637
Personality disorders, 640
Pes anserine bursitis, 624*t*
Pesticides, 408–412
Peyronie's disease, 199
Phalen maneuver, 518
Phantom limb pain, 45*t*
Pharyngitis
clinical features of, 551
description of, 240–241
emergency department care and disposition of, 551
group A β-hemolytic *Streptococcus,* 240–241, 550–551
high-altitude, 435
pathophysiology of, 550
viral, 551
Phenobarbital, 374, 377
Phentolamine with lidocaine, 65
Phenylbutazone, 392
Phenytoin, 400–401, 516
Pheochromocytoma, 111
Phimosis, 198*f,* 198–199
Phlebotomy, 190
Phlegmasia alba dolens, 103, 108
Phlegmasia cerulea dolens, 103, 108–109
Phosgene, 415
Photopsias, 536
Photosensitivity, 562
Phototherapy, 237
Physeal fractures, 287*f*–288*f,* 287–288, 593, 594*f*
Physician telephone advice, 659
Physostigmine, 366*t,* 369
Pilocarpine, 535
Pilonidal abscess, 327
Pilonidal sinus, 175
Pinworms, 175, 356
Piperacillin/tazobactam
bowel obstruction treated with, 168
cholecystitis treated with, 163
diverticulitis treated with, 166
neutropenic fever treated with, 491*t*
posttransplant pneumonia treated with, 358
shock treated with, 156
spontaneous bacterial peritonitis treated with, 180
Piriformis syndrome, 623
Pisiform, 598*t*
Pit viper bites, 429–430
Pittsburgh Knee Rules, 610, 610*f*
Pityriasis rosacea, 300–301, 315
PIVKA II, 470*t*
Placenta previa, 216, 218
Plague, 351–352
Plantar fasciitis, 636
Plantar fibromatosis, 638
Plantar interdigital neuroma, 637
Plantar puncture wounds, 64
Plantar warts, 635
Plasmodium falciparum, 342–345
Platelet count, 469*t*
Platelet defects, acquired, 471
Platelet disorders, 466
Platelet function assays, 470*t*
Platelet transfusions, 308, 471, 480
Platysma, 579
Pleural effusion, 122–123, 123*t,* 129, 156

Pneumococcal pneumonia, 125, 126*t*
Pneumocystis pneumonia, 334–335, 337, 358
Pneumonia
aspiration, 125, 127–128
bacterial, 125, 126*t*, 253
bronchial, 125
chest pain caused by, 72*t*
in children, 253–255
clinical features of, 125
community-acquired, 125, 127
cytomegalovirus, 357
diagnosis and differential of, 125–127, 126*f*–127*f*, 254–255
emergency department care and disposition of, 127–128, 255, 255*t*
epidemiology of, 125
in infants, 253–255
interstitial, 125
lobar, 125, 126*f*, 254*f*
pathophysiology of, 125
pediatric, 253–255
pneumococcal, 125, 126*t*
Pneumocystis, 334–335, 337, 358
postoperative, 182
posttransplant, 358
treatment of, 127–128, 255, 255*t*
viral, 253
Pneumothorax
chest pain caused by, 72*t*
iatrogenic, 132–134
spontaneous, 132*f*, 132–134
tension, 132, 134, 580–581
ultrasound of, 581
Podofilox, 318
Poison hemlock, 451*t*
Poisoning. *See also* Toxicology
arsenic, 413–414, 414*t*
carbamate, 409
carbon monoxide, 449–450
clinical features of, 363
cyanide, 416–418, 417*t*
DEET, 410
diagnosis and differential of, 363
epidemiology of, 363
fat-soluble vitamins, 418–419
herbicides, 410–411
lead, 412*t*, 412–413
mercury, 414–415, 415*t*
metalloids, 412–415
metals, 412–415
mushrooms, 451–453, 452*t*
organochlorines, 409–410
organophosphates, 408–409, 409*t*
pathophysiology of, 363
pyrethrins, 410
pyrethroids, 410
rodenticides, 411*t*, 411–412
Poisonous plants, 451–453
Poliomyelitis, 522–523
Polyarteritis nodosa, 630*t*
Polyarthritis, 626*t*
Polyarticular disease, 291
Polyethylene glycol, 152
Polymyalgia rheumatica, 630*t*
Polymyositis, 630*t*, 631
Polyvalent Crotalidae immune Fab, 429
Porifera, 431
Portuguese man-of-war, 431, 432*t*
Postconization bleeding, 226
Postembolization syndrome, 227
Posterior circulation stroke, 498
Posterior communicating artery aneurysm, 537
Posterior cruciate ligament injuries, 612
Posterior fossa hemorrhage, 513
Posterior tibial nerve block, 39
Posterior tibialis tendon rupture, 637
Postextraction alveolar osteitis, 546–547
Postextraction pain, 546–547
Postherpetic neuralgia, 45*t*, 331
Post-lumbar puncture headache, 495
Postobstructive diuresis, 197
Postpartum hemorrhage, 217
Postpolio syndrome, 522–523
Post-puncture wound osteomyelitis, 64
Postrenal azotemia, 184, 188, 310*t*
Postseptal cellulitis, 528
Post-streptococcal reactive arthritis, 292
Poststroke pain, 45*t*
Posttonsillectomy bleeding, 554
Posttransplant lymphoproliferative disease, 360
Post-traumatic stress disorder, 640
Potassium abnormalities
in children, 286*t*
hyperkalemia, 26*f*, 26–27, 27*t*, 286, 286*t*, 395–396, 425, 483
hypokalemia, 25, 26*t*, 286, 286*t*, 483
Potassium chloride, 25
Potassium-sparing diuretics, 399
Pralidoxime, 366*t*, 409, 409*t*
Praziquantel, 356
Precordial catch syndrome, 72*t*
Prednisolone, 151
Prednisone
anaphylaxis treated with, 35
Crohn's disease treated with, 150
idiopathic thrombocytopenic purpura treated with, 471
Preeclampsia, 111, 217
Preexcitation syndromes, 11
Pregabalin, 402
Pregnancy. *See also* Labor and delivery
abruptio placentae in, 216, 218, 568
acute appendicitis during, 165
asthma in, 214–215
cocaine abuse during, 385
deep vein thrombosis in, 214
diabetes in, 213–214
diagnostic imaging during, 215–216
domestic violence during, 215
dysrhythmias in, 214
ectopic, 210–212
emergencies during, 212–213
emergency delivery, 218–221
headaches during, 215
human immunodeficiency virus during, 215
hyperbaric oxygen therapy in, 450
hyperemesis gravidarum during, 144
hypertension in, 217
hyperthyroidism in, 214
maternal death during, 212
medication use during, 213*t*–214*t*
nausea and vomiting of, 212–213
placenta previa in, 216, 218
postpartum complications, 217–218
preeclampsia in, 111, 217
premature rupture of membranes, 216, 218
preterm labor, 216–217
pulmonary embolism in, 107, 214
pyelonephritis in, 215
seizure disorders in, 215
sickle cell disease in, 215
substance abuse during, 215
thromboembolism in, 214
trauma in, 568–569
trichomoniasis in, 314
ultrasonography evaluations, 653
urinary tract infections in, 215
vaginal bleeding in, 216
Prehn's sign, 200
Premature atrial contractions, 9–10, 10*f*
Premature infants, 233
Premature rupture of membranes, 216, 218
Premature ventricular contractions, 15–16, 15*f*, 89
Prepatellar bursitis, 624*f*, 624*t*, 629*t*
Prerenal failure, 184, 185*t*, 186–187, 309, 310*t*
Preseptal cellulitis, 528
Preterm labor, 216–217
Priapism, 199, 303
Primaquine, 344
Primary dysmenorrhea, 209
Procainamide
atrial fibrillation treated with, 14
wide-complex supraventricular tachycardia treated with, 13

Procedural sedation
  agents used in, 41*t*, 41–43
  anxiety management before, 43
  care after, 43
  in children, 43
  in critically ill patients, 43
  description of, 40–41
  in elderly, 43
  indications for, 36
  rescue agents for, 41
Prochlorperazine, 145
Proctitis, 173
Prolactin, 515
Promethazine, 43, 145, 492*t*
Proparacaine, 529*t*
Propofol, 8*t*
  ketamine and, 41*t*, 43
  procedural sedation use of, 41*t*, 42
Propoxyphene, 384
Propranolol
  narrow-complex supraventricular tachycardia treated with, 12
  thyroid storm treated with, 462*t*
Propylthiouracil, 214, 462*t*
Prostaglandin E1, 259
Prosthetic valve disease, 95–96, 338
Protamine, 366*t*
Protected health information, 660
Protein C, 108, 469*t*, 473*t*
Protein S, 470*t*, 473*t*
Prothrombin, 481*t*
Prothrombin time, 176, 469*t*
Proton pump inhibitors, 154, 159
Proximal femur fractures, 607*t*, 609*t*
Proximal fibular fractures, 610
Proximal humerus fractures, 603–604
Proximal interphalangeal joint dislocation, 596
Proximal phalanx fracture, 597
Pruritus ani, 175
Pseudocoma, 507
Pseudocyanosis, 121
Pseudo-dendrite, 530
Pseudogout, 627
Pseudohyperkalemia, 26
Pseudohyponatremia, 456
Pseudomonas aeruginosa, 64–65, 126*t*
Pseudo-obstruction, 168
Pseudotumor cerebri, 495, 537
Psilocybin, 387*t*, 451
Psoas abscess, 623
Psoriasis, 562
PSVT. *See* Paroxysmal supraventricular tachycardia
Psychiatric disorders
  amnestic disorder, 639
  brief psychotic disorder, 639
  delirium, 639
  dementia, 639
  mood disorders, 639–640
  schizophrenia, 639
Psychiatric dizziness, 513
Psychogenic coma, 507
Psychopharmacologic agents
  antipsychotics, 374–375
  atypical antidepressants, 370, 370*t*
  bupropion, 371
  cyclic antidepressants, 369–370
  lithium, 375–376
  mirtazapine, 371
  monoamine oxidase inhibitors, 373*t*, 373–374
  selective serotonin reuptake inhibitors, 371–372
  serotonin/norepinephrine reuptake inhibitors, 372
  trazodone, 370–371
Psychosis, 641*t*
Psychotherapy notes, 661
Psyllium, 152
Pthirus pubis, 561
Public safety agencies, 656
Pulmonary barotrauma, 436*t*
Pulmonary contusions, 581–582
Pulmonary edema
  acute, 88–90, 95
  acute hypertensive, 110
  high-altitude, 433–435
  immersion, 438
  noncardiogenic, 483
  pediatric, 259
  reexpansion, 134
Pulmonary embolism
  adjunctive therapy for, 108–109
  algorithm for, 106*f*
  ancillary testing for, 105–107
  chest pain caused by, 72*t*
  clinical features of, 103
  clotting disorders and, 474
  computed tomography angiography of, 107, 107*f*
  D-dimer testing for, 106
  diagnosis and differential of, 104
  emergency department care and disposition of, 107
  epidemiology of, 102
  heparin for, 108
  inferior vena cava filter for, 108–109
  low molecular weight heparin for, 108
  pathophysiology of, 103
  in pregnancy, 214
  signs and symptoms of, 103
  thrombolytic therapy for, 108
  treatment of, 107, 485
  Wells score for, 104*t*
Pulmonary embolism rule-out criteria, 104, 104*t*
Pulmonary emergencies
  asthma. *See* Asthma
  chronic obstructive pulmonary disease. *See* chronic obstructive pulmonary disease
  hemoptysis, 134–136, 135*f*
  pneumonia. *See* Pneumonia
  pneumothorax. *See* Pneumothorax
  respiratory distress. *See* Respiratory distress
  tuberculosis. *See* Tuberculosis
Pulmonary emphysema, 137
Pulmonary hypertension, 112
Pulmonary overinflation, 437
Pulpitis, 546
Pulse oximetry, 137
Pulseless electrical activity, 20
Pulsus paradoxus, 250
Puncture wounds, 64–65
PVCs. *See* Premature ventricular contractions
Pyelonephritis, 192, 194, 205, 215
Pyloric stenosis, 235, 267
Pyogenic granuloma, 548
Pyrazinamide, 131*t*
Pyrethrins, 410, 428
Pyrethroids, 410
Pyridostigmine, 520
Pyridoxine, 366*t*, 383, 418*t*, 453
Pyrimethamine, 337
Pyuria, 269

Q

QT interval, 483
Quadriceps tendon rupture, 611–612
Qualification examination, 1–2
Quincke pulse, 95
Quinidine, 345
Quinine sulfate, 344

R

Rabies, 341–342
Radial head fracture, 600
Radial head subluxation, 290–291
Radial nerve
  block of, 39
  motor testing of, 56*t*, 599*t*
  sensory testing of, 57*t*
Radial styloid fracture, 598
Radiculopathy, 617–618, 619*t*
Radius fractures, 601
Ramsay Hunt syndrome, 331, 513
Ranitidine, 35
Ranson's criteria, 161, 161*t*
Rapid-sequence intubation
  in adults, 7–8, 8*t*–9*t*, 564, 578
  in children, 21, 565

Rasburicase, 490
Rashes
bacterial infections that cause, 297*f*–298*f*, 297–299
cellulitis, 298–299
description of, 293
diaper, 299
erysipelas, 298, 299*f*
erythema infectiosum, 294*f*, 294–295
fungal, 296–297
herpes virus, 295, 295*f*
impetigo, 297, 297*f*
measles, 294
neonatal, 299
Rocky Mountain spotted fever, 347
roseola infantum, 296, 296*f*
rubella, 294
scarlet fever, 297–298, 298*f*
varicella, 295–296, 296*f*
viral, 293–296
RBBB. *See* Right bundle branch block
Reactivation tuberculosis, 130, 131*f*
Rebound tenderness, 140–141
Recombinant tissue plasminogen activator, 499*t*, 502, 503*t*
Rectal foreign bodies, 174–175
Rectal prolapse, 173–174
Red cell distribution width, 467*t*
Reentrant supraventricular tachycardia, 11*f*
Reexpansion pulmonary edema, 134
Reflex sympathetic dystrophy, 45*t*
Refusal of consent, 658–659
Regional anesthesia, 37–38, 38
Regional nerve entrapment syndromes, 623
Reiter's syndrome, 313, 629
Renal calculi, 653
Renal contusions, 589
Renal failure
acute. *See* Acute renal failure
complications of, 190–191
pathophysiology of, 190
Renal insufficiency, 631
Renal replacement therapy, 190
Renal transplantation, 360–361
Renin-angiotensin system, 109
Reperfusion injury, 118
Reserpine, 462*t*
Respiratory acidosis, 30–32
Respiratory alkalosis, 30, 32
Respiratory distress
cyanosis, 121*t*, 121–122
dyspnea, 119, 120*t*
hypercapnia, 120–121, 121*t*, 137
hypoxia, 119–120
pleural effusion, 122–123, 123*t*, 129, 156
Respiratory syncytial virus
acute bronchitis caused by, 124*t*
bronchiolitis caused by, 251
in infants, 229
periodic breathing and, 236
rapid viral antigen tests for, 254
Respiratory viruses, 123, 124*t*
Restrictive cardiomyopathy, 99
Resuscitation
of children, 20–23
do-not-resuscitation orders, 659
of neonates, 20–23
termination of, 659
Retching, 144
Reteplase, 78*t*, 79
Reticulocyte count, 467*t*
Retinal detachment, 536, 536*f*
Retinal hemorrhages, 435
Retinoblastoma, 306, 307*f*
Retinopathy, high-altitude, 435
Retrobulbar hematoma, 534
Retrocalcaneal bursitis, 636
Retroperitoneal injuries, 585
Retropharyngeal abscess, 242*t*, 247, 553, 553*f*
Reverse bite injury, 65
Reversible pulpitis, 546
Rewarming, 423, 423*t*
Reye syndrome, 296
Rh (D) immunoglobulin, 216, 569
Rhabdomyolysis, 188–190, 189*t*, 425
Rhabdomyosarcoma, 306
Rhesus sardonicus, 340
Rheumatic diseases, 629–632
Rheumatic heart disease, 94
Rheumatoid arthritis, 628–629, 630*t*
Rhinosinusitis, 544–545
Rhinovirus, 124*t*
Rib fractures, 581, 588, 602
Ribavirin, 355
Riboflavin, 418*t*, 419
Ricin, 451
Rickettsia rickettsii, 347
Rickettsial spotted fevers, 354
Rifabutin, 131*t*, 337
Rifampin, 131*t*, 337
Rifapentine, 131*t*
Rifaximin, 150
Right bundle branch block, 9, 19
Right left quadrant pain, 163
Right ventricular infarction, 74, 76*f*
Rigid chest syndrome, 42
Ring tourniquet syndrome, 59–60
Rocky Mountain spotted fever, 347–348
Rocuronium, 8*t*
Rodent bites, 66*t*, 68
Rodenticides, 411*t*, 411–412
Romaña sign, 355
Romberg sign, 509
Roseola infantum, 296, 296*f*
Rotator cuff impingement injury, 620
Rotator cuff tears, 622
Rotator cuff tendinitis, 621
Rubella, 294
Rufinamide, 402
Rule of nines, 441, 441*f*
Running sutures, 51, 51*f*
Ruptured globe, 533–534
Rust rings, 530

S

Sabah, 419*t*
Sacral fracture, 607*t*
Sail sign, 600
Salicylate toxidromes, 364*t*, 388–390
Salicylism, 390
Salivary gland disorders, 539
Salmonella spp., 264*t*
S. paratyphi, 353
S. typhi, 353
Salmonellosis, 337
Salter–Harris classification of fractures, 287*f*–288*f*, 287–288, 593, 594*f*, 595*t*
Sandifer syndrome, 270
Saphenous nerve block, 39
Sarcoma
Bone, 306–307
Ewing, 307, 307*f*
Kaposi, 336
osteosarcoma, 306–307
rhabdomyosarcoma, 306
SARS. *See* Severe acute respiratory syndrome
Satellite lesions, 299
Scabies, 428, 561
Scalp lacerations, 53–54
Scaphoid fracture, 597, 598*t*
Scapholunate dissociation, 597
Scapula fracture, 602
Scarlet fever, 297–298, 298*f*
Schistosomiasis, 355–356
Schizophrenia, 639
Schizophreniform disorder, 639
Sciatica, 45*t*, 619
Scombroid fish poisoning, 346
Scopolamine, 513
Scorpion stings, 428
Scrotal abscesses, 197–198
Scrotal skin avulsion, 590
Scrotum, 197–198
Scrub typhus, 354
Sea snake, 432*t*
Sea urchins, 431, 433*t*
Sebaceous cysts, infected, 327
Seborrheic dermatitis, 299
Secondary adrenal insufficiency, 489

Second-degree AV block, 18, 18*f*
Second-degree burn, 442*t*
Sedation
  definition of, 40
  level of, 40
  minimal, 40
  procedural, 36, 40–43
Sedative–hypnotics
  barbiturates, 376–377
  nonbenzodiazepines, 378–379
  withdrawal of, 379–380
Seidel's test, 531, 533
Seizures
  absence, 270, 514
  afebrile, 273
  atonic, 270
  benzodiazepines for, 386
  classification of, 514*t*
  clinical features of, 514
  definition of, 514
  diagnosis and differential of, 270–271
  differential diagnosis of, 515
  emergency department care and disposition of, 271–273, 515–517
  febrile, 270–272
  generalized, 270, 514
  myoclonic, 270
  neonatal, 272
  partial, 270, 514
  pediatric
    clinical features of, 270
    diagnosis and differential of, 270–271
    emergency department care and disposition of, 271–273
    epidemiology of, 270
    febrile, 270–272
    in head trauma, 273
    hypocalcemia as cause of, 273
    hypoglycemia as cause of, 273
    hyponatremia as cause of, 273
    neonatal, 272
    overview of, 270
    pathophysiology of, 270
    ventriculoperitoneal shunt, 273
  in pregnancy, 215
  secondary, 515*t*
  syncope versus, 86
  treatment of, 573
Selective serotonin reuptake inhibitors, 371–372
Self-neglect, 647
Senile gait, 509
Sepsis
  in children, 230–231, 231*t*
  definition of, 321
  diabetic ketoacidosis and, 283
  in infants, 231*t*
  severe, 321
Sepsis syndrome, 253
Septic abortion, 212
Septic arthritis, 627, 628*t*
Septic pelvic thrombophlebitis, 226
Septic shock
  in adults, 323
  in children, 323–324
  clinical features of, 321–322
  corticosteroids for, 324
  cutaneous lesions caused by, 322
  definition of, 321
  diagnosis and differential of, 322–323
  disseminated intravascular coagulation in, 322, 324
  early goal-directed therapy for, 323
  emergency department care and disposition of, 323–324
  epidemiology of, 321
Seromas, 181–182
Serotonin reuptake inhibitors, 370
Serotonin syndrome, 370, 372–373, 385
Serotonin/norepinephrine reuptake inhibitors, 372
Severe acute respiratory syndrome, 124*t*, 128
Severe sepsis, 321
Sexual abuse, 646
Sexual assault, 648–649
Sexually transmitted diseases
  chancroid, 316–317, 317*f*
  chlamydial infections, 313, 649
  genital warts, 318
  gonococcal infections, 313–314, 649
  herpes simplex infections, 315–316, 316*f*
  lymphogranuloma venereum, 317*f*, 317–318
  oral manifestations of, 548
  prophylaxis against, in sexual assault patients, 649
  recommendations for, 313
  syphilis, 314–315, 315*f*, 649
  trichomonas infections, 223, 314, 649
Shaken baby syndrome, 572
Shark bites, 431
Shiga toxin-producing *Escherichia coli*, 264*t*, 345–346
Shigella, 264*t*
Shin splints, 613
Shingles. *See* Herpes zoster
Shock
  cardiogenic, 81–82, 260
  congenital heart disease and, 258–259
  definition of, 32
  diagnosis and differential of, 33
  emergency care for, 33–34
  hypovolemic, 285, 574
  septic. *See* Septic shock
  systemic responses to, 32–33
Shoulder dystocia, 221
Shoulder injuries
  acromioclavicular joint injuries, 602, 603*t*
  glenohumeral joint dislocation, 602–603, 604*t*
  sternoclavicular joint sprains and dislocations, 601–602
Shoulder pain, 620–622, 621*f*
SIADH. *See* Syndrome of inappropriate secretion of antidiuretic hormone
Sialolithiasis, 539
Sickle cell disease
  acute central nervous system events, 303
  acute chest syndrome, 302, 302*f*, 478*t*
  acute splenic sequestration crises, 303
  aplastic episodes, 303–304
  clinical features of, 477–478
  description of, 215
  diagnosis and differential of, 478
  emergency department care and disposition of, 478–479
  epidemiology of, 301
  hematological crises associated with, 303–304
  infections, 304
  pathophysiology of, 301
  priapism, 303
  variants of, 304, 479
  vaso-occlusive crises, 301–302
Sickle cell hemoglobin-C disease, 304
Sickle cell–β-thalassemia disease, 304
SIDS. *See* Sudden infant death syndrome
Sildenafil, 435
Silibinin, 453
Silymarin, 453
Simple febrile seizures, 270
Simple interrupted percutaneous sutures, 50–51
Sin Nombre virus, 350
Sinus arrhythmia, 10, 10*f*
Sinus barotrauma, 436*t*
Sinus bradycardia, 10–11
Sinus tachycardia
  in children, 22
  description of, 11
Sinusitis, 240, 495, 544–545
SIRS. *See* Systemic inflammatory response syndrome
Sjögren's syndrome, 630*t*
Skin
  caustic exposure effects on, 406–407
  chemical burns of, 444
  hydrofluoric acid burns of, 444, 446*t*

Skin disinfectants, 49
Skin disorders
- disseminated gonococcal infection, 559
- erythema multiforme, 556
- exfoliative dermatitis, 557–558
- herpes zoster, 560
- pediculosis, 561–562
- pemphigus vulgaris, 559–560
- scabies, 428, 561
- tinea infections, 296–297, 560–561
- toxic epidermal necrolysis, 556–557
- toxic-infectious erythemas, 558–559

Skull fractures, 570–571, 573
Sleeping sickness, 355
Slipped capital femoral epiphysis, 291
Slipping rib syndrome, 72*t*
Small bowel
- injuries of, 585
- obstruction of, 144

Smith fracture, 597
Smoke inhalation injury, 442
Smoking, 136
Snail fever, 355–356
Snakebites, 429–430
Sodium abnormalities
- in children, 286*t*
- hypernatremia, 24–25, 25*t*, 286, 286*t*
- hyponatremia, 24, 24*t*, 273, 285, 286*t*, 388, 489

Sodium bicarbonate
- as antidote, 366*t*
- hyperkalemia treated with, 27
- during neonatal resuscitation, 23

Sodium polystyrene sulfonate, 27
Soft tissue foreign bodies, 62–63
Soft tissue infections
- Bartholin gland abscess, 327
- carbuncles, 327–328
- cellulitis. *See* Cellulitis
- cutaneous abscesses, 327–328
- description of, 324
- erysipelas, 298, 299*f*, 326–327, 538, 538*t*
- folliculitis, 327–328
- hidradenitis suppurativa, 327
- infected sebaceous cysts, 327
- methicillin-resistant *Staphylococcus aureus*, 64–65, 127, 297, 299, 324–325
- necrotizing, 325
- pilonidal abscess, 327
- sporotrichosis, 328

Soft tissue upper extremity injuries
- clinical features of, 56
- diagnosis and differential of, 57
- emergency department care and disposition of, 57–60
- epidemiology of, 56
- pathophysiology of, 56

Somatic abdominal pain, 140
Sorbitol, 152
Spasmodic croup, 244
Speed's test, 621–622
Spider bites, 427
Spinal cord compression, 487
Spinal cord decompression sickness, 436
Spinal cord injuries
- cervical, 574*t*
- diagnosis and differential of, 574–576
- emergency department care and disposition of, 576–577
- epidemiology of, 573
- pathophysiology of, 573–574

Spinal cord injury without radiographic abnormality, 565, 576
Spinal cord syndromes, 575*t*
Spinal cord tracts, 573
Spinal cord-related pain, 617*t*
Spinal infections, 620
Spinal shock, 574
Spine
- anatomy of, 573
- anterior column of, 573
- fractures of, 565, 575
- middle column of, 573
- posterior column of, 573
- radiographs of, 618

Spinothalamic tracts, 573
Spirometry, 137
Spironolactone, 180
Splenic infarction, 303
Splenic injuries, 585
Splinters, 63
Splints, 595
Sponges, 431, 433*t*
Spontaneous bacterial peritonitis, 179
Spontaneous pneumothorax, 132*f*, 132–134
Sporothrix schenckii, 328
Sporotrichosis, 328
Sprain
- ankle, 613–614
- sternoclavicular joint, 601–602

Spurling sign, 620*t*
Stab wounds, 587
Staghorn calculi, 202
Standard of care, 657
Staphylococcal scalded skin syndrome, 297, 558
Staphylococcus aureus
- methicillin-resistant, 64, 127, 297, 299
- pneumonia caused by, 126*t*

Staphylococcus epidermidis, 96
Staphylococcus saprophyticus, 193–194
Staples, for wound closure, 52
Status epilepticus, 215, 270–271, 272*f*, 508, 514, 516*f*
Steinstrasse, 205
Stellate laceration, 51*f*
Stem cell transplantation, 361–362
Sternoclavicular joint sprains and dislocations, 601–602
Sternocleidomastoid test, 644*t*
Sting(s)
- bee, 426–427
- jellyfish, 431
- scorpion, 428
- wasp, 426–427

Stinging ant bites, 426–427
Stingrays, 431, 432*t*
Stomas, 183
Stomatitis, 240–241
Stonefish, 432*t*
Stool culture testing, 146
Straight leg raise test, 617, 618*f*, 620*t*
Strangulation
- hernia, 169
- neck, 579

Strawberry tongue, 548
Streptococcal toxic shock syndrome, 320–321, 321*t*, 558
Streptococcus pneumoniae, 125, 126*t*, 228
Streptococcus pyogenes, 320
Streptokinase
- acute coronary syndromes treated with, 78*t*, 80
- description of, 485
- pulmonary embolism treated with, 108

Streptomycin, 350
Stridor
- bacterial tracheitis as cause of, 242*t*, 246–247
- causes of, 242*t*
- congenital causes of, 243
- epiglottitis as cause of, 242*t*, 245*f*, 245–246
- foreign body aspiration as cause of, 242*t*, 248
- laryngomalacia as cause of, 243–244
- in neonates, 236, 243–244
- peritonsillar abscess as cause of, 242*t*, 247–248
- retropharyngeal abscess as cause of, 242*t*, 247
- upper airway obstruction as cause of, 242–243
- viral croup as cause of, 242*t*, 244–245

Stroke
- anterior cerebral artery, 498
- cerebellar, 498
- classification of, 497*t*
- clinical features of, 497–498

definition of, 497
diagnosis and differential of, 498*t*, 498–502
emergency department care and disposition of, 502–504
in hemodialysis, 191
hemorrhagic, 497
ischemic, 303, 485, 494, 497, 497*t*, 503
middle cerebral artery, 498
National Institutes of Health Stroke Scale, 499, 500*t*–502*t*
pathophysiology of, 497
posterior circulation, 498
symptoms of, 498*t*
Strychnine poisoning, 340
ST-segment elevation myocardial infarction, 74, 80, 83
Stye, 528
Subacromial bursitis, 621
Subarachnoid hemorrhage, 111, 494, 496, 504, 571
Subclavian artery injury, 583
Subconjunctival hemorrhage, 531
Subdural hematoma, 494, 571
Submersion events, 439, 439*t*, 440*f*
Substance abuse
cocaine, 385–386
disorders caused by, 639
hallucinogens, 386–388, 387*t*
opioids, 383–385
in pregnancy, 215
Substance withdrawal, 639
Subtentorial lesions, 274
Subtrochanteric fracture, 607*t*
Subungual hematomas, 59
Succimer, 414*t*
Succinylcholine, 8*t*
Sudden death, 277–279
Sudden hearing loss, 541
Sudden infant death syndrome, 238
Suicide, 639, 640*t*–641*t*
Sulfasalazine, 150
Sulfhemoglobinemia, 421
Sulfonylureas, 454
Sunburn, 562
Superficial peroneal nerve
block of, 39
motor function of, 61*t*
Superior vena cava syndrome, 488
Supination technique, for radial head subluxation, 290*f*, 290–291
Suppurative parotitis, 538*t*, 539
Supracondylar fractures, 289–290, 290*f*, 600, 600*t*
Supraglottitis. *See* Epiglottitis
Supraorbital nerve block, 40
Supratentorial mass lesions, 274
Supratrochlear nerve block, 40
Supraventricular tachyarrhythmias
atrial fibrillation, 13–14, 14*f*
atrial flutter, 12–13, 13*f*
junctional rhythms, 15*f*, 15
multifocal atrial tachycardia, 14–15, 14*f*
sinus tachycardia, 11
tachycardia, 11–12, 11*f*
Supraventricular tachycardia
with aberrancy, 17
characteristics of, 11–13, 12*f*–13*f*
in children, 22
Sural nerve block, 39
Surgery
abdominal, 225–226
breast, 182
complications of, 181–182, 225–226
drug therapy complications of, 181–182
fever after, 181
gastrointestinal, 182–183
genitourinary complications of, 181
respiratory complications of, 181
vascular complications of, 181
wound complications of, 181
Sutures
absorbable, 50
continuous percutaneous, 51, 51*f*
deep dermal, 51, 52*f*
horizontal mattress, 51–52, 52*f*, 57*f*
nonabsorbable, 50
running, 51, 51*f*
simple interrupted percutaneous, 50–51
size of, 50
vertical mattress, 51, 52*f*
Suturing, 50
Swallowed foreign bodies, 156–157
Swan neck deformity, 58
Swan–Ganz catheter, 319
Sympatholytic agents, 399
Sympathomimetics, 364*t*
Symptomatic intracerebral hemorrhage, 502
Syncope
in adolescents, 277–279, 278*t*–279*t*
in adults, 85*t*, 85–86, 87*f*, 88*t*
in children, 277–279, 278*t*–279*t*
definition of, 277
heat, 425
Syndrome of inappropriate secretion of antidiuretic hormone, 24, 489
Synovial fluid, 626, 627*t*
Syphilis, 314–315, 315*f*, 649
Syrup of ipecac, 367
Systemic inflammatory response syndrome, 321
Systemic lupus erythematosus, 630*t*
Systemic sclerosis, 631*t*
Systolic dysfunction, 89

T

Tabes dorsalis, 509
Tachycardia
fetal, 569
multifocal atrial, 14–15, 14*f*
sinus, 11
supraventricular, 11–12, 11*f*–13*f*
ventricular, 16–17, 17*f*
Tachypnea, 230, 253, 256
Tadalafil, 435
Taenia saginata, 356
Taenia solium, 356
Takayasu arteritis, 631*t*
Talar injuries, 615
Tamsulosin, 204
Tapes, adhesive, 52–53
Tapeworms, 356
Tarantulas, 427
Tardive dyskinesia, 374
Tarsal tunnel syndrome, 636
Teeth
anatomy of, 545*f*
avulsed, 549, 549*f*
fractures of, 548–549, 549*f*
identification of, 545*f*
Temporal arteritis, 494–495, 495*t*, 536, 630*t*, 631
Temporomandibular joint disorder, 496, 540
Tendinitis, 634, 637
Tenecteplase, 78*t*, 79–80
Tennis elbow, 599
Tenosynovitis
DeQuervain's, 634
flexor, 632, 633*t*
foot, 637
transient tenosynovitis of the hip, 293
Tensilon test, 520
Tension headache, 44*t*–45*t*, 277
Tension pneumothorax, 132, 134, 580–581
Terbutaline sulfate, 138, 215
Tertiary syphilis, 315
Testes
torsion of, 199–200, 200*f*
trauma of, 590
Testicular appendage torsion, 199–200
Test-taking techniques, 4–5
Tet spells, 256, 258
Tetanospasmin, 339–340
Tetanus
clinical features of, 340
diagnosis and differential of, 340
emergency department care and disposition of, 340–341
epidemiology of, 339
immunizations for, 61, 69, 69*t*, 447
pathophysiology of, 339–340

Tetanus immune globulin, 340
Tetracaine, 529*t*
Tetracycline, 347
Tetralogy of Fallot, 256–257, 257*t*, 258*f*
Thalassemias, 479
Thenar muscles, 595
Theophylline poisoning, 393–394
Thermal burns
  American Burn Association classification of, 443*t*
  body surface area calculations, 441, 441*f*–442*f*
  classification of, 442, 442*t*
  clinical features of, 441–442
  depth of, 442*t*
  diagnosis and differential of, 442, 443*t*
  emergency department care and disposition of, 442–444, 443*t*
  epidemiology of, 441
  escharotomy for, 443
  first-degree, 442*t*
  fluid resuscitation for, 443, 565
  full-thickness, 441
  inhalation, 442
  Lund and Browder diagram for, 441, 442*f*
  pathophysiology of, 441
  rule of nines for, 441, 441*f*
  second-degree, 442*t*
Thiamine, 367*t*, 418*t*, 419, 460, 510
Thiazide diuretics, 398
Thigh adductor test, 644*t*
Thiocyanate, 399
Third-degree AV block, 18–19, 18*f*
Third-degree burn, 442*t*
Thompson's test, 61
Thoracic compression fractures, 619
Thoracic duct injuries, 584
Thoracic spine fractures, 576, 576*t*
Threatened abortion, 212
Thrombin clotting test, 469*t*
Thrombocytopenia, 305, 308, 471, 480
Thromboembolism, venous
  ancillary testing for, 104–107
  anticoagulation for, 107–108
  deep vein thrombosis. *See* Deep vein thrombosis
  diagnosis and differential of, 103–104
  emergency department care and disposition of, 107–109
  epidemiology of, 102
  in malignancies, 492
  pathophysiology of, 102–103
  in pregnancy, 214
  pretest probability assessment for, 103–104
  pulmonary embolism. *See* Pulmonary embolism
  risk factors for, 102, 102*t*
  thrombolytic therapy for, 108
  treatment of, 107–109
Thrombolytic therapy, 79, 108
Thrombophlebitis
  septic pelvic, 226
  superficial, 182
Thrombosis
  acute arterial occlusion caused by, 116*t*
  cavernous sinus, 546
  deep vein. *See* Deep vein thrombosis
  lateral sinus, 542
Thrombotic arterial occlusion, 115
Thrombotic thrombocytopenic purpura, 480
Thrush, 237, 336*f*, 336–337
Thumb
  dislocation of, 596
  ulnar collateral ligament rupture of, 596
Thymus, 254*f*
Thyroglossal duct cysts, 554
Thyroid disorders, 461–463
Thyroid storm, 214, 461–463
Thyrotoxicosis, 461–463, 512*t*
Tiagabine, 402
Tibial nerve, 61*t*
Tibial plafond fractures, 610
Tibial plateau fractures, 610, 611*t*
Tibial tubercle fracture, 611*t*
Tibial tuberosity fractures, 610, 611*t*
Tibialis anterior, 61*t*
Tic douloureux, 496
Ticarcillin/clavulanate
  diverticulitis treated with, 166
  spontaneous bacterial peritonitis treated with, 180
Tick paralysis, 517
Ticlopidine, 484
Tietze syndrome, 72*t*
Tinea infections, 296–297, 560–561
Tinel sign, 518
Tinidazole, 314
Tinnitus, 541
Tinzaparin, 108
Tirofiban, 78*t*
Tissue hypoperfusion, 32
Tissue plasminogen activator, 79, 108, 485
Tobramycin, 491*t*, 529*t*
Tocolytics, 217, 569
Todd paralysis, 515
Toe lacerations, 62
Toenail, ingrown, 635*f*, 635–636
Tongue
  lacerations of, 550
  lesions of, 548
  size of, 7*f*
Tonsillitis, 550–551
Tooth eruption, 545–546
Topical anesthesia, 38
Topiramate, 402
Torsades de pointes, 16*f*, 370–371, 375
Torus fractures, 288–289
Total anomalous pulmonary venous return, 257*t*
Toxic epidermal necrolysis, 556–557
Toxic megacolon, 150
Toxic shock syndrome
  antimicrobial therapy for, 320
  clinical features of, 319, 558
  definition of, 558, 558*t*
  diagnosis and differential of, 319, 319*t*
  emergency department care and disposition of, 319–320
  epidemiology of, 318
  fluid therapy for, 319
  pathophysiology of, 318–319
  risk factors for, 318
  streptococcal, 320–321, 321*t*, 558
Toxic shock syndrome toxin-1, 318
Toxic-infectious erythemas, 558–559
Toxicology
  acetaminophen, 391–392, 392*t*
  angiotensin-converting enzyme inhibitors, 399
  antihypertensive agents, 398
  arsenic, 413–414, 414*t*
  aspirin, 388–390
  beta-blockers, 396–397
  caffeine, 393–394
  calcium channel blockers, 397–398
  carbamates, 409
  carbamazepine, 401
  caustics, 406–407
  cyanide, 416–418, 417*t*
  DEET, 410
  digitalis glycosides, 395*t*–396*t*, 395–396
  diuretics, 398–399
  drugs of abuse. *See* Drugs of abuse
  fosphenytoin, 400–401
  hydrocarbons, 404–406
  industrial toxins, 415–418
  iron, 402–404
  lead, 412*t*, 412–413
  mercury, 414–415, 415*t*
  metabolic toxins, 416–418
  metalloids, 412–415
  metals, 412–415
  methylxanthines, 393–394
  nicotine, 393–394
  nonsteroidal anti-inflammatory drugs, 392–393

organochlorines, 409–410
organophosphates, 408–409, 409*t*
pesticides, 408–412
phenytoin, 400–401
sympatholytic agents, 399
theophylline, 393–394
valproate, 401–402
volatile substances, 404–406
Toxidromes
description of, 363
types of, 364*t*
Toxoplasmosis, 337, 358
tPA. *See* Tissue plasminogen activator
Tracheobronchial injuries, 582
Tracheostomy, 8
Tramadol, 385
Tranexamic acid, 209*t*
Transcutaneous cardiac pacing, 10
Transesophageal echocardiogram, 583
Transfer dysphagia, 154
"Transformed migraine," 44
Transfusion reactions, 482–483, 483*t*
Transfusion therapy
coagulation factors, 481, 481*t*
complications of, 481–482
emergency, 483
epidemiology of, 479
fresh frozen plasma, 480
intravenous immunoglobulins, 481
massive, 483
packed red blood cells, 302–303, 466, 480
pathophysiology of, 479
platelets, 308, 471, 480
whole blood, 480–481
Transfusion-related acute lung injury, 482*t*
Transient ischemic attack, 497, 503, 504*t*
Transient tenosynovitis of the hip, 293
Transplantation
cardiac, 359
hematopoietic stem cell, 361–362
immunosuppressive agents, 358–359
infectious complications of, 357*t*, 357–359
liver, 361
lung, 360
renal, 360–361
Transport dysphagia, 154
Transposition of the great arteries, 256–257, 257*t*
Transtentorial herniation, 571
Transthoracic echocardiography, 93
Transudative pleural effusions, 122, 123*t*
Transvenous pacing, 18
Trapezium, 598*t*
Trapezoid, 598*t*
Trauma
abdominal. *See* Abdominal trauma
blunt. *See* Blunt trauma
cardiothoracic. *See* Cardiothoracic injuries
in children, 564–566
clinical features of, 563
diagnosis and differential of, 563–564
ear, 542–543
emergency department care and disposition of, 564
esophageal, 584
extremity, 591–592
facial, 564, 577*t*, 577–579
focused assessment with sonography for, 563, 586, 605, 652
genitourinary. *See* Genitourinary trauma
geriatric, 566–567
great vessels, 583–584
head. *See* Head trauma
laryngeal, 555
neck, 579*t*, 579–580
orofacial, 548–550
penetrating. *See* Penetrating trauma
in pregnancy, 568–569
soft tissue, 550
thoracic duct, 584
ultrasonography of, 652
Traumatic brain injuries, 569–570
Traumatic hemarthrosis, 628
Traveler infections. *See* World traveler infections
Traveler's diarrhea, 147–148
Trazodone, 370–371
Treatment, refusal of, 658–659
Trench foot, 422
Trench mouth, 547
Trephination, 573
Treponema pallidum, 314
Triceps tendon rupture, 598–599
Trichomonas infections, 223, 314, 649
Trichomonas vaginalis, 221–222, 314
Trichomoniasis, 223, 649
Tricuspid atresia, 257*t*
Trifascicular block, 19
Trigeminal nerve, 578
Trigeminal neuralgia, 45*t*, 496, 547
Trigeminal rhythms, 15
Trigger finger, 634
Triiodothyronine, 461
Trimethoprim/sulfamethoxazole
diverticulitis treated with, 167
infectious diarrhea treated with, 148
Pneumocystis pneumonia treated with, 337, 358
urinary tract infections treated with, 194
Tripod fractures, 578
Trismus, 340
Trochanteric bursitis, 624*t*
Tropicamide, 529*t*
Troponins
acute myocardial infarction and, 72, 73*t*
I, 72
T, 72
Trousseau's sign, 27
True labor, 218
Truncus arteriosus, 257*t*
Trypanosoma cruzi, 355
Trypanosomiasis, 355
Trypsin, 159
Tube thoracostomy, 438
Tuberculin skin tests, 129–130
Tuberculosis
cavitary, 130, 130*f*
clinical features of, 129–130
diagnosis and differential of, 130
directly observed treatment of, 131
drug-resistant, 130
emergency department care and disposition of, 130–132, 337
epidemiology of, 129
extrapulmonary, 129–130
hospitalization for, 131–132
in immunocompromised patients, 130
isoniazid for, 130, 131*t*
latent, 129
miliary, 129–130
pathophysiology of, 129
pulmonary manifestations of, 335
reactivation, 130, 131*f*
referrals for, 131
transmission of, 129
treatment of, 130–132, 337
tuberculin skin tests for, 129–130
Tuberculous meningitis, 129
Tubo-ovarian abscess, 143*t*
Tularemia, 349–350
Tumor lysis syndrome, 306, 490
Tympanic membrane
description of, 238, 238*f*–239*f*
perforation of, 543
Typhoid fever, 353–354
Typhoidal tularemia, 350
Typhus, 354

U

Ulcerative colitis, 150–151
Ulnar fractures, 601
Ulnar mononeuropathy, 518
Ulnar nerve
block of, 39
motor testing of, 56*t*, 599*t*
sensory testing of, 57*t*, 599*t*
Ulnar styloid fracture, 598

Ultrasonography
abdominal aortic aneurysm findings, 113*f,* 653
abdominal pain, 142
abdominal trauma, 586
acute appendicitis, 164*f,* 165
acute renal failure, 186
acute urinary retention evaluations, 197*f*
cardiac, 653
cholecystitis, 162*f*
compression, 654
deep vein thrombosis evaluations, 105, 105*f*
ectopic pregnancy, 210*f*–211*f,* 210–211
emergency department use of, 652–654
gallbladder disease, 653
gallstones, 161
hernia, 170, 170*f*
inferior vena cava, 187*f*
intussusception, 266, 266*f*
ocular, 537
pneumothorax, 132–133, 133*f,* 581
pregnancy applications of, 653
renal colic, 653
urologic stone disease, 203, 204*f*
Ultraviolet keratitis, 435, 532
Umbilical hernia, 169
Uncal herniation, 507, 571
Unfractionated heparin
acute coronary syndromes treated with, 79
description of, 484
pulmonary embolism treated with, 108
Unstable angina, 74, 83
Upper airway
angioedema of, 555
infections of. *See* Upper airway infections
obstruction of, 242–243
Upper airway infections
epiglottitis, 552*f,* 552–553
odontogenic abscess, 553–554
peritonsillar abscess, 551*f,* 551–552
pharyngitis, 550–551
tonsillitis, 550–551
Upper gastrointestinal bleeding, 153–154, 265*t*
Urea-splitting bacteria, 202
Uremia, 190
Uremic encephalopathy, 191
Uremic pericarditis, 191
Ureteral calculi, 653
Ureteral injuries, 590
Ureteral injury, 226
Ureteral stents, 206
Ureteral valves, 193
Ureteropelvic junction, 202
Urethra
foreign bodies in, 201
male, 201
trauma of, 590
Urethral stricture, 201
Urethritis, 192, 193, 201
Uric acid, 202
Uric acid crystals, 628
Urinary catheters, 205–206
Urinary diversion, 207
Urinary extravasation, 589
Urinary retention, acute, 196–197
Urinary sphincters, artificial, 206
Urinary stones. *See* Urologic stone disease
Urinary tract infections
catheter-related, 205
in children, 230, 268–269
clinical features of, 193
complicated, 192, 193*t,* 194
definition of, 192
diagnosis and differential of, 194
emergency department care and disposition of, 194–195, 269*t*
epidemiology of, 192–193
fever caused by, 230
fluoroquinolones for, 194–195
in infants, 230, 268–269
lower, 194
pathophysiology of, 193
pediatric, 230, 268–269, 269*t*
postoperative, 181
in pregnancy, 215
risk factors for, 193*t*
stent migration or malfunction versus, 206–207
treatment of, 182, 269*t*
uncomplicated, 192–194
urologic stone disease and, 204
Urine specimens, 194
Urokinase, 108
Urologic stone disease
ancillary tests in, 204*t*
in children, 202
clinical features of, 202
diagnosis and differential of, 202–203, 203*f*–204*f*
emergency department care and disposition of, 204–205
epidemiology of, 201–202
extracorporeal shock wave lithotripsy for, 202
pathophysiology of, 202
stone composition, 202
urinary tract infection and, 204
Urushiol, 452
Uterine atony, 217
Uterine rupture, 568
Uveitis, 531

V

Vaginal bleeding, 208, 209*t,* 216
Vaginal cuff cellulitis, 225–226
Vaginitis, 193
Valacyclovir, 316, 330, 547
Valproate, 401–402
Valsalva maneuver, 11–12
Valvular disease
aortic incompetence, 94–95
aortic stenosis, 91*t,* 94, 94*f*
mitral regurgitation, 91*t*
mitral stenosis, 91*t,* 91–92, 92*f*
mitral valve prolapse, 91*t,* 93–94
overview of, 91
prosthetic, 95–96
Vancomycin
bacterial endocarditis treated with, 339
bacterial tracheitis treated with, 247
Clostridium difficile-associated diarrhea treated with, 149
epiglottitis treated with, 246
neutropenic fever treated with, 491
toxic shock syndrome treated with, 320
wound infections treated with, 65
Variceal bleeding, 154
Varicella, 295–296, 296*f,* 330–331, 336
Vascular access
in children, 21
complications of, 191–192
hemorrhage caused by, 192
infections caused by, 192
in neonates, 21
ultrasonography of, 653
Vascular syncope, 278
Vasodilators, 399–400
Vaso-occlusive crises, 301–302, 477*t*
Vasopressin, 17
Vasovagal reactions, 43
Vasovagal syncope, 86, 277
Vecuronium, 9*t,* 340
Venlafaxine, 372
Venous hum, 256*t*
Venous thromboembolism
ancillary testing for, 104–107
anticoagulation for, 107–108
deep vein thrombosis. *See* Deep vein thrombosis
diagnosis and differential of, 103–104
emergency department care and disposition of, 107–109
epidemiology of, 102
in malignancies, 492

pathophysiology of, 102–103
in pregnancy, 214
pretest probability assessment for, 103–104
pulmonary embolism. *See* Pulmonary embolism
risk factors for, 102, 102*t*
thrombolytic therapy for, 108
treatment of, 107–109
Venous ultrasonography
deep vein thrombosis evaluations, 105, 105*f*
pulmonary embolism evaluations, 107
Ventilation/perfusion mismatch, 103, 120, 249, 252
Ventilation/perfusion scanning, 107
Ventricular arrhythmias
accelerated idioventricular rhythm, 15–16, 16*f*
premature ventricular contractions, 15–16, 15*f*
Ventricular fibrillation, 17*f,* 17–18, 22
Ventricular septal defects, 256
Ventricular tachyarrhythmias, 17
Ventricular tachycardia, 16–17, 16*f*
Ventriculoperitoneal shunt, 273
Veracity, 660
Verapamil
atrial fibrillation treated with, 14
multifocal atrial tachycardia treated with, 15
narrow-complex supraventricular tachycardia treated with, 12
Vertebral artery dissection, 495, 498, 512*t,* 513
Vertebrobasilar insufficiency, 512*t,* 513
Vertical mattress sutures, 51, 52*f*
Vertigo, 510–513, 511*t*–512*t*
Vesicants, 445
Vesicovaginal fistula, 226
Vesiculopustular lesions, 627
Vestibular ganglionitis, 512
Vestibular neuronitis, 512
Vibrio spp.
marine envenomations, 431
V. vulnificus, 346
Videolaryngoscopy, 8
Vincent disease, 547
Viral arthritis, 628
Viral conjunctivitis, 529
Viral croup, 242*t,* 244–245
Viral infections
arboviral, 332
Epstein–Barr virus infection, 331–332
herpes simplex virus 1, 328–330, 329*f*
herpes zoster, 330*f,* 330–331
influenza. *See* Influenza
varicella, 295–296, 296*f,* 330–331
Viral parotitis, 539
Viral pharyngitis, 551
Viral pneumonia, 253
Virchow's triad, 473
Visceral abdominal pain, 140
Visceral injuries, 585
Visual reduction and loss
acute angle-closure glaucoma, 534*f,* 534–535
Bell's palsy, 536
benign intracranial hypertension, 537
central retinal artery occlusion, 535
central retinal vein occlusion, 535
diabetic palsies, 536
giant cell arteritis, 536
Horner's syndrome, 537
hypertensive cranial nerve palsies, 536
optic neuritis, 535
papilledema, 537, 537*f*
posterior communicating artery aneurysm, 537
ultrasonography evaluations, 537
Vitamin(s)
B, 419
fat-soluble, 418–419
Vitamin A, 418*t,* 419
Vitamin B_1, 418*t,* 419
Vitamin B_2, 418*t,* 419
Vitamin B_3, 418*t,* 419
Vitamin B_6, 418*t,* 419
Vitamin B_{12}, 418*t,* 419, 509
Vitamin B_{12A}, 417
Vitamin C, 418*t*
Vitamin D, 28, 418*t*
Vitamin E, 418*t,* 419
Vitamin K, 404, 418, 471–472
Vitamin K_1, 367*t*
Vitreous hemorrhage, 531
Vocal cord paralysis, 243–244
Volatile substances, 404–406
Volkmann's ischemic contracture, 289, 600
Volume overload, 23, 311
Volvulus, 167–168, 266
Vomiting. *See also* Nausea and vomiting
in children, 260–264, 263*t*
description of, 144
in infants, 235, 260–264, 263*t*
in neonates, 235, 263*t*
von Willebrand's disease, 475–477, 481*t*
von Willebrand's factor, 73–74, 475
Vulvovaginitis, 208, 221–223

W

Wallenberg syndrome, 513
Warfarin, 108, 503
Warts
genital, 318
plantar, 635
Wasp stings, 426–427
"Water hammer pulse," 95
Water hemlock, 451*t*
Waterborne diseases, 345–347
Wegener granulomatosis, 631*t*
Weil disease, 354
Wells score, 104*t*
Wenckebach AV block, 18*f*–19*f,* 18–19
Wernicke's encephalopathy, 380, 510
Wernicke's disease, 460
West Nile virus, 332
Westermark's sign, 106
"Wet drowning," 439
Wheezing, 249*t,* 249–250
Whole-bowel irrigation, 367, 390, 403
Wide-complex supraventricular tachycardia, 12
Wilms tumor, 306
Wolff–Parkinson–White syndrome
atrial fibrillation in, 14*f*
description of, 12, 12*f*
Woolsorter's disease, 351
Word catheter, 327
World traveler infections
African tick typhus, 354
African trypanosomiasis, 355
amebiasis, 356
ascariasis, 356
brucellosis, 354
Chagas disease, 355
chikungunya, 353
clinical features of, 352–353
Crimean–Congo hemorrhagic fever, 354–355
cysticercosis, 355
dengue fever, 353
diagnosis and differential of, 352–353
enterobiasis, 356
epidemiology of, 352
exposure risks, 352*t*
leishmaniasis, 355
leptospirosis, 354
louse-borne typhus, 354
malaria, 353
regional tropical illnesses, 352*t*
rickettsial spotted fevers, 354
schistosomiasis, 355–356
scrub typhus, 354
typhoid fever, 353–354
yellow fever, 355

Wormwood, 419*t*
Wound
antibiotic prophylaxis of, 49, 68–69
blunt force, 60
cleansing of, 49, 69
clinical features of, 48
complications of, 181
debridement of, 49
dehiscence of, 181
diagnosis and differential of, 48
healing of, 49
hemostasis of, 48
irrigation of, 49
long-term cosmetic outcome of, 70
management of, 592
pain management, 69
pathophysiology of, 48
post repair care of, 68–70
puncture, 64–65
tetanus prophylaxis for, 69, 69*t*
Wound closure
adhesive tapes for, 52–53
cyanoacrylate tissue adhesives for, 53
delayed, 52
overview of, 49
staples, 52
sutures for. *See* Sutures
suturing techniques for, 50
Wound drains, 69
Wound dressings, 68
Wound hematomas, 181–182
Wound infections
bites as cause of, 66–67
cellulitis versus, 64
clinical presentation of, 181
in lower extremity injuries, 62
treatment of, 182
WPW syndrome. *See* Wolff–Parkinson–White syndrome
Wrist
injuries of, 597–598
lacerations of, 57

X
Xanthochromia, 496
Xiphodynia, 72*t*

Y
Yellow fever, 355
Yergason's test, 621, 622*f*
Yersinia, 264*t*, 351–352
Yew, 451*t*
Yohimbe, 419*t*
Young–Burgess classification system, 605, 606*t*

Z
Zaleplon, 379
Zanamivir, 333
Zoledronic acid, 489
Zolpidem, 379
Zonisamide, 402
Zoonoses, 347
Zoonotic infections
anthrax, 350–351
Colorado tick fever, 349
description of, 347
ehrlichiosis, 349
hantavirus, 350
Lyme disease, 348–349
plague, 351–352
Rocky Mountain spotted fever, 347–348
tularemia, 349–350
Zopiclone, 379
Zoster, herpes, 330*f*, 330–331, 547, 560
Zosyn, 175
Zygoma fractures, 578